TEXTBOOK OF
Neonatal Dermatology

TEXTBOOK OF
Neonatal Dermatology

LAWRENCE F. EICHENFIELD, MD

Associate Clinical Professor of Pediatrics and Medicine (Dermatology)
University of California, San Diego School of Medicine
Chief, Division of Pediatric and Adolescent Dermatology
Children's Hospital and Health Center
San Diego, California

ILONA J. FRIEDEN, MD

Clinical Professor, Dermatology and Pediatrics
Chief, Pediatric Dermatology Clinics
University of California, San Francisco, School of Medicine
San Francisco, California

NANCY B. ESTERLY, MD

Professor of Dermatology and Pediatrics
Medical College of Wisconsin
Medical Director, Pediatric Dermatology
Children's Hospital of Wisconsin
Milwaukee, Wisconsin

W.B. SAUNDERS COMPANY
A Harcourt Health Sciences Company
Philadelphia   London   New York   St. Louis   Sydney   Toronto

W.B. SAUNDERS COMPANY
A Harcourt Health Sciences Company

The Curtis Center
Independence Square West
Philadelphia, Pennsylvania 19106

Acquisitions Editor: Liz Fathman
Developmental Editor: Kristen Mandava
Project Manager: Patricia Tannian
Project Specialist: Melissa Lastarria
Book Design Manager: Gail Morey Hudson
Cover Designer: Teresa Breckwoldt

Library of Congress Cataloging-in-Publication Data
Textbook of neonatal dermatology / [edited by] Lawrence F. Eichenfield, Nancy B.
Esterly, Ilona J. Frieden.
     p. ; cm.
  Includes bibliographical references and index.
  ISBN 0-7216-7810-6
    1. Pediatric dermatology. 2. Infants (Newborn)—Diseases. I. Eichenfield, Lawrence F.
II. Esterly, Nancy B. III. Frieden, Ilona J.
  [DNLM: 1. Skin Diseases—Infant, Newborn. WS 260 T3547 2001]
RJ511 .T48 2001
618.92'5—dc21   00-050070

TEXTBOOK OF NEONATAL DERMATOLOGY   ISBN 0-7216-7810-6

Printed in the United States of America

Last digit is the print number: 9   8   7   6   5   4   3   2   1

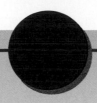

Contributors

RICHARD J. ANTAYA, MD
Assistant Professor of Dermatology and Pediatrics,
Departments of Dermatology and Pediatrics,
Yale University School of Medicine,
New Haven, Connecticut

EULALIA BASELGA, MD
Department of Dermatology,
Hospital de la Santa Creu i Sant Pau, Barcelona, Spain;
Consultant Pediatric Dermatologist, Department of
  Dermatology,
Institut Universitari Dexeus,
Barcelona, Spain

MIRIAM B. BIRGE, MD
Postdoctoral Fellow, Department of Dermatology,
New York University School of Medicine,
New York, New York

JOHN S. BRADLEY, MD
Associate Clinical Professor of Pediatrics,
University of California, San Diego;
Director, Division of Infectious Diseases,
Children's Hospital and Health Center
San Diego, California

BERNARD A. COHEN, MD
Associate Professor of Pediatrics and Dermatology,
Johns Hopkins University School of Medicine;
Director of Pediatric Dermatology,
Johns Hopkins Children's Center,
Baltimore, Maryland

BARI B. CUNNINGHAM, MD
Assistant Clinical Professor of Pediatrics and Medicine
  (Dermatology)
University of California, San Diego, School of Medicine;
Attending Physician,
Division of Pediatric and Adolescent Dermatology,
Children's Hospital and Health Center,
San Diego, California

GARY L. DARMSTADT, MD
Research Director, Saving Newborn Lives Initiative,
Office of Health, Save the Children,
Washington, D.C.
Adjunct Assistant Professor,
Department of International Health,
Division of Community Health and Health Systems,
School of Hygiene and Public Health,
The Johns Hopkins Medical Institutions,
Baltimore, Maryland

JAMES G. DINULOS, MD
Acting Instructor,
Division of Dermatology, Department of Pediatrics,
Division of Dermatology, Department of Medicine,
University of Washington School of Medicine,
  Seattle, Washington;
Assistant Professor,
Department of Medicine (Dermatology),
Department of Pediatrics, Dartmouth Medical School,
Hanover, New Hampshire

BETH ANN DROLET, MD
Associate Professor of Dermatology and Pediatrics,
Medical College of Wisconsin,
Milwaukee, Wisconsin

LAWRENCE F. EICHENFIELD, MD
Associate Clinical Professor of Pediatrics and Medicine
    (Dermatology)
University of California, San Diego School of Medicine,
Chief, Division of Pediatric and Adolescent
    Dermatology,
Children's Hospital and Health Center
San Diego, California

SUSAN S. ELLIS, MD
Fellow,
Department of Dermatology,
Washington University,
St. Louis, Missouri

ODILE ENJOLRAS, MD
Consultant, Director "Consultation de Angiomes,"
Department of Neuroradiology,
Lariboisière Hospital,
Paris, France

NANCY B. ESTERLY, MD
Professor of Dermatology and Pediatrics,
Medical College of Wisconsin,
Medical Director, Pediatric Dermatology
Children's Hospital of Wisconsin
Milwaukee, Wisconsin

ILONA J. FRIEDEN, MD
Clinical Professor, Dermatology and Pediatrics,
Chief, Pediatric Dermatology Clinics,
University of California,
San Francisco, School of Medicine,
San Francisco, California

SHEILA FALLON FRIEDLANDER, MD
Associate Clinical Professor of Pediatrics and Medicine
    (Dermatology)
University of California San Diego Medical Center,
    San Diego, California;
Attending Physician, Division of Pediatric and
    Adolescent Dermatology,
Children's Hospital and Health Center
San Diego, California

MARIA C. GARZON, MD
Assistant Professor,
Departments of Dermatology and Pediatrics,
Columbia University,
College of Physicians and Surgeons,
New York, New York;
Director, Pediatric Dermatology,
Babies and Children's Hospital of New York,
New York, New York

NEIL F. GIBBS, MD
Assistant Clinical Professor,
Departments of Medicine (Dermatology) and Pediatrics,
University of California, San Diego;
Department of Dermatology,
Naval Medical Center, San Diego,
San Diego, California;
Assistant Clinical Professor,
Department of Dermatology,
Uniformed Services University of the Health Sciences,
Bethesda, Maryland

ADELAIDE A. HEBERT, MD
Vice Chairman, Department of Dermatology,
Professor of Dermatology and Pediatrics,
The University of Texas Medical School at Houston,
Houston, Texas

PAUL J. HONIG, MD
Professor of Pediatrics and Dermatology,
University of Pennsylvania School of Medicine;
Director, Pediatric Dermatology,
Children's Hospital of Philadelphia,
Philadelphia, Pennsylvania

RENÉE HOWARD, MD
Clinical Instructor, Department of Dermatology,
University of California, San Francisco, California;
Division Chief, Department of Pediatric Dermatology,
Children's Hospital,
Oakland, California

HO JIN KIM, MD
Assistant Professor of Pediatrics and Dermatology,
Departments of Pediatrics and Dermatology,
University of Pennsylvania School of Medicine;
Assistant Professor, Department of Pediatric
    Dermatology,
Children's Hospital of Philadelphia,
Philadelphia, Pennsylvania

BERNICE R. KRAFCHIK, MB, ChB, FRCPC
Professor, Departments of Pediatrics and Medicine,
University of Toronto;
Head, Section of Dermatology,
Division of Pediatric Medicine,
Hospital for Sick Children,
Toronto, Ontario, Canada

MOISE L. LEVY, MD
Professor, Departments of Dermatology and Pediatrics,
Baylor College of Medicine, Houston, Texas;
Chief, Dermatology Service,
Texas Children's Hospital,
Houston, Texas

CYNTHIA A. LOOMIS, MD, PhD
Assistant Professor,
Departments of Dermatology and Cell Biology,
New York University School of Medicine,
New York, New York

ANNE W. LUCKY, MD
Volunteer Professor of Dermatology and Pediatrics,
University of Cincinnati College of Medicine;
Division of Pediatric Dermatology,
The Children's Hospital Medical Center;
Dermatology Associates of Cincinnati,
Cincinnati, Ohio

SUSAN BAYLISS MALLORY, MD
Professor of Dermatology and Pediatrics,
Division of Dermatology,
Washington University School of Medicine;
Director, Pediatric Dermatology,
St. Louis Children's Hospital,
St. Louis, Missouri

ANTHONY J. MANCINI, MD
Assistant Professor,
Departments of Pediatrics and Dermatology,
Northwestern University Medical School;
Attending Physician, Division of Dermatology,
Children's Memorial Hospital,
Chicago, Illinois

CATHERINE CAMERON McCUAIG, MD, FRCPC
Assistant Clinical Professor of Pediatrics
University of Montreal,
Department of Pediatrics (Dermatology Service),
Sainte-Justine Hospital,
Montreal, Quebec, Canada

DENISE W. METRY, MD
Assistant Professor,
Departments of Pediatrics and Dermatology,
Baylor College of Medicine, Houston, Texas;
Assistant Professor,
Departments of Pediatrics and Dermatology,
Texas Children's Hospital,
Houston, Texas

AMY S. PALLER, MD
Professor of Pediatrics and Dermatology,
Northwestern University Medical School;
Head, Division of Dermatology,
Children's Memorial Hospital,
Chicago, Illinois

ALICE L. PONG, MD
Assistant Clinical Professor, Department of Pediatrics,
University of California, San Diego, California;
Division of Infection, Children's Hospital and Health
    Center,
San Diego, California

JULIE S. PRENDIVILLE, MB, MRCPI, FRCPC
Clinical Associate Professor, Department of Pediatrics,
University of British Columbia;
Head, Division of Pediatric Dermatology,
Department of Pediatrics,
British Columbia's Children's Hospital,
Vancouver, British Columbia, Canada

NEIL S. PROSE, MD
Director, Pediatric Dermatology,
Duke University Medical Center,
Durham, North Carolina

MAUREEN ROGERS, MB, BS, FACD
Head, Department of Dermatology,
Royal Alexandra Hospital for Children,
Westmead, Sydney, Australia

ELAINE C. SIEGFRIED, MD
Associate Professor, Pediatrics and Dermatology,
Department of Dermatology,
St. Louis University School of Medicine;
Associate Professor, Department of Dermatology,
Cardinal Glennon Children's Hospital,
St. Louis, Missouri

ROBERT A. SILVERMAN, MD
Clinical Associate Professor, Department of Pediatrics,
Georgetown University, Washington, D.C.;
Clinical Associate Professor,
Departments of Pediatrics and Dermatology,
University of Virginia,
Charlottesville, Virginia

MARY K. SPRAKER, MD
Associate Professor of Dermatology and Pediatrics,
Emory University School of Medicine, Atlanta, Georgia;
Chief of Dermatology, Egleston Hospital for Children,
Atlanta, Georgia

VIRGINIA P. SYBERT, MD
Professor, Department of Medicine,
University of Washington School of Medicine,
Seattle, Washington

ANNETTE M. WAGNER, MD
Assistant Professor of Pediatrics and Dermatology,
Departments of Pediatrics and Dermatology,
Northwestern University;
Department of Medicine, Division of Dermatology,
Children's Memorial Hospital,
Chicago, Illinois

MARY L. WILLIAMS, MD
Adjunct Professor of Dermatology and Pediatrics,
Department of Dermatology,
University of California, San Francisco,
San Francisco, California

To

Lori, Matthew, Julia;
Mark, Sarai, Mike;
Thistle and **McTavish,**

We thank you for your love and support
during all the hours spent editing this book.
In addition,
Larry and Ilona would especially like to thank

Nancy Esterly

for the opportunity of a lifetime—
to create a neonatal textbook with the
"mother of pediatric dermatology"
and editor *par excellence.*

Foreword

Imagine—a multiauthored book with 3 editors and 37 contributors on the topic of neonatal dermatology, which is obviously now a mature field. This textbook is indeed welcome, since many of the advances in dermatology have been of relatively recent origin, and it is incumbent on the pediatrician to know what's known—even if most of us would find it an impossible assignment to memorize the information in this volume. For example, note that there are at least seven distinct types of ichthyoses. This is reason enough to realize that pediatric dermatology is a definable subspecialty, and that its content is of such breadth and depth that you either consult this book or call the pediatric dermatologist, or probably both.

A welcome attribute of this book is an extensive discussion of the many kinds of problems that are associated with the skin after preterm birth. Did you know that the barrier function of the skin of most preterm infants, regardless of gestational age, is competent by 2 to 3 weeks of postnatal age except in very low birth weight infants, who might require as long as 8 weeks for this function to mature? Statements such as, "In the care of the preterm infant, it is safest to assume that any medication applied to the skin may be absorbed systemically," and, ". . . cutaneous fluid losses are perhaps the most important destabilizing factor in fluid homeostasis in the preterm infant," demonstrate some of the valuable wisdom imparted to the reader.

Not only have the contributors presented their observations in detail, but also they have brought the story up-to-date with the latest genetic analyses, which are, of course, indispensable for communicating prognosis or recurrence in subsequent pregnancies. One of the strengths of this volume is careful identification of what is known and what is yet to be defined. It comes as no surprise, but we are reminded by the authors that, "a standard for optimized care for neonatal skin has yet to be defined" (see Chapter 5). Among the reader-friendly aspects of this text are the number of tables that describe the contents of various remedies and diagnostic tests.

Finally, this text presents a multitude of outstanding photographs of relevant conditions. Thus the reader can learn much from the pictures, but the discussion and documentation that accompany them make it far more than an atlas, but closer to a compendium of what is known in the field of neonatal dermatology. This is an appropriate time for experienced academic clinicians to bring together the essence of an enormous, carefully cited literature. Drs. Eichenfield, Frieden, and Esterly have accomplished that with skill and wisdom.

Mary Ellen Avery, MD
Thomas Morgan Rotch Distinguished Professor of Pediatrics
Harvard Medical School
Department of Pediatrics, Children's Hospital
Boston, Massachusetts

Preface

Almost 30 years have passed since the publication of a textbook devoted in its entirety to the subject of newborn skin. *Neonatal Dermatology* (by L.M. Solomon and N.B. Esterly) was published in the Saunders series *Major Problems in Clinical Pediatrics* in 1973 and, like most of those monographs, enjoyed a wide readership but has long been out of date. It was written at a time when pediatric dermatology was not yet a special discipline, and neonatal cutaneous disorders in particular often went unrecognized and untreated. Little was known about the developmental physiology of the fetus and newborn and even less about the skin as a functional organ and its properties as an effective barrier.

The past two to three decades have seen a tremendous increase in our understanding of the biochemical and molecular mechanisms involved in both normal organ function and disease processes in people of all ages. The neonate is no exception. Several excellent neonatology texts are now available, but of necessity, the pages given over to a discussion of the integument are few in number. It therefore seemed appropriate to consider organizing another textbook of neonatal dermatology.

This book is intended for clinicians. However, in addition to chapters on the various dermatologic entities, we have included information on fetal skin development, barrier function, percutaneous absorption, the skin of the premature infant, toxicology, and iatrogenic and traumatic injuries with the hope that we will pique the interest of investigators as well. Our intent was also to provide illustrations of as many skin disorders as possible, along with information about cause, course, treatment, and prognosis.

Because of the incredible amount of new knowledge, this book could no longer be a slim volume written by two or three authors. We have enlisted the help of many colleagues who generously contributed their time and expertise, making this an international effort with chapters by many distinguished pediatric dermatologists. The book has already passed the "use test" in our own practices, where we find ourselves repeatedly turning to its chapters when evaluating infants and newborns. We hope our readers will agree.

Our thanks to Aimee Rosen, Tiffany Bagalini, and Jan Conavay for their assistance and dedication in the production of this book.

Lawrence F. Eichenfield
Ilona J. Frieden
Nancy B. Esterly

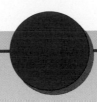

Contents

1   Fetal Skin Development, 1
CYNTHIA A. LOOMIS and MIRIAM B. BIRGE

2   Structure and Function of Newborn Skin, 18
ANTHONY J. MANCINI

3   Lesional Morphology and Assessment, 33
HO JIN KIM and PAUL J. HONIG

4   Skin of the Premature Infant, 46
MARY L. WILLIAMS

5   Neonatal Skin Care and Toxicology, 62
ELAINE C. SIEGFRIED

6   Diagnostic and Therapeutic Procedures, 73
BARI B. CUNNINGHAM and
ANNETTE M. WAGNER

7   Transient Benign Cutaneous Lesions
in the Newborn, 88
ANNE W. LUCKY

8   Iatrogenic and Traumatic Injuries, 103
NANCY B. ESTERLY

9   Developmental Abnormalities, 117
BETH ANN DROLET

10   Vesicles, Pustules, Bullae, Erosions,
and Ulcerations, 137
ILONA J. FRIEDEN and RENÉE HOWARD

11   Bacterial Infections, 179
GARY L. DARMSTADT and JAMES G. DINULOS

12   Viral Infections, 201
SHEILA FALLON FRIEDLANDER and
JOHN S. BRADLEY

13   Fungal Infections, Infestations, and Parasitic
Infections in Neonates, 223
ALICE L. PONG and
CATHERINE CAMERON McCUAIG

14   Eczematous Disorders, 241
BERNICE R. KRAFCHIK

15   Erythrodermas: The Red Scaly Baby, 260
MOISE L. LEVY and MARY K. SPRAKER

16   Disorders of Cornification (Ichthyosis), 276
AMY S. PALLER

17   Inflammatory and Purpuric Eruptions, 294
EULALIA BASELGA

18   Vascular Stains, Malformations,
and Tumors, 324
ODILE ENJOLRAS and MARIA C. GARZON

19   Hypopigmentation Disorders, 353
SUSAN S. ELLIS and
SUSAN BAYLISS MALLORY

20   Hyperpigmentation Disorders, 370
LAWRENCE F. EICHENFIELD and NEIL F. GIBBS

21   Lumps, Bumps, and Hamartomas, 395
JULIE S. PRENDIVILLE

22   Disorders of the Subcutaneous Tissue, 420
BERNARD A. COHEN

23   Neoplastic and Infiltrative Diseases, 436
NEIL S. PROSE and RICHARD J. ANTAYA

24   Selected Hereditary Diseases, 451
VIRGINIA P. SYBERT

25   Neonatal Mucous Membrane Disorders, 473
      DENISE W. METRY and ADELAIDE A. HEBERT

26   Hair Disorders, 487
      MAUREEN ROGERS

27   Nail Defects, 504
      ROBERT A. SILVERMAN

Fetal Skin Development

CYNTHIA A. LOOMIS
MIRIAM B. BIRGE

Skin is a complex tissue made up of many different cell types, derived from both embryonic mesoderm and ectoderm. Skin cells originating from embryonic mesoderm include fibroblasts, vascular cells, and adipocytes, as well as the bone marrow–derived Langherhans' cells, which reside in the epidermis. Skin cells originating from embryonic ectoderm include epidermal keratinocytes and the neural crest–derived melanocytes. Development, growth, and regional patterning of the skin are regulated by sequential and tightly regulated inductive interactions between these various cell types within the skin, as well as between skin and adjacent nonskin tissues. Genetic or teratogenic disruptions in these regulatory interactions result in serious congenital anomalies that can impact directly on the care of the infant. Moreover, premature birth before full maturation of the skin can lead to impaired thermoregulation and defective barrier function in the neonate.

The main purpose of this chapter is to provide a detailed morphologic description of normal skin development. Where appropriate, a discussion is presented on what is currently known about the molecular controls that direct these embryonic processes, focusing primarily on the clinical impact of known genetic mutations and teratogenic agents. Significant progress has been made over the last several years in our understanding of the molecular basis of skin development. For the clinician, a firm molecular and morphologic understanding of normal skin development is a requisite starting point for making the correct diagnosis, initiating appropriate parental counseling, and determining effective therapeutic strategies for infants affected by congenital skin disorders.

A time line highlighting several important morphologic events that occur during skin morphogenesis is illustrated in Fig. 1-1. In this figure and throughout the text, two distinct dating systems are indicated. We use the term *estimated gestational age (EGA)*, as it is used in basic embryology texts and by researchers, to refer to the age of the fetus.[1] In this system, fertilization occurs on day 1. However, the dating system used by obstetricians and most other clinicians as a reliable and convenient method for staging the pregnancy defines day 1 as the first day of the last menstrual period (LMP) and is synonymous with *menstrual age.*[2] In this dating system, fertilization occurs on approximately day 14. Thus a woman who is 14 weeks pregnant (LMP) is carrying a 12-week-old fetus (EGA).

From a functional point of view, fetal skin development can be divided into three temporally overlapping stages—**organogenesis, histogenesis,** and **maturation**[3]—that roughly correspond to the embryonic period (0 to 60-plus days), the early fetal period (60 days to 5 months), and the late fetal period (5 to 9 months) of development. The first stage, **organogenesis,** involves the specification of ectoderm lateral to the neural plate to become epidermis and the allocation of subsets of mesenchymal and neural crest cells to become dermis. During this stage, embryonic ectoderm and mesoderm become physically apposed, and they initiate the signaling cross-talk necessary for basement membrane and subsequent skin appendage (hair, nail, and sweat gland) formation. The second stage, **histogenesis,** is characterized by dramatic morphologic changes in the presumptive skin, including epidermal stratification, epidermal appendage involution and differentiation, mesenchymal subdivision of the dermis and hypodermis, and vascular neogenesis. The third stage, **maturation,** entails the functional evolution of these skin components so that they provide adequate thermoregula-

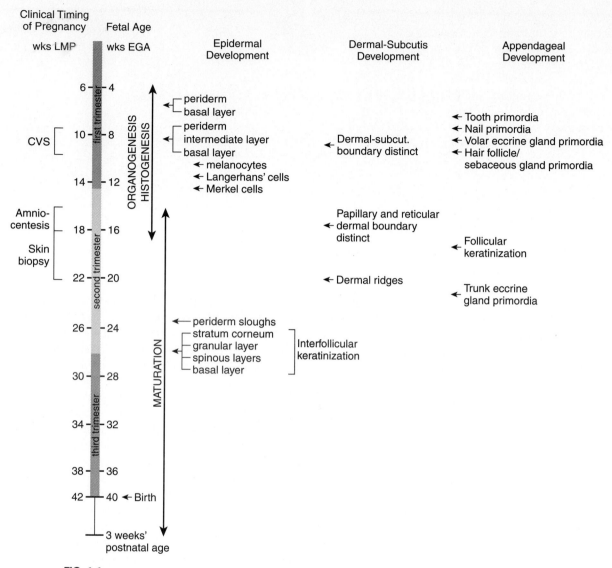

FIG. 1-1

Critical events in the development of skin and its specialized structures, indicating their times of initiation as defined by fetal age (EGA) and duration of pregnancy (LMP). Unless otherwise stated, times refer to back skin.

tory capacity, surface tensile strength, and barrier function for postnatal survival in the harsh, arid environment outside the uterus.

To simplify the discussion, development of the epidermis and the dermis/subcutis is presented in two sequential sections. In the third section, collaborative interactions of these two tissues in basement membrane and epidermal appendage formation are discussed. Finally, in the fourth section specific aspects of skin development related to prenatal diagnosis are addressed.

EPIDERMIS

Overview

The epidermis is a self-renewing stratified epithelium covering the entire surface of an individual. The predominant cell within this epithelium is the keratinocyte. In its mature form, the epidermis consists of four histologically distinct keratinocyte layers, described from deep to superficial: (1) the basal layer, (2) the spinous layers, (3) the granular layer, and (4) the stratum corneum. The proliferative basal keratinocytes are anchored to the basement membrane, an extracellular meshwork separating the epidermis from the underlying dermis. As the daughter cells produced by this layer differentiate, they down-regulate the synthesis of matrix adhesion proteins, detach from the basement membrane, and move outward into the spinous layers. In this zone, the keratinocytes expend much of their energy in the production of keratin intermediate filaments. These rigid rods insert into the numerous desmosomal adhesion junctions and through these interconnections provide tensile strength and mechanical integrity for the epidermis.[4] On further differentiation, keratinocytes accumulate large protein and lipid granules, structures that define the most superficial viable layer, the granular layer. As the cells undergo terminal differentiation, moving from the granular layer into the stratum corneum, several biochemical events occur simultaneously, including (1) cell enucleation, (2) keratin filament aggregation by the protein filaggrin, (3) transglutaminase-mediated protein cross-linking to form an insoluble cornified envelope, and (4) lamellar granule extrusion of lipid sheets to form the water-impermeable mortar surrounding the cornified envelopes.

Keratinocytes are not the only cells present within the epidermis, however. Melanocytes are pigment-producing cells interspersed among the basal keratinocytes.[5] Transport of their pigment-containing melanosomes to nearby keratinocytes provides protection from mutagenic effects of ultraviolet irradiation. Langerhans' cells are antigen-presenting cells located primarily within the suprabasal epidermal layers, and they act as immunologic sentinels responding to the invasion of skin pathogens. Merkel cells are specialized neuroendocrine cells that are important in mechanoreception. Both Langerhans' cells and melanocytes migrate into the epidermis during embryonic development, whereas Merkel cells appear to be derived from a pluripotent keratinocyte.

Embryonic Development

During the third week after fertilization the human embryo undergoes gastrulation, a complex process of involution and cell redistribution, which generates the three primary embryonic germ layers: endoderm, mesoderm, and ectoderm.[1] Shortly after gastrulation, the ectoderm is further subdivided into neuroectoderm, a medial strip parallel to the long axis of the developing embryo, and presumptive epidermis on either side of this strip. The early presumptive epidermis is a loosely associated single cell layer.[6,7] By 6 weeks EGA (8 weeks LMP), the earliest point in time that human embryos are generally available for study, the surface ectoderm covering most regions of the

body already consists of basal cells and more superficial periderm cells (Fig. 1-2), which are not attached to basement membrane.[8-10] The periderm layer is a transient embryonic layer that does not participate in the production of definitive epidermal progenitors, and the presumptive epidermis at these early stages is not considered a true stratified epithelium.

Basal cells of the embryonic epidermis display morphologic and biochemical features similar, but not identical, to basal cells of later developmental stages. Embryonic basal cells are slightly more columnar than later fetal basal cells, and they lack the morphologically distinct matrix adhesion structures, called hemidesmosomes.[11] Immunohistochemical analyses indicate that they do not express two of the hemidesmosomal components—BPA1 and BPA2[11]—and that although they express α6β4, these latter proteins fail to localize along the basal surface of basal cells.[12] Matrix adhesion of the early embryonic epidermis is probably mediated in part by the actin-associated α6β4 integrin, as suggested by expression and genetic studies in the mouse and human.[12-15]

Intercellular attachment between individual basal cells at this stage appears to be mediated by classical cadherin adhesion molecules, such as E- and P-cadherin, as well as by a few desmosomal junctions. E- and P-cadherin have both been detected on basal cell membranes as early as 6 weeks EGA, whereas E-cadherin alone is expressed on the early periderm.[16] Cytoplasmic filaments in the basal cells include both actin microfilaments and the less abundant keratin intermediate filaments, which even at these early stages are composed of K5 and K14 keratins, proteins generally restricted to definitive stratified epithelia.[17-19]

Periderm cells of the embryonic epidermis are larger and flatter than the underlying basal cells. As such, periderm cells have been termed a pavement epithelium.[8,20] Apical surfaces in contact with the amniotic fluid are studded with microvilli. Their lateral surfaces in contact with adjacent peridermal cells are sealed with tight junctions, possibly precluding passive, but not active, diffusion of fluids across this outer layer of the embryo.[10] Toward the end of the second trimester, these superficial cells are eventually sloughed and become a component of the vernix caseosa covering the newborn.[21] At this stage of fetal development, the maturing epidermis begins to form its own barrier to the external environment.[22]

Periderm cells, like the embryonic basal cells, express the stratified epithelial keratins K5 and K14, but they also express simple epithelial keratins K8, K18, and K19.[23-26] Based on this co-expression of simple epithelial keratins and other protein markers, as well as morphologic simi-

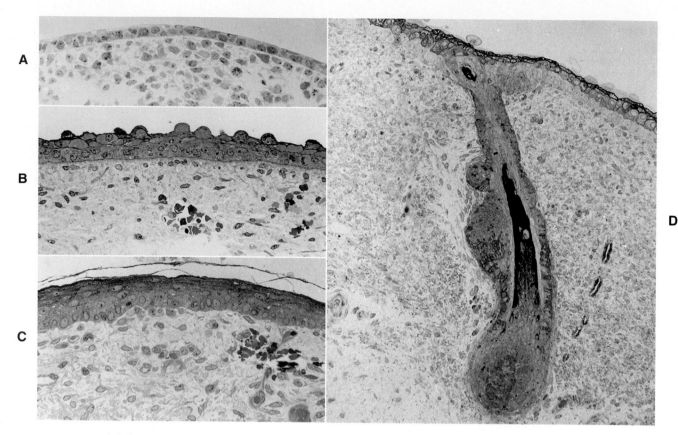

FIG. 1-2

Epidermal morphogenesis. At 36 days, **A,** the epidermis consists only of a basal layer and a superficial peri-derm layer. By 72 days, **B,** a well-formed intermediate layer is present between the basal and periderm lay-ers. By the end of the second trimester, there are several intermediate cell layers, and the stratified epidermis begins to keratinize. In neonatal skin, a distinct granular layer and stratum corneum are present **(C).** Hair follicles first begin to bud down in the dermis between 75 and 80 days. An early bulbous hair peg–stage follicle, **D,** from a mid–second trimester fetus. (Photomicrographs courtesy Dr. Karen Holbrook.)

larities, it has been posited that periderm cells are derived from migrating amnion cells.[10] Cell-labeling studies in rodents, however, provide compelling evidence that the mammalian periderm is produced by the underlying epidermal basal layer.[27]

Early Fetal Development

By the end of 8 weeks' gestation (10 weeks LMP), the basic components of most organ systems have been laid down and hemopoietic production has shifted to the bone marrow. This marks the classical division between embryonic and fetal development, and it corresponds to the timing of definitive epidermal stratification and the formation of the third "intermediate" layer between the two preexisting cell layers. Similar to cells in the spinous layers of the mature epidermis, cells in the intermediate layer of the early fetal epidermis express the K1/10 skin differentiation-type ker-atin markers, as well as the desmosomal protein, desmo-glein 3, which is also known as the pemphigus vulgaris antigen.[28,29] Moreover, intermediate filaments and desmo-somal junctions are more abundant in this layer than in the basal or periderm layers. In contrast to the spinous cells of the mature nonwounded epidermis, cells within the in-termediate layer remain highly proliferative.[30,31] Over the next several weeks, more layers are gradually added to this intermediate zone of the developing epidermis such that by 22 to 24 weeks EGA, the epidermis contains four to five layers in addition to the degenerating periderm.

After the onset of stratification, the basal layer also dis-plays characteristic morphologic and biochemical changes. Basal cells become more cuboidal and begin to synthesize other keratin peptides, including K6, K8, K19, and the K6/K16 hyperproliferative pair.[25,26] This latter keratin pair is not normally expressed in mature interfollicular epidermis but is up-regulated in response to wounding and hyperproliferative conditions.[32] During early fetal development, the basal cell layer also begins to express the hemidesmosomal proteins—BPA1 and BPA2—and to secrete collagen types V and VII, the latter being the major component of the anchoring fibrils of the dermis.[28,33-35] DNA-labeling studies indicate that by 80 to 90 days EGA, a distinct subset of slow-cycling cells exists within the basal cell population, suggesting that an epidermal stem cell population has already been set aside at these early stages.[30]

Late Fetal Development

Maturation of the epidermis during late fetal development is characterized by the generation of granular and stratum corneal layers, the formation of a water-impermeable barrier, and the sloughing of the periderm. Keratinization, which is the type of terminal differentiation mediated by granular layer and stratum corneum formation, is initiated first in the skin appendages between 11 and 15 weeks EGA and only begins to involve the interfollicular epidermis starting at 22 to 24 weeks EGA.[25] Initiation of keratinization is morphologically characterized by the marked increase in cytoplasmic density of the superficial keratinocytes and the precursor of the keratin-aggregating protein, filaggrin. The early granular layer continues to mature with the formation of more granules. More superficial layers arise, which undergo incomplete terminal differentiation, resulting in the formation of transglutaminase-mediated cross-linked envelopes that still encase remnant organelles. At slightly later stages, the terminal differentiation is more complete, resulting in the complete absence of organelles in keratinized cells of the stratum corneum. During the third trimester, the cornified cell layers increase in number, aiding in the formation of a barrier. Although the third-trimester stratum corneum is structurally similar to that of the adult, functional studies indicate that it is much less effective at preventing water loss and is less permeable to exogenous compounds.[36-40]

Clinical Relevance

Gross defects in early epidermal specification and organogenesis are rarely observed in the neonate, probably because they are incompatible with fetal survival. One such defect, aplasia cutis, generally affects focal areas of skin and might in some cases reflect inappropriate epidermal specification or development as a result of a postzygotic genetic mutation that affects only a subpopulation of epidermal cells (somatic mosaicism).

In contrast to defects in early epidermal organogenesis, congenital defects in epidermal maturation are not uncommon, since these usually do not impinge on in utero survival. Lamellar ichthyosis is usually inherited in an autosomal recessive manner and in 30% of patients is caused by mutations in the gene encoding epidermal transglutaminase,[41-44] the enzyme that cross-links submembranous proteins to form the insoluble cornified envelopes of the stratum corneum. In its absence, large polygonal dark scales form over the entire body, and at birth the infant may be transiently wrapped in a waxy, collodion-like membrane.[45] Ineffective maturation and desquamation also occur in X-linked ichthyosis, a disorder caused by deficient steroid sulfatase activity. A more severe defect in epidermal desquamation is observed in infants with harlequin ichthyosis,[46-49] who are born encased in armorlike plates of thickened, adherent stratum corneum. Although the molecular defect(s) responsible for this often fatal condition remain unknown, a striking feature is the paucity of normal lamellar granules and lack of interkeratinocyte lipids in the stratum corneum.

In contrast to the permanent manifestations of genetic defects, the inadequate epidermal keratinization and maturation of the premature epidermis are transient. Immaturity of the stratum corneum, especially in infants born before 28 weeks EGA (30 weeks LMP), places these neonates at increased risk for dehydration, excessive penetration of topical drugs or other chemicals, and infection from organisms newly colonizing the skin[36-40,50] (see Chapters 4 and 5). In general, even full-term newborns display a somewhat reduced barrier function, and continued maturation occurs over the first few weeks of life, such that by 3 weeks of age, the newborn's stratum corneum is structurally and functionally equivalent to the adult's; it is accelerated in the premature infant, although the duration may be longer in extremely premature infants.[38,51]

Specialized Cells Within the Epidermis

Two major immigrant cells—melanocytes and Langerhans' cells—populate the epidermis during early embryonic development. Melanocytes are derived from a subset of neuroectoderm cells, the neural crest, which forms along the dorsal neural tube and gives rise to a variety of cell types, including many tissues of the face and peripheral autonomic neurons.[52] Neural crest cells destined to become melanocytes migrate away from the neural tube within the mesenchyme subjacent to the presumptive epidermis. They migrate as semicoherent clones laterally and then ventrally around the trunk to the thoracoabdominal midline, anteriorly over the scalp and face, and distally along the extremities. Postnatally, the embryonic paths taken by these partially coherent clones can be readily visualized in patients with banded pigmentary dycrasias following Blaschko's lines, such as the disorders classified as hypomelanosis of Ito, and linear and whorled hypermelanosis (see Chapters 19 and 20).[53,54]

The melanocytes can be first detected within the epidermis of the human embryo at approximately 50 days EGA based on their dendritic morphology and their immunoreactivity with the HMB-45 monoclonal antibody.[55] Even at these early developmental time points, the density of melanocytes is quite high (1000 cells/mm²).[56] The density further increases around the time of epidermal stratification (80 to 90 days EGA) and initiation of appendageal development. Between 3 and 4 months EGA, depending on body site and race of the fetus, melanin (visible pigment) production becomes detectable, and by 5 months, melanocytes begin transferring melanosomes to the keratinocytes, a process that will continue after birth.[57-59] Although all melanocytes are in place at birth and melanogenesis is well under way, the skin of the newborn infant is not fully pigmented, and it will continue to darken over the first several months of life. This is most apparent in individuals with darker skin tones.

Langerhans' cells, the other major immigrant population, are detectable within the epidermis by 40 days EGA.[60] Similar to melanocytes, the early embryonic Langerhans' cells do not yet possess the specialized organelles characteristic of mature cells, but they can be distinguished from other epidermal cells by their dendritic morphology, immunopositive reaction for the HLA-DR surface antigen, and high levels of ATPase activity. After the embryonic-fetal transition, they begin to express the CD1 antigen on their surface and to produce characteristic granules of mature Langerhans' cells.[60,61] Although the extent of dendritic processes from individual Langerhans' cells increases during the second trimester, the total number of cells remains low and only increases to typical adult numbers in the third trimester.[62,63]

Another distinct subset of cells within the basal cell layer are Merkel cells, which are highly innervated neuroendocrine cells involved in mechanoreception. Merkel cells can be round or dendritic and are found at particularly high densities in volar skin. They are frequently associated with epidermal appendageal structures and are occasionally detected within the dermis. Their distinguishing morphologic and immunohistochemical features are cytoplasmic dense core granules, keratin 18, and neuropeptide expression, which can be detected as early as 8 to 12 weeks EGA in palmoplantar epidermis and at slightly later times in interfollicular skin.[17,64] Recent keratin expression data, as well as transplant studies, suggest that Merkel cells are derived from pluripotent keratinocytes, rather than neural progenitors such as neural crest, but the results are not conclusive.[64-67]

Clinical Relevance

Many clinical defects are known to affect normal pigmentation within an individual. Defects in melanoblast migration, proliferation, and/or survival occur in several clinical syndromes, and many of the genetic mutations responsible for these defects have been identified. Failure of an adequate number of melanoblasts to completely supply distal points on their embryonic migration path occurs in the different types of Waardenburg syndrome, as well as in piebaldism, resulting in depigmented patches on the central forehead, central abdomen, and extremities. These defects are associated with mutations in several different genes, including genes encoding transcription factors, such as *Pax3* and *MITF*, as well as membrane receptors and their ligands, such as endothelin 3, endothelin-receptor B, and c-kit.[68-78] In albinism, on the other hand, melanocyte development is normal, but production of pigment or melanin is inadequate. The most severe form of oculocutaneous albinism results from null mutations in the gene encoding tyrosinase, the rate-limiting enzyme in the production of melanin. Less severe forms of albinism are caused by mutations in tyrosinase alleles, which lead to partial loss of function, as well as by mutations in other genes encoding proteins important in melanin assembly in melanosomes or transport.[5]

DERMIS AND SUBCUTIS

Overview

The mature dermis is characterized by complex interwoven collagen and elastic fibers enmeshed in a proteoglycan matrix. Fibroblasts, mast cells, and macrophages are scattered throughout this mesh, and nerve fibers and vascular networks course through it, dividing it into distinct domains. In contrast, the embryonic dermis is quite cellular and amorphous, lacking organized extracellular fibers. Embryonic mesenchymal cells capable of differentiating into a wide variety of cell types are embedded in a highly hydrated gel, rich in hyaluronic acid. Moreover, only a few nerve fibers have reached this peripheral location, and vessels have not evolved into their mature patterns. During the course of fetal development, this so-called cellular dermis, which is conducive to cell migration and tissue remodeling, is transformed into the fibrillar dermis of the adult, which provides increased strength, resilience, and structural support.[79]

Embryonic Dermal Development

Specification and allocation of dermal mesenchymal cells is rather complex and not well understood. The cell of origin for the presumptive dermis depends on its anatomic location. Dermis of the face is derived from neural crest cells; dermis of the dorsal trunk is derived from the dermatomyotome portion of the differentiated somite; and dermis of the limbs is derived from the lateral plate (somatic) mesoderm.[79-81] Regional patterning of the skin and differences in the type and quality of the epidermal appendages produced in the older fetus might in part reflect these early differences in dermal cell precursors. In addition, signaling from adjacent tissues plays a critical role.[82,83]

By 6 to 8 weeks EGA, the presumptive dermal cells already underlie the epidermis. However, a sharp demarcation between cells giving rise to skin dermis and those giving rise to musculoskeletal elements does not yet exist. Electron microscopic (EM) studies of the presumptive dermis at these stages demonstrate fine filaments, but rarely fibers.[84] Although most protein components of collagen fibers and some microfibrillar components of elastin fibers (fibrillin) are synthesized by the embryonic dermal cells, the proteins are not yet assembled into large, rigid fibers.[3,35] Moreover, the ratio of collagen III to collagen I is 3:1, the reverse of what it is in the adult.[35,85,86]

Fetal Dermal Development

After the embryonic fetal transition at 60 days, the presumptive dermis is distinguishable from the underlying skeletal condensations. Moreover, within the dermis, there is a progressive change in matrix organization and cell morphology, such that by 12 to 15 weeks, the fine interwoven mesh of the papillary dermis adjacent to the epidermis can be distinguished from the deeper, more fibrillar reticular dermis.[3,35] Large collagen fibers accumulate in the reticular dermis during the second and third trimesters. Definitive elastin fibers first become detectable by EM studies around 22 to 24 weeks EGA,[87] although both the microfibrillar protein, fibrillin, as well as microfibrillar structures, which are morphologically similar to elastin-associated microfibrils of the adult, can be detected at earlier stages.[3] By the completion of gestation, the dermis is thick and well organized, but it is still much thinner than it is in the adult and contains a higher water content, reminiscent of the fetal dermis. Maturation of the dermis is marked by increasing tensile strength and the transition from a nonscarring to a scarring response after wounding. Thus fetal skin biopsies tend to heal with little evidence of the surgical event. This has obvious clinical implications, and the molecular controls critical for nonscarring fetal wound healing is an area of active research by many groups.[88-90]

Clinical Relevance

Congenital defects in the specification and development of the dermis are probably incompatible with survival to term, although there are a few exceptions. Infants with the restrictive dermopathy disorder, which is characterized by a thin, flat dermis, lack of elastic tissue fibers, and shortened appendageal structures, do survive to birth but then die in the neonatal period.[91-93] Although the underlying molecular etiology has yet to be identified, the current data suggest inadequate growth and development of the dermal mesenchyme. Another syndrome characterized by inadequate dermal development is Goltz syndrome (focal dermal hypoplasia).[45,94] This is an X-linked dominant condition in which males who inherit the mutation on their single X chromosome die in utero. In contrast, females are functional mosaics as a result of random X-inactivation early in embryogenesis, and those with Goltz syndrome display areas of dermal hypoplasia where the mutant X is active. These bands of dermal hypoplasia follow Blaschko's lines and alternate with bands of normal dermal development where the normal X is active.[54,95] Another disorder that displays patchy dermal hypoplasia and probably reflects mosaicism for an autosomal dominant mutation is Proteus syndrome.[96] In addition, other focal developmental dysplasias or hamartomas, such as nevus sebaceus, probably also reflect inappropriate inductive signaling events between the dermis and epidermis.

Specialized Components of the Dermis

The structure and organization of the cutaneous nerves and vessels begin early in gestation but do not develop into those of the adult until a few months after birth. And although the pattern of the vasculature varies among regions of the body, vessels of the endoderm-mesoderm interface form through the in situ differentiation of endothelial cells (vasculogenesis).[97,98] Originally, they form horizontal plexuses within the subpapillary and deep reticular dermis, which are interconnected by groups of vertical vessels. This vascular framework has been elegantly reconstructed by the use of computer graphics to illustrate the complexity that already exists by 45 to 50 days EGA.[99] Such structure does not remain constant even throughout fetal life, but varies depending on the body region and gestational age, as well as on the presence of hair follicles and glands that may require an increased blood supply. Furthermore, vascular emergence and development correlate directly with the particular tissue, determined specifically by the influences of pressure and function.

Regional variation depends on gestational age as well. Blood vessels have been identified in fetal skin as early as 9 weeks EGA. At this stage, they help delineate the dermal-hypodermal junction. By 3 months, the distinct horizontal and vertical networks have formed. And by the fifth month, vasculogenesis has largely ceased and the formation of the complex vascular plexus is initiated by angiogenesis, the budding and migration of endothelium from preexisting vessels. With increasing gestational age, the superficial architecture becomes more organized, culminating at birth in an extensive capillary network responsible for the redness (of the skin) often observed in the newborn. Within the first few postnatal months, the complexity decreases as skin surface area increases, lanugo hairs are lost, and sebaceous gland activity decreases. It is during this time that the rate of skin growth is greatest. By approximately 3 months of age, the vascular patterns most closely resemble those of the (mature) adult.

Development of the cutaneous innervation closely parallels that of the vascular system in terms of its pattern, rate of maturation, and organization. Nerves of the skin consist of somatic sensory and sympathetic autonomic fibers, which are predominantly small and unmyelinated. Development of these nerve fibers consists of myelination with a concomitant decrease in the number of axons and is far from complete at birth. It may in fact continue until puberty.

Clinical Relevance

Not only does the number and caliber of the blood vessels change over time, so too does the direction of blood flow. Considering the dynamic nature of this circulatory system, it is not surprising that of the congenital malformations seen in newborns, vascular defects are the most common. The Klippel-Trénaunay and Sturge-Weber syndromes are examples of these. In the former, unilateral cutaneous vascular malformations, usually involving an extremity, are seen in association with venous varicosities and hypertrophy of the associated soft tissue and/or bone. In the latter, cutaneous capillary malformations are also often unilateral and may involve the lips, tongue, and nasal and buccal mucosa. Studies of families with heritable vascular anomalies have begun to provide insights into the pathways critical for normal fetal vascular development and subsequent postnatal remodeling. Specifically, increased activity of the TIE2 receptor tyrosine kinase, one of the vascular endothelial cell-specific receptor tyrosine kinases

that have been characterized, has been described in some families with inherited venous malformations.[100,101] In addition, aberrant activities of TGF-β binding proteins, endoglin and activin receptor-like kinase 1, have been reported in patients with hereditary hemorrhagic telangiectasia (Osler-Weber-Rendu syndrome), resulting in the apparent abnormal capillary bed remodeling.[102,103]

Development of the Hypodermis

A distinct region that is the hypodermis can be delineated by 50 to 60 days EGA.[3] It is separated from the overlying cellular dermis by a plane of thin-walled vessels. Toward the end of the first trimester, the sparse matrix of the hypodermis can be distinguished morphologically from the slightly denser, more fibrous matrix of the dermis.[79,104] In the second trimester, mesenchymally derived preadipocytes begin to differentiate and accumulate lipids,[105] and by the third trimester the more mature adipocytes are aggregated into large lobules of fat divided by fibrous septae. Although the molecular pathways that direct mesenchyme cells to commit to the adipocyte pathway are not well understood, many regulators involved in the subsequent preadipocyte differentiation have been identified.[106,107] An example is the gene that encodes leptin, whose abnormal regulation has been implicated in the pathogenesis of obesity.[108-110]

COMBINED DERMAL-EPIDERMAL STRUCTURES

Dermal-Epidermal Junction

The dermal-epidermal junction (DEJ) is the region where the epidermis and dermis abut. In the broadest definition, it includes the specialized extracellular matrix on which the basal keratinocytes sit, known as the basement membrane, as well as the basal-most portion of the basal cells and the superficial-most portion of the dermis. Importantly, both the dermal and epidermal compartments contribute to the molecular synthesis, assembly, and integration of this region.

A simple basement membrane, separating the dermis and epidermis, can be discerned as early as 8 weeks EGA. The basic protein constituents common to all basement membranes can already be detected immunohistochemically at this stage.[12,34,111] These include collagen IV, laminin, and heparin sulfate and proteoglycans.

Specialized components of the DEJ do not appear until after the embryonic-fetal transition around the time of initial epidermal stratification.[12,34,111] With a few exceptions, all basement membrane antigens are in place by the end of the first trimester.[3] As discussed, the α6 and β4 integrin subunits are expressed quite early by embryonic basal cells.[12] However, they do not become localized to the basal surface until after 9.5 weeks, which is coincident with the time when bullous pemphigoid antigens are first detected immunohistochemically and hemidesmosomes are recognized ultrastructurally.[11,12,34,112] Similarly, anchoring filaments and anchoring fibrils, the basement membrane components that mediate basal cell attachment to extracellular matrix, are recognizable by 9 weeks EGA.[3,11] Collagen VII, the anchoring fibril protein, is detected slightly earlier, at 8 weeks.[11]

Recent experimental data have delineated many of the molecular interactions crucial for connecting the cytoskeletal networks of the basal cells with the extracellular filamentous networks important in matrix adhesion (Fig. 1-3). On the outer surface of the basal cell α6β4, the hemidesmosome integrin binds laminin 5, the major constituent of anchoring filaments.[113] Laminin 5 in turn binds

collagen VII, the major component of anchoring fibrils, thus indirectly connecting the hemidesmosome to the anchoring fibrils.[114] On the inner side of the basal cell membrane, the cytoplasmic tail of β4 interacts with the submembranous plaque protein plectin, which then binds with keratin intermediate filament proteins.[115] In addition, the cytoplasmic tail of BPA2 binds the hemidesmosomal plaque protein BPA1, which in turn appears to bind the keratin intermediate filaments.[116]

Clinical Applications

Several congenital disorders characterized by severe blistering of the skin occur as a result of mutations in genes encoding DEJ components[117] (see Chapter 10). The severity of the disorder, the exact plane of tissue separation, and the involvement of nonskin tissues depend in part on which proteins are affected by the genetic mutations (see Fig. 1-2). Because these blistering disorders are associated with a high morbidity and mortality postnatally, they are

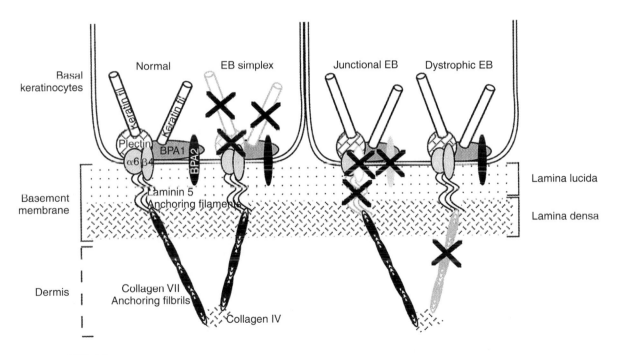

FIG. 1-3
Schematic of the dermal-epidermal junction indicating the proteins that are defective in the relevant hereditary bullous diseases *(X)*. Mutations in genes encoding keratin 5 or keratin 14 cause epidermolysis bullosa (EB simplex). Plectin function is disrupted in EB associated with muscular dystrophy. One of the subunits of laminin 5 is defective in most forms of junctional EB. However, the β4 subunit of α6β4 integrin is altered in the form associated with pyloric atresia, and bullous pemphigoid antigen 2 (BPA2) is mutated in generalized atrophic benign EB. Collagen VII is defective in all forms of dystrophic EB published to date.

frequent candidates for prenatal testing, and when the responsible genetic mutation is one that has been identified, this can be accomplished by chorionic villus sampling (CVS) or amniocentesis (see the section on Prenatal Diagnosis of Severe Congenital Skin Disorders).

Development of Appendages

Skin appendages (hair, nails, sweat and mammary glands in mammals, and feathers and scales in birds and reptiles) all consist of two distinct components: an epidermal component that elaborates the differentiated end product, such as the hair or nail, and the dermal component that regulates specification and differentiation of the appendage. Fetal development of these structures depends on rigidly choreographed, collaborative interactions between early epidermis and dermis.[79,118,119] Defects in dermal induction or specification of the overlying ectoderm or in the ectoderm's responses to these instructions result in aberrant development, as has been demonstrated in genetic studies and transplant experiments in animal model systems.[79,118-120] Moreover, the recent demonstration that defects in human homologs of mouse hairless, *LMX1B*, and tabby genes result in clinically significant developmental abnormalities in humans confirms the relevance of such animal studies to our understanding of human skin appendage development.[121-125]

Hair Follicle and Sebaceous Gland Development

Hair follicle formation begins on the head and then spreads caudally and ventrally in waves, resulting in regularly spaced rows and whorls of follicles.[126,127] The first morphologic evidence of follicle formation in humans is the focal crowding of small groups of basal keratinocytes at regularly spaced intervals, starting between 75 and 80 days on the face and scalp.[126,128-130] This ectodermal structure is called the placode of the pregerm-stage follicle. Slightly later in development, mesenchymal cell clusters are observed beneath these ectodermal placodes. Although morphologically similar to other dermal fibroblasts, these clustered mesenchymal cells are biochemically distinguishable based on their continued expression of certain molecular markers, such as nerve growth factor receptor (NGFR).[3] On the trunk at approximately 80 days EGA, a cluster of basal epidermal cells thickens and begins to bud downward into the dermis, forming the early hair germs.[130,131] Transplant studies in other species indicate that ectodermal budding requires an induction signal from the underlying mesenchymal cells. The cells of the early ectodermal bud or placode then respond with their own signal, which elicits a second mesenchymal signal. This second signal directs the species-specific type of mesenchymal appendage that will ultimately develop.[79,119]

The next stage of hair development involves further proliferation and resulting downward elongation of the ectodermal bud, forming the so-called hair peg.[126] At 12 to 14 weeks EGA, the hair peg develops a widened bulb at its base that flattens and then invaginates, engulfing the subjacent clustered mesenchymal cells, which become the follicular dermal papilla. In addition to the widened bulb at the base, two other bulges form along the length of the developing follicle, which is now termed the bulbous hair peg (see Fig. 1-2).[126,132] The uppermost bulge is the presumptive sebaceous gland, and the middle bulge, which forms at approximately one-third the distance from the follicular base, is the site of the future insertion of the arrector pili muscle. Accumulating evidence suggests that this middle bulge is also the location of multipotent hair stem cells, which give rise to all the progenitors necessary for the cycling follicle, as well as to cells capable of replenishing the overlying epidermal covering in the event of extensive surface wounds or burns.[133,134]

Maturation of the hair peg into a definitive follicle is a complex process involving the formation of a patent hair canal and the elaboration of at least six distinct concentric rings of cells.[135] The most peripheral ring of ectodermal cells makes up the outer root sheath, whose upper portion is continuous with the interfollicular epidermis and undergoes a similar process of keratinization. Its lower portion, in contrast, does not form a granular layer or classical stratum corneum. The inner root sheath forms just internal to the outer root sheath. The cells in this sheath do form a granular layer through the keratin proteins, and keratin-aggregating products produced here differ from those produced by the normal epidermis. Cells in this inner root sheath arise from multipotent matrix cells at the base of the follicle, which differentiate as they move upward toward the skin surface surrounding the hair shaft. The hair shaft is composed of three layers that also arise from the matrix cells at the base of the follicle: cuticle, cortex, and medulla (from outer to inner). These deep matrix cells sit on the basement membrane "mat," along the concavity of the hair follicle invagination, and as such are in close proximity to the dermal papillae mesenchymal cells.

By 19 to 21 weeks EGA, the hair canal has fully formed and the scalp hairs are visible just above the surface of the fetal epidermis.[127,136,137] They continue to lengthen until 24 to 28 weeks, when they shift from the active growing phase (anagen) to the short-lived degenerative phase (catagen) and then to the resting phase (telogen).[3,138] They then reenter the active growing stage (second anagen), and the first wave of hairs is shed into the amniotic fluid as the new hairs grow out. Cycling through active and inactive phases continues for all hairs throughout the life of an individual,[139] although cycles for individual hairs become asynchronous postnatally. The maintenance of a tight anatomic relationship between dermal papilla cells and the cycling ectodermal portion of the hair follicle is critical for follicular self-renewal, and the inability to maintain this relationship results in a form of inherited alopecia in which hair neogenesis is normal but after the first resting phase, cycling is aberrant.[122]

Perinatally the second wave of fine lanugo hairs is shed. With subsequent cycles, hairs increase in diameter and coarseness, forming first vellus and then adult-type terminal hair shafts on the scalp and brow.[138] During adolescence, vellus hairs of androgen-sensitive areas undergo a similar transition to terminal-type hair follicles.

Sebaceous gland maturation occurs in parallel with that of the follicle proper and begins between 13 and 16 weeks EGA.[140] Lipogenic cells produced by the outer proliferative layer of the sebaceous gland progressively accumulate lipid/sebum until they terminally differentiate, which results in their disintegration and the release of their products into the upper portion of the newly formed hair canal.[141,142] The synthesis and secretion of sebum is accelerated in the second and third trimesters under the influence of the maternal steroids, and the glands themselves become hyperplastic.[143,144] This stimulated activity by the sebaceous glands is believed to be responsible for the common condition known as neonatal acne. In the absence of exogenous maternal hormones, these glands become quiescent during the first few months of life and again increase in activity during the hormonal changes of adolescence.[143]

Nail Development

The first evidence of nail formation is the delineation of the flat surface of the future nail bed on the dorsal digit tip at 8 to 10 weeks,[10,145] slightly earlier than the initiation of hair follicle development. Along the proximal boundary of the early nail field, a wedge of ectoderm buds inward at an oblique angle to the surface, forming the proximal nail fold. The presumptive nail matrix cells, which will give rise to the differentiated nail plate, reside on the ventral (deeper) side of the proximal invagination. At around 11 weeks, the dorsal surface of the nail bed begins to keratinize, a process similar to subsequent keratinization of the embryonic epidermis.[146-149] In the fourth month, the definitive nail plate

grows out distally from the proximal fold, replacing the embryonic cornified layers. It completely covers the nail bed by the fifth month. Keratinization of the nail resembles that of the epidermis except that nail terminal differentiation, like hair shaft differentiation, involves the synthesis of distinct keratins and keratin-aggregating proteins normally not expressed in epidermis.[150-152] The keratins found in hairs and nails provide greater structural stability and rigidity than those in epidermis.

Eccrine and Apocrine Sweat Gland Development

The first morphologic indicators of palmoplantar eccrine gland development are the formation of large mesenchymal bulges or pads on the volar surfaces of the hands and feet between 55 and 65 days EGA, and the induction of parallel ectodermal ridges overlying these bulges between 12 and 14 weeks.[153,154] The curves and whorls that these ridges adopt are intimately related to the size and shape of the embryonic volar pads and result in the characteristic dermatoglyphic patterns, or "fingerprints," which can be visualized on the surface of the digit tips in the fifth month.[154,155] In contrast to those of most other animal species, the volar mesenchymal pads in humans regress by the third trimester.

Individual eccrine gland primordia bud at regularly spaced intervals along the ectodermal ridges, elongating as cords of cells into the pad mesenchyme. By 16 weeks, the glandular regions at the terminal portion of this downgrowth have formed, and the secretory and myoepithelial components become discernable. Canalization of the dermal components of the glands occurs by loss of desmosome adhesion along the innermost ectodermal surfaces with maintenance of lateral adhesion between cells of the duct and gland walls. This process is complete by 16 weeks, whereas the opening of the epidermal portion of the duct by vesicular fusion and autolysis and keratinization of the wall are not complete until 22 weeks EGA.[156,157] Although the primary ectodermal ridges are established quite early in embryonic development, secondary ridges form at later stages and the complexity of the undulating DEJ increases further at late fetal stages and postnatally with the formation of dermal papillae protruding into the overlying epidermis.

In contrast to volar eccrine glands, interfollicular eccrine glands and apocrine glands do not initiate budding until the fifth month of gestation.[136,158] Apocrine sweat glands, like sebaceous glands, usually bud from the upper portion of a hair follicle, whereas eccrine sweat glands arise independently. Over the next several weeks, the glandular cords of cells elongate. By 7 months EGA, the clear cells and mucin-secreting dark cells characteristic of apocrine glands are distinguishable. At birth, the secretory portions of non-volar sweat glands remain high in the dermis but progressively extend down to the subcutis postnatally. The apocrine gland functions transiently in the third trimester and then becomes quiescent in the neonate,[144,159] whereas the eccrine gland does not appear to function in utero but progressively reaches functional maturity postnatally.[160-164]

Ectodermal Appendages: Clinical Relevance

Genetic studies in mice have suggested that mutations in genes directing early regional patterning of the mammalian embryo can have a profound impact on later skin appendage specification and differentiation.[82,83,165,166] One such gene, LMX1B, which encodes a homeobox-containing transcription factor, acts several stages before initiation of appendageal downgrowths and is important in distal limb patterning.[166] Experimental ablation of LMX1B function in mice results in the transformation of dorsal limb musculoskeletal elements and dermal structures to a more ventral (volar side) phenotype. Viewed from the side, Lmx1b mutant mouse limbs appear perfectly symmetric, with the paw pads present on both the ventral and dorsal aspects. Mutations in LMX1B have been observed in at least some people with the autosomal dominant disease nail-patella syndrome.[121] These patients display a much less dramatic limb phenotype characterized by aberrant or absent nail and patella development (elbows). This milder effect on dorsal limb structures reflects the fact that individuals with nail-patella syndrome are heterozygotes. Thus they carry a single defective copy of LMX1B, together with a wild-type copy, resulting in only partial loss of gene function.

Several other genes have been identified that appear to regulate skin appendage formation. Positional cloning strategies have been used to identify genes affected in two different types of ectodermal dysplasias, resulting in a heterogenous group of disorders defined by their involvement of hair, nails, glands, and/or teeth. The most common type of ectodermal dysplasia, anhidrotic (hypohidrotic) ectodermal dysplasia, is caused by mutations in the EDA gene, which encodes a transmembrane protein with a collagenous extracellular domain.[125] The exact role of this gene in eccrine gland, hair, and tooth development is under investigation. The gene encoding MSX1, another homeobox-containing transcription factor, has been shown to be mutated in familial tooth agenesis, which affects not only tooth development, but also formation of nails and hair.[167,168]

Studies in mice suggest that other classical embryonic patterning genes play a direct role in epidermal appendage development, including genes encoding components of the Notched, Wnt, and Sonic hedgehog signaling pathways.[118,169] The importance of such genes in human skin homeostasis has already been demonstrated by the finding that PATCHED is the tumor suppressor gene mutated in nevoid basal cell carcinoma (Gorlin) syndrome and that it and other genes of the pathway are frequently mutated in spontaneous basal cell carcinomas.[170-174] Finally, it is important to consider potential teratogenic effects on normal skin appendage development. Dilantin, for example, can cause broadening of the nail associated with distortions in the underlying distal phalange.

PRENATAL DIAGNOSIS OF SEVERE CONGENITAL SKIN DISORDERS

A number of inherited skin disorders are compatible with in utero survival but are life threatening or result in severe morbidity after birth. Often these disorders can be diagnosed during the first or second trimesters of pregnancy. Candidates for prenatal testing include those fetuses with an affected sibling or other family member. Importantly, the need for prenatal testing depends on the familial relationship, the mode of inheritance of the disorder in question, and in some cases the sex of the fetus. DNA from parents and from both affected and unaffected siblings should be analyzed before conception to determine the exact mutational event responsible for the disorder in the relevant pedigree and the likelihood that the fetus will in fact inherit the disease.[175] With this in mind, prenatal and genetic counseling should be a critical component of early interventional care of infants affected with severe genodermatoses.

Until recently, prenatal diagnosis of inherited disorders has relied on fetal skin biopsies done between 19 and 22 weeks EGA.[176,177] The procedure is performed under ultrasound guidance, and multiple biopsies must be taken, although the number of biopsies and the sites from which they are taken depend on the disorder for which the fetus is at risk. In some disorders, such as those in which keratinization of the interfollicular dermis is not yet complete, analysis of the developing appendageal structures is required for accurate diagnosis.[177] Fortunately, because of the identification of the genetic mutations responsible for many of these disorders, diagnosis can be made using cells obtained from CVS at 8 to 10 weeks EGA or amniocentesis at 16 to 18 weeks EGA.[9] The obvious advantages of these procedures is that they can be performed early in the pregnancy with minimal risk to the mother and fetus.

Fundamental knowledge of those skin disorders whose etiologies are genetic is crucial for the practicing pediatric dermatologist. Awareness of the resources available for both diagnosis and treatment of those fetuses suspected of having an inherited disorder is equally as important and must frequently be reviewed as our understanding of the molecular bases for genetic abnormalities evolves. Data on genetic test availability, provided by both commercial and research laboratories, are provided by GeneTest (http://www.genetests.org), a database for healthcare providers. It is only through physicians' awareness of the different genodermatoses, as well as their understanding of normal fetal skin development, that the need for evaluation can be recognized, the necessary therapies and supports provided, and the patients best served.

ACKNOWLEDGMENTS

We gratefully acknowledge Angela Christiano, Karen Holbrook, and William Larsen for their thought-provoking discussions and insights into human genetics and embryology.

REFERENCES

1. Larsen WL. Human Embryology. New York: Churchill Livingstone, 1997.
2. Cunningham FG, MacDonald PC, Gant NF, et al. Williams Obstetrics. Stanford: Appleton & Lange, 1997.
3. Holbrook KA. Structural and biochemical organogenesis of skin and cutaneous appendages in the fetus and newborn. In Polin RA, Fox WW, eds. Fetal and Neonatal Physiology. Philadelphia: WB Saunders, 1998: pp 729-752.
4. Fuchs E. The cytoskeleton and disease: genetic disorders of intermediate filaments. Ann Rev Genet 1996;30:197-231.
5. Barsch GS. The genetics of pigmentation: from fancy genes to complex traits. Trends Genet 1996;12.99-305.
6. Matsunaka M, Mishima Y. Electron microscopy of embryonic human epidermis at seven and ten weeks. Acta Dermatol Venereol 1969;49:241-250.
7. Breathnach AS, Robins J. Ultrastructural features of epidermis of a 14 MM. (6 weeks) human embryo. Br J Dermatol 1969;81:504-516.
8. Holbrook KA, Odland GF. The fine structure of developing human epidermis: light, scanning, and transmission electron microscopy of the periderm. J Invest Dermatol 1975;65:16-38.
9. Holbrook KA, Odland GF. Regional development of the human epidermis in the first trimester embryo and the second trimester fetus (ages related to the timing of amniocentesis and fetal biopsy). J Invest Dermatol 1980;74:161-168.
10. Holbrook KA. Structure and function of the developing human skin. In Goldsmith LA, ed. Physiology, biochemistry, and molecular biology of the skin. New York: Oxford Press, 1991: pp 63-110.
11. Smith LT, Sakai LY, Burgeson RE, et al. Ontogeny of structural components at the dermal-epidermal junction in human embryonic and fetal skin: the appearance of anchoring fibrils and type VII collagen. J Invest Dermatol 1988;90:480-485.
12. Hertle MD, Adams JC, Watt FM. Integrin expression during human epidermal development in vivo and in vitro. Development 1991;112:193-206.
13. Thorsteinsdottir S, Roelen BA, Freund E, et al. Expression patterns of laminin receptor splice variants alpha 6A beta 1 and alpha 6B beta 1 suggest different roles in mouse development. Dev Dyn 1995;204:240-258.
14. Hodivala-Dilke KM, DiPersio CM, Kreidberg JA, et al. Novel roles for alpha3beta1 integrin as a regulator of cytoskeletal assembly and as a trans-dominant inhibitor of integrin receptor function in mouse keratinocytes. J Cell Biol 1998;142:1357-1369.
15. DiPersio CM, Hodivala-Dilke KM, Jaenisch R, et al. alpha3 beta1 Integrin is required for normal development of the epidermal basement membrane. J Cell Biol 1997;137:729-742.
16. Furukawa F, Fujii K, Horiguchi Y, et al. Roles of E- and P-cadherin in the human skin. Microsc Res Tech 1997;38:343-352.
17. Moll R, Moll I, Franke WW. Identification of Merkel cells in human skin by specific cytokeratin antibodies: changes in cell density and distribution in fetal and adult plantar epidermis. Differentiation 1984;28:136-154.
18. Sun TT, Eichner R, Nelson WG, et al. Keratin classes: molecular markers for different types of epithelial differentiation. J Invest Dermatol 1983;81:109s-115s.
19. Moll R, Franke WW, Schiller DL, et al. The catalog of human cytokeratins: patterns of expression in normal epithelia, tumors and cultured cells. Cell 1982;31:11-24.
20. Hoyes AD. Electron microscopy of the surface layer periderm of human foetal skin. J Anat 1968;103:321-36.
21. Nieland ML, Parmley TH, Woodruff JD. Ultrastructural observations on amniotic fluid cells. Am J Obstet Gynecol 1970;108:1030-1042.
22. Benzie RJ, Doran TA, Harkins JL, et al. Composition of the amniotic fluid and maternal serum in pregnancy. Am J Obstet Gynecol 1974;119:798-810.
23. Lehtonen E, Lehto VP, Vartio T, et al. Expression of cytokeratin polypeptides in mouse oocytes and preimplantation embryos. Dev Biol 1983;100:158-165.
24. Jackson BW, Grund C, Winter S, et al. Formation of cytoskeletal elements during mouse embryogenesis. II. Epithelial differentiation and intermediate sized filaments in early postimplantation embryos. Differentiation 1981;20:203-216.
25. Dale BA, Holbrook KA, Kimball JR, et al. Expression of epidermal keratins and filaggrin during human fetal skin development. J Cell Biol 1985;101:1257-1269.
26. Moll R, Moll I, Wiest W. Changes in the pattern of cytokeratin polypeptides in epidermis and hair follicles during skin development in human fetuses. Differentiation 1982;23:170-178.
27. Sanes JR, Rubenstein JL, Nicolas JF. Use of a recombinant retrovirus to study post-implantation cell lineage in mouse embryos. EMBO J 1986;5:3133-3142.

28. Lane AT, Helm KF, Goldsmith LA. Identification of bullous pemphigoid, pemphigus, laminin, and anchoring fibril antigens in human fetal skin. J Invest Dermatol 1985;84:27-30.

29. Woodcock-Mitchell J, Eichner R, Nelson WG, et al. Immunolocalization of keratin polypeptides in human epidermis using monoclonal antibodies. J Cell Biol 1982; 95:580-588.

30. Bickenbach JR, Holbrook KA. Label-retaining cells in human embryonic and fetal epidermis. J Invest Dermatol 1987; 88:42-46.

31. Bickenbach JR, Holbrook KA. Proliferation of human embryonic and fetal epidermal cells in organ culture. Am J Anat 1986;177:97-106.

32. Weiss RA, Eichner R, Sun TT. Monoclonal antibody analysis of keratin expression in epidermal diseases: a 48- and 56-kdalton keratin as molecular markers for hyperproliferative keratinocytes. J Cell Biol 1984;98:1397-1406.

33. Muller HK, Kalnins R, Sutherland RC. Ontogeny of pemphigus and bullous pemphigoid antigens in human skin. Br J Dermatol 1973;88:443-446.

34. Fine JD, Smith LT, Holbrook KA, et al. The appearance of four basement membrane zone antigens in developing human fetal skin. J Invest Dermatol 1984;83:66-69.

35. Smith LT, Holbrook KA, Madri JA. Collagen types I, III, and V in human embryonic and fetal skin. Am J Anat 1986; 175: 507-521.

36. West DP, Halket JM, Harvey DR, et al. Percutaneous absorption in preterm infants. Pediatr Dermatol 1987;4:234-237.

37. Evans NJ, Rutter N. Percutaneous respiration in the newborn infant. J Pediatr 1986;108:282-286.

38. Evans NJ, Rutter N. Development of the epidermis in the newborn. Biol Neonate 1986;49:74-80.

39. Harpin VA, Rutter N. Barrier properties of the newborn infant's skin. J Pediatr 1983;102:419-425.

40. Nachman RL, Esterly NB. Increased skin permeability in preterm infants. J Pediatr 1971;79:628-632.

41. Laiho E, Ignatius J, Mikkola H, et al. Transglutaminase 1 mutations in autosomal recessive congenital ichthyosis: private and recurrent mutations in an isolated population. Am J Hum Genet 1997;61:529-538.

42. Epstein EH, Jr. The genetics of human skin diseases. Curr Opin Genet Dev 1996;6:295-300.

43. Huber M, Rettler I, Bernasconi K, et al. Mutations of keratinocyte transglutaminase in lamellar ichthyosis. Science 1995;267:525-528.

44. Russell LJ, DiGiovanna JJ, Rogers GR, et al. Mutations in the gene for transglutaminase 1 in autosomal recessive lamellar ichthyosis. Nat Genet 1995;9:279-283.

45. Novice FM, Collison DW, Burgdorf WHC, et al. Handbook of genetic skin disorders. Philadelphia: WB Saunders, 1994.

46. Akiyama M, Kim DK, Main DM, et al. Characteristic morphologic abnormality of harlequin ichthyosis detected in amniotic fluid cells. J Invest Dermatol 1994;102:210-213.

47. Akiyama M, Dale BA, Smith LT, et al. Regional difference in expression of characteristic abnormality of harlequin ichthyosis in affected fetuses. Prenat Diagn 1998;18:425-436.

48. Dale BA, Holbrook KA, Fleckman P, et al. Heterogeneity in harlequin ichthyosis, an inborn error of epidermal keratinization: variable morphology and structural protein expression and a defect in lamellar granules. J Invest Dermatol 1990;94:6-18.

49. Milner ME, O'Guin WM, Holbrook KA, et al. Abnormal lamellar granules in harlequin ichthyosis. J Invest Dermatol 1992;99:824-829.

50. Lane AT. Development and care of the premature infant's skin. Pediatr Dermatol 1987;4:1-5.

51. Kalia YN, Nonato LB, Lund CH, et al. Development of skin barrier function in premature infants. J Invest Dermatol 1998;111:320-326.

52. Anderson DJ. Stem cells and transcription factors in the development of the mammalian neural crest. FASEB J 1994; 8:707-713.

53. Loomis CA. Linear hypopigmentation and hyperpigmentation, including mosaicism. Semin Cutan Med Surg 1997;16:44-53.

54. Loomis CA, Orlow SJ. Cutaneous findings in mosaicism and chimerism. Curr Probl Dermatol 1996;3:87-92.

55. Gown AM, Vogel AM, Hoak D, et al. Monoclonal antibodies specific for melanocytic tumors distinguish subpopulations of melanocytes. Am J Pathol 1986;123:195-203.

56. Holbrook KA, Underwood RA, Vogel AM, et al. The appearance, density and distribution of melanocytes in human embryonic and fetal skin revealed by the anti-melanoma monoclonal antibody, HMB-45. Anat Embryol 1989;180: 443-55.

57. Zimmerman AA, Cornbleet T. The development of epidermal pigmentation in the Negro fetus. J Invest Dermatol 1948;11:383-395.

58. Mishima Y, Widlan S. Embryonic development of melanocytes in human hair and epidermis. J Invest Dermatol, 1996;46:263-277.

59. Breathnach AS, Wyllie LM. Electron microscopy of melanocytes and Langerhans cells in human fetal epidermis at 14 weeks. J Invest Dermatol 1965;44:51-60.

60. Foster CA, Holbrook KA, Farr AG. Ontogeny of Langerhans cells in human embryonic and fetal skin: expression of HLA-DR and OKT-6 determinants. J Invest Dermatol 1986; 86: 240-243.

61. Berman B, Chen VL, France DS, et al. Anatomical mapping of epidermal Langerhans cell densities in adults. Br J Dermatol 1983;109:553-558.

62. Drijkoningen M, De Wolf-Peeters C, Van der Steen K, et al. Epidermal Langerhans' cells and dermal dendritic cells in human fetal and neonatal skin: an immunohistochemical study. Pediatr Dermatol 1987;4:11-17.

63. Foster CA, Holbrook KA. Ontogeny of Langerhans cells in human embryonic and fetal skin: cell densities and phenotypic expression relative to epidermal growth. Am J Anat 1989;184:157-164.

64. Moll I, Lane AT, Franke WW, et al. Intraepidermal formation of Merkel cells in xenografts of human fetal skin. J Invest Dermatol 1990;94:359-364.

65. Moll I, Kuhn C, Moll R. Cytokeratin 20 is a general marker of cutaneous Merkel cells while certain neuronal proteins are absent. J Invest Dermatol 1995;104:910-915.

66. Moll I, Moll R. Early development of human Merkel cells. Exp Dermatol 1992;1:180-184.

67. Moll I, Paus R, Moll R. Merkel cells in mouse skin: intermediate filament pattern, localization, and hair cycle-dependent density. J Invest Dermatol 1996;106:281-286.

68. Nobukuni Y, Watanabe A, Takeda K, et al. Analyses of loss-of-function mutations of the MITF gene suggest that haploinsufficiency is a cause of Waardenburg syndrome type 2A. Am J Hum Genet 1996;59:76-83.

69. Hofstra RM, Osinga J, Tan-Sindhunata G, et al. A homozygous mutation in the endothelin-3 gene associated with a combined Waardenburg type 2 and Hirschsprung phenotype (Shah-Waardenburg syndrome). Nat Genet 1996; 12:445-457.

70. Edery P, Attie T, Amiel J, et al. Mutation of the endothelin-3 gene in the Waardenburg-Hirschsprung disease (Shah-Waardenburg syndrome). Nat Genet 1996;12:442-444.

71. Attie T, Till M, Pelet A, et al. Mutation of the endothelin-receptor B gene in Waardenburg-Hirschsprung disease. Hum Molec Genet 1995;4:2407-2409.

72. Ezoe K, Holmes SA, Ho L, et al. Novel mutations and deletions of the KIT steel factor receptor gene in human piebaldism. Am J Hum Genet 1995;56:58-66.

73. Tassabehji M, Newton VE, Read AP. Waardenburg syndrome type 2 caused by mutations in the human microphthalmia MITF gene. Nat Genet 1994;8:251-255.

74. Puffenberger EG, Hosoda K, Washington SS, et al. A missense mutation of the endothelin-B receptor gene in multigenic Hirschsprung's disease. Cell 1994;79:1257-1266.

75. Spritz RA, Droetto S, Fukushima Y. Deletion of the KIT and PDGFRA genes in a patient with piebaldism. Am J Med Genet 1992;44:492-495.

76. Tassabehji M, Read AP, Newton VE, et al. Waardenburg's syndrome patients have mutations in the human homologue of the Pax-3 paired box gene. Nature 1992;355: 635-636.

77. Fleischman RA, Saltman DL, Stastny V, et al. Deletion of the c-kit protooncogene in the human developmental defect piebald trait. Proceedings of the National Academy of Sciences of the United States of America 1991;88:10885-10889.

78. Giebel LB, Spritz RA. Mutation of the KIT mast/stem cell growth factor receptor protooncogene in human piebaldism. Proceedings of the National Academy of Sciences of the United States of America 1991;88:696-699.

79. Sengal P. Morphogenesis of the skin. Cambridge: Cambridge University Press, 1976.

80. Christ B, Jacob HJ, Jacob M. Differentiating abilities of avian somatopleural mesoderm. Experientia 1979;35:1376-1378.

81. Noden DM. Vertebrate craniofacial development: novel approaches and new dilemmas. Curr Opin Genet Dev 1992; 2:576-581.

82. Loomis CA, Harris E, Michaud J, et al. The mouse Engrailed-1 gene and ventral limb patterning. Nature 1996; 382:360-363.

83. Parr BA, McMahon AP. Dorsalizing signal Wnt-7a required for normal polarity of D-V and A-P axes of mouse limb. Nature 1995;374:350-353.

84. Smith LT, Holbrook KA. Development of dermal connective tissue in human embryonic and fetal skin. Scanning Electron Microsc 1982;1745-1751.

85. Sykes B, Puddle B, Francis M, et al. The estimation of two collagens from human dermis by interrupted gel electrophoresis. Biochem Biophys Res Commun 1976;72:1472-1480.

86. Epstein EH, Jr. α[3]3 human skin collagen. Release by pepsin digestion and preponderance in fetal life. J Biolog Chemis 1974;249:3225-3231.

87. Deutsch TA, Esterly NB. Elastic fibers in fetal dermis. J Invest Dermatol 1975;65:320-323.

88. Martin P. Wound healing—aiming for the perfect skin regeneration. Science 1998;276:75-81.

89. Cass DL, Bullard KM, Sylvester KG, et al. Wound size and gestational age modulate scar formation in fetal wound repair. J Pediatr Surg 1997;32:411-415.

90. Stelnicki EJ, Bullard KM, Harrison MR, et al. A new in vivo model for the study of fetal wound healing. Ann Plast Surg 1997;39:374-380.

91. Smitt JH, van Asperen CJ, Niessen CM, et al. Restrictive dermopathy. Report of 12 cases. Dutch Task Force on Genodermatology. Arch Dermatol 1998;134:577-579.

92. Mau U, Kendziorra H, Kaiser P, et al. Restrictive dermopathy: report and review. Am J Med Genet 1997;71:179-185.

93. Holbrook KA, Dale BA, Witt DR, et al. Arrested epidermal morphogenesis in three newborn infants with a fatal genetic disorder (restrictive dermopathy). J Invest Dermatol 1987; 88:330-339.

94. Mucke J, Happle R, Theile H. MIDAS syndrome respectively MLS syndrome: a separate entity rather than a particular lyonization pattern of the gene causing Goltz syndrome. Am J Med Genet 1995;57:117-118.

95. Happle R. Lyonization and the lines of Blaschko. [Review]. Hum Genet 1985;70:200-206.

96. Happle R, Steijlen PM, Theile U, et al. Patchy dermal hypoplasia as a characteristic feature of Proteus syndrome. Arch Dermatol 1997;133:77-80.

97. Risau W, Lemmon V. Changes in the vascular extracellular matrix during embryonic vasculogenesis and angiogenesis. Dev Biol 1988;125:441-450.

98. Noden DM. Embryonic origins and assembly of blood vessels. Am Rev Respir Dis 1989;140:1097-1103.

99. Johnson CL, Holbrook KA. Development of human embryonic and fetal dermal vasculature. J Invest Dermatol 1989; 93:10S-17S.

100. Sato TN, Tozawa Y, Deutsch U, et al. Distinct roles of the receptor tyrosine kinases Tie-1 and Tie-2 in blood vessel formation. Nature 1995;376:70-74.

101. Vikkula M, Boon LM, Carraway KLR, et al. Vascular dysmorphogenesis caused by an activating mutation in the receptor tyrosine kinase TIE2. Cell 1996;87:1181-1190.

102. Johnson DW, Berg JN, Baldwin MA, et al. Mutations in the activin receptor-like kinase 1 gene in hereditary haemorrhagic telangiectasia type 2. Nat Genet 1996;13:189-195.

103. McAllister KA, Grogg KM, Johnson DW, et al. Endoglin, a TGF-beta binding protein of endothelial cells, is the gene for hereditary haemorrhagic telangiectasia type 1. Nat Genet 1994;8:345-351.

104. Smith LT, Holbrook KA, Byers PH. Structure of the dermal matrix during development and in the adult. J Invest Dermat 1982;79:93s-104s.

105. Fujita H, Asagami C, Oda Y, et al. Electron microscopic studies of the differentiation of fat cells in human fetal skin. J Invest Dermatol 1969;53:122-139.

106. Fajas L, Fruchart JC, Auwerx J. Transcriptional control of adipogenesis. Curr Opin Cell Biol 1998;10:165-173.

107. Klaus S. Functional differentiation of white and brown adipocytes. Bioessays 1997;19:215-223.

108. Skolnik EY, Marcusohn J. Inhibition of insulin receptor signaling by TNF: potential role in obesity and non-insulin-dependent diabetes mellitus. Cytokine Growth Factor Rev 1996;7:161-173.

109. Digby JE, Montague CT, Sewter CP, et al. Thiazolidinedione exposure increases the expression of uncoupling protein 1 in cultured human preadipocytes. Diabetes 1998;47:138-141.

110. Ioffe E, Moon B, Connolly E, et al. Abnormal regulation of the leptin gene in the pathogenesis of obesity. Proceedings of the National Academy of Sciences of the United States of America 1992;95:11852-11857.

111. Lane AT. Human fetal skin development. Pediatr Dermatol 1986;3:487-491.

112. Riddle CV. Focal tight junctions between mesenchymal cells of fetal dermis. Anat Rec 1986;214:113-117.

113. Giancotti FG. Integrin signaling: specificity and control of cell survival and cell cycle progression. Curr Opin Cell Biol 1997;9:691-700.

114. Rousselle P, Keene DR, Ruggiero F, et al. Laminin 5 binds the NC-1 domain of type VII collagen. J Cell Biol 1997;138:719-728.

115. Rezniczek GA, de Pereda JM, Reipert S, et al. Linking integrin alpha6beta4-based cell adhesion to the intermediate filament cytoskeleton: direct interaction between the beta4 subunit and plectin at multiple molecular sites. J Cell Biol 1998;141:209-225.

116. Guo L, Degenstein L, Dowling J, et al. Gene targeting of BPAG1: abnormalities in mechanical strength and cell migration in stratified epithelia and neurologic degeneration. Cell 1995;81:233-243.

117. Christiano AM, Uitto J. Molecular complexity of the cutaneous basement membrane zone. Revelations from the paradigms of epidermolysis bullosa. Exper Dermatol 1996; 5:1-11.

118. Oro AE, Scott MP. Splitting hairs: dissecting roles of signaling systems in epidermal development. Cell 1998;95:575-578.

119. Hardy MH. The secret life of the hair follicle. Trends Genet 1992;8:55-61.

120. Sundberg JP. Handbook of mouse mutations with skin and hair abnormalitiies: Animal models and biomedical tools. Boca Raton: CRC Press, 1994.

121. Dreyer SD, Shou G, Antonio B, et al. Mutations in LMX1B cause abnormal skeletal patterning and renal dysplasia in nail patella syndrome. Nat Genet 1998;19:47-50.

122. Ahmad W, Faiyaz ul Haque M, Brancolini V, et al. Alopecia universalis associated with a mutation in the human hairless gene. Science 1998;279:20-24.

123. Ferguson BM, Brockdorff N, Formstone E, et al. Cloning of Tabby, the murine homolog of the human EDA gene: evidence for a membrane-associated protein with a short collagenous domain. Hum Molec Genet 1997;6:1589-1594.

124. Srivastava AK, Pispa J, Hartung AJ, et al. The Tabby phenotype is caused by mutation in a mouse homologue of the EDA gene that reveals novel mouse and human exons and encodes a protein ectodysplasin-A with collagenous domains. Proceedings of the National Academy of Sciences of the United States of America 1997;94:13069-13074.

125. Kere J, Srivastava AK, Montonen O, et al. X-linked anhidrotic (hypohidrotic) ectodermal dysplasia is caused by mutation in a novel transmembrane protein. Nat Genet 1996;13:409-416.

126. Pinkus H. Embryology of hair. In Montagna W, Ellis RA, eds. The biology of hair growth. New York: Academic Press, 1958: pp 1-32.

127. Holbrook KA, Odland GF. Structure of the human fetal hair canal and initial hair eruption. J Invest Dermatol 1978; 71:385-390.

128. Carlsen RA. Human fetal hair follicles: the mesenchymal component. J Invest Dermatol 1974;63:206-211.

129. Wessells HK, Roessner KD. Nonproliferation in dermal condensation of mouse vibrissae and pelage hairs. Dev Biol 1965;12:419-433.

130. Hashimoto K. The ultrastructure of the skin of human embryos V. The hair germ and perifollicular mesenchymal cells. Br J Dermatol 1970;83:167-176.

131. Breathnach AS, Smith J. Fine structure of the early hair germ and dermal papilla in the human foetus. J Anat 1968; 102:511-526.

132. Robins EJ, Breathnach AS. Fine structure of the human foetal hair follicle at hair-peg and early bulbous-peg stages of development. J Anat 1969;104:553-569.

133. Cotsarelis G, Sun TT, Lavker RM. Label-retaining cells reside in the bulge area of pilosebaceous unit: implications for follicular stem cells, hair cycle, and skin carcinogenesis. Cell 1990;61:1329-1337.

134. Lavker RM, Sun TT. Hair follicle stem cells: present concepts. J Invest Dermatol 1995;104:8S-39S.

135. Montagna W, Van Scott E. The anatomy of the hair follicle. In Montagna W, Ellis RA, eds. The biology of hair growth. New York: Academic Press, 1958: pp 39-64.

136. Serri F, Montagna W, Mescon H. Studies of the skin of the fetus and the child. J Invest Dermatol 1962;39:99-217.

137. Smith DW, Gong BT. Scalp-hair patterning: its origin and significance relative to early brain and upper facial development, Teratology 1974;9:7-34.

138. Barth JH. Normal hair growth in children. Pediatr Dermatol 1987;4:173-184.

139. Paus R. Control of the hair cycle and hair diseases as cycling disorders. Curr Opin Dermatol 1996;3:248-258.

140. Serri F, Huber MW. The development of sebaceous glands in man. In Montagna W, Ellis RA, Silver AF, eds. Advances in biology of skin. The sebaceous glands. Oxford: Pergamon Press, 1963: pp 1-18.

141. Fujita H. Ultrastructural study of embryonic sebaceous cells, especially of their droplet formation. Acta Dermatol Venerol 1972;52:99-155.

142. Williams ML, Hincenbergs M, Holbrook KA. Skin lipid content during early fetal development. J Invest Dermatol 1988;91:263-268.

143. Pochi PE, Strauss JS, Downing DT. Age-related changes in sebaceous gland activity. J Invest Dermatol 1979;73:108-111.

144. Solomon LM, Esterly NB. Neonatal dermatology. I. The newborn skin. J Pediatr 1970;77:888-894.

145. Holbrook KA. Structural abnormalities of the epidermally derived appendages in skin from patients with ectodermal dysplasias: Possible insight into developmental errors. In Salinas C, ed. The ectodermal dysplasias, birth defects: original article series. New York: Liss, 1988: pp 15-44.

146. Zaias N. Embryology of the human nail. Arch Dermatol 1963;87:37-53.
147. Zaias N, Alvarez J. The formation of the primate nail plate. An autoradiographic study in squirrel monkey. J Invest Dermatol 1968;51:120-136.
148. Lewis BL. Microscopic studies, fetal and mature nail and surrounding soft tissue. Arch Dermatol 1954;70:732-747.
149. Hashimoto K, Gross BG, Nelson R, et al. The ultrastructure of the skin of human embryos. 3. The formation of the nail in 16-18 weeks old embryos. J Invest Dermatol 1966; 47:205-217.
150. Lynch MH, O'Guin WM, Hardy C, et al. Acidic and basic hair/nail "hard" keratins: their colocalization in upper cortical and cuticle cells of the human hair follicle and their relationship to "soft" keratins. J Cell Biol 1986;103:2593-2606.
151. O'Guin WM, Galvin S, Schermer A, et al. Patterns of keratin expression define distinct pathways of epithelial development and differentiation. Curr Top Dev Biol 1987;22:97-125.
152. O'Guin WM, Sun TT, Manabe M. Interaction of trichohyalin with intermediate filaments: three immunologically defined stages of trichohyalin maturation. J Invest Dermat 1992; 98:24-32.
153. Mulvihill JJ, Smith DW. The genesis of dermatoglyphics. J Pediatr 1969;75:579-589.
154. Hirsch W, Schweichel JU. Morphological evidence concerning the problem of skin ridge formation. J Mental Deficien Res 1973;17:58-72.
155. Okajima M. Development of dermal ridges in the fetus. J Med Genet 1975;12:243-250.
156. Hashimoto K, Gross BG, Lever WF. The ultrastructure of the skin of human embryos. I. The intraepidermal eccrine sweat duct. J Invest Dermatol 1965;45:139-151.
157. Hashimoto K, Gross BG, Lever WF. The ultrastructure of human embryo skin. II. The formation of intradermal portion of the eccrine sweat duct and of the secretory segment during the first half of embryonic life. J Invest Dermatol 1966;46:205-217.
158. Hashimoto K. The ultrastructure of the skin of human embryos. VII. Formation of the apocrine gland. Acta Derm Venereol 1970,50:241-251.
159. Montagna W, Parakkal PF. Apocrine glands. In Montagna W, Parakkal PF, eds. The structure and function of skin. New York: Academic Press, 1974: pp 332-365.
160. Foster KG, Hey EN, Katz G. The response of the sweat glands of the newborn baby to thermal stimuli and to intradermal acetylcholine. J Physiol 1969;203:13-29.
161. Green M, Behrendt H. Sweating capacity of neonates. Nicotine-induced axon reflex sweating and the histamine flare. Am J Dis Children 1969;118:725-732.
162. Bagnara JT, Ferris W, Turner WA Jr, et al. Melanophore differentiation in leaf legs. Dev Biol 1978;64:149-164.
163. Behrendt H, Green M. Nature of the sweating deficit of prematurely born neonates. Observations on babies with the heroin withdrawal syndrome. N Engl J Med 1972;286:1376-1379.
164. Sinclair JD. Thermal control in premature infants. Ann Rev Med 1972;23:129-148.
165. Loomis CA, Kimmel RA, Tong CX, et al. Analysis of the genetic pathway leading to formation of ectopic apical ectodermal ridges in mouse Engrailed-1 mutant limbs. Development 1998;125:1137-1148.
166. Chen H, Lun Y, D, O, et al. Limb and kidney defects in Lmx1b mutant mice suggest an involvement of LMX1B in human nail patella syndrome. Nat Genet 1988;19:51-55.
167. Lyngstadaas SP, Nordbo H, Gedde-Dahl T Jr, et al. On the genetics of hypodontia and microdontia: synergism or allelism of major genes in a family with six affected members. J Med Genet 1996;33:37-42.
168. Vastardis H, Karimbux N, Guthua SW, et al. A human MSX1 homeodomain missense mutation causes selective tooth agenesis. Nat Genet 1996;13:417-421.
169. Cheng-Ming C. Molecular basis of epithelial appendage morphogenesis. Austin: RG Landes, 1998.
170. Aszterbaum M, Rothman A, Johnson RL, et al. Identification of mutations in the human PATCHED gene in sporadic basal cell carcinomas and in patients with the basal cell nevus syndrome. J Invest Dermatol 1998;110:885-888.
171. Gailani MR, Stahle-Backdahl M, Leffell DJ, et al. The role of the human homologue of Drosophila patched in sporadic basal cell carcinomas. Nat Genet 1996;14:78-81.
172. Hahn H, Wicking C, Zaphiropoulous PG, et al. Mutations of the human homolog of Drosophila patched in the nevoid basal cell carcinoma syndrome. Cell 1996;85:841-851.
173. Johnson RL, Rothman AL, Xie J, et al. Human homolog of patched, a candidate gene for the basal cell nevus syndrome. Science 1996:272:668-671.
174. Xie J, Murone M, Luoh SM, et al. Activating smoothened mutations in sporadic basal-cell carcinoma. Nature 1998; 391:90-92.
175. Sybert VP, Holbrook KA. Prenatal diagnosis and screening. Dermatol Clin 1987;5:17-41.
176. Blanchet-Bardon C, Dumez Y. Prenatal diagnosis of a harlequin fetus. Semin Dermatol 1984;3:225-228.
177. Holbrook KA. The biology of human fetal skin at ages related to prenatal diagnosis. Pediatric Dermatol 1983; 1:97-111.

Structure and Function of Newborn Skin

ANTHONY J. MANCINI

The skin of the newborn serves a pivotal role in the transition from the aqueous intrauterine environment to extrauterine terrestrial life and is integral to the vital functions of mechanical protection, thermoregulation, cutaneous immunosurveillance, and maintenance of a barrier that prevents insensible loss of body fluids. The anatomy and function of skin is most easily understood by dissecting the individual compartments (stratum corneum, epidermis, dermal-epidermal junction [DEJ], dermis and subcutaneous tissue) and their component cell types. Specialized structures found within these compartments, such as pilosebaceous units, sweat glands, nerves, and vascular networks, play an essential role both anatomically and functionally in cutaneous homeostasis in the neonate. The anatomy of these compartments and structures of the skin, and the physiologic processes involved in their functions, are the focus of this chapter.

Human skin consists of three layers: epidermis, dermis, and subcutaneous fat (Fig. 2-1). All elements of skin are derived from either ectoderm or mesoderm, the former giving rise to the epidermis and other cutaneous epithelial components.[1] A brief description of fetal skin development is helpful in understanding the structure and function of newborn skin and is incorporated into some of the following discussions of the various compartments and structures. A more thorough review of cutaneous embryology is the focus of Chapter 1.

STRATUM CORNEUM AND EPIDERMIS

The most obvious clinical difference between the skin of the term newborn infant and that of an adult is the presence of the moist, greasy, yellow-white substance called vernix caseosa, which is a coating comprising a combination of sebaceous gland secretions, desquamated skin cells, and shed lanugo hairs.[2,3] This coating persists for the first several days of postnatal life, eventually disappearing completely to reveal the more typical, moderately dry newborn skin.

The structure of term newborn skin is histologically similar to that of older individuals, whereas premature infant skin reveals several unique features that have increased our understanding of fetal skin development. The outermost compartment of skin, or epidermis, arises from surface ectoderm and at about the third week of fetal life consists of a single layer of undifferentiated cells that becomes two-layered by around 4 weeks.[4] The outer layer of cells, the periderm, is found only in developing skin and is transiently present, eventually undergoing a series of apoptotic cellular events as the epidermis becomes multilayered and the stratum corneum, the outermost layer of flattened, nonnucleated skin cells, is forming.[5] By 24 weeks of gestation, the periderm is largely absent,[4,5] and the epidermis shows considerable progressive maturation, which is largely complete by 34 weeks.[6] A thin, hydrophobic layer of the periderm may persist for several days postnatally and may participate in protective and thermoregulatory functions.[7]

The epidermis is a stratified epithelium, the number of cell layers varying between different body regions. The various layers, from the dermal side toward the skin surface, are termed the stratum basale, stratum spinosum, stratum granulosum, and stratum corneum. In areas of thicker skin, such as palms and soles, the stratum lucidum is interposed between the granular and corneal layers. These epidermal layers are shown in Fig. 2-2.

Individual cells within the epidermis are referred to as keratinocytes, so named for the intermediate-sized filament

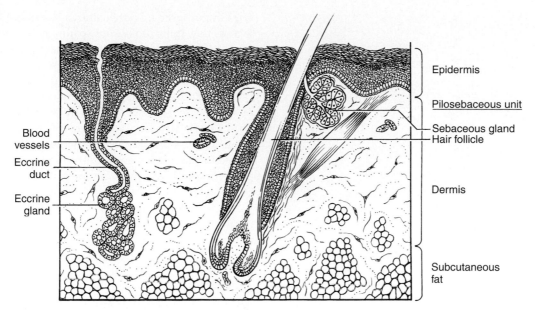

FIG. 2-1

Basic anatomy of skin, which is composed of three major divisions: epidermis, dermis, and subcutaneous fat. Adnexal structures include pilosebaceous units and eccrine ducts and glands (shown) and apocrine glands (not shown). (Courtesy Randall Hayes.)

proteins (keratins) that are synthesized within them. Keratins are the major structural proteins of the epidermis and its appendages, constituting up to 85% of the total protein of fully differentiated epidermal keratinocytes.[8] They have been divided into types I and II based on their acidic or basic nature, respectively, and are frequently configured in specific pairs of a type I and a type II protein as obligatory heteropolymers.[9] Terminal differentiation of the epidermis involves the sequential expression of different proteins, including the keratins, in the basal and spinal layers.[10] An important function of the keratins is imparting mechanical integrity to epithelial cells. Mutations in the genes encoding these proteins have been confirmed as the basis of several inherited skin defects, such as the simplex form of the mechanobullous disease, epidermolysis bullosa.[8]

The stratum basale consists of a single layer of cells, the basal portions of which are in contact with the dermis and contribute to the DEJ. The cells of the basal layer are cuboidal to columnar in shape and are anchored to the underlying dermis by cytoplasmic processes. The stratum basale has an undulating surface inferiorly, forming the projections called rete ridges, which lie interposed between the dermal papillae of the superficial (papillary) dermis (Fig. 2-3). The basal cell layer contains cells that eventually replace those continually lost from the epidermis through terminal differentiation, maturation and desquamation.

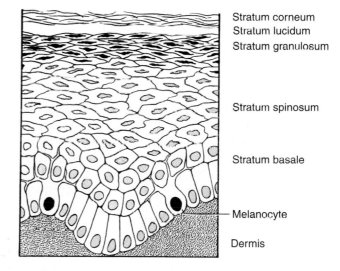

FIG. 2-2

The cell layers of the epidermis. Note the interspersed distribution of melanocytes in the basal cell layer. (Courtesy Randall Hayes.)

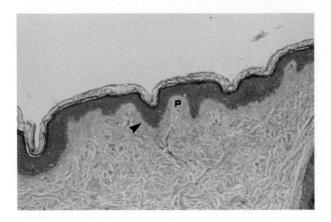

FIG. 2-3
Histologic appearance of normal skin. The basal portion of the epidermis has an undulating surface, resulting in rete ridges (*arrowhead*) interposed between dermal papillae *(p)*.

Interspersed among the cells in the basal cell layer are the dendritic, pigment (or melanin)–producing cells (melanocytes). These cells first appear between a gestational age of 40 and 50 days and migrate to the skin from the neural crest.[11] Whereas melanocytes are found in both a basal and suprabasal location during embryogenesis, neonatal skin reveals a more limited distribution restricted to the basal epidermal layer.[12,13] Melanin is manufactured within organelles called melanosomes, which are formed in melanocytes and transferred to neighboring keratinocytes via dendritic connections. Each melanocyte is in contact with roughly 36 keratinocytes, an association that is referred to as the epidermal melanin unit. The transfer of melanin from the melanocyte to the keratinocytes within this unit results in pigment distributed in the basal layer, as well as more superficially, where melanin serves a protective role by absorbing and scattering ultraviolet radiation (UVR).[14] Two forms of melanin are present in human skin: eumelanin, which is brown, and pheomelanins, which are red and yellow.[15,16] Differences in native skin pigmentation among individuals are related to the concentration, as well as distribution and retention, of melanin in the basal cell layer, rather than to the absolute number of melanocytes.[1,17,18] Although melanocytes in newborn skin are quantitatively comparable to those in older individuals, melanin production, and hence skin pigmentation, is relatively decreased during the neonatal period,[2,3] with gradual darkening over several months following birth.

The stratum spinosum consists of the cells between the stratum basale and the stratum granulosum and forms the bulk of mammalian epidermis. The keratino-cytes in this layer are polyhedral in shape and have numerous tiny, spiny projections spanning the intercellular space between contiguous cells.[16] These projections are ultrastructurally composed of desmosomes, which form communication junctions between the cells. Keratinocytes of the spinous layer become larger, flatter, and more desiccated as they progress from the basal layer toward the skin surface. Also present in this layer are Langerhans' cells, bone marrow–derived cells that are involved in cutaneous immunosurveillance through antigen processing and presentation (see Cutaneous Immunosurveillance, Langerhans Cells and Cytokines).

The stratum granulosum comprises a thin layer of darkly-stained keratinocytes at the outermost surface of the stratum spinosum. The dark appearance of these cells is due to the presence of keratohyaline granules, which are composed of an electron-dense protein (profilaggrin) and keratin intermediate filaments.[14] Profilaggrin is subsequently converted to filaggrin, a protein involved in the aggregation and disulfide bonding of keratin filaments,[19,20] and it has been suggested that keratohyaline serves to form a matrix that provides structural support by linking keratin filaments to one another.[16] The granular cell layer is also where lamellar bodies (Odland bodies, membrane-coating granules) are produced.[21] These intracellular organelles participate in the formation of the epidermal permeability barrier through the production and discharge of lipid substances into the intercellular corridors of the stratum corneum.

In areas of thicker skin, such as palms and soles, the stratum lucidum is present as a layer with a clear hyaline appearance. At this level one can visualize transitional cells that exhibit marked degeneration of the nucleus and other organelles and, ultramicroscopically, keratin filaments and keratohyaline granules, which are abundant but not yet as compact as in the stratum corneum.[16]

The stratum corneum, or cornified layer, is composed of several layers of flattened, nonnucleated keratinized cells (corneocytes) arranged in an overlapping fashion. The thickness of this layer varies by body region, being thinnest on the face (especially over the eyelids) and genitalia, and thickest on the palms and soles. It is now widely accepted that the epidermal permeability barrier resides in the stratum corneum and serves the vital functions of preventing excessive transepidermal water loss (TEWL) and preventing penetration of a variety of substances.[22-26]

The formation of the epidermal barrier is accomplished through the lipid secretions of lamellar bodies, which include free fatty acids, ceramides, and cholesterol. These lipids are deposited in the intercellular interstices within the stratum corneum. This arrangement has been likened to "bricks and mortar," where the corneocytes represent the bricks and the intercellular lipids represent the mortar.[27] Although these lipids represent only about 10% of the dry weight of the stratum corneum,[28] their location and composition are vital, and cutaneous barrier function is dependent on both the generation of sufficient quantities of these lipids and their strategic secretion and organization into lamellar bilayer unit structures.[26,27,29-31] In fact, the epidermis is equipped with the necessary machinery to autonomously regulate its lipid-synthetic apparatus in response to specific barrier requirements.[32-34] Development of a functional barrier has been demonstrated to be closely correlated with normal ontogenesis and does not appear to be disrupted by somatic growth retardation.[35] Hence, more mature infants, even those who are small for gestational age, have a competent epidermal barrier.[36]

The epidermis and stratum corneum in the full-term infant are well developed, and the barrier properties are excellent.[37] Conversely, premature infants have greater skin permeability and a more poorly functioning barrier. Histologically, the term infant has a well-developed epidermis, which is several layers in thickness, and a well-formed stratum corneum.[2,6] This maturity is lacking in preterm infants.[37-41] An acceleration of skin maturation may occur postnatally in preterm infants, although in extremely low birth weight infants (23 to 25 weeks gestational age) complete development of a fully functional barrier may require up to 8 weeks.[38,39,42] Recent studies support the long-held notion that the shift from an aqueous to air environment, and hence water flux, may be an important factor in this acceleration of barrier formation.[43] Nonetheless, during the period of postnatal maturation, large transepidermal water losses contribute to the morbidity of the preterm infant, and therefore a major focus of past studies has been the development of a therapeutic strategy to accelerate epidermal barrier maturation or augment its function, including the use of semipermeable membranes[44-47] or topical emollients.[48,49] Premature infant skin and barrier maturation are discussed in more detail in Chapter 4.

In addition to the prevention of insensible water losses across the skin by the epidermal barrier, the epidermis and stratum corneum of the newborn provide important protection against toxicity from UVR exposure, and this protective effect may be greater for ultraviolet B than ultraviolet A radiation.[50] As previously noted, melanin is primarily responsible for UVR protection, although the "protein barrier" of the stratum corneum may augment this cutaneous function.[51] Epidermal lipids may also play a role in protection from UVR. Another function of the superficial skin layers is protection against microorganisms, which are blocked from invasion across the skin by an intact stratum corneum. In addition to such physical factors,

the antimicrobial qualities of skin may be related to the relative dryness of the stratum corneum, the presence of skin surface lipids, and the degree of epidermal cellular differentiation.[51-54] Skin is also a vital participant in the process of neonatal thermoregulation (discussed in more detail later) through regulation of cutaneous blood flow and evaporative water loss.

Percutaneous absorption of substances across neonatal skin requires passage through the stratum corneum and epidermis, diffusion into the dermis, and eventual transfer into the systemic circulation. Transfer across the stratum corneum and epidermis may be through the intercellular corridors (favoring nonpolar or hydrophobic compounds) or via a transcellular route (which favors polar or hydrophilic substances).[55] Hair follicles and eccrine sweat ducts may serve as diffusion shunts for certain substances (i.e., ions, polar compounds, very large molecules), which would otherwise traverse the stratum corneum slowly (because of their large molecular weight).[56] The rate-limiting step of percutaneous absorption seems to be diffusion through the stratum corneum,[56] and hence the effectiveness of the epidermal permeability barrier correlates inversely with percutanous absorption. Percutaneous absorption, although continuously being explored in terms of its therapeutic applications, may contribute to systemic absorption and potential toxicity after topical application of some substances to newborn skin, especially in preterm infants or infants with cutaneous damage.[38] Importantly, while the barrier function of intact skin in the term infant is usually normal, the surface area-to-weight ratio is greater than in older children and adults. Caution should therefore be exercised in the use of topical agents in any newborn, with extra caution and a thorough risk/benefit analysis being employed in the case of premature infants or any neonate with a compromised skin barrier. Percutaneous absorption is discussed in more detail in Chapter 5.

DERMAL-EPIDERMAL JUNCTION

The dermal-epidermal junction is an important site of attachment in skin, occurring at the interface between the basal epidermis and the papillary dermis. It appears that the various components of the DEJ are expressed in term newborn skin in a manner similar to that in adults, without apparent differences in their quantity or associations.[2] For reasons that are poorly understood, however, skin appears to be more fragile during the newborn period, even in term infants, as evidenced by blisters or erosions developing in situations that do not cause blisters later in life (e.g., erosions due to diapering, sucking blisters on fingers and hands, and disease states such as bullous syphilis).

Specialized structures termed hemidesmosomes assist in anchoring the basal keratinocytes to the underlying plasma membrane. The DEJ can be ultrastructurally broken down into several planes, including (from the epidermal side to the dermal side) the inferior portion of the basal keratinocyte; an empty-appearing, electron-lucent clear plane known as the lamina lucida; a thin, dark, electron-dense layer known as the lamina densa; and the sublamina densa fibrillar region[14,57] (Fig. 2-4). Each of these layers of the DEJ contains individual components that harmoniously function in concert to form cohesion between the epidermis and underlying dermis. Defects in, or antibodies directed against, some of these components have been etiologically linked to cutaneous disease.

Major constituents of the DEJ include bullous pemphigoid (BP) antigens, α6β4 integrin, laminin-5, type IV collagen, and type VII collagen. The BP antigens are large glycoproteins with both intracellular (BP antigen 1) and transmembrane (BP antigen 2) components. BP antigen 2, also known as collagen type XVII, extends from the basal keratinocyte across the lamina lucida into the lamina densa,[58] and autoantibodies directed against it are found in the sera of patients with BP, and more recently in patients with linear IgA bullous disease.[59] Reduced or absent expression of BP antigen 2 is found in patients with a hereditary junctional form of epidermolysis bullosa (EB) termed generalized atrophic benign EB.[60-62]

α6β4 integrin is a membrane glycoprotein component of the hemidesmosome, and defects in this integrin have been identified in a subset of patients with junctional EB in combination with pyloric atresia.[63-66] Laminin-5 is a glycoprotein localized mainly to the lamina densa and lower lamina lucida[67] and is also associated predominantly with hemidesmosomes.[68] Mutations in the genes encoding various chains of laminin-5 have been identified in patients with the lethal (Herlitz) junctional type of EB.[69-72]

Type IV collagen predominates in the lamina densa region, whereas type VII collagen, which is also known as the epidermolysis bullosa acquisita (EBA) antigen, is situated in the zone beneath the lamina densa. EBA antigen was so named because it was first defined by circulating autoantibodies in the sera of patients with EBA, an acquired autoimmune blistering disease.[73] The dystrophic forms of inherited EB have been shown to be a result of defects in the gene encoding type VII collagen.[74]

DERMIS AND SUBCUTANEOUS FAT

The dermis of human skin consists primarily of connective tissues, including proteins (collagen and elastic tissue) and ground substance. This compartment lies between the epidermis superiorly and the subcutaneous fat inferiorly and forms a resilient and flexible layer that envelops the entire organism. It is divided into superficial (papillary) and deep (reticular) components, which are anatomically divided by a thin plexus of blood vessels. Although differentiation between these dermal compartments can be ascertained on the basis of the size of the collagen fiber bundles in adult skin, this criterion is less helpful in newborn skin, where there is a more gradual transition in fiber bundle size.[2] Structures found within the dermis, which are discussed in different sections of this chapter, include the cutaneous appendages (pilosebaceous units, eccrine and apocrine sweat glands), as well as nerves, blood vessels, and lymphatics.

Collagen is the major constituent of mammalian dermis and accounts for approximately 75% of the dry weight of the skin.[14] The collagens are a family of related, yet individually distinct, structural proteins, and in the skin they provide tensile strength and elasticity. Collagen types I and III are the major collagens found in human dermis, and smaller amounts of types IV (a primary component of the basement membrane as noted above), V, VI, and VII are also present.[75] Eighty percent to 90% of dermal collagen is type I. Type III collagen was initially termed fetal collagen because of its predominance in fetal tissues, where it accounts for over half of total skin collagen. However, synthesis of type I collagen accelerates during the postnatal period, and eventually the ratio of type I to type III collagen increases such that in adult skin it is around 5:1 to 6:1.[76]

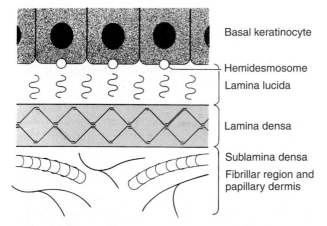

FIG. 2-4
Depiction of the ultrastructure of the dermal-epidermal junction (DEJ). Hemidesmosomes assist in anchoring the basal keratinocyte to the underlying plasma membrane. Planes of division within the DEJ include the lamina lucida, lamina densa, and sublamina densa fibrillar region. (Courtesy Randall Hayes.)

Basal keratinocyte

Hemidesmosome
Lamina lucida

Lamina densa

Sublamina densa
Fibrillar region and
papillary dermis

Abnormalities in collagen synthesis or posttranslational processing may result in clinical disease, including osteogenesis imperfecta and the Ehlers-Danlos syndromes.

Elastic fibers play an important role in the structure and function of skin, providing elasticity and resilience. They consist of two components: elastin, which is a connective tissue protein, and elastic fiber–associated microfibrillar component, a complex of glycoproteins.[75] Elastic fibers are distributed in the papillary and reticular dermis. Fibers in the papillary dermis have been subdivided into elaunin fibers, which are oriented parallel to the DEJ, and oxytalan fibers, which connect the elaunin fibers to the DEJ.[1] It has been demonstrated that elastic fibers are distributed in the term newborn dermis in a manner similar to that of the adult, albeit with a decreased elastin content in the papillary dermal bundles, and with a finer fiber diameter in the reticular dermis.[2] The most widely recognized disease related to abnormalities in elastin production is cutis laxa, a heterogeneous group of disorders featuring lax skin and occasional systemic involvement in the form of hoarseness, emphysema, hernias, and diverticulae.[77]

The ground substance of the dermis is an amorphous material that surrounds and embeds the fibrous and cellular components found in this compartment. Glycosaminoglycans (GAGs), which are long chains of aminated sugars, and proteoglycans (PGs), which are large molecules consisting of a core polypeptide linked to GAGs, are major constituents of ground substance.[1,14] Major GAGs and PGs in the dermis are chondroitin sulfate, dermatan sulfate, heparin/heparin sulfate, chondroitin 6-sulfate, and hyaluronic acid (hyaluronan).[1,14,78] These components are capable of retaining large amounts of water and may also play a role in binding growth factors and providing structural support, anticoagulation, and adhesion.[1,79,80] Hyaluronic acid has been demonstrated in large amounts in fetal dermis and amniotic fluid and is thought by some to be associated with the rapid wound healing without scarring that has been observed to occur in fetal wounds.[81] Fibronectin is a large glycoprotein also found in the dermis and is associated with a variety of putative functions, including organization of the extracellular matrix, wound healing, attachment, and chemotaxis.[1,14]

The subcutaneous fat is an important layer, providing roles in shock absorption, energy storage, and maintenance of body heat. The individual cells in the subcutaneous fat, adipocytes, form lobules that are separated by fibrous septae. The fibrous septae contain neural and vascular elements and connect deeper with the fascia of underlying skeletal muscle. In contrast, brown fat is a distinct type of adipose tissue present only in newborns that plays a vital role in neonatal thermoregulation (discussed in more detail later) through oxidation of fatty acids.[82] Brown fat makes up 2% to 6% of the neonate's total body weight and is found primarily in the scapular region, the mediastinum, around the kidneys and adrenal glands, and in the axilla.[83] The nonshivering thermogenesis that occurs in this tissue appears to be regulated by the enzyme-uncoupling protein thermogenin, which serves as a protonophore through the mitochondrial membrane, enabling high rates of cellular respiration and proton conductivity.[84] Brown fat is depleted over time and is virtually absent in adults.

PILOSEBACEOUS UNITS, APOCRINE GLANDS, AND NAILS

Hair Follicles

The earliest hair follicles begin to form at 9 to 12 weeks gestation,[85] primarily in a facial location, and the bulk of the remaining hairs start developing around 16 to 20 weeks, progressing in a cephalocaudad fashion.[85,86] Some full-term infants, and especially premature infants, have their skin surface covered with lanugo hairs, which are soft, fine hairs with limited growth potential.[2] These hairs are usually shed by term, or shortly thereafter, and are replaced by vellus hairs, which are eventually replaced on the scalp by coarse terminal hairs. The majority of hairs present at birth are synchronized in their growth phase,[3,87] although this synchrony of growth is disrupted within a few months and may result in a period of temporary alopecia.[87] The growth of a hair follicle is cyclic, the stages being divided into anagen (active growth), catagen (transitional involution), and telogen (resting) phases. The typical length of each of these phases is 2 to 5 years, 3 days, and 3 months, respectively.[86] No new hair follicles are formed after birth.

The hair follicle is organized into a series of concentric cellular compartments, the details of which are beyond the scope of this chapter. The structure of a pilosebaceous unit is depicted in Fig. 2-5. Longitudinally, the hair follicle can be divided into three zones: the infundibulum, extending from the opening of the follicle to the entrance of the sebaceous duct; the isthmus, extending from the entrance of the sebaceous duct to the insertion of the arrector pili muscle; and the inferior segment, which forms the remainder of the follicle from the insertion of the pili muscle to the base. A subpopulation of hair follicle keratinocytes that share properties with other keratinocyte stem cells has been identified in the upper follicle near the insertion site of the arrector pili muscle.[88,89] This area has been termed the bulge, and these cells may be involved

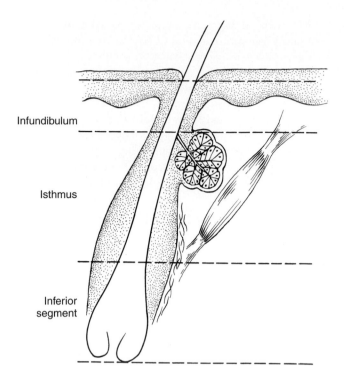

Infundibulum

Isthmus

Inferior
segment

FIG. 2-5

The pilosebaceous unit, divided into three zones: the infundibulum, extending from the opening of the follicle to the entrance of the sebaceous duct; the isthmus, extending from the entrance of the sebaceous duct to the insertion of the arrector pili muscle; and the inferior segment, extending from the insertion of the arrector pili muscle to the base. (Courtesy Randall Hayes.)

not only in the regeneration of the anagen hair follicle, but also in the long-term maintenance of the epidermis.[90] The integrity of the hair shaft is related to its protein constituents, including the intermediate filament hair keratins and high-sulfur proteins, and to the strong disulfide bonding between these proteins.[86] In neonates, hair may be a source of valuable clinical information, with the utility of neonatal hair shaft analysis as a marker for intrauterine exposure to drugs of abuse having emerged as a valuable tool over the last decade.[91-94]

Sebaceous Glands

Sebaceous glands begin to develop between 13 and 15 weeks of fetal life.[95] They are nearly always associated with hair follicles and are found diffusely in the skin except on the palms, soles, and dorsal feet.[96] The locations of the most prominent glands are the face and scalp, and they may be quite evident in term neonates over the nose, fore-

head, and cheeks. Modified glands are found in the skin of the nipples and areolae (Montgomery's tubercles), on the labia minora and prepuce (Tyson's glands), on the vermilion border of the lips (Fordyce's condition), and in the eyelids (Meibomian glands). Sebaceous glands are well formed at birth and are quite active during the neonatal period, when they are stimulated by transplacentally derived steroid hormones and possibly by endogenous steroid production.[3] This sebaceous activity in the newborn is reflected by the common finding of neonatal acne. Sebum, the substance produced by the holocrine sebaceous glands, is a composite of triglycerides, wax esters, squalane, cholesterol, and cholesterol esters and serves a role in lubrication of the follicle and epidermal surface.[1] Sebum levels sharply decline over the first year of life,[97] putatively in response to diminished levels of circulating hormones. The glands then remain relatively quiescent, producing only small amounts of sebum, until puberty.[2]

Apocrine Glands

Apocrine glands are limited in distribution and are found primarily in the axillae, areolae, mons pubis, labia minora, scrotum, perianal area, external ear canal, and eyelids (Moll's glands).[96] Their function in humans is unclear, although they may serve as scent glands. Apocrine glands remain small until puberty, when they enlarge and begin the process of secretion of a milky white fluid. Body odor in postadolescent individuals is related to bacterial action on these secretions.

The Nail

The nail acts as a hard, protective covering over the distal end of the digit and may have served a function in evolution to assist in grasping small objects. The nail unit is depicted in Fig. 2-6. The nail plate consists of cornified cells with a high protein (primarily keratin) content and is produced by the matrix, a cellular zone situated underneath the proximal nail fold at the base of the nail. The nail plate is situated on top of the nail bed, a highly vascular zone. The lateral nail folds consist of skin that envelops the lateral borders of the nail plate. The average growth rate of the human fingernail is 0.10 to 0.12 mm per day and appears to be greatest during the second decade of life.[98] Toenails, which grow at a slower rate, may appear to be abnormal or "ingrown" in newborns as a result of relative nail plate hypoplasia with a bulbous distal phalanx.[99] Despite their abnormal appearance, these nails eventually grow out and take on a more normal appearance.

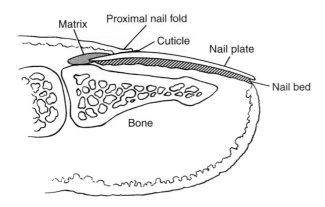

FIG. 2-6

The nail unit. The hard nail plate consists of cornified cells and is produced by the mitotically active cells of the nail matrix, which is situated underneath the proximal nail fold. (Courtesy Randall Hayes.)

ECCRINE GLANDS AND NEONATAL SWEATING

Eccrine sweating is a physiologic response to increased body temperature and is the most effective means by which humans regulate their body temperature through evaporative heat loss.[100] Gestational age, postnatal age, and body site are all important variables with regard to eccrine glands, and much of what is known about the process of neonatal sweating has been learned from studies of the normal physiologic eccrine gland responses of term and preterm neonates to various sweat-inducing stimuli.

Eccrine sweat glands first appear during fetal development at 14 weeks and are initially limited to the volar surface of the hands and feet.[101] They then appear in the axillae and eventually in a generalized distribution, with a full complement of anatomically normal glands present by the twenty-eighth week of gestation, although functionally the glands are immature until 36 weeks of gestation.[102] The total number of eccrine sweat glands is formed before birth[103] and is estimated to be between 2 and 4 million.[101]

The eccrine sweat gland consists of two segments: a secretory coil and a duct. The secretory coil is composed of secretory cells and myoepithelial cells, the latter being contractile cells with smooth muscle–like characteristics.[101] The duct is composed of two cell layers, the basal and luminal ductal cells, which are involved in secretion and reabsorption of solutes. Components of eccrine sweat include water, sodium, chloride, potassium, urea, lactate, and ammonia.[101] Although newly formed sweat is isotonic, reabsorption of water and solutes occurs in the duct such that the expelled product is hypotonic. Evaporation

of sweat from the surface of skin removes 0.58 calorie of heat for each gram of water that evaporates.[104]

Eccrine sweat glands are innervated anatomically by fibers of the sympathetic nervous system, although functionally they are under cholinergic influence, and acetylcholine is the major neurotransmitter released from the periglandular nerve endings.[101] Circulating catecholamines can also have a stimulatory effect on eccrine sweat production,[104] as can a variety of other peptides or neurotransmitters.

Sweating can be induced by pharmacologic stimulation and by emotional or thermal stress, and all mechanisms appear to be developed to some extent at birth in term infants. Levels of sweat production in response to the intradermal injection of pharmacologic agents have been demonstrated to bear a direct relation to gestational age,[105-108] as well as to birth weight.[105] Thermal stress–induced sweating, although present in infants, appears to require a greater thermal stimulus in neonates as compared with adults, and this response also appears to be less developed in premature infants,[103,108-111] with an increased response noted with increasing postnatal age.[109] However, the thermal stimulus of sweating is an important contributor to increased insensible water loss in certain infants at risk, such as those treated with phototherapy for hyperbilirubinemia[112] and those under radiant warmers.[113,114] The core temperature at which sweating begins in full-term newborns has been estimated at around 37.2° C.[115]

"Emotional sweating" also appears to be well developed at birth in full-term but not premature neonates.[102] In one study, skin conductance after heel prick for routine blood testing rose sharply, and to a greater extent, in infants of more advanced gestational ages,[116] supporting the role of postconceptual age in maturation of the sweating response to emotional stress.

The process of neonatal sweating, therefore, appears to develop early anatomically in fetal life and functionally at later stages, and the sweating response appears to be well developed at birth in term but not preterm infants. Hypotheses on the potential mechanisms for progressive postnatal maturity of the sweating response include anatomic development of the sweat gland, functional development of the gland, or nervous system maturation.[109]

NERVES, VASCULAR NETWORKS, AND THERMOREGULATION

The cutaneous neural and vascular networks both develop early in the fetus, and their architecture becomes organized into adult patterns with increasing postnatal age.[2]

Nerve networks in the skin contain both somatic sensory and sympathetic autonomic fibers and function as innervation for arrector pili muscles, cutaneous blood vessels, and sweat glands, as well as serving as receptors for touch, pain, temperature, itch, and mechanical stimuli. Large myelinated fibers, which are cutaneous branches of musculoskeletal nerves, innervate the skin in a pattern similar to that of vascular supply, whereas sensory nerves follow segmental dermatomes, which often show some overlap. Although cutaneous nerve fibers in the neonate are similar in structure and distribution to those in the adult, ultramicroscopic examination has revealed a higher percentage of unmyelinated fibers with bundling of axons, suggesting cytoarchitectural immaturity or incomplete growth.[117]

Sensory cutaneous nerves may end freely or in encapsulated terminals. Free nerve endings in skin represent the most important of sensory receptors and include penicillate fibers found in a subepidermal location in hairy skin,[118] multiple types of free endings in digital (nonhairy) skin,[119] and papillary nerve endings found at the orifice of hair follicles.[14] Free nerve endings may also be associated with Merkel cells, neurosecretory cells of uncertain biologic significance that are of epithelial derivation and become scarce in human skin after fetal development.[2,120,121] Studies suggest that Merkel cells may actually be trophic for developing nerves and therefore play an inductive role in the development of the human cutaneous nerve plexus.[122] Specialized sensory receptors are present to varying degrees at birth, including Pacinian corpuscles, which are well developed and abundant in palm and sole skin, and Meissner's corpuscles, which are not fully formed and undergo continued morphologic changes with age.[2]

The vasculature of human dermis comprises two plexuses that parallel the skin surface: one in the lower dermis (deep plexus) and one just beneath the papillary dermis (superficial plexus).[96] These two systems are connected by intercommunicating vessels, and vertical vessel arcades project superiorly from the superficial plexus toward the epidermis to form papillary loops (Fig. 2-7). This subpapillary plexus also gives rise to vessels that infuse the periadnexal structures.[96] The cutaneous vascular system also contains arteriovenous shunts, or glomi, which are specialized anastomoses that assist in the regulation of skin blood flow and thermoregulatory shunting.[3,103] The cutaneous capillary network is fairly disordered at birth and assumes a more orderly network pattern by the second week of life,[123] with continued development until around 3 months of postnatal life.[124]

Vasomotor tone is under the control of a complex series of neurogenic, myogenic, and pharmacologic mechanisms,[3] and the ability to control skin blood flow is now

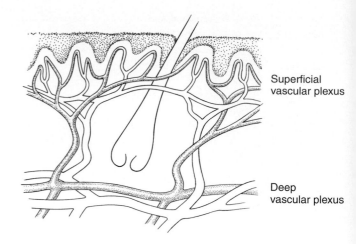

FIG. 2-7
Vasculature of the skin, which is composed of the superficial plexus and the deep plexus with intercommunicating vessels. The superficial plexus gives rise to vertical vessel arcades that project superiorly into the dermal papillae and form papillary loops. (Courtesy Randall Hayes.)

known to be well developed in neonates.[125] It was previously suggested that skin blood flow and total peripheral blood flow both correlate inversely (and decrease) with increasing birth weight, gestational maturity, and postnatal age, along with the development of increasing peripheral vascular resistance.[126] However, studies of capillary blood cell velocity (CBV) in full-term infants have demonstrated a correlation between CBV and postnatal age, making the significance of previous microvascular findings in the neonate unclear.[127]

Thermoregulation, which maintains an equilibrium between heat production and heat loss, is a crucial requirement in the neonate for maintenance of optimal core body temperature. It is a complex physiologic process under control of the nervous (most importantly the hypothalamus) and endocrine systems. Although the thermoregulatory response is present in both term and preterm neonates, it is more pronounced in term infants.[128] The primary contributors to thermogenesis are muscles (voluntary and involuntary, or "shivering" thermogenesis), sweat glands, blood vessels, and adipose tissue.[129] Heat loss, or thermolysis, is accomplished by flow of heat from the center of the body to the surface and, subsequently, flow of heat from the body surface to the environment.[129] Heat transfer to the surroundings can be accomplished through conduction (thermal exchange between the body surface and objects with which it is in contact), convection (heat loss from mass flow of moving air over the body surface), or radiation (electromagnetic heat loss to cool surfaces within the environment). Water evaporation, the fourth mechanism of heat loss, is discussed in the section on neonatal sweating.

Thermal stimuli providing information to the hypothalamus are transmitted from skin thermal receptors, as well as from deeper receptors present in the abdominal cavity and central nervous system.[129,130] In general, increased environmental temperature results in cutaneous arteriolar vasodilatation and heat dissipation, whereas cold stress leads to vasoconstriction with resultant decreased skin blood flow and reduced heat loss from the body core. Heat production in the neonate is accomplished primarily through nonshivering thermogenesis, which utilizes the increased number of mitochondria, increased glycogen stores, and abundant blood supply of brown fat.[130] The primary mechanism utilized by the overheated neonate to dissipate heat is evaporative water loss through sweating.

Although temperature regulation is developed to some extent in most infants, they are susceptible to both cold and heat stress. Transition out of the stable thermal environment of the uterus, as well as birth trauma, malformations, drugs, and respiratory deficiency, may all predispose the newborn to hypothermia, whereas birth trauma and exogenous sources of heat may lead to hyperthermia.[129] Thermoregulation is a multifaceted process, which at times may be inadequate in the maintenance of the homeothermic state in the neonate. An understanding of these processes is therefore vital for providing appropriate thermal support to such infants.

CUTANEOUS IMMUNOSURVEILLANCE, LANGERHANS' CELLS, AND CYTOKINES

Cutaneous Immunosurveillance

The skin, while participating in the important roles of physical protection, barrier function, and thermoregulation, also occupies a niche in the immunologic system of the host as a peripheral immune organ. Various models and terms have been used to describe the immunologic capacities of the skin, including skin-associated lymphoid tissues (SALT), skin immune system (SIS), dermal microvascular unit (DMU), and dermal immune system (DIS).[131,132] The SALT is composed of epidermal Langerhans' cells and keratinocytes, as well as dermal endothelial cells and the skin-draining lymph nodes, and is an important system in the induction of immunity and tolerance.[132] The broader terminology of the SIS refers to the entire complex interplay of immune response–related systems in the skin, including cellular components and humoral factors[132,133] and both dermal and epidermal components.

These immunologic systems in the skin provide cutaneous immunosurveillance, which functions in the prevention of the development of cutaneous neoplasms and mediates against persistent infections with intracellular pathogens.[134] Cellular components include keratinocytes, antigen-presenting cells (APCs), monocytes and macrophages, granulocytes, mast cells, lymphocytes, and endothelial cells, whereas humoral constituents include antimicrobial peptides, complement proteins, immunoglobulins, cytokines, and prostaglandins.[132]

Characterization of lymphocyte populations within normal human skin have revealed that they are predominantly T cells, with 90% of cells clustered around postcapillary venules or adjacent to cutaneous appendages.[133,135] Intraepidermal localization of T lymphocytes accounts for less than 2% of skin lymphocytes normally present. B lymphocytes are not present in normal human skin but may be found in mucosal locations.

Langerhans' Cells

The cell that sets the SIS apart from others is the Langerhans' cell (LC). This APC resides in the epidermis and is involved in skin allograft rejection, delayed hypersensitivity reactions, and specific T-cell responses.[136] LCs are derived from the bone marrow and migrate via a hematogenous route to the skin. They are present in the fetus as early as 16 weeks gestation, with early restriction to the basal layer and eventual distribution among suprabasal cells.[137]

The function of the LC was unclear until the 1970s, when surface Fc receptors, major histocompatability complex (MHC) class II molecules, and C3 receptors were described on its surface,[134] suggesting an immunologic role. It is now well accepted that the epidermal LC is involved in antigen processing and presentation in a variety of skin-induced immune responses against a variety of antigens, including contact allergens, alloantigens, tumor antigens, and microorganisms.[138] These cells have been found to have positive staining for other characteristic surface markers, including CD1a and S100 proteins and membrane-bound adenosinetriphosphatase (ATPase).[138] Although the exact function of the CD1a glycoprotein remains unclear, relatively weak expression of the antigen on LCs from neonatal skin has been demonstrated[139] and may partially explain why neonatal donor skin demonstrates extended survival compared with adult donor skin after transplantation in animal models.[140-142] Ultrastructurally, LCs are found to contain Birbeck granules, distinctive cytoplasmic organelles with central striations and a characteristic "tennis racket" appearance on thin sections.[136] Although the exact function of these granules is unknown, it has been suggested that they may be involved in receptor-ligand interactions and surface antigen trafficking.[143]

LCs are a member of the dendritic family of cells, which are stellate cells with cytoplasmic extensions, or dendrites. Other dendritic APCs are present in human skin, including dermal dendritic cells, which also contribute to the surveillance function of the immune system and initiation of the primary immune response. These cells were also shown to express high levels of MHC class II molecules, as well as factor XIIIa, and are isolated primarily from the dermis.[144] Some dermal dendritic cells may acquire ultrastructural characteristics of LCs and therefore may be precursors of these epidermal APCs.[144]

Cytokines

In addition to the role of such cellular components in cutaneous immunity, a complex interplay with several humoral factors is also present, including the biologic proteins known as cytokines. These autocrine, paracrine, endocrine, exocrine, and intracrine proteins include the interleukins (ILs), interferons (IFNs), colony-stimulating factors (CSFs), tumor necrosis factors (TNFs), and growth factors (GFs).[133,138] They are produced by various cell types, including keratinocytes, which have been demonstrated to be capable of secreting multiple types of cytokines.[133]

Cytokines have multiple biologic functions and act on target cells by binding to specific receptors. The result of such binding is signal transduction to the cell interior followed by activation of various second-messenger pathways and eventual altered gene expression and cell function.[138] For instance, on exposure to contact allergens, LCs may show enhanced migration after induction of local IL-1 beta production, ultimately resulting in activation and expansion of allergen-specific T cell populations,[132] whereas IL-10 inhibits the ability of LCs to stimulate T cells.[136] Cytokines are involved in many cutaneous processes, both physiologic and pathologic, the details of which are beyond the scope of this chapter. Although not clearly elucidated, the secretion, activity, and effector function of cytokines in neonates may differ from that in adults. An example is the hypothalamic response to IL-1, also known as endogenous pyrogen, in newborns. The synthesis of prostaglandins in response to this protein normally shifts the thermoregulatory set-point, resulting in fever, but this responsiveness is decreased in the neonate, which may account for the attenuated fever response in the setting of infection.[129]

REFERENCES

1. White CR, Bigby M, Sangueza OP. What is normal skin? In Arndt KA, LeBoit PE, Robinson JK, Wintroub BU, eds. Cutaneous medicine and surgery. an integrated program in dermatology. Philadelphia: WB Saunders, 1996: pp 3-45.
2. Holbrook KA. A histological comparison of infant and adult skin. In Maibach HI, Boisits EK, eds. Neonatal skin, structure and function. New York: Dekker, 1982: pp 3-31.
3. Solomon LM, Esterly NB. Neonatal dermatology. I. The newborn skin. J Pediatr 1970;77:888-894.
4. Serri F, Montagna W. The structure and function of the epidermis. Pediatr Clin N Am 1961;8:917-941.
5. Holbrook KA, Sybert VP. Basic science. In Schachner LA, Hansen RC, eds. Pediatric dermatology, 2nd edition. New York: Churchill Livingstone, 1995: pp 1-70.
6. Evans NJ, Rutter N. Development of the epidermis in the newborn. Biol Neonate 1986;49:74-80.
7. Wickett RR, Mutschelknaus JL, Hoath SB. Ontogeny of water sorption-desorption in the perinatal rat. J Invest Dermatol 1993;100:407-411.
8. Fuchs E. Keratins: Mechanical integrators in the epidermis and hair and their role in disease. Prog Dermatol 1996; 30:1-12.
9. Fuchs E, Weber K. Intermediate filaments: Structure, dynamics, function, and disease. Annu Rev Biochem 1994; 63:345-382.
10. Byrne C, Tainsky M, Fuchs E. Programming gene expression in developing epidermis. Development 1994;120:2369-2383.
11. Holbrook KA, Underwood RA, Vogel AM, et al. The appearance, density and distribution of melanocytes in human embryonic and fetal skin revealed by the anti-melanoma monoclonal antibody, HMB-45. Anat Embryol 1989;180:443-455.
12. Haake AR, Scott GA. Physiologic distribution and differentiation of melanocytes in human fetal and neonatal skin equivalents. J Invest Dermatol 1991;96:71-77.
13. Scott GA, Haake AR. Keratinocytes regulate melanocyte number in human fetal and neonatal skin equivalents. J Invest Dermatol 1991;97:776-781.
14. Haake AR, Holbrook KA. The structure and development of skin. In Freedberg IM, Eisen AZ, Wolff K, et al, eds. Dermatology in general medicine, 5th edition. New York: McGraw-Hill, 1999: pp 70-114.
15. Jimbow K, Quevedo WC, Prota G, et al. Biology of melanocytes. In Freedberg IM, Eisen AZ, Wolff K, et al, eds. Dermatology in general medicine, 5th edition. New York: McGraw-Hill, 1999: pp 192-220.
16. Bressler RS, Bressler CH. Functional anatomy of the skin. Clin Podiatr Med Surg 1989;6:229-246.
17. Boissy RE. The melanocyte. Its structure, function, and subpopulations in skin, eyes, and hair. Dermatol Clin 1988; 6:161-173.

18. Szabo G, Gerald A, Pathak MA. Racial differences in the fate of melanosomes in human epidermis. Nature 1969; 222: 1081-1082.

19. Dale BA, Holbrook KA, Steinert PM. Assembly of stratum corneum basic protein and keratin filaments in macrofibrils. Nature 1978;276:729-731.

20. Manabe M, Sanchez M, Sun TT, et al. Interaction of filaggrin with keratin filaments during advanced stages of normal human epidermal differentiation and in ichthyosis vulgaris. Differentiation 1991;48:43-50.

21. Odland GF, Holbrook K. The lamellar granules of epidermis. Curr Prob Dermatol 1981;9:29-49.

22. Elias PM. Lipids and the epidermal permeability barrier. Arch Dermatol Res 1981;270:95-117.

23. Elias PM. Epidermal lipids, barrier function and desquamation. J Invest Dermatol 1983;80(Suppl):44S-49S.

24. Proksch E, Holleran WM, Menon GK, et al. Barrier function regulates epidermal lipid and DNA synthesis. Br J Dermatol 1993;128:473-482.

25. Elias PM, Feingold KR. Lipids and the epidermal water barrier: metabolism, regulation, and pathophysiology. Semin Dermatol 1992;11:176-182.

26. Grubauer G, Feingold KR, Harris RM, et al. Lipid content and lipid type as determinants of the epidermal permeability barrier. J Lipid Res 1989;30:89-96.

27. Elias PM. Dynamics of the epidermal barrier: New implications for percutaneous drug delivery, topical therapeutics and disease pathogenesis. Prog Dermatol 1992;26:1-8.

28. Friberg SE. Micelles, microemulsions, liquid crystals, and the structure of stratum corneum lipids. J Soc Cosmet Chem 1990;41:155-171.

29. Elias PM, Goerke J, Friend DS. Mammalian epidermal barrier layer lipids: Composition and influence on structure. J Invest Dermatol 1977;69:535-546.

30. Elias PM, Friend DS. The permeability barrier in mammalian epidermis. J Cell Biol 1975;65:180-191.

31. Aszterbaum M, Menon GK, Feingold KR, et al. Ontogeny of the epidermal barrier to water loss in the rat: Correlation of function with stratum corneum structure and lipid content. Pediatr Res 1992;31:308-317.

32. Menon GK, Feingold KR, Moser AH, et al. De novo sterologenesis in the skin. II. Regulation by cutaneous barrier requirements. J Lipid Res 1985;26:418-427.

33. Grubauer G, Feingold KR, Elias PM. Relationship of epidermal lipogenesis to cutaneous barrier function. J Lipid Res 1987;28:746-752.

34. Monger DJ, Williams ML, Feingold KR, et al. Localization of sites of lipid biosynthesis in mammalian epidermis. J Lipid Res 1988;29:603-611.

35. Williams ML, Aszterbaum M, Menon GK, et al. Preservation of permeability barrier ontogenesis in the intrauterine growth-retarded fetal rat. Pediat Res 1993;33:418-424.

36. Hammarlund K, Sedin G, Stromberg B. Transepidermal water loss in newborn infants. VIII. Relation to gestational age and post-natal age in appropriate and small for gestational age infants. Acta Paediatr Scand 1983;72:721-728.

37. Barker N, Hadgraft J, Phil D, et al. Skin permeability in the newborn. J Invest Dermatol 1987;88:409-411.

38. Harpin VA, Rutter N. Barrier properties of the newborn infant's skin. J Pediatr 1983;102:419-424.

39. Evans NJ, Rutter N. Percutaneous respiration in the newborn infant. J Pediatr 1986;108:282-286.

40. Rutter N. The immature skin. Br Med Bull 1988;44:957-970.

41. Hammarlund K, Sedin G. Transepidermal water loss in newborn infants. III. Relation to gestational age. Acta Paediatr Scand 1979;68:795-801.

42. Kalia YN, Nonato LB, Lund CH, Guy RH. Development of skin barrier function in premature infants. J Invest Dermatol 1998;111:320-326.

43. Hanley K, Jiang Y, Elias PM, et al. Acceleration of barrier ontogenesis in vitro through air exposure. Pediatr Res 1997; 41:293-299.

44. Bustamante SA, Steslow J. Use of a transparent adhesive dressing in very low birthweight infants. J Perinatol 1989; 9:165-169.

45. Knauth AK, Gordin M, McNelis W, et al. Semipermeable polyurethane membrane as an artificial skin for the premature neonate. Pediatrics 1989;83:945-950.

46. Vernon HJ, Lane AT, Wischerath LJ, et al. Semipermeable dressing and transepidermal water loss in premature infants. Pediatrics 1990;86:835-847.

47. Mancini AJ, Sookdeo-Drost S, Madison KC, et al. Semipermeable dressings improve epidermal barrier function in premature infants. Pediatr Res 1994;36:306-314.

48. Lane AT, Drost SS. Effects of repeated application of emollient cream to premature neonates' skin. Pediatrics 1993; 92:415-419.

49. Nopper AJ, Horii KA, Sookdeo-Drost S, et al. Topical ointment therapy benefits premature infants. J Pediatr 1996; 128:660-669.

50. Corsini E, Sangha N, Feldman SR. Epidermal stratification reduces the effects of UVB (but not UVA) on keratinocyte cytokine production and cytotoxicity. Photodermatol Photoimmunol Photomed 1997;13:147-152.

51. Jackson SM, Elias PM. Skin as an organ of protection. In Fitzpatrick TB, Eisen AZ, Wolff K, et al, eds. Dermatology in general medicine, 4th edition. New York: McGraw-Hill, 1993:pp 241-253.

52. Wyatt JE, Poston SM, Noble WC. Adherence of staphylococcus aureus to cell monolayers. J Appl Bacteriol 1990; 69: 834-844.

53. Romero-Steiner S, Witek T, Balish E. Adherence of skin bacteria to human epithelial cells. J Clin Microbiol 1990; 28:27-31.

54. Darmstadt GL, Fleckman P, Jonas M, et al. Differentiation of cultured keratinocytes promotes the adherence of streptococcus pyogenes. J Clin Invest 1998;101:128-136.

55. Ebling FJG. Functions of the skin. In Champion RH, Burton JL, Ebling FJG, eds. Textbook of dermatology, 5th edition. Oxford: Blackwell Scientific Publications, 1992: pp 125-155.

56. Hurley HJ. Permeability of the skin. In Moschella SL, Hurley HJ, eds. Dermatology, 3rd edition. Philadelphia: WB Saunders, 1992: pp 101-106.

57. Woodley D, Sauder D, Talley MJ, et al. Localization of basement membrane components after dermal-epidermal junction separation. J Invest Dermatol 1983;81:149-153.

58. Pulkkinen L, Uitto J. Hemidesmosomal variants of epidermolysis bullosa. Mutations in the Greek $\alpha_6\beta_4$ integrin and the 180-kD bullous pemphigoid antigen/type XVII collagen genes. Exp Dermatol 1998;7:46-64.

59. Zone JJ, Taylor TB, Meyer LJ, et al. The 97 kDa linear IgA bullous disease antigen is identical to a portion of the extracellular domain of the 180 kDa bullous pemphigoid antigen, BPAg2. J Invest Dermatol 1998;110:207-210.

60. Jonkman MF, deJong MC, Heeres K, et al. 180-kD bullous pemphigoid antigen (BP180) is deficient in generalized atrophic benign epidermolysis bullosa. J Clin Invest 1995; 95:1345-1352.

61. Pohla-Gubo G, Lazarova Z, Giudice GJ, et al. Diminished expression of the extracellular domain of bullous pemphigoid antigen 2 (BPAG2) in the epidermal basement membrane of patients with generalized atrophic benign epidermolysis bullosa. Exp Dermatol 1995;4(4 Pt 1):199-206.

62. Gatalica B, Pulkkinen L, Li K, et al. Cloning of the human type XVII collagen gene (COL17A1), and detection of novel mutations in generalized atrophic benign epidermolysis bullosa. Am J Hum Genet 1997;60:352-365.

63. Vidal F, Aberdam D, Miquel C, et al. Integrin beta 4 mutations associated with junctional epidermolysis bullosa with pyloric atresia. Nat Genet 1995;10:229-234.

64. Pulkkinen L, Bruckner-Tuderman L, et al. Compound heterozygosity for missense (L156P) and nonsense (R554X) mutations in the beta4 integrin gene (ITGB4) underlies mild, nonlethal phenotype of epidermolysis bullosa with pyloric atresia. Am J Pathol 1998;152:935-941.

65. Ruzzi L, Gagnoux-Palacios L, Pinola M, et al. A homozygous mutation in the integrin alpha6 gene in junctional epidermolysis bullosa with pyloric atresia. J Clin Invest 1997; 99:2826-2831.

66. Brown TA, Gil SG, Sybert VP, et al. Defective integrin alpha 6 beta 4 expression in the skin of patients with junctional epidermolysis bullosa and pyloric atresia. J Invest Dermatol 1996;107:384-391.

67. Stanley JR, Woodley DT, Katz SI, et al. Structure and function of basement membrane. J Invest Dermatol 1982; 79(Suppl 1):69S-72S.

68. Masunaga T, Shimizu H, Ishiko A, et al. Localization of laminin-5 in the epidermal basement membrane. J Histochem Cytochem 1996;44:1223-1230.

69. Uitto J, Pulkkinen L, Christiano AM. Molecular basis of the dystrophic and junctional forms of epidermolysis bullosa: mutations in the type VII collagen and kalinin (laminin 5) genes. J Invest Dermatol 1994;103(5 Suppl):39S-46S.

70. Pulkkinen L, McGrath J, Airenne T, et al. Detection of novel LAMC2 mutations in Herlitz junctional epidermolysis bullosa. Mol Med 1997;3:124-135.

71. Kivirikko S, McGrath JA, Pulkkinen L, et al. Mutational hotspots in the LAMB3 gene in the lethal (Herlitz) type of junctional epidermolysis bullosa. Hum Mol Genet 1996; 5:231-237.

72. Kivirikko S, McGrath JA, Baudoin C, et al. A homozygous nonsense mutation in the alpha 3 chain gene of laminin 5 (LAMA3) in lethal (Herlitz) junctional epidermolysis bullosa. Hum Mol Genet 1995;4:959-962.

73. Woodley DR. Importance of the dermal-epidermal junction and recent advances. Dermatologica 1987;174:1-10.

74. Hovnanian A, Rochat A, Bodemer C, et al. Characterization of 18 new mutations in COL7A1 in recessive dystrophic epidermolysis bullosa provides evidence for distinct molecular mechanisms underlying defective anchoring fibril formation. Am J Hum Genet 1997;61:599-610.

75. Uitto J, Olsen DR, Fazio MJ. Extracellular matrix of the skin: 50 years of progress. J Invest Dermatol 1989;92(4 Suppl): 61S-77S.

76. Uitto J, Perejda AJ, Abergel RP, et al. Altered steady-state ratio of type I/III procollagen mRNAs correlates with selectively increased type I procollagen biosynthesis in cultured keloid fibroblasts. Proc Natl Acad Sci USA 1985;82:5935-5939.

77. Micali G, Bene-Bain MA, Guitart J, et al. Genodermatoses. In Schachner LA, Hansen RC, eds. Pediatric dermatology, 2nd edition. New York: Churchill Livingstone, 1995: pp 347-411.

78. Couchman JR, Caterson B, Christner JE, et al. Mapping by monoclonal antibody detection of glycosaminoglycans in connective tissues. Nature 1984;307:650-652.

79. Hardingham TE, Fosang AJ. Proteoglycans: many forms and many functions. FASEB J 1992;6:861-870.

80. Scott JE. Proteoglycan: collagen interactions and subfibrillar structure in collagen fibrils. Implications in the development and ageing of connective tissues. J Anat 1990;169: 23-35.

81. Longaker MT, Adzick NS, Hall JL, et al. Studies in fetal wound healing. VII. Fetal wound healing may be modulated by hyaluronic acid stimulating activity in amniotic fluid. J Pediatr Surg 1990;25:430-433.

82. West DP, Worobec S, Solomon LM. Pharmacology and toxicology of infant skin. J Invest Dermatol 1981;76:147-150.

83. Buczkowski-Bickmann MK. Thermoregulation in the neonate and the consequences of hypothermia. Clin Forum Nurse Anes 1992;3:77-82.

84. Nedergaard J, Cannon B. Brown adipose tissue: Development and function. In Polin RA, Fox WW, eds. Fetal and neonatal physiology, 2nd edition. Philadelphia: WB Saunders, 1998:478-489.

85. Muller M, Jasmin JR, Monteil RA, et al. Embryology of the hair follicle. Early Human Develop 1991;26:159-166.

86. Bertolino AP, Klein LM, Freedberg IM. Biology of hair follicles. In Fitzpatrick TB, Eisen AZ, Wolff K, et al, eds. Dermatology in general medicine, 4th edition. New York: McGraw-Hill, 1993: pp 289-293.

87. Barman JM, Pecoraro V, Astore I, et al. The first stage in the natural history of the human scalp hair cycle. J Invest Dermatol 1967;48:138-142.

88. Cotsarelis G, Sun TT, Lavker RM. Label-retaining cells reside in the bulge area of pilosebaceous unit: implications for follicular stem cells, hair cycle and skin carcinogenesis. Cell 1990;61:1329-1337.

89. Sun TT, Cotsarelis G, Lavker RM. Hair follicular stem cells: The bulge-activation hypothesis. J Invest Dermatol 1991; 96(5 Suppl):77S-78S.

90. Yang JS, Lavker RM, Sun TT. Upper human hair follicle contains a subpopulation of keratinocytes with superior *in vitro* proliferative potential. J Invest Dermatol 1993;101:652-659.

91. Klein J, Forman R, Eliopoulos C, et al. A method for simultaneous measurement of cocaine and nicotine in neonatal hair. Ther Drug Monit 1994;16:67-70.

92. Koren G. Measurement of drugs in neonatal hair: a window to fetal exposure. Forensic Sci Int 1995;70:77-82.

93. Kintz P, Mangin P. Determination of gestational opiate, nicotine, benzodiazepine, cocaine and amphetamine exposure by hair analysis. J Forensic Sci Soc 1993;33:139-142.

94. Eliopoulos C, Klein J, Chitayat D, et al. Nicotine and cotinine in maternal and neonatal hair as markers of gestational smoking. Clin Invest Med 1996;19:231-242.

95. Pochi PE, Strauss JS, Downing DT. Age-related changes in sebaceous gland activity. J Invest Dermatol 1979;73:108-111.

96. Stal S, Spira M, Hamilton S. Skin morphology and function. Clin Plast Surg 1987;14:201-208.

97. Agache P, Blanc D, Barrand C, et al. Sebum levels during the first year of life. Br J Dermatol 1980;103:643-649.

98. Baden HP, Kvedar JC. Biology of nails. In Fitzpatrick TB, Eisen AZ, Wolff K, et al, eds. Dermatology in general medicine, 4th edition. New York: McGraw-Hill, 1993: pp 294-297.

99. Wagner AM, Hansen RC. Neonatal skin and skin disorders. In Schachner LA, Hansen RC, eds. Pediatric dermatology, 2nd edition. New York: Churchill Livingstone, 1995: pp 263-346.

100. Mancini AJ, Lane AT. Sweating in the neonate. In Polin RA, Fox WW, eds. Fetal and neonatal physiology, 2nd edition. Philadelphia: WB Saunders, 1998: pp 767-770.

101. Sato K. Biology of the eccrine sweat gland. In Fitzpatrick TB, Eisen AZ, Wolff K, et al, eds. Dermatology in general medicine, 4th edition. New York: McGraw-Hill, 1993: pp 221-231.

102. Atherton DJ. The neonate. In Champion RH, Burton JL, Ebling FJG, eds. Textbook of dermatology, 5th edition. Oxford: Blackwell Scientific Publications, 1992: pp 382-383.

103. Green M. Comparison of adult and neonatal skin eccrine sweating. In Maibach HI, Boisits EK, eds. Neonatal skin, structure and function. New York: Dekker, 1982: pp 35-66.

104. Guyton AC: Textbook of medical physiology, 8th edition. Philadelphia: WB Saunders, 1991: pp 799-801.

105. Green M, Behrendt H. Sweating capacity of neonates. Nicotine-induced axon reflex sweating and the histamine flare. Am J Dis Child 1969;118:725-732.

106. Behrendt H, Green M. Drug-induced localized sweating in full-size and low-birth-weight neonates. Am J Dis Child 1969;117:299-306.

107. Green M, Behrendt H. Drug-induced localized sweating in neonates. Am J Dis Child 1970;120:434-438.

108. Foster KG, Hey EN, Katz G. The response of the sweat glands of the newborn baby to thermal stimuli and to intradermal acetylcholine. J Physiol 1969;203:13-29.

109. Harpin VA, Rutter N. Sweating in preterm babies. J Pediatr 1982;100:614-618.

110. Green M, Behrendt H. Sweating responses of neonates to local thermal stimulation. Am J Dis Child 1973;125:20-25.

111. Hey EN, Katz G. Evaporative water loss in the newborn baby. J Physiol 1969;200:605-619.

112. Oh W, Karecki H. Phototherapy and insensible water loss in the newborn infant. Am J Dis Child 1972;124:230-232.

113. Jones RWA, Rochefort MJ, Baum JD. Increased insensible water loss in newborn infants nursed under radiant heaters. Br Med J 1976;2:1347-1350.

114. Williams PR, Oh W. Effects of radiant warmer on insensible water loss in newborn infants. Am J Dis Child 1974;128:511-514.

115. Karlsson H, Hanel SE, Nilsson K, et al. Measurement of skin temperature and heat flow from skin in term newborn babies. Acta Paediatr 1995;84:605-612.

116. Gladman G, Chiswick ML. Skin conductance and arousal in the newborn. Arch Dis Child 1990;65:1063-1066.

117. Sato S, Ogihara Y, Hiraga K, et al. Fine structure of unmyelinated nerves in neonatal skin. J Cutan Pathol 1977;4:1-8.

118. Cauna N. The free penicillate nerve endings of the human hairy skin. J Anat 1973;115:277-288.

119. Cauna N. Fine morphological characteristics and microtopography of the free nerve endings of the human digital skin. Anat Rec 1980;198:643-656.

120. Moll R, Moll I, Franke WW. Identification of Merkel cells in human skin by specific cytokeratin antibodies: changes of cell density and distribution in fetal and adult plantar epidermis. Differentiation 1984;28:136-154.

121. Moll I, Moll R, Franke WW. Formation of epidermal and dermal Merkel cells during human fetal skin development. J Invest Dermatol 1986;87:779-787.

122. Narisawa Y, Hashimoto K, Nihei Y, et al. Biological significance of dermal Merkel cells in development of cutaneous nerves in human fetal skin. J Histochem Cytochem 1992;40:65-71.

123. Perera P, Kurban AK, Ryan TJ. The development of the cutaneous microvascular system in the newborn. Br J Derm 1970;82:86-91.

124. Mayer KM. Observations on the capillaries of the normal infant. Am J Dis Child 1921;22:381-387.

125. Beinder E, Trojan A, Bucher HU, et al. Control of skin blood flow in pre- and full-term infants. Biol Neonate 1994;65:7-15.

126. Wu PYK, Wong WH, Guerra G, et al. Peripheral blood flow in the neonate. 1. Changes in total, skin, and muscle blood flow with gestational and postnatal age. Pediatr Res 1980;14:1374-1378.

127. Norman M, Herin P, Fagrell B, et al. Capillary blood cell velocity in full-term infants as determined in skin by videophotometric microscopy. Pediatr Res 1988;23:585-588.

128. Jahnukainen T, van Ravenswaaij-Arts C, Jalonen J, et al. Dynamics of vasomotor thermoregulation of the skin in term and preterm neonates. Early Hum Dev 1993;33:133-143.

129. Risbourg B, Vural M, Kremp O, et al. Neonatal thermoregulation. Turk J Pediatr 1991;33:121-134.

130. Thomas K. Thermoregulation in neonates. Neon Network 1994;13:15-22.

131. Bos JD. The skin immune system: lupus erythematosus as a paradigm. Arch Dermatol Res 1994;287:23-27.

132. Bos JD. The skin as an organ of immunity. Clin Exp Immunol 1997;107 (Suppl 1):3-5.

133. Bos JD, Kapsenberg ML. The skin immune system: progress in cutaneous biology. Immun Today 1993;14:75-78.

134. Streilein JW, Bergstresser PR. Langerhans cells: antigen presenting cells of the epidermis. Immunobiol 1984;168:285-300.

135. Bos JD, Zonneveld I, Das PK, et al. The skin immune system (SIS): distribution and immunophenotype of lymphocyte subpopulations in normal human skin. J Invest Dermatol 1987;88:569-573.

136. Hogan AD, Burks AW. Epidermal Langerhans cells and their function in the skin immune system. Ann Allergy Asthma Immunol 1995;75:5-12.

137. Drijkoningen M, de Wolf-Peters C, Van Der Steen K, et al. Epidermal Langerhans cells and dermal dendritic cells in human fetal and neonatal skin: an immunohistochemical study. Pediatr Dermatol 1987;4:11-17.

138. Stingl G, Hauser C, Wolff K. The epidermis: an immunologic microenvironment. In Fitzpatrick TB, Eisen AZ, Wolff K, et al, eds. Dermatology in general medicine, 4th edition. New York: McGraw-Hill, 1993: pp 172-197.

139. Kowolenko M, Carlo J, Gozzo JJ. Histologic identification of cellular differences that may contribute to the reduced immunogenicity of transplanted neonatal versus adult skin tissue. Int Arch Allergy Appl Immunol 1986;80:274-277.

140. Silvers WK. Studies on the induction of tolerance of the H-Y antigen in mice with neonatal skin grafts. J Exp Med 1968;128:69-83.

141. Silvers WK, Collins NH. The behavior of H-Y-incompatible neonatal skin grafts in rats. Transplantation 1979;28: 57-59.

142. Kowolenko M, Gozzo JJ. Comparative study of neonatal and adult skin transplants in mice. Transplantation 1984; 38:84-86.

143. Hanau D, Fabre M, Schmitt DA, et al. Appearance of Birbeck granule-like structures in anti-T6 antibody-treated human epidermal Langerhans cells. J Invest Dermatol 1988; 90:298-304.

144. Nestle FO, Nickoloff BJ. Dermal dendritic cells are important members of the skin immune system. Adv Exp Med Biol 1995;378:111-116.

3

Lesional Morphology and Assessment

HO JIN KIM
PAUL J. HONIG

The skin of the newborn infant can exhibit a vast spectrum of conditions, from benign to life-threatening. A meticulous examination is essential, since skin changes may be the initial sign of internal disease or genetic alteration. A dermatologic evaluation is not unlike that of other medical disciplines in that the foundation is based on a comprehensive history and careful physical examination. However, the dermatologic evaluation is unique in that the pathologic processes are readily visible to the clinician. Therefore it is often more efficient to first assess lesional morphology and then focus one's history based on these clinical findings. A neonatal skin evaluation is similar in this respect, but presents unique challenges. A basic understanding of general newborn care is important, particularly with respect to preterm infants. Moreover, a definitive diagnosis is dependent on an understanding of the physiology of neonatal skin and its specialized reaction patterns. This chapter reviews the salient aspects of the prenatal and natal history, as well as the principles of morphologic assessment.

COMPREHENSIVE HISTORY AND ITS IMPACT

The first step of the neonatal skin examination is to obtain a comprehensive history. In the newborn setting, this includes not only prenatal and natal histories but also maternal, paternal, and family medical histories (Box 3-1). Prenatal history should focus on questions about potential exposure to medications, both prescription and over-the-counter, as well as controlled and uncontrolled substances such as tobacco, alcohol, and cocaine and other illicit drugs. Certain drugs, for example, phenytoin, val-

proic acid, coumadin, diethylstilbestrol, isotretinoin, etretinate, tetracycline, and penicillamine are known teratogens. As substance abuse among mothers has become more prevalent, our knowledge of their effects on the fetus is expanding. In some instances, such as in fetal alcohol syndrome, specific cutaneous features, including short palpebral fissure, broad and flat nasal bridge, and long upper lip with an absent or ill-defined philtrum, have been well described.[1] Other cutaneous findings of substance abuse are less specific and defined, but have been linked with premature birth and fetal growth retardation and its inherent cutaneous susceptibilities.[2] Additional factors important in the prenatal history include maternal infections, especially within the first trimester when organogenesis occurs. The TORCH infections (**to**xoplasmosis, **r**ubella, **c**ytomegalovirus, **h**erpes), syphilis, human papilloma virus, and human immunodeficiency virus (HIV) may have significant systemic and cutaneous effects on the infant, as addressed specifically in later chapters.

Maternal history should include age, medical history, and outcomes of prior pregnancies. Certain genetic disorders have been linked to increased maternal age during pregnancy, particularly chromosomal abnormalities, the most frequent being Down syndrome.[3] A prime example of pertinent maternal disease is lupus erythematosus with the anti-Ro/SSA, or U1RNP antibody, which may result in an infant with neonatal lupus erythematosus.[4] Other autoimmune disorders (such as bullous disorders), as well as chronic medical conditions requiring systemic medications, are also important in assessing the newborn. Medical conditions acquired during pregnancy, such as gestational diabetes, will also affect fetal development. Previous pregnancies, resulting in spontaneous abortions, may be evidence for X-linked dominant conditions or autosomal recessive conditions that are fatal in utero. Failure to initiate or poor progression of labor may be the first clue to X-linked icthyosis in the infant.[5] Polyhydramnios has been associated with trisomies, and junctional epidermolysis bullosa with associated pyloric atresia.[6,7] Paternal history, although less significant, may be useful. Increased paternal age has also been linked to chromosomal abnormalities, in particular Down syndrome and Apert's syndrome.[8,9] Finally, parents should be questioned for a family history of congenital anomalies or genetic disorders. Affected family members may indicate a specific pattern of inheritance. A history of consanguinity should be sought if recessive genetic disorders are suspected.

The history of labor and delivery should include approximate gestational dates. Premature, term, and post-date infants present with different cutaneous examinations, and are differentially susceptible to cutaneous disease. For instance, premature infants have a higher incidence of hemangiomas, term infants are more likely to develop erythema toxicum neonatorum, and post-date infants undergo significant desquamation shortly after birth. Premature rupture of membranes, prolonged labor, and evidence of fetal distress from hypoxia or meconium aspiration, may predispose an infant to cutaneous infection and subsequent sepsis. Low birth weight infants must be watched with particular vigilance for signs of septicemia. Other risk factors for sepsis include male sex and prematurity, with risk inversely proportional to gestational age. Apnea, bradycardia, irritability, feeding intolerance, temperature instability, abdominal distention, increased respiratory effort, and hypotonia can be subtle early signs of sepsis. Cutaneous findings of infection may include a full or bulging fontanelle, generalized erythema, petechiae, purpura, and vasomotor instability, with poor peripheral circulation (i.e., mottling and cyanosis of the acral areas).[10] The umbilical area, as well as central venous or arterial catheterization sites, should be evaluated closely as potential portals of entry. Prolonged labor, abnormal presentation, and artificial extraction measures may account for petechiae and ecchymoses, which may herald the onset of hyperbilirubinemia. In certain disorders, such as congenital melanoma, examination of the placenta may be helpful.

CUTANEOUS EXAMINATION AND EVALUATION

Although historical evidence is important, the cornerstone of dermatology remains a careful, detailed cutaneous examination. This requires both visual and tactile assessment of the skin. Special precautions must be followed in the newborn nursery, especially in the intensive care unit setting. Careful handwashing, with removal of jewelry, must be performed to reduce the risk of nosocomial in-

---

BOX 3-1

Maternal, Family, Perinatal, and Neonatal History Relevant to Neonatal Skin Evaluation

Maternal and Family History
- Parental age
- History of skin or mucous membrane disease
- History of blistering, skin fragility, ectodermal defects, or birthmarks
- History of significant systemic disease, congenital anomalies, or genetic disorders
- History of infectious diseases (e.g., herpes simplex virus)

Obstetric History
- Previous pregnancies, outcomes, miscarriages, maternal serologic status, (syphilis, rubella, HIV)
- Illnesses, surgery, fever, or rash
- Medication used during pregnancy
- Prenatal testing (amniocentesis, chorionic villus sampling)
- Timing of amniotic membrane rupture
- Labor duration/complications
- Intrauterine monitoring
- Amniotic fluid (+/− meconium)
- Fever before or after delivery
- Fetal distress
- Delivery method (e.g., vacuum extraction, forceps)
- Placental abnormalities

Neonatal History
- Gestational age, birth weight, and birth weight relative to gestational age (low, average, large)
- Resuscitation needs
- Medication—past, present
- Cutaneous history: outset, morphology, distribution, prior treatment, evolution
- Lesions/rash
- General medical/surgical history: includes structural anomalies, history of lethargy, irritability, feeding intolerance

fections.[11,12] Some infants may require incubators to maintain their temperature and fluid balance. During examination, prolonged exposure outside of the isolette can result in hypothermia. Open radiant warmers are helpful, but prolonged exposure should be avoided because open warmers will increase transepidermal water loss. When examining an infant, good lighting and adequate exposure are essential. Although natural lighting is best, this is rarely available. Fluorescent lights and bilirubin lights may mask some of the subtle contours and colors of individual lesions. The infant should have all clothing removed, including diapers, so that the entire skin surface can be examined. A great deal of similarity may occur between pathologic processes. Although some diagnoses are obvious, there is only a finite number of ways that skin can express disease. An organized approach to evaluating and describing lesions is paramount.

Examination of the skin surface must be performed systematically, separating the body into segments to ensure complete evaluation. A determination of primary and secondary lesions should be made (Table 3-1). An understanding of the significance of these primary and secondary lesions will not only help generate a differential diagnosis but also allow for concise communication of pertinent data to colleagues. We have attempted to use the most commonly used definitions for primary and

secondary lesions. Unfortunately, a review of the core dermatologic textbooks and literature reveals a great deal of inconsistency among these definitions.[13-17] Subsequently, the color, borders, configuration, and distribution of lesions are assessed (Table 3-2). When evaluating color, one should take into account the variations in different races because background color will alter the overall color of lesions. This is followed by palpation of the lesion, with particular attention to the border. Lesions may be soft, firm, fluctuant, indurated, or tender. The border should be examined for distinct or indistinct margins. Next, configuration should be assessed. Are the lesions linear, annular, nummular, targetoid, grouped, or retiform? Finally, the last step is the evaluation of distribution. Is the lesion single or multiple, localized or generalized, symmetric or asymmetric, extensor or flexural, acral, or inverse?

Mucous membranes, teeth, hair, and nails should be included in a full cutaneous examination. Teeth, hair, and nails, being ectodermal structures like the skin, can be intimately linked to cutaneous pathologic processes. Teeth are normally absent at birth, but natal teeth, which represent prematurely erupted primary incisors, can be seen. Delayed onset of eruption, absent or abnormal teeth, or enamel dysplasia can be seen in the ichthyoses, ectodermal dysplasias, and incontinentia pigmenti. Sparse to abundant

Text continued on p. 45

TABLE 3-1

Primary and Secondary Lesions

Primary Lesions

Primary lesions are defined as lesions that arise de novo and are therefore most characteristic of the disease process. The graphic representations are intended to demonstrate three-dimensional and topographic relationships and not necessarily the histology of the example shown.

Macule	*Examples*
A circumscribed, flat lesion with color change, up to 1 cm in size, although the term is often used for lesions larger than 1 cm. By definition, they are not palpable.	Ash leaf macules, café au lait macules, capillary malformations

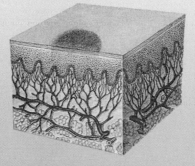

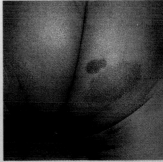

Café au lait macules

Continued

TABLE 3-1

Primary and Secondary Lesions—cont'd

Patch
A circumscribed, flat lesion with color change, greater than 1 cm in size.

Examples
Nevus depigmentosus, mongolian spots, nevus simplex

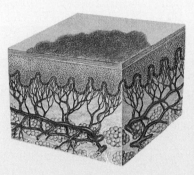

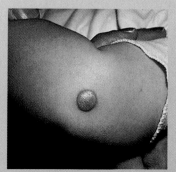

Hemangioma precursor

Papule
A circumscribed, elevated, solid lesion, up to 1 cm in size. Elevation may be accentuated with oblique lighting.

Examples
Verrucae, milia, and juvenile xanthogranuloma.

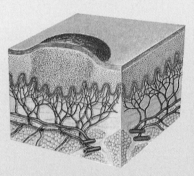

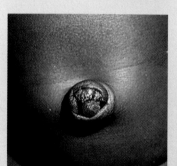

Umbilical granuloma

Plaque
A circumscribed, elevated, plateaulike, solid lesion, greater than 1 cm in size.

Examples
Mastocytoma, nevus sebaceous

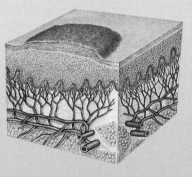

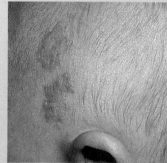

Nevus sebaceous

Nodule
A circumscribed, elevated, solid lesion with depth, up to 2 cm in size.

Examples
Dermoid cysts, neuroblastoma

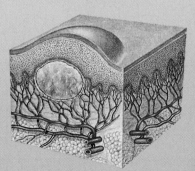

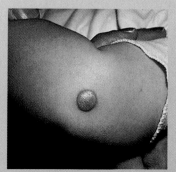

Juvenile xanthogranuloma

TABLE 3-1

Primary and Secondary Lesions—cont'd

Tumor
A circumscribed, elevated, solid lesion with depth, greater than 2 cm in size.

Examples
Hemangioma, lipoma, rhabdomyosarcoma

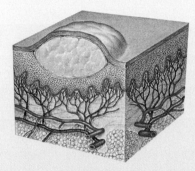
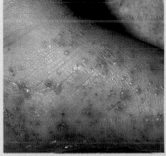

Hemangioma

Vesicle
A circumscribed, elevated, fluid-filled lesion up to 1 cm in size.

Examples
Herpes simplex, varicella, miliaria crystallina

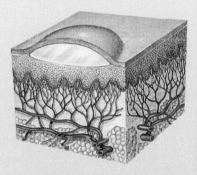
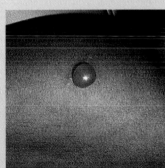

Acropustulosis of infancy

Bulla
A circumscribed, elevated, fluid-filled lesion greater than 1 cm in size.

Examples
Sucking blisters, epidermolysis bullosa, bullous impetigo

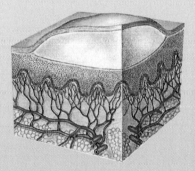
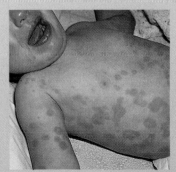

Insect bite reaction

Wheal
A circumscribed, elevated, edematous, often evanescent lesion, due to accumulation of fluid within the dermis.

Examples
Urticaria, bite reactions, drug eruptions

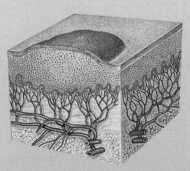

Drug eruption

Continued

TABLE 3-1

Primary and Secondary Lesions—cont'd

Pustule
A circumscribed, elevated lesion filled with purulent fluid, less than 1 cm in size.

Examples
Transient neonatal pustular melanosis, erythema toxicum neonatorum, infantile acropustulosis

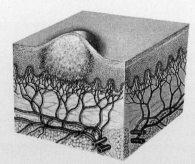

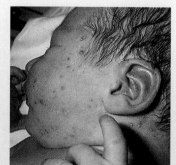

Transient neonatal pustular melanosis

Abscess
A circumscribed, elevated lesion filled with purulent fluid, greater than 1 cm in size.

Example
Pyodermas

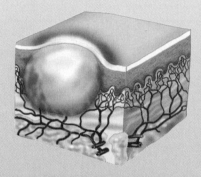

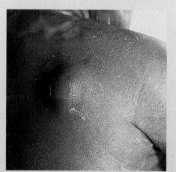

Abscess

Secondary Lesions

Secondary lesions are characteristically brought about by modification of primary lesions, either by the individual or through the natural evolution of the lesion in the environment. The graphic representations are intended to demonstrate three-dimensional and topographic relationships and not necessarily the histology of the example shown.

Crust
Results from dried exudate overlying an impaired epidermis. Can be composed of serum, blood, or pus.

Examples
Epidermolysis bullosa, impetigo

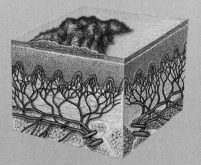

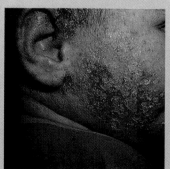

Infected atopic dermatitis

TABLE 3-1
Primary and Secondary Lesions—cont'd

Scale
Results from increased shedding or accumulation of stratum corneum as a result of abnormal keratinization and exfoliation. Can be subdivided further into pityriasiform (branny, delicate), psoriasiform (thick, white, and adherent), and icthyosiform (fish scale–like).

Examples
Ichthyoses, post-maturity desquamation, seborrheic dermatitis

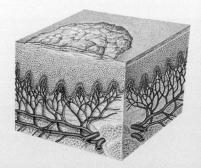

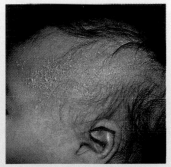
Seborrheic dermatitis

Erosion
Intraepithelial loss of epidermis. Heals without scarring.

Examples
Herpes simplex, certain types of epidermolysis bullosa

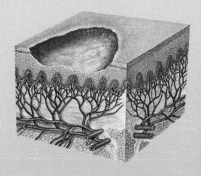

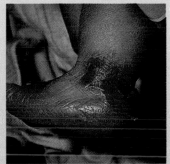
Epidermolysis bullosa

Ulcer
Full-thickness loss of the epidermis, with damage into the dermis. Will heal with scarring.

Examples
Ulcerated hemangiomas, aplasia cutis congenita

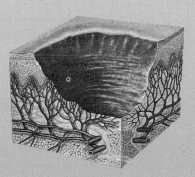

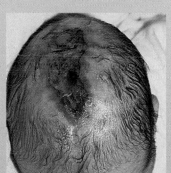
Aplasia cutis congenita

Continued

TABLE 3-1

Primary and Secondary Lesions—cont'd

Fissure
Linear, often painful break within the skin surface, as a result of excessive xerosis.

Examples
Inherited keratodermas, hand and foot eczema

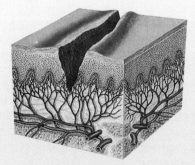

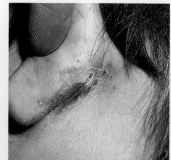

Atopic dermatitis

Lichenification
Thickening of the epidermis with exaggeration of normal skin markings caused by chronic scratching or rubbing.

Examples
Sucking callus, atopic dermatitis

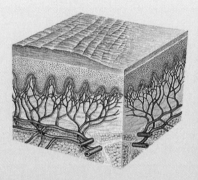

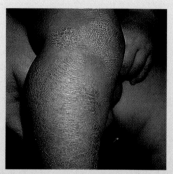

Atopic dermatitis

Atrophy
Localized diminution of skin. *Epidermal atrophy* results in a translucent epidermis with increased wrinkling, whereas *dermal atrophy* results in depression of the skin with retained skin markings. Use of topical steroids can result in epidermal atrophy, whereas intralesional steroids may result in dermal atrophy.

Examples
Aplasia cutis congenita, intrauterine scarring, and focal dermal hypoplasia.

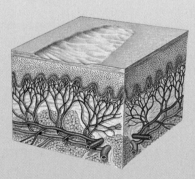

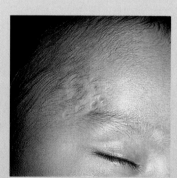

Focal dermal hypoplasia

Primary and Secondary Lesions—cont'd

Scar
Permanent fibrotic skin changes that develop as a consequence of tissue injury. In utero scarring can occur as a result of certain infections or amniocentesis or postnatally from a variety of external factors.

Examples
Congenital varicella, aplasia cutis congenita

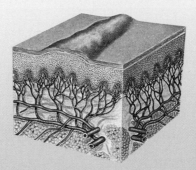

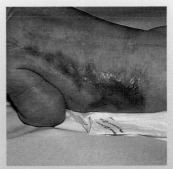

Aplasia cutis congenita

TABLE 3-2

Color, Borders, Configuration, and Distribution of Lesions

Color	To the untrained eye, the appreciation of subtle variations in color is often the most difficult concept to grasp. Fortunately, this assessment does not carry the diagnostic weight of the primary or secondary lesions. When evaluating the color, one must take into account the background pigmentation of the patient. In infants with darker skin type, subtle erythema or jaundice may be difficult to appreciate. Likewise, pigment dilution is more difficult to evaluate in lighter skin. The most prominent colors seen in cutaneous pathologic processes are described.
Red	Red color can be the result of vasodilation or hyperemia caused by inflammation. Deeper red or purple hues suggest extravasation of red blood cells. Diascopy is a diagnostic maneuver to help differentiate these possibilities. By applying pressure to the lesion, one can determine if the lesion blanches, which suggests rubor from vasodilation or inflammation. Conversely, nonblanching lesions suggest vascular damage with consequent extravasation of blood into the dermis.
White	White color can be the result of loss of pigment within the epidermis or the accumulation of white material such as purulent exudate or keratinous material. One should not use the term *white* to describe skin-colored lesions.
Yellow	Yellow coloration can be seen in lipid-containing lesions such as xanthomas, or as a result of bile accumulation, as in jaundice.
Brown/Blue/Grey/ Black	Variations in color related to increased melanin or hemosiderin in the skin. The more superficial the pigmentation in the skin, the darker the color. Melanin in the deep dermis appears blue to gray, due to the Tyndall effect.

Evaluation of hyperpigmentation and hypopigmentation must take into account the infant's genetic and racial background. Diffuse hyperpigmentation is rare and may signify systemic disease such as congenital Addison's disease and other endocrinopathies, nutritional disorders, and hepatic disease. Likewise, diffuse hypopigmentation can be seen in systemic diseases such as albinism and phenylketonuria.

Continued

TABLE 3-2

Color, Borders, Configuration, and Distribution of Lesions—cont'd

Border

The border of lesions may also help in the differential diagnosis of cutaneous lesions. Some lesions, such as acrodermatitis enteropathica, ichthyosis linearis circumflexa, and erysipelas, have distinct borders.

Examples of lesions with indistinct borders include cellulitis and atopic dermatitis. The borders of the lesion may be raised and indurated, as in granuloma annulare and neonatal lupus.

Configuration

Linear

Several lesions follow a linear pattern. If they are found to be discordant with normal lines of demarcation, one should search for an external insult. Linear lesions can be subdivided (see below).

Blaschko

These linear V- and S-shaped lines are believed to represent patterns of neuroectodermal migration. They do not follow any known vascular, nervous, or lymphatic pattern.

Examples

Linear epidermal nevus, incontinentia pigmenti

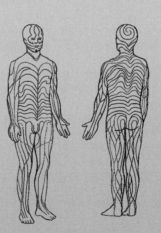

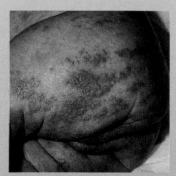

Incontinentia pigmenti

TABLE 3-2

Color, Borders, Configuration, and Distribution of Lesions—cont'd

Dermatomal/Zosteriform
Lines demarcating a dermatome supplied by one dorsal root ganglia.

Example
Herpes zoster

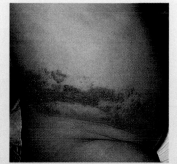

Herpes zoster

Annular
A round, ring shaped lesion, where the periphery is distinct from the center.

Examples
Tinea corporis, neonatal lupus, syphilis, annular erythema of infancy

Neonatal lupus

Nummular
A coin-shaped lesion, with homogenous character throughout.

Example
Nummular eczema

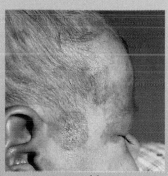

Neonatal lupus

Continued

TABLE 3-2

Color, Borders, Configuration, and Distribution of Lesions—cont'd

Gyrate/Polycyclic/Arciform/Serpiginous
Variations in the spectrum of annular lesions

Examples
Neonatal lupus erythematosus, urticaria

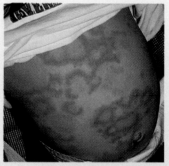
Drug eruption

Targetoid/Iris
Concentric ringed lesions, often with a dusky or bullous center. This is characteristic of erythema multiforme.

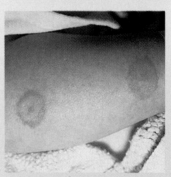
Insect bite reaction

Herpetiform
An example is herpes simplex.

Example
Herpes simplex

Corymbiform
Defined as a central cluster of lesions surrounded by scattered individual lesions.

Example
Verrucae

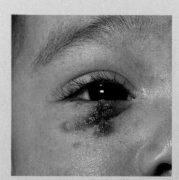
Herpes simplex infection

Retiform/Reticulate
Netlike pattern of lesions.

Examples
Cutis marmorata, cutis marmorata telangiectatica congenita

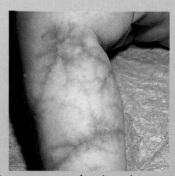
Cutis marmorata telangiectatica congenita

hairs can be seen as a variation of normal. Synchronous loss of hair followed by regrowth is a normal finding until development of an adult hair distribution, usually during the first year of life. Subtle changes in hair texture with a matted, lusterless, brittle, or unruly appearance should prompt closer evaluation by light microscopy for hair shaft abnormalities. Diffuse hypotrichosis can be seen in hidrotic and anhidrotic ectodermal dysplasia, ichthyoses, and incontinentia pigmenti. Diffuse hypertrichosis can be seen in mucopolysaccharidosis, Cornelia de Lange syndrome, and hypertrichosis lanuginosa. Nail abnormalities, in particular aplasia, hypoplasia, and dysplasia, have been associated with chromosomal disorders, ectodermal dysplasias, and epidermolysis bullosa. Absent nails or triangular lunulae have been associated with nail-patella syndrome. Finally, to complete the cutaneous examination, the lymph nodes should be palpated, particularly when there is a suspicion of infectious or neoplastic diagnoses.

REACTION PATTERNS

Reaction patterns in newborns differ significantly from those seen in children and adults, as a result of the immaturity of the skin and its components. Although the precise mechanisms are not fully deciphered, there are numerous clinical examples of these differences. Although all the known dermal-epidermal junction antigens are made by the middle of the second trimester, the lack of a developed rete ridge pattern and well-developed collagen fibrils within the papillary dermis may explain the greater propensity for vesicle formation in the newborn.[18] The epidermis, particularly in immature infants, has a relatively thin stratum corneum, which results in increased transepidermal water loss, making infants more susceptible to xerosis. Furthermore, the immature epidermis is quite fragile and prone to trauma at sites of maceration and friction, such as the neck, axillae, and groin. Even mild adhesive can strip the epidermis, causing significant damage.[19] The loss of this barrier function increases susceptibility to cutaneous infection, both with bacteria and *Candida* species. The composition of neonatal subcutaneous fat, with its greater proportion of saturated fatty acids, makes it more prone to hypoxic trauma, leading to subcutaneous fat necrosis.[20] The immaturity of the cutaneous vasculature, with its exaggerated vasomotor tone in response to hypothermia, contributes to the prevalence of cutis marmorata in infancy.[21] An understanding of these specialized reaction patterns, in conjunction with a comprehensive history and assessment of cutaneous morphology, will aid the clinician in making the proper dermatologic diagnosis.

REFERENCES

1. Clarren SK, Smith DW. The fetal alcohol syndrome. N Engl J Med 1978;298:1063-1067.
2. Buchi KF. The drug-exposed infant in the well-baby nursery. Clin Perinatol 1998;25:335-350.
3. Hansen JP. Older maternal age and pregnancy outcome: a review of the literature. Obstet Gynecol Surv 1986;41:726-742.
4. McCauliffe DP. Neonatal lupus erythematosus: a transplacentally acquired autoimmune disorder. Semin Dermatol 1995;14:47-53.
5. Bradshaw KD, Carr BR. Placental sulfatase deficiency: maternal and fetal expression of steroid sulfatase deficiency and X-linked ichthyosis. Obstet Gynecol Survey 1986;41:401-413.
6. Carlson DE, Platt LD, Medearis AL. The ultrasound triad of fetal hydramnios, abnormal hand posturing, and any other anomaly predicts autosomal trisomy. Obstet Gynecol 1992;79(5(Pt 1)):731-734.
7. Lin AN. Management of patients with epidermolysis bullosa. Dermatol Clin 1996;14:381-387.
8. McIntosh GC, Olshan AF, Baird PA. Paternal age and the risk of birth defects in offspring. Epidemiol 1995;6:282-288.
9. Moloney DM, Slaney SF, Oldridge M, et al. Exclusive paternal origin of new mutations in Apert syndrome. Nat Genet 1996;13:48-53.
10. Fanaroff AA, Korones SB, Wright LL, et al. Incidence, presenting features, risk factors and significance of late onset septicemia in very low birth weight infants. Pediatr Infect Dis J 1998;17:593-598.
11. Baltimore RS. Neonatal nosocomial infections. Semin Perinatol 1998;22:25-32.
12. Gaynes RP, Edwards JR, Jarvis WR, et al. Nosocomial infections among neonates in high-risk nurseries in the United States. Pediatrics 1996;98(3 Pt 1):357-361.
13. Fitzpatrick TB, Bernhard JD: Dermatologic diagnosis by recognition of clinical morphologic patterns. In Fitzpatrick TB, Eisen AZ, Wolff K, et al, eds. Dermatology in general medicine, 4th edition. vol 1. New York: McGraw Hill, 1993: p 55.
14. Hurwitz S: An overview of dermatologic diagnosis. In Hurwitz S. Clinical pediatric dermatology, 2nd edition. Philadelphia: WB Saunders, 1993, p 1.
15. Jackson R. Definitions in dermatology. A dissertation on some of the terms used to describe the living gross pathology of the human skin. Clin Exper Dermatol 1978;3:241-247.
16. Lewis EJ, Dahl MV. On standard definitions: 33 years hence. Arch Dermatol 1997;133:1169.
17. Ashton RE. Standard definitions in dermatology: the need for further discussion. Arch Dermatol 1998;134:637-638.
18. Solomon LM, Esterly NB. Neonatal dermatology. I. The newborn skin. J Pediatr 1970;77:888-894.
19. Harpin VA, Rutter N. Barrier properties of the newborn infant's skin. J Pediatr 1983;102:419-425.
20. Hicks MJ, Levy ML, Alexander J, et al. Subcutaneous fat necrosis of the newborn and hypercalcemia: case report and review of the literature. Pediatr Dermatol 1993;10:271-276.
21. Smales OR, Kime R. Thermoregulation in babies immediately after birth. Arch Dis Child 1978;53:58-61.

Skin of the Premature Infant

MARY L. WILLIAMS

The premature infant assumes the challenge of independent life despite immaturity of essential functions. Skin functions are primarily protective, and when those functions are immature, they contribute to the vulnerability of the preterm infant. The foremost function of the skin is to provide a permeability barrier that both protects the aqueous interior of the infant from desiccation in the xeric atmosphere and prevents massive influx of water when bathed in hypotonic solutions.[1] Other important barrier functions of skin include the barriers to percutaneous absorption of exogenous xenobiotics, to injury from mechanical trauma, to penetration by microorganisms, and to injury from ultraviolet light. In addition to its barrier functions, skin also participates in the thermoregulatory, neurosensory, and immunologic systems.

The consequences of skin immaturity for the premature infant depend on the infant's position on the maturational timetable for each cutaneous function, which is in turn dependent on the infant's gestational and postnatal ages. All skin layers (i.e., epidermis, dermis, and subcutaneous fat) are thinner in the preterm infant than at term.[2,3] Because the outermost layers of epidermis (i.e., the stratum corneum) are the primary effector of most of the barrier properties of skin, the timetable for maturation of the stratum corneum predicts the competence of many skin functions. Stratum corneum begins to form around hair follicles at about 14 weeks' gestational age and spreads to include the epidermis between hair follicles by 22 to 24 weeks' gestational age.[2] During the ensuing weeks, stratum corneum thickness increases from only a few to multiple cell layers,[3] such that by term it is actually thicker than adult stratum corneum. The "excess," outermost layers of stratum corneum are then shed during the first days of life; this process of physiologic desquamation is accentuated in postmature babies.

These histological features of skin development underlie the clinical characteristics of skin maturation embodied in the Ballad scale, widely used for assessing gestational age[4] (Fig. 4-1). In the extremely premature infant (<24 weeks) the skin is sticky, friable, and transparent; lanugo hairs are absent. As gestation progresses, the skin becomes less transparent, and, increasingly, peeling and surface cracking are seen, indicative of a thickening stratum corneum, while lanugo hair density peaks and then regresses. Despite definition of these milestones of gross and microscopic skin development, with the exception of the permeability barrier, little is known about the competency or developmental timetable of most skin functions in premature infants.

THE PERMEABILITY BARRIER IN THE PRETERM INFANT

The permeability barrier resides in the stratum corneum through its provision of a hydrophobic lipid shield over the underlying nucleated cell layers.[1] Because of their plasma and intracellular membranes, most cells are hydrophobic relative to the vascular and extracellular compartments; however, in stratum corneum this pattern is reversed. Instead, the extracellular compartment of stratum corneum is filled with a highly organized series of hydrophobic lipid membranes in the extracellular spaces, while the anucleate corneocytes form an aqueous compartment as a result of loss of their plasma and organelle membranes. This interposition of hydrophobic lipid membranes in the extracellular compartment retards the movement of water inward or outward across the stra-

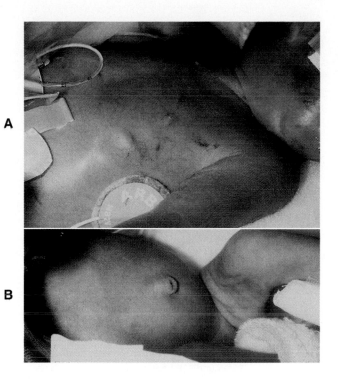

FIG. 4-1

A, Note the moist glistening surface of this ~900 g birth weight, ~29 weeks' gestational age infant on day 2 of age, reflecting an impaired barrier to TEWL. Note also the multiple abrasions, demonstrating the fragility of the newborn preterm infants' skin to trauma. **B,** This ~700 g birth weight, ~27 weeks' gestational age infant at 28 days of age exhibits the dull skin surface reflectance of a mature barrier to TEWL, illustrating the acceleration of skin maturation after birth.

tum corneum. The stacking of multiple layers of cornified cells surrounded by extracellular lipid bilayers further enhances this barrier to water movement through generation of a tortuous intercellular pathway for water movement.

As a multilayered stratum corneum develops in the third trimester,[2,3] the barrier to transepidermal water loss (TEWL) also matures, such that by 34 weeks' of gestation, TEWL rates approximate adult values.[5-7] The immaturity of permeability barrier function in infants less than 34 weeks' gestational age can be demonstrated either by directly measuring TEWL rates using a noninvasive instrument, the Evaporimeter, or by assessing the degree of vasoconstriction after application of topical phenylephrine (i.e., with a competent barrier, this small hydrophilic molecule is not absorbed, and no skin blanching occurs)[6-8] (Fig. 4-2). Other, indirect methods of assessing permeability barrier maturity during stratum corneum formation measure electrical properties of the skin, for example, capacitance[9] or electrical resistance,[10,11] as influenced by stratum corneum water and lipid content. By all of these measures, the extent of permeability barrier immaturity parallels the degree of prematurity (see Fig. 4-2). In addition to increasing stratum corneum thickness, development of a competent permeability barrier in fetal rat skin is accompanied by (1) deposition of neutral lipid in the intercellular domains of stratum corneum; (2) increasing stratum corneum cholesterol and ceramide content; and (3) the organization of these lipids into mature lamellar membrane structures, as viewed by electron microscopy.[12,13] Whether these same lipid biochemical and ultrastructural changes also underlie barrier formation during human skin development has not yet been determined.

Permeability barrier maturation accelerates following birth, such that most premature infants, regardless of gestational age, have competent barriers by 2 to 3 weeks' of postnatal age[6] (see Fig. 4-2). Thus maturation that may require approximately 10 weeks to complete in utero is accelerated following premature delivery. However, as the limits of viability have been lowered to include survivors of 25 weeks' (<750 g) to even 22 weeks' gestational age, barrier function may take as long as 8 weeks following birth to mature.[14,15] The gestational ages of these very immature infants directly abut the timetable for stratum corneum formation (see the previous discussion). It may not be surprising, therefore, that extremely premature infants do not respond as rapidly to maturational signals initiated by birth. In fetal rat skin it is air exposure with evaporation of water from the skin surface that stimulates accelerated barrier formation, because this acceleration can be prevented by covering the skin surface with a vapor-impermeable membrane.[16] This may also occur if preterm human skin is covered with occlusive materials.[17]

Permeability barrier ontogenesis is developmentally regulated; hence, small-for-dates infants exhibit barrier function that is appropriate for their gestational age.[18] In fetal rat, barrier maturation is regulated by glucocorticoids, thyroid hormone, and sex hormones, as well as activators and ligands of the PPARα and LXR nuclear hormone receptors[13] (Table 4-1). Some of these agents also regulate lung development; and glucocorticoids often are administered prepartum to mothers to accelerate fetal lung maturation when premature delivery is imminent.[19] Whether barrier maturation is also stimulated by these interventions has not been determined; however, preterm infants of glucocorticoid treated mothers have reduced insensible water losses and lower serum sodium concentrations in the first 4 days after birth, consistent with a maturational effect on the skin barrier.[19a]

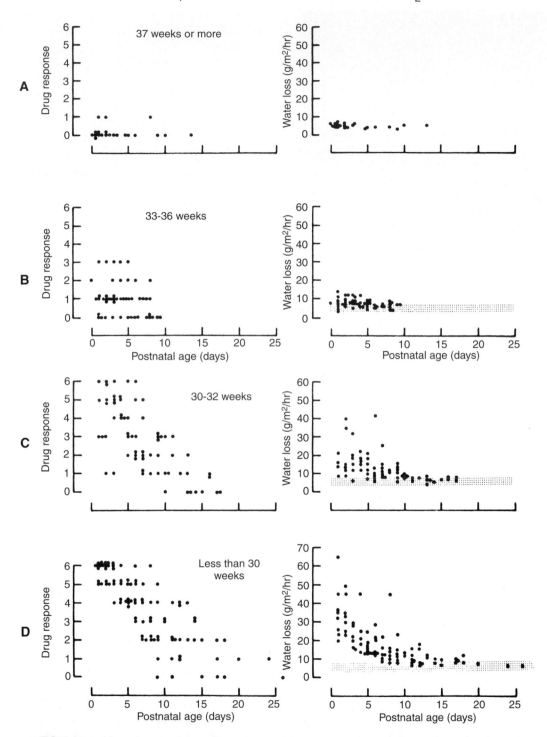

FIG. 4-2

Phenylephrine-induced blanching (*Column 1*) and TEWL (*Column 2*) in neonates of varying gestational and postgestational ages. **A,** Term infants; <37 weeks. **B,** Preterm infants 33 to 36 weeks. **C,** Preterm infants 30 to 32 weeks. **D,** Preterm infants <30 weeks. Note that preterm infants at birth (postgestational age = 0) have elevated rates of TEWL and blanch in response to topical phenylephrine. These responses are greatest in the most premature group *(D),* but normalize even in this most premature group by 2 to 3 weeks' postgestational age. (Modified from Harpin VA, Rutter N: *J Pediatr* 1983;102:419-425.)

TABLE 4-1

Regulatory Signals for Fetal Rat Skin Barrier Formation

Signal	Effect	Nuclear receptor	Class
Dexameth-asone	Accelerate	Glucocor-ticoid	I
Thyroid hormone	Accelerate	Thyroid hormone	II
Diethylstil-bestrol	Accelerate	Estrogen	I
Testosterone	Retard	Androgen	I
Linoleic acid	Accelerate	PPARα	II
Clofibric acid	Accelerate	PPARα	II
Farnesol	Accelerate	?FXR or PPARα	II
25-hydroxy-cholesterol	Accelerate	LXR	II

Class I: Steroid hormone receptors. Ligand binds in cytosol, translocates to nucleus after ligand binding; regulates gene transcription as homodimer.
Class II: RXR-interacting subfamily of receptors. Ligand binds to receptor in nucleus; regulates gene transcription as heterodimer with the RXR receptor and its ligand, 9-cis retinoic acid (e.g., RXR-T3R; RXR-Vitamin D3R).

CONSEQUENCES OF PERMEABILITY BARRIER IMMATURITY

Fluid and Electrolyte Imbalance and Evaporative Energy Loss

The primary consequences of permeability barrier immaturity are (1) increased evaporative loss of free water from the skin surface, placing the infant at risk for volume depletion, particularly hypernatremic dehydration; and (2) energy loss through heat of evaporation; that is, ~580 is calories expended for each milliliter of water that evaporates.[7] Therefore optimal care of the premature infant requires both accurate compensation for cutaneous water losses to preserve fluid and electrolyte balance and maintenance of the infant in a thermally neutral environment, such that caloric intake can be directed toward growth and not heat production.[7,20,21] Although concurrent cutaneous water losses can be directly measured (i.e., by measuring TEWL), this procedure is not standard practice in most nurseries. Instead, cutaneous water losses, along with respiratory fluid losses, together are considered *insensible* (i.e., not directly measured).[20] In term infants, TEWL accounts

for approximately two thirds of insensible losses; but cutaneous water losses are much higher in preterm infants, while respiratory fluid losses remain relatively constant.[22,23] Neonatal fluid requirements are estimated using complex formulas that take into account the following:

1. Measured losses in urine and feces
2. Estimates of insensible losses
3. Requirements to support growth (increasing with postgestational age)

Neonatal fluid requirements must be modified by postnatal age to compensate for fluid redistribution (i.e., requirements on the first extrauterine day are decreased as a result of contraction of the extracellular compartment) and adjusted, retrospectively, to compensate for excessive weight loss or gain and/or serologic parameters of fluid or electrolyte imbalance.[20]

In addition, fluid replacements must adjust for a number of environmental conditions (Table 4-2), because cutaneous losses are not merely a function of stratum corneum maturity; they are also modified by the ambient temperature and humidity (it is the vapor pressure of water at the skin surface that determines the rate of evaporation).[18]

A humidified incubator can provide a thermally neutral environment with low rates of evaporative water loss, because at a relative humidity of 80% or greater, skin surface evaporation effectively ceases.[24-26] Scrupulous antisepsis, however, is required to prevent bacterial colonization of this environment, particularly with water-loving organisms, such as *Pseudomonas.* Moreover, these devices obstruct access to extremely ill or unstable infants. Therefore these infants are commonly cared for on an open bed, where a radiant warmer provides a thermally neutral environment at the expense of greatly increased rates of TEWL.[25-28] Infants requiring care under radiant warmers are typically those who are the youngest and the most premature; that is, the population with the poorest skin barriers. Use of a plastic cover or plastic bubble blanket may increase the humidity and mitigate to some extent the adverse effects of the radiant heating on TEWL[29,30] (Fig. 4-3). Although these plastic shields are widely employed, standards for thermal stability and transmission have not been established.[31] Phototherapy, required in many preterm infants to treat hyperbilirubinemia, also increases fluid requirements, particularly when white light systems are used.[32-34] Many skin disorders also adversely affect permeability barrier competence (see the following discussion) (see Table 4-2).

There is considerable variability in TEWL among infants of the same gestational and postgestational ages (see Fig. 4-2). The timetable for maturation of barrier function

TABLE 4-2

Factors Modifying Cutaneous Water Losses in Preterm Infants

Factor	Effect on TEWL
Decreasing gestational age	Increased TEWL; rates proportional to degree of prematurity
Increasing postnatal age	TEWL decreases towards mature rates: > ~1000 g, mature by 2 to 3 weeks; < ~1000 g, mature by 4 to 8 weeks
Increasing ambient temperature	Increased TEWL; proportional to increase in temperature
Increasing ambient humidity	Decreased TEWL; proportional to increased humidity
Radiant warmer	Increased TEWL (by 40% to 100%)
Radiant warmer with heat shield	Increased TEWL (by ~20% to 40%)
Phototherapy	Increased by (up to ~50%)
Skin diseases (absent or abnormal stratum corneum)	Increased; depends on percent body surface involved and severity of defect

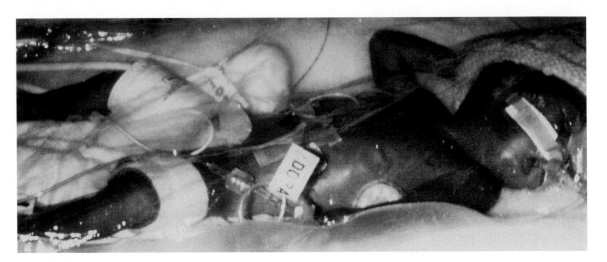

FIG. 4-3
Premature infant nursed under a radiant warmer and covered with a plastic sheet to retard evaporative water loss.

varies between infants of the same gestational age, and maturation is often quite precipitous.[7,8,14] Hence, formulas that estimate "insensible" cutaneous losses are inherently inaccurate. Moreover, these formulas rely heavily on retrospective adjustments and inevitably result in "chasing" fluids. It should not be forgotten that cutaneous losses are not inherently insensible (i.e., unmeasurable). Indeed, it has been shown that measurement of TEWL using the rapid and noninvasive Evaporimeter from as few as three body sites permits accurate estimation of total cutaneous losses in preterm infants.[35] Despite this, measurement of

TEWL has not been adopted widely by intensive care nurseries in the approach to fluid management. Clinical studies that compare outcomes using methods that incorporate direct measurement of skin losses versus traditional methods of estimating "insensible" losses are needed to determine the clinical value of more accurate, prospective determination of cutaneous losses.

Other strategies to reduce TEWL in the preterm infant include use of protective skin dressings or ointments. Semipermeable dressings (e.g., Bioclusive, Omniderm, Opsite, Tegaderm) that permit some passage of water vapor and other gases, but are impervious to water and microorganisms, can reduce TEWL rates and also are protective against trauma of adhesives from monitors.[36-40] Moreover, barrier maturation is not inhibited by these dressings, and neither have increased rate of infection nor colonization by microorganisms been observed. Nonetheless, increased bacterial colonization under such dressings is observed in other clinical settings[41] and remains a serious consideration with their use on preterm infants. In addition, many of these dressings contain adhesive materials, and even those without adhesives can cling to the moist skin surface of the preterm newborn and injure the epidermis, unless they are either removed carefully or allowed to detach spontaneously. Furthermore, partial body applications (i.e., trunk and abdomen) to very immature infants (<1000 g), may not be sufficient to decrease total fluid requirements.[36] These limitations impede widespread adoption of artificial dressings in routine skin care. It should also be remembered that the benefits of these agents have only been shown in studies with small numbers of subjects. Confirmation of these findings in larger cohorts is required before their routine use could be generally recommended.

Topical ointments, such as petrolatum[42,43] or Aquaphor,[44] also decrease TEWL, although the effect from a single application lasts only 4 to 8 hours.[44-46] Less-frequent applications do not decrease fluid requirements, but they continue to provide some protection against skin trauma and may reduce risk of systemic infection.[44] Although largely composed of nonphysiologic lipids (e.g., long-chain hydrocarbons and wax esters), these emollients have a long history of dermatologic use without associated toxicity or evidence of significant percutaneous absorption. Nonetheless, internal hydrocarbon accumulations (paraffinomas) are reported, albeit rarely,[47,48] and gastrointestinal absorption of hydrocarbons is documented.[49a] Hence, the possibility remains that these lipids may not be entirely innocuous when applied to the skin of very premature infants, whose absorptive characteristics may more closely approximate those of gastrointestinal mucosa than mature skin. (See also discussion on "Control of Transcutaneous Water Loss" in Chapter 5).

An alternate approach to barrier fortification in these infants would be use of mixtures of lipids physiologic to the skin. The extracellular membranes of the stratum corneum that provide the barrier to TEWL comprise an approximately equimolar mixture of ceramides, long-chain free fatty acids, and cholesterol.[49] The effect of various mixtures of these physiologic lipids on permeability barrier function have been examined in mature skin in experimental systems, in which the barrier is initially perturbed, (e.g., by solvent wipes to extract native stratum corneum lipids), the test lipids are then applied and the rate of barrier recovery (i.e., normalization of TEWL) determined.[46,50] Whereas applications of any one or two of the physiologic lipids (i.e., incomplete mixtures) aggravate barrier homeostasis in mature epidermis, equimolar mixtures allow normal barrier recovery. Moreover, optimized ratios of the three key physiologic lipid classes can actually accelerate barrier recovery following insult[51] and in aged skin.[52] Yet, despite the theoretic advantages of employing physiologic lipid mixtures, these are not commercially available; nor have they been examined for efficacy in treating the barrier immaturity of the preterm infant.

Increased Percutaneous Absorption of Xenobiotics

Another direct consequence of skin barrier immaturity is the increased absorption of topically applied substances (Table 4-3), sometimes with tragic consequences (see Chapter 5).[31,53-56] This vulnerability was first recognized historically when preterm infants developed methemoglobinemia through absorption of aniline dyes in the laundry marks placed on diapers.[55] Subsequently, the demonstration of neurotoxicity from percutaneous absorption of hexachlorophene, commonly in use in nurseries as an antibacterial cleanser,[52] led to broadened recognition of the vulnerability of the preterm infant to toxicity from topically applied agents.

The same factors that determine the movement of water from inside out also regulate the movement of low molecular weight substances from outside in.[56] Small (<800 daltons) hydrophilic molecules are effectively excluded by the extracellular membrane system from penetration across a mature stratum corneum, while small hydrophobic or amphipathic molecules are able to penetrate through the tortuous intercellular, lipid bilayer pathway.[1,57,58] In the preterm infant the thinner stratum corneum results in reduction in the length (tortuosity) of the intercellular pathway and would enhance percutaneous absorption of hydrophilic molecules. Whether there are also qualitative changes in the lipid composition and structural integrity of the lipid bilayers of immature stratum corneum that alter permeability function is unknown. In addition to immaturity of the permeability barrier, several other factors in premature infants may contribute to toxicity from topical xenobiotics.[53,55] First, the surface area/volume ratio is increased in all infants, but even more so in premature infants; this effectively increases the absorptive surface while decreasing the volume of distribution for the absorbed drug. Once absorbed, reduced levels of serum-binding proteins, such as albumin, may in-

TABLE 4-3

Hazardous or Potentially Hazardous Compounds that may be Absorbed Across the Skin of Preterm Infants†

Compound	Toxicity	Sources
Alcohol (methylated spirits)	Skin necrosis; neurotoxic	Topical antiseptic
Aluminum*	Neurotoxicity	Metal containers for topical ointments
Analine dyes	Methemoglobinemia	Laundry marks
Boric acid, borax	Shock, renal failure	Antifungals, talc powders
Benzocaine	Methemoglobinemia	Topical analgesics; teething products
Benzethonium chloride*	Carcinogen	Antiseptic soap
Benzoyl benzoate*	Neurotoxicity	Scabicide
Bicarbonate	Metabolic alkalosis	Baking soda for diaper dermatitis
Camphor*	Gastrointestinal toxin Neurotoxicity	Topical antipruritic; camphorated oils (Vaporub; Campho-Phenique)
Coal tars*	Carcinogen	Topical antiinflammatory products
Corticosteroid	Adrenal suppression; hyperadrenocorticism	Topical corticosteroids
Diphenhydramine	Neurotoxicity	Topical analgesics (Caladryl)
Epinephrine	High output failure	Topical vasoconstriction
Glycerin*	Hyperosmolarity	Emollients; cleansers (Aquanil)
Hexachlorophene	Neurotoxicity	Antiseptic soaps (pHisoHex)
Iodochlorhydroxyquin	Optic neuritis	Topical antibiotic (Vioform)
Isopropyl alcohol	Skin necrosis; neurotoxicity	Topical antiseptics
Lactic acid*	Metabolic acidosis	Topical keratolytics (Lac-Hydrin)
Lindane	Neurotoxicity	Scabicide (Kwell)
Mercury	Neurotoxicity; acrodynia; nephrotic syndrome	Disinfectants; teething powder (historical)
Methylene blue	Methemoglobinemia	Vital stain
Neomycin	Ototoxicity	Topical antibiotic (Neosporin)
Nystatin*	Nephrotoxicity	Topical antifungal (Mycostatin)
Phenol	Cardiac and neurotoxicity	Disinfectants (e.g., commercial laundries); local anesthetic/antimicrobials (e.g., Castellani's paint)
Propylene glycol*	Hyperosmolarity; neurotoxicity	Topical vehicles; emollients, cleansers (Cetaphil)
Povidone-iodine	Skin necrosis; hypothyroidism	Topical antiseptic (Betadine)
Prilocaine	Methemoglobinemia	Topical anesthetic (EMLA)
Resorcinol	Methemoglobinemia	Topical antiseptic
Salicylic acid	Salicylism	Topical keratolytics
Silver sulfadiazine	Kernicterus; argyria	Topical antibiotic (Silvadene)
Sulfur*	Paralysis; death	Scabicide ointment
Triclosan*	Neurotoxicity	Topical antiseptic (Lever 2000)
Urea	Elevated BUN	Topical keratolytics/ emollients

*Potentially hazardous compounds.
†References 30, 52-63, 133-144.

crease the proportion of free drug. Similarly, deficiency of an adipose reservoir to buffer against redistribution of fat-soluble drugs, such as lindane, to lipid-enriched neural tissues, may make the premature infant particularly vulnerable to central nervous system (CNS) toxicity from such agents. Immaturity of detoxification mechanisms, such as hepatic conjugation, and of renal function, also alter drug pharmacodynamics and can increase toxicity.

The increased permeability of premature skin to small hydrophilic molecules has also been exploited to enhance the percutaneous delivery of medications such as theophylline.[55,59] Transdermal drug delivery offers the theoretic advantages of (1) the avoidance of first-pass hepatic metabolism; (2) a slow and continual reservoir of release, minimizing peaks and valleys; (3) the ability to easily remove the drug source (in the case of patch delivery systems), if needed; and (4) a painless method of drug delivery with easy access.[55] A confounding factor in developing these systems for the premature infant is the variability of barrier competence, both between infants of the same gestational ages and as the dynamics of barrier competence change as these infants mature.

In the care of the preterm infant, it is safest to assume that any medication applied to the skin may be absorbed systemically. As a corollary, the ideal topical medications for preterm infants are those with low systemic toxicity. It is also necessary to consider the composition and potential toxicity of vehicles used for topical drug delivery, because components of these may also be absorbed across the immature skin barrier (See Chapter 5).[31] Provision of a safe antiseptic for use on premature infants' skin is particularly problematic, especially in the most immature infants, who have not only the most immature barriers but also the most unstable barriers, and are therefore exposed to repeated applications of antiseptics for intravenous access.[60]

Impact of Permeability Barrier Immaturity on other Organ Systems

Excluding congenital malformations and genetic diseases, the major causes of morbidity and mortality in premature infants are respiratory distress syndrome, patent ductus arteriosus (PDA), necrotizing enterocolitis (NEC), periventricular/intraventricular hemorrhage (IVH), and overwhelming infection. Maintenance of normal blood pressure and "optimal" blood volume protects against these major causes of morbidity and mortality in the preterm infant. Cutaneous fluid losses are perhaps the most important destabilizing factor in fluid homeostasis of the premature infant, and this influence is likely to be even more pronounced in the extremely premature infant. For example, overhydration contributes to the development of symptomatic PDA,[61] as larger blood volumes increase shunting through the ductus arteriosus. Conversely, systemic hypotension may increase the likelihood of an intracranial hemorrhage. Alterations in cerebral blood pressure induce hemorrhage into the periventricular germinal matrix, a gelatinous and highly vascular fetal structure, which is present up to 34 weeks' of gestational age.[62] The preterm infant may be unable to main-

tain cerebral blood flow in the presence of systemic hypotension. The period of greatest risk for IVH is in the first week of life, particularly in the first 2 days of life, which coincides not only with the time of greatest permeability barrier incompetence but also with the time when tissue fluids undergo redistribution with contraction of the extracellular fluid compartment.[63] Thus, to the extent that IVH is precipitated by fluctuations in systemic blood pressure, overcompensated or uncompensated cutaneous water losses may be an exacerbating factor.

The pathogenesis of NEC is attributed to a triad of ischemia, oral feeding, and infection[64,65]; each of these pathogenic factors may be exacerbated by skin immaturity. As in PDA and IVH, fluid imbalance resulting from skin immaturity could be a cofactor, since both overcorrection of fluids[66] and hypotensive ischemic-reperfusion injury[67] are implicated in NEC. Early initiation of oral feeds[68] is undertaken to reverse negative energy balance in the preterm infant. Caloric losses caused by increased evaporative water loss from the skin surface contribute to this caloric drain. *Staphylococcus epidermidis* has also been implicated in the pathogenesis of NEC.[69-71] An impaired cutaneous barrier to this normal skin resident could be a factor not only in the development of *S. epidermidis* septicemia (see the following discussion) but also in abnormal gastrointestinal colonization by this organism,[72] although a connection between these two phenomena is not obvious.

It seems likely, therefore, that efforts to closely monitor cutaneous losses through direct measurements of TEWL, with the goal of tight control of replacement fluids, would decrease the incidence and severity of these major complications of prematurity and would improve the outcome of these infants.[73]

IMMATURITY OF OTHER SKIN BARRIERS

Cutaneous Barrier to Mechanical Injury

The skin of the premature infant is much more vulnerable to mechanical injury than that of term infants, as a consequence of several factors. In addition to a thinner stratum, the epidermal-dermal interface is smooth, lacking interdigitations (i.e., rete ridges or dermal papillary projections) until the middle of the third trimester.[2] Both of these factors result in decreased resistance to shear forces. Moreover, the dermis is also thinner, less collagenized, and more gelatinous. Although the major structural proteins that underlie the mechanical strength of skin are expressed before the onset of keratinization, they may not be as abundant or organized into functionally mature units when compared with adult or even term infants' skin.[2] Whatever its basis, skin fragility is a major problem in the neonatal care of the preterm infant.[42] They are particularly vulnerable to abrasions and deeper wounds from adhesive tapes used to secure monitors, airways, and intravenous lines. Similarly, their threshold for irritant contact dermatitis from fecal contact (diaper dermatitis), for chemical burns from prolonged contact with antiseptics,[74] or for thermal burns is much reduced. Gentle handling, minimal use of adhesives, and use of hydrophilic gel[75] or pectin barrier[76] adhesives only when required can minimize these injuries. A regimen of emollient lubrication or use of nonadherent, semipermeable dressings may also protect against mechanical injuries (see the previous discussion).

Cutaneous Barrier to Infection

Although mature skin is colonized by a variety of bacteria and other microorganisms, these organisms are effectively excluded from the interior. The basis for the barrier to transcutaneous infection is not entirely understood but includes both the mechanical shield of the stratum corneum against invading microorganisms and specific components, such as certain lipids[77,78] and recently identified peptides, that may both inhibit the growth of microorganisms and modulate immune responses.[79] The thinner, easily abraded stratum corneum of the preterm infant constitutes an impaired mechanical shield against the ingress of microorganisms. In addition, it is possible that specific biochemical components of the cutaneous barrier to infection are also immature in preterm infants, although this has not been determined. Preterm infants' skin is colonized soon after birth with coagulase-negative staphylococci, predominantly *S. epidermidis.* Colonization with *Malassezia* and *Proprionobacteria* occurs later, that is, after 3 weeks,[72] coincident with maturation of the permeability barrier. *S. epidermidis* has become the most frequent cause of postnatally acquired systemic infections in these infants.[80-85] *Malassezia furfur,* a common colonizing yeast on human skin, and *Malassezia pachydermatitis,* a colonizer of canine skin, as well as the opportunistic fungi *Aspergillus, Candida,* and *Rhizopus,* are also systemic pathogens in this group.[86-90] Direct invasion across the preterm epidermis by fungi of low pathogenicity to the uncompromised host has been documented,[91] demonstrating that the stratum corneum barrier to infection is incompetent in these neonates. Exploitation of a portal of entry, such as site of skin injury or along transcutaneous catheter lines, may be a more common means of entry than direct stratum corneum invasion. Regardless

of the route of transcutaneous entry, immaturity of the immune system, particularly opsonic mechanisms, then permits organisms of low pathogenic potential to mature hosts to establish disease in the preterm infant.[92] The use of intravenous lipid supplements also favors establishment of a nidus of infection once entry into the circulation has been obtained.[81]

In a pilot study, topical applications of the emollient Aquaphor dramatically reduced the incidence of systemic infection in preterm infants.[44] Emollients may reduce the incidence of systemic infection either by supplying barrier lipids for the stratum corneum,[45] thereby reconstituting its barrier to transcutaneous infection, or by lubricating the skin surface, protecting the fragile stratum corneum from abrasive injuries, thereby reducing portals of entry. It is also possible that one or more components of this lipid mixture may have antimicrobial actions. If confirmed in larger trials, these findings would suggest that late-onset septicemia in the preterm infant may be caused more often by penetration of microorganisms, either across intact skin or through minor breaks in skin integrity, rather than along indwelling lines. Thus immaturity of the skin barrier may be a more important contributor to systemic infection in preterm infants than was previously appreciated.

Cutaneous Barrier to Light Injury

Energy absorbed from ultraviolet light passing through the skin may damage critical cellular functions through the generation of free radicals, principally singlet oxygen, as well as through inflammatory responses initiated by cytokine release and the generation of eicosanoids.[93,94] For example, free radical damage to deoxyribonucleic acid (DNA) may either result in cell death or initiate carcinogenic mutations. Although shorter wavelengths are more energetic and hence more damaging, they do not penetrate as deeply. In mature skin, ultraviolet B (UVB) (290 to 320 nm) does not penetrate into the dermis, but ultraviolet A (UVA) (320 to 400 nm) does, and visible wavelengths (400 to 800 nm) reach even deeper levels.[95] Hence, in considering effects of light on the skin, one must consider not only the cumulative energy of the light absorbed but also the depth of penetration. Cutaneous defenses against ultraviolet light injury include:

1. Mechanisms that absorb or reflect light (e.g., stratum corneum, melanin)
2. Enzymatic (e.g., superoxide dismutase, catalase, glutathione peroxidase) and nonenzymatic (e.g., ascorbate, beta-carotene) systems that absorb single oxy-

gen or interrupt free radical cascades initiated by superoxide and hydroxyl radicals

3. Mechanisms to repair cellular and DNA damage

In mature skin, the stratum corneum is the first line of defense, filtering out approximately 80% of incident UVB light.[95] Therefore the much thinner stratum corneum of the premature infant is one factor that must result in increased vulnerability to UV injury. In addition, rules about depth of penetration of different wavelengths based on study of mature skin may not hold for premature skin. Melanocytes are present in basal epidermis by the end of the first trimester, and melanin granules are synthesized and begin to be transferred to keratinocytes by midgestation.[2] However, inherent skin color is lighter in neonates, and melanin granule formation is not fully mature, even at term.[96] Moreover, the ability of melanocytes in preterm infants' skin to increase melanin synthesis in response to UV stress has not been examined. Although maturation of other antioxidant defenses in the epidermis has not been studied either, these antioxidant systems are immature in the lungs of preterm infants.[97] Hence, the same may also be true for skin. Taken together, it is apparent that the premature infant is particularly vulnerable to UV injury.

UVB is filtered out by window glass, but UVA is not. Therefore the preterm infant in the nursery may be exposed to solar UVA, as well as longer wavelengths from artificial light sources. UVA is implicated in certain phototoxic and photoallergic responses.[98] Although its role in carcinogenesis is still controversial, a role in the causation of melanoma has not been excluded.[99,100] It should be assumed that the cutaneous barrier to UV is immature in the preterm infant, hence they should be physically shielded from exposure to sunlight from exterior windows and other sources of ultraviolet light.

Portions of the visible light spectrum (420 to 500 nm) induce isomerization of bilirubin to compounds that can be excreted without hepatic conjugation. Hence, phototherapy with a variety of light sources is standard therapy for neonatal unconjugated hyperbilirubinemia. Because the commonly used fluorescent daylight bulbs emit UVA, interposition of a Plexiglas shield is essential to avoid burns in preterm infants.[101] No deleterious long-term effects of visible light phototherapy on skin are documented.[102,103] However, as more extremely premature infants are exposed to these modalities, the possibility that they may be unusually vulnerable should be considered. For example, severe phototoxicity occurred in a preterm infant following use of intravenous fluorescein and prolonged dye retention as a result of renal immaturity.[104] Moreover, even internal organs are potentially affected by phototherapy because light may penetrate more deeply through the skin of the preterm infant. For example, phototherapy increases symptomatic PDA in preterm infants.[105] Because merely shielding the chest wall overlying the heart can mitigate this complication, a direct photo effect on ductal tissue is likely.[105,106] Limitation on the intensity of ambient nursery lighting is recommended, largely out of concern for a contribution to the retinopathy of prematurity.[107,108] It would also seem prudent to consider the potential deleterious cutaneous and transcutaneous effects of nursery lighting on the vulnerable premature infant.

Cutaneous Contribution to Immaturity of Thermal Homeostasis

Body heat may escape through a number of mechanisms, as listed in the following:

1. Evaporative heat loss
2. Conduction, that is, direct gain or loss of heat to objects in direct contact with the infant's body
3. Convection, that is, loss of body heat to the atmosphere, a function both of ambient air temperature and airflow (increased heat transfer with increased flow)
4. Radiation (i.e., infrared energy exchanged between objects not in contact that absorb and remit radiant energy)[71]

Maintenance of a thermally neutral environment, minimizing unwanted heat loss or heat gain, is a major challenge to those who take care of premature infants. Skin participates in thermal homeostasis through several mechanisms. Evaporation of water from the skin's surface results in caloric loss (~580 cal/ml). Water loss occurs both through passage of water across the stratum corneum as a function of barrier competency (see the previous discussion) and from secreted water delivered to the skin surface by ducts (eccrine sweating) in response to neural and other stimuli.[109] Caloric losses caused by an immature skin barrier are a major contributor to the preterm infant's heat loss, particularly in the first week of life.[110] Conversely, because eccrine function is immature, the premature infant is unable to compensate for heat stress by sweating.[111] Even in term infants, sweating is not functionally mature, because the term infant's set point is higher than in mature individuals. Sweating in preterm infants matures rapidly following birth; however, the efficiency remains poor, with fewer body sites sweating in response to thermal stimuli and maintenance of a high set point.[111] Vasomotor control of cutaneous blood flow is a third component of the skin's contribution to thermal homeostasis. Both vasoconstriction or vasodilation in response to thermal stimuli are attenuated in preterm infants' skin, although these responses appear to mature within 2 to 3 weeks.[112] Finally, the subcutaneous adipose reservoir is deficient in preterm infants, reducing both their insulation against heat loss and their energy reserves for thermal conversion.

Neurocutaneous Development in the Premature Infant

Responsiveness to touch is present at a very early age; that is, by the end of the first trimester the fetus withdraws in response to skin stroking.[113] In the preterm infant, neurocutaneous responses may be immature and "globalized." Thus, in the unstable premature infant, handling is minimized to avoid adverse effects of skin stimulation, such as changes in heart rate, hypoxia, and apneic episodes.[114,115] However, older and more stable preterm infants may benefit from skin contact.[116] Originally, skin-to-skin contact was explored as a mechanism to facilitate maternal bonding with the term infant.[117] A modification of this principle, designated "kangaroo mother care," has been advocated for preterm infants in developing countries as a safe and effective mode of care for stable premature infants.[118,119] Kangaroo mother care is based on the marsupial model of transition to independent life, in which the infant is continually housed against the mothers skin and permitted *ad libitum* breast feeding. In economies that cannot provide routine nursery equipment such as incubators, adoption of kangaroo mother care can reduce both morbidity and mortality from inadequate thermal protection and infections associated with overcrowding in nurseries and formula feedings.[118] Briefer periods of maternal skin-to-skin contact during neonatal nursery residence have also been advocated in the care of the preterm infant in developed economies as a means to enhance maternal confidence and to humanize the nursery experience.[117-121] When infants are carefully selected to avoid inclusion of unstable ones, the practice does not appear to be deleterious to the babies and may be beneficial (e.g., reduce periods of purposeless activity). Long-term benefits to mother and child of skin-to-skin contact are difficult to distinguish from the benefits of more conventional maternal-infant contact but may include prolonged maternal lactation and less infant crying.[118] Although it may seem intuitively obvious that both parents and infants would benefit psychologically from the humanizing effects of skin-to-skin contact, the neurocutaneous pathways that are likely to underlie these responses are only beginning to be delineated in mature skin.[122] It will be important as this work proceeds, to examine the maturation of these pathways in the preterm infant, to better understand the capacity of the maturing infant to respond to these external stimuli and

to develop systems of care that are both rational and "humanistic."

SKIN DISEASES IN THE PREMATURE INFANT

Barrier Function of Abnormal Skin

The consequences of barrier immaturity of premature infants may be compounded if the infant also has a primary skin disorder. Infants with severe genetic skin disorders are often born prematurely.[123] Skin diseases that result in *hyperkeratosis* (scaling) or a thickened stratum corneum, such as the ichthyoses, are commonly associated with impaired barrier function[123,124]; that is, a thick stratum corneum is not necessarily a competent one. These infants are at risk for hypernatremia as a result of increased evaporative loss of free water from the skin surface.[125,126] Similarly, infants with widespread blistering diseases, whether resulting from underlying infection, as in staphylococcal scalded skin syndrome, or from one of the genetic mechanobullous diseases, e.g., epidermolysis bullosa, have increased fluid requirements as a result of loss of barrier integrity. Skin disease also increases the risk of systemic absorption of topical medication, both because of a further compromise in barrier competence and because of increased exposure to topical medications. Instances of this include prolonged use of topical steroids to dermatitic skin, resulting in adrenal suppression and other signs of hypercorticism,[127,128] and use of salicylate-containing ointments to remove excessive scale, resulting in salicylism.[129]

Scars of Prematurity

A number of nursery procedures may lead to scars; the number of scars nursery graduates bear is correlated with their degree of prematurity and duration of intensive care.[130] Although most of these scars are not of great concern, more severe scarring sequelae can occur, particularly those resulting from wounds from chest tubes, skin strippings from adhesive tapes, and extravasated intravenous fluids. In addition, very immature infants (<29 weeks) may develop atrophic scars (i.e., anetoderma[131]) most likely a result of injury from monitors and adhesives.

Hemangiomas

Hemangiomas of the involuting type are more common in preterm infants, and the frequency is related to the degree of prematurity.[132] Moreover, multiple small hemangiomas are more common among premature infants. The basis for this increased prevalence is not understood.

SUMMARY

Because skin reliably performs its life-enabling functions throughout life, it and its diseases have often been trivialized. Only in rare instances of skin failure, such as in extensive burns, drug-induced toxic epidermal necrolysis, or the severe autoimmune pemphigus vulgaris, is the importance of the skin barrier readily apparent. Yet, neonatologists have long been cognizant of the importance of fluid balance and thermal homeostasis to the care of the premature infant. Now, through advances in the care of fragile premature infants, and particularly through the advent of surfactant replacement therapy, neonates of ever-greater prematurity survive, relentlessly pushing backward the age of viability. In this context, the consequences of skin barrier immaturity emerge as a critical frontier in their management. Barrier failure contributes to the morbidity and mortality of the preterm neonate through fluid and electrolyte instability and the effects of fluid imbalance on blood volume and blood pressure, as well as an increased susceptibility to transcutaneous infections and toxicity from transcutaneous absorption of xenobiotics. As a result of the interlocking interdependence of organ systems, all of which are immature, the magnitude of the skin's contribution to neonatal morbidity cannot be presently estimated. Further study is needed to determine if direct measurement of skin losses would result in more precise, prospective fluid management and improved nursery outcomes. Insights from studies of barrier ontogenesis in experimental animals also suggest promising areas for clinical evaluation. For example, do antenatal or postnatal glucocorticoids alter barrier maturation? Can other hormones or nuclear receptor agonists be used to accelerate skin maturation, antenatally and/or postnatally?

If larger studies currently in progress confirm the observation that emollient therapy reduces rates of systemic infection, this will rapidly become standard practice in nurseries caring for premature infants. Yet, it will be important to remain vigilant to unexpected, adverse effects of emollient therapy. Are these nonphysiologic lipids absorbed systemically, and if so, what is their fate? If available, would a mixture of physiologic lipids be more efficacious and/or safer? Likewise, phototherapy for hyperbilirubinemia has been employed for years as an effective and safe treatment for hyperbilirubinemia. Phototherapy for hyperbilirubinemia is a nearly universal experience for premature infants because of their lower threshold for kernicterus and their immature hepatic function. It will be important to reconsider the issue of long-term safety in the cohort of very low birth weight survivors, who have an extremely thin stratum corneum at birth and may be particularly vulnerable to light injury.

At present it is only possible to outline broad principles for the care of the premature infants' skin.[30,41] Most of these are self-evident, such as the need to avoid exposure to topical agents of potential systemic toxicity, or for gentle handling to prevent abrogation of the skin's integrity. But the optimal application of these principles in practice is often less evident. For example, all ingredients in topical medicaments, emollients, or cleansers need to be identified and their potential for toxicity considered, yet this information may not be easily obtainable.[31] Moreover, preferred products, such as an aqueous solution of chlorhexidine for skin antisepsis, may not be commercially available.[31] In most instances skin care practices have not been systematically studied to determine optimal regimens. Just as the term infant's skin is more resilient and protective than the skin of a premature infant of 30 weeks' gestation, procedures that may not be hazardous to an infant of this gestational age may be toxic to the extremely immature "micropreemie." Therefore, in designing future studies, it will be important to consider the differences in skin function in babies of varying gestational and postnatal ages. Greater awareness of skin functions and their physiologic bases, as well as the infant's position on the maturational timetable of these functions, will be needed for the development of rational regimens of skin care in the future.

ACKNOWLEDGMENTS

The author is indebted to Dr. Khanh-Van T. Le for assistance with the literature review; to Dr. Peter M. Elias for critical review of the manuscript; and to Ms. Celia Hamilton for assistance with preparation of the manuscript.

REFERENCES

1. Elias PM, Menon GK. Structural and lipid biochemical correlates of the epidermal permeability barrier. Adv Lipid Res 1991;21:1-26.
2. Holbrook KA. Structural and biochemical organogenesis of skin and cutaneous appendages in the fetus and newborn. In Polin RA, Fox WW, eds. Fetal and neonatal physiology. 2nd edition. vol I. Phildelphia: WB Saunders, 1998: p 729.
3. Evans NJ, Rutter N. Development of the epidermis in the newborn. Biol Neonate 1986;49:74-80.
4. Ballard JL, Khoury JC, Wedig K, et al. New Ballard score, expanded to include extremely premature infants. J Pediatr 1991;119:417-423.
5. Hammarlund K, Sedin G. TEWL in newborn infants. III. Relation to gestational age. Acta Pediatr Scand 1979;68:795-801.

6. Harpin VA, Rutter N. Barrier properties of the newborn infant's skin. J Pediatr 1983;102:419-425.

7. Cartlidge PHT, Rutter N. Skin barrier function. In Polin RA, Fox WW. Fetal and neonatal physiology. 2nd edition. vol I. Phildelphia: WB Saunders, 1998: p 771.

8. Nachman RL, Esterly NB. Increased skin permeability in preterm infants. J Pediatr 1971;79:628-632.

9. Okah FA, Wickett RR, Pickens WL, et al. Surface electrical capacitance as a noninvasive bedside measure of epidermal barrier maturation in the newborn infant. Pediatrics 1995; 96 (4 Pt 1):688-692.

10. Muramatsu K, Hirose S, Yukitake K, et al. Relationship between maturation of the skin and electrical skin resistance. Ped Res 1987;21:21-24.

11. Emery MM, Hebert AA, Aguirre V-C, et al. The relationship between skin maturation and electrical skin impedance. J Dermatol Sci 1991;2:336-340.

12. Aszterbaum M, Feingold KR, Menon GK, et al. Ontogeny of the epidermal barrier to water loss in the rat: Correlation of function with stratum corneum structure and lipid content. Pediatr Res 1992;31:308-317.

13. Williams ML, Hanley K, Elias PM, et al. Ontogenesis of the epidermal permeability barrier. J Invest Dermatol (Symposium Proceedings) 1998;3:75-79.

14. Kalia YN, Nonato LB, Lund CH, et al. Development of skin barrier function in premature infants. J Invest Dermatol 1998;111:320-326.

15. Ågren J, Sjörs G, Sedin G. Transepidermal water loss in infants born at 24 and 25 weeks of gestation. Acta Paediatr 1998;87:1185-1190.

16. Hanley K, Jiang Y, Elias PM, et al. Acceleration of barrier ontogenesis in vitro through air exposure. Pediatr Res 1997; 41:293-299.

17. Williams ML, Feingold KR. Barrier function of neonatal skin (letter). J Pediatr 1998;133:467-468.

18. Hammarlund K, Sedin G. Transepidermal water loss in newborn infants. IV. Small for gestational age infants. Acta Paediatr Scand 1980;69:377-383.

19. NIH Consensus Conference. Effect of corticosteroids for fetal maturation on perinatal outcome. JAMA 1995;273:413-418.

19a. Omar SA, DeCristofaro JD, Agarwal BI, LaGamma EF. Effects of prenatal steroids on water and sodium homeostasis in extremely low birth weight neonates. Pediatrics 1999; 104:482.

20. Oh W. Fluid and electrolyte management. In Fanaroff AA, Martin RJ, eds. Neonatal-perinatal medicine: Diseases of the fetus and infant. 6th edition. vol I. St Louis: Mosby, 1997: p 622.

21. Perlstein PH. Physical environment. In Fanaroff AA, Martin RJ, eds. Neonatal-Perinatal Medicine: Diseases of the fetus and infant. 6th edition. vol I. St Louis: Mosby, 1997: p 481.

22. Fanaroff AA, Rand MB, Wald M, et al. Insensible water loss in low birth weight infants. Pediatrics 1972;50:236-245.

23. Wu PYK, Hodgman JE. Insensible water loss in preterm infants: Changes with postnatal development and non-ionizing radiant energy. Pediatrics 1974;54:704-712.

24. Harpin VA, Rutter N. Humidification of incubators. Arch Dis Child 1985;60:219-224.

25. Bell EF. Infant incubators and radiant warmers. Early Hum Dev 1983;8:351-375.

26. Williams PR, Oh W. Effects of radiant warmer on insensible water loss in newborn infants. Am J Dis Child 1974; 128:511-514.

27. Bell EF, Neidich GA, Cashore WJ, et al. Combined effect of radiant warmer and phototherapy on insensible water loss in low-birth-weight infants. J Pediatr 1979;94:810-813.

28. Kjartansson S, Arsan S, Hammarlund K, et al. Water loss from the skin of term and preterm infants nursed under a radiant heater. Ped Res 1995;37:233-238.

29. Marks KH, Friedman Z, Maisels MJ. A simple device for reducing insensible water loss in low-birth-weight infants. Pediatrics 1977;60:223-226.

30. Baumgart S. Reduction of oxygen consumption, insensible water loss, and radiant heat demand with use of a plastic blanket for low-birth-weight infants under radiant warmers. Pediatrics 1984;74:1022-1028.

31. Siegfried EC. Neonatal skin and care. Dermatol Clin 1998; 16:437-446.

32. Oh W, Karecki H. Phototherapy and insensible water loss in the newborn infant. Amer J Dis Child 1972;124:230-232.

33. Wu PYK, Hodgman JE. Insensible water loss in preterm infants: Changes with postnatal development and non-ionizing radiant energy. Pediatrics 1974;54:704-712.

34. Kjartansson S, Hammarlund K, Sedin G. Insensible water loss from the skin during phototherapy in term and preterm infants. Acta Paediatr 1992;81:764-768.

35. Hammarlund K, Nilsson GE, Oberg PA, et al. TEWL in newborn infants. I. Relation to ambient humidity and site of measurement and estimation of total transepidermal water loss. Acta Pediatr Scand 1977;66:553-562.

36. Knauth A, Gordin M, McNelis W, et al. Semipermeable polyurethane membrane as an artficial skin for the premature neonate. Pediatrics 1989;83:945-950.

37. Barak M, Hershkowitz S, Rod R, et al. The use of a synthetic skin covering as a protective layer in the daily care of low birth weight infants. Eur J Pediatr 1989;148:665-666.

38. Vernon HJ, Lane AT, Wischerath LJ, et al. Semipermeable dressing and transepidermal water loss in premature infants. Pediatrics 1990;86:357-362.

39. Donahue ML, Phelps DL, Richter SE, et al. A semipermeable skin dressing for extremely low birth weight infants. J Perinatol 1996;16:20-26.

40. Mancini AJ, Sookdeo-Drost S, Madison KC, et al. Semipermeable dressings improve epidermal barrier function in premature infants. Pediatr Res 1994;36:306-314.

41. Katz S, McGinley K, Leyden JJ. Semipermeable occlusive dressings: Effects on growth of pathogenic bacteria and re-epithelialization of superficial wounds. Arch Dermatol 1986;122:58-62.

42. Lane AT. Development and care of the premature infant's skin. Ped Dermatol 1987;4:1-5.

43. Rutter N, Hull D. Reduction of skin water loss in the newborn. I. Effect of applying topical agents. Arch Dis Child 1981;56:669-672.

44. Nopper AJ, Horii KA, Sookdeo-Drost S, et al. Topical ointment therapy benefits premature infants. J Pediatr 1996; 128:660-669.

45. Ghadially R, Halkier-Sorenson L, Elias P. Effects of petrolatum on stratum corneum structure and function. J Am Acad Dermatol 1992;26:387-396.

46. Mao-Qiang M, Brown BE, Wu-Pong S, et al. Exogenous non-physiologic vs. physiologic lipids: Divergent mechanisms for correction of permeability barrier dysfunction. Arch Dermatol 1995;131:809-816.

47. Brown BE, Diembeck W, Hoppe U, et al. Fate of topical hydrocarbons in the skin. J Soc Cosm Chem 1995;46:1.

48. Lester DE. Normal paraffins in living matter: Occurrence, metabolism, and pathology. Progr Food Nutri Sci 1979;3:1.

49. Mao-Qiang M, Feingold KR, Elias PM. Exogenous lipids influence permeability barrier recovery in acetone treated murine skin. Arch Dermatol 1993;129:728-738.

49a. Cockayne SE, Lee JA, Herrington CI. Oleogranulomatous response in lymph nodes associated with emollient use in Netherton's syndrome. Br J Dermatol 1999;141:562.

50. Yang L, Mao-Qiang M, Taljebini M. Topical stratum corneum lipids accelerate barrier repair after tape stripping, solvent treatment and some but not all types of detergent treatment. Br J Dermatol 1995;133:679-685.

51. Mao-Qiang M, Feingold KR, Thornfelt CR, et al. Optimization of physiological lipid mixtures for barrier repair. J Invest Dermatol 1996;106:1096-1101.

52. Zetterston EM, Ghadially G, Feingold KR, et al. Optimal ratios of topical stratum corneum lipids improve barrier recovery in chronologically aged skin. J Am Acad Dermatol 1997;37:403-408.

53. West DP, Worobec S, Soloman LM. Pharmacology and toxicology of infant skin. J Invest Dermatol 1981;76:147-150.

54. West DP, Halket JM, Harvey DR, et al. Percutaneous absorption in preterm infants. Pediatr Dermatol 1987; 4:234-237.

55. Rutter N. Percutaneous drug absorption in the newborn: Hazards and uses. Clinics Perinatal 1987;14:911-930.

56. Scheuplein RJ, Blank LH. Permeability of skin. Physiol Rev 1971;51:702-747.

57. Potts RO;Franceur ML. The influence of stratum corneum morphology on water permeability. J Invest Dermatol 1991; 96:495-499.

58. Menon GK, Elias PM. Morphologic basis for a pore-pathway in mammalian stratum corneum. Skin Pharmacol 1997;10:235-246.

59. Barrett DA, Rutter N. Transdermal delivery and the premature newborn. Crit Rev Ther Drug Carrier Syst 1994;11: 1-30.

60. Froman RD, Owen SV, Murphy C. Isopropyl pad use in neonatal intensive care units. J Perinatol 1998;18:216-220.

61. Bell EF, Warburton D, Stonestreet BS, et al. Effect of fluid administration on the development of symptomatic patent ductus arteriosus and congestive heart failure in premature infants. N Eng J Med 1980;302:598-604.

62. Papile L. Intracranial hemorrhage. In Fanaroff AA, Martin, RJ. Neonatal-perinatal medicine: Diseases of the fetus and infant. 6th edition. vol I. St Louis: Mosby, 1997: p 891.

63. Bauer K, Versmold H. Postnatal weight loss in preterm neonates <1500 g is due to isotonic dehydration of the extracellular volume. Acta Paediatr Scand Suppl 1989;360:37-42.

64. Musemeche CA, Kosloske AM, Bartow SA, et al. Comparative effects of ischemia, bacteria, and substrate on the pathogenesis of intestinal necrosis. J Pediatr Surg 1986;21:536-538.

65. Willoughby RE, Pickering LK. Necrotizing enterocolitis and infection. Clin Perinatal 1994;21:307-315.

66. Bell EF, Warburton D, Stonestreet BS, et al. High volume fluid intake predisposes premature infants to necrotizing enterocolitis. (Letter) Lancet 1979;2:90.

67. Nowicki PT, Nankervis CA. The role of the circulation in the pathogenesis of necrotizing enterocolitis. Clin Perinatal 1994;21:219-234.

68. Crissinger KD, Granger DN. Mucosal injury induced by ischemia and reperfusion in the piglet intestine: Influences of age and feeding. Gastroenterol 1989;97:920-926.

69. Gruskay JA, Abbasi S, Anday E, et al. Staphylococcus epidermidis-associated enterocololitis. J Pediatr 1986;109: 520-524.

70. Scheifele DW, Bjornson GL, Dyer RA, et al. Delta-like toxin produced by coagulase-negative staphylococci is associated with neonatal necrotizing enterocolitis. Infect Immun 1987; 55:2268-2273.

71. Mollit DL, Tepas JJ, Talbert JL. The role of coagulase-negative stahylococcus in neonatal necrotizing enterocolitis. J Pediatr Surg 1988;23:60-63.

72. Eastick K, Leeming JP, Bennett D, et al. Reservoirs of coagulase negative staphylococci in preterm infants. Arch Dis Child 1996;74:F99-104.

73. Williams ML, Le KVT. The permeability barrier in the preterm infant: Review of the clinical consequences of barrier immaturity and of insights derived from an animal model of barrier ontogenesis, with a call for further studies. Eur J Ped Dermatol 1998;8:101.

74. Watkins AMC, Keogh EJ. Alcohol burns in the neonate. J Pediatr 1992;28:306-308.

75. Lund CH, Nonato LB, Kuller JM, et al. Disruption of barrier function in neonatal skin associated with adhesive removal. J Pediatr 1997;131:367-372.

76. Dollison EJ, Beckstrand J, Adhesive tape vs. pectin-based barrier use in preterm infants. Neonatal Network 1995; 14:35-39.

77. Miller SJ, Aly R, Shinefeld HR, et al. In vitro and in vivo antistaphylococcal activity of human stratum corneum lipids. Arch Dermatol 1988;124:209-215.

78. Bibel DJ, Aly R, Shinefeld HR, Topical sphingolipids in antisepsis and antifungal therapy. Clin Exper Dermatol 1995; 20:395-400.

79. Gallo RL, Huttner KM, Antimicrobial peptides: an emerging concept in cutaneous biology. J Invest Dermatol 1998; 111:739-743.

80. Patrick CC, Kaplan SL, Baker CJ, et al. Persistent bacteremia due to coagulase-negative staphylococci in low birth weight neonates. Pediatrics 1989;84:977-985.

81. Freeman J, Goldman DA, Smith NE, et al. Association of intravenous lipid emulsion and coagulase-negative staphylococcal bacteremia in neonatal intensive care units. N Engl J Med 1990;323:301-308.

82. Klein JO, From harmless commensal to invasive pathogen.(Editorial) N Engl J Med 1990;323:339-340.

83. Freeman J, Epstein MF, Smith NE, et al. Extra hospital stay and antibiotic usage with nosocomial coagulase-negative staphylococcal bacteremia in two neonatal intensive care populations. Am J Dis Child 1990;144:324-329.

84. St Geme JW, Bell LM, Baumgart S, et al. Distinguishing sepsis from blood culture contamination in young infants with blood cultures growing coagualase-negative staphylococci. Pediatrics 1990;86:157-162.

85. Nataro JP, Corcoran L, Zirin S, et al. Prospective analysis of coagulase-negative staphylococcal infection in hospitalized infants. J Pediatr 1994;125:798-804.
86. Aschner JL, Punsalang A, Maniscalco WM, et al. Percutaneous central venous catheter colonization with Malassezia furfur: Incidence and clinical significance. Pediatrics 1987; 80:535-539.
87. Stuart SM, Lane AT, Candida and malassezia as nursery pathogens. Semin Dermatol 1992;11:19-23.
88. Chang HJ, Miller HL, Watkins N, et al: An epidemic of *Malassezia pachydermatis* in an intensive care nursery associated with colonization of health care worker's pet dogs. N Eng J Med 1998;338:706-711.
89. Rowen JL, Correa AG, Sokol DM, et al. Invasive aspergillosis in neonates: Report of five cases and literature review. Pediatr Infect Dis J 1992;11:576-582.
90. Linder N, Keller N, Huri C, et al. Primary cutaneous mucormycosis in a premature infant: Case report and review of the literature. Am J Perinatol 1998;15:35-38.
91. Rowen JL, Atkins JT, Levy ML, et al. Invasive fungal dermatitis in the <1000-gram neonate. Pediatr 1995;95:682-687.
92. Yoder MC, Polin RA. Developmental immunology. In Fanaroff AA, Martin RJ: Neonatal-perinatal medicine: Diseases of the fetus and Infant. 6th edition. vol II. St Louis: Mosby, 1997: p 685.
93. Granstein RD, Photoimmunology. In Fitzpatrick TB, Eisen AZ, Wolff K, et al, eds. Dermatology in general medicine. 4th edition. vol I. New York: McGraw Hill, 1993: p 1638.
94. Norris G, Gange RW, Hawk JLM. Acute effects of ultraviolet radiation on the skin. In Fitzpatrick TB, Eisen AZ, Wolff K, et al, eds. Dermatology in general medicine. 4th edition. vol I. New York: McGraw Hill, 1993: pp 1651.
95. Kohevar IE, Pathak MA, Parrish JA. Photophysics, photochemistry, and photobiology. In Fitzpatrick TB, Eisen AZ, Wolff K, et al, eds. Dermatology in general medicine. 4th edition. vol I. New York: McGraw Hill, 1993: p 1627.
96. Holbrook KA, Sybert V. Basic Science, embryogenesis of the skin. In Schachner LA, Hanson RC, eds. Pediatric dermatology, vol I. New York: Churchill Livingstone, 1988: p.3.
97. Frank L, Sosenko IRS. Development of the lung antioxidant system in late gestation: Possible implications for the prematurely born infant. J Pediatr 1987;110:9-14.
98. Hawk JLM, Norris PG. Abnormal responses to ultraviolet radiation: Idiopathic. In Fitzpatrick TB, Eisen AZ, Wolff K, et al, eds. Dermatology in general medicine. 4th edition. vol I. New York: McGraw Hill, 1993: p 1661.
99. Koh HK, Kligler BE, Lew RA. Sunlight and cutaneous malignant melanoma: Evidence for and against causation. Photchem Photobiol 1990;51:765-779.
100. Setlow RB, Woodhead AD. Temporal changes in the incidence of malignant melanoma: Explanation from action spectra. Mutat Res 1994;307:365-374.
101. Siegfried EC, Stone MS, Madison KC. Ultraviolet light burn: a cutaneous complication of visible light phototherapy of neonatal jaundice. Pediatr Dermatol 1992;9:278-282.
102. Halmek LP, Stevenson DK. Neonatal jaundice and liver disease. In Fanaroff AA, Martin RJ, eds. Neonatal-perinatal medicine: Diseases of the fetus and infant. 6th edition. vol II. St Louis: Mosby. 1997: p 1345.
103. Berg P, Lindelof B. Is phototherapy in neonates a risk factor for malignant melanoma development? Arch Pediatr Adolesc Med 1997;151:1185-1187.
104. Kearns GL, Williams BJ, Timmons OD. Fluorescein phototoxicity in a premature infant. J Pediatr 1985;107:796-798.
105. Rosenfeld W, Sadhev S, Brunot V, et al. Phototherapy effect on the incidence of patent ductus arterious in premature infants: prevention with chest shielding. Pediatrics 1986; 78:10-14.
106. Clyman RI, Rudolph AM. Patent ductus arteriosus: a new light on an old problem. Pediatr Res 1978;12:92-94.
107. Ancott SW, Walsh-Sukys MC. Reccomendations for newborn care. In Fanaroff AA, Darby RJ, eds. Neonatal-perinatal medicine. 6th edition. vol 1. St Louis: Mosby, 1997: p 408.
108. Glass P, Avery GB, Subramanian KN, et al. Effect of bright light in the hospital nursery on the incidence of retinopathy of prematurity. N Eng J Med 1985;313:401-404.
109. Mancini AJ, Lane AT. Sweating in the neonate. In Polin RA, Fox WW, eds. Fetal and neonatal Physiology. 2nd edition. vol. I. Phildelphia: WB Saunders, 1998: p 767.
110. Hammarlund K, Stromberg B, Sedin G. Heat loss from the skin of preterm and fullterm newborn infants during the first weeks after birth. Biol Neonate 1986;50:1-10.
111. Harpin VA, Rutter N. Sweating in preterm infants. J Pediatr 1982;100:614-619.
112. Jahnukainen T, van Ravenswaaij-Arts, Jalonen J, et al. Dynamics of vasomotor thermoregulation of the skin in term and preterm neonates. Early Hum Dev 1993;33:133-143.
113. Hogg ID. Sensory nerves and associated structures in the skin of human fetuses of 8 to 14 weeks of menstrual age correlate with functional capability. J Comp Neurol 1941: 75:371.
114. Long JG, Philip AG, Lucey JF. Excessive handling as a cause of hypoxemia. Pediatr 1980;65:203-207.
115. Lynch ME. Iatrogenic hazards, adverse occurences, and complications involving NICU nursing practice. J Perinatal Neonatal Nurs 1991;5:78-86.
116. Field TM, Schanberg SM, Scafidi F, et al. Tactile/Kinesthetic stimulation effects on preterm neonates. Pediatrics 1986; 77:654-658.
117. Klaus MH, Kennell JH. Care of the mother, father and infant. In Fanaroff AA, Martin RJ, eds. Neonatal-perinatal medicine: Diseases of the Fetus and Infant. 6th edition. vol I. St Louis: Mosby, 1997: p 548.
118. Cattaneo A, Davanzo R, Uxa F, et al. Recommendations for the implementation of kangaroo mother care for low birthweight infants. Acta Paediatr 1998;87:440-445.
119. Tessier R, Cristo M, Velez S, et al. Kangaroo mother care and the bonding hypothesis. Pediatrics 1998;102:e17.
120. Whitelaw A, Heisterkamp G, Sleath K, et al. Skin to skin contact for very low birthweight infants and their mothers. Arch Dis Child 1988;63:1377-1381.
121. Ludington-Hoe SM, Thompson C, Swinth J, et al. Kangaroo care: Research results and practice implications and guidelines. Neonatal Network 1994;13:19-27.
122. O'Sullivan RL, Lipper G, Lerner EA. The neuro-immuno-cutaneous-endocrine network: Relationship of mind and skin. Arch Dermatol 1998;134:1431-1435.

123. Williams ML, LeBoit PE. The ichthyoses: disorders of corni-fication. In Arndt KA, Leboit PE, Robinson JK, Wintroub BU, eds. Cutaneous medicine and surgery: An integrated program in dermatology. vol II. Philadelphia: WB Saunders, 1996: p 1681.

124. Buyse L, Graves C, Marks R, et al. Collodion baby dehydra-tion: the danger of high transepidermal water loss. Br J Der-matol 1993;129:86-88.

125. Garty BB, Metzker A, Nitzan M. Hypernatremia in congeni-tal lamellar ichthyosis. J Pediatr 1979;95:814.

126. Jones SK, Thomason LM, Surbrugg SK, et al. Neonatal hy-pernatraemia in two siblings with Netherton's syndrome. Br J Dermatol 1986;114:741-743.

127. Turpeinen M. Influence of age and severity of dermatitis on the percutaneous absorption of hydrocortisone in children. Br J Dermatol 1988;118:517-522.

128. Feinblatt BI, Aceto T, Beckhorn G, et al. Percutaneous ab-sorption of hydrocortisone in children. Amer J Dis Child 1966;112:218-224.

129. Chiaretti A, Schembri Wismayer D, Tortorolo L, et al. Sali-cylate intoxication using a skin ointment. Acta Pediatr 1997; 86:330-331.

130. Cartlidge PH, Fox PE, Rutter N. The scars of newborn in-tensive care. Early Hum Dev 1990;21:1-10.

131. Prizant TL, Lucky AW, Frieden IJ, et al. Spontaneous at-rophic patches in extremely premature infants. Arch Der-matol 1996;132:671-674.

132. Amir J, Metzker A, Krikler R, et al. Strawberry hemangioma in preterm infants. Pediatr Dermatol 1986;3:331-332.

133. Rogers SCF, Burrows D, Neill D. Percutaneous absorption of phenol and methyl alcohol in Magenta Paint B.P.C. Br J Dermatol 1978;98:559-560.

134. Segal S, Cohen SN, Freeman J, et al. Camphor: Who needs it? Pediatrics 1978;62:404-406.

135. Benda GI, Hiller JL, Reynolds JW. Benzyl alcohol toxicity: Impact on neurologic handicaps among surviving very low birth weight infants. Pediatrics 1986;77:507-512.

136. Bamford MFM, Jones LF. Deafness and biochemical imbal-ance after burns treatment with topical antibiotics in young children. Arch Dis Child 1978;53:326-329.

137. Stohs SJ, Ezzedeen FW, Anderson AK, et al. Pecutaneous ab-sorption of iodochlorhydroxyquin in humans. J Invest Der-matol 1984;82:195-198.

138. McDonald MG, Getson PR, Glasgow AM, et al. Propylene glycol: Increased incidence of seizures in low birth weight infants. Pediatrics 1987;79:622-625.

139. Bishop NJ, Morley R, Day JP, et al. Aluminum neurotoxicity in preterm infants receiving intravenous-feeding solutions. N Eng J Med 1997;336:1557-1561.

140. Barker, N, Hadgraft J, Rutter N: Skin permeability in the newborn. J Invest Dermatol 1987;88:409-411.

141. Armstrong RW, Eichener ER, Klein DE, et al: Pentacho-lophenol poisoning in a nursery for newborn infants. II. Epi-demiologic and toxicologic studies. J Pediatr 1969; 75:317-325.

142. Pramanik AK, Hansen RC: Transcutaneous gamma benzene hexachloride absorption and toxicity in infants and chil-dren. Arch Dermatol 1979;115:1224-1225.

143. L'Allemand D, Gruters A, Beyer P, et al. Iodine in contrast agents and skin disinfectants in the major cause for hy-pothyroidism in premature infants during intensive care. Hormone Res 1987;28:42-49.

144. Parravicini E, Fontana C, Paterlini GL, et al. Iodine, thyroid funtion, and very low birth weight infants. Pediatrics 1996; 98:730-734.

5

Neonatal Skin Care and Toxicology

ELAINE C. SIEGFRIED

The skin of a newborn infant differs from adult skin in several ways. A better understanding of the principles of infant skin care and a more uniform approach to skin care in the neonatal nursery can minimize risks and costs to this special population of patients.

BACKGROUND

Neonatal skin is 40% to 60% thinner than adult skin. Attenuated rete ridges formed from comparatively fewer stem cells at the basal layer provide a relatively limited area of surface attachment to an immature dermis. An infant's body surface area/weight ratio is up to five times that of an adult.[1,2] These important differences place infants at increased risk for skin damage, percutaneous infection, and percutaneous toxicity from topically applied agents. The most clinically significant difference between the skin of premature and term infants is in the structure of the stratum corneum. Infants born before 32 weeks' gestation have a very thin stratum corneum.[1,3] During the first 2 weeks of life, these infants suffer from significant insensible transepidermal water loss (TEWL) with associated thermal instability and fluid and electrolyte disturbances.[1,4] A variety of seemingly benign clinical interventions can dramatically increase these losses. Desiccated skin is even more easily injured, providing a portal of entry for invading microbes and increasing the risk of disseminated infection.[3-7] A premature infant's diminished metabolic capacity and decreased immune responses compound these problems. Optimized skin care can minimize them.[8] Pioneering work has been done in the field of skin development, but a standard for optimized care for neonatal skin has yet to be defined.

SKIN INJURY

Clinically occult skin injury accompanies routine care. Skin stripping by removal of adhesive-backed products causes acute injury and creates the potential for secondary infection and significant scarring.[9] Removal of a piece of tape, or an adhesive-backed electrode, will markedly compromise the stratum corneum.[10-12] This type of skin injury has been utilized in a positive way to facilitate transcutaneous monitoring of serum glucose in newborns[13] but is more often deleterious. Removal of hydrophilic gel-based adhesives is not accompanied by the same degree of injury.[12]

Several cases of full-thickness skin injury from presumed innocuous local application of pressure or thermal heat have been observed. The precise causes of these wounds are often difficult to identify and are underreported in the medical literature. Anetoderma of prematurity, marked by cutaneous focal depressions or outpouchings, is probably a response to mechanical or thermal injury.[14] Ultraviolet (UV) light burns have occurred in association with white-light phototherapy for jaundice, from relatively limited, inadvertent exposure to near-ultraviolet light (UVA), which is 1000 times less erythemogenic than UVB.[15] A Plexiglas safety shield, placed in front of daylight fluorescent bulbs, will filter out the UVA. However, white-light phototherapy is also a source of infrared heat, and heat stress will exacerbate TEWL. In contrast, phototherapy delivered with blue light alone does not increase TEWL.[16]

PERCUTANEOUS ABSORPTION

Increased percutaneous absorption of topically applied compounds through an immature stratum corneum has been both advantageous and hazardous to neonates. This

TABLE 5-1

Reported Hazards of Percutaneous Absorption in the Newborn

Compound	Product	Toxicity
Aniline[17]	Dye used as a laundry marker	Methemoglobinemia,* death
Mercury[85]	Diaper rinses; teething powders	Rash, hypotonia
Phenolic compounds[32]: Pentachlorophenol	Laundry disinfectant	Tachycardia, sweating, hepatomegaly, metabolic acidosis, death
Hexachlorophene	Topical antiseptic (pHisoHex)	Vacuolar encephalopathy, death
Resorcinol[32]	Topical antiseptic	Methemoglobinemia*
Boric acid[86]	Baby powder	Vomiting, diarrhea, erythroderma, seizures, death
Lindane[17,32]	Scabicide	Neurotoxicity
Salicylic acid[32,87]	Keratolytic emollient	Metabolic acidosis, salicylism
Isopropyl alcohol	Topical antiseptic	Cutaneous hemorrhagic necrosis (under occlusion)[17]
Silver sulfadiazine[88]	Topical antibiotic (Silvadene)	Kernicterus (sulfa component), Argyria (silver component)
Urea[89]	Keratolytic emollient (Carmol)	Uremia
Povidone-iodine[17,32]	Topical antiseptic (Betadine)	Hypothyroidism, goiter
Neomycin[17]	Topical antibiotic	Neural deafness
Corticosteroids[17,32]	Topical antiinflammatory (Lotrisone)	Skin atrophy, adrenal suppression
Benzocaine[90]	Mucosal anesthetic (teething products)	Methemoglobinemia*
Prilocaine[91,92]	Epidermal anesthetic (EMLA)	Methemoglobinemia*
Methylene blue[93]	Amniotic fluid leak	Methemoglobinemia*

*Heritable glucose-6-phosphate deficiencies are associated with an increased susceptibility to methemoglobinemia, as is coadministration of several drugs, including sulfonamides, acetaminophen, nitroprusside, phenobarbitol, and phenytoin.

phenomenon was described in 1971 as "raccoon facies," a visible periorbital ring of pallor from cutaneous vasoconstriction following the application of phenylephrine eye drops.[17] This effect can be quantified and is directly proportional to measurements of TEWL. Both methods have been established as useful markers of stratum corneum integrity in infants.[17,18] Transdermal delivery has been utilized for the administration for theophylline[17,19] and diamorphine[20] in premature infants. Lidocaine applied topically to premature skin is probably much more effective than after application to mature skin.[21] Even supplemental oxygen has been administered percutaneously to very small preterm infants with poor pulmonary function.[22,23]

The hazards of percutaneous absorption are documented in numerous reports of devastating systemic side effects in infants caused by absorption of topically applied agents.[17,24] Revered clinicians have historically overlooked the potential for percutaneous poisoning in designing therapy for infants. This was evidenced by Cooke's 1926 review of diaper dermatitis. Here, he recommends a rapid and permanent "cure" for "ammoniacal" dermatitis by rinsing diapers in either dilute mercuric chloride or saturated boric acid solution.[25] Over the last 70 years, published accounts have served to document only the most severe toxicities—in some cases manifesting as nursery epidemics of obvious clinical illness or deaths (Table 5-1).

SKIN CARE PRACTICES

Skin care of hospitalized infants includes bathing, emollient use, diapering, cord care, use of antimicrobial skin preparations, management of percutaneous catheter infiltration, treatment of diaper rash, and maneuvers to minimize transcutaneous water loss. Routine skin care practices in hospital nurseries vary widely and deserve further evaluation.[26]

Bathing

The once-conventional use of antimicrobial cleansing agents for routine bathing has diminished. Hexachlorophene was widely used for this purpose before 1975 and was subsequently associated with serious adverse reactions in infants, including fatal neurotoxicity.[17] Bathing products have high market visibility, but there are no products with clearly demonstrable benefits for infants. There is scant medical literature addressing the mildness of "baby" soaps,[27] and those marketed specifically for babies offer no special advantage over generic mild cleansing agents. The active ingredients in all bathing products are surfactants, and all surfactants are at least mild irritants.[28] Because these products are immediately rinsed off, their potential for cutaneous or percutaneous toxicity is very low. In efforts to create and market the mildest cleansing products, several techniques have been defined to measure the potential for causing irritation. Manufacturers emphasize the data on file that best support their product, but there is little clinical difference among the gentle cleansers in cleansing properties or potential for irritation.[29] Many mild products are now available. Regarding bathing water, at least one hospitalized term infant suffered second-degree burns after immersion in hot water tested only by touch, emphasizing the need for more careful monitoring of bath water temperature.[30]

Diapering

Cloth diapers, laundered by commercial services, are used in some hospitals. Most of these laundry services are now aware of the importance of avoiding phenolic compounds. Phenol is effectively absorbed by inhalation, skin exposure, or ingestion. Systemic toxicities have been well documented in the general population[31] and in infants, including an epidemic of percutaneous poisoning and death associated with the use of a laundry product containing pentachlorophenol in a hospital nursery.[17,32] Some laundries use sodium hypochlorite, followed by a rinse step designed to neutralize the residual chlorine. Sodium hypochlorite is used as a disinfectant, bleach, and deodorizer. Contact with a dilute solution may cause mild skin irritation; more concentrated or prolonged contact may cause skin necrosis. Sensitization dermatitis may occur in previously exposed individuals.[31]

The first disposable diapers (Pampers) were marketed in 1963. For 20 years the absorbent core was composed primarily of cellulose fluff. In the mid-1980s, a superabsorbent core material was developed, containing a cross-linked sodium polyacrylate. This material, contained in all superabsorbent disposable diapers, transforms and holds fluid within a gel and has the capacity to absorb many times its own weight. Superabsorbent diapers are clearly superior to cloth diapers in preventing irritant diaper dermatitis.[33,34] However, this condition is uncommon within the first month of life. A more important issue in the neonatal nursery is the effect of diaper type on documentation of urine output. Urine output, monitored by weighing diapers, is diminished by evaporation if diapers are allowed to remain open under a radiant warmer. Evaporative loss is greater from a regular fluff-type than from a superabsorbent diaper.[35] Pseudoanuria has been reported in an infant, the result of an inability to feel moisture on a superabsorbent diaper.[36]

Use of Emollients and Diaper Care Products

Use of topical emollients, diaper rash balms, and wipes is ubiquitous in the newborn nursery, but product selection is extremely variable, affected more by marketing than medicine.[26] Diaper wipes are typically used for the first 1 to 2 years of life, but only one published report in the medical literature evaluates the product in a 10-week comparative trial of four brands.[37] Conclusions of this limited study included correlation between the pH of skin and wipe. There were no demonstrable differences in skin integrity.

A damp diaper with a plastic coating acts as an occlusive dressing, enhancing the risk of local irritation, as well as percutaneous absorption. This relative risk is increased in infants with their twofold to fivefold greater body surface area/weight ratio and cumulative in preterm infants with immature skin. Many emollients and diaper care products contain similar ingredients. Of these, a few have documented percutaneous toxicity, especially under diaper occlusion. Even now only the more infamous compounds listed in Table 5-1 are scarce in topical products. Because there are no regulations that require disclosure of inactive ingredients in over-the-counter products, only a painstaking mission can obtain this proprietary information. An extensive list of ingredients is included in Table 5-2. Some of these ingredients may have underappreciated toxicities, as listed in Table 5-3.

There have been many studies of the mechanism of action and benefits of emollients on injured and diseased skin in adults. Synthetic skin barrier lipids such as cholesterol, free fatty acids, and ceramides may ultimately prove to be an ideal replacement, but white petroleum is currently regarded as the gold standard.[38] It acts primarily by trapping water in the epidermis.[38] Appropriate hydration of keratinocytes is essential for normal skin maturation,[39] an optimized barrier against exogenous assault and maintenance of thermal, fluid, and electrolyte balance. Oils, oil-and-water-based creams, and lotion emollients have greater tactile acceptance than greasy ointments. Some oils, such as safflower oil, contain essential fatty acids, which have the potential to greatly influence cutaneous structure and function.[40,41] However, topically applied

TABLE 5-2

Diaper Rash Products and Emollients: Composition and Cost

Product	Manufacturer	Ingredients	Cost/Oz
A&D ointment	Schering-Plough Memphis, Tenn	Cholecalciferol, fish liver oil, petroleum, fragrance, lanolin, mineral oil, paraffin	2.12
Aloe Vesta Protective Ointment	ConvaTec Princeton, NJ	Propylparaben, aloe vera gel, quaternium-15, water, hydroxylated lanolin, ozokerite, glycerin, fragrance	1.02
Aquaphor	Beiersdorf, Inc Norwalk, Conn	Petrolatum, mineral oil, mineral wax, wool wax alcohol	.68
Aquaphor Natural Healing Ointment	Beiersdorf, Inc Norwalk, Conn	Petrolatum, mineral oil, mineral wax, wool wax, alcohol, panthenol, bisabolol, glycerin	.68
Baby Magic Baby Lotion	Mennen Morristown, NJ	Water, glycerin, glyceryl stearate, cetyl alcohol, mineral oil, Peg-100 stearate, lanolin alcohol, fragrance, lanolin, methylparaben, lapyrium chloride, propylparaben, benzalkonium chloride, diazolidinyl urea	.28
Balmex Diaper Rash Ointment	Block Drug Company Jersey City, NJ	11.3% Zinc oxide, balsam of Peru, beeswax, benzoic acid, bismuth subnitrate, mineral oil, purified water, silicone, synthetic white wax	1.47
Cholysteramine in Aquaphor	Bristol-Myers Squibb Princeton, NJ; Beiersdorf Norwalk, Conn; locally compounded	15% Cholestyramine liquid (aspartame, citric acid, A&C yellow #10, FD&C red #40, flavor, propylene glycol alginate, collodial silicon dioxide, sucrose, xanthan gum), in Aquaphor	8.40
Critic-Aid	Sween Products N. Mankato, Minn	Benzethonium chloride in a soothing, occlusive moisture-resistant paste of proprietary ingredients	2.91
Desitin Diaper Rash Ointment	Pfizer New York, NY	40% Zinc oxide; BHA, cod liver oil, fragrance, lanolin, methyl paraben, petrolatum, talc, water	1.72
Dr. Danis Buttocks Cream	Compounded at St. John's Mercy Medical Center, St. Louis, Mo	32 g Zinc oxide, 32 g starch, 32 g talc, 60 ml glycerin, 112 g Aquaphor	13.50
Dyprotex	Blistex Oakbrook, Ill	40% Micronized zinc oxide, 37.6% petrolatum, 2.5% dimethicone, cod liver oil, aloe	2.85
Elase ointment	Fujisawa Deerfield, Ill	1U Fibrinolysin and 666.6 U of deoxyribonuclease in a base of petrolatum and polyethylene	52.72
Eucerin cream	Beiersdorf Norwalk, Conn	Water, mineral oil, isopropyl myristate, Peg-40 sorbitan peroleate, glyceryl lanolate, sorbitol, propylene glycol, cetyl palmitate, magnesium sulfate, aluminum stearate, lanolin alcohol, BHT, methylchloroisothiazolinone, methylisothiazolinone	.84

Continued

TABLE 5-2

Diaper Rash Products and Emollients: Composition and Cost—cont'd

Product	Manufacturer	Ingredients	Cost/Oz
Happy Hiney	Bristol-Myers Squibb Princeton, NJ; Beiersdorf Norwalk, Conn compounded at Carbondale Memorial Hospital Carbondale, Ill	12 × 4.1 g Packets of Questran powder (cholestyramine resin, acacia, citric acid, D&C yellow #10, FD&C yellow #6, flavor, polysorbate 80, propylene glycol, alginate, sucrose) compounded in 1 pound of Aquaphor	2.50
Ilex Paste	Calgon-Vestal St. Louis, Mo	Petrolatum, calcium/sodium PVM/MA copolymer, DMDM hydantoin, iodopropynyl-butycarbamate, mineral oil, peppermint oil, sodium carboxymethyl cellulose	5.75
Neosporin Plus Maximum Strength Ointment	Burroughs-Wellcome Triangle Park, NC	Polymyxin B sulfate 10,000U, bacitracin zinc 500U, neomycin 3.5 mg, lidocaine 40mg, in a special white petrolatum base	22.58
Nystatin cream	E. Fougera Melville, NJ	100,000 U Nystatin, polysorbate 60, aluminum hydroxide compressed gel, titanium dioxide, glyceryl monostearate, polyethylene glycol monostearate 400, simethicone, sorbic acid, propylene glycol, ethylenediamine, polyoxyethylene fatty alcohol ether, sorbitol solution, methyl paraben, propyl paraben, hydrochloric acid, white petrolatum, purified water	11.78
Nystatin ointment	E. Fougera Melville, NY	100,000 USP U Nystatin per gram, in a polyethylene and mineral oil base	11.78
Proshield	Health Pointe Medical Forthworth, Tex	*Cleansing foam:* purified water, glycerine, cocoamphodiacetate, polaxymer 188, cocamidopropylpeg-dimniumchloride phosphate, DMSM hydantoin, laureth-23, citric acid, fragrance *Skin protectant:* dimethicone, polyethylene glycol, copolymer broadhesive	6.09
Super Dooper Diaper Doo	Peacock Pharmaceuticals Springfield, Mo	Lanolin, petrolatum	5.75
Vaseline	Cheseborough-Ponds Greenwich, Conn	White petrolatum USP	.29
Zinc oxide ointment	E. Fogera Melville, NY	20% Zinc oxide, mineral oil, white wax, white petroleum base	.56

safflower oil does not prevent essential fatty acid deficiency in preterm infants.[42] Compared with ointments, oils, creams, and lotions provide a much less-effective moisture barrier.[43] In addition, formulation of a cream or lotion emulsion requires the addition of several potentially irritating, sensitizing, or toxic ingredients.

Eucerin Creme (Beiersdorf Inc., Norwalk, Conn) is a popular product that has been studied for use in the nursery.[43] It contains water, petrolatum, mineral oil, ceresin, lanolin alcohol, and methylchloroisothiazolinone/methylisothiazolinone (CMI/MI, also known as Kathon CG). Although susceptibility of premature infants to aller-

---

TABLE 5-3

Topically Applied Products That Should be Used With Caution in the Newborn

Compound	Product	Concern
Triclosan	Lever 2000, liquid deodorant soaps	The risk of toxicities seen with other phenolic compounds
Propylene glycol[94]	Emollients, cleansing agents (Cetaphil Cleansing Lotion)	Excessive enteral and parenteral administration has caused hyperosmolality and seizures in infants
Benzethonium chloride	Skin cleansers	Poisoning by ingestion, carcinogenesis
Glycerin	Emollients, cleansing agents (Aquanil Lotion)	Hyperosmolality, seizures
Ammonium lactate	Keratolytic emollient (Lac-Hydrin)	Possible lactic acidosis
Coal tar[95]	Shampoos, topical antiinflammatory ointments	Excessive use of polycyclic aromatic hydrocarbons is associated with an increased risk of cancer

---

gic contact sensitization is unknown, CMI/MI has been associated with allergic contact sensitization in up to 10% of exposed adults and is the third most common sensitizer in children with chronic dermatitis.[44,45] Aquaphor ointment (Biersdorf Inc., Norwalk, Conn), a petroleum wax-based emollient, contains essentially two ingredients: white petrolatum in ointment, liquid (mineral oil), and solid (mineral wax) phases, and wool wax alcohols. Wool alcohols, along with Kathon CG, thimerosal, nickel, fragrances, and neomycin rank among the most common causes of allergic contact dermatitis in children[16] (see Table 5-2).

The monetary cost of topical products used in hospitals also varies greatly. Even without considering this cost, the safest and most effective product currently available for use as an emollient is white petrolatum, and the best initial choice for diaper dermatitis is zinc oxide ointment. Ironically, these products are also available for the lowest price.

Skin Antisepsis

Skin antisepsis practices, such as cord care regimens and application of antimicrobial washes before invasive procedures, were popularized in attempts to control nursery epidemics of localized and invasive streptococcal and staphylococcal infections.[47] Prospective, controlled comparative outcome studies on the safety and efficacy of these practices are lacking. Common cord care practices include nonintervention, use of 70% isopropyl alcohol pledgettes with or without application of triple-dye, or povidone-iodine. Povidone-iodine is the most popular product for preprocedure skin antisepsis.[26]

Triple dye contains brilliant green, gentian violet, and proflavine hemisulfate. These agents all have antimicrobial activity, but efficacies have not been well studied. Although triple dye does control staphylococcal colonization of the umbilical stump, it is ineffective against group B streptococcal organisms.[48] Gentian violet is effective against some gram-positive and gram-negative bacteria, as well as some pathogenic *Candida* spp.[49] Reported toxicities to triple dye have been rare, including necrotic skin reactions following the use of brilliant green.[49] Gentian violet is infamous for deep purple staining of the skin, which is rarely permanent. Prolonged use of gentian violet has been associated with nausea, vomiting, diarrhea, and ulceration of mucous membranes[49]; carcinogenicity in mice has been reported.[50] However, this compound has enjoyed decades of widespread use with very few reported adverse events. Proflavine hemisulfate is a mutagenic photoactive aminoacridine.[2,30]

The use of povidone-iodine is a routine nursery practice that deserves further consideration. Adverse effects of topically applied iodine have been recognized in infants for at least 20 years.[51] Skin necrosis has been documented by case report, an injury most likely to occur when an excess amount of solution is inadvertently left in contact with the skin for a prolonged period of time.[52] Exposure to iodine in the perinatal or neonatal period has been associated with dramatic, prolonged elevation in plasma and urinary iodine, transient hypothyroxinemia, hypothyroidism, and goiter.[45,51,53,54] Idiopathic transient hypothyroxinemia has been estimated to occur in 50% of preterm infants delivered before 30 weeks' gestation,[55] although reference ranges for thyroid function tests of premature infants have been established without regard to iodine exposure.[56] Transient hypothyroxinemia has generally been regarded as a benign condition that does not require treatment. However, a recent historical cohort study documented a fourfold to tenfold increase in the risk of disabling cerebral palsy in premature infants with this condition.[57]

Alcohol is a commonly used topical antiseptic, which because of its volatility, rapidly evaporates before absorption. Generous application followed by occlusion can result in significant absorption and can also enhance the absorption of other concomitantly applied medications, especially through immature or diseased skin. Hemorrhagic skin necrosis due to alcohol has been reported in preterm infants. Additional potential toxicities include metabolic acidosis, central nervous system dysfunction, and hypoglycemia. Despite their comfortable familiarity, alcohol solutions should be used very sparingly in infants.[52]

Chlorhexidine gluconate is an alternative product for skin antisepsis.[17] One-half percent chlorhexidine gluconate is superior to 10% povidone-iodine in reducing the risk of peripheral intravenous catheter colonization.[58] Chlorhexidine strongly binds to skin.[59,60] Its substantivity enhances the efficacy of chlorhexidine and minimizes the risk of percutaneous absorption.[17,59] No toxic systemic effects have been attributed to chlorhexidine alone,[17] even after massive oral ingestion (Zenca Pharmaceuticals, personal communication). However, severe anaphylaxis has been rarely reported.[61] Chlorhexidine has a broad spectrum of activity against gram-positive and gram-negative bacteria and yeast,[62] but resistance to gram-negative rods is emerging, especially Serratia marcescens.[63,64]

A chlorhexidine-containing product ideally suited for infants is not commercially available in the United States. Hibistat (Zenca Pharmaceuticals, Wilmington, Del) contains 0.5% chlorhexidine and 70% isopropyl alcohol. Hibiclens (Zenca Pharmaceuticals, Wilmington, Del) and a similar product, Betasept (Xttrium Laboratories, Chicago, Ill) contain 4% chlorhexidine and 4% isopropyl alcohol. Detectable, increasing plasma chlorhexidine levels were documented in preterm infants treated with 1% chlorhexidine in an unspecified concentration of ethanol every 4 hours for 5 to 9 days. Significant absorption could not be documented in a similar group of infants treated with 1% chlorhexidine in a 3% zinc oxide dusting powder, supporting the role of alcohols in facilitating percutaneous absorption.[65] Commercially available formulations also contain the proprietary pluronics, fragrance, and red dye. Pluronics are added solely to enhance lathering and can cause serious corneal damage.

The risks and benefits of routine skin antisepsis in infants is a subject that clearly deserves further investigation.

Bacterial colonization is controlled with antiseptic cord care; chlorhexidine is superior to 70% ethanol,[66] hexachlorophene,[67] and povidone-iodine.[68] Triple dye is superior to bacitracin ointment,[69] hexachlorophene,[70] or isopropyl alcohol alone.[71] Antiseptic cord care with chlorhexidine or occlusive ointments or dressings has been associated with delayed cord detachment.[67] Although there are insufficient comparative data on the costs, risks, and benefits of skin antisepsis regimens to mandate standard practice, the use of alcohol pledgettes alone provides the least-effective antimicrobial activity. Hexachlorophene and povidone-iodine carry the most significant risks of percutaneous toxicity. The potential for subclinical toxicities must be considered by everyone caring for small newborns. When several topical therapeutic options are available, the one with the least potential for toxicity should be used. Poisindex is an extensive, frequently updated, computer-based reference source for the identification of potentially toxic compounds.[72]

Control of Transcutaneous Water Loss (See Also Chapter 4)

Evaporative losses are greatest in the youngest, most premature infants. Routine clinical interventions can exacerbate TEWL. Maintenance on an open radiant warmer bed in a nursery with low ambient humidity results in high evaporative loss of body water and heat.[73] Higher ambient temperatures are required to maintain normal body temperature under these conditions.[74] Traditional efforts to minimize these insensible water losses have centered on intravascular fluid replacement and modification of the infant's hospital bed. These approaches have inherent problems. Evaporative losses originate as free water from the extracellular compartment. Replacement has been conventionally determined by calculation based on standardized maintenance fluid requirements and measured changes in body weight and intravascular electrolytes, which have a lag time of several hours after the losses have occurred. Replacement fluids given in the form of isotonic intravenous solutions may result in sodium and glucose overload.[75]

Several alternatives are used to control transcutaneous water loss and its accompanying thermal and fluid instability in small, premature infants. Enclosed isolettes limit convective heat loss and can maintain high ambient humidity. However, this type of unit impedes easy access to patients. And although an increased incidence of infection has not been documented for infants housed in isolettes, this environment is optimal for contamination with pathogenic microbes, especially in the setting of high humidity.[73] In many high-risk nurseries, plastic barriers are placed over infants nursed on open radiant warmers. There is limited data on the safety and efficacy of this practice. A few reports have documented that blanketing an infant with a thin, pliable clear plastic wrap reduces insensible water loss and warmer power demand.[76] In direct comparison, a plastic blanket is superior to a rigid plastic hood with regard to these parameters.[77] Many adaptations to these reported techniques are currently employed. A wide variety of products and materials are used in diverse ways. The majority of these products are not manufactured or indicated for this purpose, raising several concerns, including inconsistent composition, uncertain shelf life, the possibility of degradation with prolonged exposure to heat, and the possibility of significant infrared absorption.

The majority of plastic wraps used in the hospital nursery are manufactured for food storage. Their composition varies. Saran Wrap (Dow Brands, Indianapolis, Ind) is polyvinylidone chloride sheeting. Anchor Wrap (Anchor Packaging, Senton, Mo) is a similar but not identical product of polyvinyl chloride. The composition of other generic plastic food wraps may vary from box to box. Food wraps are specifically made for use with cold storage and have not been tested for stability after prolonged heating. A rigid plastic hood-type device is used in some nurseries, either custom-made or commercially available (Baby Shield, Nova Health Systems, Inc., Blackwood, NJ). Baby Shield is made of "special formulation" polyvinyl chloride of consistent composition. Prepackaged aerosol tents (Nova Health Systems, Inc., Blackwood, NJ) are used in some nurseries for this off-label purpose. These tents are specifically manufactured and marketed for oxygen/aerosol delivery rather than thermal control. They are made from polyvinyl chloride of variable composition and weight. In some nurseries, plastic "bubble wrap" is used as a thermal blanket. This practice was introduced in 1971.[78] Two studies documented its efficacy in very specific, different settings. The first included 85 infants >2000 g during the first 40 minutes of life, with and without head cover, with and without a 750-watt overhead warmer.[79] Mean rectal temperature was best maintained for infants whose bubble wrap included a head cover. The authors assumed that "evaporation of amniotic fluid from the skin" was the major cause of heat loss, but antithetically noted no additional cooling effect in uncovered babies who were not towel dried. A second, case-controlled study included five premature infants weighing 880 to 1930 g housed in single-walled incubators. Insensible water loss (IWL) was determined from decremental weight change during 3-hour periods. The decrease in IWL was greatest for the smallest blanketed infant.[78] Plastic bubble wrap is generically manufactured and distributed as packing material; its composition is variable and difficult to reliably identify. A plastic that is translucent or opaque to infrared will acutely block heat transmission when used in the setting of an overhead infrared source. Plastics that retain heat have the potential to burn contacted skin.[73] Clearly, the use of these techniques to control thermal and fluid losses in small premature infants deserves further study.

Another strategy to limit TEWL is topical application of an occlusive dressing. Empiric use of these products has been limited by concerns about potential risks of systemic absorption and resulting toxicity, overgrowth of microbes, and secondary heat accumulation that could increase surface and core temperature. A few studies have verified the safety and efficacy of semiocclusive, polyurethane membrane barriers in preventing fluid losses from preterm infants.[80,81,82,83]

Pure white petrolatum is an effective barrier against transepidermal water loss, but has been an unpopular product in the nursery because of its greasy texture. Misconceptions are held by some nursery staff about "side effects," for example, not allowing the skin "to breathe" and causing burns if applied to infants under phototherapy or radiant warmers. A recent study documented a 67% decrease in TEWL 30 minutes after application of Aquaphor to preterm infants. Six hours after application, TEWL was only decreased by 34%, implying that a 6-hour application interval is needed to maintain the effect.[8] Routine application also improved skin integrity, did not alter skin flora, and was associated with a significant reduction the incidence of sepsis. There were no adverse effects reported. Measured skin surface temperature was stable, and there was no evidence of hyperthermia or burns following application of the petroleum-based ointment under infrared warmers, even for infants receiving concomitant white-light phototherapy, confirming the results of a previous pilot study.[84] The addition of wool wax alcohols to Aquaphor facilitates miscibility of water-soluble agents compared with white petrolatum alone. In the future, this may allow compounding of pharmacologically active agents. The benefits of this property must be weighed against the risk of contact sensitization when choosing therapy (see previous section on Use of Emollients and Diaper Care Products).

Increased understanding of the mechanisms contributing to skin development may one day provide therapy to accelerate barrier maturation in very premature infants. Prolonged maintenance in a fluid environment would be an alternate approach. Until that time, therapy should be directed toward providing a safe, temporary barrier and minimizing additional skin injury while allowing easy access and handling of infants (Box 5-1). Efforts should be directed at creating a well-defined and uniformly accepted standard of care for the skin of premature infants.

BOX 5-1

Proposed Recommendations for Basic Skin Care of the Premature Newborn

1. Use adhesives sparingly.
   - Place protective dressing at sites of frequent taping (endotrachial and nasogastric tube placement).
   - Use nonadhesive electrodes and change them only when they become nonfunctional.
2. Limit bathing.
   - Defer initial cleansing until body temperature has stabilized.
   - Avoid cleansing agents for the first 2 weeks.
   - Use warm water and moistened cotton pledgettes in a humid environment.
   - Surface cleansing is required no more than twice a week.
   - If antimicrobial skin preparation is required, use short-contact chlorhexidine (except on the face).
3. Be aware of the composition and quantity of all topically applied agents.
   - This includes antimicrobial cleansers, diaper wipes, adhesive removers, perineal products.
   - Dispense from single-use containers, if possible.

4. Ensure adequate intake of protein, essential fatty acids, zinc, biotin, and vitamins A, D, and B.
   - Be aware that erosive periorificial dermatitis is a sign of nutritional deficiency.
5. Apply an ointment emollient every 6 to 8 hours.
6. Guard against excessive thermal and UV exposure.
   - Use thermally controlled water for bathing.
   - Avoid surface monitors with metal contacts.
   - Use Plexiglas shielding over daylight fluorescent phototherapy.
7. Protect sites of cutaneous injury with the appropriate occlusive dressing.
   - Use a film dressing on nonexudative sites.
   - Use a hydrogel dressing on exudative wounds.
   - Maintain appropriate hydration at the skin-dressing interface.
   - Remove necrotic debris with each dressing change.

REFERENCES

1. Holbrook KA: Structure and function of the developing human skin. In Goldsmith LA, ed. Physiology, biochemistry and molecular biology of the skin. New York: 1991: pp 63-110.
2. Brion L, Fleischman AR, Schwartz GJ. Evaluation of four length-weight formulas for estimating body surface area in newborn infants. J Pediatr 1985;107:801-803.
3. Rutter N. The immature skin. Br Med Bull 1988;44:957-970.
4. Sedin G, Hammarlund K, Nilsson GE, et al. Measurements of transepidermal water loss in newborn infants. Clinics in Perinatol 1985;12:79-99.
5. Baumgart S. Radiant energy and insensible water loss in the premature newborn infant nursed under a radiant warmer. Clin Perinatol 1982;9:483-503.
6. Harper VA, Rutter N: Barrier properties of the newborn infant's skin. J Pediatr 1983;102:419-425.
7. Rosen JL, Atkins JT, Levy ML, et al. Invasive fungal dermatitis in the ≤1000-gram neonate. Pediatrics 1995;95:682-687.
8. Nopper AJ, Horli K, Sookdeo-Drost S, et al. Topical ointment therapy reduces the risk of nosocomial infection in premature infants. J Pediatr 1996;128:660-669.
9. Cartlidge PHT, Fox PE, Rutter N. The scars of newborn intensive care. In Early human development. Nottingham, Ireland: Elsevier Scientific Ltd, 1990: pp 1-10.
10. Harpin VA, Rutter N. Barrier properties of the newborn infant's skin. J Pediatr 1983;102:419-425.
11. Cartlidge PH, Rutter N. Karaya gum electrocardiographic electrodes for preterm infants. Arch Dis Child 1987;62:1281-1282.
12. Lund CH, Nonato LB, Kuller JM, et al. Disruption of barrier function in neonatal skin associated with adhesive removal. J Pediatr 1997;131:367-372.
13. De Boer J, Baarsma R, Okken A, et al. Application of transcutaneous microdialysis and continuous flow analysis for on-line glucose monitoring in the newborn infants. J Lab Clin Med 1994;124:210-217.
14. Prizant TL, Lucky AW, Frieden IJ, et al. Spontaneous atrophic patches in extremely premature infants. Anetoderma of prematurity. Arch Dermatol 1996;132:671-674.
15. Siegfried EC, Stone MS, Madison KC. Ultraviolet light burn: A cutaneous complication of visible light therapy for neonatal jaundice. Pediatric Dermatol 1992;9:278-282.
16. Kjartansson SK, Hammarlund K, Sedin G. Insensible water loss from the skin during phototherapy in term and preterm infants. Acta Pediatric 1992;81:764-768.
17. Rutter N: Percutaneous drug absorption in the newborn: Hazards and uses. Clin Perinatol 1987;14:911-930.
18. Plantin P, Jouan N, Karangwa A, et al. [Variations of the skin permeability in premature newborn infants. Value of the skin vasoconstriction test with neosynephrine]. Archives Francaises de Pediatrie 1992;49:623-625.
19. Cartwright RG, Cartlidge PH, Rutter N, et al. Transdermal delivery of theophylline to premature infants using a hydrogel disc system. Br J Clin Pharmacol 1990;29:533-539.
20. Barrett DA, Rutter N, Davis SS. An in vitro study of diamorphine permeation through premature human neonatal skin. Pharmac Res 1993;10:583-587.
21. Barrett DA, Rutter N. Percutaneous lignocaine absorption in newborn infants. Arch Dis Child 1994;71:F122-F124.

22. Cartlidge PH, Rutter N. Percutaneous respiration in the newborn infant. Effect of ambient oxygen concentration on pulmonary oxygen uptake. Biol Neonate 1988;54:68-72.

23. Cartlidge PH, Rutter N. Percutaneous oxygen delivery to the preterm infant. Lancet 1988;1(8581):315-317.

24. Lane AT. Development and care of the premature infant's skin. Pediatric Dermatol 1987;4:1-5.

25. Cooke JV. Dermatitis of the diaper region in infants (Jacquet dermatitis). Arch Dermatol Syphillol 1926;14:539-546.

26. Siegfried EC, Shah PY. Skin care practices in the neonatal nursery: A clinical survey. J Perinatol 1999;19:31-39.

27. Morelli JC, Weston WL. Soaps and shampoos in pediatric practice. Pediatrics 1987;80:634-637.

28. Efendy I, Maibach HI. Detergent and skin irritation. Clin Dermatol 1996;14:15-21.

29. Wolf R. Entering the 21st century: Future perspectives. Clin Dermatol 1996;14:129-132.

30. Mirowski GW, Frieden IJ, Miller C. Iatrogenic scald burn: a consequence of institutional infection control measures. Pediatrics 1996;98:963-965.

31. Sullivan JB, Krieger GR. Hazardous materials toxicology. Baltimore: Williams & Williams, 1992: p 415.

32. West DP, Worobec S, Solomon LM: Pharmacology and toxicology of infant skin. J Invest Dermatol 1981;76:147-150.

33. Lane A, Rehder P, Helm K: Evaluation of diapers containing absorbent gelling material with conventional disposable diapers in newborn infants. Am J Dis Child 1990;144:315-318.

34. Epstein E. Cantharidin treatment of molluscum contagiosum. Acta Derm Venereol 1989;69:91-92.

35. Hermansen MC, Buches M. Urine output determination from superabsorbent and regular diapers under radiant heat. Pediatrics 1988;81:428-431.

36. Barada JH. Pseudoanuria due to superabsorbent diapers. New Engl J Med 1991;325:892-893.

37. Priestley GC, McVittie E, Aldridge RD. Changes in skin pH after the use of baby wipes. Pediatric Dermatol 1996; 13:14-17.

38. Ghadially R, Elias P. Effects of petrolatum on stratum corneum structure and function. J Am Acad Dermatol 1992; 26:387-396.

39. Rawlings AV, Scott IR, Harding CR, et al. A Stratum corneum moisturization at the molecular level. In Moshell AN, ed. Progress in dermatology. Evanston, Illinois: Dermatology Foundation, 1994: pp 1-12.

40. Ziboh VA, Chapkin RS. Biologic significance of polyunsaturated fatty acids in the skin. Arch Dermatol 1987,123:1686a-1690.

41. Schurer NY, Plewig G, Elias PM. Stratum corneum lipid function. Dermatologica 1991;183:77-94.

42. Lee EJ, Gibson RA, Simmer K. Transcutaneous application of oil and prevention of essential fatty acid deficiency in preterm infants. Arch Dis Child 1993;68:27-28.

43. Lane AT, Drost SS. Effects of repeated application of emollient cream to premature neonate's skin. Pediatrics 1993; 92:415-419.

44. Frosch PJ, Lahti A, Hannuksela M, et al. Chloromethylisothiazolone/methylisothiazolone (CMI/MI) use test with a shampoo on patch-test-positive subjects. Contact Dermatitis 1994;32:210-217.

45. Linder N, Davidovitch N, Reichman B, et al. Topical iodine-containing antiseptics and subclinical hypothyroidism in preterm infants. J Pediatr 1997;131:434-439.

46. Manzini BM, Ferdani G, Simonetti V, et al. Contact sensitization in children. Pediatr Dermatol 1998;15:12-17.

47. Light IJ, Sutherland JM. Effect of topical antibacterial agents on the acquisition of bacteria by newborn infants. Antimicrobial Agents and Chemotherapy 1968;8:274-278.

48. Speck WT, Driscoll JM, Polin RA, et al. Staphylococcal and streptococcal colonization of the newborn infant. Am J Dis Child 1997;131:1005-1008.

49. Anonymous. Gentian violet. In Reynolds J, ed. Martindale: The extra Pharmacopoeia (electronic version). Englewood, CO: 1997.

50. Rosenkranz HS, Carr HS. Possible hazard in use of gentian violet. Br Med J 1971;3:702-703.

51. Pyati SP, Ramamurthy RS, Krauss MT, et al. Absorption of iodine in the neonate following topical use of povidone iodine. J Pediatr 1977;91:825-828.

52. Roberts RJ. Drug therapy in infants. Philadelphia: WB Saunders, 1984: pp. 341-349.

53. Gordon CM, Rowitch DH, Mitchell ML, et al. Topical iodine and neonatal hypothyroidism. Arch Pediatr Adolesc Med 1995;149:1336-1339.

54. Parravicini E, Fontana C, Giuseppe L, et al. Iodine, thyroid function, and very low birth weight infants. Pediatrics 1996; 98:730-734.

55. Fisher DA: Transient thyroid dysfunction in the premature infant. In Rudloph AM, Hoffman JIE, eds. Pediatrics. Norwalk, Conn: Appleton & Lange, 1987: pp 1510-1511.

56. Adas LM, Emery JR., Clark SJ, et al. Reference ranges for newer thyroid function tests in premature infants. J Pediatr 1995;126:122-127.

57. Reuss ML, Paneth N, Pinto-Martin JA, et al. The relation of transient hypothyroxinemia in preterm infants to neurologic development at two years of age. N Engl J Med 1996; 334:821-858.

58. Garland JS, Buck RK, Maloney P, et al. Comparison of 10% povidone-iodine and 0.5% chlorhexidine gluconate for the prevention of peripheral intravenous catheter colonization in neonates: a prospective trial. Pediatr Infect Dis 1995; 14:510-516.

59. AMA division of drugs. Dermatologic preparations. In Bennett DR, ed. AMA Drug evaluations. Chicago: AMA Division of Drugs, 1983: pp 1383-1384.

60. Johnsson J, Seeberg S, Kjellmer I. Blood concentrations of chlorhexidine in neonates undergoing routine care with 4% chlorhexidine gluconate solution. Acta Paediatr Scand 1987; 76:675-676.

61. Snellman E, Rantanen T. Severe anaphylaxis after a chlorhexidine bath. J Am Acad Dermatol 1999;40:771-772.

62. Reynolds J, ed. Chlorhexidine. Englewood CO: Micromedex, 1996.

63. McAllister TA, Lucas CE, Mocan H, et al. Serratia marcescens outbreak in a paediatric oncology unit traced to contaminated chlorhexidine. Scot Med J 1989;34:525-528.

64. Yasuda T, Yoshimura Y, Takada H, et al. Comparison of bactericidal effects of commonly used antiseptics against pathogens causing nosocomial infections. Part 2. Dermatology 1997;195S:19-28.

65. Aggett PJ, Cooper LV, Ellis SH: McAinsh J. Percutaneous absorption of chlorhexidine in neonatal cord care. Arch Dis Childhood 1981;56:878-891.

66. Belfrage E, Enocksson E, Kalin M, et al. Comparative efficiency of chlorhexidine and ethanol in umbilical cord care. Scand J Infect Dis 1985;17:413-420.

67. Verber IG, Pagan FS. What cord care—if any? Arch Dis Childhood 1993;68:594-596.

68. Smales O. A comparison of umbilical cord treatment in the control of superficial infection. NZ Med J 1988;101:453-455.

69. Andrich MP, Golden SM. Umbilical cord care. A study of bacitracin ointment vs. triple dye. Clin Pediatr 1984;23:342-344.

70. Wald ER, Snyder MJ, Gutberlet RL. Group beta-hemolytic streptococcal colonization. Acquisition, persistence, and effect of umbilical cord treatment with triple dye. Am J Dis Children 1977;131:178-180.

71. Paes B, Jones CC. An audit of the effect of two cord-care regimens on bacterial colonization in newborn infants. Qual Rev Bull 1987;13:109-113.

72. Editorial staff. Poisindex system. Englewood, CO: Micromedex,1996.

73. LeBlanc MH. Thermoregulation: Incubators, radiant warmers, artificial skins, and body hoods. Clin Perinatol 1991; 18:403-422.

74. Hammarlund K, Sedin G. Transepidermal water loss in newborn infants. Acta Pediatri Scand 1982;71:191-196.

75. Baumgart S, Fox WW, Polin RA. Physiologic implications of two different heat shields for infants under radiant warmers. J Pediatr 1982;100:787-790.

76. Gelman CR, Rumack BH, Hess AJ. Hyaluronidase. Englewood, CO: Micromedex, 1996.

77. Baumgart S. Reduction of oxygen consumption. Insensible water loss and radiant heat demand with use of a plastic blanket for low-birth-weight infants under radiant warmers. Pediatrics 1984;74:1022-1028.

78. Besch NJ, Perlstein PH, Edwards NK, et al. The transparent baby bag: a shield against heat loss. N Engl J Med 1971; 284: 121-124.

79. Marks KH, Friedman Z, Maisels MJ. A simple device for reducing insensible water loss in low-birth-weight infants. Pediatrics 1977;60:223-226.

80. Knauth A, Gordin M, McNeils W, et al. Semipermeable polyurethane membrane as an artificial skin for the premature neonate. J Pediatr 1989;83:945-950.

81. Vernon HJ, Lane AT, Wischerath LJ, et al. Semipermeable dressing and transepidermal water loss in premature infants. J Pediatr 1990;86:357-362.

82. Barak M, Hershkowitz S, Rod R, et al. The use of a synthetic skin covering as a protective layer in the daily care of low birth weight infants. Eur J Pediatr 1989;148:665-666.

83. Mancini AJ, Sookdeo-Drost S, Madison KC, et al. Semipermeable dressings improve epidermal barrier function in premature infants. Pediatr Res 1994;36:306-314.

84. Schwayder T, Hetzel F. Effects of emollients on skin temperature under infrared warmers. 5th International Congress of Pediatric Dermatology, Milan, Italy, July 1989; (Abstract).

85. Dinehart SM, Dillard R, Raimer SS, et al. Cutaneous manifestations of acrodynia (pink disease). Arch Dermatol 1988; 124:107-109.

86. Goldbloom RB, Goldbloom A. Boric acid poisoning. J Pediatr 1953;43:631-643.

87. Abidel-Magid EHM, El Awad Ahmed FR. Salicylate intoxication in an infant with ichthyosis transmitted through skin ointment. Pediatrics 1994;94:939-940.

88. Payne CM, Bladin C, Colchester AC, et al. Argyria from excessive use of topical silver sulphadiazine. Lancet 1992;340 (8811):126.

89. Anonymous. High plasma urea concentrations in collodion babies. Arch Dis Child 1987;62:212.

90. Gelman CR, Rumack BH, Hess AJ. Benzocaine. Englewood, CO: Micromedex, 1996.

91. Frayling IM, Addison GM, Chattergee K, et al. Methaemoglobinaemia in children treated with prilocaine-lignocaine cream. Br Med Journal 1990;301:153-154.

92. Reynolds JEF. Prilocaine hydrochloride. Englewood, CO: Micromedex, 1996.

93. Porat R, Gilbert S, Magilner D. Methylene blue-induced phototoxicity: An unrecognized complication. Pediatrics 1996; 97:717-721.

94. MacDonald MG, et al. Propylene glycol: increased incidence of seizures in low birth weight infants. Pediatrics 1987; 79:622-625.

95. van Shooten FJ, et al. Are coal-tar shampoos safe? Lancet 1994;344:1505-1506.

6

Diagnostic and Therapeutic Procedures

BARI B. CUNNINGHAM
ANNETTE M. WAGNER

Diagnostic and therapeutic procedures play an important role in the field of neonatal dermatology. Confirmation of suspected diagnoses can often be rapidly obtained with simple office-based procedures such as potassium hydroxide (KOH) preparation, Tzanck smears, hair mounts, or scabies preps. Laboratory tests such as Gram-stained smears, skin cultures, and direct fluorescent antibody testing can identify pathogenic organisms that enable directed therapy. Skin biopsy can provide invaluable information when histopathologic examination is appropriately combined with special stains, immunofluorescence, polymerase chain reactions (PCRs), immunohistochemistry, or electron microscopy.

Performing procedures in neonates can be technically challenging and requires careful attention to pediatric issues such as increased toxicity of anesthetic agents. Special dressings and postoperative wound instructions are often necessary to avert complications following procedures.

Many genetic skin diseases can be diagnosed prenatally with the aid of specific genetic and metabolic tests such as PCR or fluorescence in situ hybridization (FISH). Chromosomal analysis may be helpful in the diagnosis of certain congenital dermatologic diseases.

This chapter reviews common diagnostic and therapeutic procedures in neonatal dermatology and provides a "How To" guide for the practitioner. Appropriate use of diagnostic testing and the current status of genetic, metabolic, and prenatal diagnosis are discussed. In anticipation of rapid advances in these areas, referral sources for up-to-date information in these fields are provided.

SPECIFIC DIAGNOSTIC PROCEDURES

Potassium Hydroxide Preparation and Fungal Cultures

Potassium hydroxide examination of skin, hair, and nails for suspected fungal infection is one of the most commonly used diagnostic procedures in dermatology. Adequate specimen collection is critical and varies by diagnostic site.

Scrapings of the skin for KOH preparation and fungal culture should be collected from the margins of the lesions because this is the area of active growth of the fungus. Some authors recommend cleansing the skin with alcohol before scraping to reduce bacterial contamination.[1] Unfortunately, this procedure removes much of the scale, making collection of adequate material difficult. The use of antibacterial agents in the fungal culture media is a preferable method for preventing bacterial overgrowth of cultures.

Collection of skin scrapings is accomplished using a #15 scalpel blade, the edge of a glass microscopic slide, or a foman blade.[2] The foman blade, a two-sided, spatula-like instrument, is less likely to inadvertently cut the skin of a moving infant. An adequate specimen should be collected so that if the KOH preparation is equivocal, a fungal culture can be performed without repeating the collection procedure.[3] If blisters are present, use a curved iris scissors to remove the blister roof for examination. KOH preparation technique is outlined in Box 6-1. Hyphae should be differentiated from cell walls, fabric fibers, and small hairs (Fig. 6-1). Cell walls have an irregular linearity;

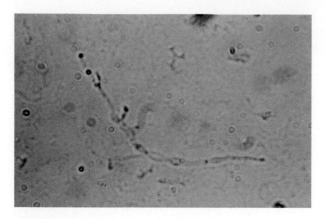

FIG. 6-1
KOH preparation for detection of dermatophytes ×100. Note branching hyphae.

BOX 6-1

KOH Preparation Technique

1. **Select an area of the lesion.** The margin of a lesion is recommended.
2. Using a #15 blade, edge of a microscopic slide, or foman blade, scrape gently across the edge of the scaling skin plaque using the motion of a knife spreading butter on bread.
3. Gently **drop the skin scrapings onto** a glass slide by tapping the edge of the blade against the glass. Material may be swept into a pile using the blade, or cover slip, and cover slip applied.
4. Apply a few drops of 10% to 20% KOH to the edge of the cover slip, and apply gentle pressure to the surface to flatten the scales.
5. **Rack down the substage condenser and put the light on low.**
6. **Scan and focus the smear** on 4-100× objectives, scanning the material at low power until suspicious areas are identified and then switching to higher power to confirm the diagnosis.

---

threads appear uniform and lack internal structures. Ink-containing KOH preparations (Swartz-Lamkin) are available to enhance the hyphae and increase the yield of positive examinations.

Scalp scrapings can be obtained in a similar manner. If culture material is needed, a toothbrush, a gynecologic viral collection brush, or a wet cotton-tipped applicator can be rubbed against the scalp surface and placed in the col-lection container or directly on the culture medium.[4] Hair samples from the scalp can be examined directly for the presence of fungus. Often, scraping with the blade is sufficient to retrieve enough hairs for a KOH preparation or culture without the trauma of "pulling."

Collection of fungal samples from nails is particularly challenging. A 2 or 3 mm skin curette may be used to scrape out subungual debris, which may be more accessible when the nail is trimmed. Alternatively, a #15 blade can be directed away from the digit toward the underside of the nail to dislodge material. If the suspected infection is on the nail surface, the blade should be used to gently scrape the superficial surface of the nail plate.

Mycosel agar (Baltimore Biological Co.) and *Mycobiotic agar* (Difco Co.) are commonly used fungal culture media composed of Sabouraud dextrose agar containing chloramphenicol and cycloheximide to reduce bacterial overgrowth. Dermatophyte test medium (DTM) is a simplified culture system for the detection of dermatophytes. When the culture is positive, dye in the media turns red. Certain nondermatophytes, such as *Aspergillus spp.* can also turn the media red, so colony morphology should also be evaluated. For most fungi, inoculated media can be kept at room temperature. The bottle caps should be kept loose to allow air into the culture bottle. Some diphasic fungi, such as *Cryptococcus spp.*, grow poorly at room temperature and should be incubated at 37° C.

For deep fungus, a skin biopsy must be performed. The collected tissue is ground into minute pieces and inoculated onto the culture media and/or stained for microscopic examination.

The yield of fungal culture is lowest for nails. This can be particularly problematic when distinction between psoriatic and fungal nails is necessary, but is not a major clinical issue in neonates or young infants. Distal nail clippings can be submitted for routine histology and periodic acid-Schiff staining to look for microscopic evidence of fungus.[5] The yield of this procedure has been demonstrated to be superior to KOH preparation and equal to fungal culture.

Bacterial Cultures and Stains

Normal skin is colonized with a variety of bacteria. Pathogenic bacteria must be identified and distinguished from "normal" flora to enable appropriate medical therapy of primary or secondary skin infection. A Gram-stained smear of material from lesions suspected of bacterial infection can allow for preliminary identification of the infecting organism and provide a guide to appropriate therapy. The presence of polymorphonuclear leukocytes, together with large numbers of bacteria, usually indicates infection.

BOX 6-2

Tzanck Smear Technique

1. **Select a lesion.** The yield for obtaining a positive smear is highest from a fresh vesicle, followed by a pustule, and then a crusted lesion.
2. **Wipe the lesion** with alcohol and allow it to dry for 1 minute.
3. Using a #15 blade, either remove the crust or **unroof the vesicle** or pustule.
4. Using a #15 blade at an angle of less than 90 degrees, **scrape the lesion** base with the edge of the blade.
5. Gently **transfer the material** from the blade to a glass slide by repeatedly and gently touching the blade to the slide. (Forceful smearing will grind the cells, resulting in crushed nuclei.)

6. Allow the smear to **air dry** (alternately, tissue may be heat fixed or fixed in methanol).
7. **Flood the slide with staining solution** for 30 to 60 seconds. Use either Giemsa, Wright, methylene blue, or toluidine blue stains.
8. **Rinse excess stain** off of the slide with tap water and allow the slide to **air dry.**
9. Apply one or two **drops of immersion oil or tap water.** Then place **cover slip** over the slide.
10. **Rack up the substage condenser** toward the stage and adjust the field diaphragm for optimal illumination and resolution.

Cultured skin specimens should be plated on blood agar and inoculated into a thioglycollate (anaerobic) broth. If infection with gram-negative rods is suspected, MacConkey or EMB agar plates should be inoculated. Suspected meningococcal and gonococcal infections should be plated on Thayer-Martin or chocolate agar plates in a CO_2 atmosphere. Anaerobic cultures for suspected anaerobic streptococcus, *Bacteroides*, and *Clostridium* should be plated on blood agar.

Early identification of infecting organisms is critical in certain rapidly progressive skin infections such as necrotizing faciitis. Gram stain and culture of overlying skin has a low yield; the growth of organisms takes several days, even when cultures are positive. Biopsy of skin for frozen section has improved the rapidity of diagnosis in this disease. The use of a rapid streptococcus test can be helpful in the early identification of streptococcal infection in necrotizing faciitis.[6]

Tzanck Preparation

Microscopic examination of cells obtained from the base of a vesicle or bulla (Tzanck smear) is used primarily for the diagnosis of viral processes, including herpes simplex and varicella zoster viruses. First introduced in 1947 as a rapid technique for evaluating cutaneous blistering, the Tzanck smear remains widely used[7] despite the development of more sophisticated, but costly techniques. This examination can be used for evaluation of other noninfectious causes of vesiculopustules in the neonate. Its use in diseases such as toxic epidermal necrolysis, staphylococcal scalded skin syndrome,[8] pem-

phigus vulgaris,[9] and Langerhans' cell histiocytosis[10] has been well documented.

The technique for performing Tzanck preparations is described in Box 6-2. The tissue can be air-dried, heat-fixed, or fixed in methanol before staining. Various commercially prepared stains can be used to provide nuclear detail, including Giemsa, crystal violet, toluidine blue, Hemacolor, thiazine-xanthene (Diff Quik, Baxter Healthcare Corp., Miami, Fla.), and others. Multinucleated giant cells are seen on high, dry power and can be diagnostic of varicella or herpes simplex infection. Examination with the oil immersion objective is often helpful in equivocal cases. Caution must be taken not to over interpret clumped epithelial or white blood cells as indicative of giant cells. To be positive, epidermal nuclei should be "molded" together with nuclear membranes that appear to be indenting each other. Homogeneous, ground-glass nucleoplasm is also characteristic of the multinucleated giant cell[11] (Fig. 6-2). Tzanck preparations, along with evaluation of free-floating blister contents by Gram or Wright stain, may display characteristic findings of a variety of diseases, as described in Table 6-1.

Direct Fluorescent Antibody Test for Diagnosis of Herpesvirus Infection

Despite its utility as a screening tool, the Tzanck preparation has limited sensitivity and specificity. The direct fluorescent antibody (DFA) test is a rapid, cost-effective, sensitive, and highly specific[12] method for detecting and distinguishing cutaneous herpes simplex virus (HSV 1 and 2) and varicella zoster virus (VZV) infections. Direct immunofluorescence is most sensitive on vesicles, less sensitive on pustules, and even less so on crusted lesions.[13] DFA testing uses monoclonal antibodies directed against type-specific glycoprotein epitopes of the herpesvirus envelope.[14] The base of a blister, erosion, or ulcer is aggressively scraped at the bedside. The material is then smeared on a glass slide and sent to the appropriate laboratory. Clinicians should consult hospital laboratories regarding requirements for obtaining samples for DFA examination. Some laboratories request commercially prepared, dual-welled glass slides to be inoculated as controls. Slides are prepared with a few drops of fluorescein-conjugated murine monoclonal antibodies against HSV 1 and 2 (prepared as a 1:1 mixture) or VZV. After approximately 30 minutes the slides are rinsed and examined by epifluorescence microscopy. Slides emitting bright-green cytoplasmic fluorescence are positive.[15] False-positive DFA results have been reported in rare instances.[16]

Viral Culture

Although Tzanck smears and DFA technique can provide rapid results in suspected viral infection, the gold standard remains viral culture. After absorbing the fluid of the vesicle with a Dacron-tipped applicator and firmly rubbing the base of the vesicle, the applicator should be placed in a sterile tube containing at least 3 ml of viral transport medium (buffered isotonic balanced salt solution, traditionally containing penicillin and streptomycin or gentamycin to prevent bacterial contamination. Recent studies suggest that less contamination occurs with the addition of vancomycin and amikacin.[17] Specimens should be refrigerated or transported on ice for best results.

Culture techniques are most useful in suspected herpes virus infection. Herpes simplex virus produces identifiable changes in culture cells in 2 to 3 days, and culture techniques are quite sensitive. Varicella-zoster is more difficult to culture and can take 7 to 14 days with frequent false-negative results.[18]

Polymerase chain reaction is now being used more widely in the diagnosis of many viral infections and in attempts to find the etiology of many common skin disorders of unknown etiology.[19, 20, 21] Studies using PCR in the identification of herpes infection in keratoconjuctivitis[22] and in primary genital herpes[23] have found the assay to be superior to viral culture in sensitivity and in ease of collection.

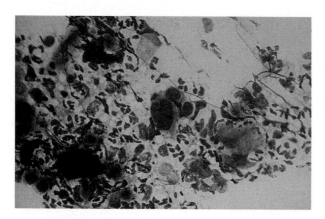

FIG. 6-2
Multinucleated giant cell on Tzanck smear.

TABLE 6-1

Findings on Tzanck Smears of Blister Scrapings and Wright/Gram Stains of Blister Fluid Contents of Selected Neonatal Cutaneous Conditions

Transient neonatal pustular melanosis	Large numbers of polymorphonuclear leukocytes
Pustular psoriasis	Large numbers of polymorphonuclear leukocytes
Acropustulosis of infancy	Large numbers of polymorphonuclear leukocytes
Incontinenti pigmenti	Large numbers of eosinophils
Erythema toxicum neonatorum	Large numbers of eosinophils
Eosinophilic pustular folliculitis	Large numbers of eosinophils
Toxic epidermal necrolysis	Cuboidal cells with high nuclear to cytoplasmic ratio; inflammatory cells present
Staphylococcal scalded skin syndrome	Broad epidermal cells without inflammation
Histiocytosis	Histiocytes with oval nuclei with longitudinal grooves or "kidney bean" shape
Varicella or herpes simplex	Multinucleated giant cells

Scabies/Ectoparasite Preparations

The most difficult part of a scabies preparation is finding the appropriate lesion to sample. A linear burrow is an excellent place to scrape but may prove hard to identify. On young infants and children, where mites abound, the palms are a highly fruitful location because hands and fingers are used for rubbing and scratching. Finger webs, wrists, feet, axillae, vesicles, and untouched pink papules are good sites for scraping.[24] The technique for scabies preparations is described in Box 6-3.

Moving mites are generally easily visible and can be viewed quickly under scanning power. Mites are 0.2 to 0.4 mm in size with four pairs of legs (Fig. 6-3). Eggs are oval and one tenth of the size of the mite. Feces are also oval but golden brown in color and usually occur in clumps (Fig. 6-4). Air bubbles are the biggest artifacts present in scabies preparations. Gently pressing on the cover slip can dislodge these. In addition, trapped air is round, whereas ova and feces are usually oval.

Epiluminescent microscopy (ELM), utilizing a handheld magnifier through which skin can be viewed through a layer of oil, can also be helpful in the identification of scabies on the skin.[25] Mites appear as dark triangular structures resulting from pigment in the anterior section of the thorax.

Microscopic Hair Examination

Various hair shaft abnormalities can be detected by simple bedside diagnostic examination. Table 6-2 lists the microscopic hair findings in certain syndromes. Hair can be examined with the light microscope, both with and without the use of polarizing lenses (see Fig. 26-31). More detailed information can be obtained from the scanning and or transmission electron microscopic examination of hair. In general, hair obtained for microscopic examination should be snipped rather than pulled. This avoids unnecessary trauma and discomfort for the infant while eliminating artifacts produced by force of epilation. A few clinical scenarios (e.g., loose anagen syndrome) involve actual abnormalities of the hair bulb, which requires that hair be pulled with its root for examination. Most hair abnormalities seen in the neonate involve scalp hair. The hair changes of Netherton syndrome, however, are variable and often absent from scalp hair. The diagnosis of Netherton syndrome can be made in these patients by sampling eye-

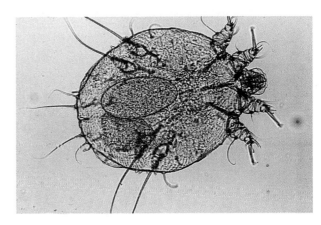

FIG 6-3
Scabies prep demonstrating mite *Sarcoptes scabeii*.

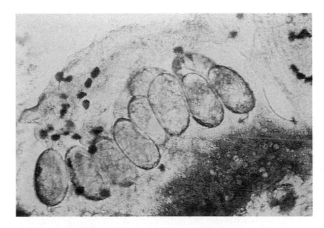

FIG. 6-4
Scabies prep demonstrating feces and eggs.

BOX 6-3

Mineral Oil Scraping for Scabies

1. **Select a good site** such as palms, web spaces, wrists, or obvious burrows that are not excoriated.
2. **Apply mineral oil to a #15 blade.** You may also want to cover the lesion to be sampled with mineral oil to reduce pain and friction.
3. **Scrape the lesion vigorously** five to six times to remove the stratum corneum. Punctate bleeding will demonstrate that you are at the correct depth.
4. **Apply mineral oil to a glass slide.**
5. Immerse the #15 blade in the oil and transfer the onto the glass slide.
6. **Add a coverslip** to the glass slide.
7. **View under microscope on low power** (4× or 10×). Mites, eggs, or feces are all recognizable (see Figs. 6-3 and 6-4).

TABLE 6-2

Hair Examination of Selected Clinical Conditions in the Newborn

Condition	Microscopic hair findings
Netherton syndrome	Light microscopy: "ball and socket" configuration or trichorrhexis invaginata[27, 28], may include golf-tee[29] or tuliplike[26] configurations. May show circumferential strictures (earliest stage of invagination)
Menkes syndrome	Light microscopy: classically reveals pili torti or twisted hair, but monilethrix and trichorrhexis nodosa[30] also reported
Trichothiodystrophy	Light microscopy: wavy, irregular outline with a flattened shaft with folded ribbon configuration. Polarized microscopy: light and dark bands or "tiger tail" pattern
Chédiak-Higashi syndrome	Light microscopy: evenly distributed small, granular melanin aggregates[31]
Griscelli syndrome	Light microscopy: large, unevenly distributed melanin aggregates, primarily located in the medulla

---

BOX 6-4

Technique for Performing A Punch Biopsy

1. Biopsy the freshest, most recent lesion.
2. Cleanse the skin with alcohol or antiseptic.
3. Anesthetize with 1% lidocaine with epinephrine using a 30-gauge needle.
4. Stretch the skin between the thumb and forefinger. Using firm, downward pressure, twist and rotate the biopsy punch back and forth until it pops through to the fat.
5. Cut the base of the specimen with a scissors. Care should be taken not to crush the tissue with forceps.
6. Place the specimen in formalin fixative for routine histopathologic examination.
7. Specimens for culture should be placed on a sterile gauze soaked with nonbacteriostatic saline in a sterile container.
8. Close the defect by placing a simple interrupted suture (using 4.O Prolene or Nylon).
9. Apply antibiotic ointment and adhesive bandage (Band-Aid).
10. Remove sutures in 7 to 10 days.

---

brow or eyelash hair.[26] The reader is referred to Chapter 26 for a detailed discussion of hair disorders in the neonate.

Skin Biopsy

One of the most useful diagnostic tests in dermatology is the skin biopsy. This simple technique allows for sampling of skin specimens for diagnostic testing, histopathologic examination, or culture. The type of biopsy performed depends on the size, the suspected depth, and the location on the skin of the lesion to be biopsied.

The **punch biopsy** is the most common method of skin sampling used in dermatology. This approach is excellent for complete removal of small lesions (<6 mm), and for skin sampling for diagnostic purposes by routine histology, immunofluorescence, electron microscopy, or culture. It may not be optimal if the suspected pathologic process is in the subcutaneous fat because of limited depth, or lesions confined to the epidermis and superficial dermis, because full-thickness skin is removed, and a more significant scar will result.

Punch biopsies are performed with reusable sterile Keyes skin punches or more commonly with inexpensive, extremely sharp, disposable punches. They can be purchased in sizes ranging from 2 to 6 mm. Typically a 3 or 4 mm punch biopsy is performed for diagnostic purposes. When specimens larger than 6 mm are required or if deeper biopsies containing fat or subcutaneous tissue are optimal for diagnosis or culture, a fusiform or excisional biopsy is indicated (Box 6-4).

Skin Biopsy/Specialized Tests

Special Stains

Routine skin biopsies are usually stained with hematoxylin-eosin (H&E), the standard staining method for tissue. In certain instances, "special staining" techniques are required to further delineate structures in the skin or pathologic organisms. Many histochemical special stains can be performed on formalin-fixed, paraffin-embedded material.

Electron Microscopy

Electron microscopy (EM) uses thin (1 micron) tissue sections to allow high-resolution images of nuclear membrane abnormalities and organelle changes, which are not routinely seen with light microscopy.[25] It may be very useful in establishing the diagnoses of several diseases, such as Langerhans' cell histiocytosis and epidermolysis bullosa (EB). Specimens for EM may be obtained by punch biopsy and placed in glutaraldehyde fixative. For EB, rotary traction may be applied to the skin just before biopsy in an attempt to elicit a microscopic cleavage plane. This can be achieved by the gentle rotary traction (pushing and twisting) of an eraser tip on the skin. The traumatized skin is then locally anesthetized, and a punch biopsy is performed. Transmission EM (TEM) allows for precise localization of the ultrastructural level of cleavage within a given specimen, thereby differentiating simplex, junctional, and dystrophic types of EB.[32] Centers vary widely, however, in their experience with the electron microscopic diagnosis of EB, and referral of the specimen to a major medical center with significant expertise and experience in the ultramicroscopic features of EB should be considered.

Immunofluorescence

Two types of immunofluorescence tests can be performed. *Direct* immunofluorescence tests for immunoreactants localized in the tissues of the patient's skin or mucous membrane, whereas *indirect* immunofluorescence testing detects circulating antibodies in the patient's serum. Although indirect immunofluorescence is less sensitive than direct immunofluorescence, it may, at times, provide valuable supplementary diagnostic information.

Direct Immunofluorescent Microscopy

Direct immunofluorescent microscopy may be useful for the diagnosis of immune-mediated vesiculobullous diseases, lupus erythematosus, and leukocytoclastic vasculitis. A perilesional biopsy (next to but not including a fresh blister) should be biopsied (Box 6-5). Frozen sections are incubated with fluorescent-linked antibodies to human IgG, IgA, IgM, and C3, as well as other antibodies. Specimens

---

BOX 6-5

Biopsy Technique for Direct Immunofluorescence

1. Biopsy the freshest, most recent lesion.
2. Perilesional (normal) skin is most desirable. Never biopsy the base of an ulcer or center of a blister.
3. If the epidermis and dermis become detached during the procedure, submit both in separately labeled containers.
4. Place specimens in transport medium (Michel's transport medium or Zeus's fixative). Never place the specimen in formalin.
5. If transport medium is not available, cover skin biopsy with saline-soaked gauze and transport immediately to immunofluorescence laboratory for processing.

---

may be frozen until testing or kept in transport medium (Michel's medium: ammonium sulfate, N-ethylmaleimide, and magnesium sulfate in a citrate buffer) for at least 2 weeks without loss of reactivity.[33]

Indirect Immunofluorescent Microscopy

Various dilutions of the patient's serum are incubated on an epithelial substrate, usually primate esophagus. The circulating antibodies are reported as the highest positive dilution, or "titer." This diagnostic technique is useful for pemphigus vulgaris, pemphigus foliaceus, bullous pemphigoid, and other autoimmune blistering disorders.

Perhaps the most common neonatal application of these techniques is in the diagnosis of epidermolysis bullosa. In this case, a skin biopsy specimen is submitted for immunofluorescent antigenic mapping. Through this modified indirect immunofluorescence technique, the ultrastructural level of a blister can be determined based on the binding of antibodies having known ultrastructural binding sites.[32] The three most commonly used antibodies are those directed against bullous pemphigoid antigen, laminin, and type IV collagen.[32] Other antibodies directed against basement membrane components may be used as well.[34]

As with specimens obtained for electron microscopy, clinically normal skin is sampled and subjected to rotary traction. The specimen should be placed in an immunofluorescence transfer medium (Michel's, Zeus's) and forwarded to a reference laboratory experienced in antigenic mapping. Immunofluorescence antigenic mapping may offer several advantages over electron microscopy for the diagnosis of epidermolysis bullosa. The transport medium used for immunofluorescence is inexpensive and readily available, and specimens can be evaluated several weeks after biopsy, if necessary. Immunofluorescence antigenic mapping can be completed rapidly, within 2 hours of receipt of a given specimen, unlike electron microscopic examination, which can take up to several weeks to complete.[32] Immunofluorescence antigenic mapping is available at no cost for any patient enrolled in the national epidermolysis bullosa registry.[32] For additional information, contact the National Epidermolysis Bullosa Registry: phone (919) 966-2007; fax (919) 966-7080; email ljohnson @med.unc.edu; Web site http://www.med.unc.edu/derm/ ebr.html.

Immunohistochemistry/Cell-typing

In general, immunohistochemical procedures require fresh tissue, since formalin fixation and subsequent tissue processing may damage antigens localized to the cell membrane.[35] However, there are several antibodies that can be utilized on formalin-fixed, paraffin-embedded tissue.[36] The use of monoclonal and polyclonal antibodies can be helpful to determine the origin of a cell, especially if the cell appears anaplastic. However, false-negative staining can occur as a result of outdated or poorly diluted antibody preparations.[37] Furthermore, a cell may be so highly anaplastic that it loses the antigenic marker and does not stain positively. There is currently no antibody that uniformly distinguishes benign from malignant cells.

SURGICAL/PROCEDURAL ISSUES IN NEONATES

EMLA

EMLA cream is an eutectic mixture of local anesthetics (2.5% lidocaine and 2.5% prilocaine) in an oil-in-water emulsion that induces topical anesthesia of intact skin. Its use in infants is well established and generally safe if caution is exercised. EMLA is very useful for decreasing the pain of local anesthetic infiltration, lumbar puncture, subcutaneous drug reservoir punctures, intravenous catheter placement, and venipuncture and as anesthesia for superficial dermatologic procedures.[38,39] It induces anesthesia at a maximum depth of 5 mm, making its use alone inadequate for excisional surgery or punch biopsy. The degree, depth, and onset of anesthesia are related to the duration of application. Mucous membranes, genital skin, and inflamed skin absorb the product more rapidly, allowing for shorter application times (5 to 40 minutes) in these anatomic areas. Patch preparations of 5% EMLA are equally as effective and avoid leakage of the cream out of the occlusive dressing.[40]

	TABLE 6-3	
Parameters for the Safe Use of EMLA in Children*		
Body weight requirements	Maximum total dose of EMLA (g)	Maximum application area (cm²)
<5 kg	1	10
5-10 kg	2	20

*These guidelines are applicable to infants with intact, nondiseased skin.

EMLA should be used cautiously in infants less than 3 months of age because of the risk of associated methemoglobinemia. The development of methemoglobinemia from prilocaine is caused by two of its metabolites, 4 hydroxy-2 methylaniline and 2 methylanaline (o-toluidine), which lead to oxidation of hemoglobin. Young infants are more susceptible to drug-induced methemoglobinemia because they have lower levels of reduced nicotinamide adenine dinucleotide (NADH)–methemoglobin reductase, catalase, and glutathione peroxidase, higher levels of hemoglobin F, which is more susceptible to oxidation, and because the dose of lidocaine and prilocaine is usually greater per kilogram of body weight.[41,42,43,44] Patients with hemoglobinopathies or glucose-6-phosphate dehydrogenase deficiency may also be at greater risk.[45] Clinical cyanosis becomes apparent with a methemoglobin level at about 15%.[46] A few small studies of EMLA use in preterm infants and those less than 3 months of age have failed to detect methemoglobinemia in the absence of the concomitant medication use.[47] Short application times, and limited quantities of EMLA (less than 2 g) lower the risk of methemoglobinemia in young infants (Table 6-3). Medications that induce a methemoglobin stress and might increase the risk of EMLA-associated methemoglobinemia include sulfonamides, acetaminophen, benzocaine, dapsone, phenobarbital, antimalarials, and phenytoin.[48,49] Use of EMLA in infants less than 3 months is therefore not advised in the presence of the above medications.

EMLA is generally safe and well tolerated. Local side effects include transient blanching, erythema, eye irritation, edema, and dermatitis. Allergic contact dermatitis has been reported, with prilocaine as the implicated allergen in most studies.[50,51] A petechial or purpuric eruption has been observed after application of EMLA, in neonates, children, and adults[52,53] (Fig. 6-5). The eruption does not seem to be related to either dose or duration of applica-

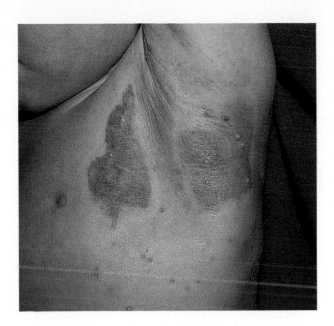

FIG. 6-5
Petechial eruption after application of EMLA cream.

TABLE 6-4		
Maximum Doses of 1% Lidocaine With and Without Epinephrine		
Type of lidocaine	Maximum dose	Maximum dose for 5 kg infant
1% Lidocaine without epinephrine	4.5 mg/kg	2.3 ml
1% Lidocaine with epinephrine	7 mg/kg	3.5 ml

tion. It appears during or immediately after EMLA application as early as 30 minutes after application. The purpura resolves spontaneously over days. Purpura may be more common in premature infants, especially those younger than 32 weeks' gestational age, and in patients with atopic dermatitis.[53] Patch testing to EMLA cream, prilocaine, lidocaine, emollient base, and Tegaderm plaster was negative in all patients tested in one study.[54] A direct toxic effect to capillary endothelium has been postulated. Rechallenge with EMLA after this reaction has been negative. Nevertheless, EMLA should be used cautiously, if at all, in infants with a history of this reaction.

To be effective, occlusive dressings for at least 1 to 2 hours are necessary to allow absorption of the lidocaine/prilocaine mixture into the skin, with the exception of genital and mucosal sites. Applications with non–airtight adhesive bandages (Band-Aids), gauze wraps, or other nonocclusive dressings will result in suboptimal anesthesia.

Lidocaine Toxicity

The two most widely used local anesthetics are lidocaine and bupivacaine (Marcaine/Sensorcaine). For most skin surgery, the recommended anesthetic is 1% lidocaine with epinephrine. Advantages of this drug combination include a negligible incidence of allergy, virtually instantaneous onset of anesthesia, and minimal bleeding caused by the epinephrine. The most common commercial preparation contains 1% lidocaine (10 mg/ml) and 1:100,000 of epi-

nephrine. Toxicity from lidocaine is extremely rare if dosed appropriately. Maximum recommended doses are listed in Table 6-4.

Although data on lidocaine pharmacokinetics in neonates are limited, it appears that the elimination half-life of lidocaine is prolonged compared with that in adults.[55,56] The volume of distribution of lidocaine in neonates is at least twofold higher than in adults partially resulting from lidocaine's diminished binding to plasma proteins.[55,56] In neonates, only 20% of lidocaine is protein bound as compared with 60% to 70% protein binding in adults.[57,58] This increased bioavailability may make neonates more susceptible to lidocaine toxicity than older patients at a given serum concentration.[59]

Lidocaine, in general, has a low incidence of systemic toxicity. Toxic reactions can occur and can range from cardiovascular or central nervous system reactions to death. Central nervous system toxicity may begin with agitation and progress to convulsions, unconsciousness, and respiratory depression. Early detection of lidocaine toxicity in infants can be difficult because of problems detecting early signs such as lightheadedness, dizziness, and confusion. The safe use of viscous lidocaine in neonates has been questioned because of reports of seizures following its use.[60,61] Furthermore, a recent report of recurrent seizures in a neonate after intravenous lidocaine administration at a standard dose suggests that lidocaine may have greater toxicity in neonates and infants with a developing central nervous system.[59] Additional pharmacokinetic studies are indicated to better define appropriate lidocaine dosing in this population.

Preoperative Care and Complications

Postoperative wound care in the neonate is usually straightforward and uncomplicated but requires adequate parental instruction. Teaching wound care to the family of the patient is best done following the surgical procedure. The family is usually preoccupied and anxious before the procedure and unable to pay attention to information pertaining to postoperative care. Written and verbal instructions for postoperative wound care should be provided. If daily cleansing of the wound is recommended, the family should be encouraged to look at the wound before application of the dressing so that they are prepared for the postoperative appearance of the wound.

There is great variability in recommendations for wound care in dermatology.[62,63,64] The need for daily cleansing of a sterilely induced sutured wound is debatable.[65] Although laboratory studies have suggested that hydrogen peroxide is toxic to epithelial cells,[66] it is unclear whether this has any clinical relevance, since most wounds cleansed with this agent heal without difficulty. Despite its global acceptance and use as a wound cleanser, hydrogen peroxide is a poor antiseptic.[67] Its benefits are likely a consequence of the debridement induced by its effervescence rather than its antimicrobial properties.[67] Therefore the use of hydrogen peroxide for wound cleansing is best reserved for those wounds that are crusted and in need of gentle debridement.

The goal of wound management is to minimize bacterial colonization while providing a moist wound environment.[68] For most surgical wounds encountered in pediatric patients, a nonsensitizing topical antibiotic, such as bacitracin or polymyxin B and bacitracin, covered by a nonadherent dressing will suffice. Because of the risk of allergic contact dermatitis, topical antibiotics without neomycin are generally recommended. Enhanced wound healing with topical antibiotics is likely a result of the moist environment provided and not a result of their antimicrobial activity. Wounds treated with petrolatum alone reepithelialize faster than untreated wounds.[69,70]

The use of topical silver sulfadiazine (Silvadene) in neonates is probably best avoided because of reports of transient leukopenia following application.[71] Because neonatal skin, especially that of young premature infants, is more fragile than that of older children or adults, adhesive dressings should be used as sparingly as possible.

OTHER DIAGNOSTIC TESTS

Nikolsky's Sign

Nikolsky first defined this clinical sign in 1927, in a description of a patient with pemphigus foliaceous.[72] It has since become a clinical tool for evaluating blistering diseases. Gentle lateral pressure is applied to the normal skin

surface, or adjacent to a bulla, vesicle, or erosion, either with the thumb or with an object such as a pencil eraser. Separation of the epidermis from the dermis with this lateral pressure is considered a positive Nikolsky's sign, indicating altered structural integrity of the skin, either at the dermal epidermal junction or within the epidermis. A similar lack of skin attachment can be demonstrated by applying vertical pressure with the thumb on the top of an intact bulla or vesicle, causing extension of the bulla into apparently normal skin.

Although Nikolsky's sign was classically applied to pemphigus, it occurs in several diseases, including toxic epidermal necrolysis, bullous erythema multiforme, staphylococcal scalded skin,[73] bullous impetigo, and epidermolysis bullosa. Some authors have suggested that several of the disorders characterized by a positive Nikolsky's sign can be further distinguished by examining the skin at the base of the bulla.[74] If the base of the skin is dry, referred to as a dry Nikolsky's sign, this implies a subcorneal blistering process such as pemphigus foliaceus or staphylococcal scalded skin. If the base of the bulla is moist, glistening, and exudative, which is referred to as a wet Nikolsky's sign, the level of split of the skin is deeper in an intraepidermal or subepidermal location such as toxic epidermal necrolysis or bullous erythema multiforme or pemphigus vulgaris. The exception to this rule is bullous impetigo, where the subcorneal split is very wet because of the presence of severe inflammation.

Darier's Sign

Gentle stroking of skin lesions in mastocytosis or urticaria pigmentosa produces edema, erythema, induration, and sometimes vesiculation of the skin surface, called a Darier's sign. Changes in the skin reflect mast cell degranulation from rubbing and the effect of potent mediators released from these cells on the blood vessels in the surrounding skin. Caution should be taken to rub gently in the case of a suspected solitary mastocytoma because blistering is not uncommon following manipulation. A history of a positive Darier's sign can often be obtained from the parents, helping to confirm the diagnosis.

Insect bites and papular urticaria can also produce a positive Darier's sign as a result of release of histamine into the skin. Recent reports have described a positive Darier's sign in non-Hodgkin's lymphoma,[75] leukemia cutis,[76] and cutaneous T-cell lymphoma.[77]

A **pseudo-Darier's sign** can be observed in patients with cutaneous smooth muscle hamartomas.[78,79,80] Smooth muscle hamartomas comprise a collection of arrector pili muscles. Rubbing of the surface of these lesions produces piloerection and temporary induration that can appear similar to a Darier's sign. This feature can be very useful in distinguishing smooth muscle hamartomas from congenital nevi because both are pigmented congenital lesions with hypertrichosis.

Darkfield Examination

Darkfield examination is an infrequently performed examination used to detect *Treponema pallidum,* the pathologic organism in syphilis. The spirochete is most likely to be detected in nasal discharge or scrapings from moist mucocutaneous lesions, but specimens from the mouth should be avoided because of the presence of normal oral spirochetes, which can be mistaken for *T. pallidum.* With a special condenser (darkfield) and a funnel stage for the lens, any microscope can be converted to a darkfield microscope. This technique uses an oblique beam of light, which refracts off small particles undetectable with conventional optics. Considerable experience is needed for mastery of this technique. The key to successful diagnosis with a darkfield examination is in the collection of the specimen. The procedure is described in Box 6-6.[81]

Wood's Light Examination

The Wood's lamp is helpful in the clinical evaluation of cutaneous pigmentary disease, selected cutaneous infections, and porphyria. Long wave ultraviolet radiation, or black light, is emitted from a high-pressure mercury lamp fitted with a filter made of nickel oxide and silica. This results in light emitted with wavelengths ranging from 320 to 400 nm. Melanin is absorbed at these wavelengths so that minor losses of melanin in skin are accentuated. Hypopigmentation appears somewhat paler than sur-

---

BOX 6-6

Technique for Darkfield Examination

1. While wearing gloves, clean the surface of the lesion with dry gauze.
2. Touch a cover slip to serous fluid expressed from a lesion.
3. Drop the cover slip on a drop of saline on a glass slide.
4. Examine immediately (if possible at the bedside); do not let the specimen dry out.
5. Spirochetes, if present, will be seen as undulating and rotating corkscrew-shaped organisms.

---

rounding normal skin, while, depending on baseline normal pigmentation, depigmentation is starkly contrasted with surrounding skin.[82]

Early subclinical hypopigmented macules of tuberous sclerosis and streaky hypopigmentation seen in hypomelanosis of Ito,[83] for example, are often detected with the Wood's lamp, making this an essential tool in the evaluation of infants with possible tuberous sclerosis and pigmentary disease. Use of the lamp is often extended to examination of the parents of infants with possible incontinentia pigmenti or tuberous sclerosis.

Wood's lamp examination can also be extended to nonpigmentary cutaneous pathology. For example, various dermatologic conditions have characteristic fluorescent patterns, including yellow-green fluorescence of hair in selected dermatophyte infections (e.g., *Microsporum canis*), yellow-green fluorescence of skin in *Pseudomonas* infection, and pinkish-red fluorescence of urine in porphyria.

Specific Genetic and Metabolic Testing

Polymerase Chain Reaction

The polymerase chain reaction is one of the most significant breakthroughs for medical diagnosis of the twentieth century.[84,85] First described in 1985,[86] PCR is an efficient, economic, and sensitive method used to detect even minute amounts of DNA. Specific DNA sequences are amplified using repetitive automated cycling.[87] At the end of one cycle, the quantity of DNA present is doubled. Expansion of a particular genetic sequence is therefore exponential (2^n, with n representing the number of cycles). Twenty cycles of PCR results in a theoretic yield of approximately 1 million copies of the original DNA sequence. This allows detection of a specific DNA sequence, even if present in minute amounts, in any specimen.[88]

Detection of foreign DNA is important in the diagnosis of infectious diseases. Practical dermatologic applications include the identification of infectious agents, which is especially helpful in neonates for whom serologic methods may be unreliable, viral cultures unproductive, and results delayed.[89,90,91,92]

PCR is also useful to detect genetic mutations for genetic disease diagnosis and for oncology. The technique has been used to detect chromosomal translocations in leukemias and lymphomas in children.[93] PCR is 100,000 times more sensitive than cytogenetic studies and 10,000 times more sensitive than flow cytometry or Southern blotting techniques in detecting chromosomal translocations.[94]

PCR is proving to be of immense value in the prenatal diagnosis of a number of genetic disorders, including dermatologic diseases. Any genetic diseases in which the defective gene is known can be potentially diagnosed using PCR technology. PCR can be used to analyze minute amounts of fetal genetic material. Because the genes for many inherited skin conditions have been or are in the process of being identified, the future applications of PCR are great. PCR has also been performed on single cells removed at the blastomere stage, allowing identification of defective genes in in vitro fertilization programs[95] (see later section, Prenatal Diagnosis).

The remarkable sensitivity of PCR makes testing under the most stringent of laboratory conditions essential. Contaminations of minute amounts of extraneous DNA can be disastrous and lead to potentially erroneous results. Appropriate positive and negative controls are essential. False-negative results can also occur. Rarely, DNA sequences may be lost because the material sought may be denatured by the use of inappropriate tissue fixatives.[96]

A major advantage of PCR is that it can be performed on minimal amounts of tissue. Both the quantity of the sample and the transport medium requirements for PCR are liberal.[97] For identification of herpes simplex virus DNA, for example, the amount of tissue used for a Tzanck smear is sufficient. Viral culture medium is effective for transport and is often readily available at the bedside.[97] Fresh, fresh-frozen, formalin-fixed, and even paraffin-embedded specimens are acceptable for PCR testing.[98]

Fluorescence in situ Hybridization

Fluorescence in situ hybridization represents a unique technology in which molecular biologic and histochemical techniques are used to evaluate gene expression in tissue sections and cytologic preparations. With FISH, specific regions of the genome can be detected by applying complementary labeled nucleic acid probes.[99] After denaturation of the DNA, the probes can hybridize to target sequences on chromosomes and form a new DNA duplex. The hybridized probes are identified using fluorescence microscopy. With this technique, also referred to as interphase cytogenetics, karyotype changes can be detected at the single cell level. This technique allows for examination of chromosomal aberrations among morphologically or immunologically deficient cell populations present within a tumor sample, for example.

FISH methods have unlimited applications for clinical medicine and diagnostic pathology. For example, DNA probes can be used to identify foreign genes, including bacteria, viruses, and fungi. Detection of infectious agents with FISH techniques has been reported for human immunodeficiency virus, cytomegalovirus, herpes simplex virus, hepatitis B virus, and Epstein-Barr virus, among others.

PRENATAL DIAGNOSIS

Knowledge of specific gene defects for many genodermatoses has led to the development of DNA-based prenatal diagnosis, which has largely superceded older techniques such as fetoscopy and fetal skin biopsy. For example, PCR-based prenatal diagnosis of dystrophic and junctional EB has been performed through analysis of type VII collagen and laminin 5 genes of dystrophic and junctional EB, respectively,[100,101] and of keratin 10 for epidermolytic hyperkeratosis[102] and others. DNA may be derived through chorionic villus sampling (CVS) at 10 to 15 weeks' gestation or by amniocentesis at 12 to 15 weeks' gestation in families at risk for recurrence of EB. Periumbilical vein blood samples during the early weeks of pregnancy may provide an even earlier source of fetal DNA without any increased fetal risk.[103] In most cases, fetal cells are also cultured, and the test can be confirmed approximately 2 weeks later from the cultured fetal cells. Thus DNA-based prenatal diagnosis offers an early, expedient, and accurate method of prenatal testing for genodermatoses with known underlying disorders. It must be emphasized, however, that use of molecular techniques for prenatal diagnosis requires that the molecular defect is known. Although prenatal cytogenetic diagnosis based on amniocytes or chorionic villus cells is accurate, the procedure carries a risk of miscarriage. Because of this iatrogenic risk, CVS- or amniocentesis-based prenatal testing should be reserved for women at high risk for chromosomal abnormalities.

Preimplantation genetic diagnosis (PGD) is an alternative to conventional approaches to prenatal diagnosis. With this technique, the genetic abnormality in question is diagnosed before implantation of the fetus, allowing for selection of nonaffected, normal fetuses. DNA analysis and in vitro fertilization are utilized to select for a normal genotype before implantation. At the 6 to 10 cell stage, one cell is removed for DNA extraction and PCR amplification. Removal of one or two cells at this stage does not affect viability or the rate of development of the embryo(s). After analysis of DNA, only the embryos with normal DNA are implanted, theoretically ensuring that the implanted fetus will be normal. This technique has been used in families at risk for cystic fibrosis[104] and EB.

The field of prenatal diagnosis is developing at an astounding pace. New molecular, enzymatic, and ultrastructural markers will be available in the future, which will aid in the accuracy and utility of in utero or preimplantation diagnosis. Readers are referred to their local genetic centers for information regarding prenatal diagnosis of specific genetic diseases. The Internet is a valuable resource for current information on specific dermatologic conditions and their prenatal diagnosis. The Online Mendelian Inheritance in Man Web site, http://www.ncbi.nlm.nih.gov/Omim, is a database of human genes and genetic disorders. The database contains textual information, pictures, and valuable reference information. It also contains extensive links to the National Center for Biotechnical Information's Entrez database of MEDLINE articles and genetic sequencing information. For more clinically based genetic information, the Web site http://www. geneclinics.org may be helpful. *Helix* is a directory of medical genetic testing laboratories for health care professionals. The reader is referred to their Web site for comprehensive listing of medical genetics counselors, testing, and laboratory services: http://www.hslib.washington.edu/helix.

REFERENCES

1. Martin AG, Kobayashi GS. Superficial fungal infections: Dermatophytosis, tinea nigra, piedra. In Fitzpatrick TB, Eisen AZ, Wolff K, et al. Dermatology in general medicine. 4th edition. New York: McGraw-Hill, 1993: pp 2337-2359.

2. Truhan AP, Hebert AA, Esterly NB. The double-edge knife. Arch Dermatol 1985; 121:970.

3. Crissey JT. Common dermatophyte infections. A simple diagnostic test and current management. Postgrad Med 1998; 103:191-2, 197-200, 205.

4. Friedlander SF, Pickering B, Cunningham BB, et al. Use of the cotton swab method in diagnosing Tinea capitis. Pediatrics 1999;104:276-279

5. Machler BC, Kirsner RS, Elgart GW. Routine histologic examination for the diagnosis of onychomycosis: an evaluation of sensitivity and specificity. Cutis 1998;61:217-219.

6. Bourgeois SD, Bourgeois MH. Use of the rapid streptococcus test in extracellular sites. Am Fam Physician 1996; 54:1634-6.

7. Tzanck A. Le cyto-diagnostic immediat en dermatologie. Ann Dermatol Venereol 1947;7:68-70.

8. Buslau M, Biermann H, Shah PM. Gram-positive septic-toxic shock with bullae. Intraepidermal splitting as an indication of toxin effect. Hautarzt 1996;47:783-789.

9. Skeete, MV. Evaluation of the usefulness of immunofluorescence on Tzanck smears in pemphigus as an aid to diagnosis. Clin Experim Dermatol 1977;2:57-63.

10. Colon-Fontanez F, Eichenfield LE, Krous HF, Friedlander SF. Congenital langerhans cell histiocytosis: The utility of the Tzanck test as a diagnostic screening tool. Arch Dermatol 1998;134:1039-1040.

11. Solomon AR, Rasmussen JE, Varani J, et al. The tzanck smear in the diagnosis of cutaneous herpes simplex. JAMA 1984; 251:633-635.

12. Zirn JR, Tompkins SD, Huie C, Shea CR. Rapid detection and distinction of cutaneous herpesvirus infections by direct immunofluorescence. J Am Acad Dermatol 1995;33:724-728.

13. Bryson YJ, Conant MA, Solomon AR, et al. Questions and answers. J Am Acad Dermatol 1988;18:222-223.

14. Solomon AR. New diagnostic tests for herpes simplex and varicella zoster infections. J Am Acad Dermatol 1988;18: 218-221.

15. Erlich KS. Laboratory diagnosis of Herpesvirus infections. Clin Lab Med 1987;7:759-776.

16. Detlefs RL, Frieden IJ, Berger TG, Weston D. Eosinophil fluorescence: a cause of false positive slide tests for herpes simplex virus. Pediatr Dermatol 1987;4:129-133.

17. Lo JY, Lim WW, Tam BK, Lai MY. Vancomycin and amikacin in cell cultures for virus isolation. Pathology 1996;28:366-369.

18. Crumpacker CS, Gulick RM. Herpes simplex. In Fitzpatrick TB, Eisen AZ, Wolff K, et al. Dermatology in general medicine. 4th edition. New York: McGraw-Hill, 1993: pp 2414-2450.

19. Chen CL, Chow KC, Wong CK, et al. A study on Epstein-Barr virus in erythema multiforme. Arch Dermatol Res 1998;290:446-449.

20. Chang YT, Liu HN, Chen CL, et al. Detection of E.B.V. and HTL V-1 in T cell lymphoma of skin in Taiwan. Am J of Dermatopath 1998;20:250-254.

21. Drago F, Ranieri E, Malaguti F, et al. Human herpesvirus 7 in patients with P.R. Electron microscopy investigations and PCR in mononuclear cells, plasma and skin. Dermatology 1997;195:374-378.

22. Hidalgo F, Melon S, de Ona M, et al. Diagnosis of herpetic keratoconjunctivitis by nested polymerase chain reaction in human tear film. Euro J Clin Microbiol Infect Dis 1998; 17:120-123.

23. Tremblay C, Coutlee F, Weiss J, et al. Evaluation of a non-isotopic polymerase chain reaction assay for detection in clinical specimens of herpes simplex virus type 2 DNA. Canadian Women's HIV Study Group. Clin Diagn Virology 1997;8:53-62.

24. Tanphaichitr A, Brodell RT. How to spot scabies in infants. Postgrad Med 1999;105:191-192.

25. Elenitsas R, Jaworsky C, Murphy GF. Diagnostic methodology: Immunofluorescence. In Murphy GF, ed. Dermatopathology a practical guide to common disorders. Philadelphia: WB Saunders, 1995: pp 29-45.

26. Rogers M. Hair shaft abnormalities: Part II. Australas J Dermatol 37:1-11, 1996.

27. Netherton EW. A unique case of trichorrhexis nodosa "bamboo hairs" Arch Derm 1958;78;483

28. Wilkinson RD, Curtis GH, Hawk WA. Netherton's disease. Trichorrhexis invaginata (bamboo hair), congenital ichthyosiform erythroderma and the atopic diathesis: A histopathologic study. Arch Derm 1964;89:106.

29. De Berker DA, Paige DG, Harper J, Dawber RPR. Golf tee hairs: A new sign in Netherton's syndrome. B J Derm 1992; 127:30.

30. Hurwitz S. Hair disorders In Schachner LA, Hansen RC, eds. Pediatric dermatology. 2nd edition. New York: Churchill Livingston, 1995: pp 583-614.

31. Mancini AJ, Chan LS, Paller AS. Partial albinism with immunodeficiency: Griselli syndrome: Report of a case and review of the literature. J Am Acad Derm 1998;38:295-300.

32. Fine JD. Laboratory tests for epidermolysis bullosa. Dermatol Clin 1994;12:123-132.

33. Nisengard RJ, Blazczyk M, Chorzelski T, et al. Immunofluorescence of biopsy specimens: Comparison of methods of transportation. Arch Dermatol 1978;114;1329-1332.

34. Fine JD, Gay S: LDA-1 monoclonal antibody: An excellent reagent for immunofluorescence mapping studies in patients with epidermolysis bullosa. Arch Dermatol 1986; 122:48-51.

35. Kurban RS, Mihm MC. Dermatopathology: Cutaneous reaction patterns and the use of specialized laboratory techniques. In Moshella SL, Hurley HJ, eds. Dermatology. 3rd edition. Philadelphia: WB Saunders, 1992: pp 125-148.

36. Hood AF, Kwan TH, Mihm MC, Horn TD. Primer of dermatopathology. Boston: Little Brown, 1993: pp 40-43.

37. Lever WF, Schaumburg-Lever, eds. Histopathology of the skin. 7th edition. Laboratory Methods. Philadelphia, Lippencott. pp 44-54.

38. Gajraj NM, Pennant JH, Watcha MF. Eutectic mixture of local anesthetics (EMLA). Anesth Analg 1994;78:574-583.

39. Halperin DL, Koren G, Attias D, et al. Topical skin anesthesia for venous subcutaneous drug reservoir and lumbar punctures in children. Pediatrics 1989;84:281-284.

40. Chang PC, Goresky GV, O'Connor G, et al. A multicentre randomized study of single-unit dose package of EMLA patch vs. EMLA 5% cream for venipuncture in children. Can J Anesth 1994;41:59-63

41. Reynolds F. Adverse effects of local anesthetics. Br J Anesth 1987;59:78-95.

42. Jakobson B, Nilsson A. Methaemoglobinemia associated with prilocaine-lidocaine cream and trimethoprim-sulphamethoxazole. A case report. Acta Anaesthesiol Scan 1985;453-455.

43. Kumar AR, Dunn N, Naqvi M. Methemoglobinemia associated with a prilocaine-lidocaine cream. Clin Pediatr 1997; 36:239-240.

44. Frayling IM, Addison GM, Chattergee K, Meakin G. Methemoglobinaemia in children treated with prilocaine-lignocaine cream. Br Med J 1990;301:153-154.

45. Olson ML, McEvoy GK, Methemoglobinemia induced by local anesthetics. Am J Hosp P 1981;38:89-93.

46. Hall AH, Kulig KW, Rumack BH. Drug and chemical induced methemoglobinemia: clinical features and management. Med Toxicol 1986;1:253-260.

47. Archarya AB, Bustani PC, Phillips JD, et al. Randomised controlled trial of eutectic mixture of local anaesthetics cream for venepuncture in healthy preterm infants. Arch Dis Child Fetal Neonat 1998;78:F138-F142.

48. EMLA: Prescribing information. Astra Pharmaceutical Products, Inc. 1998 Westborough, MA 01581.

49. Nilsson A, Engberg, Henneberg S, et al. Inverse relationship between age dependent-erythrocyte activity of methaemoglobineduetase and prilocaine-induced methaemoglobinemia during infancy. Br J Anaesth 1990;64:72-76.

50. Van Den Hove J, Decroix J, Tennstedt D, Lachapelle JM. Allergic contact dermatitis from prilocaine, one of the local anaesthetics in EMLA cream. Contact Dermatitis 1994;30:239.

51. le Coz CJ, Cribier BJ, Heid E. Patch testing in suspected allergic contact dermatitis due to Emla cream in haemodialyzed patients. Contact Dermatitis 1996;35:316-317.

52. deWaard-van der Spek FB, van den Berg GM, Oranje AP. EMLA cream an improved local anesthetic; review of current literature. Pediatr Dermatol 1992;9:126-31.

53. Juhlin L, Rollman O. Vascular effects of a local anesthetic mixture in atopic dermatitis. Acta Derm Venereol 1984; 64:439-440.

54. de Waard-van der Spek FB, Oranje AP: Purpura caused by Emla is of toxic origin. Contact Dermatitis 1997;36:11-13.

55. Mofenson HC, Caraccio TR, Miller H, Greensher J. Lidocaine toxicity from topical mucosal application: with a review of the clinical pharmacology of lidocaine. Clin Pediat 1983;22:190-192.

56. Milhaly GW, Moore CR, Thomas J, et al. The pharmacokinetics and metabolism of the anilide local anesthetics in neonates. Eur J Clin Pharm 1978;13:143-152.

57. Morselli PL. Clinical pharmocokinetics in neonates. Clin Pharmacokinet 1976;1:81-98.

58. Boyes RN, Scott DB, Jebson PJ, et al. Pharmacokinetics of lidocaine in man. Clin Pharmacol Ther 1971;12;105-116.

59. Resar LM, Helfaer MA. Recurrent seizures in a neonate after lidocaine administration. J Perinat 1998;18:193-195.

60. Rothstein P, Dornbusch J, Shaywitz BA. Prolonged seizures associated with the use of viscous lidocaine. J Pediatr 1982; 101:461-163.

61. Wehner D, Hamilton GC. Seizures following topical application of local anesthetics to burn patients. Ann Emerg Med 1984;13:456-458.

62. Marshall DA, Mertz PM, Eaglestein WH. Occlusive dressings-Does dressing type influence the growth of common bacterial pathogens. Arch Surg 1990;125:1136-1139.

63. Telfer N, Moy R. Wound care after office procedures. J Dermatol Surg Oncol 1993;19:722-731.

64. Noe, JM, Keller M. Can stiches get wet? Plast Recons Surg 1988;81:82-84.

65. Lineaweaver W, Howard R, Soucy D, et al. Topical antimicrobial toxicity. Arch Surg 1985;120:267-270.

66. Niedner R, Schopf E. Inhibition of wound healing by antiseptics. Br J Dermatol 1986;115;41-44.

67. Cunningham BB, Bernstein L, Woodley DT. Wound dressings. In Roenigk HH, Roenigk RK, eds. Dermatologic surgery principals and practice. 2nd edition. New York: Dekker, 1996: pp 131-148.

68. Zitelli J. Wound healing by first and second intention. In Roenigk HH, Roenigk RK, eds. Dermatologic surgery principals and practice. 2nd edition. New York: Dekker, 1996: pp 101-130.

69. Eaglstein W, Mertz P. Inert vehicles do affect wound healing. J Invest Derm 1980;74:90-91.

70. McGrath MH. How topical dressings salvage questionable flaps: Experimental study. Plas Recon Surg 1981;67;653.

71. Viala J, Simon L, Le Pommelet C, et al. Agranulocytosis after application of silver sulfadiazine in a 2-month old infant. Arch Pediatr 1997;4;1103-1106.

72. Doubleday CW. Who is Nikolsky and what does his sign mean? [letter]. J Am Acad Dermatol 1987;16(5 Pt 1):1054-1055.

73. Moss C, Gupta E. The Nikolsky sign in staphylococcal scalded skin syndrome. Arch Dis Child 1998;79:290.

74. Salopek TG. Nikolsky's sign: is it "dry" or is it "wet"? Br J Dermatol 1997;136:762-767.

75. Lewis FM, Colver GB, Slater DN. Darier's sign associated with non-Hodgkin's lymphoma. Br J Dermatol 1994;130: 126-127.

76. Yen A, Sanchez R, Oblender M et al. Leukemia cutis:Darier's sign in a neonate with acute lymphoblastic leukemia. J Am Acad Dermatol 1996;34(2 Pt 2):375-378.

77. Ollivaud L, Cosnes A, Wechsler J, et al. Darier's sign in cutaneous large T-cell lymphoma. J Am Acad Dermatol 1996; 34:506-507.

78. Zvulunov A, Rotem A, Merlob P, et al. Congenital smooth muscle hamartoma. Prevalence, clinical findings, and in 15 patients. Am J Dis Childr 1990;144:782-784.

79. Johnson MD, Jacobs AH. Congenital smooth muscle hamartoma. A report of six cases and a review of the literature. [Review] [22 refs]. Arch Dermatol 1989;125:820-822.

80. Berberian BJ, Burnett JW. Congenital smooth muscle hamartoma: a case report. Br J Dermatol 1986;115:711-714.

81. Felman YM, Nikitas, JA. Syphilis serology today. Arch Dermatol 1980;116;84-89.

82. Gilchrest BA, Fitzpatrick TB, Anderson RR, et al. Localization of melanin pigment on the skin with a Wood's lamp. Br J Dermatol 1977;96:245.

83. Pini G, Faulkner LB. Cerebellar involvement in hypomelanosis of Ito. Neuropediatrics 1995;26:208-10.

84. Bluestone M. Where is Roche taking PCR? Bio/Technology 1991;9:1028-1030.

85. Lo A C, Feldman SR. Polymerase chain reaction: Basic concepts and clinical applications in dermatology. J Am Acad Dermatol 1994;30:250-260.

86. Saiki RK, Scharf S, Faloona F, et al. Enzymatic amplification of beta-globin genomic sequences and restriction site analysis for diagnosis of sickle-cell anemia. Science 1985;230: 1350-1354.

87. Mullis KB, Faloona FA. Specific synthesis of DNA *in vitro* via a polymerase-catalyzed chain reaction. Methods Enzymol 1987;155;335-350.

88. Eisenstein BI. The polymerase chain reaction: a new method of using molecular genetics for medical diagnosis. N Engl J Med 1990;322:178-183.

89. Ou CY, Kwok S, Mitchell SW, et al. DNA amplification for direct detection of HIV-1 in DNA of peripheral blood mononuclear cells. Science 1988;239:295-297.

90. Rogers MF, Ou CY, Rayfield M, et al. Use of the polymerase chain reaction for the early detection of the proviral sequences of human immunodeficiency virus in infants born to seropositive mothers New York City collaborative study of maternal HIV transmission and Montefiore Medical Center HIV perinatal transmission study group. N Eng J Med 1989;320:1649-1654

91. Shoji H, Koga M, Kusuhara, T, et al. Differentiation of herpes simplex virus 1 and 2 in cerebrospinal fluid of patients with HSV encephalitis and meningitis by stringent hybridization of PCR-amplified DNAs. J Neurol 1994;241: 526-530.

92. Schlesinger Y, Tebas P, Gaudreault-Keener M, et al. Herpes simplex virus type 2 meningitis in the absence of genital lesions: Improved recognition with use of the polymerase chain reaction. Clin Infect Dis 1995;20:842-848.

93. Kawasaki ES, Clark SS, Coyne MY, et al. Diagnosis of chronic myeloid and acute lymphocytic leukemias by detection of leukemia-specific mRNA sequences amplified *in vitro*. Proc Natl Acad Sci 1988;85:5698-5702.

94. Wright PA, Wynford-Thomas D. The polymerase chain reaction: Miracle or mirage? A critical review of its uses and limitations in diagnosis and research. J Pathol 1990;162: 99-117.

95. McGrath JA, Handyside AH. Preimplantation genetic diagnosis of severe inherited skin diseases Exp Dermatol 1998; 7:65-72.

96. Goltz RW. Polymerase chain reaction in dermatology. West J Med 1994;160:362.

97. Nahass GT, Goldstein BA, Zhu WY, et al. Comparison of Tzanck smear, viral culture, and DNA diagnostic methods in detection of herpes simplex and varicella-zoster infection. JAMA 1992;268:2541-2544.

98. Greer CE, Peterson SL, Kiviat NB, et al. PCR amplification from paraffin-embedded tissues. Effects of fixative and fixation time. Am J Clin Path 1991;95:117-124.

99. Werner M, Wilkens L, Aubele M, et al. Interphase cytogenetics in pathology: principles, methods, and applications of fluorescence in situ hybridization (FISH). Histochem Cell Bio;1997 108:381-390.

100. Christiano AM, LaForgia S, Paller AS, et al. Prenatal diagnosis for recessive dystrophic epidermolysis bullosa in 10 families by mutation and heplotype analysis in the type VII collagen gene (COC 7A1). Molec Med 1996;2:59-76.

101. Christiano AM, Pulkkinen L, McGrath JA, et al. Mutation based prenatal diagnosis of Herlitz junctional epidermolysis bullosa. Prenatal Diagn 1997;17:343-354.

102. Rothnagel JA, Longley MA, Holder RA, et al. Prenatal diagnosis of epidermolytic hyperkeratosis by direct gene sequencing. J Invest Derm 1994;102:13-16.

103. Bianchi DW. Prenatal diagnosis by analysis fetal cells in maternal blood. J Pediat 1995;127:847-856.

104. Handyside AH, Lesko JG, Tarin JJ, et al. Birth of a normal girl after in vitro fertilization and preimplantation diagnostic testing for cystic fibrosis. N Engl J Med 1992;327:905-909.

Transient Benign Cutaneous Lesions in the Newborn

ANNE W. LUCKY

Transient benign cutaneous lesions in the newborn are important to recognize. Not only can parents be reassured, but unnecessary and erroneous evaluation and treatment of presumed serious diseases can be prevented. This chapter discusses the most common transient benign conditions seen in neonates. Table 7-1 summarizes eight studies of the incidences of transient benign cutaneous lesions.[1-8] In some instances, racial and ethnic background may determine significant differences in the incidence of a disorder. Several excellent reviews of these conditions are also available.[9-16]

PAPULES AND PUSTULES

Milia

Milia are common papules occurring primarily on the face and scalp (Fig. 7-1). Clinically, they are tiny (up to 2 mm), white, smooth-surfaced papules, which are usually discrete, but their numbers may vary from a few to several dozen. They may be present at birth or appear later in infancy. Although they usually occur on the face, they may be found anywhere. Milia are tiny inclusion cysts within the epidermis that contain concentric layers of trapped keratinized stratum corneum. Primary milia are associated with pilosebaceous units arising from the infundibula of vellus hairs. Secondary milia usually appear after trauma and originate from a variety of epithelial structures such as hair follicles, sweat ducts, sebaceous ducts, or epidermis.[17] Neonatal milia are presumably primary. The diagnosis is a clinical one. If confirmation is needed, a small incision with the tip of a #11 blade can release the contents, which appear either as a smooth, white ball or keratinous debris.

The most important differential diagnosis of milia is with sebaceous hyperplasia (see the following discussion),

which also presents with small white papules. However, sebaceous hyperplasia tends to be clustered around the nose and a bit more yellow and occurs in large plaques. Milia may be associated with certain syndromes, including junctional and dystrophic epidermolysis bullosa, where lesions appear in sites of healing erosions, and in the oro-facial-digital syndrome type I, which features congenital mouth malformations, distinct facial features, and brachydactyly.[18] In these cases milia are numerous and persistent.

Milia usually resolve spontaneously in several months without treatment. If persistent, lesions can be incised and expressed, but this is rarely necessary. Why they occur with increased frequency in the newborn period is unknown.

Oral Mucosal Cysts of the Newborn (Palatal Cysts or Epstein's Pearls, and Alveolar Cysts or Bohn's Nodules)

Epstein's pearls and Bohn's nodules are actually both similar to milia, being microkeratocysts[19,20,21] located in the mouth. They are 1 to 2 mm, smooth, yellow to gray-white papules found singly or in clusters, most commonly on the median palatal raphe (68% to 81%). They also occur on the alveolar ridges (22%), more on the maxillary than the mandibular ridge, but rarely on both. They occur in 64% to 89% of normal neonates and are more common in Caucasian infants.

When on the palate they have been called Epstein's pearls, and when on the alveolar ridges, Bohn's nodules. Although Bohn and others had presumed that these were mucous gland cysts, more recent studies have shown them to be keratin cysts derived from the dental lamina. Both of these epidermal cysts occur in keratinized mucous membranes and form in embryonic lines of fusion.

TABLE 7-1	
Incidence of Common Transient Benign Lesions in the Neonate*	
Milia	
Epstein's pearls	56% to 89%
Sebaceous hyperplasia	32% to 48%
Erythema toxicum	21% to 41%
Miliaria crystallina	3% to 15%
Mongolian spot	
African-American	64% to 96%
Asian	84% to 86%
Latino	46% to 65%
Caucasia	3% to 13%
Salmon patch	
African-American	59%
Asian	22%
Latino	68%
Caucasian	70%

*Summarized from references 1 through 8.

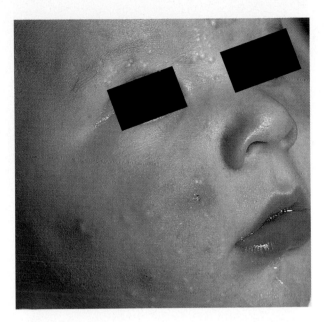

FIG. 7-1

Milia: Multiple smooth, firm, white papules are noted on the bridge of the nose; an acneiform eruption on the cheek is also evident in this young infant.

Epstein's pearls originate from epithelial remnants after fusion of palatal shelves. In a recent study of 1021 Swedish neonates,[21] most of the palatal cysts had spontaneously discharged and resolved by age 5 months. Interestingly, 17 children developed new palatal cysts postnatally. However, most of the alveolar cysts regressed.

The diagnosis is clinical. Other congenital papules in the mouth include gingival (alveolar) cysts of the newborn, dental lamina cysts, congenital epulis (granular cell tumor), lymphangiomas, mucoceles, and ranulas.[19] (See also Chapter 25.)

Perineal Median Raphe Cysts and Foreskin Cysts

Other common locations for epidermal inclusion cysts are in the foreskin and along the ventral surface of the penis and scrotum.[22] These lesions tend to be larger than the milia appearing on the head and neck and may represent a developmental abnormality of fusion with entrapment of epidermal or urethral cells. Histologically, they usually have a stratified squamous epithelial lining, but may have ciliated or mucous-secreting cells as well. They often will enlarge throughout infancy and/or seem to appear after the newborn period. They are benign and asymptomatic, although they may require surgical removal sometimes because of their large size or if they become infected.

Miliaria

Miliaria is a general term for describing obstructions of the eccrine duct.[23] Miliaria occurs in infants in warm climates or those who are being kept warm or are febrile. It is thus more common in non–air conditioned nurseries and in hot rather than in temperate climates.[4,6] The clinical manifestations of miliaria vary, depending on the level of the obstruction.

In the immediate newborn period, the most common form of miliaria is the most superficial, **miliaria crystallina** (sudamina). In miliaria crystallina, ductal obstruction is subcorneal or intracorneal. Obstruction at this level leads to very superficial trapping of sweat under the stratum corneum, producing typical small, crystal-clear vesicles resembling water droplets on the skin (Fig. 7-2). These vesicles are extremely fragile and may be wiped away on cleansing of the skin. Miliaria crystallina usually appears in the first few days of life, but there are reports of congenital lesions.[24,25] Occasionally there will be many neutrophils within the lesions, giving them a more pustular than vesicular appearance. The causes of ductal blockage or leakage are not known. Some authors, however, favor the hypothesis that the ductal occlusion is caused by extracellular polysaccharide substance (EPS) from *Staphylococcus epidermidis*.[26] Miliaria crystallina is precipitated by

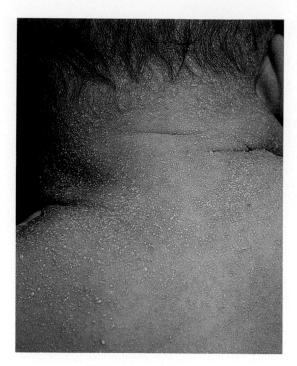

FIG. 7-2
Tiny, superficial vesicles, seen on the back and neck of this newborn, are characteristic of miliaria crystallina.

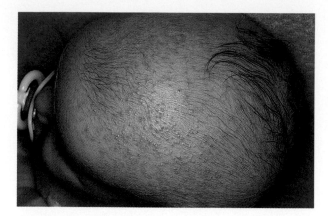

FIG. 7-3
Inflammatory papules and/or pustules of miliaria rubra are non-follicular in distribution and are seen here on the scalp of an overheated newborn infant.

environmental overheating or fever with consequent superficial retention of sweat in the obstructed ducts and surrounding epidermis. The diagnosis is clinical, although a smear of the clear fluid contents of the vesicles shows an absence of cellular material or, at most, a few neutrophils. Reducing the ambient temperature or treating the fever will prevent and/or treat miliaria. Miliaria crystallina is benign but could be mistaken for more serious vesicular or pustular disorders such as herpes simplex.

Miliaria rubra is also common in overheated or febrile infants. Other terms for this disorder include "heat rash" and "prickly heat." Miliaria rubra presents as erythematous, 1 to 3 mm papules or papulopustules on the head, neck, face, scalp, and trunk (Fig. 7-3). It can occur anywhere but has a predilection for the forehead, upper trunk, and flexural or covered surfaces. The lesions are *not* follicular. When there is inflammation with multiple neutrophils within lesions of miliaria rubra, as may be found under occlusion beneath monitor leads or bandages, miliaria rubra may look pustular and mimic worrisome conditions such as neonatal infections. Some authors subclassify this pustular form as **miliaria pustulosa.** Histologically, there is dermal inflammation around occluded eccrine ducts. The sweat duct obstruction is lower than in miliaria crystallina but still intraepidermal. The diagnosis is made clinically, but if there is any doubt, a biopsy will confirm eccrine duct occlusion. The erythematous papules of miliaria rubra may mimic a variety of neonatal conditions, such as neonatal acne, as well as candidal, staphylococcal, or herpes simplex infections. Correcting the overheating is usually sufficient for managing miliaria.

Miliaria profunda, the third and deepest level of sweat duct obstruction, has occlusion at or below the dermal-epidermal junction. It is rare in the newborn period. In older children and adults, this deep obstruction causes white papules representing dermal edema and can actually prevent adequate sweating, leading to hyperthermia.

Sebaceous Hyperplasia

Sebaceous hyperplasia is most prominent on the face, especially around the nose and upper lip, where the density of sebaceous glands is highest. Sebaceous hyperplasia appears as follicular, regularly spaced, smooth white-yellowish papules grouped into plaques (Fig. 7-4). There is no surrounding erythema. Hormonal (androgen) stimulation in utero, which comes from either the mother or infant, causes hypertrophy of sebaceous glands. Premature infants are less affected, but sebaceous hyperplasia occurs in nearly half of term newborns.[6,7] Sebaceous hyperplasia gradually involutes in the first few weeks of life. The papules differ from milia, which are epidermal inclusion cysts, and are usually discrete, solitary, and whiter in color.

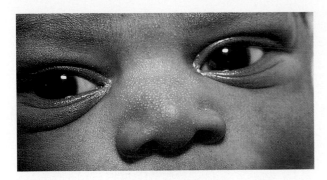

FIG. 7-4

Sebaceous hyperplasia is typically located on and surrounding the nose with sheets of tiny white-yellow follicular papules without inflammation.

Erythema Toxicum Neonatorum (Toxic Erythema of the Newborn, Flea-Bite Dermatitis)

Erythema toxicum is unquestionably the most well-known benign eruption in the newborn period, occurring in approximately half of full-term newborns.[25,26,27] Estimates of the incidence in large series range from 21% to 41%, but frequencies as high as 72% have been reported.[27] The discrepancies in estimates of incidence may be due to the length of time these infants were observed. The presence of erythema toxicum has been well correlated with birth weight and gestational age.[28] It is virtually never seen in premature infants or those weighing less than 2500 g. There is no sexual or racial predilection.[29] Congenital lesions can occur,[30,31,32] but the majority of cases have their onset between 24 and 48 hours of life. Lesions wax and wane, usually lasting a week or less, but cases lasting beyond 7 days have been reported. Occasionally very atypical presentations are seen (i.e., onset as late as 10 days of age) and pustules contain predominantly neutrophils,[29,33] but such cases require careful evaluation and skin biopsy to exclude other causes.

The classic eruption consists of barely elevated yellowish papules or pustules, measuring 1 to 3 mm in diameter, with a surrounding irregular macular flare or wheal of erythema measuring 1 to 3 cm. The irregular shape of the flare has been likened to that of a flea bite (Fig. 7-5, A). Although the characteristic lesions of erythema toxicum are usually discrete and scattered (Fig. 7-5, B), extensive cases with either clusters of pustules, confluent papules, or pustules with surrounding erythema forming huge erythematous plaques can occur and be more difficult to diagnose (Fig. 7-5, C). Lesions may appear first on the face and spread to the trunk and extremities, but may appear anywhere on the body except on the palms and soles.

Histologically, the lesions are eosinophilic pustules and characteristically intrafollicular, occurring subcorneally above the entry of the sebaceous duct.[34] This follicular location explains the absence of lesions on the palms and soles. Peripheral eosinophilia has also been associated in a minority (about 15%) of cases. The etiology of erythema toxicum is unknown: a graft-versus-host reaction against maternal lymphocytes has been postulated as a possible mechanism,[35] but there are no data to substantiate this claim.

The diagnosis of erythema toxicum can usually be made by clinical appearance alone, but simple scraping of the pustule, smearing the contents onto a glass slide, and staining with Wright or Giemsa stain will reveal sheets of eosinophils with a few scattered neutrophils. Skin biopsy is rarely needed.

The differential diagnosis of erythema toxicum includes other pustular disorders of the newborn: infantile acropustulosis has a more acral rather than truncal distribution; herpes simplex has a more vesicular character with subsequent crusting; staphylococcal impetigo has more well-developed pustules; congenital candidiasis has a positive KOH and can be more scaly. Transient neonatal pustular melanosis (TNPM) (see the following discussion) has primarily neutrophils in the infiltrate and is present at birth, and the pustules quickly disappear, leaving pigmented macules, but erythema toxicum and TNPM may appear together in some infants. Miliaria rubra can also present with erythematous papulopustules, but these favor the head and neck and are smaller lesions without the erythematous flare. No therapy is needed for erythema toxicum except for parental reassurance.

Transient Neonatal Pustular Melanosis

This disorder was first described as TNPM in 1976,[36] although it had undoubtedly occurred before that time. In fact, an abstract in 1961[37] is likely to be the first description of TNPM, which was called "lentigines neonatorum." It occurs primarily in full-term African-American infants of both sexes. In the 1976 report, 4.4% of African-American and 0.6% of Caucasian infants were affected.[36] Lesions were always present at birth.

TNPM has three phases and thus three types of lesions. First, very superficial vesicopustules, ranging in size from 2 mm to as large as 10 mm, may be present in utero and are virtually always evident at birth (Fig. 7-6, A). Because

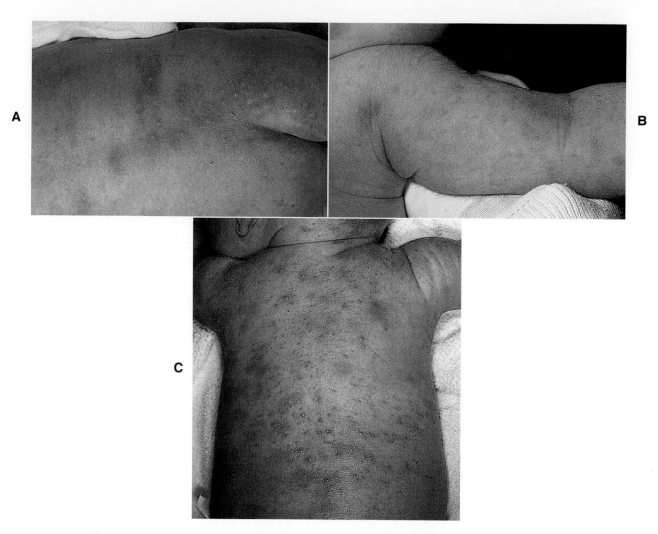

FIG. 7-5

Erythema toxicum: Erythematous macules and wheals may predominate (**A**). In some cases pustules are sparse (**B**), whereas in others extensive white to yellow papulovesicles with flares of erythema are noted (**C**).

they are intracorneal and subcorneal, and thus very fragile, the pustules may be easily wiped away during the initial cleaning of the infant to remove vernix caseosa, so that the pustular phase may not be evident (Fig. 7-6, *B*). The second phase is represented by a fine collarette of scale around the resolving pustule (Fig. 7-6, *C*). The third phase consists of hyperpigmented brown macules at the site of previous pustulation (Fig. 7-6, *D*). Although these macules have been called "lentigines" (because of their resemblance to lentils), they are not true lentigines but appear to represent transient postinflammatory hyperpigmentation. They may last for up to several months before they fade. Some infants are born with these macules, the pustular phase having presumably occurred in utero. The

most common location for TNPM has been under the chin, on the forehead, at the nape, and on the lower back and shins, although the face, trunk, palms, and soles are also affected.

The etiology of TNPM is unknown. However, some authors[38,39] have postulated that TNPM is a precocious form of erythema toxicum neonatorum, with clinical and histologic overlap. They have proposed the term *sterile transient neonatal pustulosis* to describe this overlap entity. It is more likely however, that these two conditions, which both occur commonly, may sometimes coexist. In most infants there is little confusion based either on clinical appearance or time of onset.

Smears of the contents of the pustules stained with

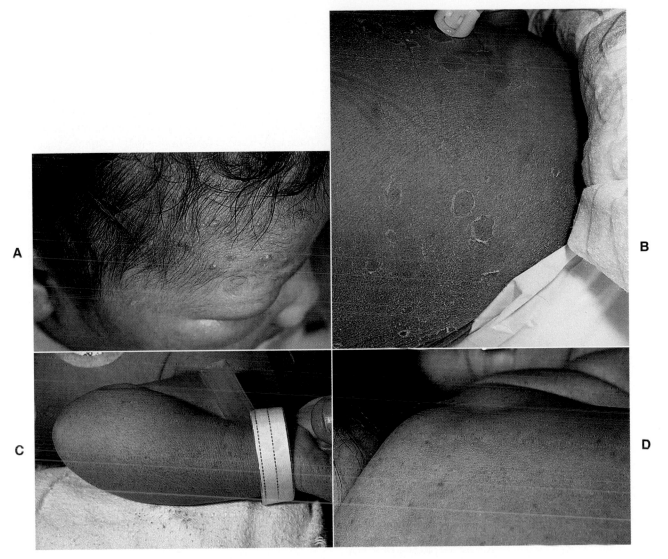

FIG. 7-6
Transient neonatal pustular melanosis first appears as small, superficial pustules without inflammation
(**A**). Collarettes of scale, typical of the second stage, are occasionally seen at birth without pustules evident
(**B**) or may develop after pustules have ruptured (**C**). The final stage is that of small hyperpigmented mac-
ules resembling lentils, which gradually fade over weeks to months (**D**).

Giemsa or Wright stain predominantly show neutrophils,
although a few eosinophils have also been reported. A
biopsy is rarely needed for diagnosis. Histologically, these
lesions consist of subcorneal pustules filled with neutrophils, fibrin, and rare eosinophils.[38] The differential diagnosis of TNPM includes the following:
- Erythema toxicum neonatorum, which appears a few
  days after birth and is inflammatory, and whose vesicles
  contain primarily eosinophils

- Staphylococcal impetigo, which shows gram-positive
  cocci on smear and positive cultures
- Neonatal candidiasis, which reveals pseudohyphae and
  spores on KOH examination
- Miliaria crystallina or rubra, which would not leave
  postinflammatory hyperpigmentation
- Acropustulosis of infancy, which usually appears later
  and predominates on the hands and feet

Although the pustules of TNPM resolve rapidly, the pigmented macules may take weeks to months to fade away. No treatment is needed except parental reassurance.

Neonatal and Infantile Acne

Neonatal and infantile acne are distinct entities distinguishable by time of onset and clinical features. **Neonatal acne** may occur at birth and usually appears within the first 2 to 3 weeks of life. This disorder is currently under close scrutiny as to its existence and/or etiology: is it acne or another pustular disorder of infancy? The term *neonatal cephalic pustulosis* has been proposed to replace the term *neonatal acne.* Classically, neonatal acne has been described as inflammatory, erythematous papules and pustules, located primarily on the cheeks but scattered over the face and often extending onto the scalp[40,41,42] (Fig. 7-7). Comedonal lesions are absent. There has been a recent hypothesis that these erythematous papulopustules seen in the first month of life may be an inflammatory reaction to *Pityrosporum* (*Malassezia*) species, both *M. furfur* and *M. sympodialis.*[43,44,45] In addition, clinical differentiation between neonatal acne and miliaria rubra may be impossible. Biopsies would aid in diagnosis, but they are not justified, since both conditions are benign and transient.

A later form of acne has been termed **infantile acne.**[40,41,42] This may be due to a persistence of neonatal acne or a later onset of true acne at 2 to 3 months of age. Infantile acne shows typical acneiform lesions, including open and closed comedones, as well as papules, pustules, and occasionally nodules (Fig. 7-8). It is found primarily on the face.

Infantile acne has been considered to be an androgen-driven condition with hyperplasia of sebaceous activity.[46] It rarely may be a sign of underlying androgen excess such as congenital adrenal hyperplasia, steroid-producing gonadal or adrenal tumor, or true precocious puberty. There is usually spontaneous resolution in the first 6 to 12 months of life. This would correlate well with what is known about neonatal androgens. The fetal adrenal gland is really an enlarged *zona reticularis,* which is the androgen-producing zone of the adrenal, producing pubertal levels of dehydroepiandrosterone (DHEA) and its sulfate (DHEAS), which wane over the first 6 months of life in both male

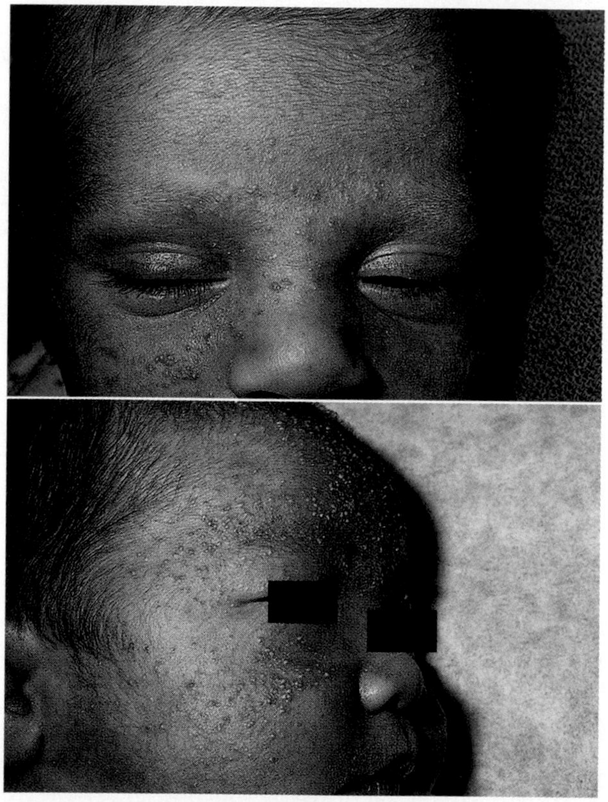

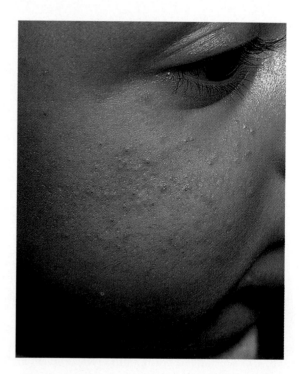

FIG. 7-7
Neonatal acne (cephalic pustulosis) (**A** and **B**) is usually found on the cheeks and scalp in the first 2 to 4 weeks of life; small red papules and pustules without comedones are evident.

FIG. 7-8
True infantile acne has the features of adolescent acne, including open and closed comedones, as seen in this 3-month-old infant.

and female infants. In the male infant, testicular testosterone is also elevated for the first 6 to 12 months of life, perhaps explaining the observation that males are more affected with infantile acne than females.

Whereas neonatal acne spontaneously resolves without treatment, infantile acne may be more persistent and even cause scarring and can benefit from treatment. Small inflammatory papules and pustules respond to topical benzoyl peroxide or erythromycin. Topical tretinoin in low concentrations (0.01% gel or 0.025% cream) can be used for open and closed comedones. Erythromycin is the only appropriate systemic antibiotic for larger papules or pustules that may scar. Tetracyclines are contraindicated because they cause permanent tooth staining. In those rare cases of severe, scarring nodular infantile acne, systemic isotretinoin has been used safely and effectively.[47,48,49,50]

SUCKING BLISTERS, EROSIONS, PADS, AND CALLUSES

Sucking blisters, erosions, and calluses on the hands and forearms are present at birth and can be solitary or bilateral.[51] Although the primary lesion from sucking is usually a tense, fluid-filled blister on normal-appearing skin (Fig. 7-9), when the blister has ruptured, an erosion may result, or if the sucking has been less vigorous and more chronic, the lesion may become a callus. These lesions appear to result from repetitive vigorous sucking in utero at one particular spot. Often when the neonate is presented after birth with the affected extremity, he/she will immediately demonstrate sucking behavior on that area. Sucking blisters on the extremities may be mistaken for other serious disorders such as herpes simplex, but their solitary, asymmetric nature and characteristic location should help to establish the correct diagnosis.

In infants who are vigorous suckers postnatally, sucking pads or calluses can also occur on the lips. These occur postnatally and should be differentiated from the lesions on the extremities. Sucking calluses appear on the mucosa caudal to the closure line of infants' lips and are hyperkeratotic pads, which eventually desquamate in 3 to 6 months.[52] Histologically, there is epithelial hyperplasia and intracellular edema secondary to friction. No therapy is required.

UMBILICAL GRANULOMA

In some neonates, granulation tissue develops at the umbilical stump after the cord dries up and falls off, usually at 6 to 8 days after birth. The raw surface of the umbilicus heals in most infants in 12 to 15 days.[53,54] Umbilical granulomata are grayish-pink papules on the umbilical stump. They are extremely friable and bleed easily to touch. They have a "velvety" feel to the surface.

The etiology of umbilical granulomas is failure of the surface of the proximal portion of the cord to heal and subsequent proliferation of endothelial cells without atypia.[55] The term *granuloma* is misleading because these lesions are composed of proliferating endothelial cells, like pyogenic granulomas, and are not true granulomas.

The diagnosis is clinical (Fig 7-10). However, it is important to distinguish umbilical granulomas from other embryonic remnants. The normal umbilical cord consists of two umbilical arteries, one umbilical vein, a rudimen-

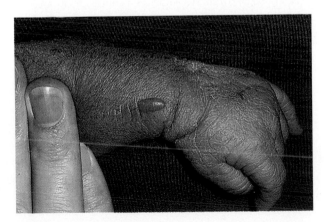

FIG. 7-9

A solitary, tense bulla arising on normal skin on the wrist of this infant is characteristic of a sucking blister. When presented with the extremity, the neonate preferentially sucked on this location.

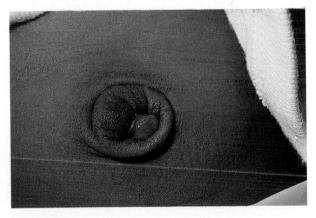

FIG. 7-10

This friable, red papule arising from the umbilical stump is a typical umbilical granuloma.

tary allantois attached to the bladder (urachus), and a remnant of the vitelline (omphalomesenteric duct) attached to the ileum.[53] The proximal end of the vitelline duct creates Meckel's diverticulum. A patent urachus will intermittently discharge urine. A persistent vitelline duct will have a malodorous discharge. An umbilical polyp is a distal remnant of the vitelline duct that creates an erythematous papule similar in appearance to an umbilical granuloma, but the surface is sticky because of mucous secreted from the intestinal mucosa. These developmental lesions all require surgical therapy. When talc-containing powders are used on the umbilical stump, talc granulomas could also form and look identical to umbilical granulomas.

The traditional treatment of umbilical granulomas is topical application of silver nitrate. Care must be taken to very lightly touch only the granulomata; otherwise burns may occur on the surrounding normal skin. If lesions fail to respond to one or two treatments, then serious consideration should be given to alternative diagnoses. Most umbilical granulomas are seen and treated by pediatricians and rarely come to the attention of the dermatologist.

COLOR CHANGES IN THE NEWBORN

Pigmentary Abnormalities Resulting From Abnormalities of Melanin

Dermal Melanosis (Mongolian Spots)
Mongolian spots are collections of melanocytes located in the dermis. They are macules or patches that may be solitary and a few millimeters or multiple and several centimeters in size. They are a distinctive slate blue, gray, or black (Fig. 7-11) and are most commonly located over the buttocks and sacrum, but often occur elsewhere.[2,56] Over the buttocks, Mongolian spots are seen in up to 96% of African-American, 86% of Asian, and 13% of Caucasian neonates (Box 7-1). In this location, on the lower back, they usually resolve over several years. Similarly appearing dermal melanosis in other locations such as the arms and shoulders (nevus of Ito) or around the cheek and eye, including the sclera (nevus of Ota), may not resolve at all. The blue color of dermal melanosis is a result of the Tyndall effect, in which red wavelengths of light are absorbed and blue wavelengths are reflected back from the brown melanin pigment located deep in the dermis. The pathogenesis is postulated to be a defect in migration of pigmented neural crest cells, which usually reside at the dermal-epidermal junction. Histologically, spindle-shaped melanocytes are dispersed within dermal collagen. No treatment is recommended for dermal melanosis. Extensive Mongolian spots have been described in infants with GM1 gangliosidosis (See Chapter 17).

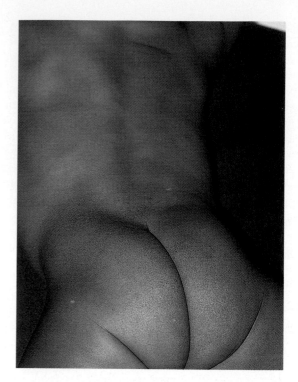

FIG. 7-11
Dermal melanosis (Mongolian spots) on the back of an African-American infant, which will most likely fade over several years.

The pigmentation of nevus of Ota has been successfully treated with the Q-switched ruby laser.[57] A small risk of melanoma exists for a nevus of Ota. It is most important to distinguish dermal melanosis from bruising, which would undergo sequential color change from blue-black to green to yellow, so that there is no confusion about possible child abuse.

Epidermal Hyperpigmentation
In more darkly pigmented neonates, transient, nearly black hyperpigmentation can be observed in the genital areas on the labia and scrotum (Fig. 7-12, A and B), in a linear fashion on the lower abdomen (linea nigra), around the areolae, in the axillae, on the pinnae, and at the base of the fingernails (Fig. 7-12, C).[13] These areas are believed to be hyperpigmented as a result of MSH stimulation in utero, but the mechanism is unclear.

Other nonhormonal patterns of brown hyperpigmentation have also been reported. Horizontal bands of hyperpigmentation corresponding to creases in the abdomen (Fig. 7-13, A)[58] or on the back seem to reflect flexion in utero. They are transient and are thought to be a result of mechanical trauma from hyperkeratosis within

---

BOX 7-1

Color Changes in the Neonate

Pigmentary
1. Melanin
   a. Dermal melanosis (Mongolian spots)
   b. Hyperpigmentation
   c. Hypopigmentation
2. Nonmelanin
   a. Bilirubin
   b. Meconium
   c. Vernix

Vascular
1. Vasomotor instability
   a. Cutis marmorata
   b. Acrocyanosis
   c. Harlequin color change
2. Rubor
3. Twin transfusion
4. Transient capillary vascular malformations

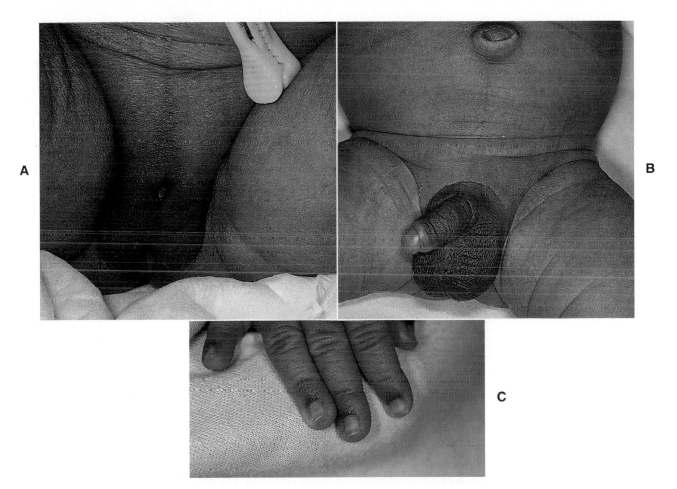

FIG. 7-12

Intense hyperpigmentation. In neonates with dark skin, transient accentuation of nearly black pigmentation can be seen in several locations on the vulva (**A**), scrotum (**B**), lower abdomen (linea nigra) (**A** and **B**), and base of the fingernails (**C**).

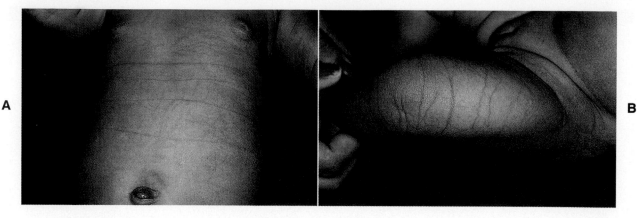

FIG. 7-13
Horizontal linear hyperpigmentation in the creases on the abdomen (**A**) or over the knees (**B**) may be related to flexed positions and hyperkeratosis in utero.

the folds. Transient reticulated or linear pigmentation on the back and knees has also been reported (Fig. 7-13, *B*),[59] presumably as a result of posttraumatic hyperpigmentation in utero.

The most important differential diagnosis of the neonate with hormonally induced hyperpigmentation is congenital adrenal hyperplasia (CAH). In this life-threatening condition, there is massive stimulation by ACTH resulting from an enzyme block in the synthesis of cortisol. The hyperpigmentation is believed to be due to cross-reactivity of ACTH with MSH receptors. Children with CAH also have ambiguous genitalia and will die if not promptly diagnosed and treated with replacement cortisol.

Hypopigmentation

African-American and Asian infants often have much lighter overall pigmentation in the newborn period, which gradually darkens over the first year of life. Generalized hypopigmentation is also seen in genetic conditions such as phenylketonuria (PKU), Menkes' syndrome, Chédiak-Higashi syndrome, and albinism (see Chapter 19).

Pigmentary Changes Not Caused By Melanin

Physiologic jaundice results from transient elevation of serum bilirubin, resulting in a generalized yellow discoloration of the skin in the first few days of life (Fig. 7-14). With jaundice, in contrast to carotenemia, which may occur later in infancy at age 1 to 2 years, there is yellow discoloration of the sclerae, as well as the skin. Physiologic jaundice fades after the bilirubin returns to normal.

Meconium staining often will darken the vernix caseosa but can also leave patchy, yellow-brown pigmentation, especially on desquamating epidermis (Fig. 7-15).

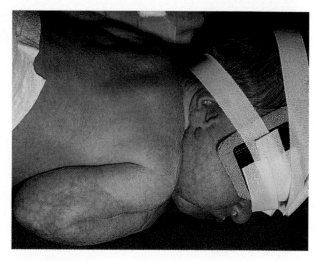

FIG. 7-14
Infant with jaundice undergoing phototherapy.

Color Changes Resulting From Vascular Abnormalities

Cutaneous Vasomotor Instability

The ability of neonates to adjust to extrauterine surroundings is at first immature, and they can exhibit distinct cutaneous blood flow abnormalities. When neonates are cold, their constricted capillaries and venules may produce a reticulated, mottled, blanchable, violaceous pattern termed **cutis marmorata** (Fig. 7-16). Exposure to cold temperatures may also induce more vasoconstriction in acral than central areas of the body, resulting in deep violaceous to blue coloration of the hands, feet and lips, termed *acrocyanosis* (Fig. 7-17). Both of these conditions

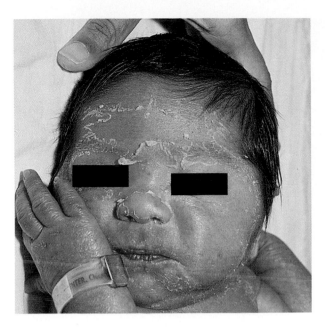

FIG. 7-15
Extensive desquamation can be a normal finding in the postmature infant.

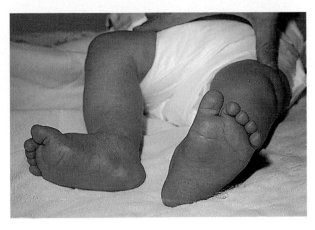

FIG. 7-17
Acrocyanosis: purplish discoloration of the feet on exposure to cold.

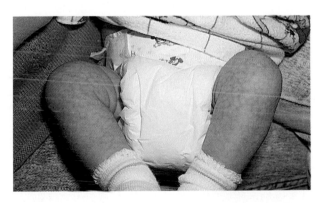

FIG. 7-16
Reticulated, violaceous pattern seen on the extremities with cutis marmorata.

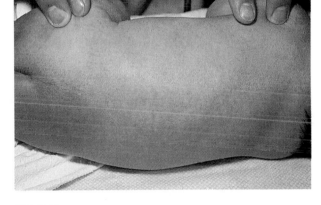

FIG. 7-18
Vasodilation of the dependent half of the body with a sharp midline cutoff is typical of a harlequin color change.

occur more often in premature infants. These transient conditions rapidly improve upon rewarming of the infant, and the tendency to occur diminishes with age. Cutis marmorata should not be confused with cutis marmorata telangiectatica congenita, a vascular malformation that persists for several years and occurs in well-defined large patches.

The so-called "harlequin" color change is a rare physiologic phenomenon whereby the amount of blood flow markedly differs on the right and left sides of the body with a sharp cutoff at the midline.[60] This is most often seen when a child is lying on one side, the dependent side, exhibiting vasodilation, and being strikingly redder than the upper half of the body (Fig. 7-18). The face and genitalia may be spared. Episodes last from seconds to minutes and are rapidly reversible with change in position or increased activity. It is more common in premature infants, but can affect up to 10% of full-term babies. Its onset is at 2 to 5 days of age, and the phenomenon lasts up to 3 weeks. There is no pathologic significance.

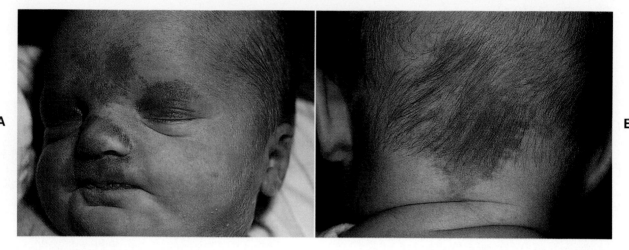

FIG. 7-19
Nevus simplex. An infant with simplex on the glabella, nevus, eyelids, nose, and upper lip (A). The nape is the most common location for a nevus simplex (B).

Rubor Resulting From Excessive Hemoglobin

Because newborns have high levels of hemoglobin in the first weeks of life, there is generalized rubor, which fades as the hemoglobin physiologically drops to normal levels. **Twin transfusion** may occur in twins as a result of shunting of blood from one twin to the other, resulting in a major color difference at birth, reflecting a marked discrepancy in hemoglobin levels between the two infants.

Capillary Ectasias (Nevus Simplex, Salmon Patch)

Erythematous macules and patches occurring over the occiput, eyelids, glabella, and, to a lesser extent, the nose and upper lip are minor vascular malformations consisting of ectatic capillaries in the upper dermis with normal overlying skin (Fig. 7-19). They occur in 70% of white, 59% of African-American, 68% of Latino, and 22% of Asian newborns[3] and have been given the common designations "angel's kisses" (eyelids) or "stork bites" (nape) (see Table 7-1). Most resolve over several months to years, but 25% to 50% of nuchal lesions and a much smaller percentage of the glabellar lesions may persist into adult life. The primary differential diagnosis of these benign transient lesions is port-wine stains, which are usually more lateral in location, do not resolve, and often continue to darken and thicken with age. These stains, particularly the glabellar ones, are often inherited as an autosomal dominant trait.

VERNIX CASEOSA

Vernix caseosa is notable on the surface of the skin at birth as a chalky-white mixture of shed epithelial cells, sebum,

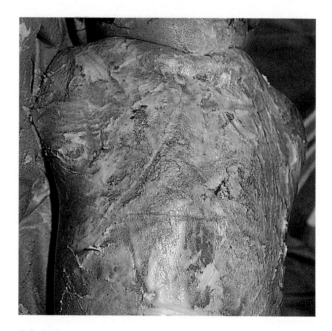

FIG. 7-20
The vernix caseosa is a white to grey, cheesy, greasy layer of sebum, keratin, and hair, which has protected the fetus in utero.

and sometimes hair (Fig. 7-20). The vernix presumably serves as a lubricant and perhaps permeability barrier to protect the infant skin from amniotic fluid. It becomes thicker with advancing gestational age, although postmature infants usually have no vernix.[12] In infants who have prepartum passage of meconium, the vernix may be stained yellow-brown, and this can be a clue to fetal distress.

DESQUAMATION

Most full-term infants will have fine desquamation of the skin at 24 to 48 hours of age. Premature infants do not show desquamation until 2 to 3 weeks of life. The post-mature infant, however, is often born with cracking and peeling of the skin of much greater intensity than the full-term or premature infant (see Fig. 7-15). The differential diagnosis of physiologic desquamation includes various forms of ichthyosis, as well as hypohidrotic ectodermal dysplasia. These are discussed in detail in Chapters 16 and 24.

REFERENCES

1. Jacobs AH, Walton RG. The incidence of birthmarks in the neonate. Pediatrics 1976;58:218-222.
2. Cordova A. The Mongolian spot: A study of ethnic differences and a literature review. Clin Pediatr Phila 1981;20:714-719.
3. Alper JC, Holmes LB. The incidence and significance of birthmarks in a cohort of 4,641 newborns. Pediatr Dermatol 1983;1:58-68.
4. Hidano A, Purwoko R, Jitsukawa K. Statistical survey of skin changes in Japanese neonates. Pediatr Dermatol 1986;3:140-144.
5. Osburn K, Schosser RH, Everett MA. Congenital pigmented and vascular lesions in newborn infants. J Am Acad Dermatol 1987;16:788-792.
6. Nanda A, Kaur S, Bhakoo ON, Dhall K. Survey of cutaneous lesions in Indian newborns. Pediatr Dermatol 1989;6:39-42.
7. Rivers JK, Frederiksen PC, Dibdin C. A prevalence survey of dermatoses in the Australian neonate. J Am Acad Dermatol 1990;23:77-81.
8. Tsai FJ, Tsai CH. Birthmarks and congenital skin lesions in Chinese newborns. J Formos Med Assoc 1993;92:838-841.
9. Hodgman JE, Freedman RI, Levine NE. Neonatal dermatology. Pediatr Clin North Am 1971;18:713-756.
10. Solomon LM, Esterly NB. Transient cutaneous lesions In Neonatal dermatology. Philadelphia: WB Saunders, 1973: pp 43-48.
11. Schachner L, Press S. New clinical, diagnostic and therapeutic aspects of vesiculo bullous disorders in infancy and childhood. Pediatr Ann 1982;11:213-224.
12. Wagner AM, Hansen RC. Neonatal skin and skin disorders. In Schachner LA, Hansen RC, eds. Pediatric dermatology. 2nd edition. New York: Churchill Livingstone, 1995: pp 263-283.
13. Rudolph AJ. Dermatology and perinatal infection. In Atlas of the newborn. Hamilton: BC Decker, 1997.
14. Treadwell PA. Dermatoses in newborns. Am Fam Phys 1997; 56:443-450.
15. Van Praag MG, Van Rooij RG, Folkers E, et al. Diagnosis and treatment of pustular disorders in the neonate. Pediatr Dermatol 1997;14:131-143.
16. Wagner A. Distinguishing vesicular and pustular disorders in the neonate. Curr Opin Pediatr 1997;9:396-405.
17. Lever WF, Schaumberg-Lever G. Histology of the skin, Philadelphia: JB Lippincott, 1990: p 536.
18. Larralde de Luna M, Raspa ML, Ibargoyen J. Oral-facial-digital type 1 syndrome of Papillon-Leage and Psaume. Pediatr Dermatol 1992;9:52-56.
19. Eisen D, Lynch DP. Developmental disorders. In The mouth: Diagnosis and treatment. St Louis: Mosby, 1998: pp 37-57.
20. Jorgenson RJ, Shapiro SD, Salinas CF, Levin LS. Intraoral findings and anomalies in neonates. Pediatrics 1982;69:577-582
21. Flinck A, Paludan A, Matsson L, et al. Oral findings in a group of newborn Swedish children. Int J Paediatr Dentis 1994; 4:67-73.
22. LeVasseur JG, Perry VE. Perineal median raphe cyst. Pediatr Dermatol 1997;5:391-392.
23. Feng E, Janniger C. Miliaria. Cutis 1995;55:213-216.
24. Straka BF, Cooper PH, Greer KE. Congenital miliaria crystallina. Cutis 1991;47:103-106.
25. Arpey CJ, Nagashima-Whalen LS, Chren MM, et al. Congenital miliaria crystallina: Case report and literature review. Pediatr Dermatol 1992;9:283-287.
26. Mowad CM, McGinley KJ, Foglia A, et al. The role of extracellular polysaccharide substance produced by *Staphylococcus epidermidis* in miliaria. J Am Acad Dermatol 1995;33:729-733.
27. Harris, JR, Schick B. Erythema neonatorum. AMA J Dis Child 1956;92:27-33.
28. Carr JA, Hodgman JE, Freedman RI, et al. Relationship between toxic erythema and infant maturity. Am J Dis Child 1966;112:129-134.
29. Chang MW, Jiang SB, Orlow SJ. Atypical erythema toxicum neonatorum of delayed onset in a term infant. Pediatr Dermatol 1999;16:137-141.
30. Levy, HL, Cothran F. Erythema toxicum neonatorum present at birth. Am J Dis Child 1962;103:125-127.
31. Marino LJ. Toxic erythema present at birth. Arch Dermatol 1965;92:402-403.
32. Maffei FA, Michaels MG. An unusual presentation of erythema toxicum: scrotal pustules present at birth. Arch Pediatr Adolesc Med 1996;150:649-650.
33. Berg FJ, Solomon LM. Erythema neonatorum toxicum. Arch Dis Child 1987;62:327-328.
34. Luders D. Histologic observations in erythema toxicum neonatorum. Pediatrics 1960;26:219-224.
35. Bassukus ID. Is erythema toxicum neonatorum a mild self-limited acute cutaneous graft-versus-host-reaction from maternal-to-fetal lymphocyte transfer? Med-Hypotheses 1992; 38:334-338.
36. Ramamurthy RS, Reveri M, Esterly NB, et al. Transient neonatal pustular melanosis. J Pediatr 1976;88:831-835.
37. Perrin E, Sutherland J, Baltazar S. Inquiry onto the nature of lentigines neonatorum: Demonstration of a statistical relationship with squamous metaplasia of the amnion. Am J Dis Child 1961;102:648-649.
38. Barr RJ, Globerman LM, Werber FA. Transient neonatal pustular melanosis. Int J Dermatol 1979;18:636-638.
39. Ferrandiz C, Coroleu W, Ribera M, et al. Sterile transient neonatal pustulosis is a precocious form of erythema toxicum neonatorum. Dermatology 1992;185:18-22.
40. Jansen T, Burgdorf WHC, Plewig G. Pathogenesis and treatment of acne in childhood. Pediatr Dermatol 1997;14:17-21.
41. Lucky AW. A review of infantile and pediatric acne. Dermatology 1998;196:95-97.
42. Lucky AW. Acne therapy in infancy and childhood. Dermatol Ther 1998;6:74-81.
43. Rapelanoro R, Mortureux P, Couprie B, et al. Neonatal *Malassezia furfur* pustulosis. Arch Dermatol 1996;132:190-193.

44. Bordazzi F. Transient cephalic neonatal pustulosis. Arch Dermatol 1997;133:528-529.
45. Niamba P, Weill FX, Sarlangue J, et al. Is common neonatal cephalic pustulosis (neonatal acne) triggered by *Malassezia sympodialis?* Arch Dermatol 1998;134:995.
46. MacFarlane JT, Davies D. Infantile acne associated with transient increases in plasma concentrations of luteinising hormone, follicle-stimulating hormone and testosterone. Brit Med J 1981;282:1275-1276.
47. Burket JM, Storrs FJ. Nodulocystic infantile acne occurring in a kindred of steatocystoma. Arch Dermatol 1987;123:432-433.
48. Arbegast KD, Braddock SW, Lamberty LF, et al. Treatment of infantile cystic acne with oral isotretinoin: a case report. Pediatr Dermatol 1991;2:166-168.
49. Horne HL, Carmichael AJ. Juvenile nodulocystic acne responding to systemic isotretinoin (letter). Br J Dermatol 1997;136:796-797.
50. Mengesha YM, Hansen R. Toddler-age nodulocystic acne. J Pediatr 1999;134:644-648.
51. Murphy, WF, Langly AN. Common bullous lesions—presumably self-inflicted—occurring *in utero* in the newborn infant. Pediatrics 1963;32:1099-1100.
52. Heyl T, Raubenheimer EJ. Sucking pads (sucking calluses) of the lips in neonates: A manifestation of transient leukoedema. Pediatr Dermatol 1987;4:123-128.
53. McCallum DI, Hall GFM. Umbilical granuloma with particular reference to talc granuloma. Br J Dermatol 1970;83:151-156.
54. Andreassi L. Diseases of the umbilicus. In Ruiz-Maldonado R, Parish LC, Beane JM, eds. Textbook of pediatric dermatology. Philadelphia: Grune and Stratton, 1989: pp 820-822.
55. Johnson BL, Honig PG, Jaworsky C. Pediatric dermatopathology. Boston: Butterworth-Heinemann, 1994: pp 16-17.
56. Levine N. Pigmentary abnormalities. In Schachner LA, Hansen RC, eds. Pediatric dermatology. 2nd edition. New York: Churchill Livingstone, 1995: pp 546-547.
57. Geronemus RG. Q-switched ruby laser therapy of nevus of Ota, Arch Dermatol 1992;128:1618.
58. Gibbs RC: Unusual striped hyperpigmentation of the torso. Arch Derm 1967;95:385-386.
59. Halper S, Rubenstein D, Prose N, Levy ML. Pigmentary lines of the newborn. J Am Acad Dermatol 1993;28:893-894.
60. Selimoglu MA, Dilmen U, Karakelleoglu C, et al. Harlequin color change. Arch Pedatr Adolesc Med 149:1171-1172, 1995.

8

Iatrogenic and Traumatic Injuries

NANCY B. ESTERLY

A variety of untoward events may befall the developing infant while in utero or postpartum. Some of these perinatal problems are inherent in the birth process. Others are related to technologic advances that have become standard obstetric and nursery practice. Although these diagnostic and therapeutic procedures have reduced morbidity and mortality, some also pose significant risk for iatrogenic complications.

PUNCTURE WOUNDS

Amniocentesis Scars

Amniocentesis is currently the most widely used diagnostic technique for the antenatal diagnosis of genetic disorders. Although routinely a second-trimester procedure, it may also be performed in the third trimester for management of isoimmunization or evaluation of fetal maturity or late in the first trimester for fetal karyotyping and DNA analysis.[1] The risk for damage to the fetus is quite low, particularly in middle trimester procedures; nevertheless, needle puncture of the skin and sometimes of the underlying structures is a possible complication. Estimates of the incidence of cutaneous scarring ranged as high as 9% in the 1970s[2,3]; however, with increased experience and the advent of real-time ultrasonography, this figure has dropped to less than 1%.[4] Despite the benignity of the procedure, the incidence of fetal injury rises dramatically with an increasing number of needle passages at amniocentesis.

Amniocentesis scars are depressed, dimplelike lesions usually measuring approximately 1 to 5 mm in diameter, although scars as large as 12 mm in diameter and 8 mm in depth have been documented[5] (Fig. 8-1). They may be solitary or multiple and are often inconspicuous. Shallow linear lesions have also been described.[3,4,6] Although sometimes present at birth, they are often not noticed until the infant is several weeks to months of age.[2,5] The most frequent sites of injury are the extremities followed by the head, neck, and chest.[6] Usually the scars are innocuous; however, the possibility of penetration of the underlying tissues must always be considered. Complications include damage to peripheral nerves, blindness secondary to ocular penetration, ileocutaneous and arteriovenous fistulization, gangrene of the arm, and exsanguination of the fetus.[5,6] Midtrimester amniocentesis has the lowest risk of fetal puncture because the fetus occupies only about 50% of the amniotic cavity; in both the first and third trimesters there is less room to maneuver, and sudden movements of the fetus may make injury unavoidable.

Amniocentesis scars must be differentiated from congenital sinus tracts, aplasia cutis, focal dermal dysplasia, amniotic band syndrome, and dimples associated with congenital rubella, diastematomyelia, Bloom syndrome, and cerebrohepatorenal syndrome.

Chorionic Villus Sampling

Chorionic villus sampling (CVS), which can be performed early in the first trimester, is the preferred procedure for patients at risk for certain single gene disorders. The technique yields mitotically active cells suitable for rapid DNA analysis and permits detection of placental mosaicism. Of concern, however, are reports of increased risk of limb and jaw malformations, particularly in fetuses undergoing CVS at less than 9 weeks of age.[1] An analysis of 138,996 outcomes in a multicenter study disputes this notion[7] but is not universally accepted,[8,9] and thus the issue remains a controversial area still under study.

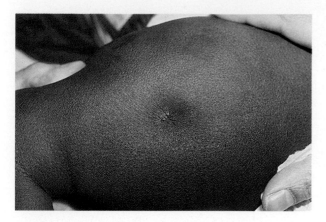

FIG. 8-1
Deep dimple and scar on the buttock of an infant whose mother had amniocentesis.

An increased incidence of hemangiomas has been noted in infants born following chorionic villus sampling as compared with those undergoing amniocentesis. In a questionnaire survey by Burton et al,[10] a threefold increase in hemangiomas occurred in the total CVS group; however, affected infants were largely confined to the subset who had CVS by the transcervical route as opposed to the transabdominal approach. One third of the infants with hemangiomas had multiple lesions, and all but one were cutaneous in location. Only one vascular malformation, a port wine stain, was reported in the CVS group. No correlation was observed between the incidence of these neoplasms and gestational age at sampling, sample size, or number of sampling attempts. Whether or not the development of hemangiomas is related to CVS limb disruption defects is currently unknown.

Fetal Monitoring

Intrauterine electronic monitoring of the fetal heart rate via a spiral electrode attached to the presenting part has become standard obstetric practice. Complications are infrequent and consist mainly of minor lacerations, ulcerations, scalp abscesses, and herpetic infections.[11,12] Herpetic infections are extremely rare; however, incidence figures for scalp abscesses in monitored infants due to other agents range from 0.1 to 5.4%,[13-17] with most in the 0.3% to 0.5% range.

Scalp abscesses are localized collections of suppurative material that present as erythematous, indurated masses with or without fluctuance in the area of electrode application. Usually solitary, they vary in size from one to sev-

eral centimeters. Onset can be as early as the first day or as late as the third week, but they are most frequently noted on the third or fourth day of life. Enlarged posterior cervical lymph nodes often accompany the abscess. Usually the inflammation remains confined to the skin; however, osteomyelitis of the underlying bone[13,14,18] and sepsis[18] have been documented in a few infants.

Contributing factors in some series, but not others, appear to be high-risk pregnancies (prematurity), prolonged rupture of the membranes, and long duration of fetal heart rate monitoring. The presence of amnionitis[11,15,17,19] does not seem to be correlated. Although an infectious cause has been disputed, because cultures obtained from some infants have been sterile, data from large series do not support the concept of a noninfectious etiology. Okada et al[15] reported on 42 infants with scalp abscess of whom 100% had positive cultures; 85% were polymicrobial, 58% grew both aerobes and anaerobes, 33% grew aerobes only, and 9% grew anaerobes only. The predominant aerobic organisms were *Staphylococcus epidermidis* and *Streptococcus*, groups A and B; the predominant anaerobes were *Streptococcus* and *Peptococcus*. A confirmatory study by Brook et al[20] demonstrated similar findings in 23 infants.

It is critical to distinguish infants with intrapartum inoculation of herpes simplex virus (HSV) from neonates with a bacterial scalp abscess. Although HSV infection as a complication of scalp monitoring is distinctly uncommon, the outcome can be devastating, with permanent neurologic damage[21] or death from systemic disease.[22] Both type 1[22] and type 2 infections[12] have been documented; unfortunately, this complication may occur with asymptomatic shedding of the virus and in the absence of a history of overt clinical disease.

Scalp abscesses usually heal uneventfully but may leave minor degrees of scarring, hypopigmentation, and alopecia, causing confusion with aplasia cutis, nevus sebaceus, or focal dermal hypoplasia in subsequent years.

Fetal Blood Gas Sampling

Scalp puncture for fetal blood gas sampling, a procedure performed more infrequently than electrode monitoring, usually causes larger lacerations in the scalp than the scalp electrode, but does not seem to be associated with abscess formation.[19]

Needle Marks and Scars

Needle marks consisting of hypopigmented pinhead-size lesions, when presenting in large numbers, may impart a speckled appearance to the skin.[23] These marks are due to

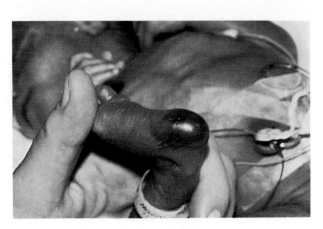

FIG. 8-2
Gangrene of the heel from repeated punctures.

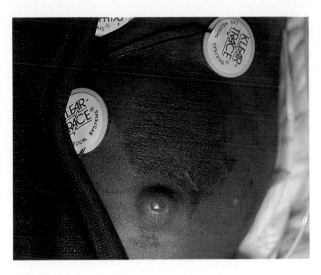

FIG. 8-3
Area of anetoderma noted at several months of age in an infant born prematurely.

venipuncture, arterial punctures, and insertion of catheters and are most commonly seen on the hands, wrists, feet, ankles, arms, and legs. Heel pricks from blood sampling may cause dimpling or, rarely, calcified nodules (see the following discussion), hypertrophic scars, or even gangrene (Fig. 8-2).

Anetoderma of Prematurity

This recently described entity consists of atrophic patches of skin that result from thinning of the dermis. Prerequisites appear to be extreme prematurity (24 to 29 weeks) and a lengthy stay in the neonatal intensive care unit,[24] although one report suggests that low birth weight may be a more important factor than young gestational age.[25] The lesions are absent at birth and lack an identifiable antecedent inflammatory phase, developing de novo between 6 weeks and 10 months of age. The patches are confined to the anterior trunk and proximal limbs, are oval or circular, appear depressed, and measure a few millimeters to several centimeters in diameter (Fig. 8-3). Often they develop at sites of application of adhesives and placement of monitoring devices. Histopathologic examination of a skin biopsy specimen demonstrates reduction or absence of dermal elastic tissue.[24]

The cause is unknown. It has been postulated that the decrease in elastic tissue might be attributable to a subclinical inflammatory reaction or, alternatively, to a transient metabolic derangement in the skin. Presumably the atrophic patches persist indefinitely, but as yet there are no long-term

observational studies. A report of congenital anetoderma in premature twins may represent the same entity.[26]

PERINATAL SOFT TISSUE INJURY

Injury to the soft tissues may occur in the setting of a prolonged labor because of cephalopelvic disproportion or in the case of a forceps delivery. Erythema, abrasions, and forceps marks are most common over the face but rarely cause significant injury and usually resolve spontaneously (Fig. 8-4).

Petechiae on the head, neck, and upper body are likely to be caused by pressure differences that occur during passage of the chest through the birth canal. It is important to exclude the possibility of an underlying infection or hematologic disorder with appropriate laboratory studies. Petechiae caused by trauma are innocuous and usually fade within 2 to 3 days.

Ecchymoses may be extensive following a traumatic or breech delivery. Large areas of bruising may result in hyperbilirubinemia, requiring phototherapy. Ecchymoses resolve gradually but may take up to several days to disappear completely.

CAPUT SUCCEDANEUM

Diffuse edematous swelling of the scalp, when it is the presenting part, is known as caput succedaneum. Extravasation of blood or serum above the periosteum occurs as a result of venous congestion as a result of pressure of the uterus,

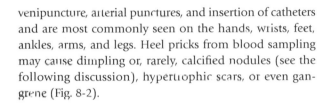

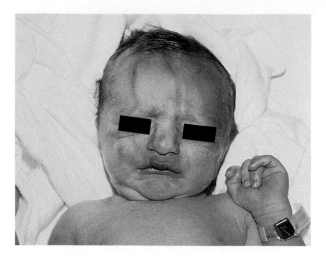

FIG. 8-4
Forceps marks over the face.

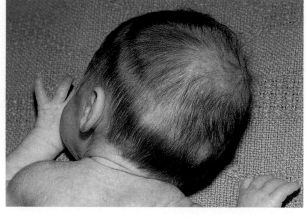

FIG. 8-5
Halo scalp ring: a band of alopecia resulting from localized injury during the birth process. (Courtesy John Hall, MD.)

cervix, and the vaginal wall on the infant's head during a prolonged or difficult labor and delivery. Because the accumulation of fluid is external to the periosteum, it crosses the midline and is not limited by the suture lines. If labor is prolonged, petechiae, purpura, and ecchymoses, as well as molding of the head and overriding sutures, may be prominent features. Unlike cephalhematoma, with which a caput is occasionally confused, the skin findings resolve within a few days. The molding may take a few weeks to disappear. Treatment is not indicated except in the rare instance when severe hemorrhage requires blood transfusions.

HALO SCALP RING

Alopecia in an annular configuration, presumably the consequence of localized injury during the birth process, has been referred to as halo scalp ring.[27] The hair loss is manifest at birth or shortly thereafter as a band of alopecia ranging in width from 1 to 4 cm and usually located over the vertex (Fig. 8-5). There is an associated caput succedaneum and in some instances frank tissue necrosis. If the injury is mild, the alopecia is usually temporary[27]; scarring alopecia may result if the injury is severe.[28,29] Correction of the defect by plastic surgery can be achieved with excellent cosmetic results.

ALOPECIA FROM ISCHEMIA

Scarring alopecia of the occipital scalp has been documented as a consequence of ischemia and compromised oxygenation or as a complication of extracorporeal mem-

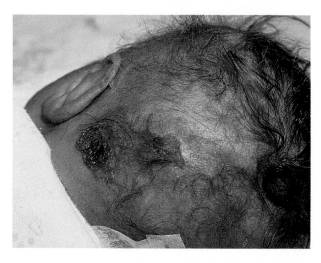

FIG. 8-6
Crusted ulcerations on the posterior scalp associated with ECMO therapy.

brane oxygenation (ECMO) therapy in neonates.[30] During a 6-month period, five infants in a neonatal intensive care unit were observed to develop erythema and edema that progressed to crusted ulcerations (Fig. 8-6) and eventuated in a patch of scarring alopecia. The ulcers were believed to be the result of prolonged pressure in a setting of hypoperfusion, acidosis, and hypoxemia. Institution of a protocol requiring frequent repositioning of the head and use of a temperature-stable gel pad as preventive measures eliminated this problem.

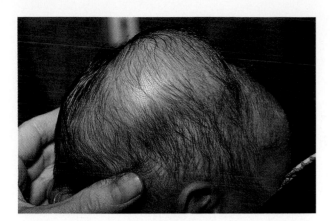

FIG. 8-7
Unilateral cephalhematoma localized to the parietal bone.

CEPHALHEMATOMA

Cephalhematoma is caused by rupture of the diploic veins of the skull during a prolonged or difficult labor or delivery. The result of subperiosteal hemorrhage, it differs clinically from caput succedaneum in that it is almost always unilateral. The hematoma is localized most often to the area over the parietal bone, and the mass is confined by the periosteum, which adheres to the margin of the bone (Fig. 8-7). Cephalhematoma less frequently involves the occipital bones and only rarely the frontal bones. If both parietal bones are involved, the hematomas are sharply delimited and separated by a midline depression corresponding to the intervening suture. The overlying scalp is not discolored.

Cephalhematomas are seen more commonly in vacuum-assisted vaginal deliveries than in forceps or spontaneous births.[31] The swelling may not become apparent until several hours to days after birth. As the hematoma ages, it develops a calcified rim and is gradually completely overlaid with bone. Estimates of underlying skull fractures have ranged from 5.4% to 25%.[32,33] Differential diagnosis includes cephalhematoma and cranial meningocele.[34] Meningoceles can be differentiated by the presence of pulsations, increased pressure when crying, and the presence of a bony defect on roentgenograms. Infection of the mass and severe hemorrhage resulting in anemia and hyperbilirubinemia are rare complications for which antibiotics, blood transfusions, and phototherapy may be required.[35] Treatment is unnecessary for uncomplicated lesions. Most cephalhematomas are resorbed during the first few weeks of life and are of no consequence.[31] Occasionally they calcify and persist for months to years.

UNTOWARD EFFECTS OF VACUUM EXTRACTION[36]

The formation of some type of hematoma is a common occurrence with the use of a vacuum extractor, although with the introduction of softer silicone cups the risk has been reduced. A "chignon," or artificial caput succedaneum, is created by adherence of the cup to the scalp and is most obvious immediately following removal of the cup. However, the swelling usually disperses relatively rapidly after birth. If a chignon is formed in the presence of a natural caput, the scalp may have a boggy sensation suggesting subgaleal hemorrhage, a potentially lethal event.[37]

Cephalhematomas, a ring of suction blisters, lacerations, and abrasions may also result from the use of the vacuum extractor.[38] The latter are usually the result of prolonged traction and sudden detachment of the cup. Scalp subcutaneous emphysema has been attributed to vacuum extraction in an infant with a coexistent scalp electrode wound.[39]

LACERATIONS

Scalpel lacerations to the infant during cesarean section represent a potential form of injury. Smith et al[40] found an incidence of fetal injury of 1.9% in a series of 896 cesarean deliveries. Lacerations were much more common in those deliveries where the indication was nonvertex presentation (breech or transverse lie). In these infants, the injuries were almost always located on the lower portion of the body, whereas infants in a vertex presentation usually sustained their lacerations on the head. Failure to recognize the injury in the delivery room was a common occurrence.

BURNS

Chemical burns from concentrated disinfectants or other solvents have been reported following use in the neonatal intensive care nursery (see Chapter 5). Isopropyl alcohol has caused second- and third-degree burns when substituted for electrode paste beneath electrocardiographic (ECG) leads[41] or used as a prep for the umbilical area.[42] Small premature infants are particularly predisposed to skin damage because of an immature epidermal barrier, and their vulnerability may be accentuated by hypoxia and hypothermia. Burns are evident as intense erythema associated with blister formation and sloughing of the damaged skin (Fig. 8-8). Tissue damage can be prevented if the skin is dried immediately and protected from prolonged contact with these substances.

Scald injury and contact burns must be considered in the differential diagnosis of bullous lesions of unknown etiology. Inadvertent immersion injury was described in

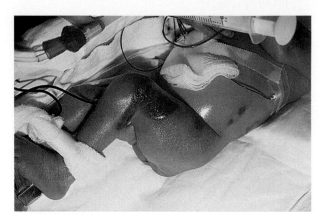

FIG. 8-8
Alcohol burn on a premature infant.

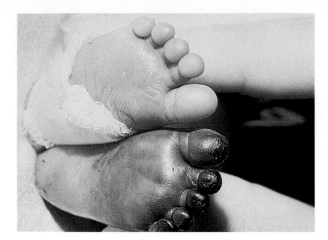

FIG. 8-9
Gangrene of the foot secondary to umbilical artery catheterization and thrombosis.

one such instance where the temperature of the hospital water supply was raised for purposes of infection control.[43] Contact with a disposable warmer causing cicatricial alopecia and a cranial defect requiring bone grafts was reported in another neonate.[44]

UMBILICAL ARTERY CATHETERIZATION

Catheterization of the umbilical arteries has become standard practice in the neonatal intensive care unit for monitoring intravascular pressures, chemistries, pH, and blood gases and for administering fluids and medications to critically ill neonates. However, this procedure is fraught with risk of serious complications, even in experienced hands. Thrombosis is the most frequent problem, as documented by aortography.[45] Other potential complications include vasospasm, blanching of the limbs, embolism, perforation of the vessels, vascular damage from hypertonic solutions, hemorrhage, infections, and ischemic and chemical necrosis of the abdominal viscera.[46,47] These untoward events are usually caused by incorrect placement of the catheter or to unduly rapid infusion of hazardous drugs or hypertonic solutions rather than vessel injury.[48]

Vasospasm may occur during placement of the catheter in the umbilical artery. It is manifest by temporary blanching or cyanosis of the leg and foot. Prompt removal of the catheter is indicated, and if this procedure is followed, sequelae are unlikely.

Thromboses and multiple small emboli can cause infarcts of the toes. Depending on the placement of the thrombus, unilateral or bilateral gangrene of the feet,

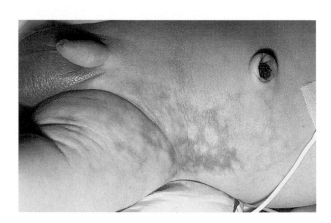

FIG. 8-10
Early skin changes of reticulated erythema resulting from attempted umbilical artery catheterization.

lower extremities, or buttocks can occur (Fig. 8-9).[47,49,50] Gangrene of the distal upper extremity with loss of fingers has also been documented secondary to similar events following percutaneous radial artery catheterization.[51] Early skin changes include erythema, transient blanching, vesicles, and bulla formation (Fig. 8-10). These lesions may abate or may progress to extensive skin and subcutaneous tissue necrosis, demarcation, and gangrene.[50]

PERINATAL GANGRENE OF THE BUTTOCK

This alarming and fortunately rare occurrence is usually attributed to iatrogenic causes[52] but has also been documented as an apparent spontaneous event.[53,54] The onset is heralded by the sudden appearance of an erythematous patch involving the buttock, perineum, and genitalia. Within hours the involved area rapidly becomes edematous and then rock hard and cold to the touch with well-defined black borders. Bullae may form on the surface. Generally the lower limbs are spared and remain warm and of normal color with palpable femoral pulses. Over the subsequent several days the necrotic tissue demarcates and sloughs leaving a deep ulcer that heals by secondary intention with scarring.

The diagnosis is made on the basis of the abrupt onset and clinical findings. The differential diagnosis is mainly that of an infectious process, but cultures are invariably negative, as are biochemical and hematologic laboratory studies. Chemical or thermal injury must also be considered.

The presumed cause is an occlusive vascular event involving the internal iliac artery. This artery, which feeds into the umbilical artery, splits into two terminal branches, the inferior gluteal and the internal pudendal arteries; these two vessels supply the buttock, perineum, vulva, and scrotum. Vasospasm followed by thrombus formation resulting from a variety of pathogenetic factors such as injury to the umbilical cord or obstruction by a misdirected umbilical catheter is thought to account for this condition. Despite the extent of the gangrenous process, generally the lesions heal without complications and the sphincters remain intact.[52,53]

COMPLICATIONS OF PHOTOTHERAPY

Visible light phototherapy has become standard therapy in the newborn nursery for infants with significant indirect hyperbilirubinemia. Visible light energy isomerizes unconjugated bilirubin to more polar forms, which are excreted into the bile and ultimately into the stool within minutes of exposure. Bilirubin absorbs light maximally in the blue portion of the spectrum (420 to 500 nm). Daylight fluorescent bulbs have an emission spectrum from 320 to 700 nm, which includes small amounts of ultraviolet A (UVA), as well as the therapeutic blue wavelengths. High-energy blue lamps emit in a narrower range and exclude light in the ultraviolet spectrum; however, they are used less frequently because the hue produced by these lamps makes it difficult to assess skin color in jaundiced infants and also may cause nausea and dizziness in nursery personnel.

Because phototherapy is not standardized, response and outcome may vary from one setting to another. Daylight, cool white, and special blue fluorescent lights can be used separately or in combination, or tungsten-halogen

lamps may be used. Likewise, the energy output, or irradiance, of the phototherapy unit may vary depending on the positioning of the lamps and the amount of skin surface area exposed to the light. Therapy may be intermittent or continuous, and most recently, fiberoptic phototherapy has been introduced using a halogen light source transmitted to a blanket that is wrapped around the infant. Adverse effects of phototherapy are few but include erythematous, purpuric, and vesicular transient eruptions (see Chapters 5 and 17), bronze baby syndrome, and rarely, ultraviolet light burns.

Ultraviolet Light Burns

Burns have been reported in only a few instances and have been a result of misadventure causing prolonged exposure to inadequately shielded phototherapy lights. Siegfried et al[55] reported two premature infants who developed generalized erythema, one with blistering, on exposure to fluorescent daylight bulbs. The burns were from the UVA wavelengths and were sustained because of inadvertent failure to place Plexiglas covers over the banks of bulbs.[55] The erythema was most intense in areas of the body closest to the light source and spared the shielded areas. The authors point out that it is important to recognize that infants cared for in beds other than Plexiglas isolettes are not protected from UVA transmission unless these shields are in place. They also caution that plastic wrap and plastic shell vapor barriers do not protect against this type of injury.

Phototherapy-Induced Drug Eruptions

Apart from burns, erythematous and vesiculobullous eruptions may be associated with phototherapy under other circumstances. Drug-induced phototoxicity eruptions have been documented in neonates receiving certain therapeutic agents (e.g., furosemide or fluorescein dye for a radiologic procedure).[56,57] These eruptions have occurred in infants given a photosensitizing drug and exposed to light of the appropriate wavelength to cause photoactivation of the chemical compound. As with true burns, these bullae develop only on light-exposed skin. Discontinuation of therapy usually results in an uneventful recovery.

Transient Porphyrinemia and Phototherapy Eruptions

Transient porphyrinemia in combination with phototherapy has also been documented as a cause of blisters and erosions,[58] as well as erythematous and purpuric

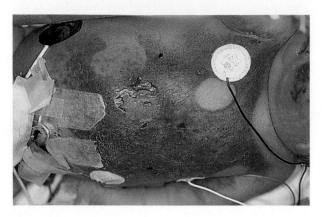

FIG. 8-11
Photosensitive eruption in a neonate with transient porphyrinemia associated with hemolytic disease of the newborn. (Courtesy Julie Prendiville, MD.)

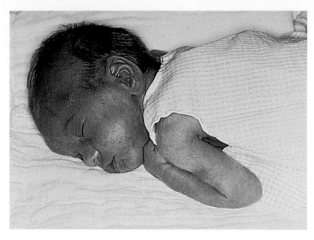

FIG. 8-12
Infant with bronze baby syndrome. (Courtesy Walter Burgdorf, MD.)

lesions[59,60] in several neonates with hemolytic disease (Fig. 8-11). The eruptions in all cases were confined to exposed areas, sparing the sites protected from the lights (e.g., skin under leads, dressings, and temperature probes). Onset was between 1 and 4 days after initiation of phototherapy, although one infant had a more delayed response.[58] Reactions ranged from violaceous discoloration resembling a sunburn[59] to frank purpura.[60] One infant had blisters with erosions and skin fragility instead.[58]

Skin biopsy specimens from the purpuric lesions showed only extravasation of erythrocytes[60] without epidermal changes, thus distinguishing the eruption from a burn. In the infant who blistered, the cleavage plane occurred at the level of the lamina lucida (subepidermal), and there was an associated minimal dermal infiltrate.[58]

The porphyrin levels in affected infants differed somewhat in that one infant had elevated free erythrocyte protoporphyrin and zinc protoporphyrin levels,[59] whereas the others had mainly increased amounts of both coproporphyrin and protoporphyrin in their plasma.[58,60] Although the cause of the elevated porphyrin levels in these infants was not clear, it was postulated that multiple factors, including cholestasis, altered hepatic function, concomitant administration of photosensitizing drugs and transfused blood products, and renal failure, might be responsible. In addition, a prolonged course of phototherapy at a relatively high level of irradiance was thought to be a contributing factor in one instance.[58]

Differential diagnosis includes infections, epidermolysis bullosa, neonatal lupus erythematosus, metabolic photosensitivity eruptions, true porphyria, and drug eruptions.

Both the cutaneous eruption and the transient porphyrinemia clear spontaneously within a few weeks, and there are no significant sequelae.

Bronze Baby Syndrome

In this rare complication of phototherapy the infant's skin, serum, and urine become a gray-brown color after several hours under the phototherapy lamps (Fig. 8-12). All of the infants who have developed this disorder have had prior evidence of hepatic dysfunction marked by conjugated hyperbilirubinemia and retention of bile acids.[61,62,63] The serum acquires a dark brown color and shows a nonspecific absorbance from 380 to 520 nm on spectroanalysis.[63] The peculiar color has been attributed to the formation of a photooxidation product of bilirubin or to copper-bound porphyrins, which yield brown photoproducts in the presence of bilirubin.[64,65] It has also been suggested that biliverdin pigments may contribute to the bronzing effect.[66] The odd hue is easily distinguished from that of cyanosis or typical neonatal jaundice. The discoloration fades over time after phototherapy is discontinued, and there are no significant sequelae.

CALCINOSIS CUTIS

Calcification of the skin occurs as a consequence of deposition of hydroxyapatite crystals and amorphous calcium phosphate in the soft tissues. Based on the pathophysiologic mechanisms, calcinosis cutis is usually classified as idiopathic (normal tissue and a normal calcium/phosphorus

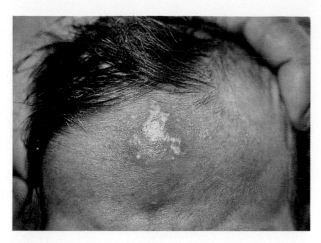

FIG. 8-13
Calcified plaque on the forehead secondary to extravasation of calcium gluconate.

ratio); dystrophic (damaged tissue and a normal calcium/phosphorus ratio); or metastatic (normal tissue and an abnormal calcium/phosphorus ratio). Iatrogenic calcinosis cutis in neonates is usually of the dystrophic type and is most often the result of an intravenous infusion of calcium gluconate or calcium chloride for treatment of neonatal hypocalcemia.[67,68,69] It may also occur following application of electrode paste containing calcium chloride for electroencephalography, electromyography, or brain stem auditory evoked potentials, particularly if applied to abraded skin,[70] and in association with subcutaneous fat necrosis.

Calcinosis Cutis from Infusion of Calcium Salts

Visible evidence of soft tissue calcification develops on average 13 days after infusion of the calcium solution, with a range of 2 hours to 24 days (Fig. 8-13). There may be marked swelling with an intense inflammatory response, even in the absence of extravasation of fluid, and occasionally there is soft tissue necrosis. The calcification takes the form of papules, nodules, an annular plaque, or a large subcutaneous plaque or may have a linear configuration conforming to the vein in which the solution is administered. The lesions are firm, erythematous, and brown, yellow, or white; when extravasation has occurred, they may be tender, warm, and fluctuant, resembling an abscess.[67]

Radiographic changes can be detected as early as 4 to 5 days following the infusion.[68,71] Three patterns have been described: (1) that of a calcified mass localized to or near the site of injection; (2) more diffuse calcification along fascial planes; and (3) a pattern of vascular or perivascular calcification.[68,72,73] Skin biopsy specimens contain calcium deposits in the dermal papillae, as well as amorphous masses of calcium intermingled with degenerated collagen and a lymphohistiocytic infiltrate in the deeper dermis. Stains for calcium (e.g., von Kossa) demonstrate focal calcium deposits in the walls of the vessels, both arteries and veins.

Several factors are believed to contribute to this reaction, which peaks at about 2 weeks. In some instances, tissue damage results from leakage of infusate from the vein at the puncture site or the development of frank phlebitis, particularly if the infusion is given over a prolonged period. However, calcinosis cutis may occur even in the absence of obvious extravasation of fluid.[69] Precipitation of calcium salts is also facilitated by an alkaline pH that results from tissue damage or when bicarbonate or certain drugs (e.g., amphotericin, prednisolone sodium phosphate) are infused through the same intravenous line.

The diagnosis of calcinosis cutis can be made clinically based on the distinctive appearance of the skin lesions and confirmed by skin biopsy and/or radiographs. Differential diagnosis includes cellulitis, osteomyelitis, periostitis, hematoma, abscess, and subcutaneous fat necrosis.[71]

Treatment is generally symptomatic, and spontaneous resolution occurs over several months by transepidermal elimination of the calcified material. An animal study has suggested that intralesional injection of triamcinolone may be effective in reducing inflammation and facilitating resorption of calcium.[74]

Calcinosis Cutis Associated With Subcutaneous Fat Necrosis

Subcutaneous fat necrosis may develop in infants who experience perinatal iatrogenic problems such as obstetric trauma, asphyxia, or hypothermia (see also Chapter 22). Hypercalcemia occasionally complicates the course in these infants.[75] Rarely, there is accompanying soft tissue calcification identifiable by biopsy or radiography.[76-80] The presence of soft tissue calcification does not seem to portend a more ominous prognosis and eventually resolves.

Calcified Nodules of the Heels

These lesions have been seen in association with heel prick marks, principally in infants of low birth weight and young gestational age who as neonates received numer-

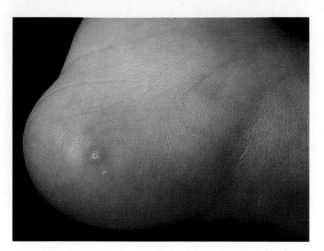

FIG. 8-14
Calcified papules nodules on the heel secondary to heel sticks.

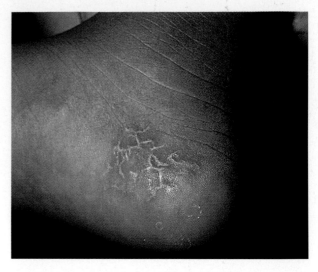

FIG. 8-15
Multiple stellate scars secondary to heel sticks in premature infant.

ous heel sticks in the nursery.[23,81] Onset is usually between 4 and 12 months after birth and is marked by the appearance of multiple tiny white or yellow specks within depressed areas on the heels (Fig. 8-14). The papulonodules enlarge and become elevated and firm but are neither inflamed nor symptomatic. The accumulated calcified material is eventually spontaneously extruded through the epidermis or can be manually expressed. There is no associated underlying biochemical abnormality, and metabolic studies are not indicated. Linear or stellate scarring without calcification may also be seen secondary to heel sticks in neonates (Fig. 8-15).

On histologic examination the nodules consist of a cystic-like space with irregular calcification around the margins but no epithelial lining. The calcification is surrounded by fibrous connective tissue and a patchy mononuclear infiltrate. The pathogenesis is poorly understood, although undoubtedly trauma plays a role. Differential diagnosis includes subepidermal calcified nodule (of Winer). The process is self-limited and does not require intervention.

COMPLICATIONS OF BLOOD GAS MONITORING

The use of noninvasive techniques for skin surface monitoring of blood gases has become routine practice in the newborn intensive care nursery.[82] Transcutaneous measurements of oxygen and carbon dioxide tension and pulse oximetry for assessment of arterial saturation levels provide accurate, reproducible information facilitating clinical management of premature and sick infants. Although these techniques are widely used, they do pose some risk for damage to the infant's skin at sites of contact with the sensors and electrodes.

Pulse Oximetry

Pulse oximetry relies on the spectrophotometric analysis of light to measure the oxygen saturation of hemoglobin. The technique employs a sensor that wraps around a hand, foot, or finger or an ear probe that clips to the antihelix. It requires no calibration and no skin heating and provides almost continuous measurement of oxygen saturation. Tight application of a probe may cause a first-degree thermal burn, skin erosion, hyperpigmentation, blister, or pressure necrosis.[83] Second- and third-degree burns have also been observed, particularly in instances where sensors and oximeters from different companies were paired and found to be incompatible.[84,85] Because pulse oximetry does not require tight contact with the skin, this complication is avoidable by frequent inspection of the probe site.[83]

Transcutaneous Oxygen Monitoring

Although also considered a noninvasive procedure, transcutaneous oxygen monitoring poses a greater risk for local skin damage because the electrode must be heated to 42° to 45° C to promote adequate blood flow.[23,82,86-88] The

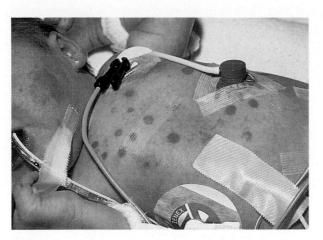

FIG. 8-16
Multiple first degree burns from transcutaneous oxygen monitoring device.

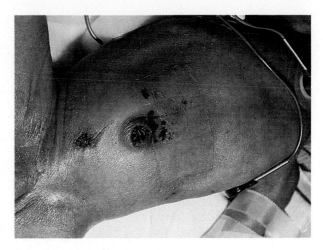

FIG. 8-17
Erosion of the abdominal skin from application and removal of adhesives.

heated electrode produces local hyperthermia and vasodilation, arterializing the vascular bed at the electrode site. As one might expect, thermal injury is a frequent problem and is directly related to the temperature of the sensor, the sensitivity of the infant's skin, and the duration of placement of the monitoring device at a single skin site. Indeed, it is usual with this device to induce a first-degree burn, although the erythema is likely to fade by 12 hours (Fig. 8-16). Second- and third-degree burns have also been documented.[82]

In a study by Boyle and Oh,[86] all infants monitored with these sensors developed blanchable erythema, the equivalent of a first-degree burn. A smaller number of infants, more often those born prematurely, sustained a more severe thermal reaction evidenced by nonblanchable erythema, which lasted from 60 hours to 6 days.[86] These reactions were interpreted as mild second-degree burns. Vesicles have been noted when the electrode is applied for extended periods.

Thermal damage caused by the electrode can be compounded by yet another type of injury from application and removal of the adhesive ring that secures the sensor in place. Stripping of the stratum corneum occurs with removal of the sensor, which is placed in a new site every 4 hours (Fig. 8-17). This epidermal damage is particularly perilous in premature infants under 30 weeks of age because it compromises an already fragile and incompetent barrier, putting the infant at increased risk for fluid and electrolyte imbalance and loss of temperature control. Furthermore, if a large surface area is denuded, these infants may be more vulnerable to infectious organisms and

chemicals placed on the skin.[82,87] Application of a copolymer acrylic dressing (Op-Site) has been shown to protect the skin from adhesive trauma and does not interfere with transcutaneous oxygen measurements.[87]

A rare complication described in two infants is the development of circular hyperpigmented macules at monitoring sites, which over several months became crateriform and remained as permanent marks. Biopsy of one affected infant revealed focal dermal cicatricial fibrosis.[88] Of interest, the craters did not develop until several months of age, a course reminiscent of that of anetoderma of prematurity.

Transillumination Blisters

Thermal burns may occur as a complication of the use of transillumination devices for detection of hydrocephalus, subdural effusions, cystic hygroma, and pneumomediastinum, or for localization of arteries and veins for blood sampling. Typical lesions are small (<5 mm), round, discrete blisters with a necrotic base that develop at sites of transillumination (Fig. 8-18).[89]

It is thought that specific wavelengths of the high-intensity fiberoptic light are converted to heat energy in the skin, causing thermal damage. Infrared and ultraviolet filters within the light source, usually a quartz halogen lamp, eliminate wavelengths of less than 570 nm, reducing the risk of thermal injury. A defect in the transilluminator unit, missing filters,[90] or failure of the filter to function properly has accounted for the occurrence of these blisters in neonates.

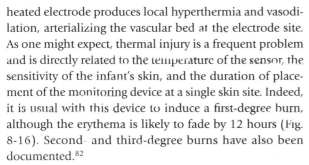

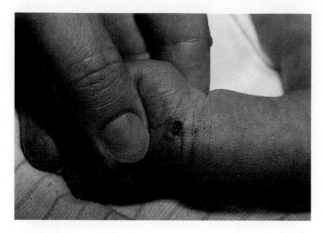

FIG. 8-18
Thermal burns from a transillumination unit causing blisters in a neonate. (Courtesy Sheila Fallon-Friedlander, MD.)

MEATAL ULCERATION FOLLOWING CIRCUMCISION

Mackenzie has proposed that meatal ulceration is a frequently unrecognized consequence of neonatal circumcision.[91] He has suggested that removal of the prepuce subjects the epithelium of the glans penis to undue irritation from the diaper, which may result in erosions followed by healing with stenosis. Because the erosions do not necessarily occur in the immediate postoperative period, the cause-and-effect relationship is not appreciated. Other rare complications include direct injury to the glans and urethra, bleeding, and infection.

REFERENCES

1. Jauniaux E, Rodeck C. Use, risks and complications of amniocentesis and chorionic villous sampling for prenatal diagnosis in early pregnancy. Early Pregnancy. Biol Med 1995; 1:245-252.
2. Karp LE, Hayden PW. Fetal puncture during midtrimester amniocentesis. Obstet Gynecol 1977;49:115-117.
3. Epley SL, Hanson JW, Cruikshank DP. Fetal injury with midtrimester diagnostic amniocentesis. Obstet Gynecol 1979; 53:77-80.
4. Cambiaghi S, Restano L, Cavalli R, et al. Skin dimpling as a consequence of amniocentesis. J Am Acad Dermatol 1998; 39:888-890.
5. Bruce S, Duffy JO, Wolf JE Jr. Skin dimpling associated with mid-trimester amniocentesis. Pediatr Dermatol 1984;2:140-142.
6. Raimer SS, Raimer BG. Needle puncture scars from mid-trimester amniocentesis. Arch Dermatol 1984;120:1360-1362.
7. Froster UG. Limb defects and chorionic villus sampling: results from an international registry, 1992-94. Lancet 1996; 347:489-1494.
8. Firth H, Boyd PA, Chamberlain P, et al. Limb defects and chorionic villus sampling. Lancet 1996;347:1406
9. Mastroiacovo P, Botto LD. Limb defects and chorionic villus sampling. Lancet 1996;347:1407-1408.
10. Burton BK, Schulz CJ, Angle B, et al. An increased incidence of haemangiomas in infants born following chorionic villus sampling (CVS). Prenat Diagn 1995;15:209-214.
11. Ashkenazi S, Metzker A, Merlob P, et al. Scalp changes after fetal monitoring. Arch Dis Child 1985;60:267-269.
12. Amann ST, Fagnant RJ, Chartrand SA, et al. Herpes simplex infection associated with short-term use of a fetal scalp electrode. J Reproduct Med 1992;37:372-374.
13. Feder HM Jr, MacLean WC Jr, Moxon R. Scalp abscess secondary to fetal scalp electrode. J Pediatr 1976;89:808-809.
14. Plavidal FJ, Werch A. Fetal scalp abcess secondary to intrauterine monitoring. Am J Obstet Gynecol 1976;125:65-70.
15. Okada DM, Chow AW, Bruce VT. Neonatal scalp abcess and fetal monitoring: Factors associated with infection. Am J Obstet Gynecol 1977;129:185-189.
16. Wagener MM, Rycheck RR, Yee RB, et al. Septic dermatitis of the neonatal scalp and maternal endomyometritis with intrapartum internal fetal monitoring. Pediatrics 1984;74:81-85.
17. Winkel CA, Snyder DL, Schlaerth JB. Scalp abscess: A complication of the spiral fetal electrode. Am J Obstet Gynecol 1976;126:720-722.
18. Overturf GD, Balfour G. Osteomyelitis and sepsis: Severe complications of fetal monitoring. Pediatrics 1975;55:244-247.
19. Cordero L, Anderson CW, Zuspan FP. Scalp abscess: A benign and infrequent complication of fetal monitoring. Am J Obstet Gynecol 1983;146:126-130.
20. Brook I, Frazier EH. Microbiology of scalp abcess in newborns. Pediatr Infect Dis J 1992;11:766-768.
21. Katz M, Greco A, Antony L, et al. Neonatal herpesvirus sepsis following internal monitoring. Int J Gynaecol Obstet 1980; 17:631-633.
22. Goldkrand JW. Intrapartum inoculationof herpes simplex virus by fetal scalp electrode. Obstet Gynecol 1982;59:263-265.
23. Cartlidge PHT, Fox PE, Rutter N. The scars of newborn intensive care. Early Hum Dev 1990;21:1-10.
24. Prizant TL, Lucky AW, Frieden IJ, et al. Spontaneous atrophic patches in extremely premature infants. Arch Dermatol 1996; 132:671-674.
25. Todd DJ. Anetoderma of prematurity. Arch Dermatol 1997; 133:789.
26. Zeyllman GL, Levy ML. Congenital anetoderma in twins. J Am Acad Dermatol 1997;36:483-485.
27. Neal PR, Merk PF, Norins AL. Halo scalp ring: A form of localized scalp injury associated with caput succedaneum. Pediatr Dermatol 1984;2:52-54.
28. Beutner KR. Halo ring scarring alopecia. Pediatr Dermatol 1985;3:83.
29. Prendiville JS, Esterly NB. Halo scalp ring: A cause of scarring alopecia. Arch Dermatol 1987;123:992-993.
30. Gershan LA, Esterly NB. Scarring alopecia in neonates as a consequence of hypoxemia-hypoperfusion. Arch Dis Child 1993;68:591-593.
31. Bofill JA, Rust OA, Davidas M. et al. Neonatal cephalohematoma from vacuum extraction. J Reprod Med 1997; 42:565-569.

32. Kendall N, Woolshin H. Cephalhematoma associated with fracture of the skull. J Pediatr 1952;41:125-127.

33. Zelson C, Lee SJ, Pearl M. The incidence of skull fractures underlying cephal hematomas in newborn infants. J Pediatr 1974;85:371-373.

34. Winter TC, Mack LA, Cyr DR. Prenatal sonographic diagnosis of scalp edema/cephalohematoma mimicking an encephalocele. Am J Roentgenol 1993;161:1247-1248.

35. Tan KL, Lim GC. Phototherapy for neonatal jaundice in infants with cephalhematomas. Clin Pediatr 1995;34:7-11.

36. Vacca A. Birth by vacuum extraction: Neonatal outcome. J Paediatr Child Health 1996;32:204-206.

37. Benaron DA. Subgaleal hematoma causing hypovolemic shock during delivery after failed vacuum extraction: A case report. J Perinatol 1993;13:228-231.

38. Metzker A, Brenner S, Merlob P. Iatrogenic cutaneous injuries in the neonate. Arch Dermatol 1999;135:697-703.

39. Birenbaum E, Robinson G, Mashiach S, et al. Skull subcutaneous emphysema - a rare complicaiton of vacuum extraction and scalp electrode. Eur J Obstet Gynecol Reprod Biol 1986;22:257-260.

40. Smith JF, Hernandez C, Wax JR. Fetal laceration injury at cesarean delivery. Obstet Gynecol 1997;90:344-346.

41. Schick JB, Milstein JM. Burn hazard of isopropyl alcohol in the neonate. Pediatrics 1981;68:587-588.

42. Weintraub Z, Iancu TC. Isopropyl alcohol burns. Pediatrics 1982;69:506.

43. Mirowski GW, Frieden IJ, Miller C. Iatrogenic scald burn: a consequence of institutional infection control measures. Pediatrics 1996;98:963-965.

44. Matsumura H, Shigehara K, Ueno T, et al. Cranial defect and decrease in cerebral blood flow resulting from deep contact burn of the scalp in the neonatal period. Burns 1996;22:560-565.

45. Neal WA, Reynolds JW, Jarvis CW, et al. Umbilical artery catheterization: Demonstration of arterial thrombosis by aortography. Pediatrics 1972;50:6-13.

46. Kitterman JA, Phibbs RH, Tooley WH. Catheterization of umbilical vessels in newborn infants. Pediatr Clin North Am 1970;17:895-912.

47. Cutler VE, Stretcher GS. Cutaneous complications of central umbilical artery catheterization. Arch Dermatol 1977;113:61-63.

48. Marsh JL, King W, Barrett C, et al. Serious complications after umbilical artery catheterization for neonatal monitoring. Arch Surg 1975;110.1203-1208.

49. deSanctis N, Cardillo G, Rega AN. Gluteoperineal gangrene and sciatic nerve palsy after umbilical vessel injection. Clin Orthop Related Res 1995;316:180-184.

50. Letts M, Blastorah B, Al-Azzam S. Neonatal gangrene of the extremities. J Pediatr Orthoped 1997;17:397-401.

51. Cartwright GW, Schreiner RL. Major complication secondary to percutaneous radial artery catherization in the neonate. Pediatrics 1980;65:139-141.

52. Rudolph N, Wang HH, Dragutsky D. Gangrene of the buttock: A complication of umbilical artery catheterization. Pediatrics 1974;53:106-109.

53. Serrano G, Aliaga A, Febrer I, et al. Perinatal gangrene of the buttock: A spontaneous condition. Arch Dermatol 1985;121:23-24.

54. Bonifazi E, Meneghini C. Perinatal gangrene of the buttock: An iatrogenic or spontaneous condition? J Am Acad Dermatol 1980;3:596-598.

55. Siegfried EC, Stone MS, Madison KC. Ultraviolet light burn: a cutaneous complication of visible light phototherapy of neonatal jaundice. Pediatr Dermatol 1992;9:278-282.

56. Kearns GL, Williams BJ, Timmons OT. Fluorescein phototoxicity in a premature infant. J Pediatr 1985;107:796-798.

57. Burry JN, Lawrence JR. Phototoxic blisters from high furosimide dosage. Br J Dermatol 1976;94:495-499.

58. Mallon E, Wojnarowska F, Hope P, et al. Neonatal bullous eruption as a result of transient porphyrinemia in a premature infant with hemolytic disease of the newborn. J Am Acad Dermatol 1995;33:333-336.

59. Crawford RI, Lawlor ER, Wadsworth LD, et al. Transient erythroporphyria of infancy. J Am Acad Dermatol 1996;35:833-834.

60. Paller AS, Eramo LR, Farrell EE, et al. Purpuric phototherapy-induced eruption in transfused neonates: Relation to transient porphyrinemia. Pediatrics 1997;100:360-364.

61. Tan KL, Jacob E. The bronze baby syndrome. Acta Pediatr Scand 1982;71:409-414.

62. Rubaltelli FF, Jori G, Reddi E. Bronze baby syndrome: A new porphyrin-related disorder. Pediatr Res 1983;17:327-330.

63. Ashley JR, Littler CM, Burgdorf WC, et al. Bronze baby syndrome. J Amer Acad Dermatol 1985;12:325-328.

64. Onishi S, Itoh S, Isobe K, et al. Mechanism of development of bronze baby syndrome in neonates treated with phototherapy. Pediatrics 1982;69:273-276.

65. Jori G, Reddi E, Rubaltelli FF. Bronze baby syndrome: An animal model. Pediatr Res 1990;27:22-25.

66. Purcell SM, Wians FH Jr, Ackerman NB Jr, et al. Hyperbiliverdinemia in the bronze baby syndrome. J Am Acad Dermatol 1987;16:172-177.

67. Ramamurthy RS, Harris V, Pildes RS. Subcutaneous calcium deposition in the neonate associated with intravenous administration of calcium gluconate. Pediatrics 1975;55:802-806.

68. Sahn EE, Smith DJ. Annular dystrophic calcinosis cutis in an infant. J Am Acad Dermatol 1992;26:1015-1017.

69. Weiss Y, Ackerman C, Shmilovitz A. Localized necrosis of scalp in neonates due to calcium gluconate infusions: A cautionary note. Pediatrics 1975;56:1084-1086.

70. Puig L, Rocamora V, Romani J, et al. Calcinosis cutis following calcium chloride electrode paste application for auditory-brainstem evoked potentials recording. Pediatr Dermatol 1998;15:27-30.

71. Berger PE, Heidelberger KP, Poznanski AK. Extravasation of calcium gluconate as a cause of soft tissue calcification in infancy. Am J Roentgenol 1974;121:109-116.

72. Lee FA, Gwinn JL. Roentgen patterns of extravasation of calcium gluconate in the tissues of the neonate. J Pediatr 1975;86:598-601.

73. Hironaga M, Fujigaki T, Tanaka S. Calcinosis cutis in a neonate following extravasation of calcium gluconate. J Am Acad Dermatol 1982;6:392-395.

74. Ahn SK, Kim KT, Lee SH, et al. The efficacy of treatment with triamcinolone acetonide in calcinosis cutis following extravasation of calcium gluconate: a preliminary study. Pediatr Dermatol 1997;14:103-109.

75. Hicks MJ, Levy ML, Alexander J, et al. Subcutaneous fat necrosis of the newborn and hypercalcemia: Case report and review of the literature. Pediatr Dermatol 1993;10:271-276.

76. Norwood-Galloway A, Lebwohl M, Phelps RG, et al. Subcutaneous fat necrosis of the newborn with hypercalcemia. J Am Acad Dermatol 1987;16:435-439.

77. Sharlin DN, Koblenzer P. Necrosis of subcutaneous fat with hypercalcemia, a puzzling and multifaceted disease. Clin Pediatr 1970;9:290-294.

78. Thomsen, RJ. Subcutaneous fat necrosis of the newborn and idiopathic hypercalcemia. Arch Dermatol 1980;116:1155-1158.

79. Duhn R, Schoen EJ, Siu M. Subcutaneous fat necrosis with extensive calcification after hypothermia in two newborn infants. Pediatrics 1968;41:661-664.

80. Gu LL, Daneman A, Binet A, et al. Nephrocalcinosis and nephrolithiasis due to subcutaneous fat necrosis with hypercalcemia in two full-term asphyxiated neonates: sonographic findings. Pediatr Radiol 1995;25:142-144.

81. Sell EJ, Hansen RC, Struck-Pierce S. Calcified nodules on the heel: A complication of neonatal intensive care. J Pediatr 1980;96:473-475.

82. Peabody JL, Emery JR. Noninvasive monitoring of blood gases in the newborn. Clin Perinatol 1985;12:147-160.

83. Miyasaka K, Ohata J. Burn, erosion, and "sun"tan with the use of pulse oximetry in infants. Anesthesiol 1987;67:1008-1009.

84. Sobel DB. Burning of a neonate due to a pulse oximeter: arterial saturation monitoring. Pediatrics 1992;89:154-155.

85. Murphy KG, Secunda JA, Rockoff MA. Severe burns from a pulse oximeter. Anesthesiol 1990;73:350-352.

86. Boyle RJ, Oh W. Erythema following transcutaneous PO_2 monitoring. Pediatrics 1980;65:333-334.

87. Evans NJ, Rutter N. Reduction of skin damage from transcutaneous oxygen electrodes using a spray on dressing. Arch Dis Child 1986;61:881-884.

88. Golden SM. Skin craters—a complication of transcutaneous oxygen monitoring. Pediatrics 1981;67:514-516.

89. Sajben SF, Gibbs NF, Fallon-Friedlander S. Transillumination blisters in a neonate. J Am Acad Dermatol 1999;41:264-265.

90. Keroack MA, Kotilainen HR, Griffin BE. A cluster of atypical skin lesions in well-baby nurseries and a neonatal intensive care unit. J Perinatol 1996;16:370-373.

91. Mackenzie AR. Meatal ulceration following neonatal circumcision. Obstetr Gynecol 1966;28:221-223.

9

Developmental Abnormalities

BETH ANN DROLET

Developmental abnormalities of the skin are a diverse group of anomalies that represent errors in morphogenesis. By definition, they are present at birth, and most are diagnosed in infancy. They vary in severity from the inconsequential to the serious, and in some instances represent a marker for significant extracutaneous problems.

SUPERNUMERARY MAMMARY TISSUE

Accessory mammary tissue (supernumerary nipples, accessory nipple, polythelia, polymastia) may consist of true glandular tissue (accessory breasts), areola, nipples, or a combination thereof. It is often bilateral and found along the course of the embryologic breast lines, which run from the axilla to the inner thigh. Accessory nipples are the most common variant and occur in as many as 2% of women, clinically manifesting as a soft, brown, pedunculated papule (Fig. 9-1). In the newborn the lesions are often very subtle, appearing as a light brown or pearly 1 to 3 mm macule. Familial occurrence has been reported.

Extracutaneous Findings. It has been suggested that renal and urogenital malformations occur with increased frequency in infants with polythelia. However, the results of published studies are conflicting; incidence figures range from zero to approximately 10%.[1-5] Ultrasound has been employed to evaluate these infants, and since this procedure is noninvasive it should be considered in infants with worrisome clinical findings or if there is concern regarding an occult developmental defect.

Diagnosis. The diagnosis is usually made clinically but can be confirmed by histologic demonstration of mammary tissue. An accessory nipple will show epidermal thickening, pilosebaceous structures, and smooth muscle, with or without true mammary glands.[6] The dif-

ferential diagnosis includes melanocytic nevus, neurofibroma, verruca, or skin tag.

Treatment. Complete surgical excision is usually recommended if there is glandular tissue because enlargement at puberty may cause pain and embarrassment. Small accessory nipples need not be excised. Breast carcinoma has also been reported in ectopic mammary tissue.[7]

PREAURICULAR PITS AND SINUSES

The auricle is formed by fusion of six tubercles derived from the first and second branchial arches. Incomplete fusion may lead to entrapment of epithelium, forming cysts that communicate to the surface through sinuses.[8] If the cyst and sinus are obliterated, a pit is left behind. Preauricular pits are common and may be inherited in an autosomal dominant fashion. They manifest as small depressions at the anterior margin of the ascending limb of the helix.

Preauricular cysts manifest as tender swellings in the preauricular region; occasionally they are bilateral. If there is a sinus tract, fluid or pus may drain from a small opening just anterior to the ascending portion of the helix (Fig. 9-2). Most patients with preauricular cysts will have a history of recurrent infections.

Extracutaneous Findings. Renal abnormalities are reported to be more common in patients with preauricular sinus, and preauricular pits have been associated with deafness, which suggests that these patients should be screened for hearing deficits.[9,10]

Diagnosis and Treatment. The diagnosis is usually apparent clinically. The sinuses and cysts are lined by stratified squamous epithelium. Surgical excision of preauricular cysts and sinuses is indicated to prevent secondary

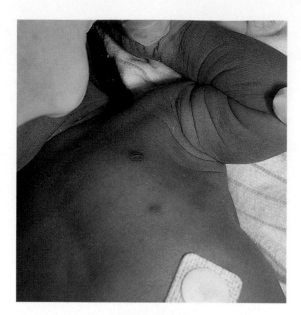

FIG. 9-1
Accessory nipple.

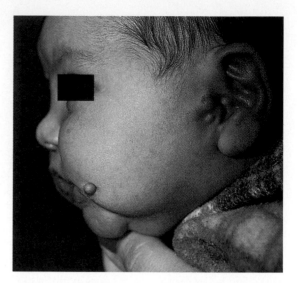

FIG. 9-3
Accessory tragus in the preauricular region and in the much less common region of the lateral commissure of the mouth.

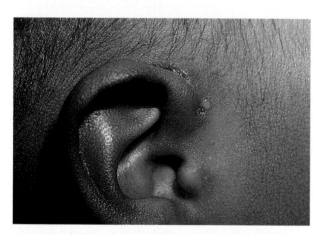

FIG. 9-2
Preauricular sinus with superinfection.

infection. An experienced surgeon should perform the excision because the procedure may be complicated by multiple cysts along a tract that ends at the periosteum of the auditory canal.

ACCESSORY TRAGI

The tragus is derived from the dorsal portion of first branchial arch. Accessory tragi are pedunculated, flesh-colored, soft, round papules usually arising on or near the tragus. They may occur anywhere from the preauricular region to the corner of the mouth following the line of fusion of the mandibular and maxillary branches of the first branchial arch (Fig. 9-3). They may be bilateral or multiple. Accessory tragi are usually isolated defects, but may be associated with other developmental abnormalities of the first branchial arch.[11] Goldenhar syndrome (oculoauriculovertebral syndrome) manifests as epibulbar dermoids, vertebral anomalies, and accessory tragi.[12]

Diagnosis and Treatment. The diagnosis is usually clinically apparent. Histologically, there are numerous tiny hair follicles with prominent connective tissue. A central core of cartilage is usually present.[13] Accessory tragi should be removed by careful surgical dissection because most contain cartilage that may extend deeply, contiguous with the external ear canal. They are not skin tags and should not be tied off with suture material.

CERVICAL TABS/WATTLES/CONGENITAL CARTILAGINOUS RESTS OF THE NECK

Cervical tabs are soft, pedunculated, irregular nodules occurring on the neck along the anterior border of the sternocleidomastoid muscle. They are thought to be remnants of branchial arches and tend to occur along branchial arch fusion lines (Fig. 9-4). Histologically they

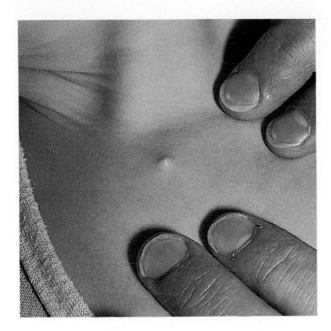

FIG. 9-4
Cartilaginous rest of the neck.

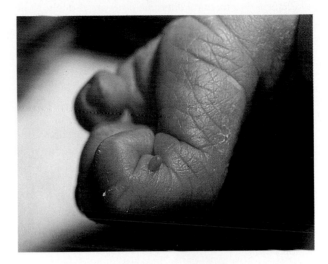

FIG. 9-5
Supernumerary digit.

show lobules of mature cartilage embedded in collagen. The lesions do not extend deeply, but complete surgical excision is the treatment of choice because ligation may result in complications.[14,15]

SUPERNUMERARY DIGITS (RUDIMENTARY POLYDACTYLY)

Supernumerary digits arise from the lateral surface of a normal digit. They are most common on the ulnar surface of the fifth digit but may occur on any finger. They may be bilateral or multiple. Some are small pedunculated papules, while others are normal-size digits containing both cartilage and nail (Fig. 9-5). These lesions should be surgically excised with dissection of the associated nerve if present. Ligation of the supernumerary digit with suture material without complete removal of the nerve may result in skin necrosis, infection, and painful neuromas in adult life.[16]

BRANCHIAL CYSTS, BRANCHIAL CLEFTS, AND BRANCHIAL SINUSES

Branchial cysts are congenital malformations; however, they are not often apparent clinically until the first or second decade of life. They are painless, mobile, cystic swellings in the neck. Most are 1 to 2 cm in size, although they maybe as large as 10 cm. Branchial cysts derived from the second

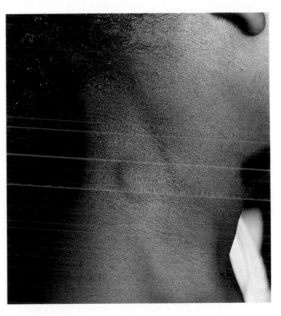

FIG. 9-6
Branchial cyst on the lateral region of the neck.

branchial arch are the most common and are found on the lateral aspect of the upper neck, along the sternocleido-mastoid muscle (Fig. 9-6). Definitive diagnosis is made by histologic examination of the lesions. Branchial cysts are lined by stratified squamous epithelium, or rarely by ciliated columnar epithelium. There is often abundant lymphoid tissue. Squamous cell carcinomas arising in these cystic lesions have been described in adults.[17]

Branchial sinuses and branchial clefts are thought to be remnants of the branchial cleft depressions. They are usually present at birth or noted during the first few years of life. The most common location is along the lateral lower third of the neck. Often a skin tag with a small amount of cartilage is associated with the pit. Branchial cleft anomalies should be surgically excised to prevent infection, with careful attention to the possibility of a true fistula connecting to the tonsillar oropharynx. Preoperative imaging may be necessary to exclude the possibility of true fistulae.

CUTANEOUS BRONCHOGENIC CYSTS AND SINUSES

Bronchogenic cysts are usually found within the chest or mediastinum but may also occasionally be found in the skin. The most common cutaneous location is in the subcutaneous tissue at the presternal notch. The cysts are congenital and usually apparent at birth. They are asymptomatic, small cystic swellings that will gradually enlarge over time and may discharge a mucoidlike material. These lesions are not usually associated with other malformations and do not connect to underlying structures.[18,19] The diagnosis is made by histologic examination of the nodule or sinus. Bronchogenic cysts are lined by lamina propria and a pseudostratified columnar ciliated epithelium with goblet cells.[20] The cyst wall may contain smooth muscle and mucous glands. Lymphatic tissue may or may not be present.

Differential diagnosis includes branchial arch cysts, thyroglossal duct cysts, teratomas, and heterotopic salivary gland tissue. The treatment is complete surgical excision to prevent infection.

MEDIAN RAPHE CYSTS

Median raphe cysts (congenital sinus and cysts of the genitoperineal raphe, mucous cysts of the penile skin, parameatal cysts) are the consequence of incomplete fusion of the ventral aspect of the urethral or genital folds. In most cases they remain asymptomatic unless superinfection occurs. They are soft, small, flesh-colored papules along the ventral aspect of the penis in the line of the median raphe (Fig. 9-7). The cysts are lined with pseudostratified columnar epithelium except at the distal penis, where they have stratified epithelium.[21]

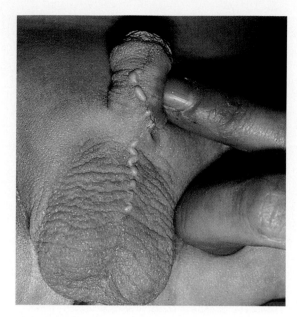

FIG. 9-7
Multiple inclusion cysts along the dorsal surface of the penis.

VENTRAL MIDLINE CLEFTS/DEFECTS

Supraumbilical Cleft

Disruption of abdominal wall fusion causes midline defects of variable degree, often involving the heart and sternum, as well as the abdominal wall. Supraumbilical raphe are linear, midline clefts that occur anterior to the umbilicus. They are frequently associated with cleft sternum and hemangiomatosis (see Chapter 18).[22-24]

Midline Cervical Clefts

This rare abnormality of the ventral neck presents as a small skin tag superiorly with a linear, vertically oriented atrophic patch. At the inferior aspect of the patch there is often a small sinus containing ectopic salivary tissue.[25] Excision with Z-plasty is the treatment of choice.

CUTANEOUS SIGNS OF NEURAL TUBE DYSRAPHISM

The skin and the nervous system share a common ectodermal origin. Separation of the neural and cutaneous ectoderm occurs early in gestational life at about the same time the neural tube is fusing. This embryologic association may explain simultaneous malformations of the skin and the nervous system. This discussion will be limited to cutaneous markers of occult neural tube dysraphic conditions in the cranial region (calvarial defects) and those along the spinal axis.

CRANIAL DYSRAPHISM

Cephaloceles

Cephalocele is the appropriate general term for congenital herniation of intracranial structures through a scalp defect. Meningoceles are congenital cephaloceles in which only the meninges and cerebrospinal fluid herniate through a calvarial defect. Large encephaloceles and meningoceles pose no diagnostic problem and are usually easily diagnosed prenatally or at birth. Smaller or atretic encephaloceles and meningoceles may be mistaken for cutaneous lesions such as hematomas, hemangiomas, aplasia cutis, dermoid cysts, or inclusion cysts. All congenital exophytic scalp nodules should be evaluated thoroughly; 20% to 37% of congenital, nontraumatic scalp nodules connect to the underlying central nervous system.[26,27]

Cutaneous Findings. Cephaloceles occur in the frontal, parietal, and occipital regions. They are usually midline, although they may also be found 1 to 3 cm lateral to the midline. Small cephaloceles are clinically heterogeneous, their appearance dictated by the type and amount of cutaneous ectoderm overlying the lesion. They may be covered with normal skin (Fig. 9-8) or have a blue, translucent, or glistening surface. There is usually a disruption of the surrounding and overlying normal hair pattern. They are soft, compressible, round, or pedunculated nodules that increase in size when the baby cries or with a Valsalva maneuver.

The association of a cephalocele with certain other cutaneous abnormalities makes the diagnosis of cranial dysraphism highly suspect. Stigmata include hypertrichosis, or the "hair collar sign," capillary malformations, hemangiomas, and cutaneous dimples and sinuses.[28,29] The hypertrichosis may overlie the nodule, surround a small sinus, or encircle the nodule (hair collar). A hair collar is defined as a congenital ring of hair that is usually denser, darker, and coarser in texture then the normal scalp hair. When found encircling an exophytic scalp nodule, it is highly suggestive of cranial dysraphism (Figs. 9-9 and 9-10).[28,29] The hair collar sign may be found in association with encephaloceles, meningoceles, atretic encephaloceles, atretic meningoceles, and heterotopic brain tissue. A hair collar may also be seen with some lesions of aplasia cutis; thus this sign is not entirely specific.[30] Cranial neural tube defects may also be associated with overlying red, blanchable

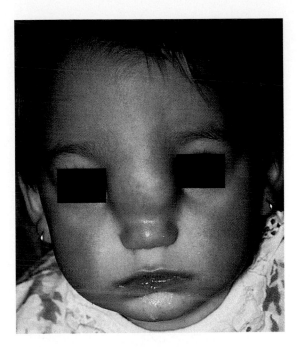

FIG. 9-8
Frontal encephalocele. (Courtesy Odile Enjolras, MD.)

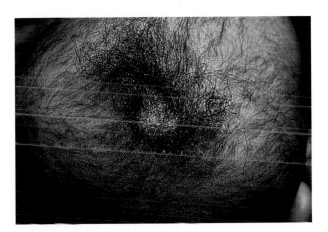

FIG. 9-9
Dense "hair collar" surrounding a vesicular scalp nodule found to be a meningocele.

patches that represent capillary malformations. The combination of a hair collar sign and capillary malformation surrounding a congenital scalp lesion is almost always indicative of a dysraphic condition (see Fig. 9-9).[29]

Extracutaneous Findings and Diagnosis. From a clinical standpoint, encephaloceles, meningoceles, atretic

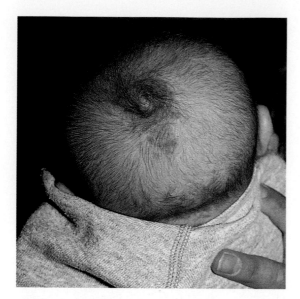

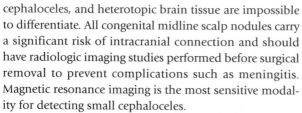

FIG. 9-10
Congenital midline nodule with hair collar and capillary malformation. MRI confirmed an atretic encephalocele.

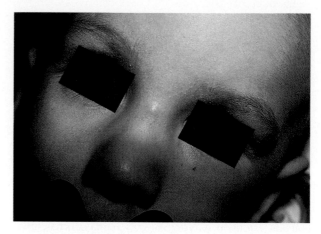

FIG. 9-11
Small midline nasal dermoid cyst.

cephaloceles, and heterotopic brain tissue are impossible to differentiate. All congenital midline scalp nodules carry a significant risk of intracranial connection and should have radiologic imaging studies performed before surgical removal to prevent complications such as meningitis. Magnetic resonance imaging is the most sensitive modality for detecting small cephaloceles.

Differential Diagnosis and Treatment. Included in the differential diagnosis of congenital scalp nodules are pilomatrixoma, epidermoid cyst, lipoma, osteoma, eosinophilic granuloma, hemangioma, sinus pericranii, dermoid cyst, leptomeningeal cyst, and cephalohematoma.[31] Surgical correction is indicated for all cephaloceles.

Nasal Gliomas

Gliomas are rests of ectopic neural tissue and differ from frontal encephaloceles in that they do not have a patent intracranial communication. The lesions maybe external, intranasal, or combined. Clinically they are firm, noncompressible, nontender, skin-colored to red-purple nodules at the root of the nose. They do not transilluminate. Gliomas may be covered with nasal mucosa or normal skin and are often associated with telangiectasia and misdiagnosed as a hemangioma. They may widen the nasal bone, giving the appearance of hypertelorism (Fig. 9-10). They are congenital and do not proliferate, which helps to differentiate them from hemangiomas. Immediate neurosurgical referral is required for surgical removal and reconstruction.

Cranial Dermoid Cyst and Sinus

Dermoid cysts are congenital subcutaneous lesions that are distributed along embryonic fusion lines. The cysts may occur within the fusion lines of the facial processes or along the neural axis. They represent faulty development and may include both epidermal and dermal elements.

Cutaneous Findings. Although dermoid cysts are always congenital, they may not be noted until early childhood, when they begin to enlarge. They can occur anywhere on the face, scalp, or spinal axis but are most frequently seen overlying the anterior fontanel, at the bregma, the upper lateral region of the forehead within or near the eyebrow, and in the submental region.[32-36] They are nontender, noncompressible, nonpulsatile, cystic blue or skin-colored nodules measuring 1 to 4 cm in size (Fig. 9-11). They do not transilluminate or enlarge with a Valsalva maneuver. The overlying skin is normal, unless there is an external connection in the form of a pit or a sinus.

Dermal sinuses are 1 to 5 mm tracts that connect a dermoid cyst to the skin surface. These usually are midline and are found on the nose, occipital scalp, and anywhere along the spinal axis. They may become clinically apparent when they become infected and drain purulent material. A small tuft of hair is often found protruding from the orifice. If the sinus and/or cyst directly communicates with the central nervous system, the patient is at risk for meningitis. The sinus serves as an occult portal of entry for bacteria, often causing a recurrent meningitis that is culture positive for skin flora. *Staphylococcus aureus* meningitis should be considered secondary to a dermal sinus until proved otherwise, and a thorough search for a cutaneous fistula should be carried out, which may necessitate shaving the scalp hair.[37] All midline dermal sinuses should have radiologic imaging prior to surgical excision. Probing these lesions is contraindicated given the potential risk of meningitis.

Extracutaneous Findings. Midline or nasal dermoid cysts are of greatest concern because 25% have an intracranial connection.[33] Nasal dermoid cysts may occur anywhere from the glabella to the nasal tip; a nasal pit or sinus is present in about half the cases.[32] The pit often leads caudally to a dermal sinus and eventuates in a cyst that may be external or within the nasal bones. If the dermoid cyst connects to the central nervous system, cerebrospinal fluid may drain from the sinus. As with nasal gliomas, the patient may have the appearance of hypertelorism if the cyst has widened the nasal bones. Nasal dermoids should always be excised, since they enlarge over time and damage the nasal bones. Dermoid cysts that are not midline should also be excised because they have the potential for infection. Dermoids of the lateral eyebrow area do not have central nervous system connections; they may be surgically excised directly or using an endoscopic approach via a scalp incision to avoid facial scarring.

Diagnosis. Definitive diagnosis is made by histologic examination of the lesions. Dermoids cysts are usually found in the subcutaneous tissue and are lined by stratified squamous epithelium that often contains hair follicles, sebaceous glands, and sweat glands. The lumen may contain keratin, lipid, and hair. Radiologic imaging is a very sensitive screening method and should be undertaken prior to surgical intervention. Currently the most sensitive study is magnetic resonance imaging (MRI). Computed tomography (CT) may better delineate bony defects and be necessary especially in the nasal region. Plain radiographs were used extensively in the past but are not sensitive and should not be used for screening.

SPINAL DYSRAPHISM

Spinal dysraphism, or incomplete closure of the spinal axis, encompasses many congenital anomalies of the spine. Larger defects are usually obvious at birth and fall within the purview of the neurosurgeon. However, small or occult malformations causing tethering of the spinal cord may be inapparent and asymptomatic. Early diagnosis is imperative since it may prevent irreversible neurologic damage in these patients. Diagnosis of occult spinal dysraphism is often suspected solely on the basis of overlying cutaneous findings, particularly in the newborn.

> ### BOX 9-1
>
> ## *Cutaneous Lesions Associated with Spinal Dysraphism*
>
> **High Index of Suspicion**
> Hypertrichosis
> Dimples (large, >2.5 cm from the anal verge, atypical)
> Acrochordons/pseudotails/true tails
> Lipomas
> Hemangiomas
> Aplasia cutis or scar
> Dermoid cyst or sinus
>
> **Low Index of Suspicion**
> Telangiectasia
> Capillary malformation (port-wine stain)
> Hyperpigmentation
> Melanocytic nevi
> Small sacral dimples <2.5 cm from anal verge
> Teratomas

Cutaneous markers are found in 50% to 90% of these patients.[38-47]

Cutaneous Findings. The cutaneous lesions that should alert the physician to an underlying occult spinal dysraphism are listed in Box 9-1. Most of these lesions are found on or near the midline in the lumbosacral region; however, similar markers in the cervical or thoracic regions may also be indicative of an underlying malformation. The literature suggests that certain skin lesions are more indicative than others of an underlying malformation.[38-48] Tavafoghi reviewed 200 cases of spinal dysraphism and found that 102 had cutaneous signs.[47] Other studies have documented an even higher incidence of cutaneous malformations (71% to 100%). Unfortunately, no prospective studies have been done to determine what percentage of children with cutaneous anomalies in the spinal axis have occult dysraphism.

These cutaneous markers should also be evaluated in the context of a full history and physical examination, particularly in the older child. The history should include questions regarding additional congenital malformations, family history of neural tube defects, weakness or pain in the lower extremities, abnormal gait, scoliosis, difficulties with toilet training or incontinence, recurrent urinary tract infections, and recurrent meningitis. The vertebrae should be palpated for any defects or abnormalities. Examination of the rectum and genitalia is also indicated, since there are often associated congenital abnormalities of the urogenital system.[49-51] The gluteal cleft should be examined carefully for small acrochordons or sinuses; it should be straight and the buttocks symmetric. If the gluteal cleft deviates, it is suggestive of an underlying mass such as a lipoma or meningocele. Examination of the lower extremities is important in older children because they may have trophic changes secondary to nerve damage.

Hypertrichosis

Localized lumbosacral hypertrichosis, or "hairy patch," is usually present at birth. The hair may be dark or light. The texture of the hair can vary but is frequently described as silky (faun tail nevus). The hypertrichosis is often V-shaped and poorly circumscribed (Fig. 9-12). Prominent hypertrichosis is commonly associated with other cutaneous stigmata of spinal dysraphism and is highly indicative of a spinal defect. Hypertrichosis in the lumbosacral region can be a normal finding; however, especially in certain racial groups, it is often difficult to decide whether or not further evaluation is indicated. Referral to a neurologist or neurosurgeon for a more complete neurologic examination may be a prudent measure in these cases.

Lipomas

Lipomas associated with spinal dysraphism are thought to be congenital and are also highly indicative of an under-lying defect. Unlike acquired lipomas, they may be poorly circumscribed and feel more like an area of increased subcutaneous fat than a discrete lesion. The lipoma may lie in the dermis or the spinal canal and often penetrates from the dermis through a vertebral defect into the intraspinal space (lipomyelomeningocele). Intraspinal lipomas are a common cause of tethered cord. Appropriate radiologic investigation of lumbosacral lipomas must be performed before surgical excision, and a neurosurgeon should be involved because small intraspinal connections may be missed, even with the most sensitive radiologic imaging.

Hemangiomas, Telangiectasia, and Capillary Malformations

Hemangiomas are proliferative vascular tumors that may be present at birth or develop in the first months of life. In 1986 Goldberg et al described five children with large sacral hemangiomas and several other associated abnormalities.[50] Three of the five children had lipomyelomeningoceles. In 1989 Albright et al reported seven infants with lumbar hemangiomas and tethered spinal cord.[38] There have been several subsequent reports supporting this association. Hemangiomas associated with spinal dysraphism are usually large (>4 cm) and overlie the midline (Fig. 9-13). There is often a skin defect or ulceration within the hemangioma. The hemangiomas may be associated with other cutaneous stigmata such as lipoma, acrochordon, or dermal sinus. These patients are difficult to manage because the hemangiomas can ulcerate, and surgical repair of the tethered cord often may have to be delayed until the hemangioma partially regresses.

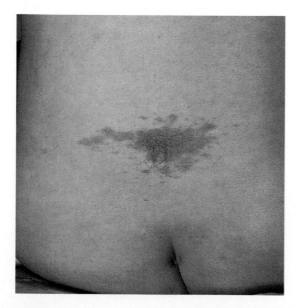

FIG. 9-12
Subtle patch of hypertrichosis with an overlying capillary malformation in a patient with a dermal sinus.

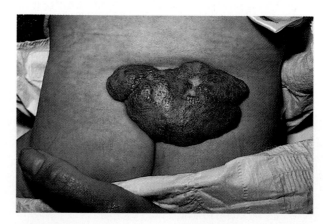

FIG. 9-13
Midline sacral hemangioma in a patient with an occult lipomyelomeningocele.

Reports of telangiectatic patches are probably describing nascent or partially regressed hemangiomas. Enjolras et al reported two patients with cervical spinal dysraphism with an overlying capillary malformation (port-wine stain), but spinal dysraphism associated with a midline, lumbosacral capillary malformation without additional clinical findings is probably uncommon.[52] Two small studies have shown a low but real incidence of spinal dysraphism associated with a solitary capillary malformation of the lumbosacral region.[53,54] Further investigation is needed to completely clarify the need for imaging in these infants. A neurologic consultation may be warranted.

Dimples, Aplasia Cutis, and Congenital Scars

Lumbosacral dimples are common, but can occasionally be a sign of spinal dysraphism.[55,56] Most infants with sacral dimples that fall within the gluteal crease are normal. Dimples that are deep, large (greater than 0.5 cm), located in the superior portion or above the gluteal crease (greater than 2.5 cm from the anal verge), or associated with other cutaneous markers should be radiologically imaged (Fig. 9-14).[54] Deep dimples may actually be dermal sinuses, communicating directly with the spinal canal. These lesions should not be probed.

Aplasia cutis has rarely been reported in the lumbosacral region and in that site may be associated with underlying spinal dysraphism.[39] Scarlike defects have also been described in patients with spinal dysraphism, and they may in fact be a variant of aplasia cutis.[50] The scarlike regions found in lumbosacral hemangiomas may represent a similar phenomenon.

Acrochordons, Tails, and Pseudotails

Acrochordons are small skin-covered sessile or pedunculated papules or nodules (Fig. 9-15). Histologically they are composed of epidermis and a dermal stalk. A true human tail (persistent vestigial tail) is a rare condition and is differentiated from a pseudotail and an acrochordon by the presence of a central core of mature fatty tissue, small blood vessels, bundles of muscle fibers, and nerve fibers. A pseudotail is a stumplike structure and is considered a hamartoma composed of fatty tissue and often cartilage. Clinically these lesions are difficult to distinguish, and all have been associated with spinal dysraphism.[41,43,47,50,57] Radiologic investigation is indicated preoperatively in all cases.

Diagnosis. Definitive diagnosis of spinal dysraphism is only made at surgery. Radiologic imaging provides a sensitive screening method. Three radiologic modalities are currently utilized for the preoperative diagnosis of spinal dysraphism. Magnetic resonance imaging remains the gold standard; however, high-resolution ultrasound is an excellent noninvasive alternative in an infant less than 6 months of age.[58-63] An infant's vertebrae are not yet completely ossified, and ultrasound serves as a relatively inexpensive screening tool. If abnormalities are found, MRI is required preoperatively.[63] Also used in the past, myelograms have been replaced by MRI. It is often useful to speak to the radiologist before ordering the examination because the technology is changing rapidly and will vary by institution.

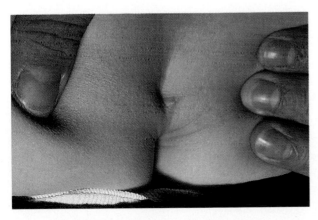

FIG. 9-14
Deep sacral dimple above the gluteal crease.

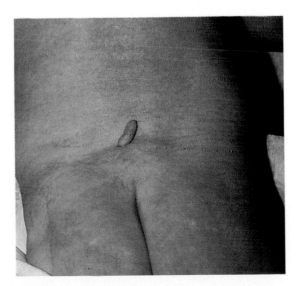

FIG. 9-15
Human tail with underlying lipoma in an infant with lipomyelomeningocele.

APLASIA CUTIS

Aplasia cutis is a general term that is used to describe focal, congenital defects of the skin. Aplasia cutis is a rare condition, and the true incidence is unknown. Several theories have been proposed as to its pathogenesis, but most authors believe that aplasia cutis has no single underlying cause but is rather a clinical finding that results from a variety of events that occur in utero. Several classifications of aplasia cutis have been proposed (Table 9-1).[64]

When evaluating a newborn with aplasia cutis, particular attention should be given to the morphology and the distribution of the defects because this may be helpful in determining the etiology, possible associated malformations, and prognosis (Table 9-2). For example, infants with large defects of aplasia cutis on the bilateral extremities have generalized increased skin fragility, the result of a genetic deficiency, and almost all have been classified as having epidermolysis bullosa. This is a lifelong affliction and will have immediate implications for the care of the infant. Large defects may be seen with trisomy 13 (Fig. 9-16). Table 9-3 correlates the clinical findings with proposed etiology and associations.

Cutaneous Findings. *Membranous aplasia cutis* is the most common form of aplasia cutis. It occurs primarily on the scalp but may also be seen on the lateral aspects of the face (focal facial dermal hypoplasia). The lesions are usually small, oval, or round defects measuring 2 to 5 cm in size. They are well circumscribed, with a "punched out" appearance (Fig. 9-17). At birth, the surface is atrophic, often with a thin, glistening, membranelike surface. Scarlike lesions in the same configuration are more common in older children. Rarely the lesions may be bullous at birth, containing a thick, clear fluid (Fig. 9-18). The bullous lesions may drain spontaneously and reform, eventually flattening to the more typical appearance. Defects of membranous aplasia cutis are often multiple, occurring in a linear

---

TABLE 9-1

A Classification of Aplasia Cutis Congenita

Category	Body area affected	Associated abnormalities	Inheritance
Group 1: scalp ACC without multiple anomalies	Scalp, usually vertex	Cleft lip and palate; tracheoesophageal fistula; double cervix and uterus; patent ductus arteriosus; omphalocele; polycystic kidney; mental retardation; cutis marmorata telangiectatica congenita	Autosomal dominant or sporadic
Group 2: scalp ACC with associated limb abnormalities (most cases are Adams-Oliver syndrome)	Midline scalp	Limb reduction abnormalities; 2-3 syndactyly; clubfoot; nail absence or dystrophy; skin tags on toes; persistent cutis marmorata; encephalocele; woolly hair; hemangioma; heart disease; cryptorchidism; postaxial polydactyly (1 family)	Autosomal dominant
Group 3: Scalp ACC with associated epidermal and organoid nevi	Membranous scalp lesions, may be asymmetric, solitary or multiple	Cephaloceles; corneal opacities; scleral dermoids; eyelid colobomas; psychomotor retardation; seizures	Sporadic
Group 4: ACC overlying embryologic malformations	Abdomen, lumbar skin, scalp; any site	Meningomyeloceles; spinal dysraphia; cranial stenosis; congenital midline porencephaly; leptomeningeal angiomatosis; ectopia of ear; omphalocele; gastroschisis	Depends on underlying condition
Group 5: ACC with associated fetus papyraceus or placental infarcts	Multiple, symmetric areas, often stellate or linear, on scalp, chest, flanks, axillae, and extremities	Single umbilical artery; developmental delay; spastic paralysis; nail dystrophy; clubbed hands and feet; amniotic bands; gastrointestinal atresia	Sporadic

ACC, Aplasia cutis congenita; *EB,* epidermolysis bullosa.
Modified from Frieden IJ. J AM Acad Dermatol 1986;14:646-660.

TABLE 9-1

A Classification of Aplasia Cutis Congenita—cont'd

Category	Body area affected	Associated abnormalities	Inheritance
Group 6: ACC associated with EB: Blistering, usually localized, without multiple congenital anomalies	Extremities	Blistering of skin and/or mucous membranes; absent or deformed nails; metatarsus varus; congenital absence of kidney (seen in cases of recessive, dystrophic EB; dominant, dystrophic EB; and EB simplex)	Depends on EB type: may be autosomal dominant or recessive
Junctional EB with pyloric atresia	Large areas on extremities and torso	Pyloric or duodenal atresia; abnormal ears and nose; ureteral stenosis; renal abnormalities; arthrogryposis	Autosomal recessive
Group 7: ACC localized to extremities without blistering	Pretibial areas; dorsal aspects of hands and feet; extensor areas of wrists	None	Autosomal dominant or recessive
Group 8: ACC caused by specific teratogens	Scalp (with methimazole); any area (with varicella and herpes simplex infections)	Imperforate anus (methimazole); signs of intrauterine infection with varicella and herpes simplex infections	Not inherited
Group 9: ACC associated with malformation syndromes (see also Table 9-2)	Scalp; any location	Trisomy 13; 4p—syndrome; many ectodermal dysplasias; Johanson-Blizzard syndrome; focal dermal hypoplasia; amniotic band disruption complex; XY gonadal dysgenesis	Varies, depending on specific syndrome

TABLE 9-2

Associated Malformations and Chromosomal Defects Reported with Aplasia Cutis

Syndrome	Clinical Phenotype	Associated Features	Inheritance
Opitz syndrome	Membranous aplasia cutis	Hypertelorism, cleft lip/palate, hypospadias, cryptorchidism	—
Adams-Oliver syndrome	Large, ill-defined, irregular scalp defects	Distal limb reduction abnormalities	Autosomal dominant
Oculocerebrocutaneous syndrome	Membranous aplasia cutis	Orbital cysts, cerebral malformations, facial skin tags, seizures, developmental delay	—
Trisomy D(13-15)	Membranous aplasia cutis	Holoprosencephaly, seizures, ocular abnormalities, deafness, neural tube defects	—
4p(-) syndrome	Not specified	Mental retardation, deafness, seizures, ocular abnormalities	—
Johanson-Blizzard syndrome	Small stellate defects of frontal scalp and membranous aplasia cutis	Dwarfism, mental retardation, deafness, hypothyroidism, pancreatic insufficiency	—
X-p22 microdeletion syndrome	Bilateral linear reticulated defects of the malar region of the face	Microphthalmia, sclerocornea	—
Chromosome 16-18 defect	Large scalp defects	Scalp arteriovenous malformation with underlying bony defect	

TABLE 9-3

Correlation of Clinical Findings with Proposed Etiology and Associations in Aplasia Cutis

Clinical phenotype	Proposed etiology	Associations
Cranial and facial membranous aplasia cutis	Developmental	Organoid nevi
Truncal, stellate aplasia cutis	Vascular disruption	Fetus papyraceus, placental insufficiency, gastrointestinal atresia
Extremity, angulated defects	Increased skin fragility	Epidermolysis bullosa
Small scarlike defects	Maternal infections	Varicella, herpes simplex virus infections
Cranial large, midline, irregular defects	Developmental, genetic	Bone defects, hydrocephalus, arteriovenous fistula, sinus thrombosis
Reticulated facial lesions	Chromosomal abnormality	X-p22 deletion syndrome

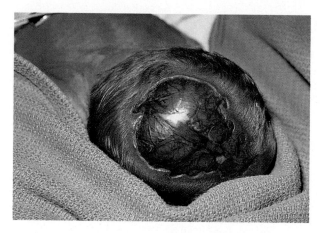

FIG. 9-16
Aplasia cutis with underlying bone defect in an infant with trisomy 13.

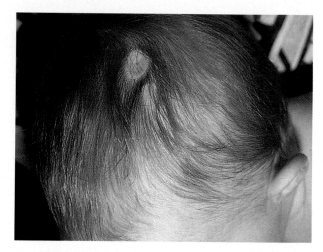

FIG. 9-17
Membranous aplasia cutis with a subtle hair collar sign.

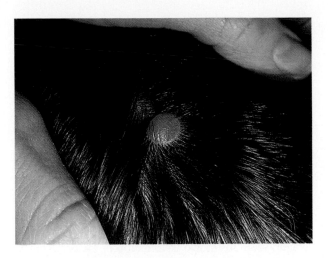

FIG. 9-18
Bullous aplasia cutis in a newborn.

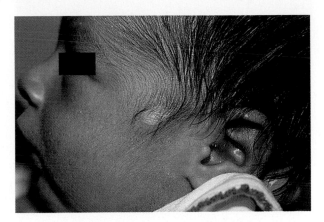

FIG. 9-19
Small, linear facial defects of aplasia cutis.

configuration. The most common location is at the vertex of the scalp, but they may also be found anterior to the vertex 1 to 2 cm off the midline on the parietal scalp, or even extending down onto the forehead along a line from the lateral forehead to the lateral edge of the eyebrows. Rarely, lesions of membranous aplasia cutis occur on the face in a line extending from the preauricular region to the angles of the mouth.[65] The term *focal facial dermal hypoplasia* has been used to describe these lesions (Fig. 9-19). Most reports of membranous aplasia cutis are sporadic; however, there are well-documented patients with autosomal dominant and autosomal recessive patterns of inheritance.[66,67] Although the exact etiology of these lesions is unknown, the configuration, distribution, and clinical appearance would suggest incomplete closure of embryonic fusion lines, rather than vascular interruption or trauma to the skin.[65] A case of membranous aplasia cutis was detected by prenatal ultrasound at 27 weeks' gestation. A protruding, round, cystic lesion was noted at the vertex of the scalp. The lesion resolved spontaneously at 37 weeks' gestation, and a small oval lesion of membranous aplasia cutis was found in the identical location at birth.[68]

Irregular, large, or stellate scalp defects are rare, but may occur along the midline of the scalp (Fig. 9-20). These defects are usually sporadic and often associated with large underlying bony defects. Abnormalities of the underlying venous system and arteriovenous malformations may be associated with these types of defects. Radiologic imaging with particular attention to the vasculature is recommended before surgical intervention, as hemorrhagic complications and death have been reported.[69]

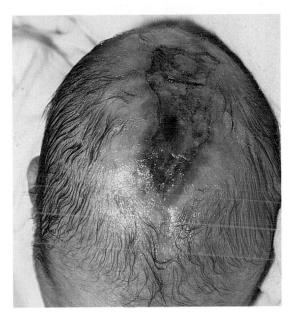

FIG. 9-20
Large, irregular scalp defect of aplasia cutis.

Aplasia Cutis of the Trunk. When the term *aplasia cutis* is used in the most literal sense, this condition is found overlying abdominal malformations such as gastroschisis and omphalocele. Extensive truncal and limb defects have been associated with fetus papyraceus.[70,71] These defects clinically differ from membranous aplasia cutis. They are large, linear, or stellate erosions involving

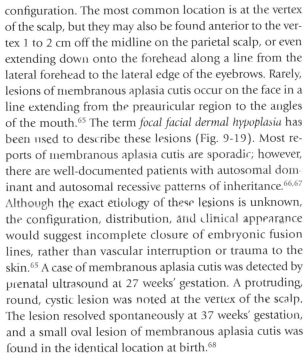

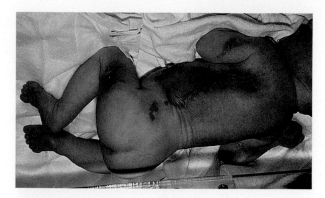

FIG. 9-21
Truncal stellate aplasia cutis associated with fetus papyraceus.

the lateral aspects of the trunk and extensor surfaces of the extremities (Fig. 9-21). Frequently they are bilateral and symmetric. It is theorized that these defects are the result of placental infarction after the death of a twin fetus, which would explain their symmetric distribution. These types of cutaneous lesions may also be associated with gastrointestinal malformations, particularly bowel atresia, which is also thought to be a consequence of early ischemia.[72] Additional extracutaneous findings include neurodevelopmental delay, intracranial hemorrhage, cardiac and arterial anomalies, renal cortical necrosis, and neonatal Volkmann ischemic contracture.[73,74] Similar truncal defects have been seen in patients with pale or small placentas, and several have also been reported without mention of the placenta.[73] Irregular defects of the extremities and trunk have been reported with blistering of the skin (Bart's syndrome); however, these are now considered to be a form of epidermolysis bullosa.[64,75]

Reticulated linear skin defects of the malar region of the face have been reported as part of the X-p22 microdeletion syndrome (see Chapter 24 and Fig. 24-9). All reported cases have been female, suggesting that the deletion may be lethal in males. Severity varies in females from relatively mild facial scarring to major organ malformations. It is associated with microphthalmia and sclerocornea.[76-78]

Pathogenesis. Several theories have been proposed as to the etiology of aplasia cutis. Incomplete closure of the neural tube may explain midline lesions, and incomplete closure of embryonic fusion lines may explain the lateral membranous aplasia cutis lesions.[65] Vascular insufficiency to the skin may result from placental insufficiency or thromboplastic material from a fetus papyraceus. Amniotic membrane adhesions, teratogenic agents, and intrauterine infections have also been implicated. The het-

erogeneity of the associated findings makes a unifying theory unlikely.

Extracutanous Findings. Lesions of membranous aplasia cutis most commonly occur as an isolated defect and usually require no further investigation. There may be small underlying bony defects that usually heal spontaneously. Larger lesions of aplasia cutis with large underlying bony defects may require surgical intervention. Interpretation of associated abnormalities is difficult because most authors do not specify the morphology of the lesion. Listed in Tables 9-2 and 9-3 are some of the associated malformations and chromosomal defects reported with aplasia cutis.[79]

Diagnosis. The diagnosis is usually based on clinical data; however, histologic examination of the defects may help to confirm the diagnosis. Membranous aplasia cutis has the most characteristic histologic findings: the epidermis is atrophic and flattened, and the normal superficial dermis is replaced by loose connective tissue.[65] The normal adnexal structures are small or completely absent.[80] If a hair collar is present, then the edge of the specimen will have clustered, hypertrophic hair follicles. Other subtypes of aplasia cutis show superficial scarring with loss of normal adnexal structures. Increased levels of acetylcholinesterase and alphafetoprotein have been reported in the amniotic fluid of mothers with children with aplasia cutis.[81,82]

Differential Diagnosis. Postnatal trauma from forceps or monitoring devices, Goltz syndrome, epidermolysis bullosa, and incontinentia pigmenti can be confused with aplasia cutis.

Prognosis and Management. If the lesion is ulcerated at birth, the area should be cleansed daily and a topical antibiotic ointment applied until complete healing has occurred. Small superficial skin ulcers usually heal in the first months of life. Likewise, small defects of the underlying bone should ossify completely without treatment.[83] Most small defects will become inconspicuous as the child's scalp grows, but larger lesions may cause significant cosmetic deformity, and almost all will result in localized alopecia. Surgical excision may be considered later in life. Very large stellate scalp defects do not heal completely and will require early surgical intervention. The large, irregular defects routinely have underlying cranial defects, often with abnormalities of the intracranial vascular system.[81,82] Radiologic investigation is required before undergoing surgical correction because severe hemorrhage and even death has been reported after repair of large defects.[84,85] The defects associated with fetus papyraceus heal remarkably well, leaving a hypopigmented scar, and usually do not require surgical correction.

BOX 9-2

Genetic Disorders Associated with Cutaneous Dimples

Dimples Associated with Aberrant Positioning During Fetal Life
Arthrogryposis
Metaphyseal chondrodysplasia
Camptomelic dysplasia
Khyphomelic dysplasia
Mesomelic dysplasia
Hypophosphatasia

Facial Dimples
Cheeks
Chin
Whistling face syndrome
Simosa craniofacial syndrome
Weaver syndrome

Shoulder Dimples
Autosomal dominant dimples
18q deletion syndrome
Trisomy 9p

Russell-Silver syndrome
Popliteal pterygium syndrome

Sacral Dimples
Spina bifida
Bloom syndrome
Carpenter syndrome
FG syndrome
Robinow syndrome
Smith-Lemli-Opitz syndrome
Dubowitz syndrome
Zellweger syndrome
X-linked dysmorphic syndrome with mental retardation

Other
Maternal rubella syndrome
Joubert syndrome
Caudal dysplasia sequence

CUTANEOUS DIMPLES

Cutaneous dimples are small, 1 to 4 mm depressions or pits in the skin. Dimples may occur at any location but are more common over bony prominences such as the elbow, knee, acromion, and sacral region.[86] Cutaneous dimples may be normal, particularly in some locations such as the face.[84,85] Symmetric shoulder dimples over the acromion or supraspinous fossae may be familial and inherited in an autosomal dominant pattern.[86-89] Cutaneous dimples have been associated with a wide variety of genetic disorders (Box 9-2).[90-93] Dimples may be the result of aberrant fetal positioning in early gestation in patients with congenital skeletal dysplasia.[93] Usually dimples do not require treatment as they are small and not cosmetically disfiguring.

ADNEXAL POLYP

Adnexal polyp is a small, congenital papule found on the chest, usually on or just medial to the areola of the nipple. The lesions are small (1 to 2 mm), flesh-colored, firm, pedunculated papules with a smooth surface (Fig. 9-22). Older lesions may have a superficial crust. Histologically

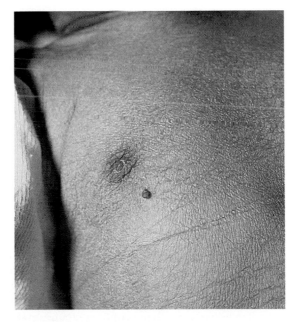

FIG. 9-22
Adnexal polyp.

the lesions are composed of adnexal structures. Hair follicles, vestigial sebaceous glands, and eccrine glands are present in the center of the lesion.[94] The lesions appear to fall
off spontaneously soon after birth.

DEVELOPMENTAL ANOMALIES OF THE UMBILICUS

The umbilicus is a scar that represents the site of attachment of the umbilical cord in the fetus. After birth it has
no function but contains embryonic remnants, the urachus, the omphalomesenteric duct, and the round liga-
ment of the liver, all of which may give rise to medical
complications.

Anomalies of the Urachus

The urachus is the remnant of the regressed allantois that
runs from the apex of the bladder to the umbilicus. If
this structure fails to regress, leaving complete patency, a
fistula forms between the bladder and the umbilicus.
This is manifest by urine draining from the umbilicus.
Partial patency of the urachus will result in a cystic dilation in which both ends are obliterated, forming a urachal cyst. Urachal cysts may occur at any point along the
course of the urachus but do not communicate with the
umbilicus or bladder. They present as tender, midline
swellings between the umbilicus and the symphysis pubis. If the urachus is only patent at the umbilicus, a
urachal sinus forms, which is usually associated with a
proximal urachal cyst presenting as a cystic swelling at
the umbilicus (Fig. 9-23).

Anomalies of the Omphalomesenteric Duct

The omphalomesenteric duct connects the ileum to the
umbilicus. This duct usually regresses during the fifth to
ninth week of gestation, leaving a fibrous cord. Failure of
normal obliteration will result in a range of congenital
anomalies, depending on the extent and the site of persistent patency. The entire duct may be patent, forming a fistula between the ileum and the umbilicus; this presents
during infancy with a red nodule at the umbilicus with a
surrounding fistula. Fecal material may discharge from the
fistula, often resulting in irritation of the surrounding skin.
If intermediate portions of the duct remain patent, an omphalomesenteric cyst forms. If the cyst is located toward
the periphery of the duct (i.e., near the umbilicus), it will
give rise to a bright red, glistening polypoid nodule usu-

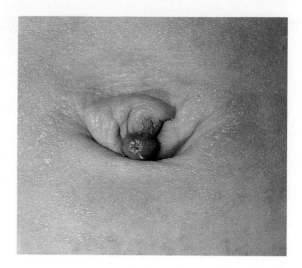

FIG. 9-23
Urachal cyst.

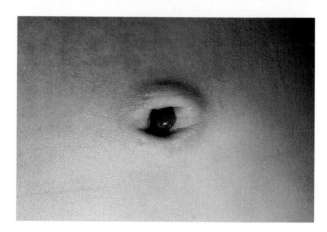

FIG. 9-24
Umbilical polyp (omphalomesenteric duct cyst).

ally referred to as a umbilical polyp (Fig. 9-24). Meckel's
diverticulum, the most common anomaly of the omphalomesenteric duct, results from incomplete regression
of the most proximal (enteric) portion.

Umbilical Granuloma (Granuloma Pyogenicum)

These are small, bright red papules that develop if the umbilicus does not reepithelialize completely; therefore they
are not usually present at birth. They can be distinguished
from umbilical polyps by the lack of serous, mucoid, or

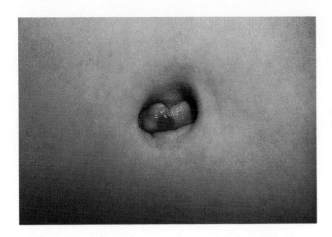

FIG. 9-25
Umbilical granuloma.

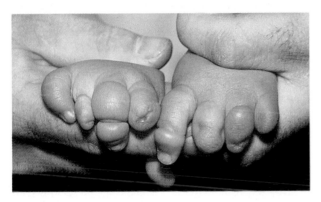

FIG. 9-26
Multiple anomalies of the feet secondary to the amniotic band sequence.

bloody discharge (Fig. 9-25), and response to treatment with topical silver nitrate.

AMNION RUPTURE MALFORMATION SEQUENCE/AMNIOTIC BANDS

A variety of disorders results from premature rupture of the amniotic sac. The clinical features will vary depending on the stage of development of the fetus at the time of rupture.[95] The defects are thought to result from early rupture of the amniotic membrane, which subsequently results in failure of growth of the amniotic sac and formation of fibrous strands from the outer surface of the amnion and the chorion. The fetus may become entangled in these strands if it passes through the defect. There may also be compression of the fetus secondary to oligohydramnios. Maternal trauma, dietary deficiencies, and teratogens have all been associated with amniotic rupture sequence.

Cutaneous Findings. The most classic cutaneous finding is that of a constriction band of the distal extremity (Fig. 9-26). The band is usually circumferential and may be deep enough to cause lymphedema, compression of nerves, or even ischemia with resultant amputation.[96] Aplasia cutis, irregular patches of alopecia, abnormal palmar creases, and alteration in dermatoglyphic pattern are also cutaneous features of the amnion rupture malformation syndrome.

Extracutaneous Findings. Rupture early in gestation, during organogenesis, will lead to the most severe deformities. Severe craniofacial abnormalities, such as neural tube defects, and facial, chest, and abdominal wall clefts, have all been reported.

Treatment. Surgical correction of the deformities is the only treatment option and is often very challenging.[96]

REFERENCES

1. Armoni M, Filk D, Schlesinger M, et al. Accessory nipples any relationship to urinary tract malformation? Pediatr Dermatol 1992;9:239-240.
2. Mimouni F, Merlob P, Reisner SH. Occurrence of supernumerary nipples in newborns. Am J Dis Child 1983;137:952-953.
3. Cohen PR. The significance of polythelia. J Am Acad Dermatol 1995;32:688.
4. Meggyessy V, Mehes K. Association of supernumerary nipples and renal anomalies. J Pediatr 1987;111:412-413.
5. Urbani CE, Betti R. Accessory mammary tissue associated with congenital and hereditary nephrourinary malformations. Int J Dermatol 1996;35:349-352.
6. Hrabovszky T, Schneider I, Zombai E. Axillare akzessorische brustdruson Hautarzt 1995;46:576-578.
7. Kao GF, Graham JH, Helwig EB. Paget's disease of the ectopic breast with an underlying intraductal carcinoma: A report of a case. 1986;13:59-66.
8. Jacobs PH, Shafer JC, Higdon RS. Congenital branchigenous anomalies. J Am Med Assoc 1959;169:442-446.
9. Leung AK, Robson WL. Association of preauricular sinuses and renal anomalies. Urology 1992;40:259-261.
10. Kugelman A, Hadad B, Ben-David J, et al. Preauricular tags and pits in newborn: The role of hearing tests. Acta Peadiatr 1997;86:170-172.
11. Resnick KI, Soltani K, Berstein JE, et al. Acessory tragi and associated syndromes involving the first branchial arch. J Dermatol Surg Oncol 1981;7:39-41.
12. Zelante L, Gasparini P, Scanderbeg AC, et al. Goldenhar complex: A further case with uncommon associated anomalies. Am J Med Genet 1997;69:418-421.
13. Satoh T, Tokura Y, Katsumata T, et al. Histologic diagnostic criteria for accessory tragi. J Cutaneous Pathol 1990;17:206-210.
14. Congenital cartilaginous rests of the neck. Int J dermatol 1986;3:186-187.
15. Hogan D, Wilkinson RD, Williams. Congenital anomalies of the head and neck. Int J dermatol 1980;19:479-486.
16. Frieden IJ, Chang MW, Lee I. Suture ligation of supernumerary digits and "tags": An outmoded practice? Arch Pediatr Adolesc Med. 1995;149:1284.
17. Maran AGD, Buchanan DR. Branchial cysts, sinuses and fistulae. Clin Otolaryngol 1978;3:77-92.
18. Muramatsu T, Shirai T, Sakamoto K. Cutaneous bronchogenic cyst. Int J Dermatol 1990;29:143-144.
19. Jona JZ, Extramediastinal bronchogenic cysts in children. Pediatr Dermatol 1995;12:304-306.
20. Patterson JW, Pittman DL, Rich JD. Presternal ciliated cyst. Arch Dermatol 1984;120:240-242.
21. Asarch RG, Golitz LE, Sausker WF, et al. Median raphe cysts of the penis. Cutis 1981;27:170-172.
22. Carmi R, Boughman JA. Pentalogy of Cantrell and associated midline anomalies: A possible ventral midline developmental field. Am J Med Genet 1992;42:90-95.
23. Hersh JH, Waterfill D, Rutledge J, et al. Sternal malformation/vascular dysplasia association. Am J Med Genet 1985;21:117-186.
24. Kaplan LC, Kurnit DM, Welch KJ, Anterior midline defects: Association with ectopic cordis or vascular dysplasia, defines two distinct entities. Am J Med Genet 1985;21:203.
25. Gargon R, McKinnon M, Mulliken J. Midline cervical cleft. Plast Reconstruct Surg. 1985;76:226-229.
26. Peter J, Sinclair-Smith C, deVilliers J. Midline dermal sinuses and cysts and their relationship to the central nervous system. Eur J Pediatr Surg 1991;1:73-79.
27. Powell K, Cherry J, Hougen T, et al. A prospective search for congenital dermal abnormalities of the craniospinal axis. J Pediatr 1975;87:744-750.
28. Commens C, Rogers M, Kan A. Heterotropic brain tissue presenting as bald cysts with a collar of hypertrophic hair; the hair collar sign. Arch Dermatol 189;125:1253-1256.
29. Drolet B, Clowry Jr L, McTigue K, et al. The hair collar sign: A cutaneous marker for neural tube dysraphaism. Pediatrics 1995;96:309-313.
30. Drolet B, Prendiville J, Golden J, et al. Membranous aplasia cutis with hair collars: Congenital absence of the skin or neuroectodermal defect? Arch Dermatol 1995;131:1427-1429.
31. Howard R. Congenital midline lesions: Pits and protuberances. Pediatr Ann 1998;27:150-160.
32. Nocini P, Barbaglio A, Dolci M, et al. Dermoid cyst of the nose: A case report and review of the literature. J Oral Maxillofac Surg 1996;54:357-362.
33. Peter J, Sinclair-Smith C, deVillies J. Midline dermal sinuses and cysts and their relationship to the central nervous system. Eur J Pediatr Surg 1991;1:73-79.
34. Paller AS, Pensler J, Tomita T. Nasal midline masses in infants and children. Dermoids, encephaloceles, and nasal gliomas. Arch Dermatol 1991;127:362-366.
35. Martinez-Lage JF, Capel A, Costa TR, et al. The child with a mass on it's head: Diagnostic and surgical strategies. Childs Nerv Syst 1992;8:247-252.
36. Hattori H, Higuchi Y, Tashiro Y. Dorsal dermal sinus and dermoid cysts in occult spinal dysraphism. J Pediatr 1999;134:793.
37. Kriss T, Kriss V, Warf B. Recurrent meningitis: The search for the dermoid or epidermoid tumor. Pediatr Infect Dis J 1995;14:697-700.
38. Albright A, Gartner J, Weiner E. Lumbar cutaneous hemangiomas as indicators of tethered spinal cords. Pediatrics 1989;83:977-980.
39. Higginbottom M, Jones K, James H, et al. Aplasia cutis congenita: A cutaneous marker of occult spinal dysraphism. J Pediatr 1980;96:687-689.
40. Anderson F. Occult spinal dysraphism: A series of 73 cases. Pediatrics 1975;55:826-835.
41. Assaad A, Mansy A, Kotb M, et al. Spinal dysraphism: Experience with 250 cases operated upon. Child's Nerv Syst 1989;5:324-329.
42. Burrows F. Some aspects of occult spinal dysraphism: A study of 90 cases. Br J Radiol 1968;41:487-491.
43. Hall D, Udvarhelyi G, Altman J. Lumbosacral skin lesions as markers of occult spinal dysraphism. JAMA 1981;246:2606-2608.
44. Lemire R, Graham C, Beckwith J. Skin-covered sacrococcygeal masses in infants and children. J Pediatr 1971;79:948-954.
45. Sattar M, Bannister C, Turnbull I. Occult spinal dysraphism—the common combination of lesions and the clinical manifestations in 50 patients. Eur J Pediatr Surg 1997;6:10-14.
46. Scatliff J, Kendall B, Kingsley D, et al. Closed spinal dysraphism: Analysis of clinical, radiological and surgical findings in 104 consecutive patients. Am J Roentgenol 1989;10:269-277.

47. Tavafoghi V, Ghandchi A, Hambrick G, et al. Cutaneous signs of spinal dysraphism: report of a patient with a tail-like lipoma and review of 200 cases in the literature. Arch Dermatol 1978;114:573-577.

48. Keim HA, Greene AF. Diastematomyelia and scoliosis. J Bone Joint Surg Am 1973;55:1425-1434.

49. Karrer F, Flannery A, Nelson, M, et al. Anorectal malformations. Evaluation of associated spinal dysraphic syndromes. J Pediatr Surg 1988;23:45-48.

50. Goldberg N, Hebert A, Esterly N. Sacral hemangiomas and multiple congenital abnormalities. Arch Dermatol 1986;122:684-687.

51. Rivosecchi M, Luchetti M, Zaccara A, et al. Spinal dysraphism detected by MRI in patients with anorectal abnormalities: Incidence and clinical significance. J Pediatr Surg 1995;30:383-388.

52. Enjolras O, Boukobza M, Jdid R. Cervical occult spinal dysraphism: MRI findings and the value of a vascular birth mark. Pediatr Dermatol 1995;12:256-259.

53. Ben-Amitai D, Davidson S, Schwartz M, et al. P16 The role of imaging in the evaluation of sacral nevus flammeus simplex: A prospective neonatal study. European J of Pediatric Dermatology International Congress of Dermatolgy 1998; 8:40.

54. Kriss VM, Desal NS. Occult spinal dysraphism in neonates: Assessment of high-risk cutaneous stigmata on sonography. AJR 1998;171:1687-1692.

55. McAtee-Smith J, Hebert A, Rapini R, et al. Skin lesions of the spinal axis and spinal dysraphism. Arch Pediatr Adolesc Med 1994;148:740-748.

56. Harrist T, Gang D, Kleinman G, et al. Unusual sacrococcygeal embryologic malformations with cutaneous manifestations. Arch Dermatol 1982;118:643-648.

57. Dao A, Netsky M. Human tails and pseudotails. Hum Pathol 1984;15:449-453.

58. Barnes P, Lester P, Yamanashi W, et al. Magnetic resonance imaging in infants and children with spinal dysraphism. AJNR 1986;7:465-472.

59. Byrd S, Darling C, Melone D, et al. MR imaging of the pediatric spine. Magn Reson Imaging Clin N Am 1996;4:797-833.

60. Rindahl M, Colletti P, Zee C, et al. Magnetic resonance imaging of pediatric spinal dysraphism. Magn Reson Imaging 1989;7:217-224.

61. Tracy P, Hanigan W. Spinal dysraphism: Use of magnetic resonance imaging in evaluation. Clin Pediatr 1990;29:228-233.

62. Raghavendra B, Epstein F, Pinto R, et al. The tethered spinal cord: Diagnosis by high-resolution real time ultrasound. Radiology 1983;149:123-128.

63. Rohrschneider U, Forsting M, Darge K, et al. Diagnostic value of spinal ultrasound: Comparative study with MR imaging in pediatric patients. Radiology 1996;200:383-388.

64. Frieden IJ. Aplasia cutis congentita: A clinical review and proposal for classification. J Am Acad Dermatol 1986;14:646-660.

65. Drolet BA, Baselga E, Gosain AK, et al. Preauricular skin defects: A consequence of a persistent ectodermal groove. Arch Dermatol 1997;133:1551-1554.

66. Pap GS. Congenital defect of the scalp and scull in three generations of one family. Plast Reconst Surg 1970:46:194-196.

67. Sybert V. Aplasia cutis congenita. A report of 12 new families and review of the literature. Pediatr Dermatol 1985;3:1-14.

68. Cambiaghi S, Gelmetti C, Nicolini U. Prenatal findings in membranous aplasia cutis. J Am Acad Dermatol 1998; 39: 638-640.

69. Singman R, Asaikan S, Hotson G, et al. Aplasia cutis congenita and arterialvenous fistula. Arch Neurol 1990;47:1255-1258.

70. Saier F, Burden L, Cavanagh D. Fetus papyraceus: An unusual case with congenital anomaly of the surviving fetus. Obstet Gynecol 1975;45:217-220.

71. Mannono F, Jones K, Benirschke K. Congenital skin defects and fetus payraceus. J Pediatr 1977;91:559-564.

72. Branspiegel N. Aplasia cutis congenita and intestinal lymphangiectasia: an unusual association. Am J Dis Child 1985; 139:509-513.

73. Dowler VB. Congenital defect of the skin in a newborn infant. Am J Dis Child 1932;44:1279-1284.

74. Leaute-Lebreze C, Depaire-Duclos F, Sarlangue J, et al. Congenital cutaneous defects as complications of surviving co-twins; aplasia cutis congenita and neonatal Volkmann ischemic contracture of the forearm. Arch Dermatol 1998; 134: 1121-1124.

75. Bart B, Garlin R, Anderson V, et al. Congenital absence of the skin and associated abnormalites resembling epidermolysis bullossa. Arch Dermatol 1966;93:296-304.

76. Al-Gazali Li, Mueller RF, Caine A, et al. Two 46, xxt(X:Y) females with linear skin defects and congenital microphthalmia: a new syndrome at Xp2.3 J Med Genet 1990;27:59-63.

77. Temple K, Hurst JA, Hings S, et al. De novo deletion of Xp22.2pter in a female with linear skin lesions on the face and neck, microphthalmia, and anterior chamber eye anomalies. J Med Genet 1990;27:56-58.

78. Allanson J, Richter S. Microphthalmia: A new syndrome at Xp22.2. J Med Genet 1991;28:143-144.

79. Evers MJ, Steijlen PM, Hamel BJ. Aplasia cutis congenita and associated disorders: An update. Clin Genet 1995;47:295-301.

80. Lever WF. Aplasia cutis. In Histopathology of the skin. 7th edition. Philadelphia:JB Lippincott 1990: pp 65-66.

81. Farine D, Maidman J, Rubin S, et al. Elevated alpha-fetoprotein in pregnancy complicated by aplasia cutis after exposure to methimazole. Obstet Gynecol 1988;71:996-997.

82. Bick DP, Balkite MS, Baumgarten JC, et al. The association of congenital skin disorders with acetylcholinesterase in amniotic fluid. Prenat Diagn 1987;7:543-549.

83. Wexler A, Harris M, Lesavoy M. Conservative treatment of cutis aplasia. Plast Reconstr Surg 1990;86:1066-1071.

84. Glasson DW, Duncan GM. Aplasia cutis congenita: Delayed closure complicated by massive hemorrhage. Plast Reconstr Surg 1985;75:423-425.

85. Schneider BM, Berg RA, Kaplan AM. Aplasia cutis complicated by sagittal sinus thrombosis. Pediatrics 1980;66:948-950.

86. Samlaska CP. Congenital supraspinous fossae. J Am Acd Dermatol 1991;25:1078-1079.

87. Weidemann Hr. Cheek dimples. Am J Med Genet 1990; 36:376.

88. Biachine JW. Achromial dimples: A benign familial trait. Am J Hum Genet 26:412-413.

89. Wood VE. Congential skin fossae about the shoulder. Plast Reconstr Surg 1990;85:798-800.

90. DiRocco, M. On Saraiva and Baraister and Joubet syndrome: A review. Am J Med Genet 732.

91. Jones KL. In Smith's recognizable patterns of human mal-formations. 4th edition. Philadelphia: WB Saunders, 1988: pp 42-44, 94-95,112-113,104-15,178-179,182-183,240-241, 370-371, 575-576.

92. Squires LA, Raymond G, Neumeyer AM, et al. Dysmorphic features of Joubert syndrome. Dysmorh Clin Genet 1991; 5:72.

93. Kozlowski K, Baca L, Brachimi L, et al. Mesomelic dysplasia of the upper extremities associated with other abnormalities: A new syndrome? Pediatr Radiol 1993;23:108-110.

94. Hidano A, Kobayashi T. Adnexal polyp of neonatal skin. Br J Dermatol 1975;92:659.

95. Higginbottom MC, Jones KL, Hall BD, et al. The amniotic band disruption complex: Timing of amniotic rupture and variable spectra of consequence of defects. 1979;95:544-549.

96. Rossillon D, Rombouts JJ, Verellen-Dumoulin C, et al. Congenital ring-constriction syndrome of the limbs; a report of 19 cases. Br J Plast Surg 1988;41:270-277.

10

Vesicles, Pustules, Bullae, Erosions, and Ulcerations

ILONA J. FRIEDEN
RENÉE HOWARD

Vesiculopustular and bullous disorders are common in the newborn period. Accurate and prompt diagnosis is essential because several of the conditions presenting with these skin findings are truly life threatening. In contrast, many of the conditions causing blisters and pustules are innocuous and self-limited, and inaccurate diagnosis of a more serious condition can lead to iatrogenic complications, expense, and parental anguish. Several recent articles have reviewed an approach to infants with these findings.[1,2,3] There is also considerable overlap in subject matter with several other chapters of this book, most notably Chapter 7 (Transient Cutaneous Lesions) and Chapters 11 through 13 (Bacterial, Viral, and Fungal Infections), with the main discussion in those chapters.

This chapter discusses not only those conditions that present with pustules, vesicles, and bullae (Boxes 10-1 and 10-2) but also many that generally present with erosions and/or ulcerations (Box 10-3). These latter morphologies can be the secondary skin manifestations of a condition that is primarily a blistering disorder. Well-known examples of this include staphylococcal scalded skin syndrome, where extremely superficial blisters erode rapidly, often without intact blisters, and *Pseudomonas* skin infection, where pustules can rapidly evolve into necrotic ulcers. A systematic approach using history, physical examination, and laboratory evaluation is essential for evaluation and treatment (Box 10-4).

BACTERIAL INFECTIONS
(See also Chapter 11)

Staphylococcus aureus Pyoderma

Skin infections caused by *S. aureus* are relatively common in newborns, and epidemic outbreaks are occasionally seen in newborn nurseries. Two forms of *S. aureus* infection can occur: direct skin infection and staphylococcal scalded skin syndrome.

Superficial skin infections with *S. aureus* (staphylococcal pyoderma) can result in crusted impetigo, bullous impetigo, and occasionally a pustular folliculitis. Infection is virtually never present at birth but often develops in the first days to weeks of life. It usually presents with vesicles, pustules, or, in the case of toxin-producing *S. aureus*, with tense, fragile bullae. Fluid inside the vesicles and bullae may be clear or yellow but often becomes turbid or purulent with time. As vesicles and bullae rupture, they leave moist superficial erosions or thinly crusted areas with a collarette of scale. Superficial staphylococcal infection can also present with crusted impetigo without clinically obvious vesicles, pustules, or bullae.[4]

Common sites of involvement include the neck folds, diaper area, and axillae.[5] Infants are usually otherwise well, without signs of more generalized infection. The diagnosis and management are discussed in Chapter 11.

Staphylococcal Scalded Skin Syndrome

Staphylococcal scalded skin syndrome (SSSS) is an acute, potentially life-threatening disease caused by exotoxin-producing *S. aureus*, usually phage types 1, 2, or 3. Only one case of congenital SSSS has been reported; the vast majority present between 3 and 7 days of age or older, with an abrupt onset of cutaneous erythema, tenderness, and widespread areas of skin fragility, superficial blistering, and/or erosions.[6] The erythema often begins on the face, especially around the mouth, and rapidly spreads. Flaccid blisters usually appear within 24 to 48 hours and quickly erode, producing areas of superficially denuded skin. These erosions are particularly prominent in areas of

137

BOX 10-1

Conditions Where Pustules and/or Vesicles Predominate

Common Causes
Superficial staphylococcal infection
Erythema toxicum neonatorum
Neonatal pustular melanosis
Miliaria crystallina and rubra
Neonatal "acne" (benign cephalic pustulosis)
Neonatal candidiasis

Uncommon Causes
Congenital candidiasis
Herpes simplex infection
Scabies
Acropustulosis of infancy
Incontinentia pigmenti

Rare Causes
Listeria monocytogenes infection
H. influenzae infection
Group A streptococcal infection
Pseudomonas infection
Neonatal varicella
Cytomegalovirus infection
Aspergillus infection
Eosinophilic pustular folliculitis
Langerhans'-cell histiocytosis
Hyperimmunoglobulin E syndrome
Pustular eruption in Down syndrome
Pustular psoriasis
Neonatal Behçet's

BOX 10-2

Conditions Where Bullae May Predominate

Common Causes
Bullous impetigo
Sucking blisters

Uncommon Causes
Staphylococcal scalded skin syndrome
Epidermolysis bullosa

Rare Causes
Group B streptococcal infection
Pseudomonas infection
Congenital syphilis
Neonatal varicella
Bullous mastocytosis
Maternal bullous disease
    Pemphigus vulgaris
    Herpes gestationis
    Pemphigus foliaceus
Chronic bullous dermatosis of childhood (Linear IgA disease)
Bullous pemphigoid
Toxic epidermal necrolysis
Epidermolytic hyperkeratosis
Acrodermatitis enteropathica
Membranous aplasia cutis congenita
Absent dermal ridge patterns, milia, and blisters of fingertips and soles

mechanical stress such as the shoulders, buttocks, body folds, feet, and hands. When firmly rubbed, the skin is easily separated from the underlying epidermis (Nikolsky's sign). A milder form of SSSS, characterized by a scarlatiniform rash with periorificial scaling, is often seen in older infants and children.

Temperature instability, irritability, and/or lethargy are common. Perioral or periocular edema and mucopurulent conjunctivitis are sometimes present. Although the primary site of *S. aureus* infection is usually not the skin, occasionally a primary skin infection, such as an abscess, purulent umbilicus, or localized area of impetigo may be the source of disease.[4,7,8,9]

Diagnosis is made by skin biopsy, which demonstrates a cleavage plane in the upper epidermis with acantholytic cells and minimal dermal inflammation. To speed diagnosis, a snip biopsy of exfoliating portions of the skin can be sent for frozen section. The differential diagnosis includes toxic epidermal necrolysis, epidermolysis bullosa, boric acid poisoning, and certain metabolic disorders such as methylmalonic acidemia.[10,11] The management of SSSS is discussed in Chapter 11.

Streptococcal Infection

Several epidemics of **group A streptococcus** (GAS) have been reported in the newborn period. Although most infants present with omphalitis or a moist umbilical cord stump, isolated pustules may be the presenting sign of GAS infection in rare cases. Generalized sepsis, cellulitis, meningitis, or pneumonia is occasionally seen.[12,13,14] Because neonatal group A streptococcal infection can result in an invasive infection, parenteral antibiotics should be considered, and infants should be observed closely for signs of systemic illness.

BOX 10-3

Conditions Where Erosions or Ulcerations May Predominate

Common Causes
Sucking blisters
Skin changes caused by perinatal/neonatal trauma
    Diaper erosions
    Scalp electrode injury
    Skin trauma due to adhesives, other causes

Uncommon Causes
Staphylococcal scalded skin syndrome
Herpes simplex, especially congenital
Epidermolysis bullosa
Aplasia cutis congenita

Rare Causes
Group B streptococcus infection
Pseudomonas (Ecthyma gangrenosum)
Intrauterine varicella infection
Congenital syphilis
Aspergillus infection
Zygomycosis/Trichosporosis
Neonatal lupus erythematosus

Rare Causes—cont'd
Toxic epidermal necrolysis
Intrauterine epidermal necrosis
Congenital erosive and vesicular dermatosis
Pyoderma gangrenosum
Noma neonatorum
Acrodermatitis enteropathica
Methylmalonic acidemia and other metabolic
    disorders
Bullous ichthyosis (epidermolytic hyperkeratosis)
Restrictive dermopathy
Hemangiomas and vascular malformations
Aplasia cutis congenita
Linear porokeratosis
Giant congenital melanocytic nevi
Focal dermal hypoplasia
Porphyrias
    Transient porphyrinemia
    Erythropoietic porphyria
Perinatal gangrene of the buttock
Congenital deficiency of protein C, S, or fibrinogen

BOX 10-4

Key Points of Obstetric and Neonatal History and Examination

Maternal, Family, and Obstetric History
Maternal history of skin or mucous membrane
    diseases
Family history of birthmarks, blistering, skin fragility,
    or ectodermal defect.
History of previous pregnancies/miscarriages
Prenatal care
Results of maternal serologies (including syphilis,
    rubella, and HIV)
History of maternal illnesses, surgery, fever, rash, or
    medications during pregnancy
History of maternal fever during delivery
Length of ruptured amniotic membranes
Method of delivery
History of intrauterine monitoring
Presence of meconium in the amniotic fluid
Placental abnormalities

Neonatal History
Apgar scores
Gestational age at birth

Neonatal History—cont'd
Birth weight relative to gestational age (i.e., small,
    average, or large)
Illnesses during the newborn period
Past history of surgery, sepsis, anatomic/structural
    abnormalities
Recent history of lethargy, irritability, temperature in-
    stability, and/or poor feeding
Medications: past or present

Neonatal Examination
Complete examination of the skin, mucous mem-
    branes, hair, and nails
Accurate definition of the morphology of skin
    lesion(s)
Head circumference (percentile for age)
Ophthalmologic abnormalities
Adenopathy
Liver or spleen enlargement
Skeletal abnormalities
Neurologic abnormalities

Infection with **group B beta-hemolytic streptococci** (GBS) is one of the most common causes of neonatal sepsis, but skin lesions resulting from GBS infection are very rare. In the few cases reported, vesicles, bullae, erosions, and honey-crusted lesions resembling GAS impetigo have been described.[4,15] These findings were present at the time of birth but could potentially occur later, since the skin and umbilicus are common sites of colonization in newborns.[16] Many areas of the body, including the scalp, face, torso, and extremities, can be affected, with lesional size varying from a few millimeters to several centimeters. Other manifestations of group B streptococcal disease (including bacteremia, pneumonia, and meningitis) should be sought.

Listeria Infection

Listeria monocytogenes is an uncommon cause of sepsis in the newborn period, but epidemic and sporadic cases of perinatal listeriosis continue to occur, often as a result of inadequately pasteurized dairy products.[17,18] Skin disease, when it occurs, is associated with an early-onset form of infection, which is present at birth or develops in the first few days of life (so-called granulomatosis infantiseptica). The rash, which is usually present at birth, consists of discrete but widespread pustules and petechiae over the trunk and extremities. In less severely affected infants, erythematous macules may progress to pustules with an erythematous halo. Salmon-colored papules concentrated on the trunk have also been described.[17,18] Typically, maternal fever, fetal tachycardia, and meconium staining of amniotic fluid are present before delivery, and premature delivery is common.[18] Affected infants are usually gravely ill with respiratory distress, meningitis, and other signs of sepsis.

The differential diagnosis includes several other infections, including congenital candidiasis, intrauterine herpes infection, and *Haemophilus influenzae* infection. Further details of diagnosis and management are discussed in Chapter 11.

Haemophilus Influenzae Infection

Haemophilus influenzae is a very rare cause of neonatal infection. Skin findings have included vesicles, pustules, crusted areas, and abscesses.[19,20] The best description of skin lesions is from the case of Halal et al,[20] who reported an infant with discrete vesicles on an erythematous base, as well as several 2 to 3 mm crusted areas, present at birth. Gram stains and culture from skin lesions confirmed the presence of *H. influenzae* type B but cultures from sites other than the ear canal were negative. Systemic infection most often causes bacteremia or meningitis. Onset of symptoms is at birth or in the first few days of life.

If *H. influenzae* is suspected, diagnostic evaluation should include Gram stain and culture of skin lesions, and cultures of the infant's blood, urine, cerebrospinal fluid (CSF), and nasopharynx. Cultures of the placenta (if available) and of the maternal cervix and lochia should also be performed. The differential diagnosis includes other infections. A Gram stain demonstrating pleomorphic gram-negative bacilli is strong evidence for *H. influenzae* infection. The treatment of *H. influenzae* infection is discussed in Chapter 11.

Pseudomonas Infection

Pseudomonas aeruginosa in newborns is primarily a late-onset nosocomial infection in very low birth weight infants who have had significant medical and/or surgical illness.[21] Skin lesions are usually a result of septicemia and hematogenous spread of infection to the skin, although in older infants, ulcerative skin lesions of *Pseudomonas* have been reported in the diaper area and in young infants in the absence of documented blood-borne infection.[22] Skin lesions may develop at any time during the newborn period, evolving from areas of erythema to hemorrhagic bullae or pustules. The pus may be green, caused by a dye produced by the bacteria. Lesions rapidly erode, becoming punched-out necrotic ulcerations with an indurated base (so-called ecthyma gangrenosum).[23]

In septicemic forms, affected neonates are usually gravely ill, and prompt diagnosis and rapid institution of treatment is necessary to prevent death from overwhelming sepsis.[23] Gram stain of fluid from a pustule or bullae will reveal gram-negative rods. If lesions are eroded, biopsy and tissue Gram stain should be performed to expedite diagnosis. Cultures of both the skin and blood will confirm the diagnosis. Treatment of suspected infection must take into account the local patterns of antibiotic resistance but often includes a semisynthetic penicillin, such as ticarcillin, and an aminoglycoside.

Congenital Syphilis

Congenital syphilis is a relatively rare neonatal infection in the United States and an even rarer cause of blisters or ulcerations. These findings occur almost exclusively in early-onset disease and are present in approximately 3% of cases, usually at the time of birth.[24] Bullae are most often located on the palms, soles, knees, or abdomen, superimposed on dusky, hemorrhagic, or erythematous skin.[25] Moist areas of eroded skin may also occur around the mouth, nose, and anogenital skin.

Because syphilis affects many organ systems, a variety of other clinical features may be present, as discussed in Chapter 11. The diagnosis can be confirmed by examining bullous or erosive skin lesions via a darkfield examination or direct FA for treponemal antigen because such skin lesions are usually teeming with spirochetes. If FA or darkfield is negative, and the skin lesions are very suggestive, a skin biopsy can be performed to demonstrate a dense inflammatory infiltrate of plasma cells. Spirochetes may be visible with a silver or Warthin Starry stain.

Blistering congenital syphilis must be differentiated from other disorders causing blistering on the palms and soles, including congenital candidiasis, acropustulosis of infancy, scabies, and epidermolysis bullosa. The clinical findings, as well as serology, darkfield examination, KOH, and skin biopsy when necessary, help in this differentiation. The details of evaluation and therapy of congenital syphilis are discussed in Chapter 11.

INFECTIOUS CAUSES—FUNGAL
(See also Chapter 13)

Congenital and Neonatal Candidiasis

Two clinical patterns of *Candida albicans* infection cause a pustular skin eruption in the newborn period: **congenital candidiasis**, where *Candida* is acquired in utero or during birth, and **neonatal candidiasis**, which is acquired postnatally.[4,26]

Congenital candidiasis, an uncommon condition, is due to exposure to *Candida albicans*, in utero or during delivery, resulting in a generalized skin eruption. The condition is usually present at birth but may have its onset any time in the first week of life. Risk factors include foreign body in the uterus or cervix (such as a retained intrauterine device or cervical suture), premature delivery, and a maternal history of vaginal candidiasis.[26,27,28]

Several types of skin lesions may be present, including erythematous papules, diffuse erythema, vesicopustules, and fine scaling. Typically, a fine erythematous papular eruption is first noted, and this evolves over time into a more pustular and scaly eruption. In milder cases, sparse papules and incipient pustules are scattered over the upper chest, back, and extremities. Virtually any part of the skin may be involved, and unlike many pustular eruptions (such as erythema toxicum and miliaria), the palms and soles are often involved.[29] Nail dystrophy and oral thrush are occasionally present. In very low birth weight infants, diffuse erythema and scaling with superficial erosions said to resemble a first-degree burn have been reported.[30]

Potassium hydroxide (KOH) preparation from involved skin demonstrates budding yeast and pseudohyphae. Organisms are usually present in large numbers even in cases where pustules are relatively sparse. *Candida* may also be present in the gastric aspirate. If the placenta is examined, characteristic yellow-white papules may be found on the umbilical cord, with evidence of infection also found at the periphery of the cord in Wharton's jelly.[4,31]

Differential diagnosis includes *Listeria* and intrauterine *herpes simplex* infections, erythema toxicum neonatorum, pustular miliaria rubra, and neonatal pustular melanosis. KOH preparation will differentiate congenital candidiasis from these conditions.

Treatment of congenital candidiasis depends on the gestational age and weight of the infant. Premature infants weighing less than 1500 g have a much greater risk for disseminated candidiasis, including involvement of the blood, lung, meninges, and urinary tract. After the blood, spinal fluid, and urine have been cultured, they should be treated with systemic therapy, as discussed in Chapter 13.

Older infants who have no evidence of disseminated disease must be observed closely because on rare occasions respiratory distress and hepatosplenomegaly may develop[32]; however, these usually are cured with topical therapy with an imidazole cream alone.

Postnatally acquired cutaneous candidiasis is common after 1 week of age in both term and preterm infants. Colonization occurs in approximately one quarter of infants less than 1500 g, and nearly one third of those colonized develop mucocutaneous disease.[33] The most common sites of involvement are the diaper area and the oral mucous membranes, but other intertriginous areas may be affected (including the face), particularly if the infant has been intubated.[4] Typically, pink-red scaly patches with satellite papules and pustules at the periphery are seen. Topical therapy with an imidazole cream or nystatin ointment is usually sufficient because dissemination does not develop in immunocompetent infants. Very low birth weight infants with evidence of postnatally acquired candidiasis should be observed closely, and blood, urine, and CSF cultures should be obtained if signs of systemic infection are present.[30]

Aspergillus Infection

Primary cutaneous aspergillosis has been reported in several neonates, most of whom were very premature.[34] The age at diagnosis ranged from 6 to 30 days, and several neonates had previously been treated with antibiotics and/or corticosteroids. Several clinical presentations were noted, including pustules and ulcerations often superimposed on indurated plaques.[34,35]

Aspergillus fumigatus, niger, and *flavus* all cause skin disease. Skin maceration and/or abrasions from adhesive tape were thought to be portals of entry in several cases, with hospital renovation or construction a risk factor in some cases. Skin biopsies, which demonstrate dermal inflammation and broad anastomosing septate hyphae on special stains, are usually necessary for diagnosis, with culture for confirmation. Management is discussed in Chapter 13. The prognosis is guarded, both because of possible dissemination of infection and because of other diseases associated with extreme prematurity.[34,35]

Trichosporosis and Zygomycosis
(See Chapter 13)

Trichosporon infection is rare in neonates, but generalized skin breakdown, peeling, and oozing without vesicles or pustules have been noted.[36] **Mucormycosis** has been reported in very ill premature infants, usually presenting with a cellulitis, which evolves into a black necrotic ulcer.[37] Both types of infections have a poor prognosis, but treatment with amphotericin B (with or without surgical debridement) has been successful in some cases.

Malazzezia Infections (See Neonatal Acne)

INFECTIOUS CAUSES—VIRAL

Herpes Simplex Infection (See Chapter 12)

Herpes simplex (HSV) infection is one of the most feared causes of blisters and pustules in the newborn. Subtle or inconspicuous skin lesions may herald the onset of infection, and the failure to promptly recognize the cause of such lesions worsens the prognosis of a potentially devastating disease. Skin lesions are present in both **intrauterine herpes simplex infection** and in **neonatal herpes simplex** infection, and although there is considerable overlap, the time of onset and many of the clinical features of the skin disease are different.

In **intrauterine HSV infection,** skin lesions are usually present at the time of birth or develop within 24 to 48 hours in 90% of affected infants. In addition to the characteristic vesicular eruption, widespread bullae and erosions resembling epidermolysis bullosa (see Fig. 10-7),[38,39] absence of skin on the scalp (resembling aplasia cutis congenita), and scars on the scalp, face, trunk, or extremities have been reported.[40] Affected infants are often premature, weighing less than 2500 g, and most have microcephaly, chorioretinitis, and diffuse abnormalities on brain computed tomography (CT) scan.

In contrast, **neonatal HSV** infection has three characteristic patterns of neonatal infection: (1) mucocutaneous disease (limited to the skin, eyes, or mouth); (2) disseminated disease (with evidence of visceral organ involvement including liver, lungs, or disseminated intravascular coagulation); and (3) central nervous system disease (where CSF or brain abnormalities are present in the absence of other visceral disease). Skin lesions may occur in all three types.[41]

Skin disease is the most characteristic finding in neonatal HSV infection, but it often lags behind other symptoms in onset and is noted in less than half of infants with disseminated and CNS disease at presentation. Feeding problems and lethargy are the most common presenting complaints.[42,43] The average age at onset of symptoms is 6 to 8 days, but the average age at diagnosis is 11 to 13 days, caused at least in part to the lack of specificity of symptoms and lack of characteristic skin lesions earlier in the disease.

Most infants will have vesicular skin lesions at some point in the course of disease. The most characteristic skin lesions are vesicles, which evolve in time into pustules, crusts, or erosions. Another important form of presentation is a poorly healing fetal scalp monitor site. Although grouped vesicles on an erythematous base are a hallmark of herpetic infection, lesions in neonatal herpes frequently lack such grouping, and in some cases a widespread vesicular exanthem or zosterlike blistering localized to one or two dermatomes may occur. Oral ulcerations are present in nearly one third of cases.[44]

A maternal history of primary herpes simplex infection (or new-onset genital ulcerations, even if not specifically diagnosed) is an important clue to infection, but the majority of cases occur in women who are either asymptomatic or whose symptoms go unrecognized.[45] Other signs and symptoms of infection in neonates include lethargy, temperature instability, jaundice, coagulopathy, hepatitis, and neurologic deterioration.[42]

If skin lesions suggest herpes infection, prompt diagnosis and institution of treatment is imperative. Skin scrapings for Tzanck preparation should be obtained. Direct fluorescent or immunoperoxidase antigen detection, as well as polymerase chain reaction (PCR), are rapid ways to obtain preliminary confirmation of HSV infection,[46] but false positive immunofluorescence has been reported.[47] Viral cultures remain the gold standard of diagnosis, and cultures of the skin, conjunctiva, throat, cerebrospinal fluid, and urine should be obtained.[44]

The differential diagnosis of herpetic skin lesions depends on the specific clinical presentation (see Boxes 10-1 and 10-2) (Table 10-1 and Table 10-2). Vesicular lesions may resemble incontinentia pigmenti, congenital varicella, and acropustulosis of infancy. Dermatomal lesions may mimic herpes zoster. Pustular lesions may resemble congenital candidiasis, erythema toxicum neonatorum, congenital self-healing histiocytosis, listeriosis, and so on. Widespread blistering may resemble epidermolysis bullosa, although a few vesicles or pustules are usually present in HSV infection.

There are some clinical presentations that are *unlikely* to represent herpes infection. In particular, a vigorous term infant with a widespread congenital onset pustular eruption is unlikely to have herpes simplex infection because its presence at birth implies intrauterine infection, which is almost invariably associated with low birth weight and other findings. A premature infant with a widespread vesiculopustular eruption involving the palms and soles could have herpes infection, but is more likely to have congenital candidiasis. Although a high index of suspicion for herpes infection is appropriate, fear of this disease should not preclude a rational and systematic approach to differential diagnosis. The management of the infant presumed to have herpes simplex infection includes strict isolation and prompt institution of intravenous antiviral therapy[44] while awaiting cultures, and is discussed in more detail in Chapter 12.

Fetal and Neonatal Varicella

Cutaneous stigmata of varicella infection may occur in the newborn period as a result of early intrauterine infection, also referred to as the "fetal varicella syndrome," "congenital varicella," and "varicella embryopathy," but varicella can also occur as a result of intrauterine infection just before delivery. This condition, which should more properly called "neonatal varicella," is often referred to in the literature as "congenital varicella."

The **fetal varicella syndrome** may occur as a result of primary varicella infection in the mother, almost always during the first trimester of pregnancy.[48] Cutaneous features include dermatomal scarring and occasional skin ulcerations, but blisters and pustules are not usually present in the neonatal period.[48-50] Herpes zoster in the newborn period can also result from exposure to varicella in utero, including infection later in pregnancy.[51-53]

Primary varicella in the neonatal period occurs in one quarter of infants exposed to maternal varicella during the last 3 weeks of pregnancy, and can be especially severe if exposure occurs between 7 days before to 2 days after delivery.[54,55] Onset is usually at 5 to 10 days of age. When maternal infection occurs between 1 and 3 weeks before delivery, partial transplacental immunity results in earlier onset of infection and milder disease.

The skin lesions in neonatal varicella begin as vesicles superimposed on an erythematous base, gradually becoming cloudy and then crusted. The clinical pattern often resembles that seen in immunocompromised hosts. Lesions may be extremely numerous, widespread, and monomorphic, with all lesions occurring at the same stage of development instead of varying stages of development. They may also be hemorrhagic and enlarge into bullae.

The most life-threatening complication of neonatal varicella is pneumonia. The diagnosis is usually obvious because of the maternal history. A positive Tzanck preparation and viral cultures are confirmatory. Management is discussed in Chapter 12.

Other Viruses

Cytomegalovirus (CMV) is a relatively common cause of intrauterine and perinatal infection, but only one case of congenital infection with vesicles has been reported.[56] The infant was premature and small for gestational age and had hepatitis at birth. Two vesicles were present on the forehead, and blister fluid, as well as saliva and urine, produced a cytopathic effect characteristic of CMV in cell culture but was not confirmed by neutralization assays, leaving some doubt about the results.

Enteroviruses are well-recognized causes of vesicular eruptions in infants and children. Enterovirus infections may occur congenitally or during neonatal life, particularly in the summer months.[57] Reports of such infections describe maculopapular rashes, but vesicular eruptions have not been mentioned in these reports. One infant with fatal neonatal echovirus 19 infection developed a hemorrhagic bulla associated with gangrene and necrosis of a portion of her hand and fingers.[58]

TABLE 10-1

Differential Diagnosis of Vesiculopustular Diseases

Disease	Usual age	Skin: morphology	Skin: usual distribution	Clinical: other	Method of diagnosis/findings
Infectious Causes					
Staphylococcal pyoderma	Few days to weeks	Pustules, bullae, occasional vesicles	Mainly diaper area, periumbilical	Boys more than girls; may be in epidemic setting	Gram stain: PMNs gram-positive cocci in clusters; bacterial culture
Group A streptococcal disease	Few days to weeks	Isolated pustules, honey-crusted areas	No specific site predisposed	Moist umbilical stump; occasional cellulitis, meningitis, pneumonia	Gram stain: gram-positive cocci in chains; bacterial culture
Group B streptococcal infection	At birth or first few days	Vesicles bullae, erosions, honey-crusted lesions	Any area	Pneumonia, bacteremia, meningitis	Gram stain: gram-positive cocci in chains; bacterial culture
Listeriosis	Birth, first few hours	Hemorrhagic pustules and petechiae	Generalized, especially trunk and extremities	Sepsis; respiratory distress; maternal fever and premature labor	Gram-positive rods; bacterial culture skin and other sites
Haemophilus influenzae infection	Birth or first few days	Vesicles, crusted areas	No specific site predisposed	Bacteremia, meningitis may be present	Gram-negative bacilli; bacterial culture
Pseudomonas infection	Days to weeks	Erythema, pustules, hemorrhagic bullae, necrotic ulcerations	Any area, but especially diaper, periorificial	History illness in neonatal period	Skin or tissue Gram stain: gram-negative rods; cultures skin, blood
Congenital candidiasis	Birth or first few days	Erythema, small papules and pustules	Any part of body; palms, soles often involved	Prematurity; foreign body in cervix, uterus are risk factors	KOH: hyphae, budding yeast; placental lesions
Neonatal candidiasis	Days or older	Scaly red patches with satellite pustules and papules	Diaper or other intertriginous area	Usually otherwise healthy	KOH: hyphae, budding yeast if pustules are present
Aspergillus infection	Few days to weeks	Pustules often clustered rapidly evolve to ulcers	Any area, especially sites of trauma, occlusion	Extreme prematurity usually present	Skin biopsy: septate hyphae; Tissue fungal culture
Neonatal herpes simplex	Usually 5 to 14 days	Vesicles, pustules, crusts, erosions	Any site; especially scalp, torso; may involve mucosa	Signs of sepsis; irritability, lethargy	Tzanck; FA or immunoperoxidase slide test, PCR, viral culture

	Age at onset	Lesion morphology	Distribution	Associated features	Diagnostic tests
Intrauterine herpes simplex	Birth	Vesicles, pustules, widespread erosions, scars, areas of missing skin	Any site, often scalp lesions	Low birth weight; microcephaly, chorioretinitis	Tzanck; FA or immunoperoxidase slide test, PCR, viral culture
Neonatal varicella	0 to 14 days	Vesicles on erythematous base	Generalized distribution	Maternal primary varicella infection 7 days before to 2 days after delivery	Tzanck, FA, viral culture
Herpes zoster	Usually 2 weeks or older	Vesicles on erythematous base	Dermatomal pattern	Maternal primary varicella infection during pregnancy or few days after delivery	Tzanck; FA, viral culture
Scabies	Usually 3-4 weeks or older	Papules, nodules, wheals, crusted areas, vesicles, burrows	Accentuated axillae, feet, wrists, may occur anywhere	Usually family members with itching, rash	Scabies prep; clinical
Transient Skin Lesions					
Erythema toxicum neonatorum	Usually 24 to 48 hours but can be birth to 2 weeks	Erythematous macules, papules, pustules, wheals	Anywhere except palms, soles	Term infants >2500 g	Clinical; Wright's stain: eosinophils
Neonatal pustular melanosis	Birth	Pustules without erythema; collarettes of scale; hyperpigmented macules	Anywhere; most often forehead, ears, back, fingers, toes	Term infants; more common in black infants	Clinical; Wright's stain: PMNs, occasional eosinophil, cellular debris
Miliaria crystallina	Birth or early infancy	Fragile vesicles without erythema	Forehead, upper trunk, arms most common	Sometimes history of overwarming, fever	Clinical; Wright, Gram and Tzanck preps negative
Miliaria rubra	Days to weeks	Erythematous papules with superimposed pustules	Forehead, upper trunk, arms most common	Sometimes history of overwarming, fever	Clinical; Wright, Gram and Tzanck preps negative
Neonatal "Acne": (Benign cephalic pustulosis)	Days to weeks	Papules and pustules on erythematous base	Cheeks, forehead, eyelids, neck, upper chest, scalp	Otherwise well	Usually clinical; Giemsa: fungal spores, neutrophils

Continued

TABLE 10-1

Differential Diagnosis of Vesiculopustular Diseases—cont'd

Disease	Usual age	Skin: morphology	Skin: usual distribution	Clinical: other	Method of diagnosis/findings
Uncommon and Rare Causes					
Acropustulosis of infancy	Birth or days to weeks	Vesicles and pustules	Hands and feet, occasional lesion elsewhere	Severe pruritus; lesions come in crops	Clinical; skin biopsy: intraepidermal vesicle/pustule
Eosinophilic pustular folliculitis	Birth or days to weeks	Pustules	Mainly scalp and face; occasionally trunk, extremities	Pruritus; Waxing and waning course with recurrent crops	Skin biopsy: dense perifollicular mixed infiltrate with eosinophils
Congenital self-healing histiocytosis	Birth to days	Vesicles, crusts, papules, nodules, petechiae	Any site	Rarely mucosal or extracutaneous involvement, but may develop later	Skin biopsy: reniform histiocytes with focal invasion epidermis; S-100 positive
Incontinentia pigmenti	Birth to days	Vesicles, hyperkeratosis in linear array	Most common trunk, scalp, extremities	Extracutaneous involvement common but often not evident at birth	Skin biopsy: eosinophilic spongiosis with dyskeratosis
Hyperimmunoglobulin E syndrome	Days to weeks	Single and grouped vesicles or pustules	Face, scalp, upper torso	IgE levels become elevated after neonatal period S. aureus infections	Skin biopsy: intraepidermal vesicle with eosinophils; eosinophilia
Neonatal Behçet's disease	First week of life	Oral and genital ulcerations and vesicles, necrotic skin lesions on hands and feet	Mucosal lesions; skin lesions mainly on hands and feet	Maternal history of Behçet's disease; diarrhea, vasculitis in 1 case	Clinical and maternal history
Pustular psoriasis	First weeks of life	Pustules on palms, soles	Generalized erythroderma	Low C3 and C4 (one case)	Skin biopsy: epidermal microabscesses and acanthosis, parakeratosis, dilated capillaries

TABLE 10-2

Differential Diagnosis of Bullae, Erosions, and Ulcerations

Disease	Usual age	Skin: morphology	Skin: usual distribution	Clinical: other	Method of diagnosis/findings
Infectious Causes					
Staphylococcal scalded skin syndrome	Few days to weeks; one congenital case	Widespread erythema, fragile bullae, erosions	Generalized with periorificial accentuation	Irritability; temperature instability	Biopsy: Epidermal separation at granular cell layer; Cultures of blood, urine or other sites demonstrate S. aureus
Group B streptococcal infection	At birth or first few days	Vesicles, bullae, erosions, honey-crusted lesions	Any area	Pneumonia, bacteremia, meningitis	Gram stain: gram-positive cocci in chains; bacterial culture
Pseudomonas infection	Days to weeks	Erythema, pustules, hemorrhagic bullae, necrotic ulcerations	Any area, but especially diaper, periorificial	History illness in neonatal period	Skin or tissue Gram stain: gram-negative rods; cultures skin, blood
Congenital syphilis	Birth or first few days	Bullae or erosions	Especially hands, feet, and periorificial	Lack of prenatal care, hepatosplenomegaly; bony lesions on radiograph	Darkfield exam of skin; FA; syphilis serologies
Aspergillus infection	Few days to weeks	Pustules often clustered rapidly evolve to ulcers	Any area, especially sites of trauma, occlusion	Extreme prematurity usually present	Skin biopsy: septate hyphae; tissue fungal culture
Zygomycosis/Trichosporosis	Days to weeks	Generalized peeling and skin breakdown or cellulitis evolving into necrotic ulcer	Any area	Extreme prematurity	Skin biopsy and tissue fungal culture
Intrauterine herpes simplex infection	Birth	Vesicles, pustules, widespread erosions, scars, areas of missing skin	Any site, especially scalp	Low birth weight; microcephaly; chorioretinitis	Tzanck; FA or immunoperoxidase slide test, PCR, viral culture
Fetal varicella infection	At birth	Scarring, limb hypoplasia, erosions	Any site but often extremity	Maternal chickenpox first trimester	Tzanck, FA, viral culture

Continued

TABLE 10-2

Differential Diagnosis of Bullae, Erosions, and Ulcerations—cont'd

Disease	Usual age	Skin: morphology	Skin: usual distribution	Clinical: other	Method of diagnosis/findings
Transient Skin Lesions					
Sucking blisters	At birth	Flaccid bulla or linear erosion—occasionally 2 symmetric lesions	Fingers, wrists, occasionally foot	Infant sucks on affected areas	Clinical
Perinatal trauma/iatrogenic injury	At birth or neonatal period	Erosions, ulcerations	Depends on cause of trauma	Perinatal history of monitoring, prolonged labor and/or vacuum or forceps delivery; other monitoring	Usually clinical
Uncommon and Rare Causes					
Epidermolysis bullosa	At birth or first few days	Bullae and skin fragility; Depending on type: mucosal erosions, aplasia cutis of anterior leg, milia, nail dystrophy, and so on	May be widespread or limited depending on type: most often extremities, especially hands, feet, other sites of friction or trauma	Pain, irritability and difficulty feeding. Occasionally corneal, respiratory tract, or gastrointestinal (pyloric atresia): anemia	Skin biopsy of blister <24 hours or induced with friction; specific type diagnosed with electron microscopy or immunofluorescent mapping
Mastocytosis	Birth or weeks to months	**Localized form:** infiltrated nodular area with intermittent superimposed wheal or bullae; **Generalized form:** Blistering usually superimposed on infiltrated skin	Any site–often on torso	Variably present: hives, flushing, irritability, sudden pallor, diarrhea	Skin biopsy: increased mast cells in dermis
Maternal bullous disease	Birth	Depends on type of maternal disease: tense or flaccid bullae or erosions	Usually generalized	Maternal history of blistering disease but occasionally inactive at time of pregnancy	Maternal history; skin biopsy and direct immunofluorescence with results depending on maternal type

Chronic bullous dermatosis of childhood	1 case at birth; Most in later infancy, childhood	Tense blisters often form rosette or sausage shapes	Generalized but often concentrated growing, buttocks, thighs; Usually spares mucosa	Usually absent	Skin biopsy: subepidermal bullae; direct immunofluorescence: linear pattern IgA DEJ
Bullous pemphigoid	2 months of age or older	Tense blisters	Often accentuated on hands and feet but may be generalized	Usually absent	Skin biopsy: subepidermal bullae; direct immunofluorescence: linear pattern IgG DEJ
Toxic epidermal necrolysis	Usually 6 weeks of age or older except for cases due to intrauterine graft vs host disease	Erythema, erosions, bullae, and cutaneous tenderness usually with mucosal involvement	Generalized, evolving rapidly over hours to days	Usually associated with gram-negative sepsis or due to intrauterine graft versus host disease in infant with congenital immunodeficiency	Skin biopsy: superepidermal blister with widespread epidermal necrosis (usually full-thickness)
Intrauterine epidermal necrosis	Birth	Widespread erosions and ulceration without vesicles or pustules	Generalized, spares mucous membranes	Prematurity and rapid mortality	Skin biopsy: Epidermal necrosis and calcification pilosebaceous follicles
Congenital erosive and vesicular dermatosis	Birth	Erosions, vesicles, crusts, erythematous areas	Generalized, usually sparing face, palms soles	Prematurity, variably: collodion membrane, transparent skin, reticulated vascular pattern	Clinical diagnosis, often retrospective. Skin biopsy: neutrophilic infiltrate; exclusion of other etiologies of erosions, vesicles
Pyoderma gangrenosum	1 case report neonate at 2 days of age	Sharply demarcated ulcerations with undermined borders	Any site, but usually groin, buttock in infancy	Many associations—mainly inflammatory bowel disease	Clinical, exclusion of other etiologies; skin biopsy with neutrophilic infiltration without vasculitis, infection, etc
Noma neonatorum	Days to weeks	Deep ulcerations, with bone loss, mutilation in some cases	Nose, lips, intraoral, anus, genitalia	Some cases due to Pseudomonas; others with malnutrition, immunodeficiency	Clinical; exclusion of other etiologies, especially infection

Continued

TABLE 10-2

Differential Diagnosis of Bullae, Erosions, and Ulcerations—cont'd

Disease	Usual age	Skin: morphology	Skin: usual distribution	Clinical: other	Method of diagnosis/findings
Acrodermatitis enteropathica	Weeks to months	Sharply demarcated crusted plaques; occasionally vesicles, bullae, erosions	Periorificial, i.e., mouth, nose, eyes, genitalia as well as neck folds, hands, and feet	Premature, breast-fed infants with low maternal milk zinc; Prolonged parenteral hyperalimentation	Low serum zinc levels (less than 50 mcg/dl)
Methylmalonic acidemia	Days to weeks	Erosive erythema	Periorificial accentuation	Lethargy, hypotonia, neutropenia, low platelets	Characteristic abnormalities plasma amino acids
Restrictive dermopathy	Birth	Rigid tense skin with erosions, linear ulcerations	Generalized skin abnormalities	Joint contractures, micrognathia, natal teeth	Clinical; distinguish from Neu-Laxova syndrome
Vascular birthmarks	Birth or first few days to weeks	Ulceration without initial vesicle or bullae	Any site, but often lip or perineum	Underlying vascular anomaly—may not always be initially evident in evolving hemangiomas	Clinical
Aplasia cutis congenita	Birth	"Bullous" form: sharply demarcated with overlying membrane; Other types with raw, full-thickness defect skin	Scalp or face most common; other sites depending on etiology	Depends on etiology: CNS defects, trisomy 13, limb-reduction abnormalities	Usually clinical; imaging studies to evaluate underlying bone, CNS

Disorder	Onset	Morphology	Distribution	Associations	Diagnosis
Linear porokeratosis	Birth—1 case report	Linear erosions	Leg, face, but any site possible	Eventual risk squamous CA skin	Skin biopsy: Coronoid lamella—may not be evident in newborn period
Erosions overlying giant nevi	Birth, first few days	Erosions, ulcerations	Superimposed on giant nevi	In some cases neurocutaneous melanosis	Clinical and biopsy to exclude melanoma if persistence or other unusual features present
Focal dermal hypoplasia	Birth	Occasional blisters, but more often hypoplasia, aplasia of skin	Linear and whorled pattern, often arms, legs, scalp	Skeletal, eye, and CNS abnormalities to varying degree	Clinical; family history; skin biopsy
Absent dermal ridges and congenital milia syndrome	Birth	Multiple bullae	Fingers, soles of feet	Absent dermal ridge patterns, multiple milia	Clinical; family history (autosomal dominant)
Porphyrias	Days to weeks	Photosensitive blistering	May be in sun-exposed areas or more generalized if exposed to phototherapy for hyperbilirubinemia	Transient form usually due to hemolytic disease; Rarer: erythropoietic porphyria (EP)	Transient: elevated plasma porphyrins; EP: pink urine; elevated urine, fecal and plasma porphyrins
Perinatal gangrene of the buttock	Days	Sudden onset erythema, cyanosis, and gangrenous ulcerations	Buttocks	Umbilical artery catheterization in some cases	Clinical
Neonatal purpura fulminans	Days	Initially purpura or cellulitis-like areas evolving to necrotic bullae or ulcers	Buttocks, extremities, trunk and scalp most common sites	Other sites of DIC	Prolonged PT, PTT, low fibrinogen, Elevated FDPs, low protein C or S levels

CUTANEOUS INFESTATIONS: SCABIES

Scabies (see also Chapter 13) is a cutaneous infestation caused by the *Sarcoptes scabiei* mite. Clinically recognizable infection in infants less than 3 to 4 weeks of age is rare, but common thereafter.[59,60,61] Vesicles and pustules are more common in infants than in older children or adults and are often concentrated on the medial feet, wrists, palms, and soles. These areas may also demonstrate erythematous papules, nodules, and burrows. The eruption may also be concentrated in the axillae, periumbilical area, and groin. Secondary bacterial infection is relatively common in young infants and should be suspected if bullae or significant honey-crusted areas are present. Young infants are often asymptomatic, without evidence of pruritus.

The diagnosis can be suspected on clinical morphology. In most cases, a history of itching or rash in other family members can be elicited. Whenever possible, the diagnosis should be confirmed with skin scrapings, which demonstrate a mite, eggs, or feces. The best lesions for scraping are burrows, intact vesicles, and pustules, but in young infants, mites are also found in crusted areas.[62] The diagnosis and management are discussed in Chapter 13.

TRANSIENT SKIN LESIONS

Erythema Toxicum Neonatorum

Erythema toxicum neonatorum (toxic erythema of the newborn) (see Chapter 7) is a common condition of term infants, but is rare in premature infants and those weighing less than 2500 g.[63,64] Most cases occur between 24 and 48 hours of age, with 11% occurring before 24 hours and 25% occurring after 48 hours of life. Rarely, the eruption is present at birth.[64,65,66] Onset as late as 10 to 14 days of life has been reported but is unusual and should prompt consideration of alternative diagnoses.[64,67]

Four distinct skin lesions occur in varying combinations: erythematous macules, wheals, papules, and pustules. Occasionally, lesions appear as vesicles before becoming pustular. The rash often begins on the face. The buttocks, torso, and proximal extremities are common sites of involvement. The palms and soles are virtually never affected. Erythematous macules and wheals may vary in size from a few millimeters to several centimeters, with papules and pustules of 1 to 2 mm in size, superimposed on erythematous macules or wheals. The rash waxes and wanes, with previously involved skin returning to normal in a few hours to 1 to 2 days, and new lesions may continue to develop for several days.[68] Mechanical irritation of the skin can precipitate the onset of new lesions.

The diagnosis of erythema toxicum is usually based on the clinical appearance of the rash in an otherwise healthy term infant. The diagnosis can be confirmed with Wright's stain of a pustule, which demonstrates numerous eosinophils. Peripheral eosinophilia is present in a small percentage of cases.[3] Skin biopsy, usually unnecessary, demonstrates eosinophilic infiltration of the outer root sheath of the hair follicle epithelium, and in pustular lesions, eosinophils coalesce into an intraepidermal or subcorneal pustule, adjacent to a hair follicle. An upper dermal and perivascular eosinophilic infiltrate is also present.[69]

The differential diagnosis of erythema toxicum includes neonatal pustular melanosis, congenital candidiasis, miliaria rubra, incontinentia pigmenti, and eosinophilic pustular folliculitis. The latter two conditions have eosinophilic inflammation, but can be differentiated by their distribution, their more chronic course, and histopathology. The associated erythema and postnatal onset may help to distinguish erythema toxicum from pustular melanosis, but both are common and can occur simultaneously.[70] Once the diagnosis has been established, no specific treatment is necessary. Parents can be reassured about the benign and noninfectious nature of the condition.

Transient Neonatal Pustular Melanosis

Transient neonatal pustular melanosis (TNPM) is a relatively common condition of unknown etiology. Like erythema toxicum, it is more common in term infants and is unassociated with other abnormalities.[71] Unlike erythema toxicum, lesions are virtually always present at birth.

Three types of lesions occur in TNPM: (1) pustules with little or no underlying erythema, (2) ruptured pustules usually manifesting as slightly hyperpigmented macules with a surrounding collarette of scale, and (3) hyperpigmented macules without scale. Lesions vary in size from 1 to 10 mm, but are typically 2 to 3 mm. They may be solitary or grouped and often small satellite pustules are evident (Fig. 10-1). More than one type of lesion may be present at the same time. Lesions may occur on virtually any part of the skin but are most common the forehead, behind the ears, under the chin, on the neck and back, and on hands and feet. The palms and soles may be affected.

The diagnosis of pustular melanosis is usually made clinically based on lesional morphology, time of onset, and the absence of other findings. Clues to clinical diagnosis are the extremely superficial nature of the pustules and the absence of underlying erythema.

Wright's stain often demonstrates polymorphonuclear neutrophils (PMNs), with an occasional eosinophil, but in rare cases eosinophils may predominate.[72] Gram stain

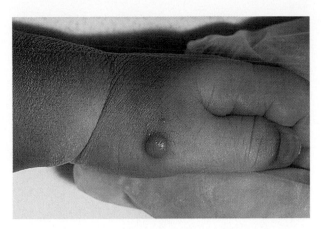

FIG. 10-1

Transient neonatal pustular melanosis: Large pustule on the hand with tiny "satellite" pustules may mimic infection. (From Frieden IJ: Blisters and pustules in the newborn. Curr Probl Pediatr 1989; 19:587.)

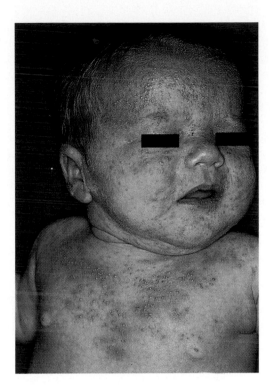

FIG. 10-2

Extensive miliaria rubra. (Courtesy Anne W. Lucky.)

demonstrates PMNs but no bacteria. Skin biopsy, rarely necessary for diagnosis, demonstrates hyperkeratosis, acanthosis, and an intracorneal or subepidermal pustule filled with PMNs, occasional eosinophils, and variable amounts of keratinous debris, serous fluid, and fragmented hair shafts.[71]

The differential diagnosis of TNPM includes erythema toxicum, staphylococcal impetigo and other bacterial infections, congenital candidiasis, acropustulosis of infancy, and miliaria. These conditions can nearly always be differentiated by time of onset, lesional morphology, and by the demonstration of PMNs on Wright's stain, and lack of organisms on Gram stain and KOH preparations.

Once the diagnosis of TPNM has been established, no treatment is necessary. Pustules usually resolve over a few days, but hyperpigmented macules may last for several weeks to months before resolving.

Sterile Transient Neonatal Pustulosis

The term *sterile transient neonatal pustulosis* has been introduced by Ferrandiz et al[70] to describe infants with clinical and histologic features of both erythema toxicum neonatorum and TNPM. They propose that a clear-cut differentiation between these two conditions is not always possible.

Miliaria

Miliaria (prickly heat) (see Chapter 7) is a relatively common finding in newborns. In warm climates without air-conditioned nurseries, miliaria may be present in up to

15% of newborns,[73,74] but it is less common in temperate climates.[75] Two types of miliaria occur in the newborn period. **Miliaria crystallina** is due to blockage of the sweat duct at the level of the stratum corneum. Sweat accumulates beneath the stratum corneum, causing tiny flaccid vesicles, resembling dewdrops. **Miliaria rubra** is also due to blockage of the sweat duct in the stratum corneum, but the obstruction leads to focal leakage of sweat into the dermis, resulting in an inflammatory response, evident in the erythematous papules, and pustules that are present clinically (Fig. 10-2).[76] Both may follow excessive warming in an incubator, fever, occlusive dressings, or dress in inappropriately warm clothing. Miliaria crystallina is occasionally present at the time of birth, whereas miliaria rubra is more common after the first week of life.[77]

The most common locations are the forehead and upper trunk. Lesions often become confluent. This, combined with location, time of onset, and a history of excessive warming, may help distinguish miliaria from other vesicular and pustular eruptions. Miliaria crystallina is also easily recognized because the dewdrop-like vesicles rupture easily with only slight pressure.

Although the precise cause of miliaria is not known, recent evidence supports the concept that an extracellular polysaccharide substance produced by some strains of *Staphylococcus epidermidis* may obstruct sweat delivery.[78]

In cases where the diagnosis is uncertain, a skin biopsy can be performed. In miliaria crystallina, subcorneal vesicles are contiguous with underlying sweat ducts. In miliaria rubra, intraepidermal vesicles are due to epidermal edema. These vesicles, which are also in contiguity with a sweat duct, have an intravesicular and dermal chronic inflammatory infiltrate.[76] No specific treatment is necessary for miliaria; the condition will disappear spontaneously if overheating is avoided.

Sucking Blisters

Sucking blisters result from vigorous sucking by the infant during fetal life. The lesions are always present at birth. They occur in approximately 1 in every 250 live births, and are not associated with other abnormalities.[79,80] These bullae are usually flaccid, vary in size from 5 to 15 mm, and may evolve rapidly to become superficial linear or round erosions. Characteristic locations include the radial forearm, wrist, and hand, including the dorsal thumb and index fingers. The lesions may be unilateral or bilateral and symmetric.

The diagnosis can be suspected if lesions are in characteristic locations and there are no vesicles or bullae on other areas of the body. The infants usually confirm the diagnosis by demonstrating "an insatiable appetite for the skin of their own forearms, wrists, and fingers."[79] The lesions resolve without specific treatment within days to weeks.

Neonatal "Acne" (Neonatal Cephalic Pustulosis)

Although neonatal acne has been considered a common condition, the term *neonatal cephalic pustulosis* (see Chapter 7) has been proposed for this condition, in large part because the hallmarks of true acne—comedones and its associated inflammatory lesions—are rare in the first month of life, developing instead between 1 and 6 months of age.

This condition is characterized by a papulopustular facial eruption usually concentrated on the cheeks, but the forehead, chin, eyelids, neck, upper chest, and scalp may also be affected (Fig. 10-3). The mean age of onset is 2 to 3 weeks, with some cases beginning as early as 1 week of life. It is usually asymptomatic and generally unassociated with other medical conditions, although prolonged

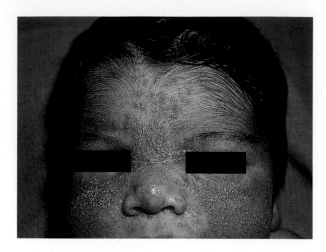

FIG. 10-3
Neonatal cephalic pustulosis.

true acne and seborrheic dermatitis have been described.[81] Several authors have proposed *Malassezia furfur* and *M. sympodialis* as causes of this condition.[81,82] Cultures of pustules have demonstrated both *Malassezia furfur* and *M. sympodialis,* especially in severe cases. Because these organisms are found on the skin under normal conditions, their role in causing this disease is still somewhat controversial.

The diagnosis is usually made clinically, but Giemsa-stained smears can demonstrate fungal spores, as well as neutrophils and occasionally other inflammatory cells.[81] Special growth media is necessary to culture *Malassezia* species. Treatment with topical imidazole creams such as ketoconazole can result in resolution of the eruption, but this condition also frequently improves with low-potency topical corticosteroids such as hydrocortisone and also remits spontaneously after several weeks.

Diaper Erosions

Rapidly healing superficial erosions have been noted in the diaper area in infants between 1 and 14 days of life in several otherwise healthy infants who were being studied prospectively as part of a study of diaper dermatitis. The erosions healed rapidly and were attributed to either perinatal trauma or the minor trauma of normal diaper care. The findings are intriguing, suggesting that term infants may have increased skin fragility when compared with older infants, where such erosions were not noted.[83]

Iatrogenic Causes of Erosions and Ulcerations

Many types of iatrogenic interventions can cause cutaneous erosions or ulceration (see Chapter 8), which is less common.[84] Scalp erosions can be due to intrauterine placement of fetal scalp electrodes for monitoring purposes. One prospective study of 535 monitored newborns found that 21% of infants had very minor superficial lacerations that healed before discharge, and 18.7% had superficial lacerations still present at discharge. A rarer finding, scalp ulcerations, was present in 1.3% of cases.[85] These lesions are usually only a few millimeters in diameter, but occasionally measure up to 1 to 1.5 cm. They are sometimes confused with lesions of aplasia cutis congenita. Persistent scalp erosions, ulcerations, or crusting should always lead to consideration of possible neonatal herpes infection.[44]

Transcutaneous pulse oximetry may rarely lead to blistering or erosions, particularly if a defective device results in overheating of the skin leading to a thermal burn, or resulting from sustained pressure from a probe left in one location for over 24 hours.[86] Erosions or crusted areas may also occur on the heel, following multiple heel sticks for blood drawing.

Scald burns represent a relatively common form of childhood injury and can occur in neonates or young infants as a result of child abuse or misinformed parenting. Localized scald burn with blistering has been reported in a 1 day old, caused by hot water, increased by the hospital as a response to an outbreak of *Legionella*.[87]

UNCOMMON AND RARE CAUSES OF VESICLES AND PUSTULES

Acropustulosis of Infancy

Acropustulosis of infancy (infantile acropustulosis) is a condition of unknown etiology, characterized by extremely pruritic vesiculopustules occurring on the hands and feet. Lesions may be present at birth, but usually develop in the first weeks or months of life.[88,89] The condition is more common in blacks, but does occur in other races.[90] An association with atopy has been reported in some patients and families.[91]

Lesions occur in crops every 2 to 4 weeks, with individual lesions usually lasting for 5 to 10 days. Boys are more commonly affected. Intensely pruritic vesicles and pustules are located on the palms and soles, dorsal hands and feet, as well as the sides of the fingers and toes (Fig. 10-4). Scattered lesions may also be located on the ankles

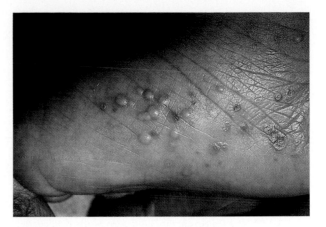

FIG. 10-4
Acropustulosis of infancy. (From Frieden IJ. Blisters and pustules in the newborn. Curr Probl Pediatr 1989;19:591.)

and wrists, and occasionally papules occur at more distant sites such as the chest, back, and abdomen. Lesions are initially tense, then begin to flatten, developing scales and postinflammatory hyperpigmentation. Infants who are too young to scratch may instead seem irritable and rub their feet together frantically.

Both clinical characteristics and direct smears or skin biopsy confirm the diagnosis. Scrapings of lesions show numerous PMNs and occasional eosinophils, but scabies mites, eggs, and feces are notably absent.[92] Skin biopsy demonstrates an intraepidermal or subcorneal pustule filled with PMNs or eosinophils or both. The earliest histopathologic changes are focal vesiculation and degeneration of keratinocytes with cell necrosis.[93] Peripheral eosinophilia is occasionally present.[94]

The condition most resembling acropustulosis of infancy is infantile scabies, and family history and multiple skin scrapings are necessary to differentiate the two. In cases with onset after the newborn period, the condition may actually be preceded by an episode of scabies, even after adequate antiscabietic treatment.[95] Other conditions in the differential diagnosis include dyshidrotic eczema and pustulosis palmaris et plantaris, which are rare in infancy; congenital candidiasis, which is usually more widespread; and neonatal pustular melanosis, which is not pruritic and does not recur.

Acropustulosis of infancy spontaneously usually remits within 1 to 2 years. Very potent topical corticosteroids are usually effective, but should be used cautiously to avoid localized atrophy or systemic absorption.[95] If symptoms are severe, oral antihistamines at maximum doses can be used to control pruritus. Dapsone 1 to 2 mg/k/day has been used for severe cases, but should be used with caution because of the risk of methemoglobinemia and other adverse effects.[88]

Eosinophilic Pustular Folliculitis

Eosinophilic pustular folliculitis is a rare pustular disorder. Several cases have been reported in young infants, including a few cases with onset at birth or in the first few days of life.[96,97,98] In the neonatal cases, the children were born with or developed pustules primarily on the scalp and face but also intermittently on the trunk or extremities (Fig. 10-5). The lesions are usually very pruritic. Recurrent crops of lesions may develop, leading to a waxing and waning course. Occasionally, scarring can develop in previous areas of involvement. Peripheral eosinophilia is present in some patients. The recurrent crops of lesions, extreme pruritus, involvement of the extremities, and similar histology has led at least one report to speculate that infantile acropustulosis and EPF may be part of the same clinical spectrum,[99] but in neither case is the etiology known.

Histopathology demonstrates a dense perifollicular and dermal infiltrate consisting of large numbers of eosinophils, as well as lymphocytes and histiocytes, with some invasion of the outer root sheath of the hair follicle.[97] The differential diagnosis in neonates includes transient neonatal pustular melanosis, erythema toxicum neonatorum, and acropustulosis of infancy. There is no specific treatment for the condition, but oral antihistamines and potent topical corticosteroids may help temporarily control symptoms.

Congenital "Self-Healing" Histiocytosis

Congenital self-healing histiocytosis (see also Chapter 23), now thought to be a subset of Langerhans' cell histiocytosis, is very rare condition that can present with papules, vesicles, pustules, and crusts.[100,101,102] It is usually caused by a proliferation of Langerhans' cells, but in one report non-Langerhans' histiocytes were also implicated.[103]

Lesions are virtually always present at birth, and new lesions may continue to erupt over the first several weeks of life. The eruption may be present on any area of the body. Multiple morphologic characteristics have been reported, including vesicles, bullae, pustules, erythematous papules, nodules, crusts, erosions, and ulcerations. Lesions vary in size from a few millimeters to several centimeters, but in most cases with vesicles or pustules, small lesions predominate. Petechiae, atrophy, and milia may occasionally be present.

If suspected, a preliminary diagnosis can be obtained via Tzanck preparation, which demonstrates histiocytes with reniform nuclei and abundant cytoplasm,[104] and can then be confirmed with skin biopsy. An infiltrate of histiocytes, with large cells and irregularly shaped vesicular nuclei and eosinophilic cytoplasm, is present in the upper dermis. The histiocytes may also invade the epidermis focally. Occasional lymphocytes and eosinophils may be present. The diagnosis should be further confirmed with an S-100 stain, immunohistochemical markers, and/or electron microscopy to evaluate for the presence of Langerhans' cells.[105] The differential diagnosis of congenital self-healing histiocytosis includes intrauterine herpes simplex infection, congenital candidiasis, neonatal varicella, and intrauterine graft versus host disease.

Most cases remain confined to the skin and resolve without treatment, but extracutaneous disease or cutaneous relapse may occur months to years later, so ongoing monitoring is necessary.[106]

Incontinentia Pigmenti

Incontinentia pigmenti (IP) (see Chapter 24) is a multisystem disease, inherited as an X-linked dominant condition that is usually lethal in males. Skin lesions are

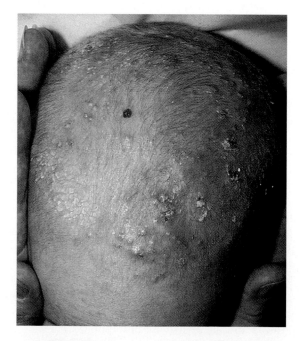

FIG. 10-5
Eosinophilic pustular folliculitis on the scalp.

present at birth in 50% of cases and occur within 2 weeks in 90%, usually beginning a vesicular eruption that evolves into linear streaks of clear or yellow confluent vesicles, following the lines of Blaschko[107] (Fig. 10-6). These lines, presumably derived from embryonal migration patterns, are not dermatomal, but instead form linear patterns on the extremities and curvilinear, whorled patterns on the torso. The eruption is most common on the trunk, extremities, and scalp. The vesicular phase may wax and wane for up to a year and occasionally recur, but individual lesions usually resolve in 1 to 2 weeks. As the initial vesicular phase subsides, a verrucous stage consisting of hyperkeratotic streaks usually occurs, followed by a pigmented stage with streaky, reticulated pigment forming a "marble-cake pattern" that fades over many years. The final stage is that of hypopigmented, atrophic areas, which may be subtle and unappreciated. Because these stages may overlap in time, as well as occur in utero, vesicular lesions may be seen in conjunction with verrucous or hyperpigmented lesions. Additional cutaneous changes include patchy, scarring alopecia, woolly hair nevus, nail dystrophy, and abnormalities in sweating.[108]

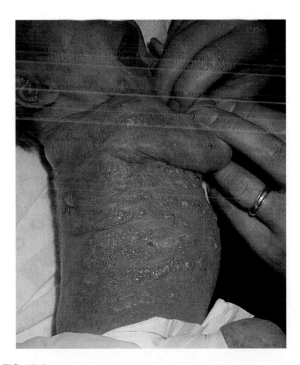

FIG. 10-6
Incontinentia pigmenti. The extensive linear blistering in this case—more pronounced than is usually seen—can resemble other causes of neonatal vesicles and bullae.

Diagnosis is made by skin biopsy, which demonstrates an edematous (spongiotic) epidermis with eosinophilic infiltration, dyskeratosis, and eosinophilic microabscesses.[76] The differential diagnosis of IP in the blistering phase includes erythema toxicum neonatorum, bullous impetigo, herpes zoster and zosteriform herpes simplex, and diffuse cutaneous mastocytosis. Extracutaneous abnormalities, evaluation, and management are discussed in Chapter 24.

Hyperimmunoglobulin E Syndrome (Job's Syndrome)

Two cases of a vesicular eruption in newborns who later were found to have hyperimmunoglobulin E syndrome have been reported.[109,110] Unfortunately, they lacked precise descriptions of the eruptions in the newborn period, but lesions were described as single, grouped, and confluent tense and umbilicated vesicles on inflamed skin, located on the face, scalp, ears, and shoulders. In one case, significant blood eosinophilia was present, but IgE levels were not markedly elevated until 1 year of age. A skin biopsy showed an intraepidermal vesicle with eosinophils. This patient also had recurrent *Staphylococcal aureus* infections.[109] Other features of hyperIgE syndrome (which generally develop after the neonatal period) include a pustular eruption on the face and scalp, cold abscesses, recurrent pneumonia, osteomyelitis, and mucocutaneous candidiasis. IgE levels are usually greater than 2000 IU/ml but may not rise until after 1 year of age.[111]

Pustular Eruption and Leukemoid Reaction in Down Syndrome

In one single case report, an extensive vesiculopustular eruption in association with a congenital leukemoid reaction and hyperbilirubinemia, was evident within 24 hours of life. Widespread papules, erosions, petechiae, and papulovesicles were present mainly on the face, but later developed on the trunk and limbs, and continued to appear for 1 week before resolving without treatment. Skin biopsy revealed an intraepidermal spongiotic vesicopustule and perivascular infiltrate. The cells were found to represent an infiltrate of immature myeloid cells, reminiscent of leukemia cutis. The infant subsequently was diagnosed with myelodysplasia and developed acute myelogenous leukemia at 2 years of age.[112]

Pustular Psoriasis

At least one case of pustular psoriasis has been described in a 20-day-old infant presenting with an exfoliative dermatitis with onset in the first few days of life. Pustules were present on the palms and soles. Skin biopsies helped confirm the diagnosis.[113]

Neonatal Behçet's Disease

A few cases of neonatal Behçet's disease, acquired transplacentally from affected mothers, have been described. The skin manifestations develop within 1 week of life and generally resolve by 2 to 3 months of age. Affected infants have oral and/or genital ulcerations and may develop pustular or necrotic skin lesions, especially on the hands and feet, as well as at sites of trauma.[114] Although most infants have no other symptoms, one infant with life-threatening disease has been described.[115] He had bloody diarrhea and vasculitis, which responded to systemic corticosteroids. Of note, his mother, who had not been diagnosed as having Behçet's disease previously, developed oral and genital ulcerations during pregnancy that resolved, but then recurred when the infant was 24 days old.[115] With this exception, the diagnosis has been evident because of the known diagnosis of Behçet's in the mother. The main disease in the differential diagnosis is neonatal HSV infection, but viral cultures and maternal history of Behçet's can help in differentiation.

EPIDERMOLYSIS BULLOSA

Epidermolysis bullosa (EB) is a large group of inherited diseases in which the skin is unable to withstand friction, resulting in skin blistering. These diseases are sometimes referred to as mechanobullous diseases. EB results from defects in the complex meshwork of proteins in the epidermis, dermis, and dermal-epidermal junction that allow the skin to adhere in the face of frictional stress. Recent advances in the understanding of the molecular biology of EB have elucidated not only the specific molecular defects of these diseases but also the role these proteins play in normal skin adhesion.

The clinical presentation and course of EB are quite variable and depend on the specific subtype. EB is classified by the clinical extent and ultrastructural level of blistering, by inheritance pattern, and more recently by specific molecular defect.[116,117,118] Although some EB subtypes tend to be severe in the neonatal period and milder later, others can be fatal in the first weeks of life as a result of severe generalized skin blistering or serious extracutaneous complications. Unfortunately, diagnosis and prognostication can be difficult in the newborn period based on clinical findings, since phenotypic features that point to a specific diagnosis may not develop until after the first year of life.[116]

Cutaneous Findings in Epidermolysis Bullosa

Friction-induced skin blistering is the cardinal cutaneous feature of all subtypes of epidermolysis bullosa. The course of this blistering over a lifetime varies significantly. Although some patients with autosomal dominant localized EB simplex may not develop blistering until puberty, others blister in the first months of life.[116] In contrast, patients with recessive dystrophic EB have pronounced fragility and severe generalized blistering throughout their lifetime. Because infants with all subtypes can present with marked blistering in the newborn period, predicting specific EB subtypes based on clinical findings can be difficult in the first weeks of life. Clinical features that may be helpful in evaluating infants with possible EB are outlined in Table 10-3.

Blisters occur in areas subjected to friction, such as the hands and feet, diaper area, and back. Blistering may also be generalized.[116] It is often worse in warm weather. The scalp and face may blister as a result of the trauma of vaginal birth. The depth of the blister depends on EB subtype. More superficial blisters may rupture easily, leaving open erosions, whereas deeper blisters may be tense or hemorrhagic (Fig. 10-7). Crusts may surmount the erosions, and foul smelling or purulent crust may develop with secondary infection. The blisters may resolve with no scarring. However, hypopigmented or hyperpigmented scarring, granulation tissue, or hypertrophic or atrophic scars may also occur. Milia suggests a dystrophic form of EB

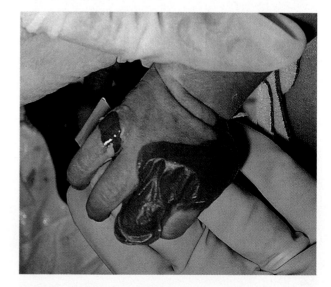

FIG. 10-7
Epidermolysis bullosa. Tense blisters are more common with dystrophic EB but are sometimes seen with other variants.

TABLE 10-3

Clinical Presentation and Diagnosis of Selected EB Subtypes in the Neonatal Period[116-118]

EB subtype (usual inheritance)	Clinical features		Diagnosis: electron microscopy (EM), immunohistochemical, and immunofluorescence antigen mapping findings (IF)
	Cutaneous	Extracutaneous	
EB Simplex, Koebner (AD)	Mild to moderate blistering, often generalized Rare scarring, milia CLAS	Occasional mucosal blistering	EM: Intraepidermal split; keratin filament changes IF: BPAG1 (BP230), BP-180 (BPAG2, collagen XVII), α6β4 integrin, laminin 10, laminin 5, type IV collagen, type VII collagen (EBA antigen) at base of blister
EB Simplex, Weber-Cockayne (AD)	Mild blistering, often localized, sometimes in first 24 mos, but often not until later infancy or childhood Rare scarring, milia	Rare mucosal involvement	EM: Intrastratum basale split IF: Same as EB simplex, Koebner
EB Simplex, Dowling-Meara (AD)	Moderate to severe blistering, starts generalized, then grouped (herpetiform) Milia Nail dystrophy, shedding CLAS	Mild mucosal blistering	EM: Intrastratum basale split; clumped keratin filaments IF: Same as EB simplex, Koebner
Junctional EB, non-Herlitz type (AR)	Moderate blistering Atrophic scars Nail dystrophy	Mild mucosal blistering Enamel hypoplasia	EM: Intralamina lucida cleavage; variable reduction in hemidesmosomes IF: Absent staining with 19-DEJ-1 (uncein); variable staining with GB3 and other laminin 5 antibodies including 46 and K140; BPAg1 (BP230) BP180 (BPAG2, collagen XVII), α6β4 integrin in blister roof Laminin 10, type IV collagen, type VII collagen (EBA antigen) at base of blister
Junctional, Herlitz type (AR)	Severe generalized blistering Heals poorly, granulation tissue Scarring, nail dystrophy, CLAS	Severe mucosal blistering GI involvement: common Laryngeal involvement with airway obstruction Urological involvement	EM: Cleavage intralamina lucida; markedly reduced or absent hemidesmosomes; absent subbasal dense plates IF: Absent staining with 19-DEJ-1 (uncein) and GB3 (laminin 5) and absent staining with other laminin 5 antibodies including 46 and K140. BPAG1 (BP230) and BP180 (BPAG2, type XVII collagen) in blister roof Laminin-10, type IV collagen and type VII collagen at base of blister
Pyloric Atresia-Junctional EB (AR)	Severe blistering CLAS	Pclyhydramnios Pyloric atresia Urological involvement: uretovesicular obstruction, hydronephrosis.	EM: Cleavage intralamina lucida and intraplasma membrane; small hemidesmosomes IF: BPAG1 (BP230) and BP180 (BPAG2, type XVII collagen) in blister roof. Laminin-10, type IV collagen and type VII collagen at base of blister Absent 19-DEJ-1 (uncein), α6β4 integrin absent or reduced
Dominant dystrophic EB (AD)	Mild to moderate blistering (but may be more severe in newborn period) Milia, scarring CLAS Nail dystrophy	Mild mucosal blistering	EM: Cleavage sublamina densa; variable reduction in anchoring fibrils IF: BPAG1(BP230) BP-180 (BPAG2, collagen XVII), α6β4, integrin laminin 10, type IV collagen at base of blister Normal, variable, or absent staining for type VII collagen (EBA antigen)
Recessive Dystrophic EB (Hallopeau-Siemens) (AR)	Severe blistering Milia, scarring CLAS	Severe muccosal blistering GI involvement common Urological involvement	EM: Cleavage sublamina densa; absent anchoring fibrils IF: BPAG1(BP230) BP-180 (BPAG2, collagen XVII), α6β4, integrin laminin 10, type IV collagen at base of blister Variable or absent staining for type VII collagen (EBA antigen)

EB, Epidermolysis bullosa; AR, autosomal recessive; CLAS, congenital localized absence of skin; AD, autosomal dominant; GI, gastrointestinal.

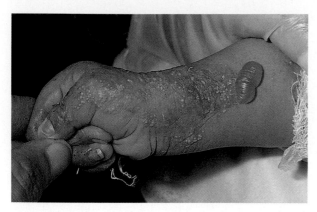

FIG. 10-8
Epidermolysis bullosa. Multiple milia and blistering in an infant
with dystrophic EB.

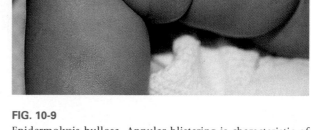

FIG. 10-9
Epidermolysis bullosa. Annular blistering is characteristic of
Dowling-Meara EB.

(Fig. 10-8), and other features may point to a specific EB
subtype, such as grouping of blisters in the Dowling Meara
type of EB simplex (Fig. 10-9).[116]

Oral involvement may develop, with open erosions or
intact vesicles on the lips, gums, and palate; these may result in pain with feeding. The nails may be absent, dystrophic, or shed in many forms of EB. Scarring alopecia
may occur.[116]

Congenital localized absence of skin (CLAS), sometimes
referred to as a form of aplasia cutis congenita, is a large
open erosion or ulcer present at birth, usually on a limb
(Fig. 10-10). Originally described in a kindred by Bart et al,
CLAS was thought to be a presenting feature of a specific
autosomal dominant EB subtype, known as Bart's syndrome.[119] Since the original description, CLAS has been reported as a presenting sign of a variety of EB subtypes, including EB simplex Dowling Meara, recessive junctional EB
with pyloric atresia, and dominant dystrophic EB.[120-124]
Bart's original kindred was reexamined with current molecular diagnostic techniques and found to have dominant
dystrophic EB.[125] CLAS is thought to result from intrauterine friction (e.g., the leg rubbing against the uterine wall)
and therefore is not specific for any one type of EB.[120] Newborns with EB can occasionally present with CLAS in the
delivery room and develop friction-induced blistering later
in the neonatal period.

Extracutaneous Findings

The nature and severity of extracutaneous involvement in
EB vary widely and must therefore be discussed by sub-

type. In general, complications involving the eye, airway
and respiratory tree, and gastrointestinal or genitourinary
systems may develop and, depending on the severity, may
be serious and impair function or may become life threatening and result in early mortality. For example, laryngeal
and airway involvement may result in airway obstruction
requiring tracheostomy.[126,127]

Although many complications occur in the neonatal
period, other long-term problems become important as
patients with more severe EB subtypes survive infancy. For
example, although not an issue in early infancy, dental involvement may ultimately become a major concern: anodontia, hypodontia, or enamel hypoplasia with excessive
caries and loss of teeth may occur.[126] Severe anemia (resulting from chronic inflammation) and iron deficiency
(from poor absorption and increased blood loss in
wounds) develop in many patients in later life with recessive dystrophic EB (RDEB) and junctional EB (JEB). This
complication has been treated successfully with intravenous iron and recombinant erythropoietin. Quality of
life improved after treatment of anemia, with patients reporting more energy, increased sense of well being, and
better tolerance of wound care regimens.[128] Attaining adequate nutrition in the face of increased demands resulting from wound healing and chronic disease is another
daunting and chronic problem in the more severe forms
of JEB and RDEB, especially when dental, oral, and gastrointestinal problems coexist. Malnutrition is common,
especially in the patients with the more severe EB subtypes.[129,130] Complications that result in mortality in early
adulthood include bacterial sepsis and the development

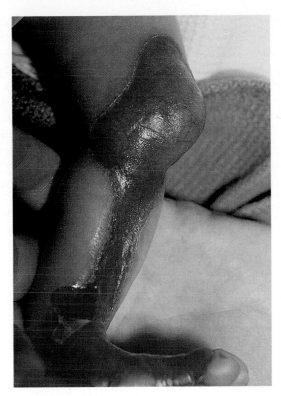

FIG. 10-10
Epidermolysis bullosa. Large defects such as this one can be present at birth in many types of EB.

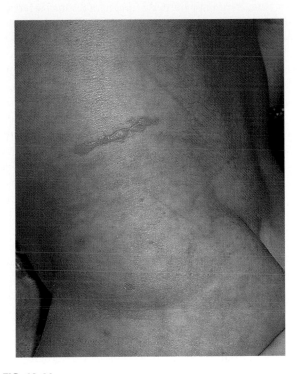

FIG. 10-11
Epidermolysis bullosa. Milder forms of EB may show blistering only at sites of friction—in this case caused by the edge of a diaper.

of cutaneous squamous cell carcinomas, particularly in RDEB.[126] Fatal cardiomyopathy was reported in two malnourished children with RDEB and was thought to be caused by selenium deficiency.[131]

Clinical Features of Specific Epidermolysis Bullosa Subtypes

Epidermolysis Bullosa Simplex

Autosomal dominant EB simplex (Koebner) is a common and relatively mild form of EB. Cutaneous blistering is located intraepidermally. EB Simplex Koebner presents with serous or serosanguinous blisters on acral sites; involvement may be more widespread and variable even within families.[116] Onset is early, at birth or infancy (Fig. 10-11).[132] Nails are normal, and scarring and milia do not usually occur. There is very little extracutaneous involvement in this type of EB, and long-term prognosis is excellent. Oral blistering may occur in infancy but is less severe than in other subtypes.[116]

In **EB simplex (Weber-Cockayne)**, the most common form of EB simplex, blisters develop later in infancy or childhood, usually on hands and feet after marked fric-

tional stress. Most cases are autosomal dominant, but autosomal recessive transmission with neonatal onset has been reported.[133]

In contrast, **autosomal dominant Dowling Meara EB simplex herpetiformis (DM-EBS)** can be severe and even fatal in the newborn period.[121,134] Blistering presents at birth or the first days of life. In the neonatal period, blisters and erosions may be generalized, or localized to acral areas, especially periungual areas. The lesions are sometimes large and hemorrhagic. Scarring is minor; milia may develop. Mucosal blistering is often present, but mild.[121,134,135]

Laryngeal involvement has been reported.[9] Nails may be thickened and ridged or may shed.[134,135] In infancy, blisters are sometimes grouped (thus the "herpetiformis" descriptor) (see Fig. 10-9). The severity of the disease decreases over time, with less marked blistering in adolescence, and rare blistering in adulthood in many cases. Itching may occur. Thickened, hyperkeratotic palms and soles develop between age 1 and 3 years, becoming more prominent throughout childhood, and persisting into adulthood.[134,135]

Other rare subtypes of EB simplex have been described and are reviewed by Fine et al.[116] **EBS with mottled pig-**

mentation (EBS-MP) is an autosomal dominant EB sub-type characterized by the development of distinctive reticulated hyperpigmentation in early infancy.[136] In one family, there was nonscarring blistering at birth or in infancy with no mucosal involvement. Hyperpigmented macules in a reticulate pattern developed in the first 6 months of life. Coleman et al reviewed other cases in the literature; blistering becomes less severe with age.[136]

Autosomal recessively inherited EB simplex has been associated with muscle disease. In this rare subtype, severe, extensive blistering (in some cases with scarring and milia) occurs in the neonatal period in association with oral and nail involvement. This is accompanied or followed by muscular dystrophy.[137,138,139] A mutation in the gene for plectin, a cytoskeleton membrane anchorage protein, has been shown to be the cause of this form of EB.[138] In one kindred, the muscular dystrophy developed early in infancy and was progressive.[140] Other cases of recessive EB simplex with severe skin involvement in infancy, but without apparent muscle involvement, have been reported.[141] Clinicians managing infants with undefined severe EB, or EB simplex that is atypically severe or autosomal recessive, should be aware of the association with muscular dystrophy and follow closely for the development of muscle weakness.

Junctional Epidermolysis Bullosa

Junctional EB (JEB) is the least common type of EB. Blisters form in the lamina lucida in the dermal-epidermal junction; thus the cleavage is deeper than in EB simplex. As with EB simplex, JEB can be autosomal recessive or dominant, localized or generalized, relatively mild or severe.[116]

Junctional EB (Herlitz type), formerly known as the gravis type, is a rare EB subtype with autosomal recessive inheritance. It has a poor prognosis due to the extent of blistering and extracutaneous involvement. Large erosions heal poorly, with formation of granulation tissue, especially in periorificial and periungual areas and the nape of the neck.[116,142,143] Nail dystrophy and shedding are common. Marked mucosal blistering occurs, with oral blisters and erosions. Extensive erosions of the laryngeal and respiratory, gastrointestinal, and urinary tract epithelium may develop, leading to life-threatening complications such as upper airway obstruction.[127] Other extracutaneous complications include dental abnormalities, failure to thrive, and anemia caused by iron deficiency and chronic disease.[142,143] Ocular problems may develop, such as blepharitis, recurrent corneal erosions leading to scarring, ectropion, and decreased visual acuity.[142,144] Urologic complications include dysuria, hematuria, meatal stenosis, hydronephrosis, and urinary tract infection (UTI) with

sepsis.[145] Early mortality in JEB gravis is due to sepsis, pneumonia, or extracutaneous complications.[143]

Autosomal recessive JEB with pyloric atresia (PA-JEB) often presents with polyhydramnios in pregnancy, and in the newborn period with blisters, as well as signs of upper GI obstruction.[123,146,147,148,149] Many of these patients also have urologic involvement, with ureterovesical obstruction and recurrent UTI.[148] A set of twins with JEB and pyloric atresia was reported; both died by 1 month of age.[150] Early mortality is usual in patients with PA-JEB.

Junctional EB (non-Herlitz type) formerly known as generalized atrophic benign epidermolysis bullosa is an autosomal recessive JEB subtype with a better prognosis. It was described by Hintner and Wolff in 1982, when they reported eight cases, most of whom were adults.[151] Marked blistering and some oral involvement is present in infancy, but skin and mucosal involvement diminishes over the years in many patients. Laryngeal involvement may occur.[152] Early infant mortality in GABEB has been reported.[153] Skin atrophy, hypopigmentation, or hyperpigmentation develop after blistering, but there is no severe scarring or granulation tissue. In some families, melanocytic nevi are seen after blistering.[153] Nail dystrophy and shedding and alopecia of scalp, brow, eyelashes, and pubic hair are prominent features.[152] Dental problems included anodontia, enamel defects, and caries.[152] Corneal abrasions may occur.[144] Multiple squamous cell carcinomas have been reported in adulthood.[154]

Dystrophic Epidermolysis Bullosa

In dystrophic EB, blistering occurs below the dermal-epidermal junction in the superficial dermis. It is inherited in an autosomal recessive or dominant fashion. Although the dominant form is often mild, **recessive dystrophic EB** (RDEB), referred to as Hallopeau-Siemens, is usually severe. In RDEB, severe blistering begins at birth and leads to joint contractures and marked scarring. On the hands and feet, scarring results in "mitten" deformities, with autoamputation of digits and marked limitation in range of motion and function.[155]

Extracutaneous involvement is the rule in RDEB. Gastrointestinal complications are the most common; there is little correlation in the severity of gastrointestinal complications with extent of skin disease.[129,155,156] Oral ulcers cause pain with eating from the newborn period, and breast feeding may be impossible.[129] Oral scarring with microstomia and dysphagia from esophageal strictures occurs in older children and adults with RDEB.[156] Chronic malnutrition and growth failure are common and contribute to other problems, such as poor wound healing, iron deficiency, and increased susceptibility to infection. Even with nutritional assessment and close monitoring, dietary intake is often inadequate to meet needs in many patients with RDEB.[129,130] One group placed gastrostomy tubes in older children and adolescents for supplemental feeding, with improved weight gain 1 year after the procedure.[157] Painful defecation and constipation are also common; in the gastrostomy study, these symptoms resolved with the use of a high-fiber enteral formula.[157]

Eye involvement results from fragility of the ocular mucosal surface, especially the cornea and conjunctiva. Many patients are asymptomatic.[158] Corneal lesions are the most common manifestations: abrasions, ulcers, and scarring occur and can lead to permanent reduction in visual acuity. Symblepharon can develop, immobilizing the globe and eyelid.[144,158] Ectropion results from blisters and scars around the eyelids. Some ocular problems can be treated surgically with improvement in acuity.[144] Most patients are able to wear glasses without adverse effects.

Urinary tract involvement may present with gross hematuria, meatal stenosis, sepsis, or dysuria. Ureterovesical obstruction and hydronephrosis can occur.[145]

Other Types of Epidermolysis Bullosa

Kindler syndrome is a rare disorder in which trauma-induced blistering begins at birth or early in infancy, then decreases with age. Photosensitivity also begins early and improves with age. Poikiloderma and cutaneous atrophy develop in childhood but persist into adulthood. The inheritance is unknown, but may be autosomal recessive.[159] In one study, clumping of tonofilaments was seen in basal keratinocytes, and the authors suggest keratin mutations similar to those seen in EB simplex may be involved.[159] **EB superficialis** is an autosomal dominant subtype of EB simplex in which the skin cleavage is in the superficial epidermis, just under the stratum corneum. It differs clinically from other forms of EB simplex in that milia, atrophic scarring, and oral and ocular involvement occur more commonly.[133]

Transient bullous dermolysis of the newborn (TBND) is a distinctive variant of dominant dystrophic EB. Blistering begins at birth or the newborn period and resolves spontaneously after early infancy, usually within the first year of life.[160-163] Type VII collagen may be temporarily stored or secreted abnormally from basal keratinocytes, resulting in lack of anchoring fibrils and fragility; as blistering resolves, so does the collagen defect.[163,164] Christiano et al reported a mutation in the type VII collagen gene (COL7A1) in a family with TBDN.[160]

Etiology/Pathogenesis

EB simplex results from defects in basal epidermal keratinocyte cytoskeleton structural proteins keratins 5 and 14.[165,166,167] Studies of the molecular pathogenesis of EB simplex have shown that the keratin cytoskeleton plays a critical role in maintaining structural integrity in the skin.[166] Specific mutations have been defined in EB simplex kindreds, and correlation of genotype to phenotype is emerging.[166,168] The position and nature of specific mutations within keratin molecules correlates with severity of disease: mutations in the more conserved regions of the gene result in more severe EB simplex phenotypes.[166] Heterozygous missense mutations have been found in both the keratin 5 (K5) and keratin 14 (K14) genes in the common forms of EB simplex: AD generalized (Koebner), localized (Weber-Cockayne), and Dowling-Meara. A mutation in the amino-terminal domain of K5 has been reported in EBS with mottled pigmentation. A homozygous premature-termination codon (PTC) mutation in K14 was found in the more severe AR EB simplex, resulting in the complete absence of keratin 14.[166]

The keratin cytoskeleton interacts with adjacent keratinocytes via desmosomes and to the basement membrane via hemidesmosomes. Mutations in molecules in these transmembrane attachment complexes result in skin fragility. For example, in autosomal recessive EB with muscular dystrophy, homozygous PTC mutations have been found in plectin, a protein involved in attachment of keratin to hemidesmosomes. Because these patients also have muscle disease, plectin is thought to be involved in structural interactions in muscle as well as skin.[166]

In PA-JEB, blistering and PA may result from altered expression of integrin α6β4, resulting in faulty formation of hemidesmosomes in the basement membrane.[174]

The pathogenesis of the GABEB subtype of junctional EB involves abnormal attachment of hemidesmosomes of epidermal basal keratinocytes in the lamina lucida. This is due to mutations in protein components of hemidesmosomes and anchoring filaments: type XVII collagen/bullous pemphigoid antigen 2 (COL17A/BPAG2, located at 10q24.3), laminin 5, and related proteins, and LAD-1.[153,167,169] Herlitz junctional EB results from PTC mutation in both laminin 5 genes. Laminin 5 is a critical protein component of the basement membrane zone; its absence results in the severe fragility of skin and other epithelial tissues in this disease.[166] Milder forms of junctional EB are due to less severe missense mutations.[166] As in EB simplex, correlation of genotype to phenotype is emerging as details of the molecular pathogenesis of junctional EB emerges.

Dystrophic EB is now known to be caused by mutations in the type VII collagen gene (COL7A1). Initial linkage studies linked both dominant and recessive DEB to the COL7A1 locus at 3p21.1. Type VII collagen is the major component of anchoring fibrils, and is secreted primarily by epidermal keratinocytes.[165,166] Many different mutations have been characterized in patients with variants of dystrophic EB, and the nature of those mutations correlate with severity of clinical phenotype.[166] For example, some dominant forms result from missense mutations, which substitute another amino acid for a glycine residue in the collagenous domain of type VII collagen. When combined with the normal collagen from the unaffected gene, the result is anchoring fibrils that are present, but morphologically altered and functionally unstable.[165,166] In other patients with severe, recessive dystrophic EB, there are PTC mutations in both alleles, with resulting absence of anchoring fibrils.[165,166]

Laboratory Evaluation

Because clinical differentiation of EB subtypes is so difficult, the development of methods for precise laboratory diagnosis has been a major advance. Skin biopsy specimens from infants with possible EB may be evaluated by the following techniques: transmission electron microscopy (EM), immunofluorescence mapping ("antigenic" mapping), and DNA mutational analysis. Light microscopy, although rapid, can result in diagnostic confusion. For example, in Dowling Meara EB, the cleavage plane in light microscopy is so deep in the epidermis that it may be mistaken for subepidermal blistering, resulting in diagnostic confusion with junctional and dystrophic forms of EB.[135,170,171] Light microscopy continues to be helpful in differentiating EB from other blistering disorders. Many dermatopathology laboratories also have one or more basement-membrane stains, such as laminin and type IV collagen, which can help to differentiate dystrophic from nondystrophic forms of EB as a preliminary form of diagnosis while awaiting results of electron microscopy and/or immunofluorescent mapping.

The basic EB classification system evolved from the location of cleavage seen on electron microscopy. In EB simplex (epidermolytic), the split is intraepidermal. In junctional EB (lamina lucidolytic), it is located in the lamina lucida of the dermal-epidermal junction, and in dystrophic EB (dermolytic), it is in the dermis.[116] One may localize the site of cleavage on EM if a blister is present in the specimen. In addition, distinctive morphologic features seen on EM may aid in making a specific diagnosis: for example, clumping of keratin tonofilaments in basal keratinocytes in Dowling Meara EB and abnormal number and appearance of hemidesmosomes in junctional EB or of anchoring fibrils in dystrophic EB. EM is the diagnostic standard for diagnosis of EB.[116] Unfortunately, a blister must be present in the specimen for a diagnosis to be made. Furthermore, because very small cleavages are

seen, overdiagnosis may occur. Finally, EM findings are not always specific to a single EB subtype.[116]

Immunofluorescence mapping uses the known ultrastructural location of skin basement membrane antigens to localize skin cleavage (see Table 10-3). These studies should be done in an experienced reference laboratory. Diagnosis can only be made if a cleft is present and large enough to be seen by light microscopy.[116] Monoclonal antibodies against type IV collagen were used in one study to rapidly diagnose EB: staining was present on the blister floor in EB simplex and on the blister roof in dystrophic EB.[172] Junctional EB also showed staining on the blister floor.

Anti–basement membrane antibody studies can be done on the same specimens submitted for immunofluorescence mapping and may provide a specific diagnosis using EB-specific monoclonal antibodies (Table 10-3).[126] These tests should also be performed at specialized reference laboratories. A major advantage is the ability to make a diagnosis in the absence of apparent skin cleavage.[116] False negatives must be excluded by using adequate controls, and binding patterns are not always specific for a particular EB subtype.

Mutational DNA analysis is most accurate when a mutation is known, but it is time-consuming and not always available. Most often, combining results of the various techniques is most helpful. This is particularly true in the differentiation of generalized JEB gravis from GABEB, the less-severe variant with a better prognosis. Immunohistochemistry and mutational analysis have been used to make this distinction.

Tissue used in these tests is acquired by skin biopsy. Punch, or shave, biopsy is done under local anesthesia after cleavage is induced by twisting a pencil eraser on the skin to apply friction or shearing stress. In some cases of milder EB variants, it is difficult to induce cleavage, since the skin is not very fragile. Biopsies of established vesicles are problematic because of degenerative or regenerative changes that may occur within blisters and confuse the morphology seen on EM.[173] Therefore fresh blisters (<24 hours old) should be used.[126] Skin specimens are divided and placed in glutaraldehyde solution for EM, and in immunofluorescence media sent to special laboratories for antigen mapping and monoclonal antibody studies.[116] Clinicians should contact reference laboratories before sending specimens for mutational analysis.

Prenatal diagnosis of EB was once available only by fetal skin biopsy. This procedure is performed relatively late in pregnancy (at 16 to 20 weeks gestation) and carries significant risk of fetal loss (up to 5%).[174] Prenatal diagnosis is now possible in families using molecular techniques.[174] Tissue is acquired by chorionic villus sampling or amniocentesis, procedures that are safer and performed earlier in gestation than fetal skin biopsy. As the molecular basis of EB is further defined, the availability and accuracy of prenatal diagnosis will expand, as will preimplantation diagnosis. Markedly elevated alpha-fetoprotein and positive acetylcholinesterase in amniotic fluid has been associated with dystrophic and junctional EB and may be helpful in prenatal diagnosis, but is not a specific enough finding to be used without confirmatory studies.[175,176,177]

Differential Diagnosis

The differential diagnosis of vesicles and bullae in the newborn is discussed in detail elsewhere in this chapter. The most critical immediate task is to exclude infection, especially intrauterine HSV infection. A positive family history is helpful in the case of autosomal dominant disease such as EB simplex Koebner, but may be unavailable or negative in some cases. In other cases when the family history is known, the diagnosis is made prenatally, and preparations can be made to minimize trauma during delivery and in the neonatal period. The infant with prenatally diagnosed EB can be delivered vaginally: cesarean section is unlikely to decrease the risk to the infant sufficiently to warrant the increased maternal risk.[176]

Management of Epidermolysis Bullosa in Infancy

No specific therapy is yet available for the treatment of EB. Therefore, general support measures, physically for the child and psychosocially for the family, are most important in the neonatal period.

EB can be a great management challenge in the neonatal period, especially when the infant has a more severe subtype with widespread or generalized blistering and extracutaneous complications. A multidisciplinary approach is ideal, with the pediatrician or neonatologist managing the infant with the dermatologist and other specialists as needed when complications develop. Goals in EB management in the neonatal period are outlined in Table 10-4. It is also critical to attend to basic issues such as fluid and electrolyte balance and temperature control. Increased insensible fluid loss results from skin erosions, and altered electrolyte balance, such as hyper- and hyponatremia, may occur. Temperature control can be aided initially by the use of an isolette; temperature probes should be secured by wrapping with gauze around the trunk and not by taping.

Neonatal intensive care nurses are skilled in prevention of trauma to newborn skin. Premature infants have fragile skin, and protocols are established in most intensive care nurseries to minimize skin trauma. However, if an infant with EB is in a normal newborn nursery or on a

hospital ward, nurses and other caretakers must be educated about basic principles of skin care for infants with EB, for example, caretakers should be instructed to avoid taping of the skin or applying adhesive bandages to the skin after procedures.

Good wound care is a major undertaking in patients with extensive skin blistering. However, providing optimal wound care is the most important aspect of managing EB and will minimize or prevent complications such as scarring and infection.[126] This step begins in the initial days of life with the first erosions and vesicles that develop after birth. Individual dermatologists have specific wound care regimens they favor, but the most important step is providing a moist wound healing environment by covering open erosions with thick emollients, such as petroleum jelly, combined with a topical antibiotic, followed by a nonstick dressing. Topical antibiotics can be rotated every few months to prevent resistance, and the choice of antibiotic may be guided by wound cultures.[126] Patients and caregivers develop preferences for specific nonstick dressings: Mepitel is one excellent choice; Vaseline gauze is also commonly used and is less expensive. Exu-dry is also favored by some patients. The dressing placed over the wound should be protected by a secondary dressing, usually a gauze wrap. The wrap is secured with tape that is placed on the dressing (not the skin). Coban, a sticky wrap, or elastic tube dressings can be used as an outside protective layer. When blisters are tense, they should be opened with a sterile needle to prevent extension of the lesion.[126] Gentle pressure should be applied with a sterile gauze to drain the fluid. The blister roof should be left in place unless it is hanging freely, when it can be cut with sharp, clean scissors. Dressings should be changed daily and should be removed gently. They can be soaked off in a tub to minimize skin trauma. The skin should be gently patted dry after bathing with a soft towel, or air-dried.[126]

The most common complication of EB in the neonatal period is sepsis, with open erosions acting as portals of entry. Therefore it is important to closely monitor the skin for signs of local infection and the infant for signs of sepsis. Topical antibiotics can be used as described previously to limit colonization of wounds, but systemic antibiotics should be reserved for severe local infection or bacteremia/sepsis.

Obtaining adequate nutrition to meet caloric needs in the newborn period, with the added stress of wound healing, is another major management challenge. This is especially true when oral erosions and ulcers render feeding painful and laborious. Bottle feeding with special high-flow nipples such as the Mead-Johnson cleft lip and palate nurser can be initiated when pain from oral blistering limits breast feeding. High-density formulas or pumped breast milk with added fortifier can be given; vegetable oil

TABLE 10-4

Management of EB in the Neonatal Period

Objective	How achieved
Minimize trauma to skin	Gentle handling
	Use wrapping or suturing of instruments and monitors instead of taping when possible; if taped, leave probes in place
Provide ideal (moist) wound-healing environment	Wound care:
	Open and drain tense vesicles with sterile needle
	Gentle daily debridement of crust in tub
	Application of emollients *and* nonstick primary dressing
	Protect wound and secure primary dressing with secondary dressing such as gauze wrap, and stockinette or Coban
	Tape dressing to itself, never to skin!
Prevent bacterial superinfection of wounds, sepsis	Observe wounds for purulence, foul smell
	Monitor colonization with weekly surveillance cultures
	Apply topical antibiotics combined with emollient on open erosions to control colonization
	If signs, symptoms of sepsis, cover gram-positive organisms with intravenous antibiotics
Maximize nutrition with minimal trauma for optimal wound healing and growth	Breast feeding if mild oral involvement and infant able to feed through pain
	If not, have mother pump breast milk and bottle feed with high flow nipple or drip feeds in
	Add breast milk fortifier to maximize caloric intake
	If formula fed, use high-calorie formulas
	Obtain dietary consult/follow up to ascertain energy needs and how to meet them
Monitor for extracutaneous complications	Eye: ophthalmology consult if redness, photophobia
	GI: if oral involvement, watch for feeding intolerance
	If polyhydramnios, look for pyloric atresia
	Respiratory: monitor airway for hoarse cry, stridor as sign of laryngeal involvement
	GU: Look for gross hematuria, meatal narrowing in boys, consider urinary source if infant febrile
Provide psychosocial support	Counseling regarding prognosis once diagnosis known. Emphasize unpredictability of course even when subtype known
	Discuss usual short-term complications in general terms
	Provide access to peer counseling through Internet sites, local chapters of national patient advocacy groups

and/or glucose polymers can also be added to increase energy density.[130] By 4 months of age, iron fortified formula should be used.[130] General guidelines are outlined in Table 10-4. The input of a pediatric gastroenterology/nutrition team can be very helpful.

Observation for extracutaneous involvement is also important, as the diagnosis is unknown in the first days of life in many cases, and the possibility exists that systemic complications may develop (see Table 10-4).

When patients with EB require reconstructive or other surgery, routine procedures can be problematic. However, surgical outcome can be excellent.[178] Preliminary data suggest that artificial skin substitutes such as Apligraft may be a helpful adjunct in healing chronic ulcers and successful reconstructive surgery.[179] Application of lubricating agents such as petroleum jelly helps minimize friction when instruments come in contact with skin. Taping should be avoided: intravenous catheters can be sutured in place, and electrocardiographic (ECG) monitors trimmed to minimize adhesive contact with skin, or gauze-wrapped.[126,178] EB patients tolerate anesthesia well, even when intubation is required; however, alternatives such as nerve blocks, face mask, and ketamine anesthesia should be used when possible.[126]

Most importantly, the medical team must provide psychosocial support for the family during the difficult period before a diagnosis is made, when prognostication is impossible. Families understandably press for more specific information, especially regarding the long-term prognosis. Even after the diagnosis is made, care should be taken to avoid setting specific expectations, as in many cases the long-term course is unpredictable. Peer support and advocacy groups, such as Dystrophic Epidermolysis Bullosa Research and Advocacy (DEBRA), provide an invaluable resource to families newly facing the daunting prospect of raising a child with EB.

The National Epidermolysis Bullosa Registry (NEBR) was established in 1986 by the National Institute of Arthritis, Musculoskeletal and Skin Diseases to enhance clinical and laboratory research in EB by identifying a large cohort of EB patients in the United States. The goal is to diagnose and enroll patients with EB; thus patients with newly diagnosed EB should be registered through the NEBR, who can by contacted by telephone (919) 966-2007 or FAX (919) 966-7080.[180]

Phenytoin was once thought to be helpful in the treatment of RDEB, but initial beneficial effect was not confirmed in further studies.[181] Although specific therapy is not yet available, gene therapy may be available in the future. Recent advances in the understanding of the molecular underpinnings of EB have led us closer to this possibility, and preliminary work has begun that may offer hope in the future for specific treatment of EB.[182]

DISORDERS (OTHER THAN EPIDERMOLYSIS BULLOSA) PRESENTING PRIMARILY WITH BULLAE, EROSIONS, OR ULCERATIONS

Mastocytosis

Mast cell disease causing blisters of the skin in infants occurs in two forms: (1) discrete nodules, or **mastocytomas** (see Chapter 23), which are uncommon, but not rare; and (2) as a diffuse, widespread infiltration of the skin, or **diffuse cutaneous mastocytosis**, which is extremely rare. Both types can develop blisters, superimposed on lesional skin, and in diffuse cutaneous masto-

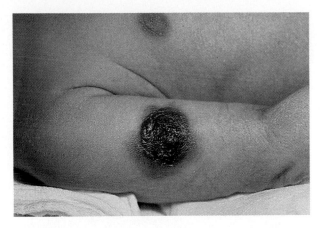

FIG. 10-12
Mastocytoma with blistering and crusting. (Courtesy Neil Prose.)

cytosis, blisters may develop on apparently uninvolved skin.

Mastocytomas may be solitary or multiple with lesions either present at birth or beginning in early infancy. Typically, lesions have an orange-red or brown color and may have a peau d'orange surface texture. They vary in size from 1 to 5 cm, and when lesions are rubbed, vasoactive substances, including histamine, are released leading to erythema, wheal formation (so-called Darier's sign), and occasionally blisters or erosions on the surface of the lesion[183] (Fig. 10-12).

Diffuse cutaneous mastocytosis is a rare condition, characterized by large collections of mast cells that infiltrate the skin over large areas of the skin. Lesions may be present at birth[104] but usually develop in the first few weeks to months of life.[185,186,187] Familial cases have been reported.[188] Initially, blisters develop on normal-appearing skin, making the clinical diagnosis difficult until thickened, leathery skin develops (Fig. 10-13). Blisters may occur anywhere on the body, including the scalp, and episodes of sudden, massive blistering may lead to erosions and desquamation. Dermographism is usually prominent. Wheezing, urticaria, diarrhea, and hypotension may also occur. Other complications include coagulation abnormalities, myeloproliferative disorder, syncope, hypotension, and shock.[186] Familial cases with apparent autosomal dominant inheritance have been reported.[188]

The differential diagnosis includes staphylococcal scalded skin syndrome and erythema multiforme. Management of mastocytosis depends on the degree of systemic symptoms and is discussed in Chapter 23.

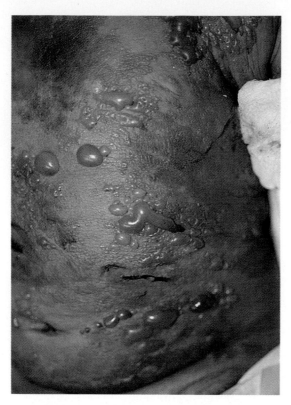

FIG. 10-13
Diffuse cutaneous mastocytosis presenting with widespread blistering. (Courtesy Sarah Chamlin.)

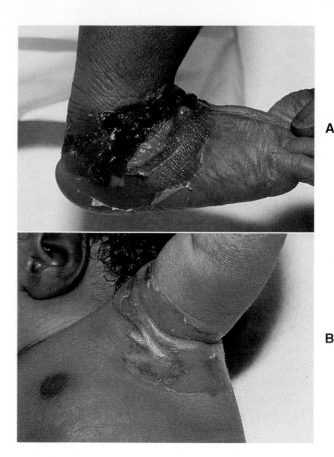

A

B

FIG. 10-14
Neonatal pemphigus vulgaris. Erosions and crusting are due to transplacental maternal autoantibodies. (Courtesy Lee Nesbit.)

Blistering Caused By Maternal Bullous Disease

Blistering may occur in the newborn whose mother has an autoimmune blistering disease mediated by IgG. IgG crosses the placenta and causes a similar disease in the fetus. This finding has been reported in three IgG-mediated diseases: **herpes gestationis, pemphigus vulgaris,** and very rarely in **pemphigus foliaceus.**[189-193]

Blistering is virtually always present at birth. Lesional morphology depends in part on which autoimmune disease affects the mother and ranges from tense or flaccid bullae to widespread areas of erosion (Fig. 10-14). There may be a few or many lesions. Infants may be born prematurely; and, before the advent of corticosteroids there was an increased incidence of stillbirths in herpes gestationis.

The diagnosis is usually obvious because of a maternal history of an autoimmune blistering disease. Although most mothers have active disease during their pregnancy, affected infants can be born to women with mild inactive disease.[194,195]

The diagnosis can be confirmed with skin biopsy and direct immunofluorescence on the infant's skin. In herpes gestationis, a subepidermal bulla with eosinophils in the bulla fluid and dermis is usually present, and direct immunofluorescence demonstrates a linear pattern of complement (C3) at the dermo-epidermal junction. Lesions in pemphigus vulgaris demonstrate an intraepidermal blister, acantholysis of keratinocytes, and a mild inflammatory infiltrate of eosinophils and occasional plasma cells,[76] and immunofluorescence shows IgG and C3 staining of the intraepidermal cement substance. In pemphigus foliaceus, intraepithelial vesicles are evident, and immunofluorescence demonstrates intracellular IgG and C3 in the superficial epidermis.

A major differential diagnosis is epidermolysis bullosa, but a maternal history of an autoimmune maternal blistering disease helps in diagnosis. Once the diagnosis is made, no specific therapy is needed, but topical petrolatum and/or antibiotics may help avoid secondary infection.[189] New blisters do not usually occur after the newborn period. If blistering is extensive, the infant should be watched closely for signs of cutaneous or systemic infection. Systemic corticosteroids should be considered only in extremely severe cases.

Chronic Bullous Dermatosis of Childhood (Linear IgA Disease)

The most common autoimmune blistering disease in children, **chronic bullous dermatosis of childhood** (CBDC), is usually not seen in the newborn period,[196] although at least one severe case in a neonate has been reported. This child had two blisters at birth and was diagnosed with CBDC at 2 weeks of age. His course was complicated by multiple infections. Other atypical features of this case included permanent ocular scarring, swallowing difficulties, and recurrent asthma.[197]

Typically, the disease is characterized by onset between 1 and 6 years of age, with widespread, tense blisters with greatest concentration on the groin, buttocks, and thighs. Blisters often form rosette or sausage-like shapes. A subepidermal bulla and linear deposition of IgA at the dermal-epidermal junction are the key diagnostic findings. Treatment options include prednisone 1 to 2 mg/kg/day, dapsone 1 to 2 mg/kg/day, and sulfapyridine 65 mg/kg/day.[198]

Bullous Pemphigoid

Bullous pemphigoid does not occur during the neonatal period, but cases with onset as young as 2 months of age have been reported.[199] Tense, generalized blisters characterize the disease, although involvement of the hands and feet appears to be more common in infancy. The diagnosis is suspected if skin biopsy demonstrates a subepidermal bulla with eosinophils; it is confirmed by demonstration of linear staining of IgG and C3 along the basement membrane zone. Treatment regimens vary—in some cases potent topical corticosteroids can control disease, whereas in others, systemic corticosteroids are necessary.

Neonatal Lupus Erythematosus

Neonatal lupus erythematosus (NLE) (see also Chapter 17) is an uncommon disorder caused by the fetal and neonatal effects of transplacental maternal autoantibodies, particularly SS-A/Ro but also SS-B/La and RNP. Blistering is virtually never seen with NLE, but the disease can present with widespread erosions.[200,201] These erosions may have resulted from the shearing of atrophic epidermis from the underlying dermis during the birth process.

The diagnosis can be suspected because, in addition to erosions, areas of atrophic or discoid skin lesions are also present. Skin biopsy shows epidermal atrophy and a vacuolar interface dermatitis, which may have associated increased dermal mucin. The mothers of affected infants are usually asymptomatic. Serology tests of both mother and infant should be obtained, looking specifically for anti SS-A/Ro, La, and RNP antibodies. If NLE is suspected, infants should be examined carefully, and an ECG, CBC, platelet count, and liver function tests should be obtained.

Toxic Epidermal Necrolysis

Toxic epidermal necrolysis (TEN) is extremely rare in the newborn period. The condition is characterized by extensive necrosis of the epidermis and is a life-threatening condition in patients of any age, because the necrosis causes the functional equivalent of a severe first- and second-degree burn. The situation is even worse in the newborn period because of decreased immune defenses and a more fragile balance of fluids and electrolytes.

The few cases reported early infancy have been in premature infants with *Klebsiella* sepsis and a young infant with *E. coli* infection on multiple antibiotics.[202-205] Graft-versus-host disease can also cause toxic epidermal necrolysis and can occur at birth because of intrauterine passage of maternal cells to an immunodeficient fetus.[206]

Infants with TEN may present with irritability, temperature instability, and diffuse cutaneous erythema. This is followed by flaccid blisters and erosions (Fig. 10-15). The diagnosis can be confirmed by skin biopsy, which demonstrates extensive, full-thickness epidermal necrosis, with minimal to absent dermal inflammation. The epidermal cleavage is located at the dermal-epidermal junction or in the mid to lower epidermis. A frozen section can be performed for rapid diagnosis.[207]

The differential diagnosis includes staphylococcal scalded skin syndrome and intrauterine epidermal necrosis.[208] Management of TEN at any age is difficult, and the mortality is high, especially in young infants. The cause of the eruption should be identified and, in the case of graft-versus-host disease or sepsis, appropriately treated. Treatment of the skin parallels that of patients with widespread

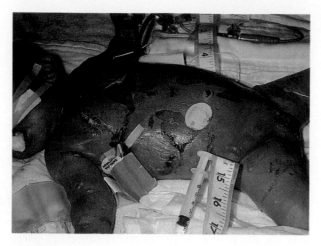

FIG. 10-15

Toxic epidermal necrolysis. Most documented cases in very young infants are due to gram-negative infections, but this case was as a result of intrauterine graft-versus-host disease. (Courtesy Mary L. Williams.)

epidermolysis bullosa (see earlier section on epidermolysis bullosa). The prognosis is extremely grave.[202]

Intrauterine Epidermal Necrosis

This rare condition is characterized by widespread epidermal necrosis. It was reported present at birth in three premature infants, all of whom died shortly thereafter.[208] Widespread areas of erosion and ulceration were noted, without vesicles or pustules present. The mucous membranes were spared. Histopathology of the skin demonstrated extensive epidermal necrosis and pilosebaceous follicular calcification. Autopsy study demonstrated brain infarcts and leukomalacia, as well as cardiomegaly and renal tubular necrosis. The etiology of this condition is unknown. The differential diagnosis includes intrauterine infection, epidermolysis bullosa, acute graft-versus-host disease with TEN, and congenital and erosive vesicular dermatosis.

Congenital Erosive and Vesicular Dermatosis

At least 10 cases of a condition characterized by erosions and vesicles at birth, healing with reticulate, and supple scarring have been reported.[209,210] Nearly all of the infants were premature. They have been described as having generalized erosions, vesicles, crusts, "scalded skin-like," and erythematous areas. Additional variably reported features include collodion membrane, transparent areas of skin, and a reticulated vascular pattern with subsequent ulcerations. In some, but not all cases, the face, palms, and soles are spared. Erosions and ulcerations heal with scarring, usually by 1 to 2 months of age. The scarring that eventuates is reticulated, and often covers the majority of the skin surface. Other, more variable mucocutaneous findings include scarring alopecia, scarring of the tongue, absent or hypoplastic nails, and heat intolerance. Mental retardation, cerebral atrophy, hemiparesis, and retinal scars have also been seen.

The cause of the condition is unknown, although some have speculated that an intrauterine infection, as yet unidentified, might result in these findings. The diagnosis has usually been made in retrospect with biopsy specimens demonstrating scar formation with loss of eccrine structures. The sole report of biopsies of the acute phase of the eruption demonstrated an eroded epidermis with a dense neutrophilic infiltrate.[211] The differential diagnosis includes the erosive form of neonatal lupus, acute intrauterine graft-versus-host disease, bullous ichthyosis, intrauterine epidermal necrosis, and a variety of intrauterine infections, especially HSV and varicella. All neonates with this clinical presentation should have biopsies, cultures, and serologic evaluations for infection and should be followed closely, especially for neurologic deficits. There is no specific treatment.

Pyoderma Gangrenosum

Pyoderma gangrenosum (PG), a disorder characterized by the spontaneous onset of skin ulcerations, has rarely been reported in children less than 1 year of age, and to date only one case with neonatal onset has been reported. In this infant, ulcers developed beginning at 2 days of age. Lesions were most prominent in the groin and buttocks, as has been the case in most other infants[212] (Fig. 10-16). The lesions are sharply demarcated ulcerations, which usually arise without prior vesiculation or pustules and have characteristically undermined borders. PG has been associated with inflammatory bowel disease, leukemia, arthritis, and less commonly immunodeficiencies. The diagnosis, one of exclusion, is made by correlating typical clinical features with histopathology demonstrating a neutrophilic infiltrate without evidence of infection, vasculitis, or other causes of ulceration. The differential diagnosis includes noma neonatorum, HSV infection, and ulcerations arising in hemangioma precursors.

The initial treatment of choice is intralesional or systemic corticosteroids, but cytotoxic agents and sulfones are sometimes needed to control disease.

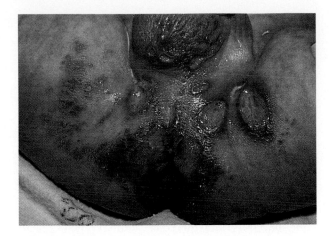

FIG. 10-16
Pyoderma gangrenosum. Multiple ulcerations in the perineum are evident.

Noma Neonatorum

Noma neonatorum is a gangrenous disease that has been described mainly in developing countries with *Pseudomonas aeruginosa* septicemia implicated as a causative agent in the majority of cases in newborns.[213] The clinical features in these cases include the abrupt onset of gangrenous, ulcerative skin lesions affecting the nose, lips, mouth, anus, scrotum, and eyelids. In severe cases the ulcerations can be mutilating, resulting in bone loss and extensive deformity. Predisposing factors include prematurity, low birth weight, malnutrition, and previous illness. Although many neonatal cases undoubtedly represent primary *Pseudomonas* infection of the skin, other etiologies may be responsible in some cases. Similar ulcerations have been described in several Native-American children with severe combined immunodeficiency.[214] The presence of oral and perineal ulcerations in newborns and young infants should prompt a thorough search for infectious and immunologic causes as possible etiologies.

Acrodermatitis Enteropathica

Acrodermatitis enteropathica (AE) (see Chapter 14) is caused by zinc deficiency, which may be due to inadequate zinc intake or because of defective transport and absorption of zinc, resulting from an autosomal recessively inherited trait. Alopecia, rash, and diarrhea are the most characteristic findings in AE. The rash is usually periorificial and acrally located, although involvement in the neck folds and inguinal creases may occur. Typically, sharply demarcated, scaly, crusted plaques are located around the eyes, nose, mouth, anus, and genitalia, and these may be erosive in some cases. Acral lesions are often bullous or vesicular. Occasional cutaneous findings include paronychia, nail dystrophy, and edema.[215] Irritability and diarrhea are almost always present.

The diagnosis is confirmed by serum zinc levels that are less than 50 μg/dl, although occasional false positive and negative results have been reported.[216]

Methylmalonic Acidemia and Other Metabolic Disorders

The term *methylmalonic acidemia* (see Chapter 15) refers to a group of defects in the metabolism of isoleucine and valine. Skin rashes can result from the metabolic perturbations or the dietary restrictions used to manage these inherited disorders of amino acid metabolism. An erosive erythema with periorificial accentuation resembling staphylococcal scalded skin syndrome, has been described as a periorificial rash resembling acrodermatitis enteropathica[10,217] and can be a presenting sign of disease or, caused by dietary restrictions. Other symptoms in early-onset disease include lethargy, hypotonia, neutropenia, and thrombocytopenia. The diagnosis is made by documenting characteristic abnormal levels of plasma amino acids. Treatment with dietary restrictions may be helpful in some cases, and intramuscular hydroxocobalamin is also helpful in some cases.[10]

Bullous Ichthyosis (Epidermolytic Hyperkeratosis)

Bullous ichthyosis (epidermolytic hyperkeratosis) (see Chapter 16) is an uncommon form of ichthyosis, which is inherited as an autosomal dominant trait. At birth, the epidermis is thickened, macerated, and erythematous, and bullae or raw denuded areas are present (Fig. 10-17). Spontaneous or mechanically induced bullae continue to form throughout infancy and early childhood, especially on the hands and feet, but generalized blistering usually resolves. Individuals with the condition are otherwise healthy.[218,219]

Restrictive Dermopathy

Restrictive dermopathy (see Chapter 16) is a rare autosomal recessive disease characterized by rigid and tense skin with erosions and ulcerations that may be linear. Infants born with this condition are often premature, have multiple joint contractures, fixed facial expression, micrognathia, and more variably blepharophimosis, absent eye-

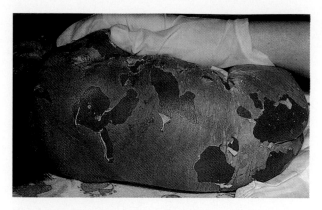

FIG. 10-17
Bullous ichthyosis (epidermolytic hyperkeratosis) presenting with widespread blistering.

lashes, natal teeth, and cardiac defects. The etiology of the condition is unknown. Most infants die in the newborn period.[220]

Hemangiomas and Vascular Malformations

In rare cases, hemangiomas (see Chapter 18) develop cutaneous ulcerations just before or at the onset of their rapid proliferative phase. In these cases, precursor lesions with macular erythema or a blanched bruised-like area are usually present as a clue to diagnosis. Such early ulcerations are most common on the pinna, the lip, and in the perineal area but can occur at other sites. The presence of an ulceration superimposed on or in direct contiguity to a vascular lesion is a key clue to the diagnosis.[221] Ulcerations are also occasionally present in fully formed congenital hemangiomas.[222]

Similarly, ulcerations may develop in affected skin in **cutis marmorata telangiectatica congenita,** a vascular malformation, without preceding blistering or other inciting event. The diagnosis can be suspected if ulcerations occur over areas of mottled and reticulated vascularity. Localized areas of cutaneous atrophy may also be present.[223]

Aplasia Cutis Congenita

Aplasia cutis congenita (ACC) (see Chapter 9) is a heterogeneous group of disorders characterized by absent areas of skin at birth. The many causes include an autosomal dominant trait; intrauterine herpes simplex or varicella infection; placental infarctions; absence of skin overlying structural malformations; chromosomal abnormalities; epidermolysis bullosa; as well as several other genetic con-

ditions. In most cases, it is easy to distinguish ACC from blistering conditions causing erosions at birth, because the absence of skin in ACC is usually full-thickness, involving both epidermis and dermis, whereas it is less deep in most blistering disorders.[224]

The scalp is the most common location of ACC. Lesions usually appear as raw, ulcerated areas, but some have a membranous covering, are fluid-filled, and thus appear blisterlike. This latter type of ACC is often associated with an increase in hair at the periphery, the so-called hair collar sign. The location on the scalp, the membranous covering, and the usual concave nature of the underlying defect help distinguish this condition from other forms of blistering. The membranous form of ACC is often a sign of an atretic cephalocele and occasionally has deeper intracranial connections and/or bony defects.[225]

Linear Porokeratosis

A case of linear porokeratosis presenting with extensive zosteriform erosions of the leg and buttock has been reported.[226] Initial biopsies were nondiagnostic but the lesions eventually healed, leaving scaling atrophic inflamed skin with threadlike areas of scale. A diagnosis of linear porokeratosis was made at 7 months of age based on typical histology, demonstrating a well-formed coronoid lamella. Infants with linear porokeratosis have a risk of eventually developing squamous cell carcinoma in affected skin, but this does not usually happen during childhood.[226] The differential diagnosis includes Goltz syndrome and intrauterine varicella infection.

Erosions and Ulcerations Overlying Giant Nevi

A case series of neonates with erosions or ulcerations overlying giant nevi has been reported. In no case did malignant melanoma develop in the affected areas but one child eventually died from primary central nervous system disease. The mechanism of these ulcerations is uncertain but possibly due to weakening of the dermal-epidermal junction as a result of the large number of melanocytes present.[227]

Ectodermal Dysplasia Syndromes

Blistering in the newborn period or early infancy has been reported in several forms of ectodermal dysplasia. In **focal dermal hypoplasia** (Goltz syndrome), blistering is an occasional feature, but the more striking cutaneous features are widespread hypoplasia and aplasia of the skin in linear and whorled patterns following Blachko's lines. Hair and nail dystrophy are common, as are skeletal and ophthalmologic abnormalities.[228] The condition is inherited as an X-linked dominant condition and is usually lethal in males.

A syndrome characterized by **absent dermal ridge patterns, congenital milia, and blisters of the fingertips and soles,** with autosomal dominant inheritance, has been described. Blistering was present at birth and was said to resemble multiple sucking blisters. Other features of the condition include decreased sweating on the hands and feet, increased heat tolerance, and painful fissures on the fingertips in affected adults.[229]

Porphyrias

Photosensitive blistering can occur the newborn period in several porphyrin disorders (see Chapters 8 and 17), including **transient porphyrinemia,** resulting from hemolytic disease in the newborn period,[230] and **erythropoietic porphyria** (Gunther's disease), an extremely rare and severe form of porphyria caused by an inborn deficiency of the enzyme, uroporphyrinogen cosynthetase. In both cases hemolytic anemia leads to hyperbilirubinemia, and the use of phototherapy to control hyperbilirubinemia can result in generalized blistering.

Perinatal Gangrene of the Buttock

Perinatal gangrene of the buttock (Chapter 8) is a rare condition characterized by the sudden onset of erythema and cyanosis of the buttocks followed by the progressive development of gangrene and ulcerations. Some cases have been attributed to therapeutic injections via an umbilical artery catheter, but other cases are apparently spontaneous.[231,232] The distribution of the cutaneous infarction suggests occlusion or spasm of the internal iliac artery.[231] The differential diagnosis includes congenital protein C deficiency and clotting disorders or forms of disseminated intravascular coagulation.

Congenital Protein C and S Deficiencies
(See Chapter 17)

Neonatal purpura fulminans due to congenital deficiency of protein in C or S is a rare condition in which severe purpura fulminans occurs within the first days of life. Bullae, when present, are always hemorrhagic, and are due to disseminated intravascular coagulation (DIC) with cutaneous infarction. Evaluation and management are discussed in Chapter 17.

REFERENCES

1. Frieden IJ. The dermatologist in the newborn nursery: approach to the neonate with blisters, pustules, erosions, and ulcerations. Curr Prob Dermatol 1992;4:123-168.
2. Wagner A. Distinguishing vesicular and pustular disorders in the neonate. Curr Opin Pediatr 1997;9:396-405.
3. van Praag MC, van Rooij RW, Folkers E, et al. Diagnosis and treatment of pustular disorders in the neonate. Pediatr Dermatol 1997;14:131-143.
4. Hebert AA, Esterly NB. Bacterial and candidal cutaneous infections in the neonate. Dermatol Clin 1986;4:3-21.
5. Speck WT, Driscoll JM, Polin RA, et al. Staphylococcal and streptococcal colonization of the newborn infant: Effect of antiseptic cord care. Am J Dis Child 1977;131:1005-1008.
6. Loughead JL. Congenital staphylococcal scalded skin syndrome: Report of a case. Pediatr Infect Dis J 1992;11:413-414.
7. Curran JP, Al-Salihi FL. Neonatal staphylococcal scalded skin syndrome: Massive outbreak due to an unusual phage type. Pediatrics 1980;66:285-290.
8. Faden HS, Burke JP, Glasgow LA, et al. Nursery outbreak of scalded-skin syndrome. Scarlatiniform rash due to phage group I Staphylococcus aureus. Am J Dis Child 1976;130:265-268.
9. Shinefield HR. Staphococcal infections. In Remington JS, Klein JO, eds. Infectious diseases of the fetus and newborn infant. Philadelphia: WB Saunders, 1995: pp 1105-1141.
10. Howard R, Frieden IJ, Crawford D, et al. Methylmalonic acidemia, cobalamin C type, presenting with cutaneous manifestations. Arch Dermatol 1997;133:1563-1566.
11. Rubenstein AD, Musher DM. Epidemic boric acid poisoning simulating staphylococcal toxic epidermal necrolysis of the newborn infant: Ritter's disease. J Pediatr 1970;77:884-887.
12. Isenberg HD, Tucci V, Lipsitz P, et al. Clinical laboratory and epidemiological investigations of a Streptococcus pyogenes cluster epidemic in a newborn nursery. J Clin Microbiol 1984;19:366-370.
13. Lehtonen OP, Kero P, Ruuskanen O, et al. A nursery outbreak of group A streptococcal infection. J Infect 1987;14:263-270.
14. Nelson JD, Dillon HC Jr, Howard JB. A prolonged nursery epidemic associated with a newly recognized type of group A streptococcus. J Pediatr 1976;89:792-796.
15. Lopez JB, Gross P, Boggs TR. Skin lesions in association with beta-hemolytic Streptococcus group B. Pediatrics 1976;58:859-861.
16. Franciosi RA, Knostman JD, Zimmerman RA. Group B streptococcal neonatal and infant infections. J Pediatr 1973;82:707-718.
17. Evans JR, Allen AC, Stinson DA, et al. Perinatal listeriosis: Report of an outbreak. Pediatr Infect Dis 1985;4:237-241.
18. Bortolussi R, Hawkins A, Evans J, Albretton WL. Listeriosis. In Feigin RD, Cherry JD, eds. Textbook of pediatric infectious diseases. Philadelphia: WB Saunders, 1999.
19. Khuri-Bulos N, McIntosh K. Neonatal Haemophilus influenzae infection. Report of eight cases and review of the literature. Am J Dis Child 1975;129:57-62.
20. Halal F, Delorme L, Brazeau M, et al. Congenital vesicular eruption caused by Haemophilus influenzae type b. Pediatrics 1978;62:494-496.

21. Leigh L, Stoll BJ, Rahman M, et al. Pseudomonas aeruginosa infection in very low birth weight infants: A case-control study. Pediatr Infect Dis J 1995;14:367-371.

22. Boisseau AM, Sarlangue J, Perel Y, et al. Perineal ecthyma gangrenosum in infancy and early childhood: Septicemic and nonsepticemic forms. J Am Acad Dermatol 1992;27:415-418.

23. Hughes JR, Newbould M, du Vivier AW, et al. Fatal Pseudomonas septicemia and vasculitis in a premature infant. Pediatr Dermatol 1998;15:122-124.

24. Wilfert C, Gutman L. Sexually transmitted diseases. In Feigin RD, Cherry JD, eds. Textbook of pediatric infectious disease. Philadelphia: WB Saunders, 1987: pp 595-621.

25. Mallory SB, Krafchik BR. Syphilis. Pediatr Dermatol 1989;6:51-52.

26. Kam LA, Giacoia GP. Congenital cutaneous candidiasis. Am J Dis Child 1975;129:1215-1218.

27. Darmstadt GL, Dinulos JG, Miller Z. Congenital cutaneous candidiasis: clinical presentation, pathogenesis, and management guidelines. Pediatrics 2000;105:438-444.

28. Rudolph N, Tariq AA, Reale MR, et al. Congenital cutaneous candidiasis. Arch Dermatol 1977;113:1101-1103.

29. Resnick SD, Greenberg RA. Autoinoculated palmar pustules in neonatal candidiasis. Pediatr Dermatol 1989;6:206-209.

30. Baley JE. Neonatal candidiasis: The current challenge. Clin Perinatol 1991;18:263-280.

31. Dvorak AM, Gavaller B. Congenital systemic candidiasis. Report of a case. N Engl J Med 1966;274:540-543.

32. Cosgrove BF, Reeves K, Mullins D, et al. Congenital cutaneous candidiasis associated with respiratory distress and elevation of liver function tests: a case report and review of the literature. J Am Acad Dermatol 1997;37:817-823.

33. Baley JE, Kliegman RM, Boxerbaum B, et al. Fungal colonization in the very low birth weight infant. Pediatrics 1986;78:225-232.

34. Groll AH, Jaeger G, Allendorf A, et al. Invasive pulmonary aspergillosis in a critically ill neonate: Case report and review of invasive aspergillosis during the first 3 months of life. Clin Infect Dis 1998;27:437-452.

35. Roth JG, Troy JL, Esterly NB. Multiple cutaneous ulcers in a premature neonate. Pediatr Dermatol 1991;8:253-255.

36. Yoss BS, Sautter RL, Brenker HJ. Trichosporon beigelii, a new neonatal pathogen. Am J Perinatol 1997;14:113-117.

37. Linder N, Keller N, Huri C, et al. Primary cutaneous mucormycosis in a premature infant: Case report and review of the literature. Am J Perinatol 1998;15:35-38.

38. Harris HH, Foucar E, Andersen RD, et al. Intrauterine herpes simplex infection resembling mechanobullous disease in a newborn infant. J Am Acad Dermatol 1986;15:1148-1155.

39. Honig PJ, Brown D. Congenital herpes simplex virus infection initially resembling epidermolysis bullosa. J Pediatr 1982;101:958-960.

40. Hutto C, Arvin A, Jacobs R, et al. Intrauterine herpes simplex virus infections. J Pediatr 1987;110:97-101.

41. Whitley R, Arvin A, Prober C, et al. Predictors of morbidity and mortality in neonates with herpes simplex virus infections. N Engl J Med 1991;324:450-454.

42. Jacobs RF. Neonatal herpes simplex virus infections. Semin Perinatol 1998;22:64-71.

43. Elder DE, Minutillo C, Pemberton PJ. Neonatal herpes simplex infection: Keys to early diagnosis. J Paediatr Child Health 1995;31:307-311.

44. Kohl S. Neonatal herpes simplex virus infection. Clin Perinatol 1997;24:129-150.

45. Riley LE. Herpes simplex virus. Semin Perintol 1998;22:284-292.

46. Cohen PR. Tests for detecting herpes simplex virus and varicella-zoster virus infections. Dermatol Clin 1994;12:51-68.

47. Detlefs RL, Frieden IJ, Berger TG, et al. Eosinophil fluorescence: A cause of false positive slide tests for herpes simplex virus. Pediatr Dermatol 1987;4:129-133.

48. Paryani SG, Arvin AM. Intrauterine infection with varicella-zoster virus after maternal varicella. N Engl J Med 1986;314:1542-1546.

49. Alkalay AL, Pomerance JJ, Rimoin DL. Fetal varicella syndrome. J Pediatr 1987;111:320-323.

50. Bai PV, John TJ. Congenital skin ulcers following varicella in late pregnancy. J Pediatr 1979;94:65-67.

51. Brunell PA, Kotchmar GS Jr. Zoster in infancy: Failure to maintain virus latency following intrauterine infection. J Pediatr 1981;98:71-73.

52. Querol I, Bueno M, Cebrian A, et al. Connatal herpes zoster. Cutis 1996;58:231-234.

53. Mogami S, Muto M, Mogami K, et al. Congenitally acquired herpes zoster infection in a newborn. Dermatology 1997;194:276-277.

54. Nathwani D, Maclean A, Conway S, et al. Varicella infections in pregnancy and the newborn. A review prepared for the UK Advisory Group on Chickenpox on behalf of the British Society for the Study of Infection. J Infect 1998;36 (Suppl) 1:59-71.

55. Miller E, Cradock-Watson JE, Ridehalgh MK. Outcome in newborn babies given anti-varicella-zoster immunoglobulin after perinatal maternal infection with varicella-zoster virus. Lancet 1989;2:371-373.

56. Blatt J, Kastner O, Hodes DS. Cutaneous vesicles in congenital cytomegalovirus infection. J Pediatr 1978;92:509.

57. Cherry JD. Enteroviruses. In Remington JS, Klein JO, eds. Infectious diseases of the fetus and newborn infant. Philadelphia: WB Saunders, 1995: pp 404-446.

58. Arnon R, Naor N, Davidson S, et al. Fatal outcome of neonatal echovirus 19 infection. Pediatr Infect Dis J 1991;10:788-789.

59. Burns BR, Lampe RM, Hansen GH. Neonatal scabies. Am J Dis Child 1979;133:1031-1034.

60. Hurwitz S. Scabies in babies. Am J Dis Child 1973;126:226-228.

61. Sterling GB, Janniger CK, Kihiczak G. Neonatal scabies. Cutis 1990;45:229-231.

62. Madsen A. Mite burrows in crusts from young infants. Acta Derm Venereol 1970;50:391-392.

63. Berg FJ, Solomon LM. Erythema neonatorum toxicum. Arch Dis Child 1987;62:327-328.

64. Carr JA, Hodgman JE, Freedman RI, et al. Relationship between toxic erythema and infant maturity. Am J Dis Child 1966;112:129-134.

65. Marino LJ. Toxic erythema present at birth. Arch Dermatol 1965;92:402-403.

66. Levy HL, Cothran F. Erythema toxicum neonatorum present at birth. Am J Dis Child 1962;103:125-127.

67. Chang M, Jiang S, Orlow S. Atypical erythema toxicum neonatorum of delayed onset in a term infant. Pediatr Dermatol 1999;16:137-141.
68. Harris JR, Schick B. Erythema neonatorum. Am J Dis Child 1956;92:27-33.
69. Luders D. Histologic observations in erythema toxicum neonatorum. Pediatrics 1960;26:219-223.
70. Ferraandiz C, Coroleu W, Ribera M, et al. Sterile transient neonatal pustulosis is a precocious form of erythema toxicum neonatorum. Dermatology 1992;185:18-22.
71. Ramamurthy RS, Reveri M, Esterly NB, et al. Transient neonatal pustular melanosis. J Pediatr 1976;88:831-835.
72. Coroleu Lletget W, Natal Pujol A, Ferraandiz Foraster C, et al. [Transient neonatal pustular melanosis]. An Esp Pediatr 1990;33:117-119.
73. Hidano A, Purwoko R, Jitsukawa K. Statistical survey of skin changes in. Pediatr Dermatol 1986;3:140-144.
74. Nanda A, Kaur S, Bhakoo ON, et al. Survey of cutaneous lesions in Indian. Pediatr Dermatol 1989;6:39-42.
75. Esterly NB. Vesicopustular eruptions in the neonate. Aust J Dermatol 1991;32:1-12.
76. Cohen LM, Skopicki BK, Harrist TJ, et al. Noninfectious vesiculobullous and vesiculopustular diseases. In Elder D, Elenitsas R, Jaworsky C, Johnson B, eds. Lever's histopathology of the skin. Philadelphia: Lippencott-Raven, 1997: pp209-252.
77. Straka BF, Cooper PH, Greer KE. Congenital miliaria crystallina. Cutis 1991;47:103-106.
78. Mowad CM, McGinley KJ, Foglia A, et al. The role of extracellular polysaccharide substance produced by Staphylococcus epidermidis in miliaria. J Am Acad Dermatol 1995;33:729-733.
79. Murphy WF, Langley AL. Common bullous lesions— presumably self-inflicted—occuring in utero in the newborn infant. Pediatrics 1963;32:1099-1101.
80. Libow LF, Reinmann JG. Symmetrical erosions in a neonate: a case of neonatal sucking blisters. Cutis 1998;62:16-17.
81. Rapelanoro R, Mortureux P, Couprie B, et al. Neonatal Malassezia furfur pustulosis. Arch Dermatol 1996;132:190-193.
82. Niamba P, Weill FX, Sarlangue J, et al. Is common neonatal cephalic pustulosis (neonatal acne) triggered by Malassezia sympodialis? Arch Dermatol 1998;134:995-998.
83. Lane AT, Rehder PA, Helm K. Evaluations of diapers containing absorbent gelling material with conventional disposable diapers in newborn infants. Am J Dis Child 1990;144:315-318.
84. Metzker A, Brenner S, Merlob P. Iatrogenic cutaneous injuries in the neonate. Arch Dermatol 1999;135:697-703.
85. Ashkenazi S, Metzker A, Merlob P, et al. Scalp changes after fetal monitoring. Arch Dis Child 1985;60:267-269.
86. Cartlidge PH, Fox PE, Rutter N. The scars of newborn intensive care. Early Hum Dev 1990;21:1-10.
87. Mirowski GW, Frieden IJ, Miller C. Iatrogenic scald burn: a consequence of institutional infection control measures. Pediatrics 1996;98:963-965.
88. Kahn G, Rywlin AM. Acropustulosis of infancy. Arch Dermatol 1979;115:831-833.
89. Jarratt M, Ramsdell W. Infantile acropustulosis. Arch Dermatol 1979;115:834-836.
90. Jennings JL, Burrows WM. Infantile acropustulosis. J Am Acad Dermatol 1983;9:733-738.
91. Lowy G, Serapiaao CJ, Oliveira MM. Childhood acropustulosis. A study of 10 cases. Med Cutan Ibero Lat Am 1986;14:171-176.
92. Lucky AW, McGuire JS. Infantile acropustulosis with eosinophilic pustules. J Pediatr 1982;100:428-429.
93. Vignon-Pennamen MD, Wallach D. Infantile acropustulosis. A clinicopathologic study of six cases. Arch Dermatol 1986;122:1155-1160.
94. Falanga V. Infantile acropustulosis with eosinophilia [letter]. J Am Acad Dermatol 1985;13:826-828.
95. Mancini AJ, Frieden IJ, Paller AS. Infantile acropustulosis revisited: History of scabies and response to topical corticosteroids. Pediatric Dermatology 1998;15:337-341.
96. Lucky AW, Esterly NB, Heskel N, et al. Eosinophilic pustular folliculitis in infancy. Pediatr Dermatol 1984;1:202-206.
97. Giard F, Marcoux D, McCuaig C, et al. Eosinophilic pustular folliculitis (Ofuji disease) in childhood: a review of four cases. Pediatr Dermatol 1991;8:189-193.
98. Larralde M, Morales S, Munoz AS, et al. Eosinophilic pustular folliculitis in infancy: Report of two new cases. Pediatr Dermatol 1999;16:118-120.
99. Vicente J, Espaana A, Idoate M, et al. Are eosinophilic pustular folliculitis of infancy and infantile acropustulosis the same entity? Br J Dermatol 1996;135:807-809.
100. Hertz CG, Hambrick GW Jr. Congenital Letterer-Siwe disease. A case treated with vincristine and corticosteroids. Am J Dis Child 1968;116:553-556.
101. Valderrama E, Kahn LB, Festa R, et al. Benign isolated histiocytosis mimicking chicken pox in a neonate: Report of two cases with ultrastructural study. Pediatr Pathol 1985;3:103-113.
102. Herman LE, Rothman KF, Harawi S, et al. Congenital self-healing reticulohistiocytosis. A new entity in the differential diagnosis of neonatal papulovesicular eruptions. Arch Dermatol 1990;126:210-212.
103. Oranje AP, Vuzevski VD, de Groot R, et al. Congenital self-healing non-Langerhans cell histiocytosis. Eur J Pediatr 1988;148:29-31.
104. Colon-Fontanez F, Eichenfield LF, Krous HF, et al. Congenital langerhans cell histiocytosis: the utility of the Tzanck test as a diagnostic screening tool. Arch Dermatol 1998;134:1039-1040.
105. Rowden G, Connelly EM, Winkelmann RK. Cutaneous histiocytosis X. The presence of S-100 protein and its use in diagnosis. Arch Dermatol 1983;119:553-559.
106. Longaker MA, Frieden IJ, LeBoit PE, et al. Congenital "self-healing" Langerhans cell histiocytosis: the need for long-term follow-up. J Am Acad Dermatol 1994;31:910-916.
107. Cohen BA. Incontinentia pigmenti. Neurol Clin 1987;5:361-377.
108. Francis JS, Sybert VP. Incontinentia pigmenti. Semin Cutan Med Surg 1997;16:54-60.
109. Kamei R, Honig PJ. Neonatal Job's syndrome featuring a vesicular eruption. Pediatr Dermatol 1988;5:75-82.
110. Blum R, Geller G, Fish LA. Recurrent severe staphylococcal infections, eczematoid rash, extreme elevations of IgE, eosinophilia, and divergent chemotactic responses in two generations. J Pediatr 1977;90:607-609.
111. Donabedian H, Gallin JI. The hyperimmunoglobulin E recurrent-infection Job's syndrome. A review of the NIH experience and the literature. Medicine 1983;62:195-208.

112. Lerner LH, Wiss K, Gellis S, et al. An unusual pustular eruption in an infant with Down syndrome and a congenital leukemoid reaction. J Am Acad Dermatol 1996;35:330-333.

113. Chang SE, Choi JH, Koh JK. Congenital erythrodermic psoriasis (letter). Br J Dermatol 1999;140:538-568.

114. Lewis MA, Priestley BL. Transient neonatal Behcet's disease. Arch Dis Child 1986;61:805-806.

115. Stark AC, Bhakta B, Chamberlain MA, et al. Life-threatening transient neonatal Behecet's disease. Br J Rheumatol 1997;36:700-702.

116. Fine JD, Eady RA, Bauer EA, et al. Revised classification system for inherited epidermolysis bullosa: Report of the Second International Consensus Meeting on diagnosis and classification of epidermolysis bullosa. J Am Acad Dermatol 2000;42:1051-1066.

117. Fine J, Bauer E, McGuire J, et al. Epidermolysis Bullosa: Clinical, epidemiologic, and laboratory advances and the findings of the National Epidermolysis Bullosa Registry. Baltimore: Johns Hopkins University Press, 1999.

118. Marinkovich MP. Update on inherited bullous dermatoses. Dermatol Clin 1999;17:473-485.

119. Bart BJ, Gorlin RJ, Anderson VE. F.W. L. Congenital localized absence of skin and associated abnormalities resembling epidermolyisis bullosa: A new syndrome. Arch Dermatol 1966;101:78-81.

120. Kanzler MH, Smoller B, Woodley DT. Congenital localized absence of the skin as a manifestation of epidermolysis bullosa. Arch Dermatol 1992;128:1087-1090.

121. Furumura M, Imayama S, Hori Y. Three neonatal cases of epidermolysis bullosa herpetiformis (Dowling- Meara type) with severe erosive skin lesions. J Am Acad Dermatol 1993; 28:859-861.

122. Puvabanditsin S, Garrow E, Samransamraujkit R, et al. Epidermolysis bullosa associated with congenital localized absence of skin, fetal abdominal mass, and pyloric atresia. Pediatr Dermatol 1997;14:359-362.

123. Maman E, Maor E, Kachko L, et al. Epidermolysis bullosa, pyloric atresia, aplasia cutis congenita: histopathological delineation of an autosomal recessive disease. Am J Med Genet 1998;78:127-133.

124. Wakasugi S, Mizutari K, Ono T. Clinical phenotype of Bart's syndrome seen in a family with dominant dystrophic epidermolysis bullosa. J Dermatol 1998;25:517-522.

125. Zelickson B, Matsumura K, Kist D, et al. Bart's syndrome. Ultrastructure and genetic linkage. Arch Dermatol 1995; 131:663-668.

126. Lin AN. Management of patients with epidermolysis bullosa. Dermatol Clin 1996;14:381-387.

127. Lyos AT, Levy ML, Malpica A, et al. Laryngeal involvement in epidermolysis bullosa. Ann Otol Rhinol Laryngol 1994;103: 542-546.

128. Fridge JL, Vichinsky EP. Correction of the anemia of epidermolysis bullosa with intravenous iron and erythropoietin. J Pediatr 1998;132:871-873.

129. Allman S, Haynes L, MacKinnon P, et al. Nutrition in dystrophic epidermolysis bullosa. Pediatr Dermatol 1992;9: 231-238.

130. Birge K. Nutrition management of patients with epidermolysis bullosa. J Am Diet Assoc 1995;95:575-579.

131. Melville C, Atherton D, Burch M, et al. Fatal cardiomyopathy in dystrophic epidermolysis bullosa. Br J Dermatol 1996;135:603-606.

132. Sedano HO, Gorlin RJ. Epidermolysis bullosa. Oral Surg Oral Med Oral Pathol 1989;67:555-563.

133. Fine JD, Johnson L, Wright T. Epidermolysis bullosa simplex superficialis. A new variant of epidermolysis bullosa characterized by subcorneal skin cleavage mimicking peeling skin syndrome. Arch Dermatol 1989;125:633-638.

134. McGrath JA, Ishida-Yamamoto A, Tidman MJ, et al. Epidermolysis bullosa simplex (Dowling-Meara). A clinicopathological review. Br J Dermatol 1992;126:421-430.

135. Puddu P, Angelo C, Faraggiana T, et al. Epidermolysis bullosa of the Dowling-Meara type: clinical and ultrastructural findings in five patients. Pediatr Dermatol 1996;13:207-211.

136. Coleman R, Harper JI, Lake BD. Epidermolysis bullosa simplex with mottled pigmentation. Br J Dermatol 1993;128: 679-685.

137. Fine JD, Stenn J, Johnson L, et al. Autosomal recessive epidermolysis bullosa simplex. Generalized phenotypic features suggestive of junctional or dystrophic epidermolysis bullosa, and association with neuromuscular diseases. Arch Dermatol 1989;125:931-938.

138. Smith FJ, Eady RA, Leigh IM, et al. Plectin deficiency results in muscular dystrophy with epidermolysis bullosa. Nat Genet 1996;13:450-457.

139. Mellerio JE, Smith FJ, McMillan JR, et al. Recessive epidermolysis bullosa simplex associated with plectin mutations: Infantile respiratory complications in two unrelated cases. Br J Dermatol 1997;137:898-906.

140. Kletter G, Evans OB, Lee JA, et al. Congenital muscular dystrophy and epidermolysis bullosa simplex. J Pediatr 1989; 114:104-107.

141. Abanmi A, Joshi RK, Atukorala DN, et al. Autosomal recessive epidermolysis bullosa simplex. A case report. Br J Dermatol 1994;130:115-117.

142. Lim KK, Su WP, McEvoy MT, et al. Generalized gravis junctional epidermolysis bullosa: Case report, laboratory evaluation, and review of recent advances. Mayo Clin Proc 1996;71:863-868.

143. Basarab T, Dunnill MG, Eady RA, et al. Herlitz junctional epidermolysis bullosa: A case report and review of current diagnostic methods. Pediatr Dermatol 1997;14:307-311.

144. Lin AN, Murphy F, Brodie SE, et al. Review of ophthalmic findings in 204 patients with epidermolysis bullosa. Am J Ophthalmol 1994;118:384-390.

145. Glazier DB, Zaontz MR. Epidermolysis bullosa: A review of the associated urological complications. J Urol 1998;159: 2122-2125.

146. Ishigami T, Akaishi K, Nishimura S, et al. A case of pyloric atresia associated with junctional epidermolysis bullosa. Eur J Pediatr 1990;149:306-307.

147. Zirn JR, Scott RA, Aronian JM, 3rd, Lin AN. Gastric outlet obstruction and gastric infarct in junctional epidermolysis bullosa. Pediatr Dermatol 1995;12:174-177.

148. Valari MD, Phillips RJ, Lake BD, et al. Junctional epidermolysis bullosa and pyloric atresia: A distinct entity. Clinical and pathological studies in five patients. Br J Dermatol 1995;133:732-736.

149. Shaw DW, Fine JD, Piacquadio DJ, et al. Gastric outlet obstruction and epidermolysis bullosa. J Am Acad Dermatol 1997;36:304-310.

150. Dennery PA, Conover PT, Kahn T, et al. Premature twins with skin lesions and gastric outlet obstruction [clinical conference]. J Pediatr 1992;120:645-651.

151. Hintner H, Wolff K. Generalized atrophic benign epidermolysis bullosa. Arch Dermatol 1982;118:375-384.
152. Paller AS, Fine J, Kaplan S, et al. The generalized atrophic benign form of junctional epidermolysis bullosa. Arch Dermatol 1986;122:704-710.
153. Darling TN, Bauer JW, Hintner H, et al. Generalized atrophic benign epidermolysis bullosa. Adv Dermatol 1997;13:87-119;discussion 120.
154. Swensson O, Christophers E. Generalized atrophic benign epidermolysis bullosa in 2 siblings complicated by multiple squamous cell carcinomas. Arch Dermatol 1998;134:199-203.
155. Lin AN, Carter DM. Epidermolysis bullosa. Annu Rev Med 1993;44:189-199.
156. Ergun GA, Lin AN, Dannenberg AJ, et al. Gastrointestinal manifestations of epidermolysis bullosa. A study of 101 patients. Medicine 1992;71:121-127.
157. Haynes L, Atherton D, Clayden G. Constipation in epidermolysis bullosa: Successful treatment with a liquid fiber-containing formula. Pediatr Dermatol 1997;14:393-396.
158. McDonnell PJ, Schofield OM, Spalton DJ, et al. The eye in dystrophic epidermolysis bullosa: Clinical and immunopathological findings. Eye 1989;3:79-83.
159. Haber RM, Hanna WM. Kindler syndrome. Clinical and ultrastructural findings. Arch Dermatol 1996;132:1487-1490.
160. Christiano AM, Fine JD, Uitto J. Genetic basis of dominantly inherited transient bullous dermolysis of the newborn: A splice site mutation in the type VII collagen gene. J Invest Dermatol 1997;109:811-814.
161. Hashimoto K, Matsumoto M, Iacobelli D. Transient bullous dermolysis of the newborn. Arch Dermatol 1985;121:1429-1438.
162. Hashimoto K, Burk JD, Bale GF, et al. Transient bullous dermolysis of the newborn: Two additional cases. J Am Acad Dermatol 1989;21:708-713.
163. Okuda C, Fujiwara H, Ito M. Transient bullous dermolysis of the newborn: New pathologic findings. Arch Dermatol 1993;129:1209-1210.
164. Fine JD, Johnson LB, Cronce D, et al. Intracytoplasmic retention of type VII collagen and dominant dystrophic epidermolysis bullosa: Reversal of defect following cessation of or marked improvement in disease activity. J Invest Dermatol 1993;101:232-236.
165. Paller AS. The genetic basis of hereditary blistering disorders. Curr Opin Pediatr 1996;8:367-371.
166. Uitto J, Pulkkinen L, McLean WH. Epidermolysis bullosa: A spectrum of clinical phenotypes explained by molecular heterogeneity. Mol Med Today 1997;3:457-465.
167. Marinkovich MP, Tran HH, Rao SK, et al. LAD-1 is absent in a subset of junctional epidermolysis bullosa patients. J Invest Dermatol 1997;109:356-359.
168. Chen H, Bonifas JM, Matsumura K, et al. Keratin 14 gene mutations in patients with epidermolysis bullosa simplex. J Invest Dermatol 1995;105:629-632.
169. Marinkovich MP. The molecular genetics of basement membrane diseases. Arch Dermatol 1993;129:1557-1565.
170. McGrath JA, Eady RA. The role of immunohistochemistry in the diagnosis of the non-lethal forms of junctional epidermolysis bullosa. J Dermatol Sci 1997;14:68-75.
171. Krous HF. Lethal Dowling-Meara-type epidermolysis bullosa simplex in a young infant. Pediatr Pathol Lab Med 1995;15:191-200.
172. Bolte C, Gonzalez S. Rapid diagnosis of major variants of congenital epidermolysis bullosa using a monoclonal antibody against collagen type IV. Am J Dermatopathol 1995;17:580-583.
173. Jaunzems AE, Woods AE, Staples A. Electron microscopy and morphometry enhances differentiation of epidermolysis bullosa subtypes. With normal values for 24 parameters in skin. Arch Dermatol Res 1997;289:631-639.
174. Christiano AM, Pulkkinen L, McGrath JA, Uitto J. Mutation-based prenatal diagnosis of Herlitz junctional epidermolysis bullosa. Prenat Diagn 1997;17:343-354.
175. Bass HN, Miranda C, Oei R, Crandall BF. Association of generalized dystrophic epidermolysis bullosa with positive acetylcholinesterase and markedly elevated maternal serum and amniotic fluid alpha-fetoprotein. Prenat Diagn 1993;13:55-59.
176. Nesin M, Seymour C, Kim Y. Role of elevated alpha-fetoprotein in prenatal diagnosis of junctional epidermolysis bullosa and pyloric atresia. Am J Perinatol 1994;11:286-287.
177. Drugan A, Vadas A, Sujov P, Gershoni-Baruch R. Markedly elevated alpha-fetoprotein and positive acetylcholinesterase in amniotic fluid from a pregnancy affected with dystrophic epidermolysis bullosa. Fetal Diagn Ther 1995;10:37-40.
178. Ciccarelli AO, Rothaus KO, Carter DM, et al. Plastic and reconstructive surgery in epidermolysis bullosa: Clinical experience with 110 procedures in 25 patients. Ann Plast Surg 1995;35:254-261.
179. Falabella A, Schachner L, Valencia I, et al. The use of tissue-engineered skin (Apligraf) to treat a newborn with epidermolysis bullosa. Arch Dermatol 1999;135:1219-1222.
180. Fine J, Johnson LB, Suchindran CM. The National Epidermolysis Bullosa Registry. J Invest Dermatol 1994;102:54S-56S.
181. Caldwell-Brown D, Ster RS, Lin AN, et al. Lack of efficacy of phyenytoin in recessive dystrophic epidermolysis bullosa. N Engl J Med 1992;327:163-167.
182. Khavari PA. Gene therapy for genetic skin disease. J Invest Dermatol 1998;110:462-467.
183. Golkar L, Bernhard JD. Mastocytosis. Lancet 1997;349:1379-1385.
184. Harrison PV, Cook LJ, Lake HJ, et al. Diffuse cutaneous mastocytosis: A report of neonatal onset. Acta Derm Venereol 1979;59:541-543.
185. Golitz LE, Weston WL, Lane AT. Bullous mastocytosis: Diffuse cutaneous mastocytosis with extensive blisters mimicking scalded skin syndrome or erythema multiforme. Pediatr Dermatol 1984;1:288-294.
186. Shah PY, Sharma V, Worobec AS, et al. Congenital bullous mastocytosis with myeloproliferative disorder and c-kit mutation. J Am Acad Dermatol 1998;39:119-121.
187. Oranje AP, Soekanto W, Sukardi A, et al. Diffuse cutaneous mastocytosis mimicking staphylococcal scalded-skin syndrome: report of three cases. Pediatr Dermatol 1991;8:147-151.
188. Oku T, Hashizume H, Yokote R, et al. The familial occurrence of bullous mastocytosis diffuse cutaneous mastocytosis. Arch Dermatol 1990;126:1478-1484.
189. Walker DC, Kolar KA, Hebert AA, et al. Neonatal pemphigus foliaceus. Arch Dermatol 1995;131:1308-1311.
190. Bonifazi E, Meneghini CL. Herpes gestationis with transient bullous lesions in the newborn. Pediatr Dermatol 1984;1:215-218.

191. Storer JS, Galen WK, Nesbitt LT Jr, et al. Neonatal pemphigus vulgaris. J Am Acad Dermatol 1982;6:929-932.

192. Merlob P, Metzker A, Hazaz B, et al. Neonatal pemphigus vulgaris. Pediatrics 1986;78:1102-1105.

193. Krusinski PA, Saurat JH. Transplacentally transferred dermatoses. Pediatr Dermatol 1989;6:166-177.

194. Tope WD, Kamino H, Briggaman RA, et al. Neonatal pemphigus vulgaris in a child born to a woman in remission. J Am Acad Dermatol 1993;29:480-485.

195. Chowdhury MU, Natarajan S. Neonatal pemphigus vulgaris associated with mild oral pemphigus vulgaris in the mother during pregnancy. Br J Dermatol 1998;139:500-503.

196. Esterly NB, Furey NL, Kirschner BS, et al. Chronic bullous dermatosis of childhood. Arch Dermatol 1977;113:42-46.

197. Hruza LL, Mallory SB, Fitzgibbons J, et al. Linear IgA bullous dermatosis in a neonate. Pediatr Dermatol 1993; 10:171-176.

198. Chorzelski TP, Jablonska S. IgA linear dermatosis of childhood chronic bullous disease of childhood. Br J Dermatol 1979;101:535-542.

199. Amos B, Deng JS, Flynn K, et al. Bullous pemphigoid in infancy: case report and literature review. Pediatr Dermatol 1998;15:108-111.

200. Crowley E, Frieden IJ. Neonatal lupus erythematosus: an unusual congenital presentation with cutaneous atrophy, erosions, alopecia, and pancytopenia. Pediatr Dermatol 1998;15:38-42.

201. Kaneko F, Tanji O, Hasegawa T, et al. Neonatal lupus erythematosus in Japan. J Am Acad Dermatol 1992;26:397-403.

202. Scully MC, Frieden IJ. Toxic epidermal necrolysis in early infancy. J Am Acad Dermatol 1992;27:340-344.

203. Hawk RJ, Storer JS, Daum RS. Toxic epidermal necrolysis in a 6-week-old infant. Pediatr Dermatol 1985;2:197-200.

204. de Groot R, Oranje AP, Vuzevski VD, et al. Toxic epidermal necrolysis probably due to Klebsiella pneumoniae sepsis. Dermatologica 1984;169:88-90.

205. Oranje AP, deGroot R. Letter to the Editor. Pediatr Dermatol 1985;3:83.

206. Alain G, Carrier C, Beaumier L, et al. In utero acute graft-versus-host disease in a neonate with severe combined immunodeficiency. J Am Acad Dermatol 1993;29:862-865.

207. Honig PJ, Gaisin A, Buck BE. Frozen section differentiation of drug-induced and staphylococcal-induced toxic epidermal necrolysis. J Pediatr 1978;92:504-505.

208. Ruiz-Maldonado R, Duraan-McKinster C, Carrasco-Daza D, et al. Intrauterine epidermal necrosis: Report of three cases. J Am Acad Dermatol 1998;38:712-715.

209. Cohen BA, Esterly NB, Nelson PF. Congenital erosive and vesicular dermatosis healing with reticulated supple scarring. Arch Dermatol 1985;121:361-367.

210. Sidhu-Malik NK, Resnick SD, Wilson BB. Congenital erosive and vesicular dermatosis healing with reticulated supple scarring: report of three new cases and review of the literature. Pediatr Dermatol 1998;15:214-218.

211. Sadick NS, Shea CR, Schlessel JS. Congenital erosive and vesicular dermatosis with reticulated, supple scarring: A neutrophilic dermatosis. J Am Acad Dermatol 1995;32:873-877.

212. Graham JA, Hansen KK, Rabinowitz LG, et al. Pyoderma gangrenosum in infants and children. Pediatr Dermatol 1994;11:10-17.

213. Ghosal SP, Sen Gupta PC, Mukherjee AK, et al. Noma neonatorum: Its aetiopathogenesis. Lancet 1978;2:289-291.

214. Rotbart HA, Levin MJ, Jones JF, et al. Noma in children with severe combined immunodeficiency. J Pediatr 1986;109:596-600.

215. Kumar SP, Anday EK. Edema, hypoproteinemia, and zinc deficiency in low-birth-weight infants. Pediatrics 1984;73:327-329.

216. van Wouwe JP. Clinical and laboratory diagnosis of acrodermatitis enteropathica. Euro J Pediatr 1989;149:2-8.

217. Bodemer C, De Prost Y, Bachollet B, et al. Cutaneous manifestations of methylmalonic and propionic acidaemia: a description based on 38 cases. Br J Dermatol 1994;131:93-98.

218. Ammirati CT, Mallory SB. The major inherited disorders of cornification. New advances in pathogenesis. Dermatol Clin 1998;16:497-508.

219. Traupe H, Kolde G, Hamm H, et al. Ichthyosis bullosa of Siemens: A unique type of epidermolytic hyperkeratosis. J Am Acad Dermatol 1986;14:1000-1005.

220. Smitt JH, van Asperen CJ, Niessen CM, et al. Restrictive dermopathy. Report of 12 cases. Dutch Task Force on Genodermatology. Arch Dermatol 1998;134:577-579.

221. Liang MG, Frieden IJ. Perineal and lip ulcerations as the presenting manifestation of hemangioma of infancy. Pediatrics 1997;99:256-259.

222. Boon LM, Enjolras O, Mulliken JB. Congenital hemangioma: Evidence of accelerated involution. J Pediatr 1996;128:329-335.

223. Mulliken JB. Capillary (port-wine) and other telangiectatic stains. In Mulliken JB, Young AE, eds. Vascular birthmarks. Philadelphia: WB Saunders, 1988: pp 170-195.

224. Frieden IJ. Aplasia cutis congenita: A clinical review and proposal for classification. J Am Acad Dermatol 1986;14:646-660.

225. Drolet B, Prendiville J, Golden J, et al. 'Membranous aplasia cutis' with hair collars. Congenital absence of skin or neuroectodermal defect? Arch Dermatol 1995;131:1427-1431.

226. Fisher CA, LeBoit PE, Frieden IJ. Linear porokeratosis presenting as erosions in the newborn period. Pediatr Dermatol 1995;12:318-322.

227. Giam YC, Williams ML, LeBoit PE, et al. Neonatal erosions and ulcerations in giant congenital melanocytic nevi. Pediatr Dermatol 1999;16:354-358.

228. Goltz RW, Henderson RR, Hitch JM, et al. Focal dermal hypoplasia syndrome. A review of the literature and report of two cases. Arch Dermatol 1970;101:1-11.

229. Reed T, Schreiner RL. Absence of dermal ridge patterns: genetic heterogeneity. Am J Med Genet 1983;16:81-88.

230. Mallon E, Wojnarowska F, Hope P, et al. Neonatal bullous eruption as a result of transient porphyrinemia in a premature infant with hemolytic disease of the newborn. J Am Acad Dermatol 1995;33:333-336.

231. Bonifazi E, Meneghini C. Perinatal gangrene of the buttock: an iatrogenic or spontaneous condition? J Am Acad Dermatol 1980;3:596-598.

232. Serrano G, Aliaga A, Febrer I, et al. Perinatal gangrene of the buttock: a spontaneous condition. Arch Dermatol 1985;121:23-24.

11

Bacterial Infections

GARY L. DARMSTADT
JAMES G. DINULOS

Bacterial skin infections vary both in their clinical presentation and their propensity for development of systemic sequelae in the neonate as a result of several factors: (1) the nature of the pathogen; (2) the developmental stage of the infant when infection is acquired, that is, early (first or second trimester) or late (third trimester) in gestation, early (first few days) or late (2 to 8 weeks) postnatal life; and, (3) the manner in which inoculation occurs (i.e., congenitally, at the time of birth via an infected mother, or postnatally). Disease present at birth resulting from hematogenous penetration of the placental barrier, for example, is often devastating, involving multiple organ systems in addition to the skin, because of the vulnerable state of the developing neonate. Even postnatally acquired infections are potentially more serious than in older children as a result of the immature immune defenses of the neonate.

Development of skin infection involves a complex interaction among environmental and local ecologic factors, such as the following:

- Alteration in the normal bacterial flora
- Predisposing tissue factors such as local trauma with breach of the epidermal barrier
- Competence of systemic and local tissue defenses of the host
- Expression of bacterial virulence factors and synergism[1-6]

Organisms that normally colonize the skin are the major agents of sepsis in very low birth weight infants, suggesting that sepsis may be a consequence of bacterial penetration at sites of skin injury or through their immature epidermal barrier.[7] Susceptibility to systemic complications of skin infection, resulting from the immaturity of immune

defenses, is especially problematic in the premature infant. Consequently, neonatal cutaneous infections mandate a prompt and thorough evaluation and aggressive treatment.[8,9] Furthermore, these infections sometimes signify the presence of congenital immunodeficiency.

GRAM-POSITIVE INFECTIONS

Staphylococcus aureus and *Streptococcus pyogenes* (group A streptococcus [GAS]) are the single most common cutaneous pathogens in the neonatal period. These gram-positive cocci can infect each of the layers of skin—epidermis, dermis, subcutaneous tissues, and fascia—and can cause a variety of skin lesions through a number of pathogenetic mechanisms.[2,6] Initiation of infection appears to require a break in skin integrity, though such a break may be inapparent clinically (e.g., arthropod bites, varicella lesions, scabies, abrasions).[5] Most primary infections are localized to the epidermis (e.g., bullous impetigo, folliculitis). Secondary infections that occur in previously diseased or wounded skin are most common in close proximity to a colonized area, such as the umbilicus or in association with eczematous dermatitis. Certain strains of *S. aureus* elaborate exotoxins, which may cause disease directly (e.g., proteolytic activity of epidermolytic toxin on desmoglein I within desmosomes to cause scalded skin syndrome), or indirectly (e.g., induction of cytokine release by monocytes and lymphocytes to cause toxic shock syndrome). *S. aureus* and GAS also are capable of penetrating to deeper dermal and subcutaneous tissues (e.g., abscess formation, cellulitis, necrotizing fasciitis) or invading the bloodstream or lymphatics to cause disseminated tertiary skin lesions, or inducing lesions as a result of coagulopathy or vasculopathy.[10]

In developed countries, *S. aureus* is usually not present on the skin of healthy newborns, but neonates may readily become colonized in neonatal wards, in situations of poor hygiene, and in association with eczematous dermatitis. Superficial skin lesions in the newborn nursery should serve as a marker for a potential infection control problem and prompt measures to isolate affected infants and identify the infectious source. Skin colonization has been shown to predispose to staphylococcal infections and may lead to nursery epidemics. Methods to curtail colonization of infant skin with pathogenic bacteria include cohorting patients, wearing barriers (e.g., gloves, gowns) and applying antiseptics to the infant. However, prevention of staphylococcal colonization is difficult despite strict adherence to these methods. Nasal carriage is an important reservoir for skin infection with *S. aureus,* and attendants' hands are thought to be the most important source for colonization of neonatal skin. As a result, handwashing is the most effective way to prevent skin colonization and avert nursery outbreaks. This method alone, however, is not sufficient to interrupt a nursery epidemic with a virulent strain of bacteria. Antiseptics applied to the umbilicus (e.g., chlorhexidine, triple dye, hexachlorophene, povidone-iodine)[11] also have decreased colonization rates in term and preterm infants, but antiseptic substances should be utilized with caution, because they may be toxic following systemic absorption through the skin, particularly in preterm infants with compromised epidermal barrier function (see Chapters 4 and 5). Intranasal (e.g., mupirocin) and/or systemic antibiotics (e.g., rifampin) are additional adjunctive treatments that may be used to quell a nursery epidemic.

Staphylococcus aureus

Superficial Infections

Impetigo

DEFINITION. Impetigo is the single most common primary skin infection in the pediatric population,[12,13,14] and impetiginous infection of atopic dermatitis is the most important secondary skin infection.[15] Nonbullous impetigo is a superficial infection localized to the subcorneal portion of the epidermis. Bullous impetigo occurs when an infant is infected with *S. aureus* from phage group 2 that elaborates toxins that cause epidermolysis and subsequent bullae formation. It has been suggested, but remains unproved, that male neonates tend to show larger areas of involvement in the diaper area and lower abdomen, whereas females may have more involvement of the face.

CUTANEOUS FINDINGS. Nonbullous impetigo is characterized by erythematous, honey-colored crusted plaques. Lesions tend to be localized in primary disease but may generalize when superimposed secondarily on diseased skin. Moist intertriginous and periumbilical areas are commonly involved in both nonbullous and bullous impetigo. Bullous impetigo often presents during the first 2 weeks of life with flaccid, transparent, subcorneal bullae. Bullae may be single or clustered, and often lack underlying cutaneous erythema. Multiple small pustules on the abdomen and diaper area are characteristic of staphylococcal pustulosis (Fig. 11-1).[16] The bullae may contain pus that layers out in the dependent portion. The lesions rupture easily, leaving a shallow erosion surrounded by a narrow rim of scale that heals without scarring. However, postinflammatory pigmentary changes may persist for weeks to months.

EXTRACUTANEOUS FINDINGS. Most cases of impetigo, including bullous impetigo in the neonate, are unaccompanied by constitutional signs of illness. Occasionally, hematogenous spread may result in osteomyelitis, septic arthritis, pneumonia, or septicemia, particularly in neonates with bullous impetigo.[12,17]

ETIOLOGY/PATHOGENESIS. *S. aureus* is isolated from approximately 85% of impetigo lesions. It is the sole pathogen in approximately 50% to 60% of cases. Bullous impetigo is always caused by coagulase-positive *S. aureus;* 80% are from phage group 2.[17,18] Locally produced exfoliative or epidermolytic toxins A and B induce bullae formation by binding to desmoglein I within desmosomes, where their effect may be mediated via proteolysis.[19] The staphylococcal organisms that cause nonbullous impetigo are variable, although generally are not from phage group 2.

DIAGNOSIS. Generally, diagnosis is made clinically. Gram stain, showing gram-positive cocci in clusters, and culture of fluid from a vesicle or pustule or from beneath the lifted edge of a crusted plaque of impetigo usually are

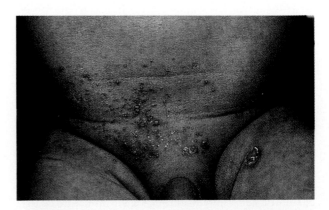

FIG. 11-1
Multiple vesicles and bullae of staphylococcal pustulosis.

sufficient to establish a diagnosis. When the diagnosis is in question, and Gram stain and culture are negative, a skin biopsy can be useful, although this is seldom necessary. Early lesions of impetigo show a vesicle or pustule in the subcorneal or granular region of the epidermis; the cavity is larger in the bullous form.

DIFFERENTIAL DIAGNOSIS. Staphylococcal impetigo is clinically indistinguishable from streptococcal impetigo.[2,12] Bullous impetigo may be confused with several other infectious vesiculobullous or pustular disorders such as herpes simplex virus (HSV) infection, varicella, enteroviral infection, congenital cutaneous candidiasis, and scabies, as well as noninfectious disorders such as erythema toxicum neonatorum, neonatal pustular melanosis, incontinentia pigmenti, epidermolysis bullosa, pemphigus, and pemphigoid (see Chapters 7 and 10).

COURSE/MANAGEMENT/TREATMENT/PROGNOSIS. The most common complication is cellulitis, which has been reported in up to 10% of cases, although this probably is an overestimation.[17] In the absence of fever or local soft-tissue involvement such as lymphadenitis or cellulitis, localized nonbullous impetigo in neonates may be managed with oral β-lactamase resistant antibiotics, such as cephalexin, cloxacillin, or dicloxacillin.[8,20] Second-line oral agents that may be considered for the treatment of uncomplicated impetigo include erythromycin, cefadroxil, cefprozil, loracarbef, clarithromycin, azithromycin, and amoxicillin/clavulanate.

Bullous impetigo may advance rapidly if not treated. Consequently, most experts recommend that therapy be initiated parenterally in neonates, usually with nafcillin, oxacillin, or methicillin. Clindamycin, a protein synthesis inhibitor, may be advantageous for decreasing epidermolytic toxin production, and a first-generation cephalosporin such as cefazolin is also suitable. Once signs of infection have begun to subside and if constitutional signs are absent, therapy may be completed orally. In older infants, oral therapy similar to that used for nonbullous impetigo may be adequate. Topical antibiotics (e.g., mupirocin) are *not* appropriate for treatment of bullous impetigo. A 7-day course of therapy may be sufficient, but because a 10-day course of treatment has been studied, it is the usual recommended length of therapy.

The antibiotic susceptibility profile must be considered when treating methicillin-resistant strains of *S. aureus* (MSRA). Vancomycin remains a reliable agent for treatment of MRSA, although other agents to which the organism is susceptible in vitro may be effective.

Bacterial Folliculitis

DEFINITION. Bacterial folliculitis is a superficial infection of the hair follicle ostium.

CUTANEOUS FINDINGS. Folliculitis presents as discrete, dome-shaped pustules with an erythematous base, located at the ostium of the pilosebaceous canals. The lesions are asymptomatic to mildly tender. Occasionally, a lesion may extend to involve deeper tissues and form an abscess (e.g., furuncle, carbuncle).

EXTRACUTANEOUS FINDINGS. Extracutaneous findings typically are lacking.

ETIOLOGY/PATHOGENESIS. Folliculitis is predominantly due to *S. aureus*, although coagulase-negative staphylococci are involved occasionally. A moist environment, maceration, poor hygiene, application of an occlusive emollient, and drainage from adjacent wounds and abscesses can be provocative factors.

DIAGNOSIS. Diagnosis usually is made on clinical grounds. The causative organism of folliculitis can be identified by Gram stain and culture of purulent material from the follicular orifice.

DIFFERENTIAL DIAGNOSIS. Both *Candida albicans* and *Malassezia furfur* can cause follicular papules and/or pustules. Diagnosis may be made by potassium hydroxide examination of scrapings from a lesion or by skin biopsy. Several other conditions that may mimic folliculitis include miliaria, eosinophilic pustular folliculitis, acne neonatorum, tinea corporis, congenital cutaneous candidiasis, scabies, and erythema toxicum neonatorum.

COURSE/MANAGEMENT/TREATMENT/PROGNOSIS. An attempt should be made to identify and eliminate predisposing factors. Oral therapy with cephalexin, dicloxacillin, or cloxacillin for 2 weeks is usually curative.

Cutaneous and Subcutaneous Abscesses

An abscess is a localized collection of pus in a cavity formed by disintegration or necrosis of tissue.[21] It is recognized clinically by the presence of a firm, tender, erythematous nodule that becomes fluctuant (Fig. 11-2). Microscopically, a cutaneous abscess is covered by normal epidermis, but the dermis contains a dense aggregate of acute inflammatory cells surrounded by a fibrinoid wall. *S. aureus* is the single most common pathogen of cutaneous and subcutaneous abscesses, but principal pathogens vary with location of the lesion on the body.[22]

A number of processes that disrupt the epidermal barrier or the integrity of local or systemic immunologic defenses are associated with abscess formation, but often no predisposing factor can be identified. Cutaneous and subcutaneous abscesses are particularly characteristic of hyper-IgE syndrome and leukocyte adhesion deficiency. Skin infections in neonates with defective neutrophil migration are most commonly due to *S. aureus*, *C. albicans*, or gram-negative bacilli. In chronic granulomatous disease, the

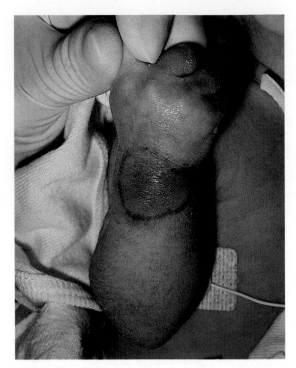

FIG. 11-2

Cellulitis and underlying abscess in a neonate. In this case the abscess was due to an intravenous line. "Inking" the margin, as was done in this case, is one way to determine response to treatment.

most common agents of cutaneous infection are *S. aureus,* gram-negative bacilli, and fungi such as *Aspergillus* spp. Identification of organisms not usually associated with abscess formation, particularly those of low virulence, should raise concerns about immunodeficiency. The causative organism(s) should be identified by Gram stain and culture.

In the neonatal period an abscess is a potentially serious infection because of the risk of dissemination. Treatment should be initiated with antimicrobial agents against a broad spectrum of gram-positive and gram-negative organisms.

Breast Abscess

DEFINITION. Breast abscess develops in full-term neonates during the first 1 to 6 weeks of life, most commonly during the second to third weeks.[23,24] The incidence is approximately equal in males and females during the first 2 weeks of life, but thereafter the incidence in girls is approximately twice that of boys.

CUTANEOUS FINDINGS. Breast abscess presents initially with breast enlargement, accompanied by varying degrees of erythema, induration, and tenderness. Fluctuance may or may not occur, depending in part on how early antibi-

otic therapy is initiated. Bilateral infection occurs in less than 5% of cases. Breast abscess caused by *S. aureus* is accompanied by cutaneous pustules or bullae on the trunk, particularly in the perineal region, in 25% to 50% of patients. The symptoms, age at presentation, and clinical findings of infants with breast abscess caused by gram-negative bacilli, or those that harbor anaerobes, are similar to those of infants infected with *S. aureus,* except that infants infected with *Salmonella* spp. generally also have gastrointestinal illness. The most common complication of breast abscess is cellulitis, which develops in approximately 5% to 10% of affected infants. The cellulitis generally is localized but can extend rapidly to involve the shoulder and/or abdomen. Scar formation leading to decreased breast size following puberty can occur as a late complication.

EXTRACUTANEOUS FINDINGS. Affected infants usually lack fever (present in approximately one third) or constitutional symptoms such as irritability or toxicity. Leukocytosis ($>15,000/mm^3$) is found in approximately half to two thirds of patients. Complications such as bacteremia, pneumonia, osteomyelitis, or sepsis are unusual.

ETIOLOGY/PATHOGENESIS. Breast abscess is usually due to *S. aureus,* but occasionally is caused by group B streptococcus, *Escherichia coli, Salmonella* spp., *Proteus mirabilis, Pseudomonas aeruginosa,* or *Ureaplasma urelyticum.*[25] Although anaerobic organisms can be isolated from up to 40% of infections, their pathogenic role in neonates is questionable, and therapy directed specifically against them is generally unnecessary. The increased incidence in girls after 2 weeks of age (when breast gland development is more pronounced in girls than boys) and the lack of the disorder in the underdeveloped breast of premature infants suggest that increased ductal tissue may be a factor in pathogenesis. Breast manipulation has also been suggested as a predisposing factor. Infants with *S. aureus* breast abscess typically are colonized with the same organism in the nose or pharynx. It seems likely that *S. aureus* spreads from the nasopharynx to colonize the skin of the nipple, moving up the ducts of the physiologically enlarged, predisposed breast, perhaps facilitated by breast manipulation, to infect deeper tissues.

DIAGNOSIS. Gram stain of material expressed from the nipple or obtained by needle aspiration or incision and drainage can help to guide initial antibiotic therapy. The presence of cutaneous vesicles or bullae may help in identifying *S. aureus* as the causal agent. Blood cultures should be obtained, but unless the infant is febrile or appears ill, cultures of urine and cerebrospinal fluid (CSF) are unnecessary.

COURSE/MANAGEMENT/TREATMENT/PROGNOSIS. If fluctuance is absent, systemic antistaphylococcal antibiotic therapy may be curative and prevent abscess development. If fluctuance is present, the abscess must be drained by needle aspiration, by gently expressing pus from the nipple, or surgically, with Gram stain and culture obtained. Antibiotic therapy with a β-lactamase-resistant antistaphylococcal antibiotic should be given systemically. If gram-negative bacilli are seen or the infant has constitutional symptoms or appears ill, initial therapy should be administered parenterally. An aminoglycoside or cefotaxime should be given while awaiting culture results. Once infection has begun to subside, oral therapy may be considered. In most instances, a total of 5 to 7 days of therapy is sufficient, although many experts continue treatment for 10 to 14 days.

Scalp Abscess (See also Chapter 8)

DEFINITION. Scalp abscess develops in neonates at the insertion site of a fetal scalp monitoring electrode. Prospective studies have reported the incidence to be 0.56% and 4.5%.[26,27]

CUTANEOUS FINDINGS. Presentation occurs most commonly on the third or fourth days of life but may be as early as the first day and as late as 3 weeks of life. The lesion initially appears as a localized, erythematous area of induration 0.5 to 2 cm in diameter. The site may become fluctuant or pustular.

EXTRACUTANEOUS FINDINGS. Regional lymphadenopathy may be present, but other more serious complications such as cranial osteomyelitis, subgaleal abscess, necrotizing fasciitis of the scalp, bacteremia, sepsis, and death are rare.

ETIOLOGY/PATHOGENESIS. Typically, scalp abscess is a polymicrobial infection, including a variety of aerobes and anaerobes. The anaerobic flora present reflects that found in the normal cervix during labor.

The most plausible hypothesis for the pathogenesis of scalp abscess is that the infection occurs through ascension of normal cervical flora into the uterus following rupture of membranes, aided by procedures that access the uterine cavity. Placement of the electrode breaks the skin barrier, providing a foreign-body nidus for infection in the subcutaneous tissue. Risk factors include longer duration of ruptured membranes; longer duration of monitoring; monitoring for high-risk indications, particularly prematurity, and nulliparous birth, possibly as a result of increased risk of infection of edematous, hypoxic caput succedaneum. However, duration of ruptured membranes and duration of monitoring have not consistently been identified as risk factors. In general, it appears that procedures that serve to provide increased access of vaginal flora to the infant or more trauma to the scalp may increase the risk of abscess development.

DIAGNOSIS. Infants who are subjected to scalp electrode monitoring in utero should be followed closely during the

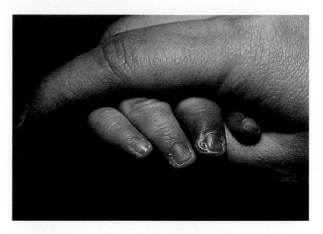

FIG. 11-3
Paronychia, presenting with erythema and edema of the lateral nail fold, was due to *Staphylococcus aureus* in this case.

first weeks of life for evidence of infection. Parents should be instructed in surveillance, and if an abscess is noted, it is advisable to remove the hair directly around the lesion to allow for closer observation. Culture for both aerobic and anaerobic organisms can be obtained by swabbing the exudate from the puncture site or by needle aspiration.

DIFFERENTIAL DIAGNOSIS. The primary differential diagnostic concern is HSV infection. The peak incidence of onset of HSV lesions (4 to 10 days) overlaps with that for scalp abscess, and they may be indistinguishable clinically. Dissemination of HSV also may occur. Consequently, if suspicion of HSV exists, therapy with acyclovir should be initiated while awaiting diagnostic test results. Aplasia cutis congenita can have clear drainage and resemble a scalp abscess.

COURSE/MANAGEMENT/TREATMENT/PROGNOSIS. Many lesions resolve spontaneously, but if fluctuance develops without spontaneous suppuration, incision and drainage are appropriate. Extensive debridement is not necessary. If surrounding cellulitis is present, a 5- to 7-day course of parenteral antibiotic therapy usually is sufficient, with culture results guiding antibiotic choice.

Paronychia. Acute paronychia, a localized inflammation of the nail fold, often follows local injury. Although the primary disorder is separation of the eponychium from the nail plate, secondary infection is common. *S. aureus* and *S. pyogenes* are the most common aerobic organisms. Occasionally, gram-negative organisms such as *Pseudomonas* spp., *Proteus* spp., and *E. coli* are involved.[28]

The lateral nail fold becomes warm, erythematous, edematous, and painful (Fig. 11-3). A purulent exudate may develop. Dermatitis often occurs around the affected area and may contribute to initiation and/or perpetuation of the problem. Extracutaneous findings generally are absent. The diagnosis is made clinically; in acute cases both aerobic and anaerobic cultures of purulent material are recommended. The differential diagnosis includes *C. albicans*, a frequent cause of acute and chronic paronychia in neonates, and HSV infection (see Chapter 27).

Attention must be directed toward eliminating or reducing predisposing factors of nailfold maceration and trauma. Warm compresses generally are curative for superficial lesions. Drainage of the abscess may be facilitated by gently pushing the nailfold away from the nail plate. Antibiotics, in addition to incision and drainage, are needed for treatment of deeper lesions. Dicloxacillin, cloxacillin, or cephalexin are the antibiotics of choice for treatment of infections caused by *S. aureus*, whereas amoxicillin plus clavulanic acid is preferred for empiric treatment as a result of the emergence of β-lactamase–producing anaerobes.

Nonnecrotizing Subcutaneous Infections

Funisitis/Omphalitis

DEFINITION. **Funisitis** is inflammation of the umbilical cord or stump characterized by increased secretions and foul odor. It may accompany chorioamnionitis. **Omphalitis** is infection of the umbilical stump. Low birth weight infants and those with complicated deliveries are at increased risk.[29]

CUTANEOUS FINDINGS. Excessive exudate from the umbilical stump, as seen in funisitis, may be a harbinger of subsequent infection. The exudate may be accompanied by bleeding from the umbilical vessels caused by a delay in closure. Omphalitis shows periumbilical erythema, edema, and tenderness with or without discharge. On average, onset occurs on the third day of life. The infection may extend subcutaneously to cause cellulitis or along abdominal wall fascial planes to cause necrotizing fasciitis. Black discoloration or crepitus of the periumbilical tissues suggest a mixed infection and more advanced disease.

EXTRACUTANEOUS FINDINGS. The umbilical cord of the newborn infant is a particularly common portal of entry for invasive bacterial pathogens. Invasion may occur directly into the peritoneal cavity with resultant peritonitis. Ascending infection along the umbilical vein is a particularly serious complication. Septic umbilical arteritis or suppurative thrombophlebitis of umbilical or portal veins, portal vein thrombosis, and liver abscesses may occur. Septic embolization from infected umbilical vessels (arteries or the vein) is uncommon, but may seed various organs, including the lungs, pancreas, kidneys, heart (i.e., endocarditis) or skin.

ETIOLOGY/PATHOGENESIS. Omphalitis is caused by a variety of organisms, but *S. aureus*, *S. pyogenes* and gram-negative organisms are most common.[30] The umbilical cord stump may become highly colonized with pathogenic bacteria shortly after birth, including vaginal flora and bacteria from caretakers hands. Candidal funisitis has been reported (see Chapter 13).

DIAGNOSIS. Gram stain and culture of moist umbilical stump material may show organisms and be helpful in the early diagnosis of omphalitis, although correlation with clinical signs is necessary to determine true infection. Culture results are helpful for guiding antimicrobial therapy.

DIFFERENTIAL DIAGNOSIS. Serous secretions of funisitis/omphalitis must be differentiated from those of a vitelline duct remnant, umbilical papilloma, or urachal remnant.

COURSE/MANAGEMENT/TREATMENT/PROGNOSIS. Most cases are responsive to broad-spectrum antimicrobial coverage against gram-positive and gram-negative organisms. Ampicillin and gentamicin is an effective therapy for initial coverage. With either suspicion or microbiologic evidence of anaerobic infection, addition of metronidazole or substitution with clindamycin for ampicillin usually is effective. Intravenous antibiotics should be continued until the erythema and drainage subside. Predictors of poor outcome include early onset of the infection, unplanned home delivery, and temperature instability. Patients should be monitored closely for signs of necrotizing fasciitis.

Cellulitis

DEFINITION. Cellulitis is characterized by infection and inflammation of loose connective tissue, with limited involvement of the dermis and relative sparing of the epidermis. A break in the skin resulting from trauma, surgery, or an underlying skin lesion predisposes to cellulitis. The condition may be seen with vascular malformations such as Klippel-Trénaunay syndrome and lymphatic malformations and in immunodeficiency disorders, but it also occurs in healthy infants.

CUTANEOUS FINDINGS. Cellulitis presents as an area of edema, warmth, erythema, and tenderness. The lateral margins tend to be indistinct because the process is deep in the skin. Application of pressure may produce pitting. Cellulitis caused by *S. aureus* tends to be more localized and may suppurate, whereas infections caused by *S. pyogenes* tend to spread more rapidly and may be associated with lymphangitis, but the distinction generally is not clear-cut.

Periorbital or preseptal cellulitis develops anterior (i.e., superficial) to an intact orbital septum.[31] It presents with swelling of the eyelid and may be associated with bacteremia, particularly when *Streptococcus pneumoniae* is involved. Cellulitis that involves structures behind the septum in the orbital space is called orbital cellulitis. It usually is associated with sinusitis or direct penetrating trauma to the orbital septum. Orbital cellulitis presents with eyelid erythema and edema, conjunctival hyperemia, chemosis, proptosis, decreased and painful extraocular movements, decreased visual acuity, fever, and constitutional signs. As the infection progresses, an abscess of the orbital tissue and subperiosteum develops. Computed tomography (CT) may define the extent of infection.

EXTRACUTANEOUS FINDINGS. Regional adenopathy and constitutional signs and symptoms of fever, chills, and malaise are common. Complications of cellulitis include osteomyelitis, septic arthritis, thrombophlebitis, and bacteremia. Glomerulonephritis also can follow infection with *S. pyogenes.* Orbital or periorbital cellulitis is a rare presenting sign of intraocular retinoblastoma.

ETIOLOGY/PATHOGENESIS. Besides *S. aureus* and *S. pyogenes,* causal organisms occasionally include group G or C streptococci, *S. pneumoniae, Haemophilus influenzae,* and group B streptococci or *E. coli.* In premature newborns or newborns with immunologic defects, a number of other bacterial or fungal agents may be involved. *Pasteurella multocida* is implicated in cellulitis that follows dog or cat bites, whereas human bites may become infected with *Eikenella corrodens.*

DIAGNOSIS. Aspirates from the leading edge of inflammation, skin biopsy, and blood cultures collectively allow for identification of the causal organism in approximately 25% of cellulitis cases. An aspirate taken from the point of maximum inflammation yields the causal organism more often than does a leading-edge aspirate.[32] Lack of success in isolating an organism stems primarily from the low number of organisms present within the lesion.

DIFFERENTIAL DIAGNOSIS. Congenital Wells syndrome, insect bites, drug reactions, contact dermatitis, and cold panniculitis may resemble cellulitis. Adenoviral conjunctivitis may mimic preseptal and septal cellulitis.

COURSE/MANAGEMENT/TREATMENT/PROGNOSIS. Empiric therapy for cellulitis should be directed by the history of the illness, the location and character of the cellulitis, and the age and immune status of the patient.[2,8,20] Cellulitis in the neonate should prompt a sepsis workup, followed by initiation of empiric therapy intravenously with a β-lactamase stable antistaphylococcal antibiotic such as methicillin, oxacillin, or nafcillin, and an aminoglycoside such as gentamicin or a cephalosporin such as cefotaxime. Once the regional erythema, warmth, edema, and fever have decreased significantly, a 10-day course of treatment may be completed on an outpatient basis provided that

other sites of infection (e.g., CSF) have been excluded. Orbital cellulitis is a medical emergency. If the response to parenteral antibiotic therapy is not prompt, or signs of optic nerve compression such as decreased vision are present, surgical decompression of the orbital space and infected sinuses must be undertaken. It is recommended that intravenous antibiotic therapy continue for at least 5 days following abscess drainage for a total of 14 to 21 days.

Necrotizing Subcutaneous Infections
Necrotizing Fasciitis
DEFINITION. Necrotizing fasciitis is a subcutaneous tissue infection that involves the deep layer of superficial fascia but largely spares adjacent epidermis, deep fascia, and muscle.[33,34]

CUTANEOUS FINDINGS. Local swelling, erythema, tenderness, and heat are typical and develop most commonly in the abdominal wall. Skin changes may progress over 24 to 48 hours as nutrient vessels are thrombosed and cutaneous ischemia develops. Because the infection advances along the superficial fascial plane, there may be few initial cutaneous signs to herald the serious nature and extent of the subcutaneous tissue necrosis that is occurring. Late cutaneous signs include formation of bullae filled initially with straw-colored and later bluish to hemorrhagic fluid, and darkening of affected tissues from red to purple to blue. Skin anesthesia and finally frank tissue gangrene and slough develop as a result of the ischemia and necrosis. Infections resulting from any one organism or combination of organisms cannot be distinguished clinically from one another, although development of crepitance signals the presence of *Clostridium* spp. or gram-negative bacilli such as *E. coli, Klebsiella, Proteus,* and *Aeromonas.*

EXTRACUTANEOUS FINDINGS. In necrotizing fasciitis, fever is usually present and pain is out of proportion to cutaneous signs.[35,36] Bacteremia is present in approximately half of patients. Significant systemic toxicity may develop, including shock and multiorgan failure. Advance of infection in this setting can be rapid, progressing to death within hours.

ETIOLOGY/PATHOGENESIS. Common predisposing conditions in neonates include omphalitis, balanitis, breast and scalp abscesses, and postoperative complications.[33,37] Most cases in newborns are polymicrobial, involving a mixture of anaerobic bacteria and aerobic and/or facultative bacteria that act together to cause tissue necrosis. Fungi of the order Mucorales, particularly *Rhizopus* spp., *Mucor* spp., and *Absidia* spp., rarely can cause necrotizing fasciitis.[35,37]

DIAGNOSIS. Fever, tachycardia, and leukocytosis can be the first signs of an evolving necrotizing fasciitis. Definitive diagnosis of necrotizing fasciitis is made by surgical exploration, which must be undertaken as soon as the diagnosis is suspected. Although magnetic resonance (MR) or CT scanning or ultrasound may aid in delineating the extent and tissue planes of involvement, these procedures should not delay surgical intervention. Frozen section incisional biopsy taken early in the course of the infection can aid management by decreasing the time to diagnosis and helping to establish margins of involvement.[38] Histopathologically, necrotizing fasciitis typically includes necrosis and suppuration of the superficial fascia; edema and an acute inflammatory infiltrate in the deep dermis, subcutaneous fat, and fascia; microorganisms within destroyed tissue; and thrombosis of arteries and veins at all levels of tissue.

DIFFERENTIAL DIAGNOSIS. Discrimination of nonnecrotizing (e.g., cellulitis) versus necrotizing infection is the most important management decision, because necrotizing soft tissue infection will not respond to antibiotics alone and requires prompt surgical removal of all devitalized tissue. Pain out of proportion to the cutaneous findings, rapidly progressive tissue necrosis, and systemic toxicity distinguish necrotizing fasciitis from cellulitis, which does not destroy subcutaneous tissue.

COURSE/MANAGEMENT/TREATMENT/PROGNOSIS. Prompt supportive care, surgical debridement, and parenteral antibiotic administration are mandatory.[36,37] All devitalized tissue must be removed to freely bleeding edges, and repeat exploration is generally indicated within 24 to 36 hours to confirm that no necrotic tissue remains. Surgery may need to be repeated on several occasions until devitalized tissue has ceased to form. Daily, meticulous wound care also is paramount. Broad-spectrum, parenteral antibiotic therapy must be initiated as soon as possible. Most experts recommend initial empiric therapy with a combination of penicillin, nafcillin, or ampicillin; clindamycin or metronidazole; and an aminoglycoside such as gentamicin.[39]

Toxin-Mediated Diseases

Exotoxin-mediated diseases are due to the effects of extracellular toxin(s) produced at a focus of infection or colonization.[10] The site of bacterial replication is typically inconspicuous in relation to the clinical effects of the toxin(s). Toxins can act locally, as in bullous impetigo; or can cause widespread clinical signs resulting from hematogenous spread, as in scalded skin syndrome.

Staphylococcal Scalded Skin Syndrome

DEFINITION. Staphyloccocal scalded skin syndrome (SSSS) is a staphylococcal epidermolytic toxin-mediated disease characterized by cutaneous tenderness and super-

ficial, widespread blistering and/or desquamation.[40] In the neonatal period, it can result in nursery outbreaks.[41]

CUTANEOUS FINDINGS. Exquisite tenderness of the skin may herald onset of SSSS. Generalized macular erythema evolves rapidly into a scarlatiniform eruption that is accentuated in flexural and periorificial areas (Fig. 11-4). The brightly erythematous skin acquires a wrinkled appearance, leading to thick flaky desquamation, particularly in the flexures, over approximately 2 to 5 days. In severe cases, the erythrodermic phase is followed by the development of diffuse, sterile, flaccid blisters and erosions, and diffuse, bullous desquamation of large sheets of skin (Fig. 11-5). At this stage, areas of epidermis may separate in response to gentle shear force (Nikolsky's sign). As large sheets of epidermis peel away, moist, glistening, denuded areas become apparent, initially in the flexures and subsequently over much of the body surface. As the exposed denuded skin dries, it develops a crusted, flaky appearance. Distinctive radial crusting and fissuring around the eyes, mouth, and nose develop approximately 2 to 5 days after the onset of erythroderma. Secondary cutaneous infection, cellulitis, omphalitis, and severe surgical wound infections may occur.

EXTRACUTANEOUS FINDINGS. Complications may include excessive fluid loss, electrolyte imbalance, faulty temperature regulation, pneumonia, endocarditis, and septicemia. Mortality, due predominantly to sepsis, is unusual but is highest in the severe generalized form of the disease.

ETIOLOGY/PATHOGENESIS. SSSS is caused predominantly by phage group II staphylococci, particularly strains 71 and 55; occasionally, a group I or III isolate is involved.[42] Foci of infection include the nasopharynx, or less commonly the umbilicus, urinary tract, a cutaneous wound, conjunctivae, or the blood. There, bacteria produce epidermolytic (i.e., exfoliative or exfoliatin) toxins A and/or B, which enter the bloodstream.[43] Rarely, the disease has also been transmitted through breast feeding.[44] Severity of the disease is related to the toxin load, rather than the nature of the focal infection, and this load may be particularly high in neonates due to reduced renal clearance.[19,42] The epidermolytic toxins appear to produce the granular layer split by binding to desmoglein I within desmosomes and exerting proteolytic activity.[19]

DIAGNOSIS. Although intact bullae on the skin are sterile, cultures should be obtained from multiple sites including the blood, cerebrospinal fluid, nasopharynx, urine, umbilicus, and any suspected sites of localized infection in an attempt to identify the source for the epidermolytic toxins. Histopathologically, subcorneal bullae formation through the granular layer without an inflammatory infiltrate is characteristic (Fig. 11-6). In cases that

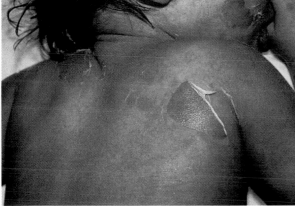
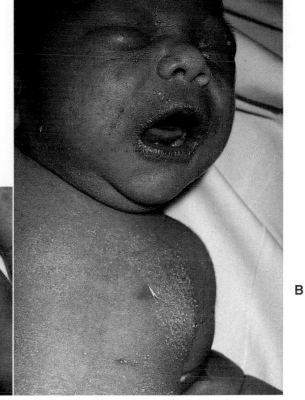

FIG. 11-4
A, Diffuse erythroderma and Nikolsky sign in staphylococcal scalded skin syndrome. B, Staphylococcal scalded skin syndrome: note the perioral accentuation which is characteristic. (A From Darmstadt GL. Staphylococcal and streptococcal skin infections. In Harahap M, ed. Diagnosis and treatment of skin infections. Oxford: Blackwell Science, 1997: p. 84. Courtesy Alfred T. Lane, MD)

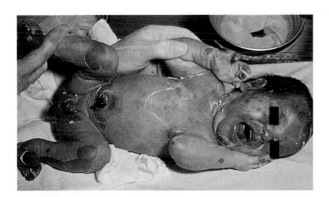

FIG. 11-5
Widespread SSSS with erosions and scaly areas of desquamation.

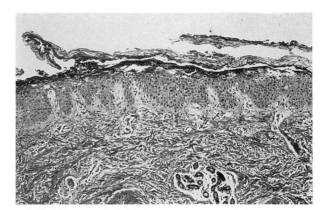

FIG. 11-6
Skin biopsy of SSSS reveals a subcorneal split at the level of the stratum granulosum.

demand a rapid diagnosis, the exfoliated corneal layer can be seen on a frozen biopsy specimen of the desquamating epidermis. Scattered acantholytic cells that are evident histopathologically in the cleftlike bullae can also be seen in a Tzanck preparation.

Differential diagnosis. SSSS may be mistaken for a number of other blistering and exfoliating disorders, including scarlet fever, bullous impetigo, epidermolysis bullosa, diffuse cutaneous mastocytosis, familial peeling skin syndrome with eosinophilia, epidermolytic hyperkeratosis, drug eruption, erythema multiforme, and drug-induced toxic epidermal necrolysis (TEN; Lyell's disease). TEN often can be distinguished by a history of drug ingestion, presence of Nikolsky's sign only at sites of erythema, and absence of perioral crusting. The differentiation of TEN from SSSS may occasionally require a skin biopsy. TEN results in full-thickness epidermal necrosis, with a blister cleavage plane in the lowermost epidermis. Distinguishing between these conditions is particularly important because mortality rates as high as 30% have been reported with TEN, and avoidance of the offending drug is crucial to preventing a recurrence.

Course/management/treatment/prognosis. Recovery usually is rapid once appropriate antibiotic therapy is begun. Parenteral therapy with nafcillin or methicillin should be given promptly. Strict isolation is imperative to avoid spread of infection. See Chapter 10 for skin care recommendations in blistering diseases. General principles include minimizing handling of the infant and use of emollients (e.g., petrolatum and petroleum jelly gauze) and semiocclusive dressings to provide lubrication and minimize pain. Corticosteroids are detrimental and should be avoided. Healing occurs without scarring in 10 to 14 days.

Group A β-Hemolytic Streptococci

S. pyogenes has been the focus of renewed interest as a result of a rise in incidence of invasive infections over the past decade.[45] This organism may be vertically transmitted from the mother.[46] In the neonatal period, *S. pyogenes* is a cause of postpartum sepsis, necrotizing fasciitis, and toxic shock syndrome, in addition to localized skin infections (e.g., impetigo, cellulitis).

Superficial Infections

Impetigo (See *S. aureus:* Impetigo). Next to *S. aureus*, *S. pyogenes* is the most important cause of nonbullous impetigo.[12] It can be isolated from approximately 30% to 40% of all lesions of impetigo and is the sole pathogen in about 5% of cases; occasionally, group B, C, G, or F strep-

tococci are present. Colonization of the skin with *S. pyogenes* occurs less frequently than with *S. aureus* but has been documented, particularly in areas with epidemics or a high endemic rate of impetigo.[17,47,48] In these instances, in contrast to *S. aureus*, *S. pyogenes* colonizes the skin an average of 10 days before development of impetigo and appears in the nasopharynx only after the appearance of impetigo, suggesting that colonized skin served as the primary source and probably the initial step for development of skin infection. Acute rheumatic fever does not occur following impetigo.

Ecthyma resembles nonbullous impetigo in onset and appearance but gradually evolves into a deeper, more chronic infection of the epidermis and dermis. Treatment of streptococcal impetigo and ecthyma is as discussed for staphylococcal impetigo.

Cellulitis (See *S. aureus:* Cellulitis). Erysipelas is a superficial form of cellulitis, involving the dermis and upper subcutaneous tissue, with prominent lymphatic involvement. A small area of burning and redness develops into a warm, shiny, bright red, confluent, indurated, tender plaque with a brawny, peau d'orange appearance and elevated, sharply demarcated margins. Vesicles, hemorrhagic bullae, petechiae, and ecchymoses may develop in the plaque, and regional adenopathy may be present. Fine desquamation and sometimes postinflammatory pigmentary changes accompany resolution of the plaque.

Given the potential involvement of a variety of organisms, empiric antibiotic therapy for erysipelas in the neonate should provide broad coverage, as for cellulitis (e.g., a β-lactamase-resistant antistaphylococcal antibiotic such as methicillin and an aminoglycoside such as gentamicin or a cephalosporin such as cefotaxime). In most cases, parenteral penicillin for 10 days is effective. In many cases, however, a longer course of therapy may be necessary to eliminate lymphatic foci of infection.

Necrotizing fasciitis (See *S. aureus:* Necrotizing fasciitis). Since the mid 1980s, there has been a resurgence of fulminant necrotizing soft tissue infections caused by *S. pyogenes*.[35,45] Most experts recommend initial empiric antibiotic therapy with penicillin, ampicillin, or nafcillin; clindamycin; and an aminoglycoside for coverage against *S. pyogenes* and the broad spectrum of potential anaerobic and gram-negative pathogens.[39] As a result of the presence of large numbers of bacteria and their entry into a slower or stationary phase of growth, *S. pyogenes* may have reduced susceptibility to the β-lactam antibiotics such as penicillin and the cephalosporins, which act by interrupting cell wall synthesis.[49] Because efficacy of the protein synthesis inhibitor clindamycin is not adversely altered by the inoculum effect and it may suppress bacterial toxin synthesis, it may be preferable to penicillin for treatment of serious soft tissue infections resulting from *S. pyogenes*.

Toxin-Mediated Diseases

Streptococcal Toxic Shock Syndrome

DEFINITION. Streptococcal toxic shock syndrome (STSS) is characterized by acute onset of shock and multisystem organ failure, caused by *S. pyogenes* infection at a normally sterile site.[50] It is very rare in newborns.

ETIOLOGY/PATHOGENESIS. STSS is associated with invasive *S. pyogenes* infection; most patients are bacteremic and/or have focal tissue infection at the time of presentation. Streptococcal toxic shock syndrome develops most often in the setting of a minor, focal skin and/or soft tissue infection, which presumably provides a portal of entry.[35,39,45,51,52] The mucous membranes also can be penetrated.[53] Lack of antibody against exotoxin appears to be a risk factor for severe, invasive disease and STSS.[54] Most isolates of *S. pyogenes* that cause STSS are M protein types 1, 3, 12, and 28 that produce streptococcal pyrogenic exotoxins A and/or B.[35,39,51,52]

CUTANEOUS FINDINGS. Most patients have localized swelling and erythema at a site of exquisite pain. Development of vesicles and bullae (5%) is a late, ominous sign of tissue devitalization.[39,55] Patients without soft tissue infection have a variety of focal infections including endophthalmitis, osteomyelitis, myositis, pneumonia, perihepatitis, peritonitis, myocarditis, and sepsis.[39] Other cutaneous signs in a minority of patients include a petechial, maculopapular, or diffuse scarlatiniform eruption.[56]

EXTRACUTANEOUS FINDINGS. Streptococcal TSS is characterized by acute onset and early, frequently fulminant progression to shock and multiorgan compromise or failure. The most common presenting sign of STSS is fever, generally accompanied by tachycardia and hypotension. Patients rapidly develop hypotensive shock, often accompanied by early renal impairment and onset of respiratory distress syndrome. Renal impairment tends to progress for the first few days regardless of therapy, often necessitating dialysis, but function generally is regained. Toxic cardiomyopathy is a life-threatening complication that is characterized by decreased contractility and cardiac output and refractory shock. Laboratory abnormalities, including hemoglobinuria, elevation of serum creatinine, and leukocytosis with a marked left shift develop early and reflect the multiorgan system dysfunction. As the disease progresses, most patients display hypoalbuminemia, hypocalcemia, anemia, and thrombocytopenia. Soft tissue infection, particularly development of necrotizing fasciitis and myositis, is reflected in an elevation of creatine phosphokinase.[35,39]

DIAGNOSIS. Definitive diagnosis of STSS requires isolation of *S. pyogenes* from a normally sterile site in a patient with hypotension and multiorgan failure.

COURSE/MANAGEMENT/TREATMENT/PROGNOSIS. Patients suspected of having STSS should be managed in an intensive care setting, due to the rapidly progressive, fulminant nature of the syndrome. Management consists of aggressive intravenous fluid resuscitation, culture of potential sites of infection, early surgical exploration of suspected deep-seated infections and debridement of devitalized tissue, and prompt administration of antibiotics. Inotropic agents may be necessary to manage refractory shock due to toxic cardiomyopathy. Use of epinephrine in patients with intractable hypotension may be complicated by gangrene of digits.

While ruling out septic shock from gram-negative bacilli or *S. aureus*, or polymicrobial necrotizing fasciitis, broad-spectrum antimicrobial therapy should be initiated as discussed for necrotizing fasciitis. Once a diagnosis of STSS is made, therapy can be tailored. Clindamycin has advantages over penicillin, although many experts recommend use of both agents concurrently for treatment of STSS.[57]

Group B Streptococcus

DEFINITION. Group B streptococcus (GBS), a gram-positive coccus, is the most common cause of septicemia in the neonate in many developed countries. Like listeriosis, there are early and late forms of GBS disease. Early-onset disease presents within the first 6 days of life, although signs of infection typically are present at birth or within hours of delivery; preterm infants are particularly susceptible. Late-onset disease occurs from 7 days to 3 months of life, with a median age at onset of 27 days.

CUTANEOUS FINDINGS. Cutaneous manifestations of GBS infection are rare.[58] Skin lesions, however, may be an early sign of bacteremia or, alternatively, may provide a focus of infection from which bacteremia may occur. Cellulitis is the most common cutaneous manifestation of GBS infection and characteristically develops in late-onset disease. It has a predilection for the face, submental, and submandibular regions in infants less than 12 weeks of age. A rapidly progressive facial cellulitis with ipsilateral submandibular adenitis and pulmonary consolidation[59]; and inguinal, scrotal, prepatellar, or retropharyngeal cellulitis also occur. This organism can cause vesicles, bullae, and erosions that resemble impetigo. The lesions may be present at birth and appear anywhere on the body. Additional cutaneous manifestations of GBS infection include abscesses of the scalp, breast, submandibular gland, and subcutaneous tissue; erythema nodosum–like lesions; conjunctivitis; necrotizing fasciitis; acute necrotizing cellulitis of the scrotum; and purpura fulminans.

EXTRACUTANEOUS FINDINGS. Early-onset disease is characterized by septicemia, respiratory distress, apnea, shock, pneumonia, and meningitis in some cases (5% to 15%). Bacteremia without a focus of infection (40% to 50%) is the most common presentation of late-onset disease, although other foci such as osteomyelitis, septic arthritis, and cellulitis/adenitis may be found. Cellulitis usually is associated with bacteremia (90%).

ETIOLOGY/PATHOGENESIS. Cutaneous manifestations of GBS infection may be due to primary infection of the skin, often in association with surgery (e.g., circumcision) or cutaneous trauma (e.g., fetal scalp monitoring), or as a result of tertiary infection of the skin during bacteremia. Colonization of the neonate as a prelude to infection is thought to occur either in utero by ascension of organisms or during delivery. Approximately 30% of women are carriers of GBS, yet only 1% to 2% of their infants develop early-onset disease, indicating that neonatal infection reflects a complex interaction between host defenses and bacterial virulence factors. In general, the likelihood of neonatal infection increases with greater bacterial inoculum, duration of exposure, and immaturity of the host.[60] A viral infection commonly precedes development of late-onset disease, suggesting that alteration of epithelial surfaces may promote transepithelial entry of GBS into the bloodstream. Infants who develop either early- or late-onset disease have low levels of antibody to type III polysaccharide, one of the organism's major virulence factors.[61]

DIAGNOSIS. The organisms may be visualized on Gram stain and recovered in cultures from skin lesions. Because skin findings may be an early indicator of occult bacteremia, evaluation should include blood and CSF cultures and a chest radiograph.

DIFFERENTIAL DIAGNOSIS. Differential diagnosis includes other bacterial infections that cause nonnecrotizing (e.g., impetigo, cellulitis, abscesses) or necrotizing (e.g., necrotizing fasciitis) soft tissue infections or purpura fulminans in the neonate. Noninfectious dermatologic diseases that may mimic the skin lesions caused by GBS (e.g., impetigo-, cellulitis-, or abscess-like) also may need to be considered (see preceding sections).

COURSE/MANAGEMENT/TREATMENT/PROGNOSIS. Parenteral penicillin remains the drug of choice for GBS infection, but initial therapy for suspected GBS infection should consist of ampicillin and an aminoglycoside such as gentamicin, because this regimen provides broad coverage for the important pathogens in neonatal septicemia and synergic action against GBS. Once GBS has been identified as

the pathogen and the bloodstream and CSF have been shown to be sterile for 24 to 48 hours, penicillin G alone can be given.[60] The length of therapy required for treatment of GBS skin infections depends on the nature and severity of the skin infection and the involvement of other sites (e.g., bloodstream, meninges), but typically will be at least 10 days. Interestingly, many infants who present with facial cellulitis have been treated previously with systemic antibiotics, suggesting there may be sanctuary sites that harbor organisms.[62]

Coagulase-Negative Staphylococcus

DEFINITION. The normal human flora includes 13 species of coagulase-negative staphylococci (CONS). The CONS colonize the skin of most neonates within 2 to 4 days of birth,[63] are of relatively low virulence, and typically do not cause infection. In the neonatal period, however, they are an important cause of sepsis in preterm infants and may cause cutaneous infection. *Staphylococcus epidermidis* is the most prevalent member of this group, making up 60% to 90% of the CONS on the skin. The most virulent and most important causes of clinical disease are *S. epidermidis* and *Staphylococcus haemolyticus.*

CUTANEOUS FINDINGS. *S. epidermidis* is the most important cause of indwelling catheter–related infections. Infection can occur at the catheter exit site, along the tunnel, or at its site of insertion into the vessel. Occurrence at the latter two sites can lead to bacteremia. Signs of catheter-related cutaneous infection include erythema, tenderness, and the presence of exudate at the exit site.

The most common cutaneous infections in neonates resulting from CONS are omphalitis and abscesses, particularly of the breast and scalp (see preceding sections). Skin abscesses have been reported in a significant proportion (e.g., 40% in one series) of low birth weight infants with septicemia due to CONS.[64] Postoperative wound infections and purulent exudative conjunctivitis also may occur.

EXTRACUTANEOUS FINDINGS. These organisms typically cause indolent disease, although they are capable of producing fulminant infections. In developed countries, the CONS are the principal agents of sepsis in premature neonates.[64-66] They also are an important cause of septicemia in neonates in many developing countries. Additional extracutaneous infections caused by CONS include infective endocarditis, CSF shunt infections, necrotizing enterocolitis, pneumonia, urinary tract infection, and osteomyelitis.

ETIOLOGY/PATHOGENESIS. Infection occurs in those with disruption of host defense mechanisms resulting from surgery, placement of an indwelling medical devise, or immunosuppression. Overall, CONS infections are most important in preterm neonates, particularly those with an indwelling medical device, and in febrile immunocompromised oncology patients. Colonization of the skin is a prerequisite for infection, and development of disease generally requires compromise of the epidermal barrier. Heavy skin colonization is a risk factor for development of catheter-related infection.[67]

DIAGNOSIS. Gram stain and cultures of the skin and blood are required. Because this organism colonizes the skin, clinical correlation is necessary to determine if it is the cause of the clinical disease.

DIFFERENTIAL DIAGNOSIS. Skin infections resulting from CONS must be differentiated from infections caused by other bacterial pathogens.

COURSE/MANAGEMENT/TREATMENT/PROGNOSIS. Strict handwashing is paramount for limiting the spread of CONS within the neonatal nursery. Vancomycin generally is begun empirically when infection is suspected or demonstrated, because resistance to penicillin, methicillin (approximately 60%), and gentamicin is common among hospital-acquired isolates. All severe infections should be treated with vancomycin. The treatment regimen can be modified appropriately once antibiotic susceptibility results are available. Infections resulting from penicillin-susceptible, β-lactamase–negative organisms can be treated with penicillin. Nafcillin is effective for treatment of penicillin-resistant strains that are susceptible to penicillinase-resistant penicillins. Penicillinase-resistant isolates should also be considered cross-resistant to cephalosporins.

Listeria Monocytogenes

DEFINITION. L. monocytogenes is an uncommon cause of infection in newborn infants, with an incidence of 5.2 cases per 100,000 live births.[68] Outbreaks of perinatal listeriosis have been described, however.[69] Similar to infection with group B streptococcus, affected infants present with early-onset disease shortly after birth or a late-onset form that generally develops between 2 and 5 weeks of life, but skin lesions have only been described in early-onset disease.

CUTANEOUS FINDINGS. Lesions usually are evident at birth. Generalized petechiae and erythematous macules progress to erythematous pustules.[69,70] Purulent conjunctivitis also may occur. Focal infection may occur from direct skin inoculation.

EXTRACUTANEOUS FINDINGS. Neonates with early-onset disease generally are delivered prematurely to mothers with a febrile illness and are septicemic (80%). They may have concomitant involvement of the liver, adrenal gland,

kidneys, lymph nodes, lungs, gastrointestinal tract, spleen, heart, bone marrow, and brain.[71] Granulomatosis infantiseptica is a disseminated form of the disease that presents with widespread microabscesses and granulomatous lesions, particularly in the liver and spleen.

ETIOLOGY/PATHOGENESIS. L. monocytogenes is a gram-positive, motile coccobacillus that may resemble diphtheroids, cocci, or diplococci. It is usually transmitted via consumption or aspiration of contaminated meat, dairy products, or raw vegetables.[68] Affected pregnant women develop an influenza-like illness that may include vertical transmission to the fetus via hematogenous spread to the placenta, from an ascending vaginal infection, or during passage through the birth canal.[69] Rarely, infection may result from cross-contamination in the delivery suite or nursery. The highest concentrations of organisms are found in the lungs and gut of the neonate, suggesting that infection may typically be acquired in utero via infected amniotic fluid. The organism has a predilection for the placenta and, once invasive disease has occurred, the central nervous system.

DIAGNOSIS. A full sepsis evaluation should be performed in infants with suspected listeriosis, including bacterial cultures of the blood, urine, and CSF. The diagnosis may be aided by obtaining Gram stains and cultures from the maternal vagina, the amniotic fluid, and the infant's meconium, gastric washings, skin, posterior pharynx, and conjunctivae. Gram stain of meconium may be particularly revealing in granulomatosis infantiseptica. Cutaneous pustules show gram-positive rods, but the organism may appear as cocci in pairs and simulate pneumococcus. L. monocytogenes also can produce white plaques on the surface of the cord. Serologic tests are not useful due to lack of sensitivity.

DIFFERENTIAL DIAGNOSIS. Other pathogens that can cause a generalized vesiculopustular eruption must be excluded (see Chapter 10). The other pathogen that characteristically shows involvement of the umbilical cord is *Candida.*[72]

COURSE/MANAGEMENT/TREATMENT/PROGNOSIS. Infection acquired in utero may result in fetal demise or congenital listeriosis. Early-onset *Listeria* infection in the first 2 days of life carries a 30% mortality rate, although mortality rates up to 38% to 60% have been reported.[69,71] Initial therapy is parenteral ampicillin and an aminoglycoside such as gentamicin, which provides synergy against *L. monocytogenes.* After an adequate clinical response has been achieved, a course of therapy (10 to 14 days for invasive disease without meningitis, 2 to 3 weeks if meningitis is present) can be completed with ampicillin or penicillin alone.[73]

Mycobacterium Tuberculosis

DEFINITION. The risk of congenital tuberculosis (CT) has increased in the 1990s because of a 41% increase in the number of tuberculosis cases in women of childbearing age. This reflects an increase in tuberculosis incidence overall, due in part to the human immunodeficiency virus (HIV) epidemic, as well as increased international adoption and denial of nonemergent medical care to illegal immigrants. An infant is considered to have CT if proven tuberculous lesions and one of the following criteria are present: (1) tuberculous lesions in the first week of life; (2) a primary hepatic complex or hepatic granulomas; (3) tuberculous infection of the maternal genital tract or placenta; or, (4) exclusion of postnatal transmission of tuberculosis by a thorough investigation of contacts.[74] It is not always possible to distinguish neonatal tuberculosis from CT. However, the distinction is not important for treatment, but identification of the person and means of infecting the infant postnatally is important to halt spread of infection in the community.

CUTANEOUS FINDINGS. Cutaneous findings in CT are unusual and include scaly, erythematous, umbilicated papules and subcutaneous nodules.[75] Infants with postnatal genital tuberculosis following circumcision may present with firm, nontender, enlarged, inguinal lymph nodes that progress to ulcerated, suppurative, bilateral, inguinal lymphadenopathy with sinus tract formation. Extensive ulceration of the penis and scrotum and varicella-like cutaneous lesions also have been described.[76]

EXTRACUTANEOUS FINDINGS. Newborns with CT frequently are premature and have low birth weight. They may be symptomatic at birth, but illness more commonly presents during the second to fourth weeks of life with poor feeding, listlessness, respiratory distress, fever, hepatosplenomegaly, abdominal distension, ear discharge, and lymphadenopathy.[74] Most have an abnormal chest radiograph (e.g., hilar lymphadenopathy, parenchymal infiltrates), and approximately 50% have a miliary pattern. Meningitis is present in about 20% of cases.

Infants with postnatally acquired tuberculosis may present with fever, lethargy, respiratory distress, cough, vomiting, weight loss, lymphadenopathy, anemia, and hepatosplenomegaly approximately 4 weeks to several months after birth.[76]

ETIOLOGY/PATHOGENESIS. Although acid-fast bacilli can be identified in the placenta of 50% of women with tuberculosis,[74] congenital infection is quite rare. Infected mothers with miliary tuberculosis are most apt to transmit the disease, although the affected infant's mother also may have tuberculous pleural effusion, meningitis, or endometritis. Women with only pulmonary tuberculosis are unlikely to infect the infant until after birth. CT is thought to be acquired primarily via transplacental spread of M. tuberculosis through the umbilical vein. This may produce a primary focus of infection in the liver, with involvement of the periportal lymph nodes and secondary hematogenous spread to the lungs, spleen, other viscera, and the central nervous system.[74]

Tuberculosis in the neonate rarely is acquired postnatally by inhalation or ingestion of infected droplets, ingestion of infected milk, or contamination of traumatized skin or mucous membranes. Inhalation is the most common route of postnatal infection, but may be impossible to distinguish from infection acquired in utero. Infection of the skin of the head and neck or the oral mucous membranes, associated with regional lymphadenopathy, may occur by kissing. In the past, tuberculosis of the skin and mucous membranes of the male genitalia was reported 1 to 4 weeks following ritual circumcision by an infected operator.[77]

DIAGNOSIS. CT should be suspected in any infant who presents with a sepsis-like syndrome, negative bacterial cultures, and lack of response to antibiotic therapy. Diagnosis is confirmed by identification of M. tuberculosis in tissue (e.g., liver, lymph node, bone marrow, skin) or fluid from the stomach, trachea, urinary tract, bone marrow, middle ear, or pleural spaces. False-positive smears from gastric aspirates in a newborn are rare. The CSF frequently is negative. Acid-fast stains are helpful if they are positive. Because M. tuberculosis is slow growing, it may take up to 10 weeks to detect the organism on solid media; use of a DNA probe may allow earlier detection. The Mantoux skin test, performed with 5 TU PPD, usually is negative and may take 3 weeks to 3 months to become positive. The placenta should be examined and cultured, and the mother evaluated for the presence of tuberculosis, including uterine infection.

COURSE/MANAGEMENT/TREATMENT/PROGNOSIS. The course of CT may vary from acute and fulminant, to subacute and insidious. The overall mortality is 38% without treatment and 22% with treatment.[74] Treatment for CT and postnatally acquired disease is the same and should be initiated promptly, regardless of skin test results, with isoniazid, rifampin, pyrazinamide, and streptomycin or kanamycin. Drug susceptibility of the isolate from the infant and/or mother will help direct therapy. Identification of the source for infection of the neonate is important to prevent infection of others.

GRAM-NEGATIVE INFECTIONS

DEFINITION. Although gram-negative infections are a frequent cause of serious bacterial illness in the newborn period, cutaneous manifestations are uncommon.

CUTANEOUS FINDINGS. Gram-negative bacteria occasionally cause a wide variety of cutaneous lesions typically associated with infections caused by *S. aureus* or *S. pyogenes* or mixed infections, including impetigo; abscesses of the breast, scalp, perirectal region, salivary glands, or subcutaneous tissue; paronychia; blepharitis; dacryocystitis; omphalitis; cellulitis; nodular cellulitis; necrotizing funisitis; and necrotizing fasciitis. *P. aeruginosa* may secondarily infect previously traumatized skin such as atopic dermatitis; characteristically, it produces a blue-green exudate and a fruity, mouselike odor. Cutaneous findings resulting from gram-negative organisms also may result from septic emboli. These tertiary lesions may appear as generalized petechiae, erythematous papules, purpuric patches, deep-seated nodules, abscesses, erythema multiform-like lesions, and nonhemorrhagic and hemorrhagic vesicles and pustules. Cellulitis and abscesses caused by *E. coli*, and ecthyma gangrenosum (see the following discussion) and other tertiary lesions caused by *P. aeruginosa*, are the most common cutaneous manifestation of gram-negative infections. *Pseudomonas* septicemia also may be associated with noma, a condition characterized by gangrenous lesions of the nose, lips, and mouth.

EXTRACUTANEOUS FINDINGS. Gram-negative organisms can cause bacteremia, sepsis, and multiorgan disease including meningitis, pneumonia, osteomyelitis, necrotizing enterocolitis, and liver abscesses.

ETIOLOGY/PATHOGENESIS. *E. coli*, *P. aeruginosa*, *Klebsiella pneumoniae*, *Serratia marcescens*, *Aeromonas spp.*, *P. mirabilis*, *Acinetobacter*, *Gardnerella vaginalis*, *Clostridium perfringens*, *Achromobacter*, and *Alcaligenes faecalis*, are a few of the gram-negative organisms responsible for infections in the neonatal period.

DIAGNOSIS. A complete sepsis evaluation including Gram stain and cultures of the blood, urine, CSF, and skin lesions is essential. Culture of the placenta, maternal cervix, and lochia also may be revealing. Histopathology is particularly helpful if ecthyma gangrenosum is a diagnostic consideration (see the following section).

DIFFERENTIAL DIAGNOSIS. Skin infections caused by gram-negative organisms must be differentiated from infections caused by gram-positive organisms such as *S. aureus*, *S. pyogenes*, and *L. monocytogenes*; viral infections such as neonatal varicella, HSV, and cytomegalovirus; and fungal infections such as congenital cutaneous candidiasis; as well as noninfectious dermatologic diseases that may mimic infectious skin lesions.

COURSE/MANAGEMENT/TREATMENT/PROGNOSIS. Development of skin lesions potentially caused by gram-negative organisms in the neonate mandates a full sepsis workup and prompt broad-spectrum parenteral antibiotic administration. Choice of antibiotics is based on the environment in which the infection was acquired (i.e., home versus hospital); the relative prevalence of pathogens in the nursery or the community; the antibiotic susceptibilities of organisms recently isolated in the nursery or the community; the CSF penetration of the antibiotics; the infant's hepatic and renal function; and the likely organism based on the patient's age and birth weight, immunologic status, prior antibiotic therapy, presence of a foreign body such as an indwelling catheter, and the clinical appearance of the patient and the skin infection. Empiric therapy for early-onset infections may be initiated with ampicillin and either an aminoglycoside (first-line) or possibly cefotaxime (second-line).[78,79] Treatment of nosocomially acquired infection may be best accomplished initially with methicillin, oxacillin, or nafcillin and cefotaxime, or with vancomycin and ceftazidime. Empiric therapy varies for late-onset infections; in general, however, nafcillin and an aminoglycoside are recommended for skin infections possibly resulting from gram-negative organisms.[79] Once the culture and susceptibility results are available, therapy may be tailored appropriately. In general, if a gram-negative enteric isolate is susceptible to both ampicillin and aminoglycosides, administration of both drugs for at least a portion of the treatment period is prudent. For treatment of *Pseudomonas* infections, combination therapy with ticarcillin, piperacillin, or ceftazidime plus an aminoglycoside should be continued for the duration of treatment. In general, antimicrobial therapy should be continued for 5 to 7 days after clinical signs and symptoms of infection have disappeared. The appropriate length of therapy will vary with the infecting organism, however, and might best be determined in consultation with infectious disease colleagues. Incision and drainage will enhance resolution of suppurative lesions.

Ecthyma Gangrenosum

DEFINITION. Ecthyma gangrenosum refers to necrotic skin lesions caused by *Pseudomonas* infection.[80,81,82]

CUTANEOUS FINDINGS. The lesion begins as a painful red or purpuric macule, which develops a pustular or vesicular center with a surrounding rim of pink or violaceous skin and then rapidly ulcerates (Fig. 11-7, *A*). The infection also may present with bullae. The ulcer develops raised edges with a necrotic, dense, black, depressed, and crusted center. Erythema multiforme–like lesions also have been described at onset. Lesions may be single or multiple and sometimes cluster around areas of moisture such as the mouth or perineum (Fig. 11-7, *B*).

EXTRACUTANEOUS FINDINGS. Most infants with ecthyma gangrenosum are septic, and skin lesions result from bacteremic spread of infection, but nonsepticemic variants have been described in newborns.

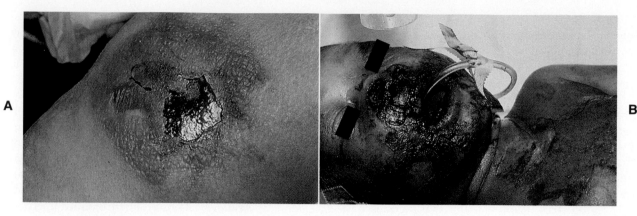

FIG. 11-7
A, Hemorrhagic, ulcerated bulla of ecthyma gangrenosum due to *Pseudomonas aeruginosa*. **B,** *Pseudomonas septicemia* with periorificial accentuation of ecthyma gangrenosum.

ETIOLOGY/PATHOGENESIS. Ecthyma gangrenosum is due to *P. aeruginosa*. Prematurity, prolonged illness, neutropenia, necrotizing enterocolitis, previous bowel surgery, and immunocompromise are risk factors in neonates and young infants. The disease can also occur de novo as a primary cutaneous infection due to direct inoculation.

DIAGNOSIS/DIFFERENTIAL DIAGNOSIS. Lesions of ecthyma gangrenosum mandate a full sepsis work-up, tissue examination for Gram stain and culture, and histopathology. Gram stain is best performed on scrapings from the base of the ulceration. Histopathologic examination allows distinction of this entity from streptococcal ecthyma. A pauci-inflammatory vasculitis particularly of the veins with surrounding edema, hemorrhage, and necrosis, is seen. Bacteria may be seen in the perivascular tissue and occasionally in the vessel walls, particularly the adventitia and media of dermal veins but not arteries; the intima and lumina generally are spared. Similar lesions rarely can develop as a result of infection with other agents such as *Aeromonas hydrophila, Enterobacter* spp., *E. coli, Proteus* spp., *Pseudomonas cepacia, S. marcescens, Xanthomonas maltophilia, Aspergillus* spp., Mucorales, and *C. albicans*.

COURSE/MANAGEMENT/TREATMENT/PROGNOSIS. Ecthyma gangrenosum in association with bacteremia is a grave sign. Aggressive empiric therapy should be initiated with an extended-spectrum penicillin (e.g., ticarcillin or piperacillin) or ceftazidime in combination with an aminoglycoside. Once the culture and susceptibility results are available, therapy may be narrowed. If the infection proves to be caused by *Pseudomonas*, combination therapy (i.e., ticarcillin, piperacillin, or ceftazidime plus an aminoglycoside) should be continued for the duration of treatment.

Neisseria Meningitidis

Purpura Fulminans

DEFINITION. Purpura fulminans (PF) is a potentially disabling and life-threatening disorder characterized by acute onset of progressive cutaneous hemorrhage and necrosis caused by dermal vascular thrombosis, and disseminated intravascular necrosis (DIC).[83] In the neonate, most cases are a result of a congenital abnormality of coagulation (see Chapter 17), but may be caused by an acute infectious illness, particularly sepsis with endotoxin-producing gram-negative bacteria such as *N. meningitidis* or GBS.[84,85]

CUTANEOUS FINDINGS. Cutaneous erythema with or without edema and petechiae develops first. Sites of involvement appear transiently to resemble ecchymoses, and up to this point the pathologic process in the skin is reversible without progression to necrosis. Lesions evolve rapidly into painful, indurated, well-demarcated, irregularly bordered purpuric papules and plaques surrounded by a thin, advancing erythematous border. Late findings in necrotic areas are the formation of vesicles and bullae, which mark the development of hemorrhagic necrosis (Fig. 11-8), and finally firm eschar, which ultimately sloughs. The distal extremities often are most severely involved, usually in a symmetric manner, probably resulting from the presence of fewer collateral channels for tissue perfusion, and the relatively greater impact of circulatory collapse on perfusion of distal vascular beds. Acute infectious PF tends to progress proximally to form purpuric plaques of various sizes and shapes in a patchy distribution.

EXTRACUTANEOUS FINDINGS. Shock is characteristic of acute infectious PF, and development of systemic con-

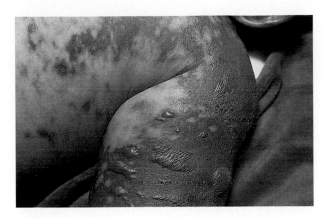

FIG. 11-8
Petechiae and purpuric plaques of purpura fulminans due to *N. meningitidis*.

sumptive coagulopathy (i.e., DIC) is a defining feature. Thrombohemorrhagic manifestations may be found in multiple vascular beds and organ systems, and multiple organ dysfunction syndrome is common. Massive nontraumatic subdural hematoma can occur in extremely premature infants. Fibrinogen, coagulation factors (e.g., factor V and factor VIII), and platelets are consumed in ongoing thrombosis and fibrinolysis. Prothrombin time (PT) and partial thromboplastin time (PTT) are prolonged; fibrin degradation products (e.g., D-dimers) are elevated; and protein C, protein S, and antithrombin III levels are reduced.

ETIOLOGY/PATHOGENESIS. Purpura fulminans develops in 15% to 25% of individuals with menigococcemia.[86] In the neonate, acute infectious PF may be caused by early- or late-onset GBS, or occasionally a number of other gram-positive and gram-negative pathogens.

The histopathologic changes in acute infectious PF are essentially identical to those of the Shwartzman reaction.[87] The local Shwartzman reaction is a hemorrhagic and necrotizing inflammatory lesion provoked by the injection of endotoxin from gram-negative bacteria. Central to the pathogenesis of the Shwartzman reaction and PF is a disturbance in the balance of anticoagulant and procoagulant activities of endothelial cells, with a shift from a quiescent state favoring anticoagulation to a disease state of overwhelming procoagulation. This disturbance, which is triggered by endotoxin, appears to be mediated by cytokines, particularly interleukin(IL)-2, interferon-γ, tumor necrosis factor (TNF)-β and IL-1, leading to consumption of proteins C and S and antithrombin III.[83]

DIAGNOSIS. Preliminary identification of *N. meningitidis* as the cause of PF can sometimes be made by finding the gram-negative diplococci on Gram stain of material obtained by needle aspiration of a petechial skin lesion,[88] or by scraping the lesion with a needle and making a smear of blood.[89]

The histopathologic hallmarks of PF are dermal vascular thrombosis and secondary hemorrhagic necrosis.[90] Vasculitis, including a perivascular neutrophilic infiltrate, is a characteristic feature.

DIFFERENTIAL DIAGNOSIS. Purpura fulminans in the neonatal period may be a manifestation of inherited, homozygous protein C, or rarely, protein S deficiency (see Chapter 17).[85] PF in the neonate must be differentiated from other causes of skin necrosis (e.g., neonatal cold injury, vascular compromise from umbilical arterial catheterization, cutaneous infiltration of substances such as calcium). Development of DIC distinguishes acute infectious PF from other forms of skin necrosis caused by dermal vascular occlusion such as warfarin- or heparin-induced skin necrosis, thrombotic thrombocytopenic purpura, cryoglobulinemia, antiphospholipid syndrome, or paroxysmal nocturnal hemoglobinuria.

COURSE/MANAGEMENT/TREATMENT/PROGNOSIS. Size of skin hemorrhage increases with disease severity,[91] and the presence of purpura, particularly when generalized, is associated with high morbidity and mortality, as it reflects a profound disturbance in hemostatic mechanisms.[92] Many who survive PF have cutaneous and/or skeletal deformities resulting from gangrene.

Initial management of the patient with acute infectious PF must be focused on preserving life through respiratory and hemodynamic support and prompt broad-spectrum intravenous antibiotic coverage. Antibiotic therapy can be adjusted after the organism has been recovered and its susceptibility profile has been determined. Penicillin remains the drug of choice for susceptible isolates of *N. meningitidis*. Surgical consultation should be sought early in the course to monitor compartment pressures and intervene in compartment syndrome. Nutritional support is also important and should be continued during the rehabilitative phase.

Therapeutic interventions that should be initiated for all patients with PF and DIC include vitamin K and fresh frozen plasma (FFP, 8 to 12 mg/kg every 12 hours) to correct possible deficiencies of vitamin K-dependent coagulation factors, antithrombin III, protein C, and protein S.

A number of other newer, nonconventional treatment modalities are available in some centers, including concentrates of protein C or antithrombin III, recombinant tissue-type plasminogen activator, prostacyclin, plasmapheresis, hyperbaric oxygen, and a host of targeted immunotherapies (e.g., IL-1 receptor antagonist, monoclonal antibody to TNF-β, anti-endotoxin antibodies, platelet-activating factor receptor antagonist, and pentoxifylline).[83] Recommendations regarding their use await the results of double-blinded, randomized, controlled studies.

Close contacts of patients with invasive meningococcal disease should receive prophylaxis with rifampin (or possibly ciprofloxacin for those 18 years or older) as soon as possible. Patients with complement or properdin deficiency should be vaccinated with tetravalent meningococcal vaccine (A/C/Y/W135) after the age of 2 years.

Treponema Pallidum

DEFINITION. Congenital syphilis (CS) occurs in infants born to mothers infected with the spirochete *T. pallidum*. In the 1980s and 1990s, the number of reported cases of CS and maternal syphilis increased in the United States. Almost half of neonates with CS had mothers who did not receive prenatal care.[93] The lack of historical and laboratory data for making a diagnosis of CS in these cases emphasizes the importance of recognizing the dermatologic features of the disease.

Congenital syphilis is divided into early and late disease. Early disease usually presents before 3 months of age, although signs can appear anytime in the first 2 years of life. Late disease appears after age 2 years.

CUTANEOUS FINDINGS. Overall, approximately half of newborns with CS are asymptomatic at birth. Cutaneous findings, although highly variable, are present in only 38% of affected newborns.[94] Palmar/plantar, perioral, and anogenital regions are classically involved. Mucous membrane involvement may present as snuffles (syphilitic rhinitis), often the first sign of CS. It begins as a clear nasal discharge that may be mistaken clinically for a viral upper respiratory infection and may become profuse, chronic, and/or bloody. Associated inflammation and ulceration of the nasal mucosae can result in perforation of the nasal septum with subsequent alteration of the nasal cartilage (saddle nose deformity). Condyloma lata refers to the highly infectious flat-topped papules and plaques that occur at the mucocutaneous junctions of the nares, angles of the mouth, and in the anogenital region; chronic induration in these areas leads to rhagades, or linear scars, which fan out from the corners of the mouth and the affected orifices. Mucous patches also may occur on the lips, tongue, and palate.[95] Other early findings include petechiae (usually from thrombocytopenia), hemorrhagic vesicles and bullae (pemphigus syphiliticus), and erythematous macular, papulosquamous, annular, or polymorphous eruptions (Fig. 11-9). The papulosquamous eruption is most common on the posterior aspects, particularly the buttocks, back, and thighs in addition to the soles. Although the papulosquamous rash resembles the coppery-red eruption of acquired secondary syphilis, pemphigus syphiliticus is unique to the newborn. Bullae form on an indurated, red base, and rupture easily, leaving a macerated base that may form crust. Changes on the palms and soles include erythema with a polished appearance; superficial peeling; indurated fissures; and oval ham-colored macules and papules that acquire a coppery-brown color as they age.[95] Nail deformities, paronychia, and alopecia may occur. Untreated skin lesions resolve in 1 to 3 months with postinflammatory hyperpigmentation and/or hypopigmentation, but dyspigmentation is infrequent in the newborn period.

EXTRACUTANEOUS FINDINGS. CS commonly presents with extracutaneous findings that include low birth

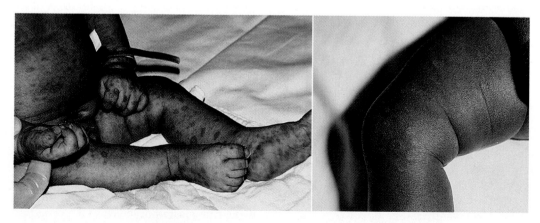

FIG. 11-9
Papulosquamous plaques in two infants with syphilis.

weight, hepatomegaly with elevation of serum alkaline phosphatase, splenomegaly, anemia, thrombocytopenia, jaundice, osteochondritis, generalized lymphadenopathy, respiratory distress, hydrops fetalis, meningitis, meningoencephalitis, nephrotic syndrome, chorioretinitis, and pseudoparalysis.[94]

Late manifestations of CS (i.e., appearing after 2 years of age) involve the central nervous system (neurosyphilis, which may be asymptomatic), bones (frontal bossing, saddle nose, concave central face, saber shins, Clutton's joints), teeth (Hutchinson peg-shaped notched central incisors, mulberry multicuspid first molars), skin (rhagades, nodular syphilides, gummata), eyes (interstitial keratitis, optic atrophy), and ears (eighth nerve deafness).[96] Hutchinson's triad of defects in the incisors, interstitial keratitis, and sensorineural hearing loss is pathognomonic.

ETIOLOGY/PATHOGENESIS. Infection occurs by invasion of the placenta by the spirochete *T. pallidum.* The organism enters the bloodstream directly and invades the liver with subsequent invasion of other organs, principally the skin, mucous membranes, bones, and central nervous system. Infection can occur at any time during pregnancy or at birth. Spirochetes preferentially adhere to endothelial cells and induce vasculitis. Nearly all neonates born to mothers with primary or secondary syphilis have congenital infection, but only about 50% are clinically symptomatic at birth.[97] A high percentage will be preterm and at high risk for neurologic complications. Up to 25% to 40% die in utero.[98] Neonates infected during the third trimester typically are normal at birth, and although they may become ill during the first weeks of life, the most common age of onset is 2 to 6 weeks of life.

DIAGNOSIS. The laboratory diagnosis of CS may be difficult because false positive and negative serologies confound interpretation and because *T. pallidum* cannot be cultured on artificial media.[96] Maternal nontreponemal and treponemal IgG antibodies are present in the fetus as a result of transplacental transfer even if the mother was adequately treated during pregnancy. Serum should be taken from the infant, rather than from cord blood, to increase the accuracy of serologic test results.[99] The diagnosis of CS can be made by demonstration of spirochetes within a clinical specimen, obtained by scraping the base of a mucocutaneous lesion, using dark field microscopy or direct fluorescent antibody testing. Specimens from mouth lesions require direct fluorescent antibody techniques to distinguish *T. pallidum* from commensal oral spirochetes. Histopathologic examination of the placenta and umbilical cord using specific fluorescent antitreponemal antibody staining also is recommended. If a serum nontreponemal titer (VDRL, RPR) in the infant is ≥ 4 times the mother's level, then the diagnosis of congenital syphilis is made; a titer ≤ 4 times that of the mother, however, does not exclude CS. Nontreponemal tests in both an infected mother and her congenitally infected infant may be falsely negative if the mother acquired the disease late in pregnancy or in the case of a prozone phenomenon. False-positive reactivity of nontreponemal tests can be caused by certain infectious diseases (e.g., hepatitis, varicella, measles, infectious mononucleosis, tuberculosis, malaria, endocarditis), malignancies (e.g., lymphoma), and connective tissue disease (e.g., systemic lupus erythematosus). The nontreponemal tests are useful for screening, and if reactive, should always be confirmed using a treponemal test. Treponemal tests (FTA-ABS, MHA-TP) also are not 100% specific for syphilis, however, since reactivity may occur in patients with other spirochetal diseases such as yaws, pinta, bejel, leptospirosis, rat-bite fever, and Lyme disease. The most helpful specific serologic test is a serum IgM against *T. pallidum* (IgM FTA-ABS).[100] A CSF VDRL test should be performed on all neonates evaluated for CS. A negative result does not exclude neurosyphilis, however; conversely, a false-positive result may occur in an uninfected newborn with a transplacentally acquired high serum VDRL titer. Newer techniques may improve our diagnostic capabilities, including immunoblotting to detect IgM against a 47 kD membrane protein and PCR amplification of the genomic region encoding this same membrane protein.[101] A skin biopsy is helpful in the evaluation of CS and shows swelling and proliferation of endothelial cells, and a predominantly perivascular infiltrate composed of lymphoid cells and plasma cells.

Radiographic abnormalities are particularly important since they are present in up to 95% of symptomatic and 20% of asymptomatic neonates with CS.[102] Multiple long bones tend to be affected symmetrically, particularly the lower extremities. The metaphyseal lesions of osteochondritis vary from radiopaque bands to punctate lucencies or mottled regions; diaphyseal lesions appear as periosteal new bone formation.

DIFFERENTIAL DIAGNOSIS. As a result of the variable morphology of the lesions and the broad differential diagnosis it engenders, syphilis has been called "the great imitator." Blistering in CS must be differentiated from other vesiculobullous conditions that involve the palms and soles, including but not limited to congenital candidiasis, acropustulosis of infancy, scabies, and epidermolysis bullosa (see Chapter 10). Congenital Lyme borreliosis has been described.[103] Nontreponemal tests can be used to differentiate Lyme disease from syphilis because the VDRL test is nonreactive in the former condition.

COURSE/MANAGEMENT/TREATMENT/PROGNOSIS. If an infant cannot be fully evaluated, or if adequate follow-up is uncertain, then empiric treatment is recommended.[104] For infants with proven or probable CS (see Centers for Disease Control and Prevention [CDC] guidelines),[98] a 10- to 14-day course of parenteral aqueous crystalline penicillin G is the treatment of choice. A sustained fourfold decrease in titer of the nontreponemal test is indicative of successful treatment; the nontreponemal test usually becomes nonreactive within 2 years of successful treatment in CS. It is recommended that infants treated for CS have follow-up examinations at 1, 2, 4, 6, and 12 months of age, including nontreponemal tests at 3, 6, and 12 months after treatment or until they become nonreactive. If the infant was not infected and nontreponemal tests initially were positive as a result of transplacentally acquired maternal antibody, then the antibody titer should decline by 3 months of age and be nonreactive at age 6 months. A fourfold increase in titer following treatment suggests reinfection or relapse; patients with persistent, stable low titers also should be considered for retreatment. Treated infants should be followed with a CSF examination at 6-month intervals until the examination becomes nonreactive. A reactive CSF VDRL at 6 months, or cell counts that are abnormal or not steadily decreasing, are indications for retreatment.[104] Positive MHA-TP and FTA-ABS treponemal tests usually remain reactive for life despite successful treatment. The prognosis in promptly treated early congenital syphilis is excellent.

REFERENCES

1. Roth R, James W. Microbiology of the skin: Resident flora, ecology, infection. J Am Acad Dermatol 1989;20:367-390.
2. Darmstadt G. Staphylococcal and streptococcal skin infections. In Harahap M, ed. Diagnosis and treatment of skin infections. Oxford: Blackwell Scientific Publications, 1997: pp 7-115.
3. Darmstadt G, Fleckman P, Rubens C. TNF-α and IL-1α decrease the adherence of *Streptococcus pyogenes* to keratinocytes. J Infect Dis 1999, 180:1718-1721.
4. Darmstadt G, Fleckman P, Jonas M, et al. Differentiation of cultured keratinocytes promotes the adherence of *Streptococcus pyogenes.* J Clin Invest 1998;101:128-136.
5. Darmstadt G, Fleckman P, Rubens C. Role of keratinocyte injury in adherence of *Streptococcus pyogenes.* Infect Immon 1999; 67:6707-6709.
6. Darmstadt G, Marcy S. Skin and soft tissue infections. In Long SS, Prober CG, Pickering LK, eds. Principles and practice of pediatric infectious diseases. New York: Churchill Livingstone, 1996: pp 476-517.
7. Williams M, Hanley K, Elias P, et al. Ontogeny of the epidermal permeability barrier. J Invest Dermatol 1998;3:75-79.
8. Darmstadt G. Oral antibiotic therapy for uncomplicated bacterial skin infections in children. Pediatr Infect Dis J 1997;16:227-240.
9. Darmstadt G. Superficial streptococcal and staphylococcal infections. Contemp Pediatr 1997;14:95-116.
10. Darmstadt G. Scarlet fever and its relatives. Contemp Pediatr 1998;15:44-63.
11. Darmstadt G, Rose V, Smith B, et al. Preventing postnatal infections in the preterm infant: a national survey of neonatal skin care practices. Submitted, 2000.
12. Darmstadt G, Lane AT. Impetigo: An overview. Pediatr Dermatol 1994;11:293-303.
13. Lookingbill D. Impetigo. Pediatr Rev 1985;7:177-181.
14. Tunnessen W Jr. A survey of skin disorders seen in pediatric general and dermatology clinics. Pediatr Dermatol 1984; 1:219-222.
15. Leyden J, Marples R, Kligman A. *Staphylococcus aureus* in the lesions of atopic dermatitis. Br J Dermatol 1974;90:525-530.
16. Hebert A, Esterly N. Bacterial and candidal cutaneous infections in the neonate. Dermatol Clin 1986;4:3-21.
17. Dillon H Jr. Impetigo contagiosa: suppurative and non-suppurative complications. Clinical, bacteriologic, and epidemiologic characteristics of impetigo. Am J Dis Child 1968;115:530-541.
18. Wannamaker L. Differences between streptococcal infections of the throat and of the skin. N Engl J Med 1970; 282:23-31.
19. Elias P, Fritsch P, Dahl M, et al. Staphylococcal toxic epidermal necrolysis: Pathogenesis and studies on the subcellular site of action of exfoliatin. J Invest Dermatol 1975;65:501-512.
20. Darmstadt G. Antibiotics in the management of pediatric skin disease. Dermatol Clin 1998;16:509-525.
21. Darmstadt G. A guide to abscesses in the skin. Contemp Pediatr 1999;16:135-145.
22. Brook I, Finegold S. Aerobic and anaerobic bacteriology of cutaneous abscesses in children. Pediatrics 1981;67:891-895.
23. Rudoy R, Nelson J. Breast abscess during the neonatal period. A review. Am J Dis Child 1975;129:1031-1034.
24. Walsh M, McIntosh K.: Neonatal mastitis. Clin Pediatr (Phila) 1986;25:395-399.
25. Brook I. The aerobic and anaerobic microbiology of neonatal breast abscess. Pediatr Infect Dis J 1991;10:785-786.
26. Wagener M, Rycheck R, Yee RB, et al. Septic dermatitis of the neonatal scalp and maternal endomyometritis with intrapartum internal fetal monitoring. Pediatrics 1984;74:81-85.
27. Okada D, Chow A: Neonatal scalp abscess following intrapartum fetal monitoring: Prospective comparison of two spiral electrodes. Am J Obstet Gynecol 1977;127:875-878.
28. Brook I. Aerobic and anaerobic microbiology of paronychia. Ann Emerg Med 1990;19:994-996.
29. Guvenc H, Aygun A, Yasar F, et al. Omphalitis in term and preterm appropriate for gestational age and small for gestational age infants. J Trop Pediatr 1997;43:368-372.
30. McKenna H, Johnson D. Bacteria in neonatal omphalitis. Pathology 1977;9:111-113.
31. Molarte A, Isenberg S: Periorbital cellulitis in infancy. J Pediatr Ophthalmol Strabismus 1989;26:232-235.
32. Howe P, Eduardo Fajardo J, Orcutt M. Etiologic diagnosis of cellulitis: Comparison of aspirates obtained from the leading edge and the point of maximal inflammation. Pediatr Infect Dis J 1987;6:685-686.
33. Goldberg G, Hansen R, Lynch P. Necrotizing fasciitis in infancy: Report of three cases and review of the literature. Pediatr Dermatol 1984;2:55-63.

34. Hsiech W, et al. A review of 66 cases of neonatal necrotizing fasciitis. Pediatrics 1999;103(4):e53.

35. Stevens D. Invasive group A streptococcus infections. Clin Infect Dis 1992;14:2-11.

36. Brogan T, Nizet V, Waldhausen J, et al. Group A streptococcal necrotizing fasciitis complicating primary varicella: A series of fourteen patients. Pediatr Infect Dis J 1995;14:588-594.

37. Sawin R, Schaller R, Tapper D, et al. Early recognition of neonatal abdominal wall necrotizing fasciitis. Am J Surg 1994;167:481-484.

38. Stamenkovic I, Lew P. Early recognition of potentially fatal necrotizing fasciitis. The use of frozen-section biopsy. N Engl J Med 1984;310:1689-1693.

39. Stevens D, Tanner M, Winship J, et al. Severe group A streptococcal infections associated with a toxic shock-like syndrome and scarlet fever toxin A. N Engl J Med 1989;321:1-7.

40. Elias P, Fritsch P, Epstein E. Staphylococcal scalded skin syndrome. Clinical features, pathogenesis, and recent microbiological and biochemical developments. Arch Dermatol 1977,113:207-219.

41. Saiman L, Jakob K, Holmes KW, et al. Molecular epidemiology of staphylococcal scalded skin syndrome in premature infants. Pediatr Infect Dis J 1998;17:329-334.

42. Melish M, Glasgow L. Staphylococcal scalded skin syndrome: The expanded clinical syndrome. J Pediatr 1971; 78:958-967.

43. Elias P, Fritsch P, Tappeiner G, et al. Experimental staphylococcal toxic epidermal necrolysis (TEN) in adult humans and mice. J Lab Clin Med 1974;84:414-424.

44. Raymond J, Bingen E, Brahimi N, et al. Staphylococcal scalded skin syndrome in a neonate. Eur J Clin Microbiol Infect Dis 1997;16:453-454.

45. Stevens D. Invasive group A streptococcal infections: The past, present and future. Pediatr Infect Dis J 1994;13:561-566.

46. Bingen E, Denamur E, Lambert-Zechovsky N, et al. Mother-to-infant vertical transmission and cross-colonization of Streptococcus pyogenes confirmed by DNA restriction fragment length polymorphism analysis. J Infect Dis 1992; 165:147-150.

47. Ferrieri P, Dajani A, Wannamaker L, et al. Natural history of impetigo. Site sequence of acquisition and familial patterns of spread of cutaneous streptococci. J Clin Invest 1972; 51:2851-2862.

48. Dajani A, Ferrieri P, Wannamaker L: Natural history of impetigo. Etiologic agents and bacterial interactions. J Clin Invest 1972,51:2863-2871.

49. Stevens D, Gibbons A, Bergstrom R, et al. The Eagle effect revisited: Efficacy of clindamycin, erythromycin, and penicillin in the treatment of streptococcal myositis. J Infect Dis 1988;158:23-28.

50. The Working Group on Severe Streptococcal Infections. Defining the group A streptococcal toxic shock syndrome. Rationale and consensus definition. JAMA 1993;269:390-391.

51. Belani K, Schlievert P, Kaplan E, et al. Association of exotoxin-producing group A streptococci and severe disease in children. Pediatr Infect Dis J 1991;10:351-354.

52. Cone L, Woodard D, Schlievert P, et al. Clinical and bacteriologic observations of a toxic shock-like syndrome due to Streptococcus pyogenes. N Engl J Med 1987;317:146-149.

53. Bradley J, Schlievert P, Peterson B. Toxic shock-like syndrome, a complication of strep throat [letter]. Pediatr Infect Dis J 1991;10:790.

54. Mahieu L, Holm S, Goossens H, et al. Congenital streptococcal toxic shock syndrome with absence of antibodies against streptococcal pyrogenic exotoxins. J Pediatr 1995; 127:987-989.

55. Wolf J, Rabinowitz L. Streptococcal toxic shock-like syndrome. Arch Dermatol 1995;131:73-77.

56. Novotny W, Faden H, Mosovich L. Emergence of invasive group A streptococcal disease among young children. Clin Pediatr (Phila) 1992;31:596-601.

57. Bisno A, Stevens D. Streptococcal infections of skin and soft tissues. N Engl J Med 1996;334:240-245.

58. Lopez J, Gross P, Boggs T. Skin lesions in association with beta-hemolytic Streptococcus group B. Pediatrics 1976; 58:859-861.

59. Baker C. Group B streptococcal cellulitis-adenitis in infants. Am J Dis Child 1982;136:631-633.

60. Baker C, Edwards M. Streptococcus agalactiae (group B streptococcus). In Long S, Pickering L, and Prober C, eds. Principles and practice of pediatric infectious diseases. New York: Churchill Livingstone, 1998: pp 812-818.

61. Martin T, Ruzinski J, Rubens C, et al. The effect of type-specific polysaccharide capsule on the clearance of groups B streptococci from the lungs of infant and adult rats. J Infect Dis 1992;165:306-314.

62. Rand T. Group B streptococcal cellulitis in infants: A disease modified by prior antibiotic therapy or hospitalization? Pediatrics 1988;81:63-65.

63. D'Angio C, McGowan K, Baumgart S, et al. Surface colonization with coagulase-negative staphylococci in premature neonates. J Pediatr 1989;114:1029-1034.

64. Patrick C. Coagulase-negative staphylococci: pathogens with increasing clinical significance. J Pediatr 1990;116:497-507.

65. Hall R, Hall S, Barnes W, et al. Characteristics of coagulase negative staphylococci from infants with bacteremia. Pediatr Infect Dis J 1987;6:377-383.

66. Sidebottom D, Freeman J, Platt R, et al. Fifteen-year experience with bloodstream isolates of coagulase-negative staphylococci in neonatal intensive care. J Clin Microbiol 1988;26:713-718.

67. St. Geme J. Staphylococcus epidermis and other coagulase-negative staphylococci. In Long S, Pickering L, Prober C, eds. Principles and practice of pediatric infectious diseases. New York: Churchill Livingstone, 1997: pp 793-801.

68. Centers for Disease Control. Update: Foodborn listeriosis—United States, 1988-1990. MMWR 1992;41:250.

69. Evans J, Allen A, Stinson D, et al. Perinatal listeriosis: Report of an outbreak. Pediatr Infect Dis 1985;4:237-241.

70. Smith K, Yeager J, Skelton H, et al. Diffuse petechial pustular lesions in a newborn. Disseminated Listeria monocytogenes. Arch Dermatol 1994;130:245-248.

71. McLauchlin J: Human listeriosis in Britain, 1967-1985, a summary of 722 cases. Listeriosis during pregnancy and in the newborn. Epidemiol Infect 1990;104:181-189.

72. Darmstadt GL, Dinulos JG, Miller Z. Congential cutaneous candidiasis: Clinical presentation, pathogenesis, and management guidelines. Pediatrics 2000;105:438-444.

73. Gordon R, Barrett F, Clark D. Influence of several antibiotics, singly and in combination, on the growth of Listeria monocytogenes. J Pediatr 1972;80:667-670.

74. Cantwell M, Shehab Z, Costello A, et al. Brief report: congenital tuberculosis. N Engl J Med 1994;330:1051-1054.

75. McCray M, Esterly N. Cutaneous eruptions in congenital tuberculosis. Arch Dermatol 1981;117:460-464.
76. Kendig E. Tuberculosis in the very young: Report of three cases in infants less than one month of age. Am Rev Respir Dis 1954;70:161-165.
77. Holt L. Tuberculosis acquired through ritual circumcision. JAMA 1913;61:99-102.
78. Saez-Llorens X, McCraken G. Septicemia and shock. In Long S, Pickering L, Prober C, eds. Principles and practice of pediatric infectious diseases. New York: Churchill Livingstone, 1997: pp 102-107.
79. Saez-Llorens X, McCraken G. Perinatal bacterial diseases. In Feign R, Cherry J, eds. Textbook of pediatric infectious diseases. 4th edition. Philadelphia: WB Saunders, 1998: pp 892-926.
80. Leigh L, Stoll BJ, Rahman M, et al. *Pseudomonas aeruginosa* infection in very low birth weight infants: a case-control study. Pediatr Infect Dis J 1995;14:367-371.
81. Boisseau A, Sarlangue J, Perel Y, et al. Perineal ecthyma gangrenosum in infancy and early childhood: Septicemic and nonsepticemic forms. J Am Acad Dermatol 1992;27:415-418.
82. Hughes J, Newbould M, du Vivier A, et al. Fatal pseudomonas septicemia and vasculitis in a premature infant. Pediatr Dermatol 1998;15:122-124.
83. Darmstadt G. Acute infectious purpura fulminans: pathogenesis and medical management. Pediatr Dermatol 1998; 15:169-183.
84. Clegg H, Todres I, Moylan F, et al. Fulminant neonatal meningococcemia. Am J Dis Child 1980;134:354-355.
85. Adcock D, Bronza J, Marlar R. Proposed classification and pathologic mechanism of purpura fulminans and skin necrosis. Semin Thromb Hemost 1990;16:333-340.
86. Wong V, Hitchcock W, Mason W. Meningococcal infections in children: A review of 100 cases. Pediatr Infect Dis J 1989; 8:224-227.
87. Bronza J. Shwartzman reaction. Semin Thromb Hemost 1990;16:326-333.
88. van Deuren M, van Dijke B, Koopman R, et al. Rapid diagnosis of acute meningococcal infections by needle aspiration or biopsy of skin lesions. BMJ 1993;306:1229-1232.
89. Periappuram M, Taylor M, Keane C. Rapid detection of meningococci from petechiae in acute meningococcal infection. J Infect 1995;31:201-203.
90. Adcock D, Hicks M. Dermatopathology of skin necrosis associated with purpura fulminans. Semin Thromb Hemost 1990;16:283-292.
91. Brandtzaeg P. Pathogenesis of meningococcal infections. In Cartwright K, ed. Meningococcal Disease. New York: John Wiley & Sons, 1995: pp 71-114.
92. Brandtzaeg P, Dahle J, Hoiby E. The occurrence and features of hemorrhagic skin lesions in 115 cases of systemic meningococcal disease. NIPH Am 1983;6:183-203.
93. Congenital syphilis New York City, 1986-1988. MMWR 1989;38:825-829.
94. Chawla V, Pandit P, Nkrumah F. Congenital syphilis in the newborn. Arch Dis Child 1988;63:1393-1394.
95. Solomon L, Esterly N. Neonatal dermatology. Philadelphia: WB Saunders, 1973: pp 158-162.
96. Darmstadt G, Harris J. Luetic hearing loss: Clinical presentation, diagnosis, and treatment. Am J Otolaryngol 1989; 10:410-421.
97. Wendel G. Gestational and congenital syphilis. Clin Perinatol 1988;15:287-303.
98. Guidelines for the prevention and control of congenital syphilis. MMWR 1988;37(Suppl)1:1-13.
99. Rawstron S, Bromberg K. Comparison of maternal and newborn serologic tests for syphilis. Am J Dis Child 1991;145: 1383-1388.
100. Stoll B, Lee F, Larsen S, et al. Clinical and serologic evaluation of neonates for congenital syphilis: a continuing diagnostic dilemma. J Infect Dis 1993;167:1093-1099.
101. Sanchez P. Laboratory tests for congenital syphilis. Pediatr Infect Dis J 1998;17:70-71.
102. Brion L, Manuli M, Rai B, et al. Longbone radiographic abnormalities as a sign of active congenital syphilis in asymptomatic newborns. Pediatrics 1991;88:1037-1040.
103. Trevisan G, Stinco G, Cinco M. Neonatal skin lesions due to a spirochetal infection: A case of congenital Lyme borreliosis? Int J Dermatol 1997;36:677-680.
104. American Academy of Pediatrics. Syphilis. In Peters G, ed. 1997 Red Book: Report of the Committee on American Academy of Pediatrics. 24th edition. Elk Grove Village, IL: American Academy of Pediatrics, 1997: pp 504-514.

Viral Infections

SHEILA FALLON FRIEDLANDER
JOHN S. BRADLEY

Viral infections can lead to a broad range of cutaneous manifestations in the neonate. Infections may occur in utero, perinatally (acquired between the onset of labor and the delivery), or postnatally. The spectrum of cutaneous manifestations is a result of the complex interaction of the virulence of the viral pathogen for tissues, the tissue tropism of the virus, and the time of gestation at which the fetal infection is acquired. Skin pathology may be a direct consequence of skin infection or an indirect consequence of viral infection of other tissues. Diagnosis of infection is based on morphology and distribution of the skin lesions in the context of the overall clinical presentation of the infant, supported by specific laboratory studies. Rapid diagnosis and appropriate antiviral therapy maximizes the possibility of a positive outcome for the infant.

HERPES SIMPLEX VIRUS

Herpes simplex virus (HSV) types 1 and 2 are pathogens for the fetus and newborn infant, leading to a spectrum of clinical disease in which manifestations depend on the time of exposure (in utero versus perinatal versus postnatal), the route of exposure, and the presence or absence of maternal immunity (primary versus recurrent maternal infection). Herpes simplex virus is a large, double-stranded DNA virus that can produce an acute primary infection in the susceptible host. In addition, HSV 1 and 2 have the capability, similar to other herpesviruses, of integrating into host DNA and establishing latency. Poorly understood host and environmental factors can cause reactivation of virus within latently infected sensory ganglia, leading to a recurrent, active infection. Neonatal infection occurs most often as a direct result of active maternal infection, either primary or recurrent. The rate of neonatal disease has been shown to parallel the rate of genital herpes in a community.[1]

Epidemiology

Neonatal infection is estimated to occur at a rate of 0.2 to 0.5 per 1000 live births. Infection of the fetus or newborn may occur during gestation (in utero), at the time of labor and delivery (perinatal), or following the delivery (postnatal). Although the majority of neonatal infections (80% to 90%) are considered to be acquired perinatally, both in utero infections (4%) and postnatal infections (10%) have been well documented.[2]

The majority of neonates acquire infection from exposure to infectious genital secretions or lesions present at the time of vaginal delivery. Although primary infection in the pregnant woman usually leads to symptomatic disease, a significant proportion of women with primary infection do not have recognizable systemic or local disease.[3] Primary maternal infection is usually associated with prolonged shedding (2 to 3 weeks) of high titers of virus from lesions while the maternal immune response develops, in contrast to the more limited viral shedding and much shorter duration of lesions (2 to 5 days) that accompanies recurrent disease in women with specific humoral and cellular immunity. Infection in the newborn occurs in up to 50% of infants born to mothers during primary infection, compared with 5% or less of infants born to mothers during recurrent infection. Active maternal infection at the time of delivery, based on viral culture, is thought to occur in approximately 1 to 7 per 1000 births. However, preliminary data based on polymerase chain reaction (PCR) techniques from genital specimens at delivery suggest that active maternal infection may occur up to eight times more frequently than previously appreciated.[4] Prospective studies have documented that the majority of women with active infection at the time of delivery are asymptomatic, suggesting that improved rapid laboratory diagnosis and careful examination will be necessary to identify the at-risk mother and infant.

Postnatal infections may be transmitted from both maternal, nongenital sites (including transmission from breast lesions), as well as from nonmaternal sources. These include other family members and nosocomial transmission from healthcare workers.

Intrauterine Infection

Congenital (intrauterine) infection was described in 1966 by Sieber et al in an infant with culture-positive lesions, seizures, and evidence of immunity at the time of a normal delivery in which the amniotic membranes were ruptured at birth.[5] In 1969 South described an infant with microcephaly, microphthalmia, seizures, and vesicular lesions present on the fingers and toes following a maternal primary HSV 2 genital infection during the first month of pregnancy.[6] Subsequent studies of congenital infection have documented the presence of specific cell-mediated immunity to HSV in the newborn at birth, whereas infants infected during labor and delivery do not usually develop cellular immunity until the second week of the infection.[7]

Infection in utero may occur either as a result of ascending infection through apparently intact membranes, or potentially as a result of viremia occurring with a primary maternal infection. Fetal infection often leads to fetal demise; however, if the fetus survives, delivery may occur at term with late sequelae in both skin and central nervous system (CNS).

CUTANEOUS FINDINGS. Skin manifestations at delivery are the result of residua from primary fetal infection in addition to latent virus reactivation at previous cutaneous sites of fetal infection. Skin lesions are common in the neonatal period (Fig. 12-1). In one study, 70% of infected infants had vesicular lesions, while 30% also had evidence of scar formation on the face, trunk, or extremities.[8] Lesions characteristic of epidermolysis bullosa have also been described, as well as aplasia cutis congenita–like lesions.[9]

EXTRACUTANEOUS FINDINGS. Infections acquired in utero in which the infant completes a normal gestation are almost invariably associated with CNS damage easily detected by computed tomography. Changes in the CNS indicate longstanding destruction of neuronal tissue without acute inflammation. Microcephaly is present in over 50%,

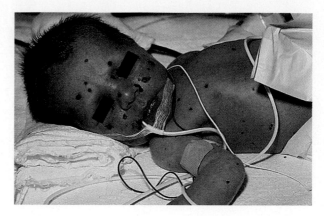

FIG. 12-1
Congenital herpes simplex. Generalized necrotic crusted papules.

and chorioretinitis is present in 60% of infants with congenital infection. Although skin and CNS abnormalities are present at birth, infected infants often do not show the signs of systemic toxicity and overwhelming sepsis that may occur with primary perinatal or postnatal infection.

DIAGNOSIS. The diagnosis of a herpes virus infection can be made by several means (Table 12-1). Histologic staining of epithelial cells obtained by scraping the base of a vesicle or mucosal ulceration (Tzanck preparation) will demonstrate multinucleate giant epithelial cells containing intranuclear viral inclusions (see Chapter 6). A biopsy is usually not required to arrive at a diagnosis, but will show the characteristic intraepidermal vesicle with ballooning degeneration of epithelial cells, resulting in acantholysis. Eosinophilic inclusion bodies may be seen in the degenerating epithelial cells. In the adjacent dermis, an inflammatory cell infiltrate of variable severity reflects the nature of the infant's response to the viral infection (primary versus recurrent).

A specific diagnosis of herpes simplex virus can be obtained rapidly by antibody-specific stains (such as direct fluorescent antibody for HSV-1 or HSV-2). Viral culture can be performed on skin or mucous membrane lesions. Cultures generally take from 2 to 7 days to develop cytopathic effects. The PCR technique for diagnosis of HSV takes several hours and is currently not well standardized for biologic samples other than cerebrospinal fluid. Attempting to identify the type of herpes simplex virus responsible for the infection is important because the epidemiology of acquisition of virus and the course of the infection differ between HSV-1 and HSV-2.

Serologic status of an infant should be obtained to assess preexisting and ongoing antibody response. In congenital infection, all antibody present at birth is maternal

TABLE 12-1

Diagnosis of Infection

Virus	Culture	Histology of skin lesion	PCR	Serology
HSV	Widely available; reliable; culture skin lesions	Tzanck stain of epithelial cells from the bottom of a vesicle: specific for herpesviruses HSV and VZV; direct fluorescent antibody stains for HSV 1 or 2 are specific	Highly sensitive; best studied on CSF (sensitivity of skin lesions not well studied)	Rising antibody titer to HSV IgG is a sensitive and specific test; HSV IgM is not a sensitive test in the newborn
VZV	Available in many reference laboratories; culture skin lesions	Tzanck stain (see above): specific stains available for VZV	Highly sensitive, but not well studied on skin lesions; not widely available	Rising antibody titer to VSV IgG is a sensitive and specific test; VZV IgM is not a sensitive test in the newborn
CMV	Widely available; reliable; culture urine, saliva; shell vial technique yields results in 48-72 hours	Skin lesions are due to extramedullary hematopoiesis, not due to viral replication in skin	Highly sensitive; well studied in plasma as a marker of disseminated CMV infection in immune compromised hosts	Rising antibody titer to CMV IgG is a sensitive and specific test; CMV IgM is not a sensitive test in the newborn
Rubella	Not usually available; culture pharynx	Skin lesions are due to extramedullary hematopoiesis, not due to viral replication in skin	Not well studied	Rising antibody titer to rubella IgG is a sensitive and specific test; rubella IgM is not a sensitive test in the newborn. Compare mother's prenatal serology test results with those at the time of birth
Enterovirus	Available in reference laboratories; culture vesicular lesions, pharynx (during the acute phase of illness), and stool (up to 6 weeks following the illness)	Nonspecific	Highly sensitive; not widely available	Not usually helpful, as no classspecific antibody response can be measured and typespecific serologies are not widely available
Parvo virus B19	Not available in standard cell culture	Placental and fetal tissues—intranuclear inclusions in nucleated erythroid cells EM and immunohistochemistry may be helful	Highly sensitive; can be used on amniotic fluid, fetal blood, and tissues	IgM or IgG seroconversion helpful in pregnant female Fetal IgM specific but not sensitive
HIV	Available; not highly sensitive in newborn, repeat culture at 1 month of age	Nonspecific	Sensitive means of diagnosis; can be repeated at 1-2 months and 4-6 months of age prn	Nonspecific passive maternal antibody present at birth persists; PCR for 18 month evaluation preferred

in origin and decreases prior to the development of the infant's humoral immunity; a response pattern that is distinct from early perinatal infection.

DIFFERENTIAL DIAGNOSIS. Other congenital infections associated with skin lesions and CNS injury should be investigated, such as congenital varicella syndrome and syphilis. Noninfectious entities such as incontinentia pigmenti and other disorders producing vesicular lesions (Chapters 10 and 24) should also be considered.

MANAGEMENT/PROGNOSIS. Infants are treated with intravenous acyclovir at 60 mg/kg/day divided every 8 hours, based on current protocols for infants with perinatal CNS infection.[10] No prospective data exist on the required treatment course for congenitally infected infants, although preexisting immunity should allow for a shorter course of therapy compared with infants with primary infection. The neurologic prognosis for infants with congenital infection is poor, with virtually all infants demonstrating significant developmental delay.

Neonatal (Perinatal) Herpes Simplex Infection

Neonatal disease occurs in three clinically recognized syndromes, all acquired in the perinatal period: disseminated infection; infection localized to the skin, eye, or mouth; and CNS infection. Exposure to maternal primary infection at the time of delivery may lead to overwhelming infection in the neonate with a high mortality rate, or a more slowly progressive, insidious disease in which the infant has only mucocutaneous manifestations or develops slowly progressive neurologic symptoms. The incubation period varies substantially, from clinical symptoms at delivery from presumed ascending infection through nonintact membranes, to infection presenting as late as 3 weeks of age. The variability of the incubation period is dependent on the integrity of the amniotic membranes, the inoculum of virus, the tissue site inoculated (e.g., skin, mucous membrane), and the presence or absence of transplacental specific antibody.

CUTANEOUS MANIFESTATIONS. The infection may manifest clinically with cutaneous or mucosal lesions (mouth, nose, eye), with or without signs of sepsis or encephalitis. Infants with skin, eye, or mouth disease account for 40% of all neonatal cases of HSV infection. The skin lesions appear as small, 2 to 4 mm vesicles, with surrounding erythema, often in herpetiform (zosteriform) clusters (Fig. 12-2). The skin lesions usually occur on the part of the body in prolonged contact with the cervix. Often, lesions will occur at sites where the skin integrity has been breached. One of the most common sites of cutaneous in-

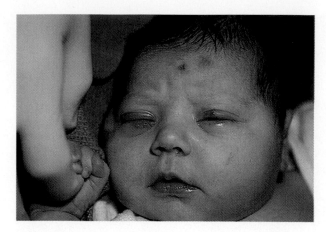

FIG. 12-2
Neonatal herpes simplex. Cluster of vesicles on the forehead and periocular area.

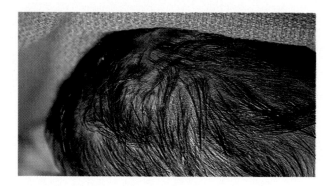

FIG. 12-3
Neonatal herpes simplex. Vesicles with central necrotic plaque at site of fetal monitor electrode placement.

fection is on the scalp vertex at the site of fetal scalp monitor electrode placement (Fig. 12-3). Vesicular lesions usually develop within the first 1 to 2 weeks of life following inoculation at this site. They may progress locally, or disseminate (Fig. 12-4). In areas of mucosal involvement, a shallow ulceration with moderate inflammation is most often seen. The ulceration may be focal, with the lesion size closely resembling that of a cutaneous vesicle, or ulcerations may spread irregularly, coalescing over a much larger area. Lesions tend to follow the clinical stages of vesicle resolution seen in the older child, with pustulation 24 to 72 hours after the appearance of the vesicle, followed by eschar formation. Skin lesions are present in most neonates with disseminated disease (77%), and in 60% of infants who present with CNS disease. In any new-

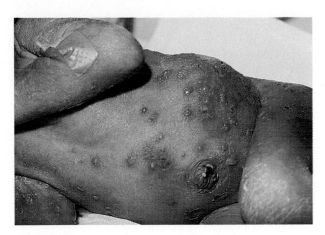

FIG. 12-4
Neonatal herpes simplex virus. Multiple vesicles and crusted papules on an erythematous base in the periumbilical area, and left flank.

born with skin or mucosal lesions of HSV, even without a history of symptomatic illness, an investigation must be undertaken to rule out disseminated or CNS disease.

EXTRACUTANEOUS MANIFESTATIONS. Dissemination is the most devastating manifestation, presenting in the more premature infant (average gestational age at birth of 36.5 weeks) at an average chronologic age of 11 days. Multisystem involvement is analogous to overwhelming bacterial sepsis. Shock, disseminated intravascular coagulation, and multiple organ system failure are characteristic. Involvement of the lung, liver, and brain is common. The mortality is high. Without antiviral therapy approximately 75% of infants will die, and even with specific antiviral therapy, mortality is 50%. Neurologic sequelae in survivors are also common, occurring in approximately 40%. Statistically, these infants have the lowest average circulating concentration of antibody to HSV.

In as many as 40% of infants ultimately diagnosed with disseminated or CNS infection, clinical disease begins with skin lesions only. Clinical and laboratory evidence of dissemination or CNS involvement not obvious at the time of presentation may develop during the first days of therapy despite antiviral therapy.

Infants with encephalitis present at a slightly older age (mean 17 days) and tend to be full term, in contrast with newborns with other clinical presentations. Antibody titers are higher in this group of infants, leading to speculation that antibody may modify the progression of disease, with virus inoculated at delivery producing a clinically undetectable initial infection with retrograde spread from mucosal sites to the CNS. Subtle neurologic symptoms are of-

ten present for days before recognition by the parent that the infant requires medical attention. As the child becomes more irritable and seizures become more pronounced, infants are hospitalized and evaluated. Skin lesions are only present in 60% of infants with HSV encephalitis, making the diagnosis in many infants difficult.

DIAGNOSIS. Rapid diagnosis of herpes virus infection can be made on the basis of a Tzanck, but for infants without skin or mucous membrane lesions, the diagnosis is more difficult. Laboratory and radiographic evidence of multisystem involvement is supportive, but not diagnostic. Viral cultures of cutaneous lesions, nasopharynx, conjunctiva, urine, plasma, and CSF can provide a specific diagnosis but take several days for results. Direct fluorescent antibody testing can provide a more rapid analysis but is not 100% sensitive. Cerebrospinal fluid examination is important because pleocytosis, elevated protein, and a high CSF red blood cell count can suggest necrotizing encephalitis. Culture of CSF is positive for HSV in up to 20% of infants with encephalitis. Rapid diagnosis of encephalitis by HSV PCR may be attempted, although the sensitivity of this assay has not been well studied in the newborn.

Computed tomography (CT) of the brain may be helpful in the diagnosis of encephalitis but is not considered sensitive until after 5 days of CNS symptoms. Magnetic resonance imaging (MRI), which is more sensitive for CNS inflammation of the temporal lobes, may be diagnostic within 3 days of onset of symptoms. EEG can also be helpful in CNS infections localized to the temporal lobe and may be positive earlier than any imaging study.

DIFFERENTIAL DIAGNOSIS. Disseminated infection with HSV produces a clinical picture similar to early onset neonatal sepsis caused by group B streptococcus, enteric gram-negative bacilli, and *Listeria*. Empiric therapy with antibiotics, standard management for the hospitalized ill neonate, will have no effect on the progression of HSV disease. For infants with progressive clinical symptoms of sepsis and sterile bacterial cultures of blood, urine, and CSF, HSV should be considered as a potential pathogen.

Other viral infections in the newborn period may also be confused with HSV. Enteroviral infection can cause a wide spectrum of clinical signs in the neonate, from fever and irritability to overwhelming sepsis with multiple organ system failure, to aseptic meningoencephalitis with minimal symptoms of systemic toxicity. Enteroviral infections may be associated with cutaneous vesiculopustular lesions. Neonatal seizures caused by enteroviral infections are the result of diffuse CNS irritation in contrast to the focal temporal lesions of early HSV disease. Destructive changes of HSV that are appreciated on serial imaging studies of the CNS (by either CT or MRI) are not generally seen with enteroviral disease.

Perinatal varicella may produce overwhelming sepsis in the newborn. The density of cutaneous lesions in neonatal varicella usually far exceeds that seen with HSV infections, which characteristically produce a focal cluster of lesions at the site of inoculation with minimal cutaneous dissemination. However, both demonstrate the identical findings of multinucleate giant cells on Tzanck preparations. Only virus-specific staining techniques, PCR or culture will be able to differentiate between these viruses.

Other viral pathogens occasionally cause severe acute disease in the newborn, including influenza A and B, parainfluenza 1, 2, and 3, and adenovirus. In general, the seasonal context of the infection, exposure history, and a predominance of respiratory tract symptoms help differentiate these infections. Viral cultures of the respiratory tract will assist in the identification of these pathogens.

Incontinentia pigmenti may present with localized vesicles, which may be mistaken for herpes simplex infections. These infants often have peripheral eosinophilia. Biopsy will reveal increased numbers of eosinophils, and cultures will be negative. Vesicular lesions that appear herpetic can occur in Langerhans' cell histiocytosis. Tzanck prep will reveal histiocytes, and biopsy will show large numbers of histiocytes and an absence of multinucleate giant cells.

MANAGEMENT AND PROGNOSIS. The treatment of choice in neonatal herpes infections is acyclovir administered intravenously, regardless of the clinical presentation.[11] Although the dose of acyclovir originally studied for skin or mucosal surface infection was 15 mg/kg/day divided into 8-hourly doses, data collected in infants treated at 30 mg/kg/day for disseminated infection and encephalitis suggest that this dose may safely be used in mild to moderate neonatal herpes simplex infections.[12] Ongoing clinical trials of 60 mg/kg/day for dissemination and encephalitis suggest a small incremental improvement in efficacy, with safety that is equivalent to the 30 mg/kg/day dose.[10] In infants with renal failure, the doses should be adjusted accordingly.

Varicella

Varicella (chicken pox) is usually a benign, self-limited disease when it occurs in immunocompetent individuals during childhood. Unfortunately, the developing fetus and neonate are at higher risk for adverse outcome following infection. Approximately 95% of women have acquired varicella infection before childbearing years and are immune, conferring immunity to the fetus. The exact

incidence of varicella during pregnancy is unknown; 3 to 10 cases per 10,000 pregnancies have been documented in the United States.[13,14,15] Fetal or early neonatal exposure may result in a variety of manifestations ranging from minimal cutaneous lesions to significant morbidity and death. Three distinct disorders may occur following intrauterine or neonatal exposure to VZV: fetal varicella syndrome, neonatal varicella, and infantile herpes zoster.

Fetal Varicella Syndrome

Congenital defects predominantly involving the skin, nervous system, and musculoskeletal system can occur following fetal exposure to varicella virus. Other terms for the fetal varicella syndrome include *varicella embryopathy* and *congenital varicella syndrome*.

CUTANEOUS FINDINGS. Specific anomalies include cicatricial skin lesions that correspond to a dermatomal distribution, often with hypoplasia of underlying tissues. These skin lesions may initially appear as denuded areas and subsequently develop stellate or angular scars (Fig. 12-5).

EXTRACUTANEOUS FINDINGS. Low birth weight is a common finding in affected infants. The varied extracuta-

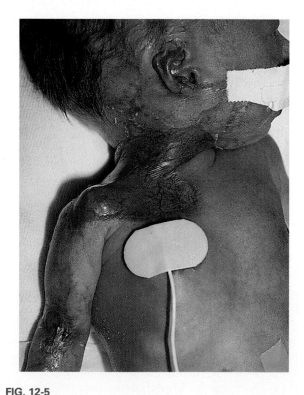

FIG. 12-5
Congenital varicella. Segmental and stellate-shaped deep scars on the right ear, head, shoulder, and arm, which appear to follow a dermatome.

neous manifestations of this syndrome can be grouped as neurologic, musculoskeletal, ophthalmologic, gastrointestinal, and genitourinary. Limb paresis and hypoplasia of the extremities are common findings, as is chorioretinitis. Less common findings include microphthalmia, cataracts, nystagmus, hydrocephalus, and mental retardation[16] (Table 12-2).

ETIOLOGY AND PATHOGENESIS. Varicella zoster is a herpes virus consisting of double-stranded DNA. The incubation period is usually 14 days but extends from 10 to 21 days after exposure. Most fetuses exposed to VZV during gestation will have no discernible sequelae. Retrospective studies documented an incidence of fetal varicella syndrome of zero to 9% after maternal infection during pregnancy, with a first trimester attack rate of 2.2%.[17,18,19] The greatest risk for fetal varicella syndrome occurs in the first 20 weeks of gestation, with the highest risk between 13 and 20 weeks

gestation (2%).[20] A lower rate before 13 weeks gestation (0.4%) may reflect underreporting or a higher rate of spontaneous abortion. Rare cases in the second half of pregnancy have been reported.[21]

It has been postulated that the severe segmental anomalies that can be seen in fetal varicella syndrome are the result of reactivation of primary varicella in the developing fetus at a time when the immune system is not sufficiently developed to modify the severity of infection. Maternal herpes zoster does not appear to pose a significant risk to the fetus. No cases of congenital varicella occurred in a prospective study of 366 women who had zoster during pregnancy, and no serological evidence of transplacental transmission was noted.[20]

Approximately 18 cases of congenital anomalies occurring in association with maternal herpes zoster infection have been reported; however, it is not clear that these

TABLE 12-2

Features of Varicella Syndrome

Characteristic organ system	Common (>50%)	Uncommon (<50%, >10%)	Rare (<10%)
Skin	Cicatricial Lesions	Hydrocephalus and cortical atrophy	Cerebellar hypoplasia
Neurologic	Limb paresis	Seizures	Auditory nerve palsy
		Horner syndrome	Facial nerve palsy
		Bulbar dysphagia	
		Mental retardation	
		Optic nerve atrophy	
		Anal sphincter malfunction	
		Microcephaly	
		Phrenic nerve palsy	
Eye	Chorioretinitis	Anisocoria	Corneal opacity
		Nystagmus	Heterochromia
		Microphthalmia	
		Cataract	
Skeletal	Hypoplasia of upper or lower extremities	Hypoplasia of fingers or toes	Hypoplasia of mandible
		Equinovarus or calcaneovalgus	Scoliosis
		Hypoplasia of scapulae or clavicles	Lacunar skull
		Hypoplasia of ribs	
Gastrointestinal			Gastroesophageal reflux
			Duodenal stenosis
			Dilated jejunum
			Small left colon
			Sigmoid atresia
Genitourinary			Absence of kidney
			Hydronephrosis
			Hydroureter
			Undescended testes
			Bladder abnormalities

anomalies were a result of maternal zoster infection.[22] A case of cutaneous lesions and limb hypoplasia in a fetus whose mother developed disseminated herpes zoster at 12 weeks gestation did appear consistent with fetal varicella syndrome, but localized maternal zoster has not been clearly implicated as a cause of fetal disease.[23]

DIAGNOSIS. The denuded or scarred areas seen with fetal varicella syndrome may be mistaken for aplasia cutis congenita or Bart syndrome. Other congenital viral infections should be considered in any infant presenting with microcephaly, ophthalmologic, or neurologic abnormalities.

Prenatal diagnosis of fetal varicella syndrome using viral or immunologic methods is unreliable.[24] IgM may be undetectable, even in infants with classic clinical findings. Infection before 18 weeks' gestation may lead to a suboptimal or altered immune response resulting from immaturity of the fetal immune system. Prenatal diagnosis of intrauterine exposure to varicella may be accomplished by means of cordocentesis, amniocentesis, and chorionic villus sampling.[24] IgM may be detected in cord blood as early as 19 to 22 weeks' gestation. Virus can be grown from amniotic fluid and fetal blood samples, and DNA probes can be utilized to evaluate placental tissue.[25,26] However, transplacental transfer of virus can occur without any significant sequelae to the fetus, and degree of fetal involvement cannot be determined by immunologic or viral evaluation. Thus, although the above-mentioned evaluations may be useful in diagnosing fetal varicella syndrome, they are neither sensitive nor specific enough to accurately determine with certainty which fetuses will suffer untoward effects.

High quality ultrasound at 20 to 22 weeks' gestation has been utilized as a means of surveying at-risk fetuses. Sonographic abnormalities include fetal hydrops, polyhydramnios, abnormal foci within the liver, microcephaly, and limb hypoplasia.[27] Unfortunately, some findings may not be apparent until later in pregnancy.

Varicella virus is not usually isolated from live-borne infants with congenital infection, and other findings must be utilized to confirm the diagnosis. Criteria useful in confirming the diagnosis include clinical, virologic, or serologic evidence of maternal varicella infection during pregnancy; skin lesions in a dermatomal distribution; and immunologic evidence of varicella infection in the infant, including IgM antibody or persistence of IgG antibody beyond 1 year of life in the absence of clinical varicella infection.[24] The development of herpes zoster in the first year of life without a prior history of varicella infection is also good evidence that the infant was exposed to varicella zoster during gestation. In rare instances, herpes virus particles have been detected by means of electron microscopy in skin samples obtained at or near birth.[25]

TREATMENT. Prevention by the elimination of natural infection during pregnancy is the best approach to this disease, and should be facilitated by the increasing use of the varicella vaccine in childhood. Ideally, preconception evaluation should identify at-risk females, who should then receive the varicella vaccine before conceiving. No fetal anomalies have been reported in the infants born to pregnant women who have received the vaccine inadvertently. Nonetheless, the vaccine, which is a live attenuated virus, is contraindicated in pregnancy.

Therapeutic abortion is not automatically recommended to at-risk mothers, since the risk of a fetal anomaly following exposure is so small.[28] At-risk mothers known to have recent exposure to varicella during the first 20 weeks of pregnancy should have varicella serologic evaluation performed. Complement fixation tests are insensitive; however, latex agglutination (LA), immunofluorescent (IFA), fluorescent antibody-to-membrane antigen assays (FAMA), and enzyme-linked immunoabsorbent assays (ELISA) are sensitive and specific.[24] The LA test is also a rapid, simple test, making it quite useful in evaluating at-risk pregnant females.[24] Varicella zoster immunoglobulin (VZIG) may be administered within 5 days of exposure, but is most efficacious within the first 48 hours following exposure. It does not reliably prevent maternal illness, but does appear to modify severity of the infection. It is unclear if VZIG prevents fetal varicella syndrome or neonatal infection; however, there were no cases of fetal infection in 97 pregnancies complicated by maternal exposure and treated with VZIG.[20,29] Because fetal varicella syndrome is so rare, larger studies will be required to determine if VZIG is definitely protective. Exposed pregnant women who are seropositive for VZV do not require VZIG.

Treatment with acyclovir should be considered in any pregnant women with varicella, particularly those in the third trimester because of the risk of severe maternal disease, and to minimize the risk of neonatal disease in case delivery occurs during or soon after acute infection. The drug is usually well tolerated with little toxicity to the mother, but the risks and benefits to the mother and fetus have not yet been clearly delineated.[30] The International Registry of Acyclovir Use During Pregnancy has followed at least 746 fetal exposures to the drug thus far, and an increased incidence of fetal abnormalities in exposed infants has not been noted.[31] It has not been determined if such treatment will eliminate the risk of varicella embryopathy or infantile zoster in exposed fetuses.

Treatment of an affected infant is supportive if no active viral lesions are present. Ophthalmologic and neurologic evaluation is indicated, as is careful examination of the musculoskeletal, genitourinary, and gastrointestinal system for underlying anomalies.

Neonatal Varicella

Neonatal varicella may result if a mother develops chickenpox before or immediately following delivery. If maternal varicella occurs from 5 days before to 2 days after delivery, the fetus is at high risk for severe disseminated disease.

CUTANEOUS FINDINGS. The clinical course of neonatal varicella can be quite variable. Those who are more likely to develop severe illness generally develop skin lesions within 5 to 10 days after delivery. Some children will develop a few cutaneous lesions, but otherwise remain well. Lesions often initially appear as small pink to red macules that relatively rapidly become papular and subsequently develop a teardrop–shaped vesicle. Other patients initially develop crops of cutaneous lesions that may evolve into hemorrhagic and/or necrotic vesicles (Fig. 12-6).

EXTRACUTANEOUS FINDINGS. Disseminated infection with widespread cutaneous and visceral involvement may develop and lead to severe morbidity. The mortality rate for neonatal varicella before the use of acyclovir has been estimated at 10% to 30%.[28,29] Death from severe pneumonitis and respiratory distress often occurs 4 to 6 days after onset of lesions. Hepatitis and encephalitis may also develop. A study from Thailand in 1999, evaluating 26 children with neonatal varicella, reported no mortality in this group. Twelve of the 26 children received intravenous acyclovir.[32]

ETIOLOGY/PATHOGENESIS. Infants may develop lesions from 1 to 16 days after birth if the mother experiences active disease near the time of birth (Fig. 12-7). Administration of VZIG may prolong the incubation period to 28 days.[31] The usual onset of rash is 9 to 15 days after onset of maternal rash. Infection later in gestation is more likely to lead to zoster in infancy or neonatal chickenpox. In aggregate data from two studies, 23% to 62% of infants whose mothers developed varicella in the last 3 weeks of pregnancy developed neonatal varicella.[20] The risk of severe neonatal varicella is clearly related to the time maternal infection occurs, presumably because of a critical time period when transmission of virus to the infant occurs without time for transplacental transfer of maternal antibodies, which would help modify expression of the infection in the neonate.

DIAGNOSIS. Smears of vesicles will demonstrate multinucleate giant cells and margination of the nucleoplasm (Tzanck preparation). Direct fluorescent antibody testing and PCR evaluation are also helpful and not as subject to inter-rater variability. Fluorescent antibody tests are occasionally false positive in disorders such as incontinentia pigmenti and Langerhans' cell histiocytosis; therefore positive viral culture remains the best, most reliable means of diagnosis.[33] A history of maternal varicella infection during pregnancy is also helpful but not necessary to confirm the diagnosis because infants may also contract the disease from siblings, caretakers, and other close contacts.

The differential diagnosis of vesiculopustular lesions is discussed in Chapter 10.

TREATMENT. Prevention is the optimal intervention. Delaying delivery until sufficient time has elapsed for transplacental transfer of maternal antibody is one approach;

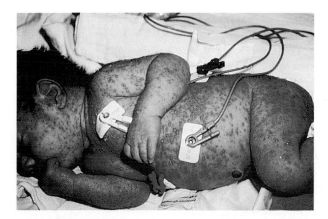

FIG. 12-6
Neonatal varicella. Generalized crusted papules. (Courtesy Gerald Goldberg.)

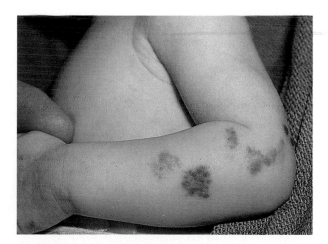

FIG. 12-7
Early varicella zoster in an infant whose mother contracted varicella during pregnancy.

this generally occurs 5 to 7 days after onset of maternal illness. Neonates born to mothers who have developed varicella from 5 days before to 2 days after delivery should receive VZIG at a dose of 125 units.[31] Direct contact between maternal skin lesions and infant should be avoided, but breast feeding is not prohibited if contact with lesions can be avoided. Approximately 50% of at-risk infants will develop varicella despite VZIG therapy, but disease is generally milder.[29] Such children should be treated with intravenous acyclovir, 20 mg/kg every 8 hours for a minimum of 5 days and receive appropriate and aggressive supportive therapy as required. The use of prophylactic acyclovir therapy in high-risk infants has also been suggested by some authors.[31]

Famciclovir and valacyclovir are therapeutic options in adults with zoster, and may have a role in treatment of neonatal varicella in the future. There are presently insufficient data on safety and efficacy in infants and children to recommend their use in pregnancy.

It should be kept in mind that any infant born to a woman who has had varicella within 3 weeks of delivery may be infectious at birth or shortly thereafter. If onset of maternal infection is within 1 to 2 weeks of delivery, many experts recommend that the child be isolated (from at risk hospital personnel and other babies) from birth. If onset of disease occurs in the mother within 1 week of delivery, or following birth of the infant, isolation of the infant should occur 7 days after onset of maternal disease.[31]

If a mother develops a varicella rash 3 or more days after delivery, the infant may well contract varicella, but it will more likely be via the respiratory route, which theoretically leads to a smaller systemic inoculum and less-severe disease. However, serious illness has been reported in the first 4 weeks of life when infants contract disease from their mother or siblings during this period. Severe infantile disease may occasionally occur even in infants born to immune mothers.[34] If the mother is seronegative and the infant is exposed to an infectious sibling, many would recommend VZIG treatment for the infant and mother.[31] Although the mortality rate following noncongenital infantile varicella (0.008%) is higher than that of the older child, it is still lower than the rate in the immunocompromised individual (7%) or following intrauterine exposure (10% to 30%).[29] VZIG and/or acyclovir therapy should be considered in exposed infants, particularly if they are premature.

Infantile Herpes Zoster

Following primary infection, the varicella zoster virus persists in the sensory dorsal root ganglia and is kept in check by cell-mediated host immune mechanisms. Reactivation of the virus can occur and generally leads to localized involvement of skin and nerves in a dermatomal pattern corresponding to the ganglion in which reactivation took place. This disease, termed *herpes zoster*, has been recognized since antiquity. The term *zoster* (girdle in Greek) refers to the tendency of the lesions to involve the trunk in a "girdle-like" pattern. Infants may develop classic herpes zoster without prior evidence of primary varicella if exposed to varicella virus in utero. This is generally a benign disease without significant morbidity or sequelae for the infant.

CUTANEOUS FINDINGS. Affected infants usually have discrete papular lesions that predominantly involve the thoracic dermatomes. The lesions initially appear as a group of small pink to erythematous papules that subsequently vesiculate and crust. Occasionally lesions become hemorrhagic and develop necrotic eschars. Scarring may occur in the involved area. Although the disease may disseminate, immunocompetent children usually have a benign course and excellent outcome.

DIAGNOSIS. The diagnosis is usually straightforward when the lesions assume a dermatomal distribution. A Tzanck preparation is the most rapid means to evaluate suspicious vesicular lesions. Zoster lesions may be initially mistaken for arthropod bites or impetigo. Herpes simplex infections may mimic herpes zoster but are usually more localized, with the potential to recur. Direct fluorescent antibody testing and PCR evaluation are also relatively rapid diagnostic techniques (see discussion in infantile varicella). Varicella virus can be isolated from vesicular lesions of herpes zoster.

ETIOLOGY/PATHOGENESIS. The risk of infantile herpes zoster increases if exposure to varicella zoster virus occurs in the second half of pregnancy.[20] Approximately 2% of fetuses exposed to VZV during the second half of pregnancy will develop herpes zoster during infancy.[20]

TREATMENT. Many infectious disease experts treat zoster in neonates with systemic acyclovir. Immunocompetent infants with zoster generally do well and do not require antiviral therapy. Patients who develop severe hemorrhagic disease, as well as those with disseminated lesions, are likely to benefit from systemic therapy. Supportive therapy in all cases should include good hygiene at the blister sites, compresses as needed, and treatment for secondary bacterial infection if indicated.

Special Concerns for the Neonatal Nursery and Intensive Care Unit

VARICELLA EXPOSURE IN THE NEONATAL INTENSIVE CARE UNIT. Recommendations regarding prophylaxis vary. The UK Advisory Group on Chickenpox recommends routine administration of VZIG to all neonates following exposure.[21] If sensitive and rapid testing is available, exposed infants may be tested, and unnecessary use of VZIG and isolation thus avoided. Others recommend concentrating prophylactic measures on those infants less than 30 weeks old and weighing less than 1 kg. The *Red Book Report of the Committee on Infectious Diseases* of the AAP recommends VZIG for all exposed, hospitalized premature infants >28 weeks old or weighing ≥1000g. In addition, those exposed, hospitalized premature infants <28 weeks with mothers who are seronegative or lacking a history of varicella should also be given VZIG.

CYTOMEGALOVIRUS

Cytomegalovirus (CMV), one of the most common viral infections of the newborn, is acquired either congenitally, perinatally, or postnatally. CMV is a double-stranded DNA virus, a member of the herpesvirus family. It represents the most frequently recognized cause of congenital infection, occurring in 1% to 2% of all births.[36]

CUTANEOUS FINDINGS. The principal cutaneous manifestations of CMV infection are similar to those of congenital rubella syndrome and consist of skin lesions of extramedullary hematopoiesis ("blueberry muffin" spots) and petechiae secondary to thrombocytopenia, which resolves during the first weeks of life.

EXTRACUTANEOUS FINDINGS. Other manifestations of congenital CMV infection syndrome include intrauterine growth retardation, microcephaly with chorioretinitis, hepatosplenomegaly, and pneumonitis.

ETIOLOGY/PATHOGENESIS. Congenital infection occurs most often following reactivation of a latent maternal infection during pregnancy, resulting in viremia and/or transplacental transmission of lymphocyte-associated virus to the fetus. The vast majority of infected infants born to immune mothers with reactivation of CMV are normal and have no stigmata of congenital infection. However, seronegative mothers may acquire a primary CMV infection during pregnancy, leading to a far greater incidence of symptomatic disease in the neonate.[37] The severity of infection depends on the trimester in which fetal infection has occurred, with infections early in gestation leading to more pronounced clinical findings and a poorer prognosis than those sustained during the third trimester. Infection may also occur at the time of delivery following exposure to infectious secretions during the process of vaginal birth. The infection is acquired perinatally in 40% of infants born to culture-positive mothers. Postnatal transmission has also been well documented in breast fed infants following ingestion of culture-positive breast milk.

DIAGNOSIS. Viral culture of urine or saliva is the easiest, most widely available method of diagnosis. Infants with congenital infection are, by definition, culture-positive at the time of birth. For diagnosis of congenital infection, cultures should be obtained within the first 2 weeks of life. If cultures are positive in the infant beyond 1 to 2 weeks of age, it is not possible to differentiate between congenital and perinatal CMV infection. This distinction is often critical, as the prognosis for perinatal CMV is uniformly good, while that of congenital CMV is not. Biopsies of skin do not usually reveal evidence of active CMV infection, although specimens from liver, lung, or kidney will show clear evidence of CMV inclusions in infected parenchymal tissues. A spun sample of urine may demonstrate viral inclusions in tubular epithelial cells in up to 50% of culture-positive samples and may demonstrate CMV by electron microscopy in up to 93% of culture-positive urine samples.[38] Serologic studies can also be used to make a diagnosis of congenital/perinatal CMV infection either by demonstrating specific CMV-IgM antibody produced by the neonate or by documenting a persistent, increasing titer of IgG antibody during the first 4 to 6 months of life. Although the presence of specific CMV-IgM in cord blood will verify congenital infection, the sensitivity of this test as currently performed in reference laboratories may be less than 50%. PCR testing for CMV-DNA is accepted as a very sensitive diagnostic technique for plasma and certain tissue fluids in immunocompromised hosts and should prove to be a highly sensitive test in the newborn.[39]

THERAPY. Vaccines have been in development for several years but have not demonstrated sufficiently adequate protection from CMV infection to justify extensive use. Currently, treatment of CMV infections is primarily accomplished with ganciclovir, a nucleoside analogue with potent activity against most strains of CMV. The antiviral is available in both intravenous and oral formulations but is associated with significant bone marrow toxicity. Clinical trials of intravenous ganciclovir for congenital CMV are ongoing, and it is hoped that the drug will offer some benefit to severely affected neonates. Unfortunately, congenital CMV infections cannot be cured but only suppressed during the period of antiviral administration. No data exist on the use of oral ganciclovir in the neonate.

RUBELLA

The association of maternal rubella infection with congenital disease of the newborn was first recognized in 1941. Extensive investigations have resulted in delineation of the congenital rubella infection syndrome, typified by a small-for-gestational age infant with microcephaly, chorioretinitis, hepatosplenomegaly, and a papular rash on the face, trunk, and extremities.

CUTANEOUS FINDINGS. The rash can be mild or extensive and is a manifestation of intradermal sites of extramedullary hematopoiesis (EMH). It often becomes hemorrhagic secondary to thrombocytopenia present at birth in these infants. The initial "cranberry muffin" character of these 2 to 20 mm, raised, erythematous, soft, spongy lesions changes to the more characteristic appearance of "blueberry muffin" spots following intralesional hemorrhage. Petechiae may also be present in addition to the lesions of EMH. The lesions of EMH are not specific for rubella infection, and may also occur with congenital cytomegalovirus and toxoplasma infections. Petechial and purpuric lesions are evident in up to 60% of infants with congenital rubella.

EXTRACUTANEOUS FINDINGS. Associated clinical findings, beyond those listed previously, include congenital heart disease (patent ductus arteriosus, pulmonic stenosis, and aortic stenosis), cataracts, and pneumonia, which may actually develop and progress after birth. Psychomotor retardation and deafness occur in up to 50% of infants with documented congenital rubella syndrome.[40]

ETIOLOGY/PATHOGENESIS. Maternal infection gives rise to viremia, which is transmitted to the fetus, affecting rapidly dividing fetal tissues most prominently during the first 12 weeks of gestation. This single-stranded RNA virus usually causes a noncytolytic infection of cells, leading to cell dysfunction and defects in organogenesis. Although fetal infection may occur at any time during gestation, visible consequences of infection are most common following first-trimester infection, rare with a second-trimester infection, and virtually nonexistent following infection late in pregnancy.[41]

DIAGNOSIS. Viral culture of the pharynx is the definitive method of confirming the diagnosis of rubella infection (see Table 12-1), as shedding of virus continues for several weeks to months after birth. Assessing the maternal serologic status can be helpful, but many "prenatal" serologies are actually performed at the end of the first trimester and therefore do not truly represent the mother's immune status before pregnancy and cannot rule out infection at week 12 of gestation. If the infant is believed to have been infected, acute (cord blood) and convalescent (obtained at 4 to 6 months of age) blood samples should be obtained to determine antibody titers for rubella. These titers are diagnostic, since virtually all maternal transplacental antibody will have disappeared from the infant by 6 months of age. Evaluation of the cutaneous lesions will lead only to the nonspecific diagnosis of EMH.

PREVENTION AND THERAPY. No specific antiviral therapy exists for rubella virus. Universal immunization of children is specifically designed to prevent congenital rubella infection in the United States. Prenatal screening of women during early pregnancy should detect susceptible individuals and immunization immediately following the pregnancy is indicated.

ACQUIRED IMMUNODEFICIENCY SYNDROME

Acquired immunodeficiency syndrome (AIDS) is a multisystem disorder characterized by T-lymphocyte depletion and recurrent opportunistic infections. It results from infection with the human immunodeficiency virus (HIV). Characteristics of the infection include a variable latency period and an extremely high mortality rate. Perinatal transmission from infected mothers is the most common cause of childhood infection.[42] Most infants are asymptomatic in the first few months of life, but severe disease can occur within this time frame. Cutaneous abnormalities are among the earliest findings, and may be of an infectious, inflammatory or neoplastic nature.

CUTANEOUS FINDINGS. Cutaneous and mucous membrane disease is very common in infants with symptomatic HIV infection. Frequently the first indication that an infant is infected is the development of a severe or recurrent bacterial or fungal infection. In other instances, widespread and protracted seborrheic dermatitis may be the first clue to the patient's underlying immunodeficiency. Cutaneous infections that are extensive, progressive, or difficult to treat should raise suspicion for HIV infection. The type of cutaneous involvement that occurs with disease is generally related to the degree of immunosuppression.

INFECTIOUS DISORDERS. Mucocutaneous candidiasis is the most common dermatologic manifestation of pediatric HIV infection and occurs in the overwhelming majority of infected symptomatic children.[43] The disease is more severe and chronic than in the immunocompetent host and frequently persists beyond the first 6 months of life. White, cheesy patches or plaques overlying an erythematous base are found on the buccal mucosae, tongue, and palate. The lesions are friable and in severe cases may extend to involve the esophagus. The diaper area is commonly involved, with a beefy red erythema involving the convex surfaces and creases, along with satellite papules or pustules. Angular cheilitis and extensive, generalized, cutaneous involvement may also occur. Severe dermatophyte infections of the nails, hair, and skin may develop, and other unusual fungi such as cryptococcus and *Aspergillus* may cause systemic, as well as cutaneous disease.[44]

Bacterial infections of the skin may take the form of severe and recurrent staphylococcal impetigo, folliculitis, cellulitis, or abscesses. Other more unusual pathogens may be noted, particularly when the patient is severely immunosuppressed. Although PMN function against bacteria is not altered, T-B cell cooperation leading to opsonizing antibacterial function may be severely affected.

Viral infections are also atypical in course and lesion morphology. The lesions of varicella zoster infection may become chronic, hemorrhagic, ulcerating, and/or hypekeratotic.[45] Herpes zoster occurs earlier and more frequently in HIV-infected children. Herpes simplex infections may also be severe, prolonged, and/or recurrent. Molluscum contagiosum and papillomavirus infections are more frequent and may be relatively refractory to therapy.

Scabies can occur in early infancy and may present in a severe crusted form, often referred to as Norwegian scabies. Such cases are highly infectious because the affected infant usually possesses numerous generalized crusted papules that harbor large numbers of organisms.

Neoplastic Disease

Cancer is the presenting sign for AIDS in only 2% of children, as compared with 15% of adults.[46] Kaposi's sarcoma is significantly less common in childhood than adult AIDS. However, a recent report from Zambia noted a significant increase in the incidence of pediatric KS since 1987.[47] Kaposi's sarcoma has been described in a 6-day-old infant, but is rare in the neonatal period.[48] Non-Hodgkin's lymphomas, which are sometimes limited to the CNS, occur with increased frequency in the pediatric AIDS population, as do leiomyomas and leiomyosarcomas.[49]

Inflammatory Disease

Confluent beefy erythema with superimposed greasy thin scale first noted on the scalp and face is characteristic of seborrheic dermatitis in children with AIDS. It spreads to involve the axillae and diaper area and occasionally may progress to a severe generalized erythroderma. Atopic dermatitis and psoriasis can also occur in HIV-infected patients, but are not commonly diagnosed in the neonatal period. Drug eruptions, particularly from trimethoprim-sulfamethoxazole, are more frequent in children with AIDS.[50] The rash usually develops within 7 to 10 days after initiating therapy and is a pink papular or morbilliform eruption. Evolution to TEN may occur, but most eruptions resolve following discontinuation of the offending agent.

EXTRACUTANEOUS MANIFESTATIONS. An HIV-related embryopathy described in 1986, and characterized by microcephaly and dysmorphic facial features has not been substantiated. The papular exanthem/enanthem which develops shortly after HIV infection in adults has not been noted in perinatally acquired disease.[51]

Clinical conditions that should raise suspicion for HIV infection include failure to thrive, recurrent severe bacterial or opportunistic infections, hepatitis, lymphoid interstitial pneumonia, parotitis, lymphadenopathy, and hepatosplenomegaly. *Pneumocystis carinii* pneumonia is the most common serious opportunistic infection in HIV-infected children but usually does not develop until 3 to 6 months of age. Patients may also develop severe wasting, encephalopathy, developmental delay, nephropathy, cardiomyopathy, and diarrhea.

ETIOLOGY/PATHOGENESIS. HIV is a human retrovirus containing RNA. Two forms exist: HIV-1, most prevalent in the United States, and HIV-2, a related virus more commonly seen in West Africa. The virus has a predilection for CD4 lymphocytes, glial cells, macrophages and monocytes, and infection generally leads to significant impairment in cell-mediated immunity.

HIV is transmitted by contaminated blood, semen, human milk, and cervical secretions. The virus has also been isolated from saliva, tears, urine, cerebrospinal fluid, and pleural fluid, but these body fluids have not been shown to routinely transmit infection.

Perinatal transmission of HIV accounts for 90% of pediatric cases in the United States.[52] Infection may be transmitted to the infant in utero, at the time of delivery, or through breastfeeding. It is thought that the majority of infections are transmitted close to or at the time of delivery. Routine prenatal screening for HIV infection and treatment of infected women and their infants with antiviral agents such as zidovudine are recommended. Cesarean section may decrease the risk of HIV transmission to the fetus, presumably because the infant has decreased exposure to maternal blood and cervical secretions.[53]

The incubation period for HIV infection is quite variable. Infants are generally asymptomatic during the first few months of life. The median age of onset for perinatally acquired disease is 3 years, but some children may be asymptomatic for 5 or more years.[54] Conversely, severe illness can develop in the first few months of life. Approximately 10% to 15% of children will succumb before 4 years of life.[55]

DIAGNOSIS. Children born to HIV-infected mothers are almost always seropositive secondary to transplacentally acquired antibody, which may persist for up to 18 months. It is therefore necessary to document infection utilizing other methods in the newborn and young infant. A positive viral culture is diagnostic; however, only 25% to 50% of infected children will be identified at birth by means of culture. PCR evaluation is a very sensitive and widely available method for the detection of HIV infection in the neonatal period, and is the most commonly used means of diagnosis. If initial evaluation within the first 48 hours of life is negative, repeat tests should be performed at 1 to 2 months of life, and then again at 4 to 6 months of age if necessary.[55]

Laboratory findings suspicious for HIV infection include a decreased helper to suppressor T cell ratio and hypergammaglobulinemia. One study suggested that elevated IgG levels and oral candidiasis in children less than 15 months had a high (98%) specificity for the diagnosis, but low sensitivity (37%).[55] Lymphopenia is not usually seen in infants and children. Microcytic, hypochromic anemia is common, and thrombocytopenia may also be present. Because cutaneous disease in HIV-infected patients often presents in an atypical fashion, culture and biopsy of any suspicious lesion should be obtained if the diagnosis is in doubt.

TREATMENT. Treatment of the HIV-infected pregnant woman and the newborn infant with zidovudine can significantly decrease perinatal transmission. Short-term adverse effects of the drug include anemia, neutropenia, and hepatitis. No long-term adverse side effects have been noted.[56] Infected infants should be referred to an HIV specialist as recommendations for therapy are in evolution.

Chemoprophylaxis with TMP/SMX decreases the risk of infection with *Pneumocystis carinii* and may decrease the incidence of cutaneous bacterial infections. Cutaneous infections with fungi, bacteria, and viruses should be treated as appropriate for each disease. Candidiasis usually requires systemic therapy, and fluconazole has proved particularly useful for this purpose. Acyclovir therapy is appropriate for the treatment of herpes simplex and zoster infections, but chronic use may lead to acyclovir resistance, which is more common in the AIDS population. Foscarnet and ganciclovir have both proved to be efficacious antiviral agents in immunocompromised patients.

HUMAN PARVOVIRUS B19 INFECTIONS

Parvovirus is classically associated with a benign viral exanthem of childhood (erythema infectiosum), but can also cause transient aplastic crisis, chronic anemia, and petechial/purpuric cutaneous eruptions, as well as disease in the developing fetus.[57] The entire range of clinical manifestations caused by parvovirus B19 continues to expand, and the list of associated findings is remarkable for its diversity. This virus has a particular propensity for red blood progenitor cells, but can also affect skin, liver, and myocardial cells.[58] Although the majority of healthy individuals who are infected have few or no symptoms, the fetus is at particular risk for significant morbidity. Infection during pregnancy has been associated with an increased risk of miscarriage and fetal hydrops of 1% to 9%.[58] Symptomatic neonatal disease is rare and usually consists of persistent anemia following congenital infection.[59]

Fetal/Congenital and Neonatal Disease

CUTANEOUS FINDINGS. The most common findings in affected abortuses are pallor, maceration, and subcutaneous edema, all consistent with the diagnosis of hydrops. Blueberry muffin lesions showing extramedullary hematopoiesis have been reported as well.

EXTRACUTANEOUS FINDINGS. Increased fluid may develop in the peritoneal and pleural cavities. The exact risk of congenital anomalies following B19 infection is controversial. Significant ocular abnormalities involving the globe, retina, and cornea have been reported in one case.[60] Bilateral cleft lip and palate, micrognathia, subcutaneous hemorrhage, and congestion of internal organs have been found in fetuses in association with characteristic nuclear inclusions within erythroid precursor cells, endothelial, and smooth muscle cells.[61] Three live-born infants with severe neurologic defects whose mothers had serologically documented parvovirus infection during pregnancy have also been described.[62] Large prospective studies have failed to note significant risk of congenital abnormalities following maternal parvovirus infection.[63] Consensus at this time is that the risk of congenital infection from parvovirus is less than 1% and is not yet clearly determined.[64]

Most cases of documented neonatal infection consist of persistent anemia following congenital infection.[59] Isolated congenital red cell aplasia, which may mimic Diamond Blackfan anemia, may be caused by parvovirus B19 infection.[64] Relapsing erythroid hypoplasia in a 2-month-old infant has also been attributed to parvoviral infection. Multisystem disease in an infant who presented at birth with petechiae and thrombocytopenia and developed edema, cardiomegaly, bradycardia, and hypotension on day 2 has also been reported.[65] True neonatal disease is thought to be rare, but it is possible that it may be unrecognized and underreported. Unfortunately, technical problems in identifying neonatal infection make it difficult to ascertain the true incidence (see the following discussion).

ETIOLOGY/PATHOGENESIS. Parvovirus is one of the smallest known DNA viruses to infect humans. It is a global pathogen with increased prevalence in the late winter and early spring in temperate climates. Periodic epidemics occur.[66] The most common mode of transmission of B19 disease is person-to-person contact via respiratory secretions. The incubation period is 4 to 14 days, but can be as long as 21 days.[67] B19 can also be transmitted vertically from mother to fetus, and during transfusion with contaminated blood products.[67]

Infection is rare in the first year of life, and the highest rate of infection occurs among school-age children. The prevalence of IgG antibodies in pregnant women is approximately 65%.[59] Secondary attack rates are highest with household contact. Pregnant women with a child in the household age 5 to 7 years appear to have a higher risk of becoming infected than do those with children under 2 years of age. Of particular concern is the risk to seronegative women in day care and school settings because infection in the first 20 weeks of gestation can lead to increased fetal wastage and fetal hydrops. The greatest risk occurs during epidemics, and nursery school teachers appear to have a threefold increased risk of acute infection as compared with other pregnant women.[59]

Parvovirus B19 propagates in human erythroid cells. In normal hosts, the cytotoxic effect of the virus leads to cessation of red blood cell production for approximately 4 to 8 days, creating a significant stress in patients with a rapidly expanding red cell mass (e.g., second-trimester fetus), or decreased red cell survival (e.g., underlying hemolytic anemia). The cellular receptor for parvovirus B19 (globoside or blood group P antigen) is located predominantly on the surface of erythroid precursor cells, thus explaining the virus's affinity for this cell line. It is also present on myocardial cells, megakaryocytes, and endothelial cells, which may explain the thrombocytopenia, vasculitis, and myocarditis that is occasionally noted in affected fetuses and individuals.[58] Immunocompromised hosts, presumably including fetuses, may have persistent viral infection and resultant chronic anemia.

The pathogenesis of hydrops secondary to parvovirus may be multifactorial. Severe anemia is almost always present and may lead to hypoxic injury and high output cardiac failure. Ascites, effusions, and skin edema may result. Myocarditis and diminished fetal cardiac output have also been noted in some cases, and may contribute to hydrops.

The exact risk to any pregnant woman (and her fetus) following exposure is not precisely known, although risk appears to occur only if infection develops within the first 20 weeks of gestation. Various studies have estimated the risk of adverse fetal outcome following maternal infection to be from 1% to 9%.[59] Prospective studies have shown an excess rate of fetal loss of 9%, confined to exposure during the first 20 weeks of gestation, and an incidence of fetal hydrops of 2.9% with maternal infection between 11 and 18 weeks gestation.[63,68] No significant risk for congenital anomalies has

been noted. Spontaneous resolution of hydrops has been documented and complicates the issue of when and if intrauterine transfusion should be carried out (see Treatment).

DIAGNOSIS. The diagnosis of acute parvovirus infection in pregnant women using IgM antibodies or IgG seroconversion is straightforward. Using radioimmunoassay or ELISA, over 90% of cases can be documented at the time of rash.[67] However, fetuses, neonates, and immunocompromised patients may not mount an appropriate immune response following infection, and other methods may be required to document infection in these patients.

Virus may be identified using DNA hybridization techniques and PCR assays for B19.[63] Routine histopathologic evaluation may reveal the presence of characteristic intranuclear inclusions in nucleated erythroid cells in placental or fetal tissue. Immunohistochemistry may detect viral antigen by staining techniques. Electron microscopy has been used to detect virus particles in serum and prenatally in amniotic fluid, fetal blood, and ascitic fluid, as well as in postmortem tissue.[58]

Serologic evidence of infection in infants may be reevaluated at 1 year of age, at which time maternal antibody should have disappeared and immunoglobulin detection will indicate true fetal or neonatal infection. Viral studies may fail to reveal acute infection if carried out subsequent to resolution of the infection. Viremia persists only 2 to 4 days in the immunocompetent host and is generally absent by the time the classic rash develops.

DIFFERENTIAL DIAGNOSIS. Nonimmune fetal hydrops can result from a number of diverse etiologies. It has been associated with many cardiac, infectious, hematologic, and genetic abnormalities, including anemias of diverse origin, CMV, toxoplasmosis, and syphilis.

TREATMENT

Management of the exposed pregnant woman: Serologic evaluation should be offered; if the woman has high IgG titers to parvovirus B19 and lacks IgM, she is immune and not at risk. If she is seronegative, titers should be rechecked in 2 weeks for the presence of specific IgM. If evidence of acute infection exists, serial ultrasonographic evaluation is suggested.[69,70] Alpha fetoprotein levels have also been used as a screening tool.[69,70] The risk of adverse outcome is minimal if infection occurs after 20 weeks gestation, and low even if the mother becomes infected in the first two trimesters.

Management of fetal hydrops: Fetal intrauterine transfusion may be useful if significant fetal hydrops is observed.[70] Although studies have shown decreased mortality with transfusion, its use is controversial because cases of spontaneous resolution of intrauterine hydrops can occur, and the procedure poses some risk to the fetus.

Congenital and neonatal infection: Neonates with congenital infection attributed to parvovirus may respond to intravenous immunoglobulin therapy. Supportive care, including transfusion, may be required.

Prophylaxis: A candidate recombinant vaccine for human parvovirus B19 has been developed using empty capsid particles generated in a recombinant baculovirus-insect cell expression system and is under investigation.[71]

ENTEROVIRUS

The enteroviruses are a group of common, single-stranded RNA viruses that include the polioviruses, coxsackieviruses A and B, and echoviruses. Enteroviral infection in the neonate occurs most frequently during summer and early fall.

CUTANEOUS FINDINGS. Perinatal disease occurs within the first few weeks of life and results in the nonspecific clinical symptoms of sepsis (fever, irritability, poor feeding), accompanied by skin findings in approximately one third to two thirds of infants.[72,73] The rash is most often maculopapular (morbilliform), macular, or petechial (Fig. 12-8). The vesicopustular lesions that occur on intact skin (lesions analogous to those seen in hand, foot, and mouth disease) develop secondary to viremia, not from local inoculation as is seen in HSV infections. The pharynx is often erythematous, but usually without lesions. However, ulcers consistent with herpangina may appear on the soft palate. These early lesions may be indistinguishable from those of HSV infection. With progression of the infection, oral lesions remain circular (2 to 4 mm in diameter), confined to the soft palate, and exhibit a "punched-out" appearance surrounded by a rim of erythema. Unlike those of HSV, they do not continue to enlarge or involve the hard palate, buccal mucosa, or gingival sulci.

EXTRACUTANEOUS FINDINGS. Systemic manifestations of infection may be mild or severe. Disseminated infection involving lung, liver, and CNS (in addition to the upper respiratory tract and skin) occurs more often in the premature than in the full-term infant. The degree of transplacental antibody present is likely to affect the severity of the infection; therefore the most overwhelming infections occur in premature infants who lack significant amounts of specific maternal antibody for the infecting type of enterovirus.

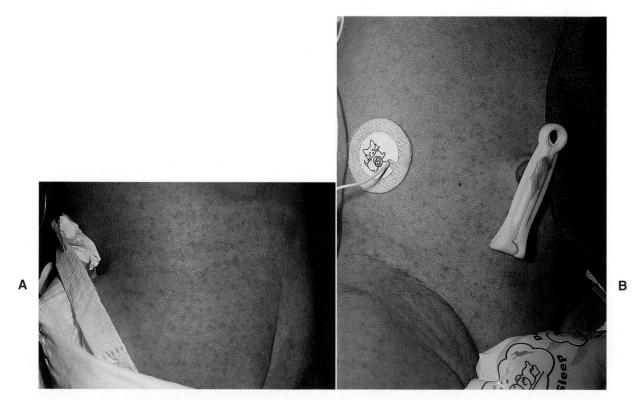

FIG. 12-8
Generalized erythematous papular eruption associated with enterovirus infection.

In utero disease may occur rarely, with insufficient numbers of cases reported to consider a "congenital infection syndrome." Findings in the neonate appear to result from residual damage to heart, gastrointestinal tract, urogenital tract, muscle, or cutaneous tissue, rather than ongoing infection or latent infection with reactivation of virus.

ETIOLOGY/PATHOGENISIS. Estimated rates of neonatal infection are between 2 and 38 cases per 1000 births.[74] Modes of transmission to the infant are similar to HSV. Acquisition from maternal sources at the time of delivery occurs in the majority of neonatal infections, with congenital infection being reported only rarely.[75] Postnatal infection from sources other than the mother is also very common, leading to illness and frequent hospitalization of symptomatic infants during the first few months of life.

DIAGNOSIS. Definitive diagnosis of enteroviral infection is most often achieved by viral culture of the pharynx or stool (see Table 12-1). During acute infection, cultures of the pharynx are the most likely to yield the pathogen, whereas intestinal excretion of virus from gut-associated lymphoid tissue increases following clinical recovery. Fecal shedding of virus may continue for up to 6 weeks following acute infection, despite the presence of neutralizing antibody in serum. The PCR technique has been exceptionally useful in the diagnosis of enteroviral meningitis and may be performed on the CSF of an infant whose rash is suspected to be of enteroviral origin.[76] PCR of material from the pharynx, stool, or lesions has not been systematically evaluated. Histologic examination of the morbilliform skin eruptions does not yield specific cytologic information on the viral etiology of the rash. Serologies are not usually helpful, since no class-specific antibody response occurs with enteroviral infections, and at least 72 serotypes of enterovirus have been identified to date.

TREATMENT. Traditionally, only supportive care has been given; however, some experts recommend administration of intravenous immunoglobulin to infants with overwhelming systemic infection.[77] Specific antiviral therapy with a novel antipicorna agent, pleconaril, is currently in clinical trials in newborn infants and has the potential to offer effective therapy for serious enteroviral infections.

HUMAN PAPILLOMA VIRUS INFECTIONS

Infection with the human papilloma virus (HPV) can lead to cutaneous infections that commonly manifest as warts on the skin or mucous membranes. Lesions may be spread by direct sexual or nonsexual contact, or from mother to infant in the prenatal or perinatal period. There is some evidence that fomite spread may be possible. The incubation period for HPV has been estimated at 1 to 20 months, but latency periods may be in excess of 2 years.[78,79] Although the vast majority of HPV disease results in transient lesions with a benign course, infection with certain subtypes of HPV can eventually lead to malignant metaplasia of the infected tissue.

Clinical lesions associated with HPV infections are only rarely present at birth or during the early neonatal period. Such lesions include anogenital warts (condyloma acuminata) and laryngeal papillomatosis. These lesions are more likely to become evident from 6 months to 2 years of life, and are believed to result from perinatal infection with a long latency period preceding clinical expression.

CUTANEOUS FINDINGS. Condyloma acuminata favor the mucocutaneous junctions and are papillomatous pink to flesh-colored soft lesions that may be discrete or confluent, pedunculated or flat-topped (Fig. 12-9). Areas most frequently affected in infants include the perianal skin, glans penis, vulva, and vaginal introitus (Fig. 12-10). The usual interval between exposure and development of lesions appears to be 1 to 8 months, with an average of 3 months.[80,81] Lesions presenting in the neonatal period may represent in utero or perinatal exposure. Laryngeal papillomas may affect the larynx, and less commonly the trachea, bronchial, and pulmonary epithelium. Such lesions usually present in infancy with hoarseness and respiratory distress.

ETIOLOGY/PATHOGENESIS. HPV is a small, 55 nm, nonenveloped, circular, double-stranded DNA virus. It is expressed exclusively in fully differentiated keratinocytes and

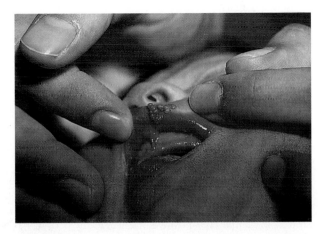

FIG. 12-9
Human papillomavirus infection. Congenital verrucous, filiform papules of the upper lip.

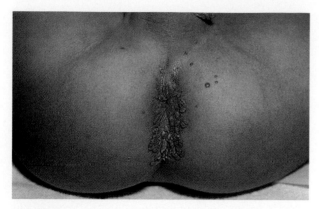

FIG. 12-10
Human papillomavirus infection. Multiple flesh-colored, discrete, and coalescent verrucous papules in the perianal region. Several smaller, ovoid flat lesions can be seen periperal to the perianal site.

cannot be perpetuated in tissue culture. Over 130 different subtypes possessing varied oncogenic potential and tissue trophism have been identified.[82] Although the papillomaviruses are categorized as to mucosal or cutaneous trophism, this classification is not strict, since genital types may be found on the skin, and cutaneous subtypes have been identified in anogenital lesions, particularly in children.[82] The viruses have also been classified as to their malignant potential. HPV 6 and 11 are considered low-risk subtypes, while HPV 16, 18, 31, and 33 have been associated with anogenital cancer. HPV 30 has been associated with oral and laryngeal carcinoma, as well as anogenital carcinoma.[82]

HPV is currently one of the most common sexually transmitted diseases, and the increasing incidence in infants and children that has been noted by clinicians probably reflects the increasing prevalence in the adult population.[83] Most anogenital warts are subclinical and asymptomatic. The prevalence of genital lesions (condyloma) in the adult population is 0.6% to 13%, but molecular diagnostic studies show evidence of HPV infection in 11% to 80% of asymptomatic, sexually active young women.[84,85] Transmission of infection may occur through vertical, innocent, and sexual contact. Subclinical infection of the cervix or vagina of a pregnant woman may lead to infection in her infant.[86] The virus can be transmitted from mother to fetus before or during birth, and the rate of perinatal transmission from genital HPV-positive mothers to the pharyngeal mucosa of their infants is approximately 30% to 50%.[87,88] However, studies of maternal-infant newborn pairs have demonstrated that even when there is transmission of virus,

it is most often only transiently positive, and clinical disease is unlikely to occur.[87,88,89]

Neonates appear to be at higher risk for exposure to HPV during vaginal delivery than during cesarean section delivery.[88] However, infants born by cesarean section have been found to be HPV DNA positive for the same type as their mothers.[90] Rare cases of anogenital warts present at birth following cesarean section delivery would support the possibility of ascending infection.[87] Transplacental exposure would explain such findings, as would small amniotic tears or leaks. The risk of a child contracting laryngeal papillomatosis is quite small.

HPV DNA has been identified in hepatic tissue from four infants with extrahepatic biliary duct atresia and three infants with neonatal giant cell hepatitis. Concordant HPV types were found in the infants' mothers, supporting vertical transmission of the virus and its role in the pathologies noted in these infants.[91]

DIAGNOSIS. The clinical appearance of anogenital warts is usually diagnostic. A careful maternal history, including prior genital lesions and abnormal PAP smears, should be obtained. However, a negative history and normal maternal examination do not rule out the possibility of HPV disease. A spontaneous remission rate as high as 67% has been reported for HPV infections,[83] and subclinical infection of the cervix or vagina may be present.

Histopathologic examination of anogenital HPV lesions demonstrates a slightly thickened stratum corneum, papillomatosis, and acanthosis of the epithelium, and thickening and elongation of the rete ridges. The presence of large vacuolated cells (koilocytes) in the epithelium is a characteristic sign, but is absent in approximately 50% of biopsies. HPV typing utilizing probes against the most commonly encountered types (6, 11, 16, 18, and 33) may be useful. Such typing can now be performed using paraffin sections from routinely fixed tissue samples. PCR evaluation of suspicious areas has also been performed utilizing specimens obtained by swabbing the site with a simple cotton swab.[92]

DIFFERENTIAL DIAGNOSIS. Sexual abuse must be considered in childhood HPV disease but is much less likely in the small infant. Condyloma lata should always be considered in the differential diagnosis. Syphilitic lesions are usually more moist, more wide-based, and frequently larger than the anogenital HPV lesions. Infantile pyramidal protrusion consists of a soft tissue swelling covered by smooth erythematous skin on the perineal median raphe. These may be congenital, tend to be larger than anogenital HPV lesions, and possess a smoother surface and a broad base. Molluscum contagiosum lesions are generally smoother, with a dome-shaped configuration, and central umbilication. Pseudoverrucous papules and nodules occur following a chronic irritant diaper dermatitis and can be mistaken for condylomata. Skin tags may resemble condyloma acuminata, but are uncommon in the neonatal period, are flesh-colored, discrete, and do not spread.

TREATMENT. Many experts believe that treatment may not always be necessary because warts are relatively asymptomatic, the spontaneous remission rate is quite high, and the cure rate with therapy low.[93] No easy, universally effective treatment exists. A number of therapeutic modalities have been used in adults and older children. These include liquid nitrogen, podophyllin resin, trichloroacetic acid, cantharidin, podofilox, imiquimod cream, and interferon. Physical destruction, including electrodesiccation, laser therapy, and simple excision are also alternative therapies. The failure rate for treatment of HPV infections has been estimated at 25% to 50%, regardless of the method used.[93]

Most experts opt for simple, less painful means of treatment in infants and young children. Topical agents frequently used include podophyllin resin, trichloroacetic acid and imiquimod cream. The family must be aware that frequent treatments are often required and that subclinical lesions in surrounding skin may become evident over time despite eradication of currently existing lesions. Prophylactic and therapeutic HPV vaccines, as well as gene therapy, are all under investigation at the present time.[93]

MOLLUSCUM CONTAGIOSUM

Molluscum contagiosum is a viral infection of the skin that most commonly affects young children but can occur at any age. This disease is only rarely noted in the neonatal period, but lesions have been documented within the first week of life.[94]

CUTANEOUS FINDINGS. Molluscum lesions initially appear as small pink or flesh colored pinpoint papules, which gradually enlarge and assume a pearly or white dome-shaped appearance. The papules are usually 1 to 5 mm in size, but giant lesions in excess of 1 cm can occur. The lesions tend to cluster and more commonly appear on the trunk and in intertriginous areas such as the antecubital and popliteal fossae and axillae. Rarely lesions may develop on the palms, soles, or mucous membranes. An eczematoid, red, scaling patch may surround the papules and is termed *molluscum dermatitis*. Autoinoculation from scratching or shaving may occur.[94]

There are rare reports of neonatal disease in the literature. Mandel and Lewis[94] reported an infant who developed two thigh papules at one week of life, and another author documented multiple scalp lesions in a 6-week-

old.[95] Wilkin[96] described five women who had genital lesions at the time of delivery; none of their infants developed molluscum.

ETIOLOGY/PATHOGENESIS. Molluscum contagiosum is caused by a large, approximately 300 nm, brick-shaped poxvirus, which contains double-stranded DNA. Three types of molluscum virus have been identified, but there are no clinically significant differences among the three. The entire genetic sequence of MCV type 1 has been determined, and there appears to be considerable protein homology with the smallpox virus.[97] The virus does not grow in tissue culture, and an animal model does not exist.

Molluscum has a worldwide distribution, but is most common in tropical countries. Spread is through contact with infected persons, contaminated items, or by means of autoinoculation. The incubation period is estimated at 2 weeks to 6 months. The duration of disease is quite variable and may last just a few weeks or more than a year.[98] Two peaks in incidence occur, one in early childhood and the other in young adults as a result of sexual transmission. An increased incidence has been noted in wrestlers and swimmers, and outbreaks have occurred in pools and water parks.[99] The disease has only rarely been noted in neonates, and it has been hypothesized that transplacental maternally derived antibody may be protective. The immunocompromised, especially those with HIV infection, are subject to particularly extensive and prolonged infections that commonly involve the face. Patients with atopic dermatitis also appear to have more prolonged infections.

DIAGNOSIS. The diagnosis is easily established when classic dome-shaped opalescent lesions with central umbilication are present. A curdlike material can be expressed from the central core and examined for the presence of molluscum bodies. These appear as monomorphous ovoid granular structures, and are best visualized with Wright's or Giemsa stain. Histopathologic evaluation of a lesion will reveal large intracytoplasmic inclusion bodies within suprabasalar epithelial cells and lobular proliferation of the epidermis.

DIFFERENTIAL DIAGNOSIS. Cutaneous cryptococcal lesions are occasionally mistaken for molluscum contagiosum in immunocompromised patients. Small lesions may be mistaken for common or flat warts. Giant molluscum lesions can resemble juvenile xanthogranuloma or Langerhans' cell histiocytosis. Large inflamed lesions may resemble furuncles. The differential diagnosis for atypical giant lesions includes a number of neoplastic disorders, and biopsy is indicated in such cases.

TREATMENT. Molluscum is generally self-limited and frequently does not require therapy.[100] Instances where intervention may be necessary include conjunctival lesions, which may damage the cornea, irritated, bleeding, or rapidly spreading lesions, and cosmetically disfiguring lesions, particularly in the immunosuppressed patient. Genital lesions are usually treated to prevent spread. A number of therapeutic modalities are used, including physical agents such as cryotherapy and curettage. Chemical treatments include cantharidin, podophyllin, salicylic acid, tretinoin, and silver nitrate. Adhesive tape occlusion and systemic cimetidine therapy have been utilized, all with variable results. A local anesthetic, lidocaine plus prilocaine (EMLA), may be applied prior to curettage. Families should be counseled that multiple visits and treatments may be required and that spread of infection may occur through shared baths, towels, and swimming pools. Genital lesions are not uncommon in young children and are thought to be the result of autoinoculation. The issue of sexual abuse may be raised, but supporting evidence should be documented prior to referral, as nonsexually transmitted genital involvement is often seen in childhood infections.[100]

REFERENCES

1. Sullivan-Bolyai J, Hull HF, Wilson C, et al. Neonatal herpes simplex virus infection in King County, Washington. JAMA 1983;250:3059-3062.
2. Overall JC. Herpes simplex virus infection of the fetus and newborn. Pediatr Ann 1994;23:131-136.
3. Brown ZA, Benedetti J, Ashley R, et al. Neonatal herpes simplex virus infection in relation to asymptomatic maternal infection at the time of labor. N Engl J Med 1991;324:1247-1252.
4. Cone RW, Hobson AC, Brown Z, et al. Frequent detection of genital herpes simplex virus DNA by polymerase chain reaction among pregnant women. JAMA 1994;272:792-796.
5. Sieber OF, Fulginiti VA, Brazie J, et al. In utero infection of the fetus by herpes simplex virus. J Pediatr 1966;69:30-34.
6. South MA, Tompkins WAF, Morris CP, et al. Congenital malformation of the central nervous system associated with genital (type 2) herpes virus. J Pediatr 1969;75:13-18.
7. Sullender WM, Miller JL, Yasukawa LL, et al. Humoral and cell-mediated immunity in neonates with herpes simplex virus infection. J Infect Dis 1987;155:28-37.
8. Hutto C, Arvin A, Jacobs R, et al. Intrauterine herpes simplex virus infections. J Pediatr 1987;110:97-101.
9. Honig PJ, Brown D. Congenital herpes simplex infection initially resembling Epidermolysis bullosa. J Pediatr 1982; 101:958-960.
10. Kimberlin DW, Jacobs RF, Powell DA, et al. The safety and efficacy of high-dose (HD) acyclovir (ACV) in neonatal herpes simplex virus (HSV). Presented at The American Pediatric Society/The Society for Pediatric Research. May, 1999.
11. Englund JA, Fletcher CV, Balfour HH. Acyclovir therapy in neonates. J Pediatr 1991;119:129-135.
12. Whitley R, Arvin A, Prober C, et al. A controlled trial comparing vidarabine with acyclovir in neonatal herpes simplex virus infection. N Engl J Med 1991;324:444.
13. Sever J, White LR. Intrauterine viral infections. Annu Rev Med 1968;19:471-486.
14. Dufour P, de Bievre P, Vinatier D, et al. Varicella and pregnancy. Eur J Obstet Gynecol Reprod Biol 1996;66:119-123.
15. McIntosh D, Isaacs D. Varicella-zoster virus infection in pregnancy. Arch Dis Child 1993;68:1-2.
16. Kellner B, Kitai I, Krafchik B. What syndrome is this? Congenital varicella syndrome. Pediatr Dermatol 1996;13:341-344.
17. Paryani SG, Arvin AM. Intrauterine infection with varicella-zoster virus after maternal varicella. N Engl J Med 1986; 314:1542-1546.
18. Enders G. Varicella-zoster virus infection in pregnancy. Prog Med Virol 1984;29:166-196.
19. Pastuszak AL, Levy M, Schick B, et al. Outcome after maternal varicella infection in the first 20 weeks of pregnancy. N Eng J Med 1994;330:901-905.
20. Enders G, Miller E, Craddock-Watson J, et al. Consequences of varicella and herpes zoster in pregnancy: Prospective study of 1739 cases. Lancet 1994;343:1548-1551.
21. Salzman MB, Sood SK. Congenital anomalies resulting from maternal varicella at 25 1/2 weeks of gestation. Pediatr Infect Dis J 1992;11:504-505.
22. Birthistle K, Carrington D. Fetal varicella syndrome—a reappraisal of the literature. A review prepared for the UK Advisory Group on Chickenpox on behalf of the British Society for the Study of Infection. J Infect 1998;36:25-29.
23. Harris RE, Rhoades ER. Varicella pneumonia complicating pregnancy: Report of a case and review of literature. Obstet Gynecol 1965;25:734-740.
24. Chapman SJ. Varicella in pregnancy. Semin Perinatol 1998;22:339-346.
25. Hartung J, Enders G, Chaoui R, et al. Prenatal diagnosis of congenital varicella syndrome and detection of varicella-zoster virus in the fetus: A case report. Prenat Diagn 1999; 19(2):163-166.
26. Mouly F, Mirlesse V, Meritet JF, et al. Prenatal diagnosis of fetal varicella-zoster virus infection with polymerase chain reaction of amniotic fluid in 107 cases. Am J Obstet Gynecol 1997;177:894-898.
27. Pretorius DH, Hayward I, Jones KL, et al. Sonographic evaluation of pregnancies with maternal varicella infection. J Ultrasound Med 1992;11:459-463.
28. Gershon AA. Chicken Pox, measles, and mumps. Infect Dis Fetus Newborn 1995;4:578-583.
29. Miller E, Cradock-Watson JE, Ridehalgh MK. Outcome in newborn babies given anti-varicella zoster immunoglobin after perinatal maternal infection with varicella zoster virus. Lancet 1989;2:371-373.
30. Eldridge R, Tillson HH. Pregnancy outcome following systemic prenatal acyclovir exposure. Arch Dermatol 1994; 130:153-154.
31. Prober CG, Gershon AA, Grose C, et al. Consensus: varicella-zoster infections in pregnancy and the perinatal period. Pediatr Infect Dis J 1990;9:865-869.
32. Singalavanija S, Limpongsanurak W, Horpoapan S, et al. Neonatal varicella: a report of 26 cases. J Med Assoc Thai 1999;82:957-962.
33. Frieden IJ, Berger TG, Westrom D. Eosinophil fluorescence: A cause of false positive slide tests for herpes simplex virus. Pediatr Dermatol 1987;4:129-133.

34. Bendig JA, Meurisse EV, Anderson F, et al. Neonatal Varicella despite maternal immunity. Lancet 1998;352:1985-1986.

35. American Academy of Pediatrics. 1997 Red Book: Report of the Committee on Infectious Diseases. 24th edition. Elk Grove Village, Ill: American Academy of Pediatrics, 1997: p 578.

36. Saigal S, Luny KO, Larke R, et al: The outcome in children with congenital cytomegalovirus infection. Am J Dis Child 1982;136:896-901.

37. Stagno S, Pass RF, Dworsky ME, et al. Congenital cytomegalovirus infection: the relative importance of primary and recurrent maternal infection. N Engl J Med 1982; 306: 945-949.

38. Demmler GJ. Summary of a workshop on surveillance for congenital cytomegalovirus disease. Rev Infect Dis 1991; 13:315-329.

39. Nelson CT, Istas AS, Wilkerson MK, et al. Polymerase chain reaction detection of cytomegalovirus DNA in serum as a diagnostic test for congenital cytomegalovirus infection. J Clin Microbiol 1995;33:3317-3318.

40. Cooper LZ, Preblud SR, Alford CA, et al. Rubella. In Remington JS, Klien JO, eds. Infectious diseases of the fetal and newborn infant. 4th edition. Philadelphia: WB Saunders, 1995.

41. Overall JC, Feigin RD, Cherry JD. Viral infections of the fetus and neonate. In Feigin RD, Cherry JD, eds. Textbook of pediatric infectious diseases. 4th edition. Philadelphia: WB Saunders, 1998.

42. Centers for Disease Control. HIV/AIDS surveillance report. August 1990;1-18.

43. Pahwa S, Kaplan M, Fikrig S, et al. Spectrum of human T-cell lymphotropic virus type III infection in children. Recognition of symptomatic, asymptomatic, and seronegative patients. JAMA. 1986, 255.2299 2305.

44. Shetty D, Giri N, Gonzalez CE, et al. Invasive aspergillosis in human immunodeficiency virus-infected children. Pediatr Infect Dis J 1997;16:216-221.

45. Prose NS. Cutaneous manifestations of HIV infection in children. Dermatol Clin 1991;9:543-550.

46. Centers for Disease Control. HIV/AIDS surveillance report. Cancer as AIDS-defining illness. Oct 1993;1-18.

47. Athale UH, Patil PS, Chintu C, et al. Influence of HIV epidemic on the incidence of Kaposi's sarcoma in Zambian children. J Acquir Immune Defic Syndr Hum Retrovirol 1995;8:96-100.

48. Gutierrez-Ortega P, Hierro-Orozco S, Sanchez-Cisneros R, et al. Kaposi's sarcoma in a 6-day-old infant with human immunodeficiency virus. Arch Dermatol 1989;125:432-433.

49. Mueller BU, Butler KM, Higham MC, et al. Smooth muscle tumors in children with human immunodeficiency virus infection. Pediatrics 1992;90:460-463.

50. Straka BF, Whitaker DL, Morrison SH, et al. Cutaneous manifestations of the acquired immunodeficiency syndrome in children. J Am Acad Dermatol 1988;18(5 Pt 1):1089-1102.

51. Marion RW, Wiznia AA, Hutcheon RG, et al. Fetal AIDS syndrome score. Correlation between severity of dysmorphism and age at diagnosis of immunodeficiency. Am J Dis Child 1987;141:429-431.

52. Centers for Disease Control. HIV/AIDS surveillance report. 1998;10:1-40.

53. Gelber RD, Shapiro DE. Mode of delivery and the risk of vertical transmission of HIV-1.N Engl J Med 1999;15: 341:206-207.

54. American Academy of Pediatrics [Leishmaniasis]. In Peter G, ed. 1997 Red Book:Report of the Committee on Infectious Diseases. 24th edition. Elk Grove Village, IL: American Academy of Pediatrics, 1997: p 286.

55. Meyer MP, Latief Z, Haworth C, et al. Symptomatic HIV infection in infancy—clinical and laboratory markers of infection. S Afr Med J 1997;87:158-162.

56. Culnane M, Fowler M, Lee SS, et al. Lack of long-term effects of in utero exposure to zidovudine among uninfected children born to HIV-infected women. Pediatric AIDS Clinical Trials Group Protocol 219/076 Teams. JAMA 1999; 13:281:151-157.

57. Vogel H, Kornman M, Ledet SC, et al: Congenital parvovirus infection. Pediatr Pathol Lab Med 1997;17:903-912.

58. Valeur-Jensen AK, Pedersen CB, Westergaard T, et al. Risk factors for parvovirus B19 infection in pregnancy. JAMA 1999;281:1099-1105.

59. Brown KE, Green SW, Antunez de Mayolo J, et al. Congenital anaemia after transplacental B19 parvovirus infection. Lancet 1994;343(8902):895-896.

60. Van Elsacker-Niele AM, Salimans MM, Weiland HT, et al. Fetal pathology in human parvovirus B19 infection. Br J Obstet Gynaecol 1989;96:768-775.

61. Tiessen RG, van Elsacker-Niele AM, Vermeij-Keers C, et al. A fetus with a parvovirus B19 infection and congenital anomalies. Prenat Diagn 1994;14:173-176.

62. Conroy JA, Torok T, Andrews PI. Perinatal encephalopathy secondary to inutero human parvo B19 infection (absract 7365) Neurology 43 (suppl) A346, 1993.

63. Miller E, Fairley CK, Cohen BJ, et al. Immediate and long-term outcome of human parvovirus B19 infection in pregnancy. Br J Obstet Gynaecol 1998;105:174-178.

64. Auerbach AD, Verlander PC, Brown KE, et al. New molecular diagnostic tests for two congenital forms of anemia.J Clin Lab Anal 1997;11:17-22.

65. Minowa H, Nishikubo T, Uchida Y, et al. Neonatal erythema infectiosum. Acta Paediatr Jpn 1998;40:88-90.

66. Brown KE, Young NS. Parvovirus B19 in human disease. Annu Rev Med 1997;48:59-67.

67. American Academy of Pediatrics [Leishmaniasis]. In Peter G, ed. 1997 Red Book:Report of the Committee on Infectious Diseases. 24h edition. Elk Grove Village, IL: American Academy of Pediatrics, 1997: pp 383 385.

68. Prospective study of human parvovirus (B19) infection in pregnancy. Public Health Laboratory Service Working Party on Fifth Disease. BMJ 1990;300(6733):1166-1170.

69. Levy R, Weissman A, Blomberg G, et al. Infection by parvovirus B 19 during pregnancy: A review. Obstet Gynecol Surv 1997;52:254-259.

70. Fairley CK, Smoleniec JS, Caul OE, et al. Observational study of effect of intrauterine transfusions on outcome of fetal hydrops after parvovirus B19 infection. Lancet 1995; 346(8986):1335-1337.

71. Bansal GP, Hatfield JA, Dunn FE, et al. Candidate recombinant vaccine for human B19 parvovirus. J Infect Dis 1993; 167:1034-1044.

72. Lake AM, Lauer BA, Clark JC, et al. Enterovirus infections in neonates. J Pediatr 1976;89:787-791.

73. Abzug MJ, Levin MJ, Rotbart HA. Profile of enterovirus disease in the first two weeks of life. Pediatr Infect Dis J 1993; 12:820-824.

74. Overall JC, Feigin RD, Cherry JD. Viral infections of the fetus and neonate. In Feigin RD, Cherry JD, ed. Textbook of pediatric infectious diseases. 4th edition. Philadelphia: WB Saunders, 1998.

75. Modlin JF. Update on enterovirus infections in infants and children. Adv Pediatr Infect Dis 1997;12:155-180.

76. Sawyer MH. Enterovirus infections: Diagnosis and treatment. Pediatr Infect Dis J 1999;18:1033-1040.

77. Abzug MJ, Keyserling HL, Lee ML, et al. Neonatal enterovirus infection: Virology, serology, and effects of intravenous immune globulin. Clin Infect Dis 1995;20:1201-1206.

78. Siegfried EC. Warts on children: An approach to therapy. Pediatr Ann 1996;25:79-90.

79. Frasier LD. Human papillomavirus infections in children. Pediatr Ann 1994;23:354-360.

80. Barrett TJ. Genital warts: A venereal disease. J Am Acad Dermatol 1954:333-334.

81. Oriel JD. Natural history of genital warts. Br J Vener Dis 1971;47:1-13.

82. Majewski S, Jablonska S. Human papillomavirus-associated tumors of the skin and mucosa. J Am Acad Dermatol 1997; 36(5 Pt 1):659-85; quiz 686-688.

83. Allen AL, Siegfried EC. The natural history of condyloma in children. J Am Acad Dermatol 1998;39:951-955.

84. Schneider A, Koutsky LA. Natural history and epidemiological features of genital HPV infection. IARC Sci Publ 1992; 265:472-477.

85. Moscicki AB. Human papillomavirus infections. Adv Pediatr 1992;39:257-281.

86. Mazzatenta C, Fimiani M, Rubegni P, et al. Vertical transmission of human papillomavirus in cytologically normal women. Genitourin Med 1996;72:445-446.

87. Tseng CJ, Liang CC, Soong YK, et al. Perinatal transmission of human papillomavirus in infants: Relationship between infection rate and mode of delivery. Obstet Gynecol 1998; 91:92-96.

88. Sedlacek TV, Lindheim S, Eder C, et al. Mechanism for human papillomavirus transmission at birth. Am J Obstet Gynecol 1989;161:55-59.

89. Tenti P, Zappatore R, Migliora P, et al. Perinatal transmission of human papillomavirus from gravidas with latent infections. Obstet Gynecol 1999;93:475-479.

90. Puranen MH, Yliskoski MH, Saarikoski SV, et al. Exposure of an infant to cervical human papillomavirus infection of the mother is common. Am J Obstet Gynecol 1997;176:1039-1045.

91. Drut R, Gomez MA, Drut RM, et al. Acta Gastroenterol Latinoam. 1998;28:27-31. Spanish.

92. Siegfried EC, Frasier LD. Anogenital warts in children. Adv Dermatol 1997;12:141-66; discussion 167.

93. Hines JF, Ghim SJ, Jenson AB. Prospects for human papillomavirus vaccine development: Emerging HPV vaccines. Curr Opin Obstet Gynecol 1998;10:15-19.

94. Mandel MJ, Lewis RJ. Molluscum contagiosum of the newborn. Br J Dermatol 1971;84:370-372.

95. Young WJ. Molluscum Contagiosum with unusual distribution. Kentucky Med J 24:467, 1926.

96. Wilkin JK. Molluscum contagiosum venereum in a women's outpatient clinic: A venereally transmitted disease. Am J Obstet Gynecol 1977;128:531-535.

97. Senkevich TG, Bugert JJ, Sisler JR, et al. Genome sequence of a human tumorigenic poxvirus: Prediction of specific host response-evasion genes. Science 1996;273:813-816.

98. Lewis EJ, Lam M, Crutchfield CE III. An update on molluscum contagiosum. Cutis. 1997;60:29-34.

99. Castilla MT, Sanzo JM, Fuentes S. Molluscum contagiosum in children and its relationship to attendance at swimming-pools: An epidemiological study. Dermatology 1995; 191:165.

100. Highet AS. Molluscum contagiosum. Arch Dis Child 1992; 67:1248-1249.

13

Fungal Infections, Infestations, and Parasitic Infections in Neonates

ALICE L. PONG
CATHERINE CAMERON McCUAIG

FUNGAL INFECTIONS

Infections caused by fungus and yeast are common in neonates and infants. Of these, the most frequent is *Candida* infection, presenting as thrush and diaper dermatitis. More extensive manifestations, such as congenital and systemic candidiasis, are less common. Significant fungal infections are being seen more often in very low birth weight (VLBW), preterm infants. *Malassezia furfur* can colonize the skin or manifest as neonatal cephalic pustulosis, tinea versicolor, or fungemia. *Aspergillus* is second only to *Candida* as a cause of opportunistic fungal infections in these hosts. Zygomycosis and trichosporonosis are seen almost exclusively in premature infants. Dermatophyte infections include tinea capitis, tinea corporis, and less commonly, onychomycosis.

Candidiasis

Epidemiology and Pathogenesis

Candida is the most common fungal pathogen in newborns.[1] Infection may be acquired vertically from the mother or horizontally by nosocomial transmission in the nursery. *C. albicans* is responsible for approximately 75% of neonatal fungal infections.[2] Other *Candida* species associated with neonatal disease include *C. tropicalis, C. parapsilosis, C. lusitaniae,* and *C. glabrata (Torulopsis glabrata)*. Normally these yeasts are saprophytes, inhabiting the skin or gastrointestinal tract without invasion unless host defenses are altered. *Candida* spp. may also colonize endotracheal tubes and catheters without causing systemic illness.[3]

Virulence mechanisms associated with *Candida* infections include fungal proteinase, increased adherence of yeast to epithelial cells due to similarity to mammalian cell ligands, and resistance to neutrophil ingestion of hyphal forms.[4] Secretory IgA, functional T lymphocytes, and phagocytic cells are important in defense of *Candida* infections, hence the increased susceptibility to these infections in patients with secretory IgA deficiency, primary T cell deficiency such as DiGeorge syndrome, severe combined immunodeficiency, chronic granulomatous disease, myeloperoxidase deficiency, and human immunodeficiency virus (HIV) infection. Recurrent or persistent yeast infections can be presenting symptoms of immunodeficiency. Host resistance to fungal infections also depends on activated macrophages, which in turn rely on T lymphocyte release of interferon-gamma (IFN). Incomplete activation of macrophages by IFN in neonates[5] contributes to increased susceptibility to invasive fungal disease.

Predisposing factors for *Candida* (monilial) infections include excessive humidity, maceration, diabetes, and broad-spectrum antibiotics. Risk factors for systemic candidiasis in neonates include low birth weight, prematurity, broad-spectrum antibiotic therapy, indwelling catheters, prolonged endotracheal intubation, tracheostomy, immunosuppression, defective neutrophil function or neutropenia, and steroid therapy.[2,6,7]

Various techniques in addition to culture techniques are used to evaluate the epidemiology of fungal pathogens. They include polymerase chain reaction (PCR), restriction fragment endonuclease digestion of chromosomal DNA, electrophoretic karyotyping, and Southern blot hybridization analysis using DNA probes.[1]

Clinical presentations of candidal infections are discussed in the following section, followed by diagnostic and treatment recommendations.

223

Congenital Candidiasis

Congenital candidiasis (CC) refers to *Candida* infection acquired in utero and presenting with symptoms in the first days of life.[8] Classic congenital candidiasis presents as a diffuse cutaneous infection, presumed to arise from an ascending intrauterine chorioamnionitis. The typical patient is an otherwise healthy term neonate who, within the first 12 hours of life, develops a monomorphous papulovesicular eruption that is intensely erythematous (Figs. 13-1 and 13-2). The papular rash progresses to pustules followed by late crusting and desquamation. Any area of the body surface, including the face, palms, and soles, can be involved, and widespread involvement is often evident (Fig. 13-3). *Candida* paronychia and onychodystrophy have been reported.[8,9] Congenital candidiasis is surprisingly uncommon given the 33% *Candida* vaginal colonization rate in pregnant women.[2] The presence of a foreign body in the maternal uterus or cervix is a risk factor for CC. In the majority of term infants with CC, systemic dissemination of yeast is rare, and the prognosis is excellent with rapid clearance of the rash with topical treatment alone. Occasionally CC can present as pneumonia and sepsis without a rash.[10] CC with systemic involvement is more commonly seen in premature, low birth weight infants (<1500 g).[11,12] Skin

findings in these infants may be variable, with ecchymoses and necrosis in addition to the usual maculopapular eruption. A widespread rash in a premature or ill-appearing infant should alert the physician to the possibility of systemic candidiasis despite negative blood cultures.[13,14]

Systemic Candidiasis

Systemic candidiasis (SC), defined as *Candida* infection in an otherwise sterile body fluid such as blood, urine, or cerebrospinal fluid, affects 2% to 4% of VLBW newborns.[6,15] Skin manifestations occur in 50% to 60% of these infants.[14] These infections can be acquired in utero

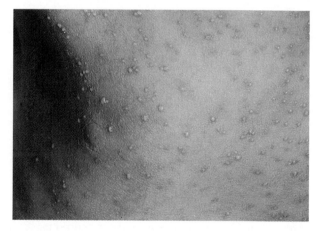

FIG. 13-2
Congenital candidiasis: Diffusely distributed, distinct pustules.

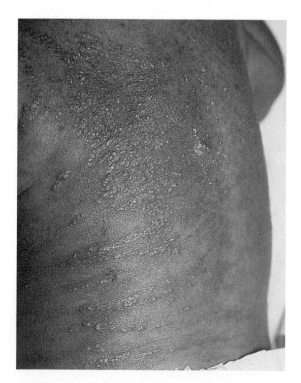

FIG. 13-1
Congenital candidiasis: Diffuse, erythematous, pustular eruption.

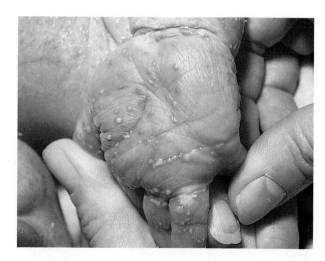

FIG. 13-3
Congenital candidiasis: Palmar pustules with erythema.

(CC) or postnatally. Baley et al[15] described skin manifestations of VLBW infants with SC. Included were an extensive burnlike dermatitis followed by desquamation, progressive diaper dermatitis involving papules and pustules, and isolated diaper rash with or without thrush (Fig. 13-4).[15] Cutaneous abscesses at the site of intravascular catheters may also be seen.[2] Systemic signs include apnea, bradycardia, abdominal distension, guaiac-positive stools, hyperglycemia, temperature instability, leukemoid reaction, and hypotension.[2,6,16]

Invasive Fungal Dermatitis

Invasive fungal dermatitis (IFD) is a clinicopathologic entity of erosive crusting lesions in VLBW infants. It is described by Rowen et al[17] as a primary skin condition that leads to secondary systemic disease. It is primarily due to *Candida albicans* or other *Candida* species. *Aspergillus, Trichosporum beigelii,* and a *Curvularia* sp. are also etiologic agents of invasive fungal dermatitis. Skin biopsy demonstrates fungal invasion beyond the stratum corneum, well into the epidermis, and at times extending into the dermis. Onset several days after birth, the presence of erosions and crusts, and typical histologic findings help to differentiate IFD from congenital candidiasis. Risk factors include extreme prematurity (<25 weeks gestational age), vaginal birth, steroid administration, and hyperglycemia.[17]

Localized Neonatal Candidiasis

Oral candidiasis (thrush). Acute oral candidiasis appears on the oropharyngeal mucosa as white adherent curdlike plaques, resembling milk or formula (Fig. 13-5). Plaques can be scraped off only with difficulty, leaving a bright erythematous base (pseudomembranous and ery-thematous forms, respectively). Extensive infection can lead to feeding difficulties, particularly if the esophagus is involved.[2]

***Candida* diaper dermatitis.** *Candida* infection of the diaper area may occur alone or in conjunction with thrush. Bright, erythematous plaques, papules, and pustules affect the moist intertriginous areas of the perineum, with a predilection for inguinal creases. White scale and satellite pustules are common along the periphery, often prominent at the border of involved and uninvolved skin (Fig. 13-6). Perianal involvement is common. Pustules may be very superficial and rupture easily. Candidal dermatitis may be seen in 4% to 6% of term newborns, with the incidence peaking at 3 to 4 months of age.[2] Similar bright erythema may be seen in napkin psoriasis. Further

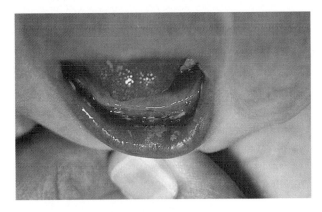

FIG. 13-6
White plaques of oral thrush.

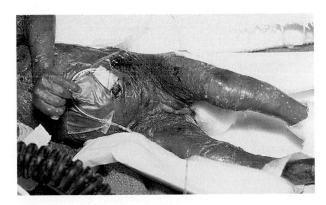

FIG. 13-4
Congenital candidiasis in a premature (<700 g) infant presenting with diffuse erythema and a scaldlike appearance.

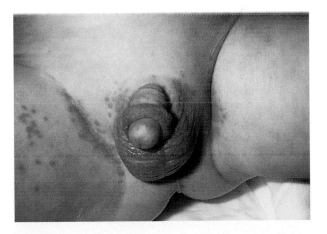

FIG. 13-6
Candidal diaper dermatitis: red plaque with inguinal crease involvement and satellite pustules.

differential diagnoses include infectious and noninfectious entities outlined in Chapter 14.

Candida infection of the nail. Candidal infection of the nail may occur alone or in conjunction with systemic and congenital candidiasis. Finger sucking is a potential predisposing event. Erythema and swelling in proximal and lateral nail folds may resemble bacterial paronychia, and separation of the cuticle from the nail plate may be seen (Figs. 13-7 and 13-8). The resultant onychodystrophy may lead to proximal-, distal-, and lateral-subungual, superficial white, or total dystrophic onychomycosis. The latter condition presents with a crumbling nail and abnormal thickened nail bed. It is frequently seen in patients with chronic mucocutaneous candidiasis and other immunodeficiency states.[18] Tinea unguium, hereditary onychodystrophy, ectodermal dysplasia, epidermolysis bullosa, psoriasis, and acrodermatitis may present with similar nail findings.

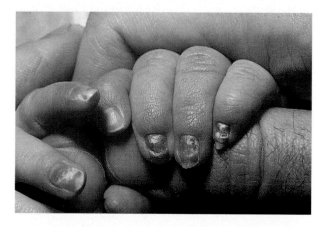

FIG. 13-7
Nail changes secondary to congenital candidiasis

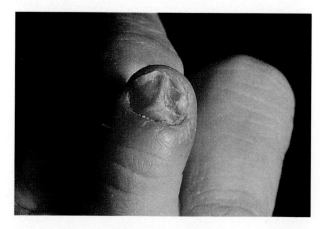

FIG. 13-8
Candidal paronychia.

Diagnosis of Candida Infections

Skin scrapings from pustules or peripheral scale should be examined using KOH solution or Giemsa, Gram, or calcofluor stains. Pseudohyphae and spores may be visualized with direct staining. Satellite pustules are most likely to yield positive results. Cultures from multiple sites, including skin, blood, cerebrospinal fluid, and urine should be collected if systemic disease is suspected. Culture yield is inconsistent,[7] and negative cultures do not rule out systemic disease in the symptomatic infant.[2] Buffy coat smear microscopy, a rapid bedside test with 100% specificity, can confirm candidemia within 1 to 2 hours. Sensitivity is 62%, compared with 44% for peripheral blood smear examination.[19] In some centers, buffy coat culture may yield results faster than whole blood cultures.[19] A skin biopsy specimen may reveal a subcorneal pustule with neutrophils, and periodic acid-Schiff (PAS) staining will highlight the organisms. Invasive fungal dermatitis demonstrates invasion and inflammation of the epidermis and possibly invasion of the dermis.

Treatment of Candida Infections

Localized forms of candidiasis can be treated topically in most infants. For thrush, nystatin solution (100,000 units/ml) is applied to the oral mucosa four times per day for at least 1 week. Resistant thrush may respond to oral fluconazole (2 to 3 mg/kg/day)[20] or itraconazole,[21] particularly in immunocompromised children. Oral amphotericin B is being studied for treatment of recurrent thrush.[22] Imidazole creams are useful for diaper dermatitis and nail infection. Nystatin, allylamines (including naftifine and terbinafine), or aqueous solutions of 1% gentian violet or 2% eosin are alternatives for localized disease. Diaper dermatitis may require a combination of the above with a 1% hydrocortisone cream or ointment and barrier paste containing zinc oxide. Oral nystatin may also be a useful adjunct for treatment of diaper dermatitis, especially for recurrent disease or concurrent oral candidiasis, reducing the load of gastrointestinal *Candida*.

Congenital candidiasis in term infants can be treated with topical agents alone. However, for ill and VLBW preterm infants, systemic treatment is recommended.

The drug of choice for systemic antifungal therapy is amphotericin B, a polyene macrolide antibiotic.[2] Intravenous doses of 0.5 to 1 mg/kg/day are recommended.[2,23] It should be diluted in dextrose water to <0.2 mg/ml and delivered over 4 to 6 hours to avoid infusion-related reactions. Treatment is usually continued for a minimum of 14 to 21 days, depending on the degree of systemic illness.[24] Associated nephrotoxicity is seen less commonly in neonates than in adults treated with amphotericin;

however, renal function should be monitored. Hepatotoxicity and bone marrow suppression are also potential side effects.[23] Lipid-associated amphotericin B formulations have been developed to deliver greater dosages, limit infusion volume, and minimize toxicity.[25] Successful treatment of systemic fungal disease in neonates with these products has been reported.[26]

5-Fluorocytosine (5-FC) is a pyrimidine antimetabolite that acts synergistically with amphotericin B against fungal pathogens such as *Cryptococcus* and *Candida* spp. 5-FC is given orally (50 to 150 mg/kg/day) and penetrates well into CSF. Potential toxicity includes bone marrow suppression and gastrointestinal side effects. Bone marrow suppression is associated with serum 5-FC concentrations greater than 100 mg/l.[23]

Systemic fluconazole has been used successfully for treatment of systemic candidiasis in neonates.[27,28] The recommended daily dose is 6 mg/kg/day for infants greater than 4 weeks of age, with less-frequent dosing for infants with compromised renal function and for those less than 4 weeks of age. Given in the first trimester of pregnancy, fluconazole has been reported to be teratogenic, leading to multiple malformations.[29]

Resistance to fluconazole can be seen especially in non-albicans *Candida* species such as *C. krusei,* and susceptibility testing can be performed to document utility of these agents.[30] Oral itraconazole administered at 5 mg/kg/day has been safe and well tolerated in infants and children[31,32]; however, only one report documents its use in a newborn with candidiasis.[33] Oral ketoconazole (3 to 6.5 mg/kg/day) has been largely supplanted by the newer triazoles for candidiasis, because of the risk of fulminant hepatitis.[34]

Malassezia Infections

Malassezia (previously *Pityrosporum* species) are saprophytic yeasts found on 90% of adults as normal skin flora. Skin colonization of newborns usually occurs in the first 1 to 3 months of life.[35,36] Although *M. furfur* is the most commonly associated species, *M. pachydermatis* and *M. sympodialis* have also been associated with neonatal infection.[37,38] Three clinical forms of *Malassezia* infection may present in neonates: tinea versicolor, cephalic pustulosis, and catheter-associated sepsis without cutaneous lesions.

Skin Colonization with Malassezia Species
Malassezia furfur is the main species responsible for human skin colonization and infection, but other Malassezia species, including *M. sympodialis* and *M. pachydermatis,* have been implicated in human disease. *M. furfur* colonizes the skin of adults who are usually asymptomatic. Skin colonization begins in infancy, and the prevalence of colonization increases with age. The organism is found more frequently on premature infants in neonatal intensive care units than on term infants, and colonization increases with duration of hospitalization.[39,40] Other risk factors for colonization include mechanical ventilation and multiple episodes of suspected sepsis. Fungal growth from skin and catheter cultures is not always associated with clinical sepsis.

Tinea Versicolor
Tinea versicolor (pityriasis versicolor) is less common in infants than in older children, adolescents, and young adults. Facial involvement is very typical in affected infants and young children, although lesions may also be seen on the neck and upper trunk.[41,42] Tinea versicolor presents with multiple, 0.3 to 1 cm oval-shaped macules or plaques with fine scaling (Fig. 13-9). Lesions may be hypopigmented, skin-colored, or hyperpigmented relative to normal skin. Woods light examination highlights the pigmentary changes and may produce a golden fluorescence. Differential diagnoses include pityriasis alba and postinflammatory hypopigmentation and hyperpigmentation.

Neonatal Cephalic Pustulosis
Neonatal cephalic pustulosis is a new term, which may represent what has been previously called neonatal acne.[43] During the second or third week of life, multiple, tiny,

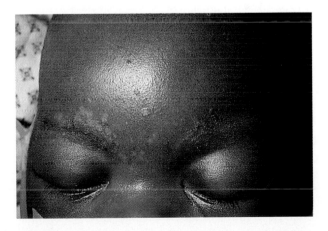

FIG. 13-9
Tinea versicolor: hypopigmented, scaling plaques on the face in this premature infant revealed hyphae and spores on KOH preparation.

monomorphous papulopustules on an erythematous base begin to cover the face, scalp, and neck. Contrary to classic acne, comedones are not a feature, and follicular accentuation is absent. Both *M. furfur* and *M. sympodialis* have been reported in association with neonatal cephalic pustulosis.[43,44,45] Diagnosis is suggested by age at onset, cephalic distribution, microscopic findings of yeast forms suggestive of *Malassezia*, exclusion of other pustular eruptions, and response to topical ketoconazole. The differential diagnosis of this pustular eruption is discussed more extensively in Chapters 6 and 10.

Malassezia Sepsis

Malassezia fungemia is seen primarily in premature infants receiving intralipids through intravenous catheters. Skin colonization rates are much higher in premature infants than in full-term newborns, and the pathogenesis of disease likely involves organisms on the skin gaining venous access through indwelling catheters.[45] Although in one study of very low birth weight infants (<1250 g), skin colonization with *M. furfur* was not predictive of catheter infection, the skin colonization rate was 70%, and positive blood cultures were common in infants with central venous catheters.[3] Clinical presentation ranges from asymptomatic colonization of the indwelling catheter to sepsis and death.[45] Fever, apnea, bradycardia, and thrombocytopenia in the presence of negative routine bacterial cultures suggest fungal disease. Clusters of cases of infantile bronchopneumonia in neonatal units have been attributed to *M. furfur* as well.[40,45]

Diagnosis and Treatment of Malassezia Infections

Malassezia can be identified by KOH preparation or Giemsa stain examination of the fine scales or pus; this examination will reveal clusters of spherical yeast and associated filaments. *Malassezia* is differentiated from *Candida* and other yeasts by a broader budding base. *Malassezia furfur* is a lipophilic yeast that requires fatty acid supplementation for growth. Modified Dixon agar or an olive oil overlay on routine fungal media is used for isolation of these fungi from blood specimens.

Cutaneous infections can be treated with an imidazole cream.[34] A high level of suspicion for *Malassezia* sepsis is appropriate in premature infants with clinical sepsis with negative bacterial and viral cultures, especially if intravenous lipid emulsions are being infused through venous catheters. Removal of the catheter and cessation of intravenous lipids, without systemic antifungal therapy, is usually sufficient therapy for catheter associated sepsis, although systemic antifungals may be considered if the infant does not clinically improve rapidly.[45]

Trichosporonosis

Trichosporon beigelii (cutaneum), a yeast found in soil, causes superficial mycoses in healthy persons (white piedra). Invasive disease is possible in immunocompromised hosts and has emerged as a cause of systemic fungal disease in very premature infants. The cutaneous manifestation of trichosporonosis in neonates is persistent generalized skin breakdown with epidermal peeling, and slight oozing of a serous fluid; neither erythema nor pustules are present.[46] Neutropenia and hemophagocytosis may be seen in systemically affected infants and can be resistant to therapy. Both colonization of central venous lines without evidence of disease, and sepsis associated with fungal dissemination are reported in VLBW infants.[46] Treatment is with a systemic antifungal agent. *T. beigelii* can exhibit tolerance to amphotericin B,[47,48] and lack of fungicidal activity has been associated with treatment failure and death.[47,49] Successful treatment of disseminated neonatal trichosporonosis with liposomal amphotericin B has been reported.[50]

Aspergillosis

Aspergillus species are ubiquitous saprophytic fungi found in decaying vegetation and are infrequently pathogenic in healthy people.[51] The conidia can spread through the air, and there are reports of acquisition in immunosuppressed patients following hospital construction.[52] The pathogenesis of disease with systemic *Aspergillus* infection involves invasion of blood vessels with subsequent thrombosis and necrosis of tissue. Macrophage and neutrophil function are important immunologic defense mechanisms against *Aspergillus* infection.[53] Risk factors for invasive aspergillosis include extreme prematurity, neutropenia or neutrophil incompetence, immunosuppression from severe disease such as malnutrition or bacterial sepsis, and induced immunosuppression with steroids.[53,54,55]

Aspergillosis in neonates presents with a spectrum of diseases, including primary cutaneous aspergillosis, single-system involvement such as pulmonary or gastrointestinal aspergillosis, and disseminated aspergillosis. Mortality rates increase with more invasive disease. There can be overlap in clinical symptoms, and cutaneous lesions can be either primary or a manifestation of dissemination.

Primary Cutaneous Aspergillosis

Primary cutaneous aspergillosis (PCA) with infection limited to the skin is being reported more frequently in premature infants.[51,52,53,55] PCA is often associated with breaks in normal skin integrity, such as occur with intravenous catheter insertion, or skin erosion or maceration secondary to adhesive tape, monitor leads, or dressings. Occlusive dressings and tape presumably enhance fungal growth. Lesions are often confused with skin trauma and contact dermatitis, and diagnosis can be delayed unless a high level of suspicion is maintained. PCA may begin as a localized zone of erythema, evolving into a dark-red plaque with pustules on the edge.[52] Clustered, erythematous papules or pustules, or a necrotic plaque or nodule with an eschar, are characteristic lesions (Fig. 13-10). The differential diagnosis includes ecthyma gangrenosum, zygomycosis, noninfectious vasculitis, and pyoderma gangrenosum.[51] Histologic evaluation and culture of a biopsy specimen from the affected area can be diagnostic. Microscopically, vesicular surface erosion of a granuloma with infiltrating dichotomously branched septate hyphae is apparent.[52] Growth of *Aspergillus* is supportive of a diagnosis, but lack of a positive culture does not rule out disease, especially if hyphal elements are seen on histologic examination.

Systemic Aspergillosis

Isolated pulmonary, gastrointestinal, and central nervous system aspergillosis may not be associated with skin findings; however, disseminated aspergillosis can have cutaneous manifestations, and cutaneous aspergillosis may disseminate. A maculopapular eruption that may become pustular[54] is described with systemic aspergillosis. This often represents embolic phenomena from fungal dissemination. Mortality from systemic aspergillosis in neonates is high compared with that of primary cutaneous aspergillosis (100% versus 27%, respectively).[55]

Systemic antifungal therapy is recommended for all forms of neonatal aspergillosis. Amphotericin B is the standard antimicrobial agent prescribed, either alone or in conjunction with flucytosine. Lipid formulations of amphotericin B have been used in adults with aspergillosis,[53] but data in neonates are lacking. It is unclear if complete surgical excision of cutaneous lesions is necessary for cure because there are reports of cure with debridement and/or biopsy alone.[55] Progression of the lesion while on therapy may warrant surgical intervention.

Cutaneous Zygomycosis (Mucormycosis, Phycomycosis)

Zygomycosis is the term for infection caused by fungi in the class Zygomycetes. There are six fungal genera causing disease in humans: *Rhizopus, Cunninghamella, Mucor, Rhizomucor, Saksenea,* and *Absidia.*[56] These fungi are found in soil, decaying food, and other organic matter. Although infections may follow ingestion or inhalation of spores, direct inoculation into skin is the cause of primary cutaneous zygomycosis, which is seen predominantly in premature infants. Immunocompromise from prematurity, immunosuppressive drugs, and metabolic acidoses are risk factors.[57] Similar to aspergillosis, zygomycosis can involve the skin alone (primary cutaneous) or may involve other organ systems, including the gastrointestinal, pulmonary, and central nervous system. Skin lesions may represent dissemination, or primary cutaneous infection may disseminate. Zygomycosis in immunocompetent hosts includes cutaneous zygomycosis and sinusitis. The cutaneous lesions present as erythematous cellulitis that may develop pustules and can evolve into a sharply defined, black, necrotic plaque producing a pathognomonic black pus (Fig. 13-11)[57]

In a review of 31 cases of neonatal zygomycosis, 22 were in premature infants, and in 12 the skin was the

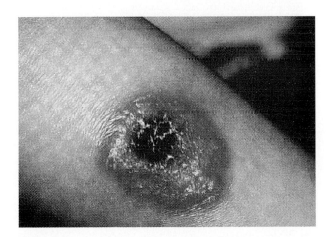

FIG. 13-10
Primary cutaneous aspergillosis: an indurated, erythematous plaque with central eschar.

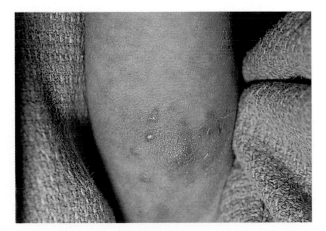

FIG. 13-11
Cutaneous rhizopus.

initial site of infection.[56] Reports include an association with contaminated dressings and tongue depressors used as splints for intravenous and arterial cannulation sites.[57,58] The Centers for Disease Control and Prevention (CDC) recommends that skin dressings be treated with cobalt irradiation as a preventive measure.[57]

Diagnosis is made by tissue biopsy and culture. Histologic examination shows large, nonseptate hyphae with right-angle branching. The fungus invades downward into tissue and blood vessels, frequently leading to thrombosis with dermal edema and minimal inflammatory infiltrate.[59] Vascular invasion results in cutaneous ischemia and necrosis.

Zygomycosis is treated with intravenous amphotericin B. As with aspergillosis, lipid formulations of amphotericin B can be used to deliver higher concentrations of drug, and other agents such as rifampin may be of use for antimicrobial synergy.[56] In vitro data reveal resistance to azoles (except *Absidia*), flucytosine, and naftifine.[60] Although one successful case of medical treatment alone is reported,[57] surgical debridement is often imperative in the treatment of cutaneous zygomycosis, and wide excision with clean margins of involved tissue is recommended.[56,61]

Dermatophytosis

Dermatophytes are fungal pathogens responsible for the cutaneous infection known as tinea. Clinical conditions are named according to the affected anatomic location: tinea capitis, tinea faciei (face), tinea corporis (body), tinea diaper dermatitis (diaper area), and tinea unguium (nails); tinea cruris (groin) and tinea pedis (feet) are uncommon in infants.

Dermatophytosis in neonates may be acquired from infected caregivers, or infected animals. Dermatophyte invasion of the stratum corneum is mediated by keratinase and other proteases.[62] Cell-mediated immunity and evidence of delayed type hypersensitivity response are important in host resistance.[62]

In North America, **tinea faciei** and **corporis** in infants are most often due to *Trichoplyton tonsurans*, *Trichophyton rubrum*, or *Microsporum canis*.[63-68] In West African newborns, *Microsporum landeronii* is a common cause.[69,70] The most common cause of **tinea capitis** in North America is *Trichophyton tonsurans*, which may also cause tinea faciei and corporis secondary to cutaneous spread. Fungal invasion in tinea capitis extends to the hair follicle, where infection may be either within the hair shaft (endothrix) or on the surface of the hair shaft (ectothrix).[62] Neonatal tinea capitis has also been re-

ported with other fungal species, including *T. rubrum* and *T. mentagrophytes*.[66,67] **Tinea diaper dermatitis** is primarily due to *T. rubrum* and *Epidermophyton floccosum*. **Tinea unguium** in childhood has been caused by *T. mentagrophytes* and *T. rubrum*.[68]

Tinea in babies occurs most commonly on the exposed scalp and face (Fig. 13-12)[63-72] Tinea capitis often presents as erythematous, scaling areas with partial alopecia.[63-67,71,72] Clinical manifestations vary from noninflammatory "black dot" alopecia to a scaling, seborrheic, dermatitis-like eruption without obvious hair loss.[63,69,70] Pustules may be present. Kerion can be seen in conjunction with tinea capitis. Kerions consist of pustules, nodules, and crusting with underlying bogginess of scalp tissue. The inflammatory nature mimics bacterial infection and may lead to unsuccessful therapy with antibacterial agents. Tinea capitis associated with kerion formation has been reported in a neonate.[72] Posterior cervical lymphadenopathy is usually present.

Tinea infection on other parts of the body usually presents as elevated, annular lesions with superficial scaling and/or tiny pustules.[63,65,67,71] These may be mistaken for dermatitis, and facial tinea may mimic neonatal lupus. Cases of tinea faciei and tinea corporis have been reported in neonates.[64,67,73,74] Cases of resistant diaper dermatitis in

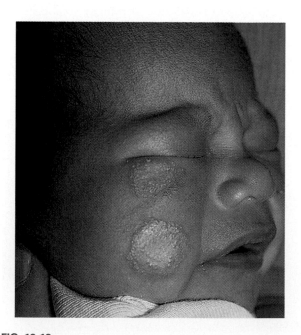

FIG. 13-12
Annular, scaling plaques on this 2-week-old infant from *T. tonsurans* infection. The 4-year-old sibling was evaluated and had evidence of tinea capitis.

infants as a result of dermatophytes have been described.[75] In **tinea diaper dermatitis,** the presence of an annular patch with a scaling peripheral border is a clue to the diagnosis (Fig. 13-13).

Onychomycosis is a fungal infection of the nail that may be caused by dermatophytes, nondermatophyte molds, and *Candida*. **Tinea unguium,** caused by dermatophytes, is uncommon in prepubertal children,[68] the youngest reported case being a 10-week-old infant.[76] Nails may have white opaque superficial patches, or yellowish discoloration with subungual hyperkeratosis. Hereditary onychodystrophy, acquired trachyonychia, psoriasis, lichen planus, and trauma may cause similar findings.

Diagnosis of dermatophytosis can be confirmed by several tests. A Wood's light examination may have limited usefulness in the diagnosis of **tinea capitis;** positive fluorescence is seen in ectothrix hair infections, but it is absent in the more common endothrix infections such as those caused by *Trichophyton*. All suspected tinea infections should be confirmed by culture, or lesional scale or hair microscopically examined under 10% potassium hydroxide (KOH) solution or alternative stains (see Chapter 6). Although KOH preparations may demonstrate spores and hyphae, false-negative examinations are common. Scrapings of scales, brush or cotton-tipped applicator swabbings of the affected skin, or collections of hair are cultured on fungal media. Dermatophytes are slow-growing and may take up to 1 month to grow in culture, although common pathogens generally grow within 2 weeks. Skin biopsy, although rarely necessary for diagnosis, may reveal hyperkeratosis with parakeratosis and a mixed inflammatory perivascular dermal infiltrate. Staining with periodic acid-Schiff (PAS) or Grocott-Gomori methenamine silver nitrate reveals fungal elements in the stratum corneum and possibly the hair follicle.[34]

Treatment of tinea capitis usually requires systemic antifungal therapy. Griseofulvin is the most commonly used agent, and successful treatment in neonates has been reported.[66,72,74] Griseofulvin doses of 15 to 20 mg/kg/day for 6 to 8 weeks may be needed. Fluconazole (6 mg/kg/day) may also be effective.[77] Alternative medications include itraconazole and terbinafine, although experience in neonates is limited. Although topical therapy alone was successful in treatment five of six mostly preterm infants (four with tinea capitis) during a nursery outbreak of *Microsporum canis,* it is not generally recommended for scalp tinea infection.[64]

Tinea faciei and **tinea corporis** can be successfully treated with topical applications of azoles such as clotrimazole, econazole, and miconazole. Ciclopirox, as well as allylamines such as terbinafine or naftifine and amorfoline, may also be used.[78,9] If persistent, systemic griseofulvin or fluconazole[77,80] for a period of 4 to 8 weeks may be required.[80]

It is important to identify the potential source of the fungal infection in family members. The prognosis for dermatophyte infections is excellent.

INFESTATIONS (ECTOPARASITIC INFESTATIONS)

Mites, flea larvae, protozoa, and helminth worms cause a variety of cutaneous lesions.[34] Mites are classified in the order Acari, class of arthropods Arachnida. The prototype is **scabies,** which is the most common parasitic infection in humans, including newborns. Flea larvae (myiasis) and other mites (demodicidosis) can occasionally cause disease in infants.

Scabies

Scabies is a common ectoparasitic infestation caused by the mite *Sarcoptes scabiei* ssp. *hominis.* Initial infestation by scabies may be asymptomatic, a carrier state being well recognized. A primary symptom of scabies is generalized pruritus, most intense at night. Infants however, may not manifest symptoms despite extensive infection. Pruritus in a neonate unable to scratch may manifest as irritability, insomnia, and poor feeding. Congenital scabies is not seen, but infestation can develop in very young infants.[81]

Skin findings include a generalized erythematous vesiculopapular eruption, with lesions commonly concentrated on the axillae, neck, palms, soles, and some-

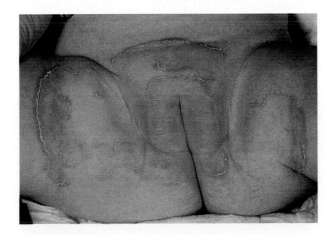

FIG. 13-13
Dermatophyte diaper dermatitis (note scaling edge).

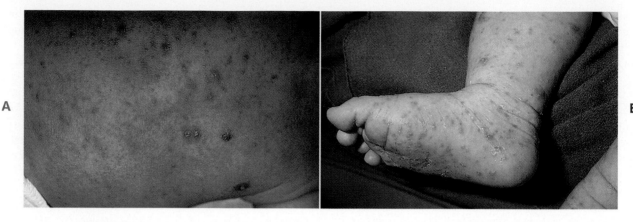

FIG. 13-14
Scabies: **A,** Diffuse erythematous papules, pustules, crusted lesions, and scattered nodules, and **B,** papules, vesicles, and pustules on the feet and legs, particularly on the instep of the foot, are characteristics in young infants.

times the head (Fig. 13-14). The head and neck are usually spared in older children and adults.[81,82] A burrow is the pathognomonic sign of scabies. Burrows appear as a small thin line with a tiny black dot at one end, indicating the location of the female mite.[83] They are found primarily on the hands, the flexural aspect of the wrists, and the medial or lateral aspects of the feet; visualization may be difficult because of secondary eczematous changes.[82]

In babies, vesicles and pustules are characteristically found on the palms and soles. Nodules may also appear during active infection, primarily in intertriginous areas, and these scabietic nodules may persist for some time after scabies has been successfully treated. Recurrent vesicular lesions similar to scabietic nodules may be manifestations of ongoing hypersensitivity response to the initial infestation.

A form of infantile scabies clinically resembling crusted scabies (Norwegian scabies) is associated with prior topical corticosteroid therapy. In addition to the generalized eruption, crusted and hyperkeratotic lesions on the palms and soles are described.[83] Unlike classic Norwegian scabies in adults, which is characterized by intense infestation of *Sarcoptes* mites, these infants lacked subungual hyperkeratosis and high mite counts.[83] There has also been a report in immunosuppressed children of a unique form of scabies consisting of fine scaling and minimal to absent pruritus, mimicking seborrheic dermatitis.[84]

The scabies mite is an obligate human ectoparasite unable to survive more than a few days without a host.[81] The microscopic adult female mite with eight legs measures 400 μm. Throughout its life span of up to 30 days, the mite burrows into the stratum corneum, laying 1 to 3 eggs per day. Larvae hatch in 3 to 4 days, and mature into adult

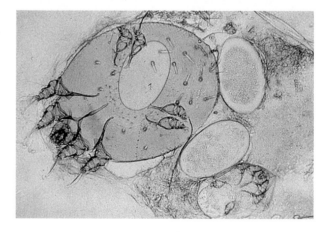

FIG. 13-15
Scabies: *Sarcoptes scabiei* mite and eggs.

mites within 10 to 14 days.[81] Although hundreds of skin lesions may develop, only a few mites are present. Other lesions appear due to hypersensitivity.[81]

Diagnosis is based on the clinical findings, as well as a history of contact with persons with a similar pruritic eruption. Definitive diagnosis is based on microscopic visualization of scrapings from a burrow or papule, demonstrating the mite, eggs, or scybala (feces) (see Chapter 6) (Fig. 13-15).[83] Skin biopsy is rarely necessary. Histopathologic examination shows a mixed dermal inflammatory infiltrate with eosinophils and epidermal spongiosis. The mites, ova, and nymphs may also be seen.

The treatment of choice for neonatal scabies is permethrin 5% cream. It is approved for use in infants as young as 2 months old, with a recent report of safety and efficacy in a 23-day-old infant.[81] Permethrin is a neurotoxin that causes paralysis and death of ectoparasites; it has low potential for toxicity in humans and there is no evidence of resistance to date.[81] Efficacy is superior to that of lindane, crotamiton, benzyl benzoate, and sulfur.[81] Permethrin applied to the entire body surface, including the scalp, and left on for 8 to 12 hours is 89% to 92% effective.[81] Reapplication is advisable 1 week later. Critical to success is the simultaneous treatment of all family members, even if asymptomatic, and close contacts. Whereas adults are treated from the neck down, children younger than 2 years of age should have the head treated as well. In addition, bedding and clothing of patients and all contacts should be washed the following day in hot water for at least 5 minutes or dry cleaned. Antihistamines such as hydroxyzine (2 mg/kg/day in divided doses every 6 to 8 hours) and a mild corticosteroid cream such as 1% hydrocortisone may help control the residual pruritus and eczematous dermatitis that can persist for several weeks following successful eradication of the parasite. Ivermectin, an avermectin with antiparasitic and antinematode properties, has been used orally in cases of refractory scabies in adults.[85] Topical formulations are currently being studied.

Demodicidosis

Demodicidosis presents as perioral dermatitis, pustular folliculitis, and blepharitis.[86] Pruritic erythematous papules, pustules, nodules, and scaling occur primarily on the face, neck, upper thorax, and extremities. *Demodex folliculorum* and *D. brevis* are human ectoparasites that are normal inhabitants of the pilosebaceous ducts and glands. *D. canis* causes mange in animals. The role of the mite *Demodex* in human cutaneous disease is controversial,[86] and its specific role in neonatal disease has yet to be determined. To date, the youngest reported case is that of a 10-month-old infant.[87] Demodicidosis is found mainly in immunosuppressed children,[86,88] although disease in healthy hosts has been described.[87] Numerous mites are seen when skin scrapings are examined using KOH or when a skin biopsy is performed. A dramatic response may be seen within 2 to 3 weeks after application of 5% permethrin cream.

Myiasis

Myiasis is a parasitic infestation of dipterous larvae in mammals, found worldwide but primarily in the tropics and subtropics.[89] Cutaneous myiasis may occur in preexisting wounds or present as a furuncle. Passage of maggots, discharge, foul smell, and pain may be reported. Myiasis is classified clinically according to the body site affected as cutaneous, nasopharyngeal, ocular, aural, intestinal, and genital. There have been reports of myiasis in infants and children chiefly in rural settings,[90] although cases have been reported in urban centers as well.[91,92] Diagnosis is made clinically and confirmed by identification of larvae, which can be preserved in 80% ethanol. Treatment involves extraction of the larvae by irrigation, manipulation, or ideally with surgery followed by debridement, cleansing, and possible primary suture closure.[89]

PARASITIC INFECTIONS

Parasitic infections with cutaneous manifestations are more commonly seen in developing countries and are infrequently reported in neonates. Table 13-1 presents summary of cutaneous diseases due to parasites. *Toxoplasma* are autonomous, single-cell organisms that are acquired in utero more frequently than postnatally in neonates. Cutaneous manifestations of helminth worms are discussed minimally here but are treated in depth by Stein.[34] Toxoplasmosis and leishmaniasis are discussed in greater detail.

Toxoplasmosis

Toxoplasmosis is caused by the intracellular protozoa *Toxoplasma gondii*. Found worldwide in many animal species, cats are the only species in which the sexual stage (sporozoite) occurs.[93,94] Infection commonly occurs through consumption of undercooked meats containing *Toxoplasma* cysts or oocysts excreted by cats.[95] Toxoplasmosis may be acquired congenitally or postnatally. Congenital toxoplasmosis is a sequela of acute maternal infection or reactivation, with risk of transmission being 15% in the first trimester, 30% in the second, and 60% in the third.[94] Severity of fetal disease varies inversely with gestational age at the time of infection. Thus early infection more likely leads to fetal death or severe neurologic and ophthalmologic disease. Most newborns infected in the second or third trimester have mild or subclinical manifestations. In at least 40% of cases, infection is discovered late, manifesting as chorioretinitis, visual impairment, and neurologic sequelae.[94] Risk of fetal infection is estimated to be 1 per 1000 to 8000 live births.[95]

Congenital toxoplasmosis has no specific cutaneous manifestations,[93,94] but in a report by Roizen et al,[96] petechial and nonpetechial rashes were seen in 17% and 14%, respectively, of affected infants. Neurologic conditions such as seizures, hydrocephalus, microcephaly, and

TABLE 13-1

Parasitic Cutaneous Infections in Neonates

Parasite	Name	Source	Clinical findings	Therapy
Mite				
Sarcopies scabiei ssp. *hominis*	Scabies	Human	Classical burrow; vesicles on palms and soles; nodules, papules, and pustules on face and extensors	Permethrin 5% cream or lotion, including scalp, Tx contacts
Demodex folliculorum	Demodicidosis	Human saprophyte	Papules and pustules on face and extensors	Permethrin 5% cream or lotion
Protozoa				
Toxoplasma gondii	Toxoplasmosis	Cats	Acquired: variable Congenital: chorioretinitis, hydrocephalus, intracranial calcifications, ± petechial rash	Pyrimethamine and sulfonamide, or spiramycin, or trimethoprim-sulfamethoxazole
Entamoeba histolytica	Amebiasis	Humans 10% worldwide GI tract colonized	Ulcer, draining sinus, vegetative plaque in the inguinal, perineal area, abdomen	Metronidazole and iodoquinol or paromomycin
L. major, L. tropica, L. aethiopica (Old World) *L. mexicana, L. braziliensis* (New World)	Cutaneous leishmaniasis	Female sandfly Mammal reservoir	Single or multiple papules and nodules ± ulcer resolving to leave scars	Sodium stibogluconate, Meglumine antimonate ± allopurinol, ketoconazole, itraconazole, amphotericin B, cryotherapy, heat
L. braziliensis	Mucocutaneous leishmaniasis		Destructive oral, nasopharyngeal lesions	
L. donovani	Visceral leishmaniasis (Kala-azar)		Gray skin color, nodules	
Myiasis: (fly larvae) order Diptera	Myiasis	Flies, gnats, mosquitos	Furuncle or infested ulcer	Surgical removal
Helminths: Platyhelminthes (tapeworms) Trematodes Cestodes	Rare in newborns			

chorioretinitis are the main clinical manifestations. Neurologic abnormalities range from CSF abnormalities with no symptoms to severe encephalitis with mental retardation, spasticity, palsies, and deafness. Intracranial calcifications and increased CSF protein may be seen. Eye abnormalities include microphthalmia, glaucoma, and retinal detachment. The most common presentation of eye involvement is strabismus in infants. Disease may be limited to the central nervous system or may include systemic findings of hepatosplenomegaly, lymphadenopathy, hyperbilirubinemia, and thrombocytopenia. Prognosis of congenital toxoplasmosis has improved with therapy; however, many cases of congenital toxoplasmosis are not recognized in the newborn period.[93]

Postnatally acquired toxoplasmosis is asymptomatic in the majority of patients. However, in an immunocompromised host, the disease can be serious. Symptomatic toxoplasmosis can involve the central nervous system and also disseminate to other organs.[94] Fever, malaise, and arthralgia are frequent symptoms, mimicking infectious mononucleosis.[34] Cutaneous manifestations are variable and include macular, papular, pustular, or vesiculobullous eruptions. They may be hemorrhagic and may resemble roseola or erythema multiforme.[34] Lymphadenopathy and hepatosplenomegaly may accompany these eruptions.

Diagnosis of toxoplasmosis is based on isolation of the organism, characteristic histopathology of lymphadenitis, detection of *Toxoplasma* antigens in tissues and body fluids, and detection of *Toxoplasma* nucleic acid by polymerase chain reaction (PCR). The most commonly used diagnostic tool is serology. Early diagnosis may be difficult due to delay in antibody response and the presence of maternal IgG. Both the enzyme-linked immunosorbent assay (ELISA) and immunosorbent agglutination assay (ISAGA) are useful tests.[94] The Sabin-Feldman dye test entails the uptake of methylene blue by *Toxoplasma* trophozoites lysed in the presence of specific antibody and complement. It is very specific but only available through reference laboratories.[94] PCR testing of amniotic fluid has now replaced cordocentesis for the prenatal diagnosis of fetal infection.[97] Ultrasound abnormalities are found in up to 40% of congenitally infected infants, the most common being ventriculomegaly.[94]

Symptomatic acquired or congenital toxoplasmosis should be treated with pyrimethamine, sulfadiazine, and folinic acid.[94] Therapeutic abortion may be offered as an alternative. In some cases, vertical transmission has been prevented by administration of spiramycin to the mother.[97] Antibiotic therapy to reduce subsequent disease is recommended for symptomatic and asymptomatic neonates. Treatment should be continued for at least 1 year.

Leishmaniasis

Leishmaniasis is a parasitic infection due to *Leishmania* species (family *Trypanosomatidae*). There are 400,000 new cases each year in Asia, Africa, the Mediterranean, and the Americas. The flagellated, extracellular promastigote is transmitted by female phlebotomine sandflies[98] to animal reservoirs, including rodents and dogs. There it becomes an obligate intracellular amastigote. Recent reports of infants with leishmaniasis living in nonendemic areas emphasize the need to consider this diagnosis when unusual skin lesions are present[98,99,100,101] Leishmaniasis is classified into the following categories: visceral (*L. donovani, L. infantum*), mucocutaneous (*L. braziliensis*), Old World cutaneous (*L major, L. tropica, L. ethiopica*), and New World cutaneous (*L. mexicana, L. braziliensis*)[102] (see Table 13-1).

Visceral leishmaniasis due to *L. donovani* presents with fever, wasting of the face and extremities, hepatosplenomegaly, ascites, pancytopenia, and earth gray skin pigmentation of the temples, perioral area, hands, and feet.[98] There may be a papular lesion seen early at the site of the sandfly bite. Mucocutaneous leishmaniasis due to *L. braziliensis* invades the mid face, nose, and upper respiratory tract. A sporotrichoid lymphatic form has been described with *L. braziliensis* and *L. major*.

In countries where leishmaniasis is prevalent, infants and children are frequently affected by cutaneous leishmaniasis. The initial lesion is an erythematous papule derived from an insect bite that evolves to form a relatively painless crusted ulcer.[98] It is typically on an exposed site (primarily on the face and hands), paired or clustered, with a volcanic or iceberg appearance, and oriented to the skin creases. Satellite papules or nodules may be present with surrounding erythema. Secondary bacterial infection is common. The lesions generally heal spontaneously in 3 to 12 months, although they may also evolve into chronic, treatment-resistant forms that are localized, lupoid, or disseminated.

Diagnosis is based on smears or skin biopsy specimens that permit visualization of the amastigote, culture, or animal inoculation that produces characteristic lesions.[98] The leishmanin skin test evaluates the degree of induration after an intradermal injection of antigen. Positive findings are seen 1 to 3 months following the initial lesion in cutaneous leishmaniasis. Serologic studies are most valuable in visceral leishmaniasis.[98]

Although visceral leishmaniasis is usually fatal if untreated, spontaneous resolution is the rule in cutaneous forms of the disease. Indications for treatment include lesions that are early, multiple, mucosal, or in cosmetically sensitive sites. Disseminated disease in an immunodeficient host also warrants treatment. If treatment is needed, there is no single ideal drug. Primary treatment is with pentavalent antimonials such as intramuscular or intravenous sodium stibogluconate (10 to 20 mg/kg/day) or meglumine antimonate (not available in the United States).[103] Ketoconazole and amphotericin B may also be effective, and temperature-sensitive Leishmania may respond to cryotherapy or heat.

ARTHROPOD BITES AND STINGS

Arthropod bites and stings may cause a variety of skin lesions, as well as be vectors from disease. Erythematous, urticarial papules and pustules with a central puncta can be seen, most commonly on exposed surfaces (Fig. 13-16). Vesicular lesions may be a manifestation of a hypersensitive response and not indicative of bacterial infection, particularly in infants. These pink raised lesions are typically arranged in groups. Persistence of lesions for weeks to months (papular urticaria) is rarely seen in the first year of life.[104] Specific lesions and subsequent diseases are outlined in Table 13-2.

Skin lesions are caused by four of the nine classes of arthropods: Insecta, Chilopoda, Diplopoda, and Arach-

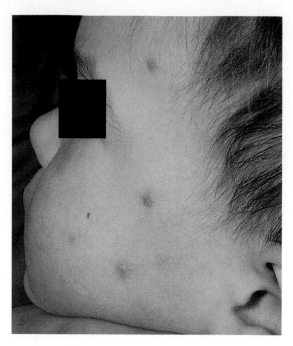

FIG. 13-16
Insect bites: urticarial papules secondary to flea bites.

TABLE 13-2					
Arthropod Bites and Stings					
Class	Order	Source	Lesions	Treatment	Disease
Insecta (three pairs of legs)	Anoplura	Lice: *Pediculus humanus Pnthirus*	Nits, pruritic bites, maculae, caeruleae	5% permethrin; Tx fomites	
	Coleoptera	Beetles	"Kissing" or touching blisters and dermatitis	Topical corticosteroid, systemic antihistamine	Secondary bacterial infection
	Diptera	Mosquitos	Pruritic papules	Topical corticosteroid, systemic antihistamine	Vector for: Encephalitis Malaria Yellow fever Dengue fever
		Flies (blood-sucking):	Pruritic, painful papules	Topical corticosteroid, systemic antihistamine	Filariasis
		Tabanae: horseflies, deerflies, etc.	± angioedema	Topical corticosteroid, systemic antihistamine	Vector for: Tularemia

TABLE 13-2

Arthropod Bites and Stings—cont'd

Class	Order	Source	Lesions	Treatment	Disease
		Simulidae: black flies Midges: sand flies	± malaise		
	Hemiptera	*Cimicidae* (bedbugs)	Pruritic papules	Topical cortico-steroid, systemic antihistamine	
		Reduviidae (kissing bugs)	Painful bites	Topical cortico-steroid, systemic antihistamine	Vector for: *Trypanosoma cruzi*
	Hymenoptera	*Apidea* (bees) *Vespidea* (wasps, hornets) *Formicoidea* (ants)	Urticarial papule Angioedema	Quick removal of stinger, SQ epinephrine, corticosteroid, antihistamine	
	Lepidoptera	Caterpillars Moths	Urticarial linear papules	Topical cortico-steroid, systemic antihistamine	
	Siphonoptera	Fleas: *Pulicidae* (human, cat, dog, bird)	Grouped papules	Topical cortico-steroid, systemic antihistamine	Vector for: Plague Typhus
		Sarcopsyllidae (sand fleas)	Necrotic abscess	Topical cortico-steroid, systemic antihistamine	
Arachnida (four pairs of legs)	Acari	Ticks: *Argasidae* *Ixodidae*	Papule, granuloma	Remove tick	Vector for: Lyme disease Rocky mountain spotted fever Colorado tick fever Tularemia
		Mites: Follicle, food, fowl, grain, harvest (chigger), murine, scabies	Pruritic papules	Topical cortico-steroid, systemic antihistamine	Vector for: Rickettsialpox
	Araneae	Spiders	Painful bite ± necrosis ± systemic reaction	Ice, elevation, antihistamine, analgesic	
	Scorpiones	Scorpions	Bite and neurotoxin		
Chilopoda Diplopoda		Centipedes Millipedes			

nida.[105] Although the terms *bite* and *sting* are often used interchangeably, in the strict sense, a "bite" involves venom injected via structures of the mouth, such as fangs or mandibles, whereas a "sting" connotes the injection of venom via a tapered posterior structure called the sting.[106] Secondary bacterial infection must be considered in infants with bites and stings. The presence of fever and wound drainage are suggestive of infection and may warrant antibiotic therapy.

REFERENCES

1. Ruiz-Diez B, Martinez V, Alvarez M, et al. Molecular tracking of *Candida albicans* in a neonatal intensive care unit: Long-term colonizations versus catheter-related infections. J Clin Microbiol 1997;35:3032-3036.

2. Baley JE. Neonatal candidiasis: The current challenge. Clin Perinatol 1991;18:263-280.

3. Shattuck KE, Cochran CK, Zabransky RJ, et al. Colonization and infection associated with *Malassezia* and *Candida* species in a neonatal unit. J Hosp Infect 1996;34:123-129.

4. Maródi L. Local and systemic host defense mechanisms against *Candida:* Immunopathology of candidal infections. Pediatr Infect Dis J 1997;16:795-801.

5. Maródi L, Káposzta R, Campbell DE, et al. Candidacidal mechanisms in the human neonate. Impaired IFN-γ activation of macrophages in newborn infants. J Immunol 1994; 153:5643-5649.

6. Baley JE, Kliegman RM, Fanaroff AA. Disseminated fungal infections in very low-birth-weight infants: Clinical manifestations and epidimiology. Pediatrics 1984;73:144-152.

7. Stuart SM, Lane AT. *Candida* and *Malassezia* as nursery pathogens. Sem Dermatol 1992;11:19-23.

8. Darmstadt GL, Dinulos JG, Miller Z. Congenital candidiasis: clinical presentation, pathogenesis, and management guidelines. Pediatrics 2000;105:438-444.

9. Raval DS, Barton LL, Hansen RC, et al. Congenital cutaneous candidiasis: case report and review. Pediatr Dermatol 1995;12:355-358.

10. Gerberding KM, Eisenhut CC, Engle WA, et al. Congenital Candida pneumonia and sepsis: A case report and review of the literature. J Perinatol 1989;IX:159-161.

11. Johnson DE, Thompson TR, Ferrieri P. Congenital candidiasis. Am J Dis Child 1981;135:273-275.

12. Waguespack-LaBiche J, Chen SH, Yen A. Disseminated congenital candidiasis. Arch Dermatol 1999;135:510-512.

13. Cosgrove BF, Reeves K, Mullins D, et al. Cutaneous congenital candidiasis associated with respiratory distress and elevation of liver function tests: A case report and review of the literature. J Am Acad Dermatol 1997;37:817-823.

14. Santos LA, Beceiro J, Hernandez R, et al. Congenital cutaneous candidiasis: Report of four cases and review of the literature. Eur J Pediatr 1991;150:336-338.

15. Baley JE, Silverman RA. Systemic candidiasis: Cutaneous manifestations in low birth weight infants. Pediatrics 1988; 82:211-215.

16. Pradeepkumar VK, Rajadurai VS, Tan KW. Congenital candidiasis: Varied presentations. J Perinatol 1998;18:311-316.

17. Rowen JL, Atkins JT, Levy ML, et al. Invasive fungal dermatitis in the <1000-gram neonate. Pediatric 1995;95:682-687.

18. Hay RJ, Baran R. Fungal (onychomycosis) and other infections of the nail apparatus. In Baran R, Dawber RPR, editors. Diseases of the nails and their management. Oxford: Blackwell Scientific, 1984: pp 121-156.

19. Reddy TCS, Chakrabarti A, Singh M, et al. Role of buffy coat examination in the diagnosis of neonatal candidemia. Pediatr Infect Dis J 1996;15:718-720.

20. Flynn PM, Cunningham CK, Kerkering T, et al. Oropharyngeal candidiasis in immunocompromised children: A randomized, multicenter study of orally administered fluconazole suspension versus nystatin. J Pediatr 1995;127: 322-328.

21. Crutchfield CE, Lewis EJ. The successful treatment of oral candidiasis (thrush) in a pediatric patient using itraconazole. Pediatr Dermatol 1997;14:246.

22. Stevens DA. Oral amphotericin B as an antifungal agent. J Mycol Méd 1997;7:241-242.

23. Van den Anker JN, van Popele NL, Sauer PJ. Antifungal agents in neonatal systemic candidiasis. Antimicrob Agents Chemother 1995;39:1391-1397.

24. Rowen JL, Tate JM. Management of neonatal candidiasis. Pediatr Infect Dis J 1998;17:1007-1011.

25. Friedlich PS, Steinberg I, Fujitani A, et al. Renal tolerance with the use of intralipid-amphotericin B in low-birth-weight neonates. Am J Perinatol 1997;14:377-383.

26. Scarcella A, Pasquariello MB, Giugliano B, et al. Liposomal amphotericin B treatment for neonatal fungal infections. Pediatr Infect Dis J 1998;17:146-148.

27. Fasano C, O'Keeffe J, Gibbs D. Fluconazole treatment of neonates and infants with severe fungal infections not treatable with conventional agents. Eur J Clin Microbiol Infect Dis 1994;13:351-354.

28. Schwarze R, Penk A, Pittrow L. Administration of fluconazole in children below 1 year of age-review. Mycoses 1998; 41:61-70

29. Aleck KA, Bartley DL. Multiple malformation syndrome following fluconazole use in pregnancy: Report of an additional patient. Am J Med Genet 1997;72:253-256.

30. Warren NG, Hazen KC. *Candida, Crytococcus,* and other yeasts of medical importance. In Murray PR, Barron EJ, Pfaller MA, et al, eds. Manual of clinical microbiology, 6th edition. Washington DC: ASM Press, 1995: pp 723-737.

31. de Repentigny L, Ratelle J, Leclerc JM, et al. Repeated dose pharmacokinetics of an oral solution of itraconazole in infants and children. Antimicrob Agen Chemotherap 1998; 42:404-408.

32. Tosti A, Piraccini BM, Vincenzi C, et al. Itraconazole in the treatment of two young brothers with chronic mucocutaneous candidiasis. Pediatr Dermatol 1997;14:146-148.

33. Sciacca A, Betta P, Cilauro S, et al. Oral administration of itraconazole in a case of neonatal hepatic candidiasis (Italian). Pediatr Med Chir 1995;17:173-175.

34. Stein DH. Fungal, protozoan, and helminth infections. In Schachner LA, Hansen RC, ed. Pediatric dermatology. 2nd edition. New York: Churchill Livingstone, 1995: pp 1295-1345.

35. Niamba P, Weill FX, Saralangue J, et al. Is common neonatal cephalic pustulosis (neonatal acne) triggered by *Malassezia sympodiali?* Arch Dermatol 1998;134:995-998.

36. Leeming JP, Sutton TM, Fleming PJ. Neonatal skin as a reservoir of *Malassezia* species. Pediatr Infect Dis J 1995;14:719-720.

37. Welbel SF, McNeil MM, Pramanik A, et al. Nosocomial *Malassezia pachydermatis* blood stream infections in a neonatal intensive care unit. Pediatr Infect Dis J 1994;13:104-108.

38. Chang HJ, Miller HL, Watkins N, et al. An epidemic of *Malassezia pachydermatis* in an intensive care nursery associated with colonization of health care workers' pet dogs. New Engl J Med 1998;338:706-711.

39. Aschner JL, Punsalang A Jr, Maniscalco WM, Menegus MA. Percutaneous central venous catheter colonization with Malassezia furfur: Incidence and clinical significance. Pediatrics 1987;80(4):535-539.

40. Marcon MJ, Powell DA. Human infection due to *Malassezia* spp. Clin Microb Rev 1992;5:101-119.

41. Terragni L, Lasagni A, Oriani A, et al. Pityriasis versicolor in the pediatric age. Pediatr Dermatol 1991;8:9.

42. Di Silverio A, Zeccara C, Serra F, et al. Pityriasis versicolor in a newborn. Mycoses 1995;38:227-228.

43. Rapelanoro R, Mortureux P, Couprie B, et al. Neonatal *Malassezia furfur* pustulosis. Arch Dermatol 1996;132:190-193.

44. Shattuck KE, Cochran CK, Zabiansky RJ, et al. Colonization and infection associated with *Malassezia* and *Candida* species in a neonatal unit. J Hosp Infect 1996;34:123-129.

45. Dankner WM, Spector SA, Fierer J, et al. *Malassezia* fungemia in neonates and adults: Complication of hyperalimentation. Rev Infect Dis 1987;9:743-753.

46. Yoss BS, Sautter RL, Brenker HJ. *Trichosporon beigelii*, a new neonatal pathogen. Am J Perinatol 1997;14:113-117.

47. Walsh TJ, Melcher GP, Rinaldi MG, et al. *Trichosporon beigelii*, an emerging pathogen resistant to amphotericin B. J Clin Microbiol 1990;28:1616-1622.

48. Perparim K, Nagai H, Hashimoto A, et al. In vitro susceptibility of *Trichosporon beigelii* to antifungal agents. J Chemother 1996;8:445-448.

49. Fisher DJ, Christy C, Spaford P, et al. Neonatal Trichosporon beigelii infection: report of a cluster of cases in a neonatal intensive care unit. Pediatr Infect Dis J 1993;12:149-155.

50. Sweet D, Reid M. Disseminated neonatal *Trichosporon beigelii* infection: successful treatment with liposomal amphotericin B. J Infect 1998;36:120-121.

51. Mowad CM, Nguyen TV, Jaworsky C, et al. Primary cutaneous aspergillosis in an immunocompetent child. J Am Acad Dermatol 1995;33:136-137.

52. Papouli M, Roilides, Bibashi E, et al. Primary cutaneous aspergillosis in neonates: case report and review. Clin Infect Dis 1996;22:1102-1104.

53. Denning DW. Invasive aspergillosis. Clin Infect Dis 1998;26:781-805.

54. Van den Anker JN, Wildervanck de Blecourt-Devilee M, Sauer PJ. Severe endophthalmitis after neonatal skin lesions with positive cultures of *Aspergillus fumigatus*. Eur J Pediatr 1993;152:699-702.

55. Groll AH, Jaeger G, Allendorf A, et al. Invasive pulmonary aspergillosis in a critically ill neonate: Case report and review of invasive aspergillosis during the first 3 months of life. Clin Infect Dis 1998;27:437-452.

56. Robertson AF, Joshi VV, Ellison DA, et al. Zygomycosis in neonates. Pediatr Infect Dis J 1997;16:812-815.

57. Linder N, Keller N, Huri C, et al. Primary cutaneous mucormycosis in a premature infant: Case report and review of the literature. Am J Perinatol 1998;15:35-38.

58. Holzel H, Macqueen S, MacDonald A, et al. *Rhizopus microsporus* in wooden tongue depressors: A major threat or a minor inconvenience? J Hosp Infect 1998;38:113-118.

59. du Plessis PJ, Wentzel LF, Delport SD, et al. Zygomycotic necrotizing cellulitis in a premature infant. Dermatol 1997;195:179-181.

60. Amin SB, Ryan RM, Metlay LA, et al. *Absidia corymbifera* infections in neonates. Clin Infect Dis 1998;26:990-992.

61. Hughes C, Driver SJ, Alexander KA. Successful treatment of abdominal wall *Rhizopus* necrotizing cellulitis in a preterm infant. Pediatr Infect Dis J 1995;14: 336.

62. Weitzman I, Chin NX, Kunjukunju N, Della-Latta P. A survey of dermatophytes isolated from human patients in the United States from 1993 to 1995. J Am Acad Dermatol 1998;39(2 Pt 1):255-261.

63. Virgili A, Corazza M, Zampino MR. Atypical features of tinea in newborns. Pediatr Dermatol 1993;10:92.

64. Snider R, Landers S, Levy ML. The ringworm riddle: An outbreak of *Microsporum canis* in the nursery. Pediatr Infect Dis J 1993;12:145-148.

65. Johnson ML, Anderson LL. Papulosquamous plaques in a mother and newborn son. Pediatr Dermatol 1995;12:281-284.

66. Ungar SL, Laude TA. Tinea capitis in a newborn caused by two organisms. Pediatr Dermatol 1997;14:229-230.

67. Singal A, Baruah MC, Rawat S, et al. *Trichophyton rubrum* infection in a 3-day-old neonate. Pediatr Dermatol 1996;13:488-489.

68. Ploysangam T, Lucky AW. Childhood white superficial onychomycosis caused by *Trichophyton rubrum*: Report of seven cases and review of the literature. J Am Acad Dermatol 1997;36:29-32.

69. Cabon N, Moulinier C, Taïeb A, et al. Dermatophytie à *Microsporum langeroni* chez un nouveau-né contaminé en France. Ann Dermatol Venereol 1994;121:247-248.

70. Cabon N, Moulinier C, Taïeb A, et al. Tinea capitis and faciei caused by *Microsporum langeroni* in two neonates. Pediatr Dermatol 1994;11:281.

71. Ghorpade A, Ramanan C. Tinea capitis and corporis due to *Trichophyton violaceum* in a six-day-old infant. Int J Dermatol 1994;33:219-220.

72. Weston WL, Morelli JG. Neonatal tinea capitis. Pediatr Infect Dis J 1998;17:257-258.

73. Alden ER, Chernila SA. Ringworm in an infant. Pediatrics 1969;44:261-262.

74. Weston WL, Thorne EG. Two cases of tinea in the neonate treated successfully with griseofulvin. Clin Pediatr 1977;16:601-602.

75. Baudraz-Rosselet F, Ruffieux P, Mancarella A, et al. Diaper dermatitis due to *Trichophyton verrucosum*. Pediatr Dermatol 1993;10:368-369.

76. Kurgansky D, Sweren R. Onychomycosis in a 10-week-old infant. Arch Dermatol 1990;126:1371.

77. Mercurio MG, Silverman RA, Elewski BE. Tinea capitis—fluconazole in trichophyton tonsurans infection. Pediatr Dermatol 1998;15:229-232.

78. Piérard GE, Arrese JE, Piérard-Franchimont C. Treatment and prophylaxis of tinea infections. Drugs 1996;52:209-224.

79. Rabinowitz LG, Esterly NB. Naftifine (naftin) in pediatrics. Pediatr 1992;90:652.

80. Friedlander SF, Suarez S. Pediatric antifungal therapy. Dermatol Clin 1998;16:527.
81. Peterson CM, Eichenfield LF. Scabies. Pediatr Ann 1996; 25:97-100.
82. Hurwitz S. Scabies in babies. Am J Dis Child 1973;126:226-228.
83. Camassa F, Fania M, Ditano G, et al. Neonatal scabies. Cutis 1995;56:210-212.
84. Duran C, Tamoyo L, Orozco ML. Scabies of the scalp mimicking seborrheic dermatitis in immunocompromised patients. Pediatr Dermatol 1993;10:136-138.
85. Huffam SE, Currie BJ. Ivermectin for *Sarcoptes scabiei* hyperinfestation. Int J Infect Dis 1998;2:152-154.
86. Castanet J, Monpoux F, Mariani R, et al. Demodicidosis in an immunodeficient child. Pediatr Dermatol 1998;14:219-220.
87. Patrizi A, Neri I, Chieregato C, et al. Demodicidosis in immunocompetent young children: Report of eight cases. Dermatol 1997;195:239-42.
88. Sarro RA, Hong JJ, Elgart ML. An unusual demodicidosis manifestation in a patient with AIDS. J Am Acad Dermatol 1998;38:120-121.
89. Noutsis C, Millikan LE. Myiasis. Dermatol Clin 1994; 12:729-736
90. Singh I, Gathwala G, Yadav SP, et al. Myiasis in children: The Indian perspective. Int J Pediatr Otorhinolar 1993;25:127-131.
91. Rao S, Berkowitz FE, Metchock B. External ophthalmomyiasis in an urban infant. Pediatr Infect Dis J 1990;9:675-676
92. Rao R, Nosanchuk JS, Mackenzie R. Cutaneous myiasis acquired in New York State. Pediatr 1997;99:601-602.
93. Boyer KM. Diagnosis and treatment of congenital toxoplasmosis. Adv Pediatr Infect Dis 1996;11:449-467.
94. Lynfield R, Guerina NG. Toxoplasmosis. Pediatr Rev 1997; 18:75-83.
95. Remington JS, McLeod R, Desmonts G. Toxoplasmosis. In Remington JS, Klein JO, eds. Infectious disease of the fetus and newborn infant. 4th edition. WB Saunders: Philadelphia, 1995: pp 140-267.
96. Roizen N, Swisher CN, Stein MA, et al. Neurologic and developmental outcome in treated congenital toxoplasmosis. Pediatrics 1995;95:11-20.
97. Alger LS. Toxoplasmosis and parvovirus B19. Infect Obstetr 1997;11:55-75.
98. Kubba R, Al-Gindan Y. Leishmaniasis. Dermatol Clin 1989; 7:331-351.
99. Di Rocco M, Vignola S, Borrone C, et al. Cutaneous leishmaniasis in a 6-month-old girl. J Pediatr 1998;132:748.
100. del Giudice P, Marty P, Lacour JP, et al. Cutaneous leishmaniasis due to *Leishmania infantum*. Arch Dermatol 1998; 134:193-198.
101. Chaliasos N, Bourantas C, Kritikou E, et al. A 7-month-old girl with fever and bleeding. Lancet 1996;347:1086
102. Wittner M. Leishmaniasis. In Feigin RD, Cherry JD, eds. Textbook of pediatric infectious diseases. 4th edition. vol 2. Philadelphia: WB Saunders, 1998: pp 2452-2458.
103. Nelson JD, ed. 1998-1999 Pocket book of pediatric antimicrobial therapy. 13th edition. Baltimore: Williams & Wilkins, 1998: p 62.
104. Brimhall CL, Esterly NB. Summertime, and the critters are biting. Contemp Pediatr 1994;11:62-77
105. Rees RS, King LE Jr. Arthropod bites and stings. In Fitzpatrick TB, et al. Dermatology in general medicine. 3rd edition. New York: McGraw-Hill, 1987: pp 2495-2506.
106. Vetter RS, Vischer PK. Bites and stings of medically important venomous arthropods. Int J Dermatol 1998;37:481-496.

14

Eczematous Disorders

BERNICE R. KRAFCHIK

Eczematous eruptions represent a significant portion of the skin diseases seen in the neonate. The most common is atopic dermatitis (AD). Seborrheic dermatitis (SD) and irritant diaper dermatitis (IDD) are now seen less frequently. Contact dermatitis is rare in infants, and many less-common eczematous disorders that result from nutritional, metabolic, and immunologic diseases have clinical manifestations that may be difficult to differentiate from AD.

Dermatitis is an all-inclusive term for inflammation of the skin that appears clinically as erythema, erythema and scaling, or erythema and scaling with crusts. The term *eczema* (boiling over) refers either to the infantile form of AD or to the morphology of erythema, scaling, and crusts.

ATOPIC DERMATITIS

Atopic dermatitis was described by Besnier[1] as prurigo diasthetique in 1892. In 1933 Wise and Sulzberger[2] coined the term *atopic dermatitis*, and Hill and Sulzberger[3] characterized the clinical entity in 1935. The term *atopy* means without place or a strange thing. Atopic dermatitis is an inherited, chronic, relapsing, pruritic skin condition characterized clinically by xerosis, inflammation, and lichenification and immunologically by an overproduction of IgE. The disease imposes an enormous burden on the social, personal, emotional, and financial resources of patients and families.[4] In the United States $364 million is spent annually on the care of AD in children.[5]

The exact incidence of AD is difficult to establish, since many of the milder cases are not seen by physicians; in the past 4 decades an increase in both the incidence and preva-

lence of AD has been reported.[6,7] Atopic dermatitis is particularly common in Caucasians and Chinese[8] and occurs with a greater frequency in highly industrialized countries.[9] It is slightly more common in girls, with a female-to-male ratio of 1.4 to 1, and in higher social classes.[10] There may also be an increased association with maternal smoking[11] but a lower incidence in preterm infants.[12]

Atopic dermatitis is usually the first manifestation of atopic disease,[13] which includes AD, asthma, and allergic rhinitis. Thirty-eight percent of cases start before 3 months, 85% occur during the first year of life, and 95% before 5 years of age.[14,15]

Cutaneous Findings

The disease is characterized by three distinct age-related clinical phases in which both the site and the morphology of the lesions change.[15,16] The infantile phase lasts for 2 to 3 years. The childhood phase, which persists into puberty, is characterized by typical, exudative, excoriated, and lichenified lesions in a flexural distribution. In adults, the face, neck, and body are diffusely involved with erythema and scaling.

The major symptom is severe pruritus that interferes with normal sleep patterns. Although many of the signs may appear earlier, parents usually seek advice when the "itch-scratch" cycle matures; the infant starts scratching and clawing at his or her skin or rubbing against hard objects.

The eruption in infancy characteristically starts on the cheeks (Figs. 14-1 and 14-2) and scalp (Fig. 14-3) and evolves over days to weeks to involve the lateral and extensor aspects of the legs and arms (Fig. 14-4).[17] Other areas of the face and body may also develop eczematous changes,

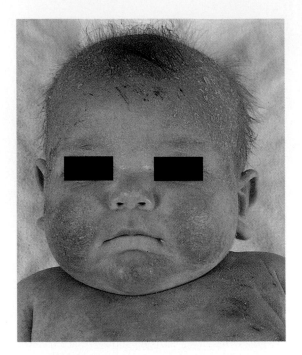

FIG. 14-1
Atopic dermatitis typical cheek involvement.

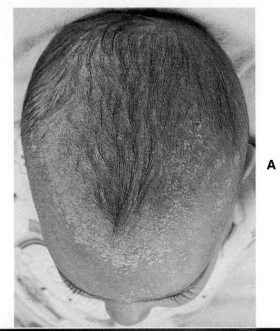

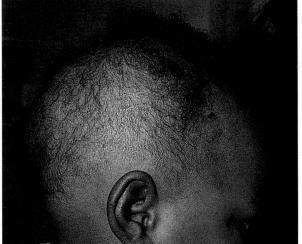

FIG. 14-3
A, Typical "cradle cap" is often the first manifestation of atopic dermatitis. **B,** Temporary alopecia may result when an infant rubs the sides of the head against bedding in order to alleviate itching.

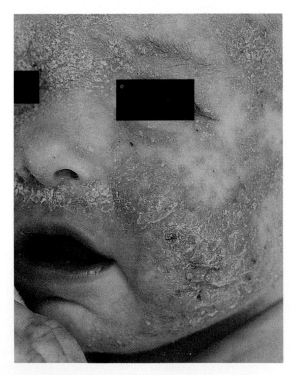

FIG. 14-2
Crusted lesions of atopic dermatitis on the face.

but the diaper area is often spared. Lesions are usually symmetric, scaly, erythematous patches and plaques within which crusting is common. Ichthyosis vulgaris affects 20% to 37% of infants on the lower legs[18] and is seen together with hyperlinearity of the palms and soles. In African-American infants, the eruption is often papular. Postinflammatory hypopigmentation or hyperpigmen-

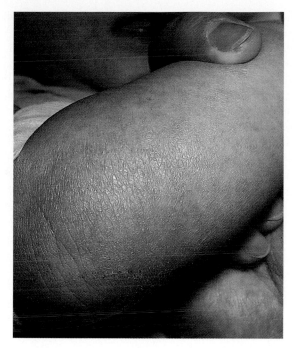

FIG. 14-4

Lichenification of extensor surfaces such as the elbow (shown here) can be seen in early infancy but is more common in older infants.

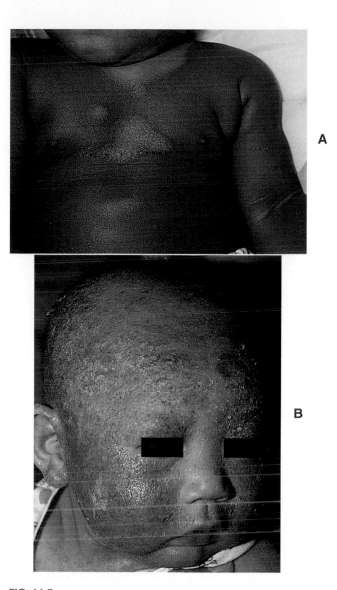

FIG. 14-5

A, Note the marked postinflammatory hypopigmentation, which is common in darkly pigmented infants. B, This young infant was initially thought to have seborrheic dermatitis, but over time the diagnosis of atopic dermatitis became evident.

tation is common and disappears weeks to months after the dermatitis has resolved (Fig. 14-5, A). In the absence of severe secondary infection, scarring is rare. A little recognized feature of AD in the neonatal period is the presence of an erythematous, scaly intertrigo that resembles SD but has a dry instead of greasy feel. Intertrigo is the presence of erythematous patches in the creases of opposing skin folds. It may be seen in both neonatal AD and SD and may also occur in normal infants as a result of skin friction. Lichenification is not seen in neonatal AD.

The Dennie-Morgan fold, a double crease found beneath the lower eyelid of patients and once thought to be pathognomonic of AD, may be present at birth or soon after. This finding occurs in normal children and in other inflammatory conditions affecting the periorbital area. Williams[19] found it to be more common in non-AD African-American children than in those with AD.

It is often difficult to establish the diagnosis of AD in early infancy, and particularly to differentiate it from SD (see Figs. 14-3, A, and 14-5, B).[20] Criteria have been formulated and subsequently modified for infants.[21,22] The most practical diagnostic criteria come from the United Kingdom Working Party.[23] An individual must have an itchy skin eruption (or parental report of scratching or rubbing in a child) plus three of the following:

1. History of flexural involvement: folds of the elbows, behind the knees, front of the ankles, or around the neck (including the cheeks in children under 10 years)
2. A personal history of asthma or hay fever (or history of atopic disease in a first-degree relative in children under 10 years)

3. A history of generalized dry skin in the last year
4. Visible flexural eczema (or eczema involving the cheeks/forehead and outer limbs in children under 4 years)
5. Onset under the age of 2 years (not used if the child is under 4 years)

These criteria disregard the minor signs, which are inconstant findings,[24,25] and serum IgE levels, which are not always high.

Extracutaneous Findings

Lymphadenopathy from chronic inflammation of the skin is common and often severe, in some cases leading to an erroneous suspicion of lymphoma or immunodeficiency.

Etiology/Pathogenesis

The etiology and pathogenesis of AD is unknown. Genetic, chemical, and immunologic abnormalities probably interact with one another and with environmental stimuli to initiate the inflammation.

There is evidence that AD is genetic: it is clustered in families; monozygotic twins are concordant, whereas dizygotic twins are discordant for AD[26]; and transfer of AD by bone marrow transplantation[27] has been reported. Although attempts to isolate an atopic gene on chromosome 11q13 and on 6p major histocompatibility complex (MHC)[28,29] have yielded inconclusive results,[30,31,32] many of the immunologic abnormalities seen in AD may be under the influence of genetic factors. These include high levels of IgE,[32] abnormal T-cell clones,[33] high levels of IL-4, low levels of interferon-gamma, and elevated phosphodiesterase (PDE) activity, which may represent a primary defect of intracellular regulation.[34] Until a suitable marker is found for diagnosing the disease, it will be impossible to characterize the exact genetic inheritance.[32]

Cytokine abnormalities are common, and their interaction may represent another pathogenetic mechanism underlying the inflammation of AD. It has recently been recognized that Th-2 responses predominate in AD and lead to the overproduction of numerous cytokines (IL-4, IL-5, IL-6 and IL-10), which inhibit Th-1 cytokine production of IFN-gamma.[35] This promotes B cell proliferation, as well as increased serum[36] and skin IgE.[37] IL-4 stimulates mast cells to produce mediators[38] such as histamine, which play a key role in the development of pruritus. Neuropeptides (substance P) stimulate histamine release from skin mast cells and may link the central nervous system with cutaneous inflammation.[39] The repeated stimulation and abnormal biochemical responsiveness and mediator release by AD

monocytes, mast cells, and eosinophils may sustain and initiate a vicious cycle, contributing to the inflammation.[40]

Xerosis may also be a primary event in the pathogenesis of AD.[41] It is associated with a reduction of lipids, notably the ceramide fraction of the stratum corneum (SC)[42] and an abnormal amino acid content of SC cells, resulting in increased transepidermal water loss and skin dehydration.[43] Irritation and breakage in the SC from the xerosis may potentiate access of environmental allergens.

Antigens are thought to activate and trigger the immune response in AD. The most common of these are foods, aeroallergens, and S. aureus. The antigens may be presented to the allergen-specific IgE receptors on Langerhans' cells (LC), and these complexes may interact with allergen-specific T cells.[44] In neonates, the evidence supporting the role of food includes the following: reports that prolonged breast feeding protects against the development of AD[45]; maternal avoidance of allergens during early lactation reduces the incidence of AD[45]; the early introduction of solid food increases the incidence of AD[46]; and immediate skin test reactions can be elicited to a variety of antigens.[47] The house dust mite, *Dermatophagoides pteronyssinus,* and the yeast *Pityrosporum ovale,* have both been cited in the pathogenesis of AD.[48] Numerous studies have refuted an association with both food and house dust mites, although there have never been studies of house dust mite elimination in the neonatal period .[49,50,51]

S. aureus colonization on the skin[52] and nares is more common in AD than in other skin diseases (or in the normal population), and the further finding of S. aureus enterotoxin B producing superantigens suggests it may play a role in pathogenesis.[53]

Diagnosis

The diagnosis of AD is usually made clinically. Skin biopsies may be helpful in distinguishing atopic dermatitis from other diseases, but biopsy findings alone are not diagnostic. The histology varies from an acute dermatitis with spongiosis and a lymphocytic infiltrate, to chronic changes in lichenified skin showing acanthosis, hyperkeratosis, parakeratosis, and a perivascular lymphocytic infiltrate around blood vessels and an accumulation of Langerhans' cells,[54] phagocytes, and mast cells.[55] The superficial venular plexus has endothelial cell hypertrophy, basement membrane thickening,[56] and increased numbers of immunoreactive nerve fibers[57] with nerve demyelination. The histologic appearance suggests a classical type IV cell-mediated hypersensitivity reaction.[58]

Patients with AD often have positive prick tests produced by specific IgE antibodies to antigens. However, these reactions do not correlate with clinical sensitivity and are of little value as a positive predictor of antigen intolerance in AD.[59] Specific antibodies in the serum tested against known antigens (RAST) have not provided better or different information.

Differential Diagnosis

The main differential diagnosis of AD in neonates includes SD, contact dermatitis, psoriasis, and scabies. Seborrheic dermatitis may be virtually indistinguishable from AD, due to the similarity in sites of involvement and morphology (see the following discussion). Contact dermatitis is rare in the newborn period. A configuration suggesting an external source of irritation may be evident and helpful in differentiating between the two.

Psoriasis is not commonly recognized in infants, although it may occur at birth or during the first year of life. Both psoriasis vulgaris and pustular psoriasis may occur in the neonate. The diaper area is most commonly affected in the former, where lesions are erythematous, well-demarcated plaques surmounted by scale, which is less silvery in the diaper area than in other areas (see the following discussion).

Scabies may be difficult to distinguish from AD because both diseases are extremely pruritic. Scabies is rarely considered in the newborn. The face is not usually involved in scabies, whereas the eczematous patches on the cheeks and xerosis are typical of AD. Moreover, the eruption of scabies is polymorphous, with burrows, papules, nodules, and eczematous and urticarial lesions, as well as typical pustules on the palms and soles. A recent onset of itching in family members is also helpful in differentiating the two conditions. When the skin lesions are associated with failure to thrive, diarrhea, infection, and other systemic signs, it is important to consider rarer possibilities such as nutritional, metabolic, or immunologic disorders (see the following discussion).

Occasionally, atopic dermatitis may be so severe that the whole body becomes erythrodermic, causing confusion with other causes of erythroderma, particularly Netherton syndrome, and nutritional deficiencies.

Prognosis

Atopic dermatitis is a disease of exacerbations and remissions. Data from follow-up surveys show enormous variation in the prognosis, owing to differences in patient sampling techniques. The degree of severity of AD and its persistence into adolescence are both predictors that the disease is more likely to continue into adult life.[60,61,62]

Other risk factors for adult disease include the presence of other atopic diseases such as asthma and allergic rhinitis, female sex, and early age of onset.[62]

Vickers[61] reported that AD cleared by age 20 in 90% of patients, but the inclusion of patients with SD, which has an excellent prognosis and clears within weeks, biased his results. Nevertheless, there is a steady decline in AD, with the highest prevalence being in those under 2 years of age (9.8%); in adulthood AD affects only 0.2% of those over 40 years of age.[63]

Figures on the incidence of asthma and hay fever following or associated with AD vary from 10% to 30%.[13,60] In one survey, 48% suffered from respiratory atopy (36% from rhinitis, 28% from asthma, and 15% from both).[13] Atopic dermatitis and asthma may be inherited together,[64] but through separate genetic pathways. There is an added risk of developing either asthma or AD if there is a family history of either.[65] Asthma can start at any time, but AD often occurs earlier than other atopic diseases.[13]

Treatment

Presently there is no cure for AD. Until the basic defect is recognized, management should be aimed at treating the pruritus, the xerosis, and the inflammation. It is extremely important to establish an honest relationship with the parents and to explain at the first meeting the goals that can be attained and the nature of the disease. It is most reassuring to a distraught, guilt-ridden parent with a sleepless infant who is unable to stop scratching, that something can be done. Because parents are inundated with so much information, attention to detail and repetition of advice can improve treatment results.[66] Parents should be warned that despite good control and meticulous care, children may flare at any time.

Environmental Control

Infants with AD do not tolerate heat or extreme cold well[67]; maintaining a cool, humid environment is helpful. In the winter, the heat should be adjusted at night so that the temperature is lowered to ensure that the infant does not sweat excessively. In the summer, a cool breeze when outdoors and air conditioning when indoors is helpful. Both heating and air conditioning dry the air; use of a humidifier is advised. Fluctuations in temperature, including fevers, may cause flares. Neonates with AD are irritated by nylon and wool; 100% cotton clothing is recommended and may be layered in the winter months to provide additional warmth.

Pruritus

One of the major challenges of treatment is controlling the intense pruritus. Pruritus causes sleep deprivation in both patients and their families. Evidence for antihistamine effectiveness is contradictory.[68,69] Although a good effect with traditional H1 antihistamines has been reported, this may be due to drowsiness from central nervous system (CNS) depression.[70] One reason for the lack of efficacy of antihistamines is that the prescribed dose is often too low. Side effects of antihistamines are unusual. Hydroxyzine is safe to use at a dose of 2 to 3 mg/kg/day (beginning at lower doses, particularly in very young infants). Diphenhydramine may also be used as an alternate option in a dose of 5 mg/kg/day. Topical treatment with steroids is more effective than antihistamines, which at best are an added benefit.

Xerosis (Dry Skin)

Xerosis is the first manifestation of AD and is worse in northern climates during the dry winter months. A humidifier in the newborn's room counteracts the drying effect of heating and air conditioning. Bleach, fabric softeners, and perfumed products should be avoided. Soaps may be eliminated, since bath oils with emulsifiers contain cleansing agents. Harsh soaps should be avoided (see Chapter 5).

The frequency of bathing is controversial. Recent evidence suggests that bathing, followed by the immediate application of an emollient while wet, has an excellent hydrating effect, is steroid sparing, and is the single most useful treatment in AD patients.[71] The water should be lukewarm. One-half to one capful of oil is sufficient; the oil should contain an emulsifier that keeps the water and oil in solution, thus preventing the water from evaporating. Alpha-Keri, Aveeno, and other oil products have emulsifiers that allow dispersion of oil in water (see Chapter 5). Parents should ensure that accidents are avoided because the infant is slippery and harder to handle. Bathing for 5 minutes is sufficient, and it is beneficial to bathe two or even three times daily.

Ideally, moisturizing agents should be safe, effective, inexpensive, and free of additives and other potential sensitizing agents. Petrolatum, Eucerin, and Aquaphor all provide good barriers and spread easily over wet skin. In hot, humid climates petrolatum may cause miliaria and itching, and a less-occlusive cream can be substituted. Products containing urea, lactic acid, and alpha-hydroxy acids should not be used because they may sting and their toxic effects are unknown. Emollients should be applied all over the body when the skin is wet and after topical corticosteroids have been applied to lesional skin. Regular applications of emollients should be continued even after the dermatitis has improved to prevent further exacerbations.

Inflammation

Topical corticosteroids were first introduced by Sulzberger and Witten[72] in 1952 and are the mainstay of treatment in AD because of their excellent antiinflammatory effect. They are grouped according to their potency into seven classes from very weak (VII) to superpotent (I). The early indiscriminate use of topical corticosteroids resulted in a number of local and systemic side effects, which has led to an unfounded fear and reluctance on the part of parents and physicians to use them appropriately. Yamamoto[73] noted that most parents do not use the prescribed medications because they fear side effects, despite the extremely small number of reported side effects in those treated.[74] The majority of adverse effects occur in patients who have received inappropriate treatment.[75] Physicians should encourage the correct use of topical corticosteroid preparations on affected inflamed areas. Close monitoring and follow-up during treatment is mandatory.

Precise information should be given to the parents regarding the manner of application. In the newborn period, it is often difficult to make a diagnosis of AD. Mild cases may be treated with low-potency steroids, such as hydrocortisone 1% ointment. In moderate and severe cases, a thin layer of a mid-strength fluorinated steroid ointment, such as betamethasone-17-valerate 0.05% or triamcinolone acetate 0.1%, should be applied to the inflamed body areas. A weaker preparation (hydrocortisone 1% to 2.5% ointment) may be applied to the face, diaper area, and folds 2 to 3 times a day, until resolution of the inflammation occurs. An ointment base is preferred, but in hot, humid weather, creams may be better tolerated. Scalp lesions should be treated with a corticosteroid cream because topical steroid lotions often contain alcohol that may burn inflamed, open areas. Steroids should always be discontinued and moisturizers substituted when the inflammation disappears, and restarted when new areas develop.

Prescriptions should be given for enough medication. Depending on the extent of the eruption and the size of the infant, 100 g will usually last for about a month. Maintenance therapy with topical corticosteroids is inappropriate. Areas should be treated two to three times a day until the inflammation disappears. Systemic corticosteroids are not indicated for the treatment of AD in neonates.

Infections

As noted, *S. aureus* frequently colonizes the skin and nares of atopic individuals. Topical corticosteroids alone can reduce bacterial counts.[76] Oral antibiotics may be necessary to treat obvious secondary bacterial infection, presenting as pustules and honey-colored crusts. Antibiotics may also be used if the AD flares for no apparent reason. The usual first-line treatments are cephalexin or cephradine 25 to 50 mg/k/day, or dicloxacillin, 12.5 to 25 mg/kg/day, in divided doses QID for 7 to 14 days. Erythromycin 25 to 50 mg/kg/day may also be effective; however, significant antibiotic resistance (25% to 40%) is reported in some geographic areas. Methicillin-resistant *S. aureus* (MRSA) is another growing concern. Bacterial culture and sensitivities may be needed to guide antibiotic therapy. Although prolonged oral antibiotic therapy is alleged to reduce the *S. aureus* superantigens,[53] resistant bacteria may develop. Because colonization is so common in this setting, antibiotics should not be used to treat culture results alone.

Mupirocin (pseudomonic acid) decreases the carrier rate of *S. aureus* on the skin,[77] but application in large areas is impractical. Antibacterial scrubs reduce the staphylococcal colony count, but irritation and potential toxicity limits their use in neonates. *S. aureus* colonization is impossible to eradicate from the nose and skin even with long-term antibiotic use.[78]

Allergen Avoidance

Some studies demonstrate a benefit from dietary manipulation in lactating mothers, but food elimination diets in both mother and/or infant and removal of aeroallergens from the environment should only be considered as a last resort. The effort to implement such changes is not worth the small success rate.

New Therapies

Treatment with topical tacrolimus 0.03% to 0.1% twice a day is the most promising new treatment for AD and may prove to be an effective alternative to topical steroids. Lesions recur when the treatment is stopped, and studies to date have not included infants.[79] Other therapies such as topical doxepin and gamma-interferon are not appropriate for use in neonates.

SEBORRHEIC DERMATITIS

First described by Unna in 1887,[80] SD is a disease of unknown etiology that affects infants with a distinct inflammatory eruption that primarily involves the scalp and intertriginous areas. The disease affects both sexes and is most common within the first 4 to 6 weeks of life, but may occur up to 1 year of age. Severe SD is not seen by dermatologists as frequently as in the past; primary care physicians may feel more comfortable in treating SD, or the true incidence may have decreased.

Cutaneous Findings

The scalp is the first area to be involved with "cradle-cap," which is a greasy, yellow scale on the vertex. Hair loss is uncommon, and erythema is variable (Fig. 14-6). The retroauricular creases are commonly affected. Lesions commonly involve the face, primarily the central forehead, glabella, eyebrows, malar eminences, nasolabial folds, and external ears with erythema and a yellow greasy scale (Fig. 14-7). Other commonly affected areas include the diaper area, with well-demarcated, erythematous plaques and a variable degree of scale; the axillary area and other creases (Fig. 14-8); and the presternal and interscapular area where eczematous patches are common. After a few days, *Candida albicans* commonly invades the affected areas, causing maceration and crusting.

Secondary bacterial infection may rarely occur with crusting and pustules on the existing lesions. Postinflammatory hypopigmentation is common in dark-skinned infants. It improves in the weeks after the dermatitis resolves.

Etiology and Pathogenesis

The etiology and pathogenesis are unknown. It is unlikely that infants with SD are more prone to suffer from the

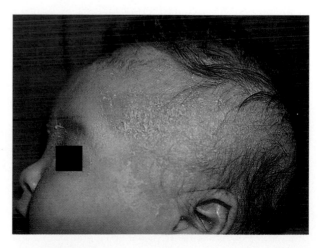

FIG. 14-6
Seborrheic dermatitis: greasy, white scalp scaling.

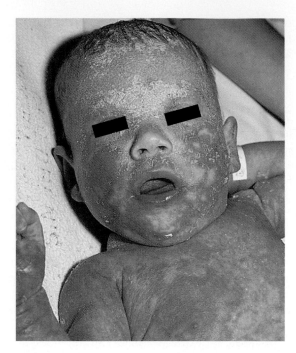

FIG. 14-7
Seborrheic dermatitis: this infant had unusually widespread disease.

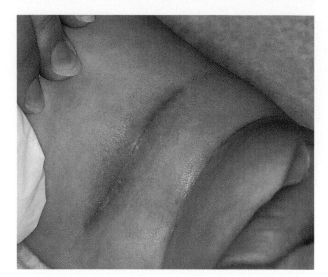

FIG. 14-8
Seborrheic dermatitis with typical involvement in body fold.

adult disease. Theories of increased sebaceous gland activity as a result of maternal hormones and nutritional factors have not been validated.[81]

Two studies have implicated *Pityrosporum ovale* (*Malassezia furfur*) in the etiology of SD in infants.[82,83] The organism was detected in the majority of infants with SD, but in only a few of the controls.[83] In the other study, treatment of the SD group with ketoconazole 2% resulted in a clinical cure in two thirds of infants within 2 weeks and a mycologic cure in almost all of them.

An abnormality of essential fatty acids has also been reported, related to a transient impairment of the enzyme activity of delta-6-desaturase, but this has yet to be validated.[84,85]

Diagnosis

The diagnosis is usually a clinical one. Histology of the lesions is not diagnostic and consists of a subacute dermatitis with elongation of the epidermal rete ridges. The presence of neutrophils is more suggestive of SD than other forms of dermatitis. There are no laboratory markers for diagnosing this condition.

Differential Diagnosis

Seborrheic dermatitis may be very difficult to distinguish from psoriasis. Psoriasis may occur in infants and often starts in the diaper area with persistent, well-demarcated, erythematous plaques surmounted by a scale (Fig. 14-9). The greasy scale in the scalp and creases that is typical of SD is not seen in psoriasis. Similarly, AD in newborns is easy to confuse with SD,[86] particularly during the first few weeks of life. The scalp is often involved in both. Cradle cap is caused by the retention of keratin and is often found in normal infants. It is also commonly seen in AD, where the scale is dry rather than greasy, as is seen in SD. The term *seboatopic* is used for cases fitting both patterns, but the diagnosis usually becomes clear early on; the majority of cases represent AD. The morphology of the lesions and the presence or absence of pruritus and xerosis is helpful in differentiation between the two. The diagnosis of SD is more likely when the axillae are affected, and AD is more likely to be diagnosed when the shins and forearms are involved.[86]

Persistent, hemorrhagic, atrophic, or ulcerative lesions should alert physicians to consider the diagnosis of Langerhans' cell histiocytosis (LCH), which in neonates

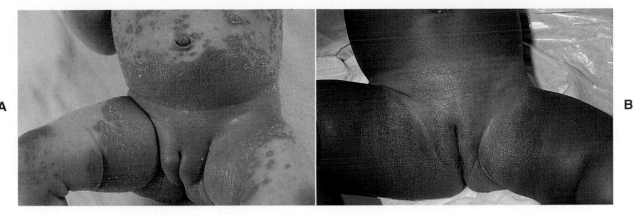

FIG. 14-9
Psoriasis: typical diaper involvement.

and young infants can resemble SD with a similar distribution in the scalp and the retroauricular and diaper areas. Well-demarcated, erythematous patches and crusts are evident, but the presence of petechiae and purpura is typical of LCH. Lesions of LCH may also involve other areas of the body with varying morphologies, including erythematous papules, vesicles, and nodules. Skin biopsy easily differentiates between the two conditions (see Chapter 23).

Leiner's disease is a rare disorder that has lesions similar to SD, but with the additional features of severe generalized erythroderma, diarrhea, and failure to thrive. This disorder is due to immunodeficiency (see Chapter 15).

Course, Management, Treatment, and Prognosis

Follow-up studies of patients with infantile SD have produced a variety of findings. Vickers classified both AD and SD as one disease.[61] Others[82,87] have concluded that many of the cases of infantile SD eventuated into AD. These reports may have based their diagnosis of SD on the finding of cradle cap, which was thought to be diagnostic of SD but is now known to frequently occur in AD. Reports of SD evolving into psoriasis may reflect the previous lack of recognition of psoriasis in infancy.[88]

Treatment consists of using a mild tar shampoo daily and oatmeal baths once or twice daily, followed by a mild steroid cream (hydrocortisone 1%) three times a day; this usually produces full recovery in a few weeks. Recurrence of SD is rare. Salicylic acid preparations should not be used because absorption can cause salicylism and irritation.

PSORIASIS

Psoriasis is a common, chronic inflammatory skin disease characterized clinically by a typical, scaly eruption and pathogenetically by an accelerated epidermal cell turnover. It affects 1% to 2% of the population,[89,90] and one third of cases occur before the age of 20.[91] Two percent of cases present before age 2 years.[91] There is a slight female preponderance[92] Although rare, psoriasis may present at birth. When psoriasis occurs in children, a family history is easier to ascertain.[91] Development of psoriasis in childhood does not imply a poor prognosis.[91]

Cutaneous Findings

There are two forms of psoriasis that may be seen in infants. The first commonly presents in the diaper area (see Fig. 14-9) or in the scalp. It may, however, involve any area and, unlike the adult form, commonly affects the face. Lesions may be pruritic and consist of erythematous, well-demarcated plaques with a silvery scale, a feature that is often absent in the diaper area.[93] In infancy the Koebner phenomenon (isomorphic response) is common. Nail changes are present in 10% of infants with psoriasis. The findings may include pitting, onycholysis, oil spots, and subungual hyperkeratosis. Severe, inflammatory nail changes (acrodermatitis continua of Hallopeau) may accompany pustular psoriasis.

A second form of psoriasis that may present in infancy, albeit much more rarely, is pustular psoriasis. This may have its onset at birth or in the ensuing few weeks. The eruption often presents with fever and sheets of small pustules that may also be arranged in a circinate or annular pattern. In this instance, pustules are located at the peripheral edge of an erythematous scale.[94] Associated findings in this pustular variety include geographic tongue, sterile osteomyelitis, and very rarely lung involvement with the capillary leak syndrome.

Etiology and Pathogenesis

The etiology of psoriasis is unknown. There is a strong family history, which is even more evident in the younger cases. This appears to be associated with certain HLA types, such as Cw6. The gene defect is not inherited in a simple autosomal dominant or recessive pattern. In older children, it is well recognized that guttate (teardrop) lesions may be related to infection with beta-hemolytic streptococcus. Guttate psoriasis has been described after a perianal streptococcal infection. The ultimate pathogenesis of psoriasis is unknown and may represent a polygenic inheritance pattern that manifests after multifactorial environmental events.

Diagnosis

The diagnosis of "napkin psoriasis" is often difficult. A biopsy may be necessary to confirm the diagnosis. Characteristic histology includes parakeratosis, loss of the granular layer, Munro microabscesses, and spongiform pustules of Kogoj. A lymphocytic infiltrate is present within the dermis. A repeated sterile culture from the pustules should alert physicians to the diagnosis of pustular psoriasis, and a biopsy is helpful.

Differential Diagnosis

It is extremely difficult to differentiate psoriasis in the diaper area and scalp from SD. The absence of intertriginous involvement, a greasy yellow scale, and nail changes may be helpful in the differentiation. Other causes of eruptions in the diaper area, including LCH and Netherton syndrome, as well as nutritional and metabolic disorders, are relatively easy to exclude with the appearance of the lesions and the biopsy findings. It is important to rule out infectious etiologies in pustular psoriasis, particularly when osteomyelitis is present.

Prognosis

The prognosis in infancy is variable. In a follow-up study of nine patients, most were still affected but had mild disease and did not require constant follow-up.[95] The more extensive the disease, the more likely lesions will persist.

Treatment

Many treatments are available for psoriasis in adults. Most of these are inappropriate for neonates. A mild to mid-strength steroid preparation with a tar shampoo is often all that is required for the plaque variety. The pustular form is more difficult to treat. A conservative approach with the use of topical corticosteroid preparations is often the first line of treatment. The addition of LCD (liquor carbonis detergens) to the topical corticosteroid is often necessary to control the disease. If this is not achieved, then oral medications should be considered. Systemic medications such as methotrexate, retinoids, and cyclosporine may be considered in refractory.

Candidiasis with Psoriasiform Id

Candidiasis with psoriasiform id is rarely seen in the neonatal period. Lesions of *Candida* in the diaper area are treated with topical corticosteroids, and after days to weeks, an explosive psoriasiform eruption occurs on the cheeks and trunk. Treatment of the candidal eruption with topical antifungal agents and mild to mid-strength corticosteroids to the psoriasiform areas results in remission in a few weeks. Whether the appearance of these lesions is associated with a psoriatic diathesis is not known.

DIAPER DERMATITIS

Diaper dermatitis encompasses all eruptions covered by the diaper, including those that are caused directly by the wearing of diapers, such as an irritant diaper dermatitis; those that are aggravated by diapers, such as psoriasis; and those that occur whether diapers are worn or not, such as zinc deficiency.[96]

The incidence and morphologies of diaper rash have changed over the years as a result of an evolution in diapering practices. Initially, diapers were home-laundered with harsh chemicals to remove the excreta. In the 1930s diaper services were started. Parents are provided with diapers, which are cycled through multiple wash and rinse cycles. Nondisposable diapers are cotton rectangles with a double layer and a multi-ply or fiber-filled center strip. The diaper is secured with safety pins or self-adhering closures. A plastic pant is used over the cloth diaper.[97]

Since the 1960s disposable diapers have been used extensively in North America, with frequent improvements over their original structure.[98] The inner surface is a top sheet that comes in contact with the infant's skin. The inner structure, or core, contains cellulose pulp, which absorbs moisture from the urine and feces. The outer layer is composed of waterproof polyethylene material. Superabsorbent diapers contain an absorbable gel material in the inner structure, which holds up to 80 times its weight in liquid when hydrated, thereby considerably decreasing skin wetness. This material also maintains pH control by providing a buffer, and decreases skin irritation by separating the urine and feces.[97] A recently marketed diaper product provides a sustained low level of a petrolatum-based emollient for further protection.[99] The environmental impact of disposable diapers has caused much concern and debate: these diapers cause 1% to 2% of the nonbiodegradable waste in North America, but cloth diapers, with their attendant repeated washing and drying, use natural resources.

Irritant Diaper Dermatitis

Irritant diaper dermatitis (IDD) was first described by Jacquet[100] in 1905. In Great Britain in the 1970s, diaper dermatitis accounted for 20% of all skin consultations in children less than 5 years of age.[101] Severe cases of diaper dermatitis seem to be less prevalent with the widespread use of superabsorbable disposable diapers.[102] Nevertheless, about 50% of infants have some degree of mild diaper dermatitis during the first year of life. Irritant diaper dermatitis is the most frequent diaper eruption, followed by candidiasis. Both SD and psoriasis are rarer causes of dermatitis in the diaper area, and other rarer causes include nutritional and metabolic diseases.

The incidence of IDD is equal between the sexes and usually occurs from a few weeks to 18 months, peaking between 6 and 9 months of age. Irritant diaper dermatitis is uncommon during the neonatal period because fecal enzymes, which are partially responsible for its development, are initially only present in low concentrations but increase after the first month of life.

Cutaneous Findings

Erythema and scaling are noted on the convex surfaces of the inner, upper thigh and buttock areas. The creases and the mons pubis in boys are generally spared (Fig. 14-10). The eruption subsequently becomes deeply erythematous with a typical glistening or glazed appearance (Fig. 14-11) and a wrinkled surface.

A specific eruption that occurs particularly on the labia or more rarely the penis and consists of well-demarcated, punched-out ulcers and erosions is Jacquet's erosive diaper dermatitis (Fig. 14-12). The ulcers heal

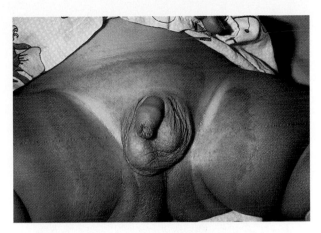

FIG. 14-10
Irritant diaper dermatitis with characteristic sparing of the folds.

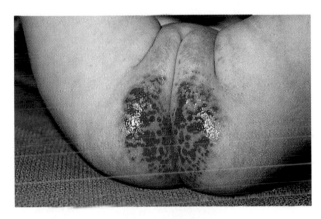

FIG. 14-11
Glazed appearance of severe irritant diaper dermatitis. Involvement of apposing areas of the buttock is often due to severe diarrhea.

quickly with a mild corticosteroid preparation three times a day and the use of thick emollients, which act as a barrier. This type of eruption is mostly associated with the use of home-laundered diapers and is now seen less frequently.

Etiology and Pathogenesis

The exact pathogenesis of IDD is only partially understood. Some infants seem constitutionally more susceptible to the development of IDD, and the ingestion of antibiotics[103] and diarrhea are both risk factors.[104] The plastic diaper covering forms an impervious layer, which with

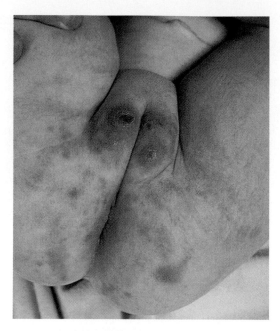

FIG. 14-12
Jacquet's erosive diaper dermatitis.

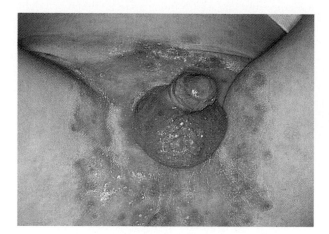

FIG. 14-13
Diaper rash resulting from *Candida albicans*.

urine causes overhydration of the skin. This worsens the friction from movement under the diaper.[105] Feces, when mixed with urine, produces a rise in the pH,[106] activating fecal lipases and proteases,[107] which, together with *Candida albicans*, cause damage to the epidermis, resulting in the loss of its normal barrier function and fostering increased susceptibility to irritation.[108]

Course, Management, Treatment, and Prognosis

Crucial factors in preventing IDD relate to the frequency of diaper changes and the use of diapers containing absorbable gel material. Mild dermatitis may be treated with emollients or pastes, such as zinc oxide or petrolatum, by providing protection from urine and feces. In moderate or severe cases, a nonfluorinated corticosteroid (hydrocortisone 1%) should be applied several times a day to the inflamed skin, followed by the emollient. After the inflammation has resolved, only an emollient should be applied. Strong corticosteroid preparations should not be used in the diaper area, as occlusion by the diaper enhances the potential for systemic absorption and causes local cutaneous atrophy and striae.

Candida Diaper Dermatitis

Candida albicans dermatitis is a frequent cause of diaper dermatitis. Some infants are particularly prone to candidal infection. Candidiasis is common in the diaper area, with 3% of infants affected from the second to the fourth month.[109] This is possibly due to the more frequent use of oral antibiotics in the neonatal period. Even without the typical morphology, *Candida albicans* may be recovered from the diaper area of any inflamed skin condition after 72 hours.[110] It may even be grown in small amounts from normal skin. *Candida* is recovered in much larger numbers from the skin and feces when candidal diaper dermatitis occurs.[111] The organism has the ability to penetrate the epidermal barrier by liberating keratinases.

Cutaneous Findings

The clinical picture of candidiasis takes two forms: it may present with a diffuse erythematous patch extending over the vulval and perineal area with a peripheral scale and satellite lesions, or with small pink papules surmounted by scale that may coalesce in some areas (Fig. 14-13). The anterior perineal area and inguinal creases are commonly involved, unlike IDD where the creases are spared. The more classic picture of a beefy red diaper area with satellite pustules is rarely seen.

Treatment with topical antifungal agents such as nystatin, clotrimazole, and ketoconazole two or three times daily is very effective. Adding hydrocortisone 1% as an antiinflammatory agent may promote more rapid healing. Potent corticosteroids should be avoided. Oral nystatin in conjunction with topical treatment is no better than topical nystatin alone.[112] Susceptible infants may have repeated infections with *Candida albicans* (see Chapter 13).

CONTACT DERMATITIS

Contact dermatitis is an inflammatory process caused by the application of an irritating substance to the skin or by a substance causing an allergic reaction. Although irritant contact dermatitis occurs in many individuals who are exposed to the irritating substance, allergic contact dermatitis (ACD) occurs only in a small number of individuals who become sensitized. Patients with AD are more predisposed to irritant contact dermatitis because of their disordered barrier function.

Both irritant and ACD are rare in infants. Although infants are able to mount an immunologic response to a sensitizing substance, nickel is the only substance causing ACD seen with any frequency. The incidence of nickel allergy appears to be increasing.

Cutaneous Findings

Nickel sensitivity in neonates is almost exclusively caused by wearing of undershirts with nickel snaps. The involved areas are on the center of the chest and upper abdomen where there is a pruritic, linear dermatitis, corresponding to the areas where the nickel snaps are in contact with the skin. Id reactions are common, particularly in the antecubital fossae, but they can affect other areas as well. Infants with nickel sensitivity are often misdiagnosed as having AD; nickel sensitization may be more common in patients with AD who may have both conditions. Another possible source of nickel allergy is ear-piercing, which in some cultures is performed in very young infants.

Pathogenesis

The pathology is that of any acute dermatitis. Immunohistochemical stains show predominance of helper cells with some suppressor cells, although only a small number of the T cells in the infiltrate have specificity for the antigen.

Allergic contact dermatitis is produced by a T-lymphocyte cell-mediated type IV immune response. There are two distinct phases in the development of ACD: the afferent or induction phase and the efferent or elicitation phase.[113] The sensitization following first exposure with an allergen takes 5 to 25 days. On repeat exposure the eruption develops within 24 to 48 hours.

Management of Nickel Dermatitis

Everything containing nickel should be eliminated, including nickel zippers and underwear with nickel snaps. Parents should be reminded that the allergy is life long. Topical corticosteroids are helpful until the inflammation has subsided.

OTHER ETIOLOGIES OF ECZEMATOUS ERUPTIONS

Zinc deficiency can result from inadequate intake, malabsorption, excessive loss, or a combination of these factors caused by inherited and acquired conditions.[114] The skin may have widespread involvement. Zinc is an essential nutrient involved in numerous biologic functions necessary for growth and development.[115]

Acrodermatitis enteropathica is a rare, autosomal recessive disorder caused by an inborn error of metabolism resulting in zinc malabsorption and deficiency. It typically presents when the child is weaned from breast to cow's milk or, in the case of formula-fed infants, after 4 to 10 weeks, when stores of zinc have been depleted. Both cow and breast milk contain adequate amounts of zinc, but in acrodermatitis enteropathica, the transport mechanism for absorbing zinc in the intestine is defective and the cow's milk lacks the ligand necessary for the transfer of zinc across the Paneth cells of the small intestine.[116]

Zinc deficiency can also result from inadequate intake of zinc. In the past, this was described in infants receiving parenteral alimentation without adequate zinc supplementation, but the routine addition of zinc to parenteral feeds has eliminated this problem. Zinc deficiency is still seen in premature infants who are exclusively breast fed. The most common cause is when the nutritional needs of premature infants rise in the first few months of life, at a time when the mother's breast milk zinc is decreasing. There is also increased secretion into the gut during the first few months and poor zinc absorption.[115] It may also be rarely seen in term breast fed infants resulting from low or completely absent zinc in the mother's breast milk, despite normal maternal plasma zinc levels. Thus the transfer of zinc from plasma to breast milk is defective.[115] This may be inherited, since there are reports of absence of breast milk zinc in numerous members of one family.[117]

The skin eruption is usually the first clinical sign of zinc deficiency. Lesions are present on the cheeks and chin in a horseshoe distribution with erythematous dermatitic erosions (Fig. 14-14, *A*). Initially bullae may be present, but these rapidly erode. Over time, a more psoriasiform eruption develops. Periorbital involvement is common. The fingers and toes may have similar erosions and can be accompanied by nail dystrophy. They often become secondarily infected with *S. aureus* and *Candida*. A typical eruption occurs in the diaper area consisting of a sharply-demarcated area of erythema with accentuation of scale at the margin (Fig. 14-14, *B*). Occasionally this may occur without facial involvement. Irritability, diarrhea, hair loss, and failure to thrive are additional features but may be difficult to recognize in a neonate.

Low levels of zinc in the plasma is the characteristic finding, and levels of zinc-dependent alkaline phosphatase may also be low. Care should be taken to use a plastic syringe when drawing zinc levels and to prevent zinc contamination from rubber stoppers on glass tubes. High levels of zinc are due to laboratory error, since the body excretes zinc and limits absorption when the levels get too high.[118]

Treatment with zinc sulfate 1 to 3 mg/kg/day (the latter dose being appropriate for acrodermatitis enteropathica), leads to rapid improvement, with irritability being the first symptom to respond.[119] The inherited condition (acro-dermatitis enteropathica) may require long-term therapy. Occasionally zinc sulfate causes gastrointestinal symptoms and zinc gluconate may be substituted.[120]

Biotin deficiency (multiple carboxylase deficiency) is an autosomal recessive disorder that becomes apparent in the neonatal period or in late infancy. Systemic signs and symptoms include vomiting, seizures, developmental delay, hypotonia, and later ataxia. Cutaneous lesions resemble those of zinc deficiency, affecting the area around the eyes, face, and perianal area. The lesions are eczematous or psoriasiform and are unresponsive to topical treatment with steroids. Secondary candidal infection is common and remains unresponsive to treatment until the biotin deficiency is corrected.

The etiology of the condition in the neonate can be attributed to the decreased activity of any or all of three carboxylases: 3-methylcrotonyl CoA carboxylase, propionyl CoA carboxylase, and pyruvate carboxylase. All are biotin-dependent enzymes in which biotin acts as a cofactor. The defect is in holocarboxylase synthetase. In the juvenile form of the disease biotinidase is absent.[121]

The absence of carboxylase enzymes leads to an accumulation of carboxyls in the urine, resulting in lactic acidosis or ketosis. Treatment consists of biotin 5 to 20 mg/day, leading to rapid improvement.[122] The biotin is well absorbed and does not accumulate in tissues. A dose of 10 mg is usually given empirically.[123]

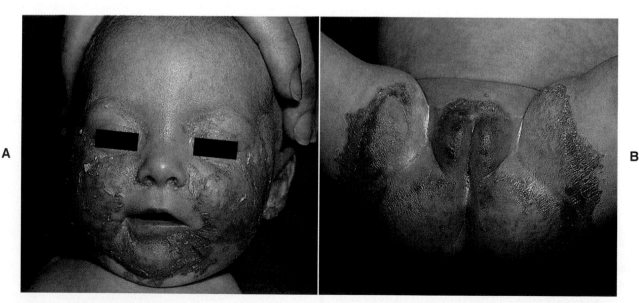

A   B

FIG. 14-14
A, Periorificial eruption and B, diaper rash: The skin findings are typical of zinc deficiency, in this case caused by low levels of zinc in breast milk.

Cystic fibrosis is an autosomal recessive disorder with widespread dysfunction of the exocrine glands resulting in chronic pulmonary disease, pancreatic insufficiency, and elevated sweat electrolytes. It can present in neonates or young infants with an erythematous, scaly rash with periorificial and/or perineal accentuation, closely resembling that of zinc deficiency.[124] Pedal edema is common. The usual presentation of failure to thrive, malabsorption, hepatosplenomegaly, and frequent pulmonary infections without symptoms may be associated with the rash. The cause of the skin eruption is unknown, and a combination of essential fatty acid deficiency, low zinc levels, and protein deficiency may all be involved.[125]

Hartnup disease is an extremely rare heterogeneous autosomal/recessive disorder characterized by a pellagra-like photosensitive eruption and cerebellar ataxia, emotional instability, encephalopathy, seizures, and aminoaciduria. The defect involves the disordered metabolism of tryptophan associated with the intestinal and renal transport of certain neutral alpha-amino acids. The disease is usually associated with consanguinity in the parents; it is extremely rare in the Western hemisphere.[126]

Omenn syndrome (see Chapter 15) presents in the neonatal period with an intensely pruritic generalized eczematous eruption that is difficult to distinguish from AD.[127] Failure to thrive, alopecia, eosinophilia, diarrhea, and repeated infections accompany the skin eruption. Organomegaly, which involves the liver, spleen, and lymph nodes, is common. Bone marrow transplantation has resulted in a complete cure.[128]

Phenylketonuria[129] is a rare autosomal recessive disorder involving the metabolism of phenylalanine. Infants may appear normal at birth, although most infants have blond hair and blue eyes or, if African-American, are fairer than their parents. About 50% of patients develop dermatitis indistinguishable from AD. Neurological signs become evident later. At birth, all babies in North America are screened for phenylketonuria, which is due to the absence of phenylalanine hydroxylase. This enzyme is required for the conversion of phenylalanine to tyrosine. To prevent the accumulation of phenylalanine in the blood, a low phenylalanine diet is instituted as soon as possible after birth to prevent the resultant mental retardation.

Wiskott-Aldrich syndrome is an X-linked recessive disease, almost always affecting male children. It presents in the first few months of life with petechiae, ecchymoses, and an associated bloody diarrhea caused by both quantitative and qualitative abnormalities of platelets. The skin eruption, which usually develops after the bleeding diathesis, is characterized by an extremely pruritic, generalized eczematous eruption with sanguinous crusts. Apart from its hemorrhagic component, the eruption is indistinguishable from atopic dermatitis (Fig. 14-15). Skin abscesses from recurrent bacterial infections with pneumococci, meningococci, and *Haemophilus influenzae*, as well as molluscum contagiosum, verrucae, and herpes simplex, are common. There is a tendency to develop nephropathy and lymphoreticular malignancies in adults. The cell surface marker, CD43 or sialophorin,[130] is absent from most cells but does not account for the Wiskott-Aldrich pheno-

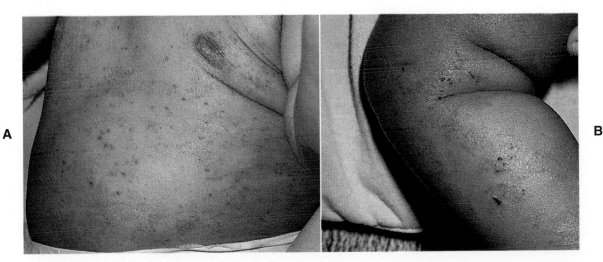

A   B

FIG. 14-15
Wiskott-Aldrich syndrome: eczematous dermatitis with crusts.

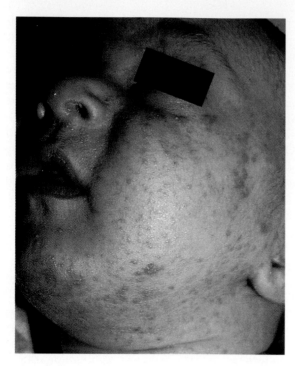

FIG. 14-16
Hypoimmunoglobulin-E syndrome: papular facial eruption.

type. The Wiskott-Aldrich–associated gene and its gene product, the Wiskott-Aldrich–associated protein, have recently been identified.[131] This gene is present on Xp11.23. Bone marrow transplantation has cured many patients.

Hyper-IgE syndrome and Job syndrome are immunodeficiency diseases characterized by chronic dermatitis, somewhat similar to AD, skeletal, and dental abnormalities. The rash has often been described as similar to atopic dermatitis, but inflammatory facial papules may predominate (Fig. 14-16). The skeletal abnormalities consist of repeated fractures. The dental abnormalities include retained primary teeth. There are also recurrent infections with cold abscesses, eosinophilia, and extremely elevated levels of IgE. Coarse facies and cranial synostosis have been reported.[132] Job syndrome occurs mainly in females with red hair and fair skin and is a variant of the hyper-IgE syndrome. The inheritance pattern is not well established, with reports of both autosomal dominant and recessive forms. Mucocutaneous candidiasis has been reported in the hyper-IgE syndrome, although its significance remains unclear. Very high levels of IgE, associated with an IgA deficiency and cutaneous hypersensitivity reactions of *S. aureus* and *Candida albicans* are noted. The cause may be related to a defect in granulocyte chemotaxis.[132]

REFERENCES

1. Besnier E. Premiere note et observations preliminaires pour servir dintroduction a letude diathesques. Ann Dermatol Syphiligr 1892; 4:634.
2. Wise F, Sulzberger MB. Editorial remarks. In Year book of dermatology and syphilology. Chicago: Year Book Medical Publishers, 1933: p 59.
3. Hill LW, Sulzberger MR. Evolution of atopic dermatitis. Arch Derm Syphilol 1935;32:451-463.
4. Su JC, Kemp AS, Varigos GA, Nolan TM Atopic eczema: its impact on the family and financial cost. Arch Dis Child 1997; 76:159-162.
5. Lapidus CS, Schwarz DF, Honig P. Atopic dermatitis in children: who cares? Who pays? J Am Acad Dermatol 1993; 28(5):699-703.
6. Walker RB, Warin RP. The incidence of eczema in early childhood. Br J Dermatol 1956;68:182.
7. Kay J, Gawkrodger DJ, Mortimer MJ, Jaron AG. The prevalence of childhood atopic eczema in a general population. J Am Acad Dermatol 1994;30:35-39.
8. Rajka G. Some aetiological data on atopic dermatitis. Presented at Second International Symposium on Atopic Dermatitis. Norway, 1984.
9. Williams HC, Pembroke AC, Forsdyke H, et al. London-born black Caribbean children are at increased risk of atopic dermatitis. J Am Acad Dermatol 1995;32:212-217.
10. Williams HC, Strachan DP, Hay RJ. Childhood eczema: disease of the advantaged? Br Med J 1994;308:1132-1135.
11. Schafer T, Dirschedl P, Kunz B, et al. Maternal smoking during pregnancy and lactation increases the risk for atopic eczema in the offspring. J Am Acad Dermatol 1997;36:550-556.
12. David TJ, Ewing CI. Atopic eczema and preterm birth. Arch Dis Child 1988;63:435-436.
13. Kuster W, Peterson M, Christophers E, et al. A family study of atopic dermatitis: Clinical and genetic characteristics of 188 patients and 2,151 family members. Arch Dermatol Res 1990;282:98-102.
14. Queille-Roussel C, Raynaud F, Saurat J-H. A prospective computerized study of 500 cases of atopic dermatitis in childhood. Acta Dermatol Venereol [Suppl 1] 1985;114: 87-92.
15. Rajka G. Essential aspects of atopic dermatitis. Berlin: Springer-Verlag, 1989; p 21.
16. Fredriksson T, Faergemann J. The atopic thigh: a "starting school" symptom? Acta Derm Venereol 1981;61:452-453.
17. Aoki T, Fukuzumi T, Adachi J, et al. Re-evaluation of skin lesion distribution in atopic dermatitis. Analysis of cases 0 to 9 years of age. Acta Derm Venereol [Suppl] 1992;176:19-23.
18. Uehara M, Hayashi S. Hyperlinear palms. Arch Dermatol 1981;117:490-491.
19. Williams HC, Pembroke AC. Infraorbital crease, ethnic group, and atopic dermatitis. Arch Dermatol 1996;132: 51-54.
20. Seymour JL, Keswick BH, Hanifin JM, et al. Clinical effects of diaper types on the skin of normal infants and infants with atopic dermatitis. J Am Acad Dermatol 1987;17:988-997.
21. Hanifin JM, Lobitz WC. Newer concepts of atopic dermatology. Arch Dermatol 1977;113:663-670.
22. Hanifin JM. Atopic dermatitis in infants and children. Ped Clin North Am 1991;38:763-789.

23. Williams HC, Burney PG, Pembroke AC, Hay RJ. The UK Working Party's diagnostic criteria for atopic dermatitis. III. Independent hospital validation. Br J Dermatol 1994;131:406-416.

24. Nagaraja, Kanwar AJ, Dhar S, Singh S. Frequency and significance of minor clinical features in various age-related subgroups of atopic dermatitis in children. Pediatr Dermatol 1996;13:10-13.

25. Kanwar AJ, Dhar S, Kaur S. Evaluation of minor clinical features of atopic dermatitis. Pediatr Dermatol 1991;8:114-116.

26. Schultz Larsen F. Atopic dermatitis: a genetic-epidemiologic study in a population-based twin sample. J Am Acad Dermatol 1993;28:719-723.

27. Bellou A, Kanny G, Fremont S, et al. Transfer of atopy following bone marrow transplantation. Ann Allergy Asthma Immunol 1997;78:513-516.

28. Cookson WOCM, Sharp PA, Faux JA, Hopkin JM. Linkage between immunoglobulin E responses underlying asthma and rhinitis and chromosome 11q. Lancet 1989;10:1292-1295.

29. Shirakawa T, Hashimoto T, Furuyama J, et al. Linkage between severe atopy and chromosome 11q13 in Japanesse families. Clin Genet 1994;46:228-232.

30. Marsh DG, Meyers DA. A major gene for allergy-fact or fancy? Nat Genet 1992;2:252-254.

31. Coleman R, Trembath RC, Harper JI. Chromosome 11q13 and atopy underlying atopic eczema. Lancet 1993;341:1121-1122.

32. Blumenthal MN. The role of genetic factors in determining atopic conditions. Can J Allergy Clin Immunol 1997;2:69.

33. Juto P, Strannegard O. T lymphocytes and blood eosinophils in early infancy in relation to heredity for allergy and type of feeding. J Allergy Clin Immunol 1979;64:38-42.

34. Butler JM, Chan SC, Stevens S, Hanifin JM. Increased leukocyte histamine release with elevated cyclic AMP-phosphodiesterase activity in atopic dermatitis. J Allergy Clin Immunol 1983;71:490-497.

35. Jujo K, Renz H, Abe J, et al. Decreased interferon gamma and increased interleukin-4 production in atopic dermatitis promotes IgE synthesis. J Allergy Clin Immunol 1992;90:323-331.

36. Ogawa M, Berger PA, McIntyre OR, et al. IgE in atopic dermatitis. Arch Dermatol 1971;103:575-580.

37. Jansen CT, Haapalahti J, Hopsu-Havu VK. Immunoglobulin E in the human atopic skin. Arch Dermatol Forsch 1973;246:209-302.

38. Hanifin JM. Immunobiochemical aspects of atopic dermatitis. Acta Derm Venereol [Suppl] 1989;144:45-47.

39. Giannetti A, Fantini F, Cimitan A, Pincelli C. Vasoactive intestinal polypeptide and substance P in the pathogenesis of atopic dermatitis. Acta Derm Venereol [Suppl] 1992;176:90-92.

40. Cooper KD. Atopic dermatitis: Recent trends in pathogenesis and therapy. Moshell AN, (Ed.) Progress in Dermatology, Evanston, IL 1993;27:1-16.

41. Imokawa G, Abe A, Jin K, et al. Decreased level of ceramides in stratum corneum of atopic dermatitis: an etiologic factor in atopic dry skin? J Invest Dermatol 1991;96:523-526.

42. Schafer L, Kragballe K. Abnormalities in epidermal lipid metabolism in patients with atopic dermatitis. J Invest Dermatol 1991;96:10-15.

43. Watanabe M, Tagami H, Horii I, et al. Functional analyses of the superficial stratum corneum in atopic xerosis. Arch Dermatol 1991;127:1689-1692.

44. Taylor RS, Baadsgaard O, Hammerberg C, et al. Hyperstimulatory CD1a+CD1b+CD36+ Langerhans cells are responsible for increased autologous T lymphocyte reactivity to lesional epidermal cells of patients with atopic dermatitis. J Immunol 1991;147:3794-3802.

45. Sigurs N, Hattevig G, Kjellman B. Maternal avoidance of eggs, cow's milk, and fish during lactation: effect on allergic manifestations, skin-prick tests, and specific IgE antibodies in children at age 4 years. Pediatr 1992;89:735-739.

46. Fergusson DM, Horwood LJ. Early solid food diet and eczema in childhood: a 10-year longitudinal study. Pediatr Allergy Immunol 1994;5 (Suppl):44-47.

47. Sampson HA, Metcalfe DD. Food allergies. JAMA 1992;268:2840-2844.

48. Clark RA, Adinoff AD. The relationship between positive aeroallergen patch test reactions and aeroallergen exacerbations of atopic dermatitis. Clin Immunol Immunopathol 1989;53:S132-140.

49. Hanifin JM. Critical evaluation of food and mite allergy in the management of atopic dermatitis. J Dermatol 1997;24:495-503.

50. Kramer MS, Moroz B. Do breast-feeding and delayed introduction of solid foods protect against subsequent atopic eczema? J Pediatr 1981;98:546-550.

51. Midwinter RE, Morris AF, Colley JR. Infant feeding and atopy. Arch Dis Child 1987;62:965-967.

52. Dhar S, Kanwar AJ, Kaur S, et al. Role of bacterial flora in the pathogenesis & management of atopic dermatitis. Indian J Med Res 1992;95:234-238.

53. Leung DY, Harbeck R, Bina P, et al. Presence of IgE antibodies to staphylococcal exotoxins on the skin of patients with atopic dermatitis. J Clin Invest 1993;92:1374-1380.

54. Uno H, Hanifin JM. Ultrastructural and L-DOPA histofluorescent observations of Langerhans cells in atopic dermatitis. Clin Res 1979;27:538A.

55. Montgomery H. Dermatopathology. vol. 1. New York: Harper & Row, 1967;pp 186-190.

56. Soter NA, Mihm MC Jr. Morphology of atopic eczema. Acta Dermatol Venereol [Suppl] 1980;92:11.

57. Tobin D, Nabarro G, Baart de la Faille H, et al. Increased number of immunoreactive nerve fibers in atopic dermatitis. J Allergy Clin Immunol 1992;90:613-622.

58. Mihm MC, Soter NA, Dvorak HF, Austen KF. The structure of normal skin and the morphology of atopic eczema. J Invest Dermatol 1976;67:305-312.

59. Sampson HA, Albergo R. Comparison of results of skin tests, RAST and double-blind, placebo-controlled food challenges in children with atopic dermatitis. J Allergy Clin Immunol 1984;74:26-33.

60. Lammintausta K, Kalimo K, Raitala R, Forsten Y. Prognosis of atopic dermatitis. A prospective study in early adulthood. Int J Dermatol 1991;30:563-568.

61. Vickers CFH. The natural history of atopic eczema. Presented at International Symposium on Atopic Dermatitis 1979. Acta Dermatol Venerol [Suppl] 1980;92:113.

62. Sampson HA. Atopic dermatitis. Ann Allergy 1992;69:469-479.

63. Herd RM, Tidman MJ, Prescott RJ, Hunter JA. Prevalence of atopic eczema in the community: the Lothian atopic dermatitis study. Br J Dermatol 1996;135:18-19.

64. Fergusson DM, Horwood LJ, Shannon FT. Parental asthma, parental eczema and asthma and eczema in early childhood. J Chronic Dis 1983;36:517-524.

65. Lubs ML. Empiric risks for genetic counseling in families with allergy. J Pediatr 1972;80:26-31.

66. Broberg A, Kalimo K, Lindblad B, Swanbeck G. Parental education in the treatment of childhood atopic eczema. Acta Derm Venereol 1990;70:495-499.

67. Roth HL, Kierland RR. The natural history of atopic dermatitis, a 20-year follow-up study. Arch Dermatol 1961; 89:209.

68. Wahlgren CF, Hagermark O, Bergstrom R. The antipruritic effect of a sedative and a non-sedative antihistamine in atopic dermatitis. Br J Dermatol 1990;122:545-551.

69. Berth-Jones J, Graham-Brown RA. Failure of terfenadine in relieving the pruritus of atopic dermatitis. Br J Dermatol 1989;121:635-637.

70. Simons FER, Simons KJ, Becker AB, Haydey RP. Pharmacokinetics and antipruritic effects of hydroxyzine in children with atopic dermatitis. J Pediatr 1984;104:123-127.

71. Lucky AW, Leach AD, Laskarzewski P, Wenck H. Use of an emollient as a steroid-sparing agent in the treatment of mild to moderate atopic dermatitis in children. Pediatr Dermatol 1997;14:321-324.

72. Sulzberger MB, Witten VH. The effect of topically applied compound F in selected dermatoses. J Invest Dermatol 1952;101-102.

73. Yamamoto K. How doctor's advice is followed by mothers of atopic children. Acta Derm Venereol [Suppl] 1989; 144:31-33.

74. Akers WA. Risks of unoccluded topical steroids in clinical trials. Arch Dermatol 1980;116:786-788.

75. Feiwel M, Kelly WF. Adrenal unresponsiveness associated with clobetasol propionate. Lancet 1974; 27(872):112-113.

76. Nilsson EJ, Henning CG, Magnusson J. Topical corticosteroids and Staphylococcus aureus in atopic dermatitis. J Am Acad Dermatol 1992;27:29-34.

77. Lever R, Hadley K, Downey D, Mackie R. Staphylococcal colonization in atopic dermatitis and the effect of topical mupirocin therapy. Br J Dermatol 1988:119:189-198.

78. Dahl MV. Staphylococcus aureus and atopic dermatitis. Arch Dermatol 1983;119:840-846.

79. Alaiti S, Kang S, Fiedler V, et al. Tacrolimus (FK506) ointment for atopic dermatitis: a phase I study in adults and children. J Am Acad Dermatol 1998;38:69-76.

80. Unna PG. Seborrhoeae eczema. J Cutan Dis 1887;5:499.

81. Erlichman M, Goldstein R, Levi E, et al. Infantile flexural seborrhoeic dermatitis. Neither biotin nor essential fatty acid deficiency. Arch Dis Child 1981;56:560-562.

82. Ruiz-Maldonado R, Lopez-Matinez R, Perez Chavariea EL, et al. Pityrosporum ovale in infantile seborrheic dermatitis. Pediatr Dermatol 1989;6:16-20.

83. Broberg A, Faergemann J. Infantile seborrhoeic dermatitis and Pityrosporum ovale. Br J Dermatol 1989;120:359-362.

84. Tollesson A, Frithz A, Berg A, et al. Essential fatty acids in infantile seborrheic dermatitis. J Am Acad Dermatol 1993; 28:957-961.

85. Tollesson A, Frithz A, Stenlund K. Malassezia furfur in infantile seborrheic dermatitis. Pediatr Dermatol 1997;14: 423-425.

86. Yates VM, Kerr RE, Mackie RM. Early diagnosis of infantile seborrhoeic dermatitis and atopic dermatitis—clinical features. Br J Dermatol 1983;108:633-638.

87. Podmore O, Burrows D, Eedy DJ, Stanford CF. Seborrheic eczema—a disease entity or a clinical variant of atopic eczema? Br J Dermatol 1986;115:341-350.

88. Neville EA, Finn OA. Psoriasiform napkin dermatitis a follow-up study. Br J Dermatol 1975;92:279-285.

89. Nall L. Epidemiologic strategies in psoriasis research. Int J Dermatol 1994;33:313-319.

90. Elder JT, Nair RP, Guo SW, et al. The genetics of psoriasis. Arch Dermatol 1994;130:216-224.

91. Farber EM, Nall L. Epidemiology: Natural history and genetics. In Roenigk HH Jr, Maibach HI, eds. Psoriasis. 3rd edition. New York: Dekker, 1998.

92. Ivker RA, Grin-Jorgensen CM, Vega VK, et al. Infantile generalized pustular psoriasis associated with lytic lesions of the bone. Pediatr Dermatol 1993;10:277-282.

93. Farber EM. Juvenile psoriasis. Early interventions can reduce risks for problems later. Postgrad Med 1998;103:89-100.

94. Juanqin G, Zhiqiang C, Zijia H. Evaluation of the effectiveness of childhood generalized pustular psoriasis treatment in 30 cases. Pediatr Dermatol 1998;15:144-146.

95. Farber EM, Mullen RH, Jacobs AH, Nall L. Infantile psoriasis: a follow-up study. Pediatr Dermatol 1986;3:237-243.

96. Koblenzer PJ. Diaper dermatitis—an overview with emphasis on rational therapy based on etiology and pathodynamics. Clin Pediatr 1973;12:386-392.

97. Wong DL, Brantly D, Clutter LB, et al. Diapering choices: a critical review of the issues. Pediatr Nurs 1992;18:41-54.

98. Levin S. Diapers. S Afr Med J 1970;44:256-263.

99. Odio MR, O'Connor RJ, Sarbaugh F, Baldwin S. Continuous topical administration of a petrolatum formulation by a novel disposable diaper? Effect on skin condition. Dermatology 2000;200:238-243.

100. Jacquet L. Traitae des maladies de l'enfance. In Grancher J, Comby J, Marfan AB, eds. Paris: Masson & Co, 1905: p 714.

101. Verbov JL. Skin problems in children. Practitioner 1976; 217:403-415.

102. Wilson PA, Dallas MJ. Diaper performance: maintenance of healthy skin. Pediatr Dermatol 1990;7:179-184.

103. Campbell RL, Bartlett AV, Sarbaugh FC, Pickering LK. Effects of diaper types on diaper dermatitis associated with diarrhea and antibiotic use in children in day-care centers. Pediatr Dermatol 1988;5:83-87.

104. Seymour JL, Keswick BH, Milligan MC, et al. Clinical and microbial effects of cloth, cellulose core, and cellulose core/absorbent gel diapers in atopic dermatitis. Pediatrician 1987;14(supp 1):39-43.

105. Boisits EK, McCormack JJ. Diaper dermatitis and the role of predisposition. In Maibach HI, Boisits EK, eds. Neonatal skin: Structure and function. New York: Dekker, 1982: p 191-204.

106. Berg RW, Milligan MC, Sarbaugh FC. Association of skin wetness and pH with diaper dermatitis. Pediatr Dermatol 1994;11:18-20.

107. Leyden JJ, Katz S, Stewart R, Kligman AM. Urinary ammonia and ammonia-producing microorganisms in infants with and without diaper dermatitis. Arch Dermatol 1977;113: 1678-1680.

108. Jordan WE, Blaney TL. Factors influencing infant diaper dermatitis. In Maibach HI, Boisits EK, eds. Neonatal skin: Structure and function. New York: Dekker, 1982: p 205-221.

109. Bound JP. Thrush napkin rashes. Br Med J 1956;1:782.

110. Beare JM, Cheeseman EA, Mackenzie DW. The association between *Candida albicans* and lesions of seborrhoeic eczema. Br J Dermatol 1968;80:675-681.

111. Hoppe JE. Treatment of oropharyngeal candidiasis and candidal diaper dermatitis in neonates and infants: review and reappraisal. Pediatr Infect Dis J 1997;16:885-894.

112. Munz D, Powell KR, Pai CH. Treatment of candidal diaper dermatitis: a double-blind placebo-controlled comparison of topical nystatin with topical plus oral nystatin. J Pediatr 1982;101(6):1022-1025.

113. Mozzanica N. Pathogenetic aspects of allergic and irritant contact dermatitis. Clin Dermatol 1992;10:115-121.

114. Stevens J, Lubitz L. Symptomatic zinc deficiency in breast-fed term and premature infants. J Paediatr Child Health 1998;34:97-100.

115. Prasad AS. Zinc: an overview. Nutrition 1995;11:93-99.

116. Lonnerdal B, Stanislowski AG, Hurley LS. Isolation of a low molecular weight zinc binding ligand from human milk. J Inorg Biochem 1980;12:71-78.

117. Zimmerman AW, Hambidge KM, Lepow ML, et al. Acrodermatitis in breast-fed premature infants: Evidence for a defect of mammary zinc secretion. Pediatrics 1982;69:176-183.

118. Van Wouwe JP. Clinical and laboratory diagnosis of acrodermatitis enteropathica. Eur J Pediatr 1989;149:2-8.

119. Goskowicz M, Eichenfield LF. Cutaneous findings of nutritional deficiencies in children. Curr Opin Pediatr 1993; 5:441-445.

120. Walsh CT, Sandstead HH, Prasad AS, et al. Zinc: health effects and research priorities for the 1990s. Environ Health Perspect 1994;102 [Suppl 2]:5-46.

121. Wolf B, Heard GS. Screening for biotinidase deficiency in newborns: worldwide experience. Pediatrics 1990;85:512-517.

122. Nyhan WL. Inborn errors of biotin metabolism. Arch Dermatol 1987;123:1696-1698a.

123. Zempleni J, Mock DM. Bioavailability of biotin given orally to humans in pharmacologic doses. Am J Clin Nutr 1999; 69:504-508.

124. Darmstadt GL, Schmidt CP, Wechsler DS, et al. Dermatitis as a presenting sign of cystic fibrosis. Arch Dermatol 1992; 128:1358-1364.

125. Schmidt CP, Tunnessen W. Cystic fibrosis presenting with periorificial dermatitis. J Am Acad Dermatol 1991;25:896-897.

126. Wilcken B, Yu JS, Brown DA. Natural history of Hartnup disease. Arch Dis Child 1977;52:38-40.

127. Omenn GS. Familial reticuloendotheliosis with eosinophilia. New Eng J Med 1965;273:427.

128. Gomez L, Le Deist F, Blanche S, et al. Treatment of Omenn syndrome by bone marrow transplantation. J Pediatr 1995; 127:76-81.

129. Lee EB. Metabolic diseases and the skin. Pediatr Clin North Am 1983;30:597-608.

130. Remold-O'Donnell E, Kenney DM, Parkman R, et al. Characterization of a human lymphocyte surface sialoglycoprotein that is defective in Wiskott-Aldrich syndrome. J Exp Med 1984;159:1705-1723.

131. Ochs HD. The Wiskott-Aldrich syndrome. Semin Hematol 1998;35:332-345.

132. Grimbacher B, Holland SM, Gallin JI, et al. Hyper-IgE syndrome with recurrent infections—an autosomal dominant multisystem disorder. N Engl J Med 1999;340:692-702.

15

Erythrodermas: The Red Scaly Baby

MOISE L. LEVY
MARY K. SPRAKER

The term *erythroderma* is used in dermatology to describe a skin eruption characterized by diffuse erythema, usually in association with scaling. Infantile erythroderma is caused by or associated with a large number of disorders (Box 15-1). The differential diagnosis includes inflammatory, infectious, inherited, and immunologic diseases (many of which have a hereditary basis). Some of these diseases are potentially life threatening, and erythroderma itself can cause serious medical complications, such as electrolyte imbalance, sepsis, and temperature instability resulting from heat loss. Therefore it is important that the physician accurately diagnose and treat the problem. This chapter focuses on the differential diagnosis of these disorders with an emphasis on the metabolic diseases associated with erythroderma.

INFLAMMATORY DISEASES

Atopic Dermatitis

Severe generalized atopic dermatitis is unusual in neonates, but because atopic dermatitis is such a common problem, it is the most common cause of acquired or noncongenital erythroderma in infants (see Chapter 14). Classic infantile atopic dermatitis involves the scalp, cheeks, and extensor surfaces of the extremities and does not appear until the infant is 2 to 3 months of age.[1] When the distribution is generalized and the onset is early, diagnosis can be more difficult.

The presence of pruritus, an almost invariable feature of this condition, is not always apparent in neonates and young infants.[2] Typically, the diaper region is spared even in cases of widespread atopic dermatitis, as a result of the moist, occlusive environment of diapered skin. In contrast to infants with severe metabolic or immunologic disease, infants with atopic dermatitis usually grow normally and thrive, assuming the disease is recognized and treated promptly. There is often a family history of atopy. Atopic dermatitis generally responds rapidly to appropriate therapy with topical corticosteroids and emollients. Skin biopsy in atopic dermatitis demonstrates acanthosis (thickening of the epidermis) and varying degrees of spongiosis (epidermal edema), as well as lymphohistiocytic inflammatory infiltrates, often with scattered eosinophils and plasma cells.

Seborrheic Dermatitis

Seborrheic dermatitis is a common problem during the neonatal period and is generally easily recognized (see also Chapter 14). Typically there is scaling and erythema involving seborrheic areas such as the scalp and body folds.[3] The yellow, greasy, scalp scale may encompass the entire forehead, including the eyebrows, and there are erythema and maceration involving body folds such as the retroauricular areas, neck, axillae, and groin. When the disease is mild, only the scalp is affected and body fold involvement is either focal or absent entirely. Occasionally, however, a more diffuse pattern of seborrheic dermatitis can occur, which must be distinguished from atopic dermatitis, neonatal candidiasis, and other causes of infantile erythroderma (Fig. 15-1) (see Box 15-1).

The distribution of the dermatitis is more helpful than any other criterion in differentiating between atopic and seborrheic dermatitis,[2] but it can be difficult and sometimes impossible to accurately differentiate the two conditions early in their course. Although the scalp can be red

---

Erythrodermas: Red Scaly Baby— Differential Diagnosis

Inflammatory Diseases
Atopic dermatitis
Seborrheic dermatitis
Psoriasis
Boric acid poisoning
Diffuse mastocytosis

Infectious Diseases
Staphylococcal scalded skin syndrome
Candida/other fungal infections
Herpes simplex virus
Syphilis

Inherited Diseases
Ichthyosis
Netherton's syndrome
Nonbullous ichthyosiform erythroderma
Bullous ichthyosis (epidermolytic hyperkeratosis)
Sjögren-Larsson syndrome
Chondrodysplasia punctata
Ectodermal dysplasia
Cobalamin deficiency
Maple syrup urine disease
Carbamoyl phosphate synthetase deficiency
Argininosuccinicaciduria
Methylmalonic aciduria
Propionic acidemia
Cystic fibrosis
Essential fatty acid deficiency
Biotinidase deficiency

Immunologic Diseases
Leiner's phenotype
Omenn's syndrome
Graft versus host disease
Severe combined immunodeficiency
Bruton's hypogammaglobulinemia
Common variable hypogammaglobulinemia
Eosinophilic gastroenteritis

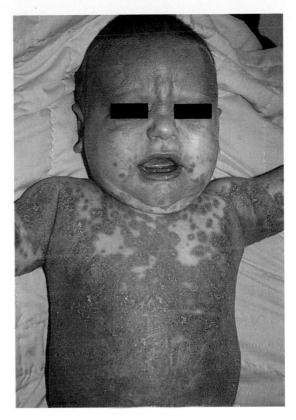

FIG. 15-1
Seborrheic dermatitis: widespread erythema and scale.

ease differs: seborrheic dermatitis usually resolves in several months, whereas atopic dermatitis often persists for several years. Skin biopsy findings in seborrheic dermatitis are similar to those in atopic dermatitis. There is mild acanthosis, spongiosis, and a mild lymphohistiocytic inflammatory infiltrate; parakeratotic scale may be present.

If clinical features suggest widespread seborrheic dermatitis in an infant who is otherwise well and thriving, and the skin readily clears after the application of low- to mid-potency topical corticosteroids without chronic rebound when therapy is tapered, the diagnosis of seborrheic dermatitis is probably accurate. Otherwise, alternative diagnoses should be considered.

Psoriasis

Less than 1% of all cases of psoriasis are said to occur in infants under 1 year of age.[3] Infantile psoriasis can be a difficult disorder to diagnose because of its clinical similarity to both seborrheic dermatitis and atopic dermatitis.

and scaly in both conditions, seborrheic dermatitis tends to involve the groin and other body folds, which are generally spared in atopic dermatitis because they are better hydrated. Since treatment of both conditions in infancy is similar, from a practical standpoint, accurate differentiation can be an academic exercise. But the course of this dis-

Infantile psoriasis can look like that seen in older individuals with discrete oval erythematous plaques with white scale involving the trunk, extremities, and face. Psoriatic plaques of infants usually have less white scale than the typical hyperkeratotic plaque seen in the adult. Facial involvement may be more common in the infant, and the scalp, palms, and soles may have diffuse erythema and scale. A periumbilical distribution may be helpful in distinguishing psoriasis from either seborrheic or atopic dermatitis. Pustular psoriasis, either in a diffuse distribution or limited to the palms and soles, may be seen rarely. In contrast to atopic dermatitis, psoriasis in young infants often involves the diaper area because it develops in areas of injured skin (the Koebner phenomenon), e.g., after a prior irritant or candida diaper dermatitis.[4]

Rarely, infantile psoriasis is generalized, a presentation that has been reported in young infants and can even be present at birth.[5] Erythroderma can evolve into and even alternate with pustulosis. Infantile generalized pustular psoriasis can be associated with lytic bone lesions,[6] and be complicated by the acute respiratory distress syndrome (pulmonary capillary leak syndrome) that can also be seen in adults with acute generalized pustular psoriasis.[7]

Skin biopsy can be helpful in diagnosis and in some cases is diagnostic. Biopsy usually shows psoriasiform hyperplasia with elongated rete ridges and parakeratotic scale often containing neutrophils. Occasionally, the diagnostic finding of a spongiform micropustule or microabscess in the upper epidermis is seen. Skin biopsies of erythrodermic psoriasis are often indistinguishable from that of a chronic dermatitis, and it may take several biopsies and close observation over time to confirm the diagnosis.

Localized psoriasis may be treated with emollients and low potency topical corticosteroids, but often clears only partially or recurs. Cases of infantile psoriasis may prove to be mild and occasionally even clear completely as the child gets older.[8] The prognosis of generalized erythrodermic or pustular psoriasis in infancy is more guarded, and treatment usually requires systemic retinoid therapy, as well as supportive care.

Boric Acid Poisoning

Boric acid poisoning is now very rare, but was seen in the past as a result of the frequent use of boric acid containing powders and lotions for the treatment of diaper dermatitis. It presents with a maculopapular eruption that can evolve into a generalized erythroderma, the appearance of which has been likened to a boiled lobster. A positive Nikolsky sign and desquamation are additional features.[9] Like staphylococcal scalded skin syndrome, accentuation in periorificial and intertriginous areas may be present. Alopecia may also develop. Affected infants are usually ill with fever, irritability, vomiting, and diarrhea, which can progress to shock and even death.

Diffuse Mastocytosis

The various forms of cutaneous mastocytosis are fully discussed in Chapter 23. Only the rare diffuse form of the disease is associated with neonatal erythroderma.[10] The affected infant usually has generalized thickening of the skin, which can be subtle. The thickening is due to infiltration of the dermis by mast cells. Because these mast cells release histamine and other vasoactive substances, they cause the skin to be very reactive, with a tendency to develop erythema, flushing, and wheals. Urtication with minor trauma (the Darier sign), and blisters, which develop either spontaneously or superimposed upon wheals, may be seen. The absence of scale and the presence of the above findings differentiate mastocytosis from other causes of erythroderma.

Skin biopsy is diagnostic—there is a dense, bandlike infiltrate of mast cells in the upper dermis, which can be confirmed with Giemsa stain.

INFECTIOUS DISEASES

Staphylococcal Scalded Skin Syndrome

Staphylococcal scalded skin syndrome (SSSS) is an uncommon cause of neonatal erythroderma (see Chapter 11). It is characterized by the abrupt onset of diffuse erythema, which rapidly evolves to erosive desquamation involving most skin surfaces. Although there is often periorificial accentuation, the staphylococcal toxin requires keratinizing epithelium and therefore spares mucous membrane surfaces. Epidermal sloughing, occurring with minor trauma, helps distinguish SSSS from the other causes of infantile erythroderma, with the exception of toxic epidermal necrolysis (TEN)[11] (see Chapter 10) and boric acid poisoning (see the previous discussion). Rarely, a widespread form of staphylococcal pustulosis can occur acutely in an otherwise healthy infant.[12,13] The pustules develop on an erythematous macular base and are small and superficial. They subsequently desquamate, thereby mimicking a true erythroderma.

Candidiasis

Candidal infection can cause neonatal erythroderma in two clinical settings: intrauterine acquisition with the development of congenital candidiasis and postnatal onset in very premature infants. **Congenital candidiasis** typically presents either at birth or within the first few days of life with generalized erythema, vesicles, pustules, papules, and scaling. The pustules can be subtle at first, with erythroderma predominating. The palms and soles are often involved, which may be a helpful clue to diagnosis. The condition can occur in either term or preterm infants. *Candida albicans* can also cause a diffuse burn-like erythema within the first 2 weeks of life in premature infants[14]; we have seen a number of cases in which the diffuse scaling and erythema were most pronounced over the back.[15] The diagnosis is made by examination of skin scrapings (KOH preparation) and/or surface culture for *Candida,* or by skin biopsy. The latter will show fungal elements within the epidermis and/or dermis, mixed inflammatory infiltrates, and occasional areas of necrosis and hemorrhage.

The risk of extracutanous disease and the prognosis depends on the gestational age of the infant. In term infants, the prognosis is excellent, and topical antiyeast therapies are usually curative. In infants less than 1500 g with either congenital or acquired generalized cutaneous candidiasis, there is a significant risk of disseminated disease, and parenteral antifungal agents are recommended. Skin biopsies of affected areas in such infants may be used to predict ultimate dissemination of disease. In one series, the finding of subcorneal invasion of *Candida* on skin biopsy was associated with a 69% risk for disseminated disease.[15] Both conditions are discussed in more detail in Chapter 13.

Herpes Simplex

Although most cases of herpes simplex virus have characteristic lesions localized on the presenting part, the so-called intrauterine variant of HSV can present at birth with either isolated or diffuse erythema, and scaling or crusted erosions on an erythematous base (see Chapter 12). It may be difficult to recognize clinically because vesicles may not be present.[16,17] This type of widespread involvement is generally associated with very severe neurologic disease. Multinucleated giant cells should be demonstrable on Tzanck smears of vesicular lesions. A skin biopsy, scrapings for direct fluorescent antibody staining, and viral cultures will help confirm the diagnosis.

Syphilis

Congenital syphilis may cause diffuse erythema and scaling (see Chapter 11). This presentation is most typically seen in infants at 6 to 8 weeks of age, in whom exposure to syphilis occurred either very late in pregnancy or at the time of delivery.[18] Superficial erosions or bullae over the

hands or feet of a newborn, together with a diffuse scaling dermatitis (Fig. 15-2), should alert the practitioner to the possibility of syphilis. Infiltrated mucosal papules and plaques (condyloma lata) may be seen in a perianal location and are similar to the mucous patches seen on other mucous membrane sites in older patients with secondary syphilis. Periosteal changes of long bones, such as the clavicles, as well as hepatosplenomegaly are additional features. Appropriate serologies are generally diagnostic and dark field examination of mucous membranes lesions should reveal spirochetes.

INHERITED DISEASES

Ichthyosis

The ichthyoses are a group of genetic disorders characterized by generalized skin scaling; generalized erythroderma is a common presentation for some types of ichthyosis (see Chapter 16). Many infants with this presentation have the **congenital ichthyosiform erythroderma** (CIE) phenotype,[19] which is notable for the diffuse erythematous appearance of the skin and overlying fine white scale (Fig. 15-3). Ectropion can occur but is less common, and when present is less severe than in patients with classic **lamellar ichthyosis.** In these patients, there is less erythema and thicker, darker, more platelike scale. Infants with autosomal dominant **bullous ichthyosis** (bullous CIE; epidermolytic hyperkeratosis) typically present with diffusely erythematous skin and mild hyperkeratosis, often in association with areas of denuded skin. The lack of mucous membrane involvement in bullous CIE helps distinguish it from epidermolysis bullosa. Over subsequent weeks and months, the blistering subsides and is replaced by varying degrees of an ichthyosiform erythroderma. Ultimately, marked hyperkeratosis is evident diffusely, with accentuation on flexural surfaces. The characteristic histopathologic findings of epidermal cytolysis of the upper spinous and granular layers helps confirm the diagnosis of bullous ichthyosis.

The ichthyosis most likely to be confused with other causes of erythroderma is **Netherton's syndrome,** a rare disorder of unknown etiology, marked by severe diffuse erythroderma, scaling, and varying degrees of alopecia, including sparse eyebrows (Fig. 15-4).[20,21] Affected infants often fail to thrive as a result of the extreme metabolic demands presented by their skin disease, and they can also develop hypernatremic dehydration. Most have a markedly elevated IgE level. The diagnosis of Netherton's syndrome is often delayed because of the late presentation of the diagnostic hair shaft abnormality, trichorrhexis invaginata (bamboo hair).

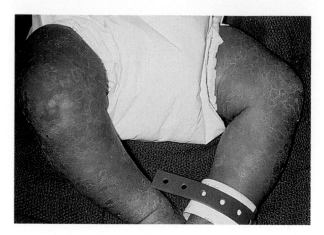

FIG. 15-2
Diffuse superficial scaling and mild erythema involving the skin of an infant with congenital syphilis.

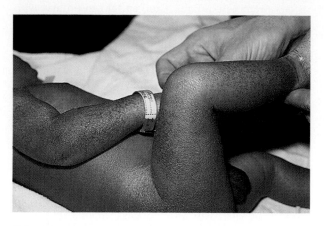

FIG. 15-3
Diffuse erythema with fine scale in an infant with nonbullous congenital ichthyosiform erythroderma.

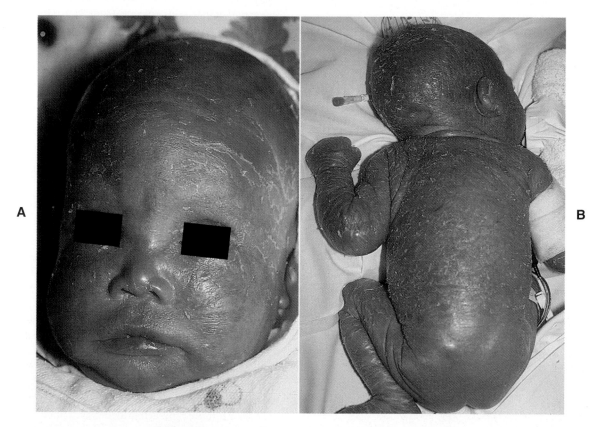

A

B

FIG. 15-4
Netherton's syndrome: diffuse erythema, scale, and alopecia.

Such hairs, when examined by routine light microscopy, will appear to have telescoped into themselves along the length of the shaft of the hair. Small bulbous areas of thickening at the site of the telescoping correspond to the areas of increased fragility and ultimate breakage of affected hairs. Plucking eyebrow hairs and evaluation of multiple areas of the scalp over time may be required to visualize the characteristic hair changes. Later in the course, patients may show a distinctive skin finding, ichthyosis linearis circumflexa. This is an erythematous scaling eruption with polycyclic and/or serpiginous morphology and elevated borders.

Sjögren-Larsson syndrome is due to a deficiency of fatty acid aldehyde dehydrogenase and can present with varying degrees of erythroderma.[22] A collodion membrane at birth is unusual. Affected infants may have a phenotype consistent with either CIE or lamellar ichthyosis. Nonprogressive spasticity and mental retardation become apparent during the early years of life. After the first year of life many, but not all, affected patients have distinctive glistening dots seen on careful retinal examination.

Chondrodysplasia punctata (Conradi-Hünermann syndrome) presents with either diffuse erythroderma or bands of erythema, and a patterned ichthyosis occurring along Blaschko's lines (Fig. 15-5).[23,24] These areas of ichthyosis typically resolve and may be replaced by a follicular atrophoderma. This syndrome is also marked by skeletal defects (dwarfism), cataracts, and other features. Plain radiographs at the time of birth may show stippling of the epiphyseal areas of bones. Some cases have been found to be caused by a peroxisosomal deficiency.

Infantile erythroderma can also be seen in keratosis-ichthyosis-deafness (KID) syndrome,[25,26] neutral lipid storage disease with ichthyosis (Chanarin-Dorfman syndrome),[27] and in newborns with trichothiodystrophy (Tay syndrome).[28]

Occasionally, males affected with **X-linked hypohidrotic ectodermal dysplasia** may present at birth with a mild diffuse erythroderma and fine superficial scaling (Fig. 15-6).[29] Such infants have the typical facial features of ED and sparse hair, lashes, and eyebrows. Periorbital hyperpigmentation and fine wrinkling can be seen at birth, and lateral plain films of the skull will demonstrate no or few

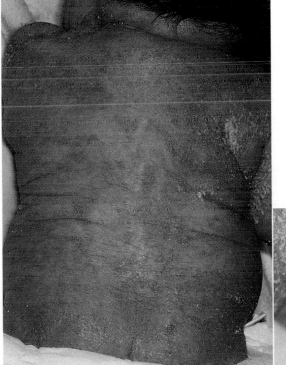
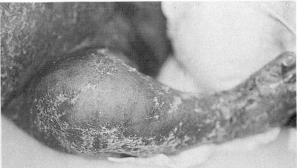

A B

FIG. 15-5
A, Diffuse cutaneous erythema with patterned hyperkeratosis over the back of a female with Conradi's syndrome. B, The same infant showing more pronounced hyperkeratosis over the right lower extremity.

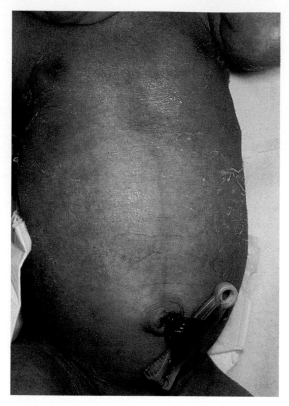

FIG. 15-6
Mild diffuse cutaneous erythema and very superficial scaling on a child with X-linked hypohidrotic ectodermal dysplasia. These findings were present at birth.

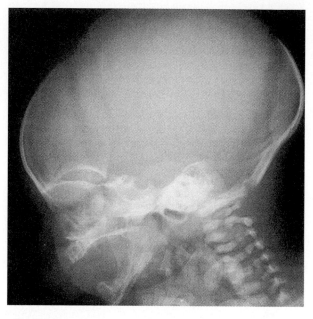

FIG. 15-7
A lateral skull film from the same male neonate in Fig. 15-6, showing the absence of tooth buds.

tooth buds (Fig. 15-7). One of us (MKS) has seen a family with the ectrodactyly–ectodermal dysplasia–cleft lip/palate syndrome in whom affected persons were erythrodermic and scaly during infancy only.

METABOLIC DISEASES

Rarely, metabolic diseases are associated with erythroderma, either shortly after birth, or later resulting from subsequent therapeutic dietary restrictions. Methylmalonic acidemia (MMA) is an inborn error of metabolism inherited in an autosomal recessive manner.[30,31] It is a group of diseases caused by a defect in the metabolism of branched-chain amino acids, which results in the accumulation of methylmalonic acid. Although some cases of methylmalonic acidemia, especially those caused by a cobalamin F and cobalamin C type of defect, have presented with a dermatitis similar to that seen in acrodermatitis enteropathica,[30,31] more commonly the dermatitis

begins after the institution of dietary restrictions.[32] In either case, the appearance is similar and in a primarily periorificial location. There are erythema and ulceration in the corners of the mouth and genital areas. A more diffuse dermatitis resembling SSSS has also been described. Extracutaneous manifestations can include poor feeding, vomiting, hypotonia, and acidosis often leading to coma and death.

Assays for serum amino acid and metabolic analysis of cultured skin fibroblasts from affected patients confirm the diagnosis. Urinary organic acids should also be examined for elevations of methyl malonate and homocystine. Skin biopsy shows vacuolar dermatitis with dyskeratotic keratinocytes, mild psoriasiform changes, and epidermal pallor as seen in acrodermatitis enteropathica. There is a lymphocytic perivascular infiltrate within the dermis, as well as areas of orthokeratosis and parakeratosis with spongiosis of the epidermis. The differential diagnosis of this disease includes other metabolic and nutritional defi-

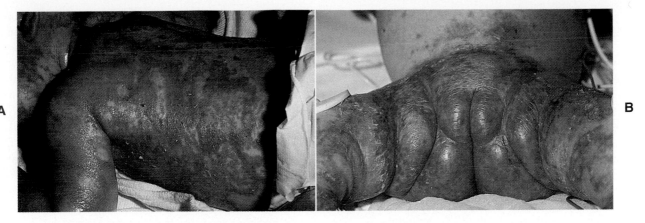

FIG. 15-8
A, Diffuse erythroderma and scaling on an infant later diagnosed with cystic fibrosis. B, A different infant with periorificial erythema and scale. This child was later diagnosed with cystic fibrosis.

ciency states such as acrodermatitis enteropathica, other aminoacidurias, and biotinidase deficiency. Management of this disorder consists of dietary restrictions of branched-chain amino acids, specifically isoleucine and valine, and in those cases marked by cobalamin deficiency, supplementation with cobalamin. The prognosis of MMA is guarded, with many patients remaining severely impaired neurologically in spite of aggressive dietary support.

In **maple syrup urine disease** (MSUD),[33-37] diffuse exfoliative erythroderma has been well described. MSUD is another inborn error of metabolism in which the metabolism of branched-chain amino acids is defective. There is an abnormality in the degradation of the branched-chain amino acids causing diagnostic elevations of isoleucine, leucine, and valine in the serum, as well as in urine and cultured tissue fibroblasts. An erythematous scaling eruption that becomes erosive begins in a primarily periorificial distribution within days after initiating dietary therapy. The eruption is similar to that seen in acrodermatitis enteropathica. It can generalize, however. Such infants may also present with poor feeding, vomiting, lethargy, and seizures. Death may occur if this disorder is not promptly recognized. The problem may be caused by low isoleucine levels from the dietary restrictions required for the disease. A similar, albeit milder dermatitis has been induced in infants fed diets deficient in isoleucine,[38] and similar eruptions have also been noted in citrullinemia,[39] carbamoyl phosphate synthetase deficiency,[40] and argininosuccinicaciduria.[40] The cause of the dermatitis in each of these cases is also presumed to be caused by an abnormality of branched-chain amino acids, such as isoleucine. Histopathology of skin

biopsies may show a very superficial perivascular lymphohistiocytic infiltrate with erosion of the outer epidermis, again as may be seen in skin biopsies of patients with other inborn errors in metabolism. The differential diagnosis includes other inborn errors of metabolism in which periorificial dermatitis may occur after initiation of dietary therapy, such as propionic acidemia and methylmalonic acidemia.[41] Treatment requires diligent attention to dietary restrictions. The diet must be liberalized so that sufficient branched-chain amino acids are delivered to raise plasma concentrations above the subnormal range.

Infants with **cystic fibrosis** (CF) can develop widespread, scaly erythematous lesions as a manifestation of global malnutrition during the first 3 or 4 months of life, and they are occasionally the initial presentation of CF.[42,43,44] The dermatitis is variable. A diffuse erythematous papular dermatitis, diffuse desquamating erythema or erythroderma, or a distinctly periorificial erythema and scaling may be seen (Fig. 15-8). However, in the author's experience, most infants present with impressive generalized desquamative erythroderma. The dermatitis does not respond to treatment with topical corticosteroids or antifungals. In contrast to infants affected with classic acrodermatitis enteropathica, infants with cystic fibrosis typically lack paronychial involvement. Affected infants often have mild depressions of zinc levels, increased liver transaminases, and normal or slightly depressed levels of alkaline phosphatase. The dermatitis of CF occasionally clears with zinc therapy, but does so more reliably with appropriate enzyme replacement and nutritional supplements.

Essential fatty acid (EFA) deficiency was seen more frequently before 1975, in patients on parenteral hyperalimentation, before the need for EFA supplementation was recognized.[45] It is now an extremely unusual condition. It presents with a diffuse fine desquamation and mild or even absent erythema. The condition sometimes occurs in patients with severe fat malabsorption and may be one of the causes of the dermatitis of cystic fibrosis.

IMMUNOLOGIC DISEASES

Leiner's Phenotype

A chapter on infantile erythroderma would not be complete without a discussion of Leiner's disease, or what we prefer to call Leiner's phenotype. Leiner's disease or syndrome was initially described in 1908 by a pediatrician, Dr. Carl Leiner.[46,47] He reported a distinctive dermatitis he had seen in 43 children at a children's hospital in Vienna over 5 years. These infants developed a generalized erythematous desquamative dermatitis that appeared during the first few weeks of life but was not present at birth. Most had diarrhea and weight loss, and the disease did not respond to any known topical or oral medication. Many improved when their diet was changed to rice water and cow's milk, but one third died from their illness. Because all but two of these infants had been breastfed, he hypothesized that breastfeeding was causative. Similar patients were seen in Prague and Belgrade during and after World War II in a time of serious food shortages.[48] Many of these infants improved when fed cow's milk, so it was postulated that the disease was caused by a deficiency of biotin, since the biotin content in cow's milk was higher than that of human milk.

Subsequently, the term *Leiner's disease* was often used to describe any infant with widespread dermatitis in association with diarrhea and/or failure to thrive. In 1968 two sibling infants with erythroderma, diarrhea, and failure to thrive, who also had an increased susceptibility to infection, were shown to have a yeast opsonization defect[49]; the dermatitis cleared in one of the children after an infusion of fresh frozen plasma. It was hypothesized that a yeast opsonization defect resulting from a dysfunction of the fifth component of complement was the cause of Leiner's disease. Additional patients were then studied, and most did not have this opsonization defect, which was subsequently shown to be quite common in the general population. Moreover, not all improved with fresh frozen plasma.[50]

In 1988 Glover et al reported a group of five infants with erythroderma, diarrhea, and failure to thrive.[51] None had a yeast opsonization defect, but instead a variety of other immunologic abnormalities, including elevated IgE levels and hypogammaglobulinemia, were found. Some were subsequently diagnosed as having Netherton's or Omenn's syndromes.[51] This paper established the need to consider the diagnosis of immunodeficiency when evaluating erythrodermic infants, and established the multiple etiologies of what had formerly been called Leiner's disease.

Leiner's disease, if the term is used today, should be used to describe a clinical phenotype defined as an infant with (1) noncongenital or acquired erythroderma (Fig. 15-9); (2) diarrhea; and (3) failure to thrive. Infants with these findings need thorough investigations searching for the underlying cause of their disorder. Most of the diseases listed in Box 15-1 need to be considered, especially immunodeficiencies, Netherton's syndrome, Omenn's syndrome, and eosinophilic gastroenteritis (see the following discussion). Baseline immune studies of such infants should include chest radiograph, CBC, quantitative im-

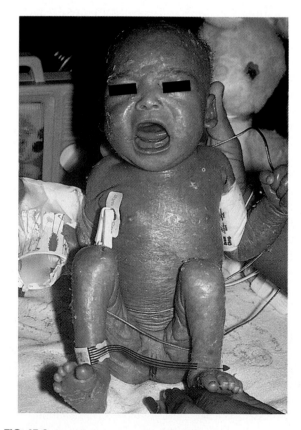

FIG. 15-9
Diffuse erythroderma and scaling with failure to thrive in an infant with hypogammaglobulinemia.

munoglobulins, and skin testing before or after specific immunizations. More detailed testing should be pursued, as indicated.

The prognosis and treatment of this condition are entirely dependent on the specific diagnosis. The associated diarrhea and failure to thrive must be treated aggressively with adequate nutritional support up to and including parental hyperalimentation as indicated.

Omenn's Syndrome

Omenn's syndrome is a T-cell deficient state marked by abnormal histiocytic cells and extreme elevations of eosinophils in affected tissues and in the peripheral blood. During early infancy, these patients develop generalized erythroderma associated with diffuse papules (Fig. 15-10), marked lymphadenopathy, recurrent infections, and failure to thrive.[52] Alopecia may be seen as well. This disorder is autosomal recessive in inheritance and was originally described as familial reticuloendotheliosis with eosinophilia. Although the condition is primarily one of T-cell dysregulation, both humoral and cellular immune defects are seen.[53] Abnormal antibody production and elevated IgE levels occur. There is usually a marked leukocytosis with eosinophilia, anemia, hypogammaglobulinemia, and depressed T-cell medicated immunity. A gene defect has been identified that maps to chromosome 11.[54] The disorder is often difficult to distinguish from graft versus host disease (GVHD). The only known effective treatment is bone marrow transplantation.

Graft-Versus-Host Disease

Graft-versus-host disease (GVHD) is caused by the interaction between immunocompetent lymphoid cells and immunodeficient host cells.[55] Nearly all cases in neonates and young infants are caused by severe T-cell immunodeficiency states (such as severe combined immunodeficiency) with maternal engraftment either in utero or at the time of delivery.[56] Clinically, affected infants typically present with a scaly erythematous rash that often begins on the scalp and face and moves downward. Fine erythematous papules may also occur. The findings may be patchy or diffuse, in some cases progressing to frank erythroderma (Figs. 15-11 and 15-12).[56,57] The most severe cutaneous manifestation of GVHD is toxic epidermal necrolysis, a finding that may rarely be evident at the time of delivery. Diffuse alopecia is a common finding and often involves eyebrows, as well as scalp hair. Although milder forms of GVHD sometimes respond (at least partially) to emollients or topical corticosteroids, recurrences are the rule. If unrecognized and untreated, GVHD progresses and may affect a variety of organ systems.

The diagnosis should be suspected in any young infant with erythroderma and frequent infections, chronic diarrhea, and/or failure to thrive. If present, a family history of prior early infant deaths is helpful because many forms of immunodeficiency are familial. Skin biopsy can be very useful in confirming the diagnosis of GVHD. The histopathologic changes of GVHD are usually graded by severity (from I to IV).[58] Most authors agree that minimum criteria for the histopathologic diagnosis of GVHD include the presence of epidermal lymphocytes, dyskeratosis, and satel-

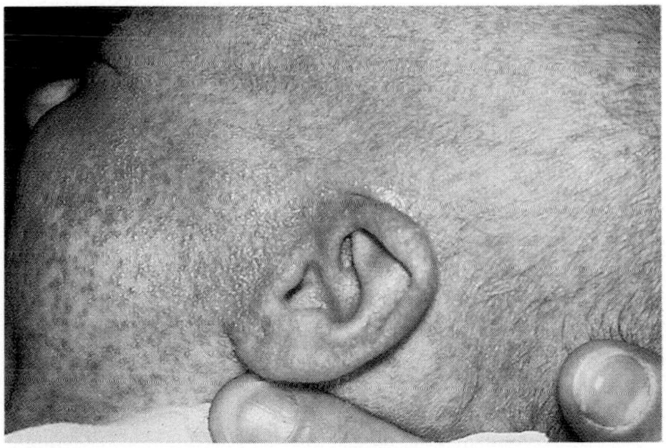

FIG. 15-10
A child diagnosed with Omenn's syndrome, illustrating diffusely distributed, scaling, erythematous papules. These findings were present over the entire skin surface.

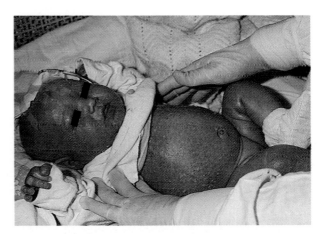

FIG. 15-11
Erythema and scaling is seen in the exfoliative phase of GVHD.

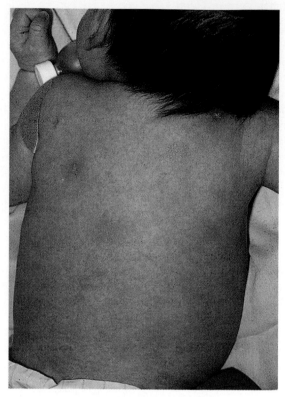

FIG. 15-12

A male child diagnosed with SCID. He manifested a diffusely distributed blanching erythema. The skin eruption was caused by post–bone marrow transplant GVHD.

lite cell necrosis. The latter refers to the finding of a lymphocyte apposed to an eosinophilic keratinocyte (dyskeratotic epidermal cell) within the epidermis. Similar changes may also result from the conditioning therapy utilized for some patients before bone marrow transplantation, as well as from the effect of certain viruses.[59,60] In some cases of GVHD caused by maternal engraftment, a spongiotic dermatitis may predominate.[61] Multiple skin biopsies obtained over days or weeks may be necessary if the diagnosis is strongly suspected, but without confirmatory histopathology. The use of immunophenotyping of skin biopsies has been used to complement the characteristic findings on routine histopathology described previously.[62] The finding of strong staining for HLA-DR within the epidermis is strongly suggestive of GVHD. It should be emphasized, however, that immunophenotyping alone should not be considered diagnostic of GVHD and that the lack of such features should not discount the presence of compatible clinical and histopathologic findings of this condition.

Since the diagnosis of GVHD in the absence of a known organ or bone marrow transplant implies a severe immunodeficiency, a complete evaluation of the immune system should be undertaken. Although lymphopenia is characteristic of severe T-cell or severe combined immunodeficiency, the lymphocyte count in the blood may be normal or even elevated because of the presence of circulating maternal lymphocytes. Eosinophilia is often present. Although small numbers of circulating maternal cells are considered a normal finding in the first few weeks of life, the presence of large numbers of maternal lymphocytes is highly suggestive of an underlying immunodeficiency, and in the setting of erythroderma strongly suggests the diagnosis of GVHD. Maternal engraftment can be documented by demonstrating extra circulating HLA haplotypes or by demonstrating an XX genotype in the blood of a male infant.[61,63]

The differential diagnosis is generally confined to other more common conditions such as seborrheic dermatitis, infantile eczema, or the unusual viral or drug eruptions.

The course of this condition can be variable and depends on the degree of organ involvement, as well as the severity of the immunodeficiency. In most instances, the skin can be treated with bland emollients, as well as low- or mid-potency topical corticosteroid preparations. More severe reactions, particularly those with systemic manifestations, may require systemic corticosteroid therapy, cytotoxic drugs, or monoclonal antibodies.[55] For subacute or chronic skin disease, in the absence of systemic involvement, PUVA therapy has proved useful both as a primary therapy and as a means to decrease or discontinue altogether the use of systemic therapies.[64,65,66] Such therapy is reserved for older patients.

The skin manifestations of GVHD occurring after transplantation, or rarely resulting from transfusions, have been well characterized and include an acute phase with a morbilliform erythema, a papular dermatitis, diffuse erythroderma, or in severe cases, diffuse bullae or frank necrosis such as seen in toxic epidermal necrolysis. Often, such skin changes begin on the head and neck and extend in a caudal fashion. The palms and soles are usually predominately involved. Chronic changes (greater than 100 days posttransplantation) may include oral mucous membrane changes, nail dystrophy, and localized or diffuse lichenoid (flat-topped) papules. Extracutaneous features of the disease are primarily gastrointestinal. A hepatitis may be found, as well as varying degrees of diarrhea. Skin biopsies of representative lesions will generally reveal features of GVHD such as vacuolization of the basal cell layer and dyskeratosis within the epidermis.

Additional Primary Immunodeficiency Syndromes

All reported forms of **severe combined immunodeficiency** (SCID) can present with a diffuse erythroderma (see Fig.

15-11) associated with failure to thrive and severe diarrhea.[67] Infants with **DiGeorge syndrome** can have a maculopapular or eczematous dermatitis that can generalize.[68,69] Other forms of primary immunodeficiency such as **Bruton's hypogammaglobulinemia and common variable hypogammaglobulinemia** may have similar findings.[51]

Eosinophilic gastroenteritis was first reported by Waldman et al, who called the condition allergic gastroenteropathy. Cutaneous features included edema, particularly over the face, as well as generalized atopic dermatitis.[70,71] The extracutaneous manifestations are striking and include growth retardation, extreme hypoalbuminemia, hypogammaglobulinemia, anemia, and eosinophilia, as well as mild gastrointestinal symptoms consisting of intermittent diarrhea or vomiting after the ingestion of certain foods, and excessive loss of protein into the gastrointestinal tract. Asthma and allergic rhinitis may also be present. Diagnosis is confirmed with intestinal biopsies, which reveal mucosal eosinophilia. The disease is now subclassified into a protein-sensitive and idiopathic form.[72] The protein-sensitive form is more common, responds to dietary restriction of cow's milk or soy protein, and ultimately resolves with time. The idiopathic form requires steroid therapy to control symptoms. The dermatitis improves rapidly and dramatically with resolution of the other symptoms when the dermatitis is aggressively treated.

EVALUATION AND MANAGEMENT OF THE RED SCALY BABY

The history and physical examination may provide important diagnostic clues to the etiology of erythroderma. Specific parameters that may be of value in determining an underlying cause include congenital onset, skin induration, and the presence of large scaling plaques, alopecia with or without hair dysplasia, evolution, response to corticosteroid therapy, presence of infections, and failure to thrive.[73] If the infant appears to have atopic or seborrheic dermatitis, then appropriate therapy can be instituted. If there is no response to therapy, or if the infant appears to be systemically ill, has failure to thrive, or shows other evidence of a more generalized disease, a more comprehensive evaluation should be undertaken (Boxes 15-1 and 15-2). Laboratory tests useful in evaluating erythroderma in neonates and infants are outlined in Box 15-2. The selection of which tests to perform depends on which disease(s) are most suspect. Appropriate smears and cultures for fungal, bacterial, or viral disease should be performed if infection is suspected. A chest radiograph may be useful to evaluate the thymic shadow, which may be absent in neonates with SCID. IgG levels, if obtained during the first months of life, are reflective of maternal

---

BOX 15-2
Red Scaly Baby—Laboratory Evaluation

Gram stain ⎫
Fungal smear ⎬ If infection suspected
Tzanck smear ⎭
Appropriate cultures (e.g., nasopharynx/rectum for viruses or staph)
Chest radiograph (may reveal absence thymic shadow in neonate with SCID)
CBC, platelets
Quantitative immunoglobulins
Isohemagglutinins
Liver function tests
Electrolytes
Plasma zinc
Biotinidase
RPR
HIV
Sweat chloride
Serum amino/urine organic acids
Trichogram
Skin biopsy

---

values. These may, however, be useful in infants older than 6 months of age. Liver function tests may be indicated in primary or secondary nutritional disease, such as cystic fibrosis. In the latter, one would expect elevations of the transaminases and severely decreased serum albumin. Serum amino and urine organic acids are necessary to screen for suspected cases of primary metabolic diseases, such as the aminoacidurias or biotin deficiencies. A biotinidase level can be obtained if biotin deficiency is suspected. Lastly, skin biopsy can be useful for direct histopathologic examination of representative lesions, and fibroblast culture can help in definitive diagnosis of several metabolic diseases.

When confronted with an infant presenting with erythroderma, immediate attention to fluid and electrolytes is paramount. For example, infants with ichthyosis can develop life-threatening hypernatremic dehydration. Infectious complications, primarily bacterial or fungal, must also be considered. These infants need a warm, humid environment to minimize their metabolic demands. Topical therapy consisting of bland emollients such as petrolatum or Aquaphor is helpful in minimizing transepidermal water loss and may decrease potential infectious complications.[74]

A summary of the evaluation and management of many of the disorders is found in Table 15-1.

TABLE 15-1

Evaluation and Management of Disorders

Diagnosis	Usual onset	Clinical features	Associated features	Management
Inflammatory Diseases				
Atopic dermatitis	Birth-6 months	Pruritus, xerosis, scaling, and erythema	Skin biopsy: acanthosis, spongiosis (infiltrate)	Emollients Topical corticosteroids
Seborrheic dermatitis	Birth-1 month	Greasy scale: Scalp, face, body Erythema of body folds and diaper region	Skin biopsy shows features of mild dermatitis and is generally nonspecific	Routine cleansing; occasionally mild topical corticosteroids for short courses
Psoriasis	Birth-adulthood	Mild or thick scale over the scalp and, diaper areas as well as the abdomen. Periumbilical involvement is typical	Skin biopsy often shows features of chronic dermatitis; spongiotic pustules may rarely be seen	Emollients, low potency, corticosteroids, cold tar/petrolatum
Diffuse mastocytosis	Birth-2 months	Absence of scale Flushing Positive Darier's	Skin biopsy: dense dermal infiltrate of mast cells. Some infants may show severe syncope, diarrhea, or shock	Prevention of degranulation is important Counseling regarding direct mast cell degranulators should be offered Oral antihistamines may be used for a period
Infectious Diseases				
Staphylococcal scalded skin syndrome	Anytime	Diffuse cutaneous erythema followed by superficial desquamation. Mucous membranes are spared	Skin culture of nasopharynx, rectum, or pustule should show *S. aureus* Skin biopsy shows superficial epidermal split	Appropriate antibiotics Superficial wound care
Candida	Birth or neonatal	Generalized erythema, papules, scaling, pustules, diffuse erythema	KOH examinations of scraping should be positive Cervical culture for yeast Skin biopsy should show typical fungal elements	Topical therapy for limited disease Systemic antifungal therapy for invasive/ disseminated disease
Herpes simplex	Birth or later	Grouped vesicles on erythematosus base over presenting part: erosions, scaling, erythema (intrauterine variant)	Tzanck smears showing multiple nucleated giant cells; skin biopsy will show intra-epidermal vesicles with ballooning degeneration of keratinocytes	Viral culture should be diagnostic Direct fluorescent antibody of scrapings may also be done

TABLE 15-1

Evaluation and Management of Disorders—cont'd

Diagnosis	Usual onset	Clinical features	Associated features	Management
Infectious Diseases—cont'd				
Congenital syphilis	Birth or 6-8 weeks	Bullae, erythema, scaling, eroded papules and plaques over anogenital areas	Dark field examination of mucous membrane lesions: spirochetes specific serology positive	Appropriate antibiotic therapy
Inherited Diseases				
Ichthyosis	Birth or later	Diffuse scale, bullae with hyperkeratosis, patterned hyperkeratosis (depending on particular disorder)	Skin biopsy showing epidermolysis with (EHK); retinal changes (Sjögren-Larsson Syndrome); bone radiographs showing epiphyseal stipling (chondrodysplasia punctata)	Supportive, emollients, hydration
Immunologic Diseases				
Leiner's phenotype	Weeks to months	Erythematous scaling, desquamative dermatitis, diarrhea, failure to thrive, alopecia	Immunoglobulin abnormalities, hair shaft abnormalities (Netherton's), T cell abnormalities	Definitive therapy depends on ultimate diagnosis; attention to fluid and electrolytes

REFERENCES

1. Bonifazi E, Meneghini CL. Atopic dermatitis in the first six months of life. Acta Derm Venereol Suppl 1989;144:20-22.
2. Yates VM, Kerr R, Frier K, et al. Early diagnosis of infantile seborrheic dermatitis and atopic dermatitis–total and specific IgE levels. Br J Dermatol 1983;108:639-645.
3. Puissant A. Psoriasis in children under the age of ten: A study of 100 observations. Gazetta Sanitaria 1970;19:191.
4. Farber EM, Jacobs AH. Infantile psoriasis. Am J Dis Child 1977;131:1266-1269.
5. Beylot C, Puissant A, Bioulac P, et al. Particular clinical features of psoriasis in infants and children. Acta Derm Venereol Suppl 1979;87:95-97.
6. Ivker RA, Grim-Jorgensen CM, Vega VK, et al. Infantile generalized pustular psoriasis associated with lytic lesions of the bone. Pediatr Dermatol 1993;10:277-282.
7. Personal communication. Dr. Bernice Krafchik.
8. Farber EM, Mullen RH, Jacobs AH, et al. Infantile psoriasis: A follow-up study. Pediatr Dermatol 1986;3:237-243.
9. Valdes-Dapena MA, Arey JB. Boric acid poisoning. J Pediatr 1962;61:521.
10. Oranje AP, Soekanto W, Sukardi A, et al. Diffuse cutaneous mastocytosis mimicking staphylococcal scalded-skin syndrome, report of three cases. Pediatr Dermatol 1991;8:147.
11. Hawk RJ, Storer JS, Daum RS. Toxic epidermal necrolysis in a six-week old infant. Pediatr Dermatol 1985;3:197-200.
12. Personal observation, Dr. Mary K Spraker, 1997.
13. Personal observation, Dr. William L. Weston, 1997.
14. Balay JE, Silverman RA. Systemic candidiasis: Cutaneous manifestations in low birth weight infants. Pediatrics 1988;82:211-215.
15. Rowan JL, Atkins JT, Levy ML, et al. Invasive fungal dermatitis in the < or 1000gm neonate. Pediatrics 1995;95:682.
16. Hutto C, Arvin A, Jacobs R, et al. Intrauterine herpes simplex infections. J Pediatr 1987;110:97-101.
17. Honig PJ, Brown D. Congenital herpes simplex infection initially resembling epidermolysis bullosa. J Pediatr 1982;101:958-960.
18. Chawla V, Pandit PB, Nkrumah FK. Congenital syphilis in the newborn. Arch Dis Child 1988;63:1393-1394.
19. Williams ML, Elias PM. Heterogeneity in autosomal recessive ichthyosis: Clinical and biochemical differentiation of lamellar ichthyosis and non-bullous congenital ichthyosiform erythroderma. Arch Dermatol 1985;121:477-488.
20. Greene SL, Muller SA. Netherton's syndrome. Report of a case and review of the literature. J Am Acad Dermatol 1985; 13:329-337.

21. Judge MR, Morgan G, Harper JI. A clinical and immunological study of Netherton's syndrome. Br J Dermatol 1994;131:615-621.

22. Williams ML, Shwayder TA. Ichthyosis and disorders of cornification. In Schachner LA, Hansen RC, eds. Pediatric dermatology. New York: Churchill Livingstone, 1995: p 413-418.

23. Kalter DC, Atherton DJ, Clayton PT. X-linked dominant Conradi-Hunermann syndrome presenting as congenital erythroderma. J Am Acad Dermatol 1989;21:248-256.

24. Corbi MR, Conejo-Mir JS, Linares M, et al. Conradi-Hunermann syndrome with unilateral distribution. Pediatr Dermatol 1998;15:299-303.

25. Nazzaro V, Blanchet-Burdon C, Lorette G, et al. Familial occurrence of KID (keratosis, ichthyosis, deafness) syndrome. Case reports of a mother and daughter. J Am Acad Dermatol 1990;23:385-388.

26. Kone-Paut I, Hesse S, Palix C, et al. Keratosis, ichthyosis, and deafness (KID) syndrome in half siblings. Pediatr Dermatol 1998;3:219-221.

27. Srebrnik A, Tur E, Perluk C, et al. Dorfman-Chanarin syndrome: A case report and a review. J Am Acad Dermatol 1987; 17:801-808.

28. Happle R, Traupe H, Grobe H, et al. The Tay syndromes (congenital ichthyosis with trichothiodystrophy). Eur J Pediatr 1984;147-152.

29. Executive and scientific advisory boards of the National Foundation for Ectodermal Dysplasia: Scaling skin in the neonate: A clue to the early diagnosis of x-linked hypohidrotic ectodermal dysplasia (Christ-Siemens-Touraine syndrome). J Pediatr 1989;114:600-602.

30. Shih VE, Axel SM, Tewksbury JC, et al. Defective lysosomal release of vitamin B12 (cbIF): A hereditary cobalamin metabolic disorder associated with sudden death. Am J Med Genet 1989; 33:555-563.

31. Howard R, Frieden IJ, Crawford D, et al. Methylmalonic aciduria, cobalamin c type, presenting with cutaneous manifestations. Arch Dermatol 1997;133:1563-1566.

32. Koopman RJ, Happle R. Cutaneous manifestations of methylmalonic aciduria. Arch Dermatol Res 1990;282:272-273.

33. DiLiberti JH, DiGeorge AM, Ayerback VH. Abnormal leucine/isoleucine ratio and acrodermatitis enteropathica-like rash in maple syrup urine disease (MSUD). Pediatr Res 1973;7:382.

34. Spraker MK, Helminski MA, Elsas LJ. Periorificial dermatitis secondary to dietary deficiency of isoleucine in treated infants with maple syrup urine disease (abstr). J Invest Dematol 1986;86:508.

35. Koch SE, Packman S, Koch TK, et al. Dermatitis in treated maple syrup urine disease. J Am Acad Dermatol 1993;28: 289-292.

36. Northrup H, Sigman ES, Hebert AA. Exfoliative erythroderma resulting from inadequate intake of branched-chain amino acids in infants with maple syrup urine disease. Arch Dermatol 1993;129:384-385.

37. Giacoia GP, Berry GT. Acrodermatitis enteropathica-like syndrome secondary to isoleucine deficiency during treatment of maple syrup urine disease. Am J Dis Child 1993;147:954-956.

38. Snyderman SE, Boyer A, Norton PM, et al. The essential aminoacid requirements of infants; isoleucine. Am J Clin Nutr 1964;15:313.

39. Theone J, Batshaw M, Spector E. Neontal citrullinemia: Treatment with ketoanalogues of essential aminoacids. J Pediatr 1977;90:218-224.

40. Kline JJ, Hug G, Schubert WK, et al. Arginine deficiency syndrome: Its occurrence in carbamoyl phosphate synthetase deficiency. Am J Dis Child 1981;135:437-442.

41. DeRaeve L, DeMeirlier L, Ramet J, et al. Acrodermatitis enteropathica-like cutaneous lesions in organic aciduria. J Pediatr 1994;124:416-420.

42. Hansen RC, Lemen R, Rersin B. Cystic fibrosis manifesting with acrodermatitis enteropathica-like eruption: Associated with essential fatty acid and zinc deficiencies. Arch Dermatol 1983;119:51-55.

43. Darmstadt GL, Schmidt CP, Wechsler DS, et al. Dermatitis as a presenting sign of cystic fibrosis. Arch Dermatol 1992; 128:1358-1364.

44. Hansen RC. Dermatitis and nutritional deficiency: Diagnostic and therapeutic considerations (editorial). Arch Dermatol 1992;128;1389-1390.

45. Hansen AE, Wiese HF, Boelsche AR, et al. Role of linoleic acid in infant nutrition. Pediatrics 1963;31:171-192.

46. Leiner C. Über erythrodermia disquamativa, eine eingenartige universalle dermatose der brustlkinder. Arch Dermatol Syphilol 1908;89:163-189.

47. Leiner C. Erythodermia desquamation (universal dermatitis of children at the breast). Br J Child Dis 1908;5:244-251.

48. Vujasin J, Petrovic D. Biotin in some erythemato-squamous dermatoses of babies. Dermatologica 1952;105:180-183.

49. Miller ME, Seals J, Kaye R, et al. A familial, plasma-associated defect of phagocytosis. Lancet 1968;ii:60-63.

50. Weston WL, Humber JR. Failure of fresh plasma in Leiner disease. Arch Dermatol 1977;113:233-234.

51. Glover MT, Atherton DJ, Levinsky RJ. Syndrome of erythroderma, failure to thrive and diarrhea in infancy: A manifestation of immunodeficiency. Pediatrics 1988;81:66-72.

52. Pupo RA, Tyring SK, Raimer SS, et al. Omenn's syndrome and related combined immunodeficiency syndromes: Diagnostic considerations in infants with persistent erythroderma and failure to thrive. J Am Acad Dermatol 1991;25:442-446.

53. Omenn GS. Familial reticuloendothiliosis with eosinophil. N Engl J Med 1965;273:427.

54. Villa A, Sautagata S, Bozzi F, et al. Partial V(D) J recombination activity leads to Omenn syndrome. Cell 1998;93:885-896.

55. Dinulos JG, Levy ML. Graft-versus-host disease in children. Semin Dermatol 1995;14:66-69.

56. Alain G, Carrier C, Beaumier L, et al. In utero acute graft-versus-host disease in a neonate with severe combined immunodeficiency. J Am Acad Dermatol 1993;29:862-865.

57. Farrell A. Scerri L, Stevens A, et al. Acute graft-versus-host disease with unusual cutaneous intracellular vacuolation in an infant with severe combined immunodeficiency. Pediatr Dermatol 1995;12:311-313.

58. Lerner KG, Kao GF, Storb R, et al. Histopathology of graft-vs-host reaction (GVHR) in human recipients of marrow from HLA matched sibling donors. Transplant Proc 1974;6:367-371.

59. Sale GE, Lerner KG, Barker EA, et al. The skin biopsy in the diagnosis of acute graft-versus-host disease in man. Am J Pathol 1977;89:621-635.

60. Fujinami RS, Nelson JA, Walker L, et al. Sequence homology and immunologic cross-reactivity of human cytomegalovirus with HLA-DR ® chain: A means for graft rejection and immunosupression. J Virol 1988;62:100-105.
61. Appleton AL, Curtis A, Wilkes J, et al. Differentiation of materno-fetal GVHD from Omenn's syndrome in pre-BMT patients with severe combined immunodeficiency. Bone Marrow Transplant 1994;14:157-159.
62. Paller AS, Nelson A, Steffan L. T-lymphocyte subsets in the lesional skin of allogeneic and antologous bone marrow transplant patients. Arch Dermatol 1988;124:1795-1801.
63. Katz F, Malcolm S, Strobel S, et al. The use of locus-specific minisatellite probes to check engraftment following allogenic bone marrow transplantation for severe combined immunodeficiency disease. Bone Marrow Transplant 1990;5:199-204.
64. Hymes SR, Morison WL, Farmer ER, et al. Methoxsalen and ultraviolet A radiation in treatment of chronic cutaneous graft-vs-host reaction. J Am Acad Dermatol 1985;12:30-70.
65. Eppinger T, Ehninger G, Steinert M, et al. 8-Methoxypsoralen and utraviolet A therapy for cutaneous manifestations of graft-vs-host disease. Transplantation 1990;50:807-811.
66. Vogelsa GB, Wolff D, Altomonte V, et al. Treatment of chronic graft-versus-host disease with ultraviolet irradiation and psoralen (PUVA). Bone Marrow Transplant 1996;17:1061-1067.
67. Hague RA, Rassam S, Morgan G, et al. Early diagnosis of severe combined innunodeficiency syndrome. Arch Dis Child 1999;70:260-263.
68. Conley ME, Beckwith JB, Mancer JFK, et al. The spectrum of the DiGeorge syndrome. J Pediatr 1979;94:883-890.
69. Archer E, Chuan T-Y, Hong R. Severe eczema in a patient with DiGeorge syndrome. Cutis 1990;45:455-459.
70. Waldman TA, Wochner RD, Laster L, et al. Allergic gastroenteropathy—a cause of excessive gastrointestinal protein loss. N Engl J Med 1967;276:761-769.
71. Jenkins HR, Walker-Smith JA, Atherton DO. Protein-losing enteropathy in atopic dermatitis. Pediatr Dermatol; 1986; 3:125-129.
72. Katz AJ, Twarog FJ, Zeiger RS, et al. Milk sensitive and eosinophilic gastroenteropathy: Similar clinical features with contrasting mechanisms and clinical course. J Allergy Clin Immunol 1984;74:72-78.
73. Pruszkowski A, Bodemer C, Fraitag S, et al. Neonatal and infantile erythrodermas. Arch Dermatol 2000;136:875-880.
74. Nopper AJ, Horii KA, Sokdeo-Drost S, et al. Topical ointment therapy benefits premature infants. J Pediatr 1996;128:660-669.

16

Disorders of Cornification (Ichthyosis)

AMY S. PALLER

Several ichthyotic conditions first manifest in the neonatal period (Table 16-1), usually either as a collodion baby or scaling erythroderma, or more rarely as a harlequin fetus. In some situations, such as the harlequin fetus or Netherton's syndrome, associated complications are life threatening. For most of these ichthyotic conditions, therapy during the neonatal and early infantile period is standard, involving frequent application of bland emollients and monitoring for evidence of infection or fluid and electrolyte imbalance. Use of topical medications with keratolytic agents during the neonatal period and first 6 months of life is usually unnecessary and leads to the risk of significant absorption of potentially toxic substances (e.g., absorption of lactic acid, salicylic acid). Our recent understanding of the underlying causes of several of these disorders improves patient management and allows for the possibility of prenatal diagnosis based on molecular techniques.

HARLEQUIN ICHTHYOSIS

Harlequin ichthyosis is a rare autosomal recessive disorder in which the neonate is born with a thick covering of armorlike scales, severe ectropion and eclabium, and underdeveloped nose and ears (Fig. 16-1). Despite these consistent phenotypic features, a variety of biochemical and structural characteristics have been described, suggesting that the molecular basis for harlequin ichthyosis is heterogeneous. The finding of increased epidermal triglyceride content suggests a lipid defect,[1] but alterations in keratinization have also been described.[2,3] In addition, type 2 protein phosphatase, which converts profilaggrin to filaggrin, has been altered in some cases.[4] It is likely that the harlequin ichthyosis phenotype may result from sev-

eral underlying mutations. Dale et al[4] have classified the disease into three subtypes, based on the presence or absence of profilaggrin, the size and number of lamellar granules in the granular layer, and the expression of epidermal keratins.

Regardless of the possible molecular mechanism, all patients have hyperkeratosis, lipid accumulation within corneocytes, and absence of normal lamellar granules.[5] The basic defect is thought to be the abnormal lamellar granules, leading to a defect in stratum corneum desquamation in vivo[6] and in terminal differentiation in vitro.[4] At this time, harlequin ichthyosis can be diagnosed in utero by morphologic analysis of amniotic fluid cells obtained by amniocentesis.[7]

In general, harlequin babies require vigorous supportive therapy, including a humid environment, the aggressive use of emollients, and careful monitoring of fluid and electrolyte needs. Patients with harlequin ichthyosis rarely survive the neonatal period because of complications such as systemic infection through fissured skin, difficulties with feeding and respiration, and distal gangrene. As a result, harlequin ichthyosis is the only ichthyotic condition in the neonate that may justify the usage of systemic retinoid therapy at this age. Treatment of harlequin ichthyosis with retinoids was first undertaken in 1985.[8] Infants can survive, and therapy with retinoids may improve the clinical appearance, with the condition evolving into a severe form of generalized ichthyosiform erythroderma.[9-13] Evaluation of biopsy specimens from a survivor of harlequin ichthyosis showed normal expression of keratins and cornified envelope proteins.[13,14] The decision to administer retinoids should only be considered in babies who survive the first few weeks with intensive nursing support, with the

TABLE 16-1

Disorders of Cornification That Usually Present During the First Weeks

Disorder	Inheritance	Clinical features	Mutation	Visual method of diagnosis
Harlequin ichthyosis	AR	Thick, armor-like scale with fissuring	Unknown	Clinical
Collodion baby	Usually AR	Shiny collodion membrane	Various	Clinical
Recessive X-linked ichthyosis	Recessive X-linked	Collodion membrane May have genital anomalies	Steroid sulfatase	Plasma cholesterol sulfate
Lamellar ichthyosis	Usually AR	Collodion membrane	Transglutaminase I Other	Clinical
Congenital ichthyosiform erythroderma	AR	Collodion membrane	Unknown	Clinical
Epidermolytic hyperkeratosis	AD	Scaling and blistering	Keratins 1, 10, 2e	Clinical and histologic
Ichthyosis hystrix	AD	Plaques of hyperkeratosis	Unknown	Clinical
Familial peeling skin	AR	Superficial peeling	Unknown	Clinical and histologic
Sjögren-Larsson	AR	Variable skin thickening Mental, developmental retardation Spastic diplegia Seizures "Glistening dots"	Fatty aldehyde Dehydrogenase (FAD)	Clinical and fibroblast cultures for FAD
Neutral lipid storage disease	AR	Collodion membrane or ichthyosiform erythroderma	Recycling of triacyl-glycerol to diacylglycerol	Blood smear for vacuolated PMNs
Netherton's	AR	Ichthyosiform erythroderma Scant hair, often failure to thrive	SPINK5	Clinical; hair exam later in infancy
Trichothiodystrophy	AR	Collodion membrane Broken hair	Unknown DNA transcription, repair gene in some	Clinical and hair microscopy; hair sulfur content
KID syndrome	May be AD, AR	Erythrokeratodermatous or thick, leathery skin with stippled papules	Unknown	Clinical; auditory evoked potentials
CHILD syndrome	X-linked dominant	Alopecia Unilateral yellow, waxy scaling Hemidysplasia Limb defects	3 β-hydroxysteroid dehydrogenase Emopamil binding protein	Clinical
Conradi-Hunermann	X-linked dominant	Thick, psoriasiform scale over erythroderma, pat-terned along Blaschko's lines Proximal limb shortening	Emopamil binding protein	Clinical
Ichthyosis follicularis	Usually X-linked recessive	Prominent follicular hyperkeratoses Alopecia Photophobia	Unknown	Clinical
CHIME syndrome	AR	Ichthyotic erythematous plaques Cardiac defects; typical facies Retinal colobomas	Unknown	Clinical
Gaucher's	AR	Collodion membrane Hepatosplenomegaly	β-Glucocerebrosidase	Clinical; fibroblast cultures

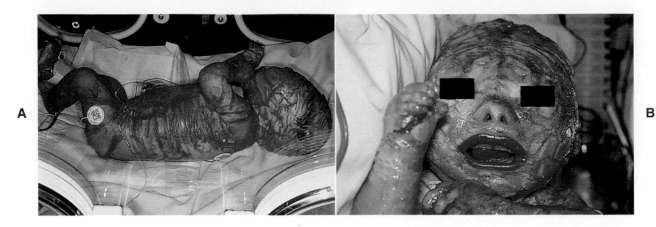

FIG. 16-1

A, Thick armorlike scaling and fissures in a neonate with harlequin ichthyosis. **B,** Note the severe ectropion, eclabion, and digital contractures. (Courtesy of Dr. Sylvia Suarez, Alexandria, VA).

knowledge that the persistent resultant ichthyotic condition is severe and associated with a poor quality of life.

COLLODION BABY

The collodion baby is the phenotype at birth of several ichthyotic disorders, but autosomal recessive congenital ichthyosiform erythroderma or lamellar ichthyosis of variable severity are the eventual phenotype in 60% of patients.[15] Others include autosomal dominant lamellar ichthyosis, Sjögren-Larsson syndrome, Conradi-Hunermann syndrome, trichothiodystrophy, and neonatal Gaucher's disease.[16] It should be recognized, however, that babies with ichthyosiform erythroderma may be erroneously labeled as collodion babies, and this has resulted in some confusion in the literature.[17] In 5% to 6% of collodion babies, normal-appearing skin replaces the collodion membrane, an autosomal recessive disorder called *lamellar ichthyosis of the newborn* or *spontaneously healing collodion baby.*[17]

Collodion babies are encased in thickened, shiny, variably erythematous skin that resembles cellophane (Fig. 16-2). Despite the thickening of the stratum corneum, the membrane is a poor barrier, leading to excessive transcutaneous fluid and electrolyte loss with hypernatremic dehydration[18,19] increased metabolic requirements, and temperature instability owing to increased evaporative cooling.

Collodion babies are often premature, and the skin disorder and prematurity increase the risk of complications. The poor barrier and numerous fissures increase the risk of the skin being a site of entry for bacteria and subsequent sepsis, a condition that may be more difficult to diagnose in view of the temperature instability and fluid imbalances

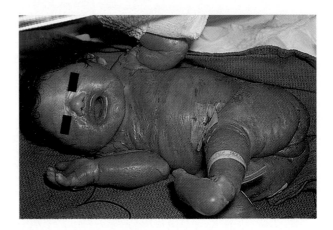

FIG. 16-2

Shiny collodion membrane of a 1-day-old collodion baby. Note the eclabion and tightened skin of the hands.

associated with the underlying skin condition. Aspiration of squamous material in the amniotic fluid may lead to neonatal pneumonia.[20] Additionally, the thickening of the skin may restrict movement, making sucking, eye closure, and rarely respiration, difficult.

Collodion babies should be placed in high humidity environments to increase hydration, and bland emollients should be applied. Electrolytes should be monitored,[19] as should fluid intake and output. The membrane sloughs during the first month of life (Fig. 16-3). Application of topical keratolytic agents should be avoided in view of the increased potential for toxicity resulting from absorption through the compromised permeability barrier.[19]

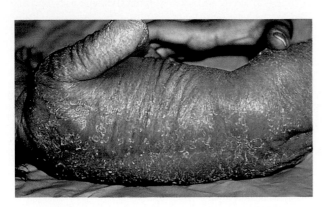

FIG. 16-3

One week after birth, this collodion baby with congenital ichthyosiform erythroderma is showing desquamation of scale. Despite the severity of the early phenotype, this infant had very mild congenital ichthyosiform erythroderma at 6 months of age. (From Paller AS. Ichthyosis in the neonate. In Dyall-Smith D, Marks R, eds. Dermatology at the millennium: Overview of past achievements, current knowledge and future trends. London: Parthenon Publishing Group, 1998: p. 580.)

ICHTHYOSIS VULGARIS

Ichthyosis vulgaris, an autosomal dominant disorder, is one of the most common genetic disorders of skin, occurring in approximately 1:250 individuals. In contrast to other forms of ichthyosis, ichthyosis vulgaris does not manifest during the neonatal period. The condition usually appears after 3 months of age as fine, light-colored scales that are larger and coarser on the lower extremities. Palmoplantar markings are accentuated. In affected boys, ichthyosis vulgaris in the young infant may need to be distinguished from X-linked recessive ichthyosis (see the following discussion).

X-LINKED RECESSIVE ICHTHYOSIS

X-linked recessive ichthyosis (RXLI), a disorder that affects 1:6000 to 1:2000 males, is present by 3 months of age in 84% of patients, although only 17% of patients show evidence of thickened skin at birth. Extensor surfaces, the preauricular areas, and the sides of the neck are most severely affected by the large, dark, adherent scales (Fig. 16-4). Occasionally, affected boys have hypogonadism with undescended testes, hypoplasia of the penis and scrotum, and failure to undergo normal sexual maturation. Development of testicular cancer has been described in one patient, without undescended testes. The condition results from muta-

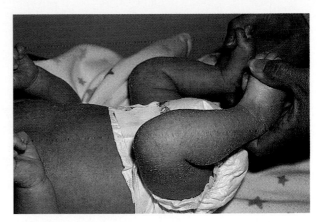

FIG. 16-4

Diffuse scaling of the trunk and extremities is seen in this 2-week-old infant with X-linked ichthyosis.

tions of the gene for steroid sulfatase (arylsulfatase C), particularly deletions (90% of patients). Approximately 10% of affected boys have a contiguous gene deletion syndrome, a larger deletion that encompasses genes that are contiguous on the terminal short arm of the X chromosome to the steroid sulfatase gene. Deletion of surrounding genes results in mental retardation, hypogonadism, and anosmia (Kallmann syndrome), and a bone dysplasia characterized radiographically by stippled epiphyses (X-linked recessive chondrodysplasia punctata).

The decrease in cholesterol and increase in cholesterol sulfate in skin is thought to result in the retention of scale. Absence of steroid sulfatase activity during fetal life also leads to increased fetal production of DHEAS and decreased placental estrogen production, which may delay the progression of parturition.

X-linked recessive ichthyosis in the neonate needs to be distinguished from other ichthyotic disorders associated with collodion membranes and early skin thickening, and from ichthyosis vulgaris in older male infants by measurement of cholesterol sulfate levels in plasma. Babies with the rare autosomal recessive disorder, **multiple sulfatase deficiency,** manifest with scaling typical of RXLI and decreased steroid sulfatase because of a global deficiency of sulfatases. Affected patients also show neurologic abnormalities characteristic of metachromatic leukodystrophy, and features of storage diseases because of the deficiency of several additional sulfatases. Prenatal diagnosis of RXLI can be performed using molecular techniques, or by the demonstration of decreased placental sulfatase activity in amniotic fluid cells and increased DHEAS levels in amniotic fluid. Corrective gene therapy has been per-

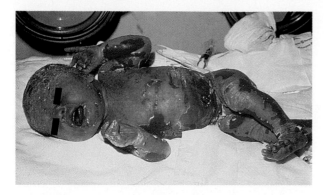

FIG. 16-5
Thick platelike scales of a 2-month-old baby with lamellar ichthyosis, born as a collodion baby. (From Paller AS. Ichthyosis in the neonate. In Dyall-Smith D, Marks R, eds. Dermatology at the millennium: Overview of past achievements, current knowledge and future trends. London: Parthenon Publishing Group, 1998: p 580.)

formed in an animal model by transplantation to mouse skin of grafts of RXLI keratinocytes that have been stably transfected with the normal steroid sulfatase gene.[21]

LAMELLAR ICHTHYOSIS

Lamellar ichthyosis (LI) is usually inherited as an autosomal recessive disorder, although an autosomal dominant form has been described.[22] Babies with lamellar ichthyosis are usually born with collodion membranes (see the previous discussion). After shedding of the collodion membrane the scales are large and platelike (Fig. 16-5) and are hyperpigmented, particularly in patients with darker skin.[23] Underlying erythroderma is minimal, but ectropion and alopecia may be severe. Biopsies from patients with LI have massive thickening of the stratum corneum, mild acanthosis, and a normal granular layer. The epidermis in LI may show papillomatosis with regular psoriasiform blunting and broadening of the rete ridges. Patients with classical lamellar ichthyosis have normal cell kinetics.[24]

The molecular basis for LI has recently been determined to be mutations in keratinocyte transglutaminase I,[25,26] an enzyme that is involved in cornified envelope formation by cross-linking precursor proteins, such as involucrin. However, the genetic basis for lamellar ichthyosis is heterogeneous, and several families have been described with normal keratinocyte transglutaminase.[27] In three consanguineous Moroccan families, the transglutaminase I gene locus was excluded and the mutant gene was instead

strongly linked to 2q33-35.[28] Prenatal diagnosis by molecular analysis of fetal DNA, obtained by chorionic villus sampling, is a preferred method of prenatal diagnosis, but is only possible in families in which the molecular defect is known.[29] Based on the discovery of the underlying gene defect in some families with LI, gene therapy has been performed in mouse models of LI, generated by transplantation of cultured LI keratinocytes that have been transfected with the normal transglutaminase I gene onto immunodeficient mice. Although the expression of the normal transglutaminase I is transient in vivo, it restores not only the transglutaminase but also normal involucrin cross-linking and involucrin expression.[30]

CONGENITAL ICHTHYOSIFORM ERYTHRODERMA

Patients with congenital nonbullous ichthyosiform erythroderma (CIE) also usually present as collodion babies. Underlying erythroderma is common, and the scales tend to be finer and lighter in color than those of infants with lamellar ichthyosis. Alopecia and ectropion may be associated.[23] Not uncommonly, patients with CIE have associated neurologic abnormalities, and the CIE phenotype may be part of other multisystem conditions, such as the neutral lipid storage disease (Chanarin-Dorfman syndrome)[31] or Netherton's syndrome. Patients with CIE show marked acanthosis of the epidermis with a moderately thickened stratum corneum and variable focal parakeratosis.[23] The cause of CIE is unknown. Further distinction between CIE and LI awaits the discovery of an underlying molecular defect in patients with CIE.

EPIDERMOLYTIC HYPERKERATOSIS (BULLOUS CONGENITAL ICHTHYOSIFORM ERYTHRODERMA, BULLOUS ICHYHYOSIS)

This autosomal dominant disorder manifests in the neonate as widespread areas of denuded skin, and the hyperkeratosis may be subtle (Fig. 16-6). Confusion with other blistering disorders in the neonate is common, particularly with epidermolysis bullosa, and secondary cutaneous bacterial infection caused by *Staphylococcus aureus* often occurs. As patients age, scaling becomes more verrucous with large dark scales, particularly at intertriginous sites, and the propensity towards blistering tends to decrease.

The histologic appearance of lesional skin confirms the diagnosis, showing vacuolization of the granular and upper spinous layers. Hyperkeratosis, acanthosis, and papillomatosis are variable, but the granular layer is thickened.

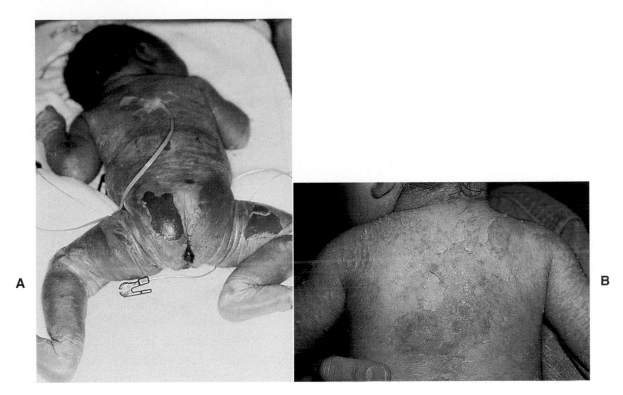

FIG. 16-6
Epidermolytic hyperkeratosis. **A,** Blistering is prominent and can be extensive at birth. **B,** In this older infant, erythema and fine scale are more prominent. Scaling becomes more verrucous especially in intertriginous areas and overlying joints as the patient becomes older. (**A,** Courtesy of Dr Anne Lucky, Cincinnati, Oh.)

By electron microscopy, tonofilaments are clumped in the lower epidermal layers and form perinuclear shells in the granular cell and upper spinous layers. These tonofilaments associate with desmosomes abnormally, resulting in the acantholysis.

The gene defects of bullous CIE involve abnormalities of keratins 1 or 10,[32] the major differentiation-specific keratins of the upper epidermis. These mutations cause formation of defective keratin filaments, which are functionally responsible for the tonofilament clumping and the blistering of this disorder.

Prenatal diagnosis has been performed at 20 to 24 weeks of gestation by fetal skin biopsy, based on the abnormal clumping of keratin filaments,[33] but also by molecular analysis of keratin 10 in an affected family.[34]

ICHTHYOSIS HYSTRIX

Ichthyosis hystrix (Curth-Macklin) is a rare autosomal dominant ichthyotic disorder characterized by plaques of spiny hyperkeratosis. The extent of involvement varies from patchy to generalized and severe. In patients with patchy involvement, the distribution is not along the lines of Blaschko. Usually the face, palms, and soles are not affected, but involvement of the penis and scrotum has been described. Affected infants tend to show cutaneous changes within the first weeks of life, with subsequent progression of involvement, although the onset during childhood has been described in some patients. Erythroderma may be present at birth but disappears with time.

Microscopic examination of skin biopsy specimens shows orthokeratosis, papillomatosis, and acanthosis of the granular and upper spinous layers with perinuclear vacuolization. Keratinocytes may have two nuclei. Ultrastructural examination shows concentric shells of tonofibrils that encase the nuclei with perinuclear vacuoles, lamellar body abnormalities, and binuclear keratinocytes.[34] Tonofilament clumping is not observed. Linkage to the keratin gene clusters has been excluded,[36] although the underlying molecular mechanism of ichthyosis hystrix is unknown.

Ichthyosis hystrix can be confused with epidermolytic hyperkeratosis. The lack of erythroderma, blistering, and typical ultrastructural characteristics distinguish these conditions. Epidermal nevi, although they may resemble ichthyosis hystrix clinically and histologically, are distinguishable by their distribution along the lines of Blaschko.

FAMILIAL PEELING SKIN SYNDROME

This rare autosomal recessive condition is characterized by spontaneous superficial peeling of skin, sometimes accompanied by pruritus and occasionally by erythema or vesiculation. Skin involvement is usually generalized, but the palms, soles, face, and scalp may be unaffected. Nikolsky sign tends to be positive, and a skin biopsy often shows psoriasiform epidermal changes and shedding of the stratum corneum just above the granular layer. Two subgroups have been noted, based on the ultrastructural level of cleavage. Type A, which begins either at birth or at 3 to 6 years of age, shows a split through the corneocyte cytoplasma. Type B, which always begins at birth, shows cleavage along the intercellular spaces.[37] Transient eosinophilia and elevation of IgE levels may be associated.

SJÖGREN-LARSSON SYNDROME

This autosomal recessive disorder usually manifests in the neonatal period with slight or moderate widespread ichthyosis,[38,39,40] although rarely, features may not occur until the infant is older than 6 months. Mild erythema is occasionally present at birth, which clears within months. Only one baby with Sjögren-Larsson syndrome has had a collodion membrane at birth. Affected babies usually show thickening of skin, especially at the umbilicus, neck, and flexural areas, that resembles lichenification. Scaling, if present, is fine and lamellar, so that some neonates have been misdiagnosed as being postmature. Some neonates with Sjögren-Larsson syndrome have had taut, shiny fingers and toes. By 1 year of age, the ichthyosis is fully developed, with generalized thickening, lamellar scaling, and relative sparing of the central face and often the palms and soles. The hair and nails are normal. Histopathologic examination of biopsied skin shows significant hyperkeratosis and papillomatosis with abnormal lamellar or membranous inclusions.[41]

Mental and developmental retardation and spastic diplegia or tetraplegia are the most common extracutaneous features. Many patients have speech abnormalities, seizures, short stature, and kyphosis. Pathognomonic retinal "glistening dots" are not present in all patients. The neurologic disease usually becomes apparent by 3 months of age with failure to reach normal developmental milestones and the onset of spasticity. Phenotypic variability may be seen, and some patients have been described with mild neurologic features of Sjögren-Larsson syndrome without associated skin disease.[42]

Sjögren-Larsson syndrome results from mutations in fatty aldehyde dehydrogenase, a component of fatty alcohol: nicotinamide adenine dinucleotide oxidoreductase (FAO), which converts fatty alcohol to fatty acid.[39,43] Fatty alcohol is used for the biosynthesis of wax esters, which are largely produced in skin, and of glycerol ether lipids, which are prominent in myelin. Prenatal diagnosis of Sjögren-Larsson syndrome is possible by measurement of FAO activity in cultured aminocytes or chorionic cells, histologic analysis, and/or analysis of fetal DNA if the gene defect is known.[44]

NEUTRAL LIPID STORAGE DISEASE (CHANARIN-DORFMAN SYNDROME)

This autosomal recessive disorder is characterized by the multisystemic accumulation of neutral lipids (triglycerides).[45] Approximately 65% of affected patients have associated ichthyosis, which is always present at birth as congenital ichthyosiform erythroderma, or occasionally as a collodion baby. Hepatomegaly occurs in 46% of patients, although fatty liver may be universal. Liver transaminase levels are often elevated. Almost 70% of patients have either elevated serum creatine kinase activity or muscle weakness or both, usually mild and first symptomatic in adulthood. Other features may include ataxia, mental retardation, neurosensory hearing loss, and cataracts. Sections of skin show accumulation of neutral lipids, and these non–membrane-bound cytosolic triacylglycerol droplets are also found in liver, muscle, intestinal mucosae, and neutrophils. The vacuolated neutrophils are considered the most consistent marker for neutral lipid storage disease. The biochemical defect involves a recycling block in the conversion of stored triacylglycerol to diacylglycerol as a substrate for phospholipid synthesis.[46] A low-fat diet, including medium-chain triglycerides, may improve liver function and the skin,[47] especially if begun in early childhood.

NETHERTON'S SYNDROME

Netherton's syndrome should be suspected in the neonate with generalized scaling erythroderma, especially with failure to thrive (Fig. 16-7).[48] Affected infants are often born prematurely and develop the eruption in utero or during

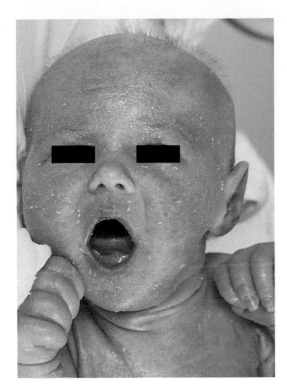

FIG. 16-7

A 32-day-old infant with failure to thrive, hypernatremic dehydration, and ichthyosiform erythroderma was determined to have Netherton's syndrome by microscopic examination of one of just a few sparse hair. Note the sparse hair secondary to trichorrhexis invaginata. The infant died of sepsis at 3 months of age. (Courtesy of Dr. Bernice Krafchik, Toronto, Canada).

the first weeks of life. A collodion baby phenotype is not associated. The failure to thrive is often profound, requiring hospitalization for nutritional support and correction of the hypernatremic dehydration that may be associated.[49,50,51] Patients may have diarrhea, and occasionally demonstrate villus atrophy if intestinal biopsy is performed. Most patients have increased levels of IgE, but other laboratory and clinical evidence of immune dysfunction may be present as well. The increased risk of sepsis occurs as a result of both the abnormal skin barrier and the associated immune defects that are only in part owing to malnutrition.

The classic hair shaft abnormality, trichorrhexis invaginata ("bamboo hairs," "ball-and-socket deformity"), is thought to result from a defect in keratinization of the internal root sheath. Multiple hairs from different areas should be examined, since only 20% to 50% of hairs may

be affected. Although trichorrhexis invaginata may be present in the neonatal period, delayed and sparse hair growth at this time, as well as the easy breakage of these hairs, makes demonstration of the hair defect in the neonatal period difficult. Skin biopsy sections show subacute or chronic seborrheic or psoriasiform dermatitis with spongiosis. The stratum corneum is thin and focally parakeratotic, and the granular layer is decreased.[49] Hair shaft abnormalities have been considered the only pathognomonic features, but recently electron microscopic studies have revealed features in skin biopsy specimens that are specific to Netherton's, particularly the premature secretion of lamellar body contents, foci of electron-dense material separating lipid membranes, and disturbed maturation of lamellar membrane structures.[52] Netherton's must be distinguished in the neonatal period from several other disorders with extensive scaling erythroderma, failure to thrive, and increased risk of infection, particularly several immunodeficiency disorders,[53] congenital psoriasis,[54] and acrodermatitis enteropathica.

Ichthyosis linearis circumflexa, the characteristic skin change associated with Netherton's, is not seen before 2 years of age, and only occurs eventually in 70% of patients.[55] It manifests episodically, often lasting for a few weeks, then clearing for weeks or months. The ichthyosiform erythroderma, however, frequently improves with increasing age. The atopic diathesis becomes problematic in two thirds of patients, with the development of pruritic atopic dermatitis and commonly urticaria, angioedema, asthma, and/or anaphylaxis.

The underlying molecular basis for Netherton's syndrome is mutations in SPINK5, a serine protease inhibitor.[56] Therapy of Netherton's syndrome is extremely difficult. Despite their pruritic, erythematous skin, patients with Netherton's syndrome tend to respond poorly to topical steroids. The application of keratolytic agents or administration of systemic retinoids often worsens the severity of the disorder, and their use is inappropriate during the neonatal period. Most patients prefer to use bland, thick emollients as the only therapy throughout life.

TRICHOTHIODYSTROPHY (TAY SYNDROME, IBIDS SYNDROME, PIBIDS SYNDROME, SIBIDS SYNDROME)

Three autosomal recessive subsets of trichothiodystrophy (TTD) are associated with ichthyosis: IBIDS (ichthyosis with brittle hair, intellectual impairment, decreased fertility, and short stature), PIBIDS (IBIDS with photosensitivity; Tay syndrome), and SIBIDS (IBIDS with osteosclerosis). Of these, PIBIDS is the most common, comprising approximately 50% of cases of TTD. Several other clinical features may be associated, including low birth weight, nail dystrophy, increased susceptibility to infection, neutropenia, hypothyroidism, nystagmus, optic atrophy, cataracts, and hypertonia.[57] Not uncommonly, patients die of sepsis during childhood.

Neonates with TTD and ichthyosis are usually born with a collodion membrane. The severity of the ichthyosis after the membrane is shed is variable, ranging from a mild to severe lamellar ichthyosis phenotype. In trichothiodystrophy, the hair has a 10% to 50% decrease in sulfur content, leading to brittle hair that shows transverse fractures (trichoschisis), a decreased cuticular layer with twisting, and a nodular appearance that mimics trichorrhexis nodosa. Polarizing microscopy shows a "tiger-tail" pattern of alternating light and dark bands consistent with the alternating content of sulfur in the hair. Examination of hairs at birth by polarizing microscopy may not reveal the tiger-tail pattern, and repeated examinations may be necessary later in the first months of life.[58]

Cells from patients with PIBIDS show decreased DNA repair levels similar to those of patients with xeroderma pigmentosum (XP), but the development of skin cancer has not been described. Most repair-deficient TTD patients have been assigned to XP complementation repair group D,[59] which also includes patients with both xeroderma pigmentosum and Cockayne syndrome. The mutated gene, ERCC2, is important for transcription, as well as DNA repair, so that the brittle hair of PIBIDS syndrome may result from decreased transcription of the genes that encode the sulfur-rich matrix of hair and nails. Prenatal diagnosis of PIBIDS has been performed by DNA repair measurements in amniotic fluid cells with confirmation by polarizing microscopic analysis of fetal hair.[60]

KID SYNDROME

The constellation of vascularizing keratitis, ichthyosiform hyperkeratosis, and neurosensory deafness are the characteristic features of KID syndrome. The underlying defect is unknown. Vertical transmission suggests an autosomal dominant disorder, but the description of KID syndrome in two children of consanguineous unaffected parents and most recently in two half siblings[61] would be consistent with either autosomal recessive inheritance or autosomal dominant transmission with parental mosaicism. Patients with KID syndrome are usually born with erythematous or erythrokeratodermatous skin that is mildly scaling; in 7% of patients these skin features develop during the first 4 weeks of life.[62] The characteristic thick, leathery skin

with tiny stippled papules develops during the first year of life, particularly during the first 3 months (Fig. 16-8), Well-defined verrucous hyperkeratotic plaques develop in 90% of patients, often localized to the face and limbs. Diffuse palmoplantar hyperkeratosis with a stippled or leathery pattern also occurs in almost all patients. Alopecia occurs overall in 80% of patients, ranging from minimal loss of eyebrows or eyelashes to total scalp alopecia; in 25% of patients, the alopecia is congenital. An additional 17% of patients have sparse, fine hair without frank alopecia. Nails are dystrophic in the majority of patients. Sweating may be decreased or absent. Biopsy of skin shows nonspecific acanthosis with papillomatosis and basket weave hyperkeratosis. Hair follicles may be atrophic.

The hearing loss tends to be neurosensory, congenital, and nonprogressive. It can be detected in the neonate by brainstem-evoked auditory potential testing. Unlike the auditory changes, ophthalmologic features are progressive and develop in childhood or early adolescence most commonly, although photophobia from birth has been de-

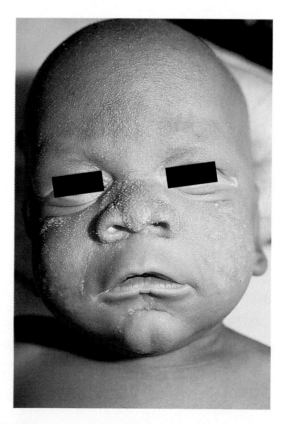

FIG. 16-8
Thick, leathery skin with tiny papules in an infant with KID syndrome.

scribed. The keratoconjunctivitis sicca with corneal vascularization leads to pannus formation and markedly decreased visual acuity.

Approximately 45% of patients have recurrent infections, especially bacterial and candidal infections of the skin, auditory canals, and eyes. Some patients have shown evidence of immunodeficiency, with moderate increases in IgE levels, defective chemotaxis, and absent lymphocyte proliferative responses to *Candida albicans*.[63] Squamous cell carcinoma of the skin and of the tongue has been described in more than 10% of patients, and may occur during childhood. Therapy is supportive, but corneal transplant and cochlear implants[64] have been successfully performed to treat corneal vascularization and the hearing loss, respectively. Oral fluconazole therapy of recalcitrant fungating candidiasis can result in complete resolution and remission for at least a year.[65]

CHILD SYNDROME

The term *CHILD syndrome* is an acronym for congenital hemidysplasia with ichthyosiform nevus and limb defects. The condition occurs almost exclusively in girls, and is presumed to be lethal in affected males. The only case in a boy is thought to represent early postzygotic mosaicism.[66] The inflammatory ichthyosiform skin lesion of CHILD syndrome may be present at birth or develop during the first few months of life.[66,67] It is characterized by yellow, waxy scaling and is strikingly unilateral, generally with a sharp demarcation at the ventral and dorsal midline regions (Fig. 16-9). Streaks of inflammation and scaling can also follow Blaschko's lines, with involvement of the apparently unaffected side of the body. Similarly, streaks of normal skin may be interspersed within the area of the CHILD nevus. With increasing age, the skin lesions may improve or clear spontaneously, but lesions in intertriginous areas tend to persist and be the most severely affected sites (ptychotropism).[68] The skin lesions of CHILD syndrome nevus can occur without any other abnormalities, but the occurrence of all features of CHILD syndrome in a sibling of a patient with only the CHILD nevus suggests variable expressivity within the spectrum of CHILD syndrome.[69]

Ipsilateral skeletal hypoplasia of a variable degree is an important feature of CHILD syndrome. As with the skin changes, unilaterality is not absolute, and slight changes may be present on the contralateral side. Punctate epiphyseal calcifications may be demonstrable by roentgenograms but tend to disappear after the first few years of life. Cardiovascular and renal abnormalities are the major viscera affected in CHILD syndrome, although anomalies of other viscera have been described.[67]

Biopsy of skin lesions shows epidermal acanthosis with marked parakeratosis alternating with orthokeratosis. Basophilic ghost cells of the granular layer are common. The papillary dermis is often filled with histiocytes showing foamy cytoplasm, resulting in the characteristic histopathologic pattern of verrucous xanthoma. Most patients with CHILD syndrome have mutations in 3β-hydroxysteroid dehydrogenase;[70] a mutation in emopamil binding protein (3β-hydroxysteroid-Δ^8, Δ^7-isomerase) has also been described.[71]

The nevus of CHILD syndrome needs to be distinguished from inflammatory linear verrucous epidermal nevus and linear psoriasis by the histopathologic features and the constellation of other clinical manifestations, if present. CHILD syndrome shares features with Conradi-Hünermann syndrome (see the following discussion), including the prevalence in girls with a presumed X-linked dominant inheritance pattern, ichthyosiform erythroderma,

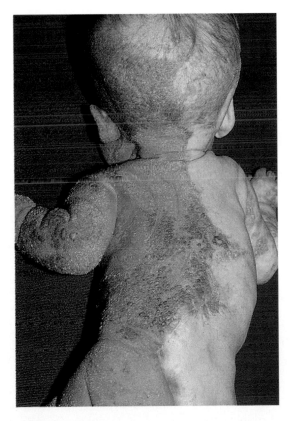

FIG. 16-9
Sharply demarcated, erythematous ichthyosiform lesions with mostly unilateral distribution are seen in this infant with hemidysplasia and CHILD syndrome. Thickened, yellow-brown scale in a whorled pattern is seen within areas of the CHILD nevus.

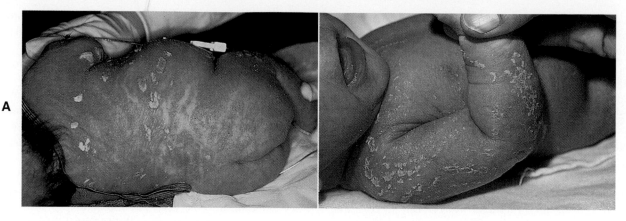

FIG. 16-10

A, Thick, psoriasiform scaling overlying erythema in a 1-month-old baby girl with chondrodysplasia punctata. Note the shortened forelimbs. As the scaling desquamated, the underlying erythema along Blaschko's lines became more apparent. **B,** The pattern of scale along Blaschko's lines is more evident in this neonate with chondrodysplasia punctata. (From Paller AS. Ichthyosis in the neonate. In Dyall-Smith D, Marks R, eds. Dermatology at the millennium: Overview of past achievements, current knowledge and future trends. London: Parthenon Publishing Group, 1998: p 582.)

limb reduction defects, stippled epiphyses, and peroxisomal defects. The unilateral nature of the nevus and limb deformities helps to distinguish these conditions but CHILD syndrome may represent a mosaic form of Conradi's.[71]

CONRADI-HÜNERMANN SYNDROME (X-LINKED CHONDRODYSPLASIA PUNCTATA)

Most cases of chondrodysplasia punctata seen by dermatologists are the X-linked dominant Conradi-Hünermann form.[72] Affected neonates are usually female, because the disorder is considered lethal to male fetuses. However, Conradi's syndrome has been described in a few male patients with and without Kleinfelter's syndrome.[73] At birth, patients most commonly have patterned erythroderma with overlying thin to thick psoriasiform scale (Fig. 16-10). In severe cases, generalized ichthyosiform erythroderma[72] occurs, and later evolves into the typical patterning along Blaschko's lines. Involvement may be predominantly unilateral. Additional features are limb reduction, typically asymmetric, and facies with frontal bossing, saddle nose, and malar hypoplasia. Asymmetric, focal stippled calcifications of the epiphyseal regions are common. With advancing age, the ichthyosiform erythroderma and stippling improves, leaving finer scaling without underlying erythema and follicular atrophoderma. Cicatricial alopecia occurs as scalp scaling resolves. Cataracts usually develop later during childhood but may be present at birth.[73]

The underlying molecular basis is mutations in empopamil binding protein (3β-hydroxysteroid-Δ^8, Δ^7-isomerase), which is involved in plasmalogen synthesis.[74] Chondrodysplasia punctata can be inherited by both autosomal and X-linked patterns, and also as a result of environmental insults, particularly fetal exposure to warfarin.[72] The differential diagnosis usually includes two other forms of chondrodysplasia punctata: autosomal recessive rhizomelic chondrodysplasia punctata[75] and X-linked recessive chondrodysplasia punctata with steroid sulfatase deficiency.[76] The rhizomelic form is also associated with peroxisomal defects, although multiple. The ichthyosis occurs in approximately one third of patients and is poorly described. Affected patients have developmental retardation and tend to die as infants. The X-linked recessive form occurs as a contiguous gene deletion syndrome of Xp, not at the site of chondrodysplasia punctata. The ichthyosis is consistent with recessive X-linked ichthyosis, but stippled epiphyses are associated. Affected infants are deficient in steroid sulfatase activity, and have no peroxisome defects.

ERYTHROKERATODERMA VARIABILIS

This autosomal dominant disorder manifests as two types of skin changes. Some patients have migratory patches of

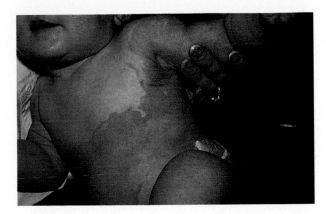

FIG. 16-11
Sharply demarcated, erythematous hyperkeratotic plaques lesions on the trunk in a child with erythrokeratoderma variabilis.

erythema, which are often targetoid or circinate and last for days to months. With time, these lesions become more fixed, erythematous, and hyperkeratotic (Fig. 16-11). In other patients, the disorder manifests as sharply demarcated, fixed hyperkeratotic plaques. Both types of lesions may be seen in the same patient. The typical areas of involvement are the extensor surfaces of the extremities, trunk, buttocks, and face. The palms and soles are not usually involved.

Lesions are present at birth in up to one third of patients.[77,78] Most patients begin to show evidence of involvement during the first year of life, with progression during childhood and stabilization at puberty. Later improvement has been described, including clearing with fevers. There are usually no extracutaneous features, although ataxia has been described.[79] Mutations in the gene for connexin 31 have recently been shown to cause erythrokeratodermia variabilis.[80] Treatment with systemic retinoids has resulted in improvement or clearing.

ERYTHROKERATODERMA PROGRESSIVE SYMMETRICA

This autosomal dominant disorder is characterized by symmetric erythematous scaling plaques that may spare the trunk, but are commonly found on the knees, buttocks, and groin region.[81,82] The palms and soles are affected in approximately 50% of patients, and the face is occasionally involved. Features are usually present during the first few years of life. Skin biopsies show acanthosis with perinuclear vacuolization of granular cells. Ultrastructural studies show lipid vacuoles in the stratum corneum, and increased numbers of swollen mitochondria in granular cells.[81]

ICHTHYOSIS FOLLICULARIS (IFAP SYNDROME)

The underlying gene defect in patients with IFAP is unknown. The predominance of the disorder in male patients suggests an X-linked recessive disorder, although an autosomal recessive disorder is also possible. Patients are born with thickening of the skin, including the palms and soles, with generalized prominent follicular keratoses and mild erythema.[83,84] The scalp is hairless, and severe photophobia is noted from birth. The nails may be dystrophic, and follicular pustules may be present. Some patients have had short stature, psychomotor delay, and/or seizures. Biopsies show a hyperkeratotic stratum corneum with a thinned dermis. The hair follicles are atrophic and shortened with abnormal localization of the bulbs to the deep portion of the dermis, rather than a subcutaneous location. There are no normal hair shafts, and sebaceous glands are absent.

CHIME SYNDROME

The acronym CHIME derives from coloboma, heart defects, ichthyosiform dermatosis, mental retardation, and ear anomalies, including conductive hearing loss. The skin is thick and dry at birth. Pruritic ichthyotic erythema develops during the first month of life, sometimes as sharply marginated plaques, and is typically migratory. Examination of biopsied skin specimens shows nonspecific changes.[85] The hair may be fine and sparse, with trichorrhexis nodosa seen by light microscopic examination. The colobomas are most commonly retinal, although choroidal colobomas have been described.[86] A variety of heart defects have been associated, including tetralogy of Fallot, transposition of the great vessels, pulmonic stenosis, and ventricular septal defect.[85] Typical facial features include hypertelorism with a broad, flat nasal root, upslanting palpebral fissures, epicanthal folds and ptosis, macrostoma with a long columella but short philtrum, and full lips. The ears tend to be cupped with rolled helices. Brachydactyly is a constant feature. Other frequent characteristics include seizures and a wide-based gait. Cleft palate and renal or urologic anomalies have been described. The underlying defect is unknown. CHIME syndrome must be distinguished from other ichthyotic disorders of infancy with retardation and seizures, particularly Sjögren-Larsson syndrome, Netherton's syndrome, KID syndrome, and IBIDS syndrome. The characteristic ocular, cardiac, ear, and dysmorphic features help confirm the diagnosis.

GAUCHER'S DISEASE

Gaucher's disease (β-glucocerebrosidase deficiency) is an autosomal recessive disorder that results from the deficient activity of lysosomal glucocerebrosidase. The acute infantile cerebral form, type 2 of three subsets, is characterized by the onset during infancy of neurologic symptoms and hepatosplenomegaly. Several infants with this form of Gaucher's have been born with a collodion membrane.[16,87,88] The enzyme deficiency with resultant abnormalities in glucocerebrosidase degradation appears directly responsible for the abnormal skin of these infants. Glucosylceramide and ceramide are components of the intercellular bilayers in the stratum corneum that participate in skin permeability barrier function, so that the absence of glucocerebrosidase leads to abnormal skin thickening and increased transepidermal water loss.

PALMOPLANTAR KERATODERMAS

The keratoderma of many forms of hereditary palmoplantar keratoderma is first apparent during the first months of life, while in others the keratoderma is not seen until early to late childhood (e.g., punctate keratoderma, keratoderma striata, Howell-Evans).[89] In the neonatal period, the affected areas may appear hyperhydrated (Fig. 16-12). The majority of types of palmoplantar keratoderma are autosomal dominant. In the Unna form of palmoplantar keratoderma (nonepidermolytic), the palms and soles are usually red at birth or soon thereafter. The skin progressively thickens on the palms and soles, starting at the margins and extending centrally, with red borders that usually disappear after several years. Keratotic lesions may occasionally be found on the dorsum of the hands and feet, the volar wrists, and the knees and elbows. The overall extent of involvement is variable. In Greither syndrome (transgrediens form), the onset of thickening tends to be later, but the diffuse palmoplantar keratoderma extends onto the dorsum of the hands and feet. The knees, elbows, shins, and forearms are often involved. Palmoplantar hyperhidrosis is commonly associated with the nonepidermolytic form. A mild defect of keratin 1 and defects in keratins 6a and 16 have been described in families with nonepidermolytic palmoplantar keratoderma.

Vorner palmoplantar keratoderma (epidermolytic palmoplantar keratoderma) can also begin at an early age, and is clinically indistinguishable from the nonepidermolytic form during the first years of life when the keratoderma is confined to the palms and soles. Epidermolytic palmoplantar keratoderma results from mutations in keratin 9, a gene that is only expressed in the skin of the palms and soles, limiting its distribution of expression.[32] It should be noted that descendants of the family described by Thost as having nonepidermolytic palmoplantar keratoderma actually have keratin 9 mutations,[90] demonstrating that the epidermolytic hyperkeratosis found in biopsy sections is an inconstant feature that may require several biopsies for detection.

The keratoses of Vohwinkel syndrome also are first noted shortly after birth, and gradually develop into the typical

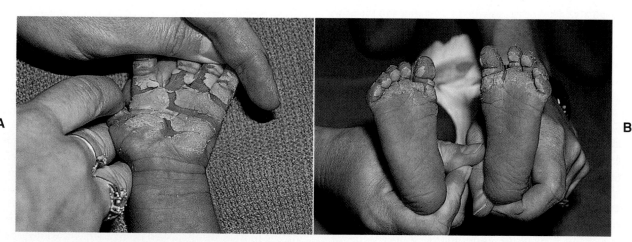

A   B

FIG. 16-12
Palmar-plantar keratoderma. Note hyperhydrated skin with cracking and peeling.

honeycombed diffuse hyperkeratoses with starfishlike keratoses on the backs of the hands, fingers, and toes. The constricting bands of the digits (pseudoainhum) first develop at 5 years of age or after, and can lead to autoamputation, as well as decreased motility of the hands. Some patients with Vohwinkel syndrome have alopecia, and an erythrokeratoderma has been described as well. The gene defect involves mutations in the gene that codes for loricrin.[91] Patients with deafness and the palmoplantar changes of Vohwinkel have connexin 26 mutations not loricrin gene mutations.

Mal de Meleda, an autosomal recessive form of palmoplantar keratoderma, is not congenital but is present during the first 6 months of life as a diffuse palmoplantar keratoderma. The dorsal surface of the hands and feet are involved, and keratotic plaques tend to be present on the knees and elbows as well.[92] Constricting bands surrounding the digits are typical and may result in autoamputation. Koilonychia, nail thickening, and subungual hyperkeratosis are usually associated. Mild perioral erythema and hyperkeratosis may be present.

OLMSTED SYNDROME

This extremely rare disorder usually presents with progressive thickening of the palms and soles during the first few years of life.[93] These begin as discrete lesions that become more confluent with time. The borders of keratoderma are erythematous. Autoamputation from progressive digital constriction is typical. The periorificial areas become hyperkeratotic with fissured plaques after the onset of palmoplantar keratoderma. This involvement of periorificial areas, particularly perioral, perianal, perinasal, pericrural, and periumbilical, distinguishes this condition from other forms of palmoplantar keratoderma. Oral leukokeratosis, alopecia, and nail dystrophy have been described in association. The cause of this disorder is unknown. While most cases are sporadic, autosomal dominant inheritance has been described.

TYROSINEMIA II

Tryosinemia II (Richner-Hanhart syndrome) is an autosomal recessive disorder, caused by a deficiency of hepatic tyrosine aminotransferase,[94] that results in elevated tyrosine levels in the plasma and urine. The ocular manifestations of the disorder appear soon after birth.[95] The early cutaneous lesions may be seen during the first year of life as sharply demarcated, yellowish keratotic papules of the palmar and plantar surfaces, but more commonly appear later, sometimes as late as the second decade. The lesions become more erythematous, erosive, and painful with time. Nail dystrophy may be associated. Photophobia and bilateral tearing commonly occur within the first 3 months of life, and progress to corneal erosions. Ocular lesions are typically transitory, and are subject to intermittent relapses. The corneal lesions are frequently misdiagnosed as herpetic keratitis, and remissions may be misinterpreted as response to antiviral therapy. The eye changes occasionally develop after the skin manifestations. Retardation to varying degrees has been described in less than half of affected patients. The treatment of choice is dietary restriction of tyrosine with a low-phenylalanine, low-tyrosine diet.

RESTRICTIVE DERMOPATHY

Neonates with this lethal autosomal recessive disorder of unknown cause are born with rigid skin, attributed to fetal akinesia or hypokinesia deformation sequence.[96,97,98] Polyhydramnios with decreased fetal movements usually eventuates in premature delivery at approximately 31 weeks' gestational age. Premature rupture of the membranes and an enlarged placenta with a short umbilical cord are often associated. The skin typically is thin, shiny, and red with prominent vessels. Scaling and erosions are frequently seen (Fig. 16-13). The facies are characterized by micrognathia, a small open mouth (O-shaped), pinched nares with choanal atresia or stenosis, and flattened or low-set pinnae. The constraint of movement in utero also leads to the flexion contractures of the joints, and bony changes such as poor ossification of the clavicle; overtubulation of the radius, ulna, and distal phalanges; and widened sutures and large fontanelles. Natal teeth have been described in 25% to 50% of the patients with restrictive dermopathy. Most

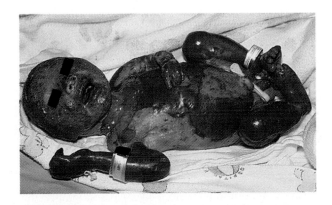

FIG. 16-13
Eroded, shiny skin is seen in this neonate with restrictive dermopathy.

patients die of pulmonary hypoplasia with respiratory insufficiency or sepsis.

Histopathologic examination of skin biopsy sections shows a thick epidermis, and a thin dermis with a paucity and hypoplasia of cutaneous appendages. Collagen bundles are abnormally arranged, and elastic fibers are almost absent. Most patients die during the neonatal period; the longest survivor with restrictive dermopathy survived until 4 months of age. The cause of restrictive dermopathy is unknown. Prenatal diagnosis is difficult, in that the skin biopsy at 20 weeks' gestational age may be normal.[99] In addition, the onset of intrauterine growth retardation, restricted fetal movement, and polyhydramnios may occur late in gestation.

NEU-LAXOVA SYNDROME

Neu-Laxova syndrome is a rare, lethal, autosomal recessive trait characterized by severe intrauterine growth retardation, microcephaly with abnormal brain development, edema and ichthyosis.[100,101] The lack of brain development is characterized by lissencephaly and agenesis of the corpus callosum. Characteristic facial features include a slanted forehead, protuberant eyes, a flattened nose, deformed ears, micrognathia, and a short neck. Microphthalmia and cleft palate are occasionally associated. The limbs, fingers, and toes are abnormal, with syndactyly, hypoplasia, and contractures. Skeletal roentgenograms often show poor mineralization. The craniofacial and limb abnormalities are related to the reduced intrauterine movement and therefore defined as fetal akinesia/hypokinesis sequence, as has been described in other syndromes. The ichthyosis is present at birth, but varies from mildly scaling skin to a harlequin fetus appearance. Histologic findings are nonspecific and show the acanthosis and orthokeratosis of lamellar ichthyosis. Excessive subcutaneous adipose tissue and myxomatous connective tissue may contribute to the characteristic edema.

ECTODERMAL DYSPLASIAS (see Chapter 24)

Scaling of the skin during the newborn period has been described in 70% of patients with X-linked hypohidrotic ectodermal dysplasia.[102] Skin has been described as "like plastic," peeling off in sheets, and "like a snake peeling." Some infants have been described as very dry at birth, and others as collodion membrane-like. Later in infancy, the typical facial features, sparsity of hair, decreased ability to sweat, and eventually dental abnormalities allow the diagnosis to be confirmed. Patients tend to have an increased

risk of upper respiratory tract infections and atopy, particularly manifesting as asthma and atopic dermatitis. The gene defect for X-linked hypohidrotic ectodermal dysplasia has recently been identified as dyskerin, which codes for a protein of keratinocytes, hair follicles, and sweat glands that appears to be important in epithelial-mesenchymal signaling.[103]

REFERENCES

1. Buxman MM, Goodkin PE, Fahrenbach WH, et al. Harlequin ichthyosis with epidermal lipid abnormality. Arch Dermatol 1977;115:189-193.
2. Craig JM, Goldsmith LA, Baden HP. An abnormality of keratin in the harlequin fetus. Pediatrics 1970;46:437-440.
3. Baden HP, Kubilus J, Rosenbaum K, et al. Keratinization in the harlequin fetus. Arch Dermatol 1982;18:14-18.
4. Dale BA, Kam E. Harlequin ichthyosis. Variability in expression and hypothesis for disease mechanism. Arch Dermatol 1993;129:1471-1477.
5. Dale BA, Holbrook KA, Fleckman P, et al. Heterogeneity in harlequin ichthyosis, an inborn error of epidermal keratinization: Variable morphology and structural protein expression and a defect in lamellar granules. J Invest Dermatol 1990;94:6-18.
6. Milner ME, O'Guin WM, Holbrook KA, et al. Abnormal lamellar granules in harlequin ichthyosis. J Invest Dermatol 1992;99:824-829.
7. Akiyama M, Kim D-K, Main DM, et al. Characteristic morphologic abnormality of harlequin ichthyosis detected in amniotic fluid cells. J Invest Dermatol 1994;192:210-213.
8. Lawlor F, Peiris S. Harlequin fetus successfully treated with etretinate. Br J Dermatol 1985;112:585-590.
9. Ward PS, Jones RD. Successful treatment of a harlequin fetus—a case report. Arch Dis Child 1989;64:1309-1311.
10. Roberts LJ. Long-term survival of a harlequin fetus. J Am Acad Dermatol 1989;21:335-339.
11. Rogers M, Scraf C. Harlequin baby treated with etretinate. Pediatr Dermatol 1989;6:216-221.
12. Prasad RS, Pejaver RK, Hassan A, et al. Management and follow-up of harlequin siblings. Br J Dermatol 1994;130:650-653.
13. Haftek M, Cambazard F, Dhouailly D, et al. A longitudinal study of a harlequin infant presenting clinically as non-bullous congenital ichthyosiform erythroderma. Br J Dermatol 1996;135:448-453.
14. Akiyama M, Yoneda K, Kim SY, et al. Cornified envelope proteins and keratins are normally distributed in harlequin ichthyosis. J Cutan Pathol 1996;23:571-575.
15. Larregue M, Gharbi R, Daniel J, et al. Le bébé collodion évolution a propos de 29 cas. Ann Dermatol Venereol 1976;103:31-56.
16. Lui K, Commens C, Choong R, et al. Collodion babies with Gaucher's disease. Arch Dis Child 1988;63:854-856.
17. Frenk E, de Techtermann F. Self-healing collodion baby: Evidence for autosomal recessive inheritance. Pediatr Dermatol 1992;9:95-97.
18. Garty BZ, Wiseman Y, Metzger A, et al. Hypernatremic dehydration and hypothermia in congenital lamellar ichthyosis. Pediatr Dermatol 1985;3:65-68.

19. Buyse L, Graves C, Marks R, et al. Collodion baby dehydration: The danger of high transepidermal water loss. Br J Dermatol 1993;129:86-88.

20. Perlman M, Bar-Ziv J. Congenital ichthyosis and neonatal pulmonary disease. Pediatrics 1974;53:573-575.

21. Freiberg R, Choate KA, Deng H, et al. A model of corrective gene transfer in X-linked ichthyosis. Hum Molec Genet 1997;6:927-933.

22. Traupe H, Kolde G, Happle R. Autosomal dominant lamellar ichthyosis: A new skin disorder. Clin Genet 1984;26:457-461.

23. Williams ML, Elias PM. Heterogeneity in autosomal recessive ichthyosis: Clinical and biochemical differentiation of lamellar ichthyosis and non-bullous congenital ichthyosiform erythroderma. Arch Dermatol 1985;121:477-488.

24. Hazell M, Marks R. Clinical, histologic and cell kinetic discriminants between lamellar ichthyosis and non-bullous congenital ichthyosiform erythroderma. Arch Dermatol 1985;121:489-493.

25. Huber M, Rettler I, Bernasconi K, et al. Mutations of keratinocyte transglutaminase in lamellar ichthyosis. Science 1995;267:525-558.

26. Russell LJ, DiGiovanna JJ, Rogers GR, et al. Mutations in the gene for transglutaminase 1 in autosomal recessive lamellar ichthyosis. Nat Genet 1995;9:279-283.

27. Huber M, Rettler I, Bernasconi K, et al. Lamellar ichthyosis is genetically heterogeneous-cases with normal keratinocyte transglutaminase. J Invest Dermatol 1995;105:653-654.

28. Parmentier L, Lakhdar H, Blanchet-Bardon C, et al. Mapping of a second locus for lamellar ichthyosis to chromosome 2q33-35. Hum Molec Genet 1996;5:555-559.

29. Schorderet DF, Huber M, Laurini RN, et al. Prenatal diagnosis of lamellar ichthyosis by direct mutational analysis of the keratinocyte transglutaminase gene. Prenatal Diagn 1997;17:483-486.

30. Choate KA, Medalie DA, Morgan JR, et al. Corrective gene transfer in the human skin disorder lamellar ichthyosis. Nat Medicine 1996;2:1263-1267.

31. Srebrnik A, Tur E, Perluk C, et al. Dorfman-Chanarin syndrome. J Am Acad Dermatol 1987;17:801-808.

32. Paller AS. Unravelling the classic concepts of patterns of inheritance: Lessons from the molecular bases for skin blistering. Am J Pathol 148:727-731, 1996.

33. Golbus MS, Sagebiel RW, Filly RA, et al. Prenatal diagnosis of congenital bullous ichthyosiform erythroderma (epidermolytic hyperkeratosis) by fetal skin biopsy. N Engl J Med 1980;302:93-95.

34. Rothnagel JA, Longley MA, Holder RA, et al. Prenatal diagnosis of epidermolytic hyperkeratosis by direct gene sequencing. J Invest Dermatol 1994;102:13-16.

35. Kanerva L, Karvonen J, Oikarinen A, et al. Ichthyosis hystrix (Curth-Macklin). Light and electron microscopic studies performed before and after etretinate treatment. Arch Dermatol 1984;120:1218-1223.

36. Bonifas JM, Bare JW, Chen MA, et al. Evidence against keratin gene mutations in a family with ichthyosis hystrix Curth-Macklin. J Invest Dermatol 1993;101:890-891.

37. Janin A, Copin M-C, Dubos JP, et al. Familial peeling skin syndrome with eosinophilia: Clinical, histologic, and ultrastructural study of three cases. Arch Pathol Lab Med 1996;120:662-665.

38. Jagell S, Liden S. Ichthyosis in Sjogren-Larsson syndrome. Clin Genet 1982;21:243-252.

39. Rizzo WB. Sjögren-Larsson syndrome. Semin Dermatol 1993;12:210-218.

40. Lacour M. Update on Sjögren-Larsson syndrome. Dermatology 1996;193:77-82.

41. Ito M, Oguro K, Sato Y. Ultrastructural study of the skin in Sjögren-Larsson syndrome. Arch Dermatol Res 1991;283:141-148.

42. Nigro JF, Rizzo WB, Esterly NB. Redefining Sjögren-Larsson syndrome: Atypical findings in three siblings and implications regarding diagnosis. J Am Acad Dermatol 1996;35:678-684.

43. DeLaurenzi V, Rogers GR, Hamrock DJ, et al. Sjögren-Larsson syndrome is caused by mutations in the fatty aldehyde dehydrogenase gene. Nat Genet 1996;12:52-57.

44. Sillen A, Holmgren G, Wadelius C. First prenatal diagnosis by mutation analysis in a family with Sjogren-Larsson syndrome. Prenatal Diagn 1997;17:1147-1149.

45. Igal RA, Rhoads JM, Coleman RA. Neutral lipid storage disease with fatty liver and cholestasis. J Pediatr Gastroenterol Nutr 1997;25:541-547.

46. Igal RA, Coleman RA. Acylglycerol recycling from triacylglycerol to phospholipid, not lipase activity, is defective in neutral lipid storage disease fibroblasts. J Biol Chem 1996;271:16644-16651.

47. Kakourou T, Drogari E, Christomanou H, et al. Neutral lipid storage disease-response to dietary intervention (letter). Arch Dis Child 1997;77:184.

48. Judge MR, Morgan G, Harper JI. A clinical and immunological study of Netherton's syndrome. Br J Dermatol 1994;131:615-621.

49. Hausser I, Anton-Lamprecht I. Severe congenital generalized exfoliative erythroderma in newborns and infants: A possible sign of Netherton's syndrome. Pediatr Dermatol 1996;13:183-199.

50. De Wolf K, Ferster A, Sass U, et al. Netherton's syndrome: A severe neonatal disease. A case report. Dermatology 1996;192:400-402.

51. Garty B-Z. Hypernatremia in Netherton's syndrome (letter). Br Med J 1987;117:672.

52. Fartasch M, Williams ML, Elias PM. Altered lamellar body secretion and stratum corneum membrane structure in Netherton's syndrome: Differentiation from other infantile erythrodermas and pathogenic implications. Arch Dermatol, 1999 (in press).

53. Glover MT, Atherton DJ, Levinsky RJ. Syndrome of erythroderma, failure to thrive and diarrhea in infancy: A manifestation of immunodeficiency. Pediatrics 1988;81:66-72.

54. Shwayder T, Banerjee S. Netherton syndrome presenting as congenital psoriasis. Pediatr Dermatol 1997;14:473-476.

55. Greene SL, Muller SA. Netherton's syndrome: Report of a case and review of the literature. J Am Acad Dermatol 1985;13:329-337.

56. Chavanas S, Bodemer C, Rochat A, et al. Mutations in SPINK5, encoding a serine protease inhibitor, cause Netherton syndrome. Nat Genet 2000;25:141-142.

57. Hersh JH, Klein LR, Joyce MR, et al. Trichothiodystrophy and associated anomalies: A variant of SIBIDS or new symptom complex? Pediatr Dermatol 1993;10:117-122.

58. Brusasco A, Restano L, Cambiaghi S, et al. The typical "tiger tail" pattern of the hair shaft in trichothiodystrophy may not be evident at birth. Arch Dermatol 1997;133:249.

59. Kleijer WJ, Beemer FA, Boom BW: Intermittent hair loss in a child with PIBI(D)S syndrome and trichthiodystrophy with defective DNA repair-xeroderma pigmentosum group D. Am J Med Genet 1994;52:227-230.

60. Sarasin A, Blanchet-Bardon C, Renault G, et al. Prenatal diagnosis in a subset of trichothiodystrophy patients defective in DNA repair. Br J Dermatol 1992;127:485-491.

61. Koné-Paut I, Hesse S, Palix C, et al. Keratitis, ichthyosis, and deafness (KID) syndrome in half sibs. Pediatr Dermatol 1998;15:219-221.

62. Caceres-Rios H, Tamayo-Sanchez L, Duran-Mckinster C, et al. Keratitis, ichthyosis, and deafness (KID syndrome): Review of the literature and proposal of a new terminology. Pediatr Dermatol 1196;13:105-113.

63. Harms M, Gilardi S, Levy PM, et al. KID syndrome (keratitis, ichthyosis, and deafness) and chronic mucocutaneous candidiasis: Case report and review of the literature. Pediatr Dermatol 1984;2:1-7.

64. Hampton SM, Toner JG, Small J. Cochlear implant extrusion in a child with keratitis, ichthyosis and deafness syndrome. J Laryngol Otol 1997;111:465-467.

65. Shiraishi S, Murakami S, Miki Y. Oral fluconazole treatment of fungating candidiasis in the keratitis, ichthyosis and deafness (KID) syndrome. Br J Dermatol 1994;131:904-907.

66. Happle R, Effendy I, Megahed M, et al. CHILD syndrome in a boy. Am J Med Genet 1996;62:192-194.

67. Hebert AA, Esterly NB, Holbrook KA, et al. The CHILD syndrome: Histologic and ultrastructural studies. Arch Dermatol 1987;123:503-509.

68. Happle R. Ptychotropism as a cutaneous feature of the CHILD syndrome. J Am Acad Dermatol 1990;23:763-766.

69. Poiares-Baptista A, Cortesao JM. Nevus épidermique inflammatoire variable (NEVIL atypique? entité nouvelle?). Ann Dermatol Vénéréol 1979;106:443-450.

70. Konig A, Happle R, Bornholdt D, et al. Mutations in the NSDHL gene, encoding a 3β-hydroxysteroid dehydrogenase, cause CHILD syndrome. Am J Med Genet 2000;90:339-346.

71. Grange DK, Kratz LE, Braverman NE, et al. CHILD syndrome caused by deficiency of 3β-hydroxysteroid-Δ^8, Δ^7-isomerase. Am J Med Genet 2000;90:328-335.

72. Kalter DC, Clayton PT, Atherton DJ, et al. The X-linked dominant Conradi-Hünermann syndrome, presenting as congenital erythroderma. J Am Acad Dermatol 1989;21:248-256.

73. Happle R. X-linked dominant chondrodysplasia puctata/ichthyosis/cataract syndrome in males. Am J Med Genet 1995;57:493.

74. HasC, Bruckner-Tuderman L, Mullen D, et al. The Conradi-Hunermann-Happle syndrome (CDPX2) and emopamil binding protein: novel mutations, and somatic andgonadal mosalcism. Hum Mol Genet 2000;9:1951-1955.

75. Poulos A, Sheffield L, Sharp P, et al. Rhizomelic chondrodysplasia punctata: Clinical. pathologic, and biochemical findings in two patients. J Pediatr 1988;113:685-690.

76. Bick D, Curry CJR, McGill JR, et al. Male infant with ichthyosis, Kallmann syndrome, chondrodysplasia punctata, and an Xp chromosome deletion. Am J Med Genet 1989;33:100-107.

77. Knipe RC, Flowers FP, Johnson FR, et al. Erythrokeratoderma variabilis: Case report and review of the literature. Pediatr Dermatol 1995;12:21-23.

78. Armstrong DKB, Hutchinson TH, Walsh MY, et al. Autosomal recessive inheritance of erythrokeratoderma variabilis. Pediatr Dermatol 1997;14:355-358.

79. Giroux J-M, Barbeau A. Erythrokeratodermia with ataxia. Arch Dermatol 1972;106:183-188.

80. Richard G, Smith LE, Bailey RA, et al. Mutations in the human connexin gene GJB3 cause erythrokeratodermia variabilis. Nat Genet 1998;20:366-369.

81. Nazzaro V, Blanchet-Bardon C. Progressive symmetric erythrokeratodermita. Histological and ultrastructural study of a patient before and after eretinate. Arch Dermatol 1986;122:434-440.

82. Macfarlane AW, Chapman SJ, Verbov JL. Is erythrokeratoderma one disorder? A clinical and ultrastructural study of two siblings. Br J Dermatol 1991;124:487-491.

83. Hamm H, Meinceke P, Traupe H. Further delineation of the ichthyosis follicularis, atrichia, and photophobia syndrome. Eur J Pediatr 1991;150:627-629.

84. Eramo LR, Esterly NB, Zieserl EJ, et al. Ichthyosis follicularis with alopecia and photophobia. Arch Dermatol 1985;121:1167-1174.

85. Tinschert S, Anton-Lamprecht I, Albrecht-Nebe H, et al. Zunich neuroectodermal syndrome: Migratory ichthyosiform dermatosis, colobomas, and other abnormalities. Pediatr Dermatol 1996;13:363-371.

86. Shashi V, Zunich J, Kelly TE, et al. Neuroectodermal (CHIME) syndrome: An additional case with long term follow up of all reported cases. J Med Genet 1995;32:465-469.

87. Fujimoto A, Tayebi N, Sidransky E. Congenital ichthyosis preceding neurologic symptoms in two sibs with type 2 Gaucher disease. Am J Med Genet 1995;59:356-358.

88. Sidransky E, Sherer DM, Ginns EI. Gaucher disease in the neonate: A distinct Gaucher phenotype is analogous to a mouse model created by targeted disruption of the glucocerebrosidase gene. Pediatr Res 1992;32:494-498.

89. Lucker GPH, Van de Kerhof PCM, Steijlen PM. The hereditary palmoplantar keratoses: An updated review and classification. Br J Dermatol 1994;131:1-14.

90. Kuster W, Zebender D, Mensing H, et al. Vorner keratosis palmoplantaris diffusa. Clinical, formal genetic and molecular biology studies of 22 families. Hautarzt 1995;46:705-710.

91. Maestrini E, Monaco AP, et al. A molecular defect in ioricrin, the major component of the cornified cell envelope, underlies Vohwinkel's syndrome. Nat Genet 1996;13:70-77.

92. Lestringant GG, Frossard PM, Adeghate E, et al. Mal de Meleda: A report of four cases from the United Arab Emirates. Pediatr Dermatol 1997;14:186-191.

93. Perry HO, Daniel-Su WP. Olmsted syndrome. Semin Dermatol 1995;14:145-151.

94. Natt E, Kida K, Odievre M, et al. Point mutations in the tyrosine aminotransferase gene in tyrosinemia type II. Proc Natl Acad Sci USA 1992;89:9297-9301.

95. Benoldi D, Orsoni JB, Allegra F. Tyrosinemia type II: A challenge for ophthalmologists and dermatologists. Pediatr Dermatol 1997;14:110-112.

96. Sillevis Smitt JH, van Asperen CJ, Niessen CM, et al. Restrictive dermopathy: Report of 12 cases. Arch Dermatol 1998;134:577-579.

97. Welsh KM, Smoller BR, Holbrook KA, et al. Restrictive dermopathy: Report of two affected siblings and a review of the literature. Arch Dermatol 1992;128:228-231.

98. Mau U, Kendziorra H, Kaiser P, et al. Restrictive dermopathy: Report and review. Am J Med Genet 1997;71:179-185.

99. Hamel BCJ, Happle R, Steylen PM, et al. False-negative prenatal diagnosis of restrictive dermopathy. Am J Med Genet 1992;44:824-826.

100. Meguid NA, Tetamy SA. Neu Laxova syndrome in two Egyptian families. Am J Med Genet 1991;41:30-31.

101. Naveed MCS, Sreenivas V. New manifestations of Neu-Laxova syndrome. Am J Med Genet 1990;35:55-59.

102. The Executive and Scientific Advisory Boards of the National Foundation for Ectodermal Dysplasias. Scaling skin in the neonate: A clue to the early diagnosis of X-linked hypohidrotic ectodermal dysplasia (Christ-Siemens-Touraine syndrome). J Pediatr 1989;114:600-602.

103. Kere J, Srivastava AK, Montonen O, et al. X-linked anhidrotic (hypohidrotic) ectodermal dysplasia is caused by mutation in a novel transmembrane protein. Nat Genet 1996;13:409-416.

Inflammatory and Purpuric Eruptions

EULALIA BASELGA

This group of eruptions is composed of lesions of variable morphology and diverse etiology. However, all share erythema as a common feature, a reflection of their inflammatory nature. Several disorders appear to represent hypersensitivity reactions but for most the etiologic agents are unknown. The differential diagnosis of purpura is extensive in neonates, and includes hematological disorders, infections, trauma, and iatrogenic disorders.

ANNULAR ERYTHEMAS

Annular erythema is a descriptive term that encompasses several entities of unknown etiology characterized by circinate polycyclic lesions that extend peripherally from a central focus.[1,2] Because of subtle differences in clinical features, age of onset, duration of individual lesions, and total duration of the eruptions, a variety of descriptive terms have been coined for these disorders (Table 17-1). For prognostic reasons, it is useful to subdivide annular erythemas into transient and persistent forms.[3] Transient forms include annular erythema of infancy and the less well-established entity, erythema gyratum atrophicans transient neonatale. Persistent annular erythemas include erythema annulare centrifugum, familial annular erythema, and erythema gyratum perstans. Other annular erythemas known to be a manifestation of well-defined diseases (e.g., neonatal lupus) or with distinctive clinical or histologic features (e.g., erythema multiforme, erythema chronicum migrans, erythema marginatum rheumaticum, and erythema gyratum repens) are not considered under this heading.

Annular Erythema of Infancy

Annular erythema of infancy is a benign disease of early infancy characterized by urticarial papules that enlarge peripherally, forming 2- to 3-cm rings or arcs with firm, raised, cordlike or urticarial borders.[4-6] Adjacent lesions become confluent, forming arcuate and polycyclic lesions (Fig. 17-1). Neither vesiculation nor scaling is present at the border. The eruption is asymptomatic. Individual lesions resolve spontaneously without a trace within several days, but new lesions continue to appear in a cyclical fashion until complete resolution within the first year of life.

The cause of annular erythema is unknown, and there are no associated systemic findings. Histologic studies reveal a superficial and deep, dense, perivascular infiltrate of mononuclear cells and eosinophils. No flame figures are observed. The epidermis is normal or mildly spongiotic.

Laboratory studies are normal. Peripheral eosinophilia does not accompany tissue eosinophilia. Immunoglobulin levels including IgE levels are normal. The differential diagnosis should include other annular lesions of infancy (see the following discussion). No treatment is warranted because of the self-limited nature of the eruption.

Erythema gyratum atrophicans transiens neonatale is a less well-defined entity,[7] clinically characterized by annular plaques with an erythematous border and an atrophic center. The lesions appear in the newborn period and resolve within the first year of life. Histologic findings include epidermal atrophy and a mild perivascular mononuclear infiltrate. Immunofluorescence studies reveal granular deposits of IgG, C3, and C4 at the dermoepidermal junction and around capillaries. Erythema gyratum atrophicans transiens neonatale possibly represents a variant of neonatal lupus erythematosus.

Erythema Annulare Centrifugum

Erythema annulare centrifugum is a more persistent type of annular erythema that usually affects adults[8] but may

TABLE 17-1

Annular Erythemas

	Age of onset	Clinical features	Duration of individual lesions	Duration of eruption	Healing	Histopathology
Transient Forms						
Annular erythema of infancy[4]	Early infancy	Annular plaques Nc scaling or vesiculation	Days	Transient (5-6 wk; cyclic course)	No residual lesions	Perivascular infiltrate of eosinophils
Persistent Forms						
Erythema annulare centrifugum[11]	Adulthood, newborn period possible	Mild scaling may be seen at borders	Weeks	Persistent (months or years, with new lesions developing continuously)	Residual hyperpigmentation	Superficial and deep perivascular cuff of lymphocytes
Familial annular erythema[22]	Early infancy to puberty Autosomal dominant	Possible vesiculation or scaling Geographic tongue may be associated Pruritus	Days	Persistent (lifelong, short remissions)	Transient hyperpigmentation	Superficial perivascular cuff of lymphocytes Spongiosis and parakeratosis
Erythema gyratum perstans[12]	Early infancy	Scaling, constant Vesiculation possible Central atrophy	Weeks	Persistent (lifelong)	Transient hyperpigmentation	Perivascular cuff of lymphocytes Spongiosis and parakeratosis

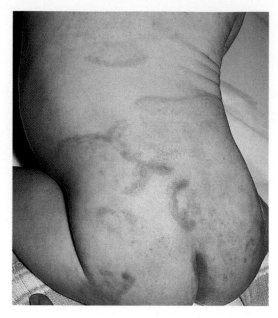

FIG. 17-1
Annular erythema of infancy. The eruption was congenital and resolved completely at 14 months of age.

also occur in children and rarely in newborns.[3,9-11] The lesions are clinically somewhat similar to annular erythema of infancy; however, scaling or vesiculation is seen at the border. The scales lag behind the advancing border, which, in contradistinction to annular erythema of infancy, is not indurated. Individual lesions resolve spontaneously after a few weeks, but new plaques continue to develop for years or may be a lifelong condition. There is no associated pruritus.

Erythema gyratum perstans falls within the spectrum of erythema annulare centrifugum.[12-15] Some authors defend the distinctness of erythema gyratum perstans and consider distinctive features of this disorder its early onset, a duration of more than 15 years, the presence of slight to severe pruritus, and especially the presence of vesiculation.[12]

Erythema annulare centrifugum is thought to represent a hypersensitivity reaction to several trigger factors, including infectious agents (*Candida*,[16,17] Epstein-Barr virus,[10] and ascaris[18]), drugs or foods,[19,20] and neoplasia, especially in adults. Intradermal injection of candidin or trichophytin may reproduce the clinical lesions.[9,21]

Histologic features consist of a dense, superficial, perivascular mononuclear infiltrate. Parakeratosis or epidermal spongiosis may be present. No therapy has been successful in all cases. Treatment agents include oral nystatin,[17] oral amphotericin B,[16] topical antifungals, antihistamines, disodium cromoglycate, and interferon alpha.[9]

Familial Annular Erythema

Familial cases of annular erythema with autosomal dominant inheritance have been described.[22,23] The onset is in early infancy. Scaling, vesiculation, and pruritus may be more common than in erythema annular centrifugum. Pruritus is usually present. Lesions resolve with residual hyperpigmentation. Chronicity is the rule. Geographic tongue may be associated.[12,22]

Differential Diagnosis of Annular Erythemas

Differential diagnosis includes other eruptions with ring-like lesions such as neonatal lupus, erythema multiforme, urticaria, urticarial lesions of pemphigoid, fungal infections,[24] erythema chronicum migrans, and congenital Lyme disease.[25] Serum antibody determinations (antinuclear, SS-A, and SS-B) are recommended to exclude neonatal lupus.

NEONATAL LUPUS ERYTHEMATOSUS[26-29]

Neonatal lupus erythematosus (NLE) is a disease of newborns caused by maternally transmitted autoantibodies. The major manifestations are dermatologic and cardiac. Skin findings are transient. Cardiac disease, which is responsible for the morbidity and mortality of NLE, begins in utero and affects the cardiac conduction system permanently. Other findings include hepatic and hematologic abnormalities. Mothers of infants with neonatal lupus have anti-Ro/SS-A autoantibodies in 95% of cases. Anti-La/SS-B and anti-U1RNP autoantibodies have also been implicated in the pathogenesis of NLE in a minority of patients.[30,31]

Cutaneous Findings

Fifty percent of infants with NLE have skin lesions, and congenital heart block is present in about 10%.[27] Lesions commonly develop at a few weeks of age but may be apparent at birth. Clinically, skin lesions are analogous to those of subacute cutaneous lupus in its two variants: papulosquamous and annular. Papulosquamous lesions are more common and are characterized by erythematous, nonindurated scaly plaques (Fig. 17-2). In contrast to discoid lupus, scarring and follicular plugging are absent. The annular variant, occurring almost exclusively in Japan,

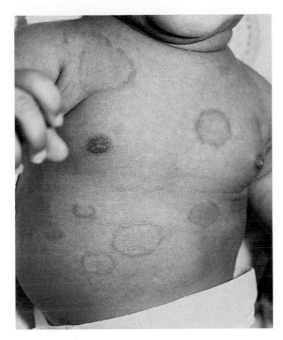

FIG. 17-2
Annular scaly plaques of neonatal lupus erythematosus resembling tinea corporis.

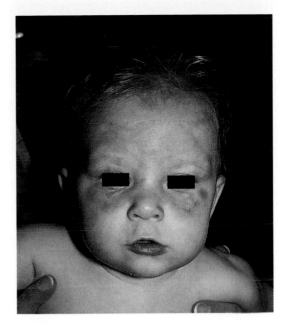

FIG. 17-3
"Raccoon eyes" eruption of neonatal lupus erythematosus.

consists of annular, more inflammatory plaques. Lupus profundus and generalized poikiloderma with erosions and patchy alopecia are rare manifestations.[32,33]

NLE lesions may be widespread but are most common on the face and scalp, predominantly affecting the periorbital and malar areas and often causing a "raccoon eyes" appearance (Fig. 17-3). The eruption is frequently precipitated or aggravated by sun exposure. Sun exposure is not strictly required, since NLE lesions may occur in sun-protected areas such as the diaper region, palms, and soles. Skin lesions are transient and cease to appear around the age of 6 months, after the disappearance of maternal antibodies. Transient hypopigmentation and epidermal atrophy may result (Fig. 17-4). Telangiectasia is a more permanent sequela. Telangiectasia also may be an initial sign of NLE, occurring without preceding identifiable inflammatory lesions; features of cutis marmorata telangiectasia congenita have been observed.[29,34]

Extracutaneous Findings

The most significant manifestation is isolated complete congenital heart block. More than 90% of the cases of isolated complete congenital heart block are due to NLE. Most patients have third-degree block, but progression from a second-degree block has been reported.[35] Heart block can often be detected as early as 20 weeks of gestation.

Transient liver disease, manifesting as hepatomegaly (with a picture of cholestasis) or elevation of liver enzymes,[29,36] and thrombocytopenia or other isolated cytopenias may occur. Petechiae and purpura have been described as presenting signs of NLE.[37] Less common findings include thrombosis associated with anticardiolipin antibodies, hypocalcemia, spastic paraparesis, pneumonitis, and transient myasthenia gravis.[38-40]

Between 30% and 50% of mothers of infants with NLE have a connective tissue disease, most commonly SLE or Sjögren syndrome. Most mothers, however, are asymptomatic. The risk for developing overt connective tissue disease in these mothers is highly debated, with estimates ranging from 2% to more than 70%.[41,42]

Etiology and Pathogenesis

Strong evidence implicates placentally transmitted maternal IgG autoantibodies in the pathogenesis of NLE. The most commonly implicated autoantibodies have been anti-Ro/SS-A and anti-La/SS-B. More than 95% of NLE infants have anti-Ro antibody, and 60% to 80% have anti-La antibodies. A small subset of affected infants do not have

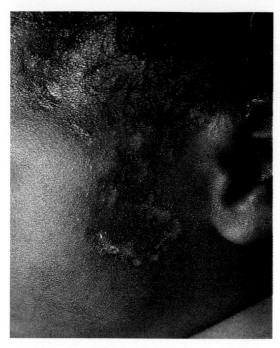

FIG. 17-4
Atrophy and pigmentary changes in an infant with neonatal lupus erythematosus. This boy also had congenital A-V block.

detectable anti-Ro or anti-La antibodies but have instead anti-U1RNP.[30,31] Mothers with high titers of anti-Ro and anti-La antibodies are at greater risk of delivering an infant with NLE. Moreover, the mean level of anti-La seems to be higher in mothers of infants with congenital heart block than in mothers of children with cutaneous NLE.[43,44]

Many questions concerning the pathogenesis of NLE remain unanswered. It is not clear why mothers of affected infants are often asymptomatic despite having the same antibodies, why fraternal twins do not necessarily develop NLE, or why NLE does not occur in every pregnancy.

Laboratory Tests and Histopathology

Serologic studies for autoantibodies in the mother and infant demonstrate anti-Ro, anti-La, and/or anti-U1RNP. Anti-nDNA, anticardiolipin antibodies, antinuclear antibody, and rheumatoid factor may also be present. Anti-Sm antibody, highly specific for systemic lupus erythematosus, is not found in NLE. The maternal antibody titer is usually higher than the infant titer, which may even be negative if only immunodiffusion techniques are used. More sensitive methods such as ELISA or immunoblotting should be used in such instances. Skin biopsy, which is usually not necessary for diagnosis, shows changes characteristic of lupus erythematosus, that is, epidermal atrophy and vacuolization of the basal layer with a sparse lymphohistiocytic infiltrate at the dermoepidermal junction and in a periappendageal distribution. Direct immunofluorescence is positive in 50% of cases, demonstrating granular deposits of IgG, C3, and IgM at the dermoepidermal junction. Histopathologic examination of the heart shows replacement of the atrioventricular node by fibrosis or fatty tissue. Endomyocardial fibroelastosis and patent ductus arteriosus may also be seen,[45,46] as well as deposits of IgG and complement.[47]

Differential Diagnosis

The differential diagnosis includes congenital rubella, cytomegalovirus infection, annular erythema of infancy, tinea corporis, and seborrheic dermatitis. Congenital syphilis should also be considered, but mucosal lesions are not a feature of NLE. False positive serologic tests for syphilis may occur in NLE. Telangiectasia and photosensitivity may suggest Bloom syndrome or Rothmund-Thomson syndrome. Serologic studies for autoantibodies both in infant and mother help to confirm the diagnosis. Skin biopsy for histologic and direct immunofluorescence studies is seldom necessary.

Course, Management, Treatment, and Prognosis

Neonates with suspected NLE should receive a complete physical examination, electrocardiogram, complete blood count with platelet count, and liver function tests.

Skin lesions are transient. Treatment of skin disease consists of sun protection and application of topical steroids. Pulsed dye laser therapy may be considered for residual telangiectases. Congenital heart block is permanent. Half of newborns with complete congenital heart block require implantation of a pacemaker in the neonatal period.[26,41] The average mortality from complete congenital heart block in the neonatal period is 15%; another 10% to 20% die of pacemaker complications.[26]

For mothers with anti-Ro or anti-La antibodies, the risk of delivering an infant with NLE is 1% to 20%, depending on whether they have asymptomatic or symptomatic SLE.[26,27] The risk of recurrence of congenital heart block in subsequent pregnancies may be as high as 25%.[41] Such pregnancies should be monitored closely with repeated fetal echocardiograms. If signs of intrauterine congestive heart failure are detected, dexamethasone or plasmapheresis, or both, have been given.[26,48,49]

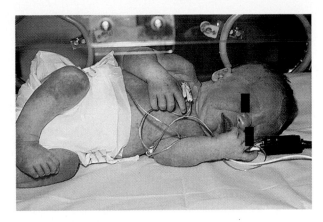

FIG. 17-5
Drug eruption resulting from procainamide.

Although NLE is usually self-limited, SLE may develop subsequently in a small subset of patients.[50] The exact risk is unknown.

DRUG ERUPTIONS[51]

Cutaneous drug reactions are extremely rare in the neonatal period because the ability to generate a drug-induced immune response appears to be lower in infants.[32-34] Cutaneous adverse reactions to drugs may be classified according to the clinical characteristics of the eruption (Box 17-1). Whenever a suspect eruption is observed, a detailed history of medications should be obtained, including drugs administered to the mother, which may be present in breast milk. Morbilliform (Fig. 17-5) or maculopapular eruptions are the most frequent type of drug reaction in neonates, and antibiotics are commonly implicated (Fig. 17-6). Distinguishing a drug eruption from a viral exanthem is often difficult.

EMLA cream, a local anesthetic that is being used with greater frequency in neonatal units, has been noted to produce a localized purpuric eruption.[55] This type of reaction is seen preferentially in neonates.[56] Subsequent applications of EMLA cream do not always reproduce the purpuric lesions. Methemoglobinemia is another complication of EMLA usage in this age group.[55] Therefore EMLA cream should be used with caution in infants who are taking methemoglobin-inducing medications such as sulfonamides, acetaminophen, nitroglycerin, nitroprusside, and phenytoin and particularly those with a history of methemoglobinemia.

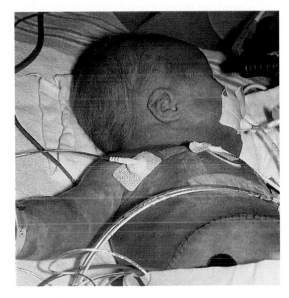

FIG. 17-6
Extensive erythematous eruption caused by a systemic antibiotic.

Vancomycin, an antibiotic frequently administered to premature newborn infants for *Staphylococcus epidermidis* nosocomial infections, may produce shock and rash in newborns (red-man syndrome).[57-59] This reaction is characterized by the appearance of an intense, macular, erythematous eruption on the neck, face, and upper trunk shortly after the infusion is completed. It may be accompanied by hypotension and shock. The reaction resolves rapidly in a matter of hours. It is frequently associated with rapid infusion; however, lengthening the infusion to more than 1 hour does not completely eliminate the risk.[58]

Newborns with AIDS have an increased susceptibility to drug reactions.[60,61] Reactions to trimethroprim/sulfamethoxazole in patients with HIV infections can be severe and life threatening.[62]

Fixed drug reactions of the scrotum and penis, with erythema and edema resulting from hydroxyzine hydrochloride, have been described in early infancy.[63] However, hydroxyzine hydrochloride is administered infrequently in the neonatal period because of the risk of antimuscarinic effects such as restlessness and excitation.

Serum sickness–like reaction is a type of drug reaction that occurs predominantly in children but has not been reported in neonates. It is characterized by fever, an urticarial eruption, and arthralgias. Lymphadenopathy may be present. In contrast to true serum sickness, there are no immune complexes, vasculitis, or renal impairment. The most commonly implicated drug has been cefaclor.[64]

Hypersensitivity syndrome reaction is a serious drug reaction characterized by fever, skin rash, lymphadenopathy, and internal organ involvement, especially the liver.[65] The most commonly implicated drugs are anticonvulsants, and therefore it is not rare in children.[66]

URTICARIA

Urticaria (hives) occurs frequently in childhood but is uncommon in children younger than 6 months of age and is even rarer in the neonatal period.[67-70] Urticaria is usually sporadic; however, familial forms with autosomal dominant inheritance have been described for many of the physical urticarias such as dermographism, heat urticaria, cold urticaria, and vibratory urticaria.

Urticaria can be divided into acute (lasting less than 6 weeks) and chronic (lasting more than 6 weeks) types. Nevertheless, this arbitrary division has prognostic and etiopathogenic significance. In infants, chronic urticaria is very rare.[73] Physical urticarias represent a special subgroup of urticaria in which wheals are elicited by different types of physical stimuli. These include dermographism, cold, pressure, cholinergic, aquagenic, vibratory, and solar urticaria.

Cutaneous Findings

Urticaria is characterized by transient edematous pruritic plaques (Fig. 17-7). By definition, individual lesions last less than 24 hours. Hives may occur on the skin and mucous membranes. Angioedema or giant urticaria is a closely related entity in which there is swelling of the deep subcutaneous tissues and diffuse swelling of the eyelids, genitalia, lips, and tongue. It may be seen alone or more often in association with "common" urticaria. Ur-

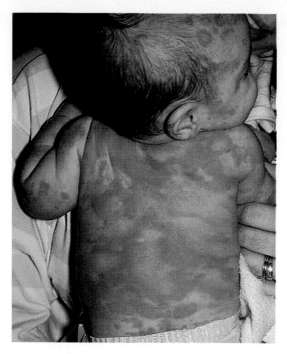

FIG. 17-7
Generalized urticaria following DPT and polio immunizations.

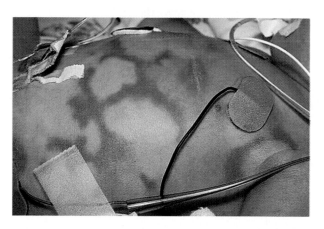

FIG. 17-8
Polycyclic lesions of urticaria associated with prostaglandin E2 infusion.

ticaria in children has certain characteristic features. The hives tend to coalesce, forming bizarre polycyclic, serpiginous, or annular shapes (figurative urticaria, Fig. 17-8; or annular urticaria, Fig. 17-9) and may become hemorrhagic.[67,74] Edema is often pronounced and painful. These features confer a dramatic appearance to the eruption. Itching may be absent in children. Urticaria may be more common and recurrent in atopic patients.[67,69]

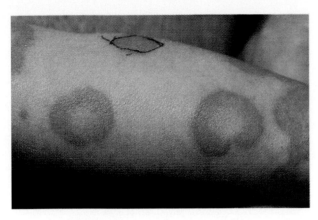

FIG. 17-9
Annular urticaria of unknown etiology.

Extracutaneous Findings

Acute urticaria may be accompanied by signs of anaphylactic shock. In cases of angioedema, abdominal pain, diarrhea, vomiting, respiratory compromise, and joint pain may occur.

Etiology and Pathogenesis[71]

Urticaria develops as a result of an increased permeability of capillaries and small venules, which leads to leakage of fluid into the extravascular space. Mast cell activation and subsequent mediator release are responsible for these changes. Histamine is the best known mediator. Many triggers (secretagogues) initiate mast cell degranulation through receptors on mast cell membranes by an IgE-dependent mechanism or through complement activation (immunologic secretagogues) or by acting directly without the need for receptors (nonimmunologic secretagogues).

The most common provocative agents in children are drugs, foods, and infections, which account for 40% of the cases of acute urticaria.[67,69,74] Antipyretics (primarily aspirin) and antibiotics (amoxicillin, macrolides, and oral cephalosporins) are the most frequently incriminated drugs. Food-related urticaria is associated with atopy.[67] Cow's milk allergy is one of the main causes of urticaria in infants, being present in 6% to 35% of cases of cow's milk intolerance.[69,75-77]

Diagnosis

The diagnosis of urticaria is made on clinical grounds. Histopathologic examination of a skin biopsy specimen shows vascular dilation, edema, and a perivascular inflammatory infiltrate composed of lymphohistiocytic cells, polymorphonuclear cells, and more specifically eosinophils. Neutrophils may predominate.

Laboratory tests are not usually necessary for the evaluation of acute urticaria. IgE levels can be elevated in some patients. An exhaustive search for an underlying cause not elicited by history alone is not warranted. An erythrocyte sedimentation rate may suffice as a screening test in cases of chronic urticaria because it is usually elevated in diseases associated with chronic urticaria (e.g., collagen-vascular diseases). No cause is identified in 10% to 15% of patients. Intradermal skin tests to discover suspected allergens are not reliable.

Differential Diagnosis

Urticaria in infants is often misdiagnosed as erythema multiforme, acute hemorrhagic edema, annular erythema of infancy, or Kawasaki disease. In an infant with urticaria and dermographism, the possibility of diffuse cutaneous mastocytosis without visible cutaneous lesions should also be considered.[78]

Course, Management, Treatment, and Prognosis

Urticaria in early infancy, despite its alarming symptoms, is usually a benign disease. Exceptions are neonatal onset multisystemic inflammatory disease (NOMID) (see below) and the inherited physical urticarias, which may have a lifelong course. If medication is required, antihistamines such as diphenhydramine or hydroxyzine are the mainstay of therapy. However, newborns have an increased susceptibility to antimuscarinic side effects, such as central nervous system (CNS) excitation that causes convulsions. Systemic corticosteroids should be reserved for cases of intractable urticaria.

Familial Physical Urticarias

Autosomal dominant variants have been described for many of the physical urticarias. Although rare, these familial cases begin early in life, even immediately after birth, and have a lifelong course usually with increased severity. The exact pathogenic mechanism for many of the physical urticarias is unknown.

Familial cold urticaria is an autosomal dominant disorder characterized by the development of burning wheals and frequently pain and swelling of joints, stiffness, chills, and even fever after exposure to cold, especially in combination with damp and windy weather.[79-81] The skin lesions appear on exposed areas and generalize afterwards.

Leukocytosis may be present during the attacks. The reaction may be delayed for up to 6 hours after cold challenge. In contrast to acquired cold urticaria, the reaction cannot be elicited by an ice cube test; rather the patient must be subjected to cold environmental temperatures or cold water immersion. On skin biopsy a neutrophilic infiltrate predominates. The symptoms tend to improve with age. Responses to H1 and H2 blockers and ketotifen are poor. Stanozolol has been of limited benefit.[82] Familial cold urticaria has also been described along with amyloidosis and deafness as Muckle-Wells syndrome.[83]

Familial dermographism (autosomal dominant) has been described in a single large family.[84] In neonates dermographism can also be a manifestation of "silent" diffuse cutaneous mastocytosis.[85] Vibratory urticaria is an autosomal dominant physical urticaria in which wheals develop after repetitive vibratory stimulation or stretching.[86] The need for repetitive trauma differentiates it from dermographism. Familial aquagenic urticaria and familial heat urticaria[87,88] usually have onset in childhood.

NEONATAL ONSET MULTISYSTEMIC INFLAMMATORY DISEASE

NOMID is a chronic, systemic, inflammatory disease of neonatal onset characterized by skin rash, arthropathy, and CNS manifestations.[89] Cutaneous findings are the presenting signs. The disease follows a chronic course with acute febrile exacerbations, lymph node enlargement, and hepatosplenomegaly. Two thirds of the patients are born prematurely.

Cutaneous Findings

A skin eruption is usually the first manifestation of the disease and is present at birth or develops during the first 6 months of life. It is characterized by generalized, evanescent, urticarial macules and papules that migrate over the course of a single day and wax and wane in intensity (Fig. 17-10). The rash is persistent, although recrudescence of the skin lesions is noted at flare-ups. Skin lesions may be pruritic, especially after sun exposure, but are usually asymptomatic.[89,90] Geographic tongue and oral ulcers have been noted in a single patient.[91]

Extracutaneous Findings

Symmetric or asymmetric arthropathy is another constant finding and is severe in half of patients. It is often absent in the first few weeks of life but usually develops during the first year.[89,91,92] The severity of the arthropathy correlates with an early onset of joint symptoms. The knees are

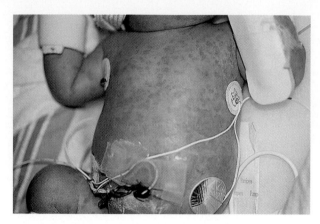

FIG. 17-10
Neonatal onset multisystemic inflammatory disease.

most frequently affected, followed by ankles and feet, elbows, wrists, and hands. Joint swelling and pain are more severe during febrile flare-ups. On palpation, a bony consistency is characteristic as a result of epiphyseal and growth cartilage involvement and overgrowth of the patellas. Joint contractures and severe deformities result.

Neurologic signs and symptoms such as headache, vomiting, and seizures develop at a variable age. Intellectual impairment is also common. Both spasticity and hypotonia have been described. Eye involvement is an inconstant finding. Papilledema with or without optic nerve atrophy is the most common feature. Other ocular manifestations include uveitis, keratitis, conjunctivitis, and chorioretinitis. These changes may lead to complete blindness in adulthood. Progressive sensorineural hearing loss and hoarseness are also common.

Affected children have a characteristic phenotype. There is progressive growth retardation and increased head circumference with frontal bossing. Fontanel closure is retarded. Icterus may be present in the neonatal period, especially in patients with severe arthropathy.[89]

Etiology and Pathogenesis

The etiology and pathogenesis are unknown. The possibility of a persistent neonatal infection has been considered but never proved. A defect in neutrophil function or migration has not been identified.[91]

Laboratory Tests, Radiologic Findings, and Histopathology

Nonspecific findings typical of a chronic inflammatory process include microcytic anemia; leukocytosis with high neutrophil and eosinophil counts, elevated platelet counts, sedimentation rates, and acute-phase reactants; and polyclonal hyperglobulinemia G, A, or M. Rheumatoid factor and antinuclear antibodies are usually absent. Liver enzymes may be mildly elevated. CSF examination shows pleocytosis and high protein levels.

Radiologic studies of the affected joints show irregularly enlarged, bizarre, spiculated epiphyses with a grossly coarsened trabecular appearance.[89,90] There is periosteal new bone formation, and growth cartilage abnormalities are frequent. With time, bowing deformity of long bones and shortening of the diaphyseal length occur. Computed tomography scans of the head have demonstrated hydrocephalus and cerebral atrophy.

Histopathologic examination of the skin reveals interstitial and perivascular neutrophilia.[90,91] Neutrophilic eccrine hidradenitis has been described.[91] Biopsies of lymph nodes, liver, and synovium show nonspecific signs of chronic inflammation.

Differential Diagnosis

NOMID must be differentiated from systemic onset juvenile arthritis. The main differences are its neonatal onset, persistent rash, the short duration of bouts of fever, absence of morning stiffness, and central nervous system involvement. The arthropathy is more deforming, and the radiographic findings of enlarged and disorganized epiphyses are distinctive. In addition, the response to NSAIDs is poor.

Course, Management, Treatment, and Prognosis

The disease follows a chronic course with acute febrile exacerbations. Occasionally the disease causes death in the first or second decade. Nonsteroidal antiinflammatory drugs may be effective for pain relief but do not alter the course of the disease. Prednisone has been palliative in doses ranging from 0.5 to 2.0 mg/kg/day.[90,93] Chlorambucil and penicillamine have been tried with limited success.[92,94]

ERYTHEMA MULTIFORME

Erythema multiforme (EM) is an acute, self-limited disorder of skin and mucous membranes.[95] It has been considered a spectrum of disorders, designated as EM minor, which consists of skin involvement only or the skin and mouth, and as EM major (Stevens-Johnson syndrome [SJS]), which involves at least two mucous membranes with variable cutaneous lesions. Some authors include toxic epidermal necrolysis within this spectrum. Recent ev-

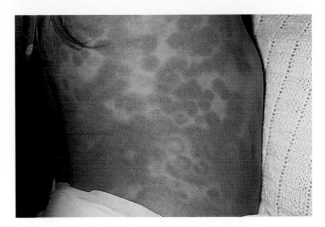

FIG. 17-11
Erythema multiforme.

idence suggests that EM and SJS have distinct clinical features and different precipitating factors, so perhaps the terms *erythema multiforme major* and *erythema multiforme minor* are best avoided.[96,97] EM is a common disease in children,[98,99] but it is extremely unusual in the neonatal period.[61,98,100] Toxic epidermal necrolysis, considered by some to be a severe form of SJS, is discussed in Chapter 10.

Cutaneous Findings

The prototypic lesion of EM is a 1- to 3-cm, erythematous, edematous papule that develops a dusky vesicular, purpuric, or necrotic center. A raised edematous ring of pallor surrounded by an erythematous outer ring is often present. These concentric color changes produce the typical target, or iris, lesion. In many cases only two zones are seen with a single ring around the central papule (atypical target lesions). The lesions are distributed symmetrically and acrally on the extensor surface of the extremities. They may extend to the trunk, flexural surfaces, palms, and soles. In children, lesions on the face and ears are common but are rare on the scalp[101] (Fig. 17-11).

In SJS, the lesions are more centrally located, predominating on the trunk. The targets are atypical and are usually flat. Individual lesions tend to coalesce in large patches. Areas of epidermal detachment may occur but usually affect less than 10% of the body surface area. Mucosal lesions occur frequently in EM and are requisite for diagnosis of SJS. Mucous membrane involvement is characterized by erythema or blisters that rapidly evolve to confluent erosions with pseudomembrane formation. The oral mucosa and conjunctiva are most commonly involved, but genital, anal, pharyngeal, and upper respiratory tract involvement may be seen.

The number of mucous membranes involved has been considered one of the main distinguishing features of EM and SJS.

Extracutaneous Findings

Mild, nonspecific, prodromal symptoms of cough, rhinitis, and low-grade fever are occasionally present in EM. Fever, arthralgias, and prostration are common in SJS.

Etiology and Pathogenesis

EM has been considered a hypersensitivity phenomenon to multiple precipitating factors such as infectious agents or drugs. Three etiologic factors have been well documented: herpes simplex for erythema multiforme and *Mycoplasma* infections and drugs for SJS. Herpes simplex, HSV-1 or HSV-2, is considered to be responsible for more than 80% of EM in children, even if clinical infection is inapparent.[102] HSV-associated EM follows the lesions of herpes by 1 to 3 weeks and is often recurrent. However, not every episode of recurrent herpes is followed by EM. HSV-specific DNA has been detected by polymerase chain reaction and in situ hybridization in lesional skin of a large number of children with EM, whether "idiopathic" or clearly HSV related.[102]

Cow's milk intolerance has been described as a cause of erythema multiforme in a neonate.[100] Drugs are the most common cause of SJS. Sulfonamides, phenylbutazone, diphenylhydantoin, and penicillin derivatives are implicated most frequently.[103]

Laboratory Tests and Histopathology

In cases of extensive involvement an elevated sedimentation rate, leukocytosis, and mild elevation of transaminases may be seen. Electrolyte imbalance and hypoproteinemia may be encountered in SJS. Eosinophilia may be seen in drug-related cases.

Histopathologic examination of early lesions reveals a lymphocytic bandlike infiltrate at the dermoepidermal junction with exocytosis and individual necrotic keratinocytes in close proximity to lymphocytes ("satellite cell necrosis").[104] There is vacuolization of the basal layer with focal cleft formation at the dermoepidermal junction. The upper dermis is edematous. Over time, more extensive confluent necrosis of the epidermis supervenes, resulting in subepidermal blister formation. In EM a lichenoid infiltrate predominates, whereas in SJS epidermal necrosis predominates.[105]

Differential Diagnosis

In typical cases EM or SJS is rarely confused with other entities. Urticarial vasculitis may be considered in some cases. Kawasaki disease may produce targetlike lesions; however, associated findings should allow differentiation.

Course, Management, Treatment, and Prognosis

Erythema multiforme is usually self-limited. Individual lesions heal in 1 to 2 weeks with residual hyperpigmentation. Conservative supportive care is the preferred form of treatment. Possible underlying causes should be sought. Treatment of underlying infection and discontinuation of nonessential drugs are indicated. Corticosteroids are unnecessary and may even worsen a concurrent infection.[106] In HSV-associated EM, early intervention or even prophylactic treatment with oral acyclovir may be beneficial.[107]

SJS has a less favorable prognosis, with a mortality rate of 5% to 15% if untreated. Use of corticosteroids in SJS is more controversial.[106,108] No controlled study has proved the efficacy of corticosteroids, and in some studies patients treated with corticosteroids have had a worse prognosis.[109] Corticosteroids may predispose to secondary infection while suppressing the signs of sepsis. Supportive care is extremely important.

SWEET SYNDROME

Sweet syndrome, or acute febrile neutrophilic dermatosis, is a benign disease characterized by tender, raised erythematous plaques, fever, peripheral leukocytosis, histologic findings of a dense dermal infiltrate of polymorphonuclear leukocytes, and a rapid response to systemic corticosteroids.[110-112] Only a few pediatric cases have been reported, [113-119] the youngest being 7 weeks of age.[114]

Cutaneous Findings

The lesions of Sweet syndrome have an acute, explosive onset and are characterized by indurated, tender, erythematous plaques or nodules that vary in size from 0.5 to 4 cm (Fig. 17-12). Tiny pustules may appear at a later stage. The borders may be raised, mammillated, or even vesicular. Some of the lesions may show central clearing, forming annular or gyrate plaques (Fig. 17-13). The lesions are usually multiple and distributed over the face and extremities or, more rarely, the trunk. Without treatment, the lesions tend to heal spontaneously within a few months. In some pa-

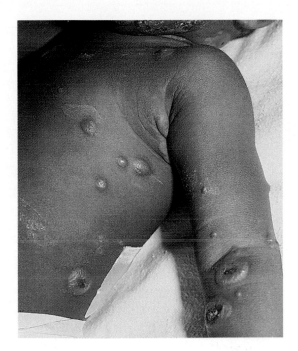

FIG. 17-12
Nodular lesions of Sweet syndrome with central crusting.

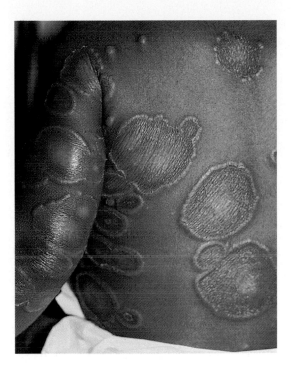

FIG. 17-13
Progression of lesions of Sweet syndrome in patient depicted in Fig. 17-12. Plaques and nodules have flattened and are clearing centrally.

tients, especially children, the lesions heal with areas of secondary cutis laxa, also known as *Marshall syndrome*.[116,117,120]

Extracutaneous Findings

High spiking fever is characteristic but may be absent in up to 50% of patients.[112] Arthralgias or asymmetric arthritis may be associated, and conjunctivitis or iridocyclitis may be seen in one third of patients.[112] Renal involvement manifesting as proteinuria or hematuria, as well as lung involvement with infiltrates visible on chest radiographs, has also been described.[121]

Etiology and Pathogenesis

The pathogenesis is unknown. Many of the patients reported have had a preceding respiratory tract infection or elevated antistreptolysin O titers.[112] Ten percent of the cases have been seen in the setting of a variety of hematologic malignancies, particularly acute myeloid and myelomonocytic leukemias.[122] Sweet syndrome has also been associated with solid tumors, inflammatory bowel disease,

connective tissue diseases, and chronic granulomatous disease,[113,122] or it may occur as an adverse reaction to drugs,[123] particularly granulocyte colony–stimulating factor.[124] Because of these associations and the rapid response to systemic corticosteroids, Sweet syndrome is thought to represent a hypersensitivity reaction to infectious agents or tumoral antigens.

Laboratory Tests and Histopathology

An elevated erythrocyte sedimentation rate and peripheral leukocytosis are frequent accompanying abnormalities. Eosinophilia, microcytic anemia, mild elevation of liver enzymes, and urinalysis abnormalities may be present occasionally. Antineutrophil cytoplasmic antibodies have been detected in some cases.[112] Alpha-1-antitrypsin deficiency has been documented in one case of Marshall syndrome.[120]

The histopathologic findings are diagnostic.[125,126] There is a dense perivascular infiltrate composed almost entirely of neutrophils. The dermis appears edematous, and subepidermal blisters may form. Spongiosis, exocytosis, and intraepidermal vesiculation may be seen. There is endothelial swelling and nuclear dust, but true vasculitis is characteristically absent.

Differential Diagnosis

Lesions of Sweet syndrome may initially resemble erythema multiforme or acute hemorrhagic edema. Lesions on the lower extremities may resemble erythema nodosum, but more characteristic lesions of Sweet syndrome are usually present in other locations.

Course, Management, Treatment, and Prognosis

Sweet syndrome is a benign disease but may be a marker of malignancy. If left untreated, it resolves spontaneously in weeks to months. Recurrences are common. Marshall syndrome may have a poorer prognosis, with development of elastolysis in the lungs or cardiovascular involvement.

Oral corticosteroids are the treatment of choice and usually elicit a prompt response. Potassium iodide administration has been successful in a few cases,[127] as has colchicine,[128] dapsone,[129] and clofazimine.[116]

KAWASAKI DISEASE

Kawasaki disease is a systemic vasculitis involving the small and medium-sized muscular arteries, especially the coronary arteries. In the past, many cases in young infants were called *infantile polyarteritis nodosa*. The disease is characterized by fever lasting at least 5 days, nonpurulent conjunctivitis, a polymorphous exanthem, erythema and swelling of the hands and feet, inflammatory changes of the lips and oral cavity, and acute nonpurulent cervical adenopathy.[130]

Kawasaki disease occurs predominantly in children under 5 and has a peak incidence between 1 and 2 years of age. It is infrequent before 6 months of age, although it has been reported in patients as young as 1 month.[131,132] Boys are affected 1.5 times as often as girls. Attacks are more frequent in winter and spring. Familial cases in household contacts have been described.[133] The incidence is highest in Japan, where the annual incidence is increasing steadily.[134,135] The recurrence rate is 3%, with some patients having two or more recurrences.

Cutaneous Findings

The skin is involved in 99% of patients. A polymorphous exanthem usually appears within 5 days of onset of fever (Fig. 17-14). The first sign often consists of diffuse ery-

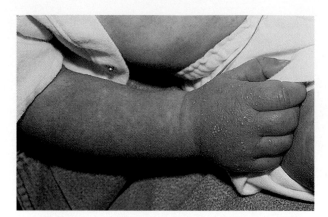

FIG. 17-14
Morbilliform eruption in an infant with Kawasaki disease.

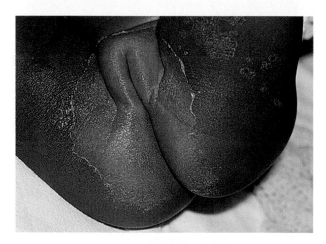

FIG. 17-15
Early perineal desquamative eruption of Kawasaki disease.

thema and painful induration of the hands and feet. Confluent macular erythema or erythematous papules in the perineum are present in 67% of patients. The perineal rash, a distinctive feature at this early stage, desquamates in 48 hours, preceding finger-tip and toe-tip desquamation[136] (Fig. 17-15). A more extensive eruption, which is most commonly macular or morbilliform but may be urticarial, scarlatiniform, targetoid, or even pustular, occurs on the trunk and proximal extremities. Between 1 and 3 weeks after onset of the disease, the eruption characteristically begins to desquamate beneath the distal nail plates, and peeling may extend to involve the entire palm and sole. Horizontal depressions in the nail plates (Beau lines) usually result.

Intermittent acrocyanosis has been observed in infants younger than 6 months of age.[131] Inflammatory changes with necrosis at the site of a previous BCG inoculation have been reported. Changes in the lips and oral mucosa include erythema, swelling and fissuring of the lips, strawberry tongue, and erythema of the oropharynx.

Extracutaneous Findings[138]

Prolonged fever for at least 5 days is the cardinal and initial feature of the disease. It begins abruptly and is high, with several spikes each day (remittent fever). It is not well controlled with antipyretics, and without treatment it lasts for 1 to 2 weeks.

Bilateral nonexudative conjunctival injection, involving mainly the bulbar conjunctivae, begins shortly after disease onset. Anterior uveitis is frequently noted. Cervical lymphadenopathy is the least common diagnostic sign. It is usually unilateral, firm, and slightly tender.

Cardiac conditions are the main cause of long-term morbidity and mortality. The pericardium, myocardium, endocardium, and coronary arteries may be involved. Pericardial effusion may be detected by an echocardiogram in 30% of patients. Myocarditis may manifest in the acute phase, and arrhythmias due to ischemia, congestive heart failure, and valvular involvement, usually mitral, may occur.

Without treatment, coronary artery aneurysms develop in 20% and are most commonly detected 10 days to 4 weeks after onset. Risk factors for the development of coronary aneurysms include age younger than 1 year, male gender, fever for more than 2 days, recurrent fever, and delayed treatment. Aneurysms may also develop in systemic medium-sized arteries and result in peripheral gangrene.[139]

Polyarticular arthritis and arthralgias may occur in the first weeks of the illness. Lethargy, irritability, and other signs of aseptic meningitis, as well as vomiting, diarrhea, and abdominal pain, are common. Mild hepatitis occurs frequently, as does acute distention of the gallbladder (hydrops). Respiratory symptoms may also be observed.

Etiology and Pathogenesis[140]

Many infectious organisms have been proposed as etiologic agents, but none has been proved.[140,141] Some cases of *Yersinia pseudotuberculosis* infection fulfill the diagnostic criteria for Kawasaki disease.[142] Regardless of the cause, evidence points to a generalized immune activation with production of various proinflammatory cytokines that are capable of damaging endothelial cells.[143-145]

BOX 17-2

Diagnostic Criteria of Kawasaki Disease

Fever of at least 5 days' duration
Presence of at least four of the following features:
    Changes in the extremities
    Polymorphous exanthem
    Bilateral conjunctival injection
    Changes in the lips and oral cavity
    Cervical lymphadenopathy of at least 1.5 cm in
        diameter.
Exclusion of other diseases with similar findings

Laboratory Tests and Histopathology

In the acute phase, laboratory studies show leukocytosis with a left shift, normochromic normocytic anemia, increased sedimentation rate and other acute phase reactants, depressed albumin, and elevated IgM and IgE levels. There may be mild elevation of transaminases and polyclonal hypergammaglobulinemia. In the subacute stage there is a marked and almost universal thrombocytosis. Antineutrophil cytoplasmatic antibodies may be detectable as a nonspecific epiphenomenon. There may be sterile pyuria with mild proteinuria. Cerebrospinal fluid shows a mononuclear pleocytosis with normal protein and glucose levels. Skin biopsy findings are not specific. There is edema in the papillary dermis with a mild perivascular mononuclear cell infiltrate. Vasculitis of medium and large arteries is observed.

Diagnosis

Clinical criteria for diagnosing Kawasaki disease have been established[138] (Box 17-2). Patients with fever and less than four principal features can be diagnosed as having Kawasaki disease when coronary artery aneurysms are detected. Patients who do not fulfill the classic criteria are categorized as having "incomplete" or "atypical" Kawasaki disease.[146] Incomplete forms are common in children younger than 1 year of age, and a high index of suspicion is needed to establish the diagnosis.[146]

Differential Diagnosis

Many diseases mimic Kawasaki disease, including viral infections, streptococcal infection, juvenile rheumatoid arthritis, erythema multiforme, staphylococcal scalded skin syndrome, and toxic shock syndrome.

Course, Management, Treatment, and Prognosis

The morbidity and mortality of Kawasaki disease depend primarily on coronary artery lesions.[134,147] Baseline and serial cardiac ultrasound studies are necessary to follow up coronary artery morphology. With early treatment, the risk of developing coronary artery aneurysms is around 5% to 12%.[134] Small aneurysms resolve completely within the first 2 years after disease onset in 30% to 60% of these patients.[147] However, coronary aneurysms, especially if giant (>8 mm), may persist and be complicated by thrombotic occlusion or development of stenosis at the outlet of the aneurysm. Stenotic lesions may develop gradually over several years, so long-term follow-up is warranted.[148-150]

Treatment in the acute phase of the disease is directed to reducing inflammation. Intravenous gamma globulin (IVGG) in combination with high-dose aspirin (100 mg/kg/day) is the treatment of choice.[138,151] High-dose intravenous methylprednisolone has been given for treatment failures.[152] Treatment of incomplete or atypical Kawasaki disease should be guided by clinical judgment.

ACUTE HEMORRHAGIC EDEMA

Acute hemorrhagic edema (AHE), purpura en cockade, or Finkelstein disease is an acute, benign leukocytoclastic vasculitis of limited skin involvement occurring in children under 2 years of age.[153-156] AHE has been considered an infantile variant of Henoch-Schönlein purpura; however, because of clinical and prognostic differences it is sometimes regarded as a separate entity.

Cutaneous Findings

The disease is characterized by the abrupt onset of fever; tender edema of the face, eyelids, ears, scrotum, and acral extremities; and ecchymotic purpura on the face and extremities. The trunk is usually spared. Individual lesions often have a darker center and expand centrifugally, giving them a cockade or targetlike configuration. Lesions range in size from 0.5 to 4.0 cm and may become confluent, forming polycyclic, annular plaques (Fig. 17-16). Necrotic[157,158] and bullous lesions may be seen.[157,159] Petechiae in the mucous membranes have also been described.[160]

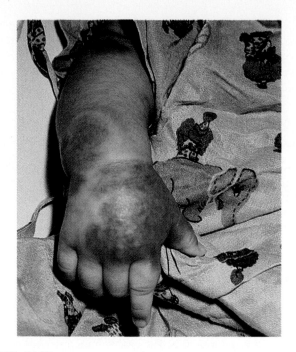

FIG. 17-16
Typical lesions of acute hemorrhagic edema on the arm of an infant.

Extracutaneous Findings

Except for fever, there are no other associated manifestations. In many patients, there is a preceding upper respiratory tract infection. The dramatic cutaneous findings contrast with the general well-being of the patient.

Etiology and Pathogenesis

The cause of AHE is unknown. It is thought to represent an immune complex–mediated disease precipitated by a preceding infection, particularly an upper respiratory tract infection, drug intake, or immunization. *Staphylococci* and *Streptococci* spp. and adenoviruses have been implicated most commonly.

Laboratory Tests and Histopathology

Leukocytosis (both lymphocytic and granulocytic), thrombocytosis, eosinophilia, and an elevated erythrocyte sedimentation rate may be present. Urinalysis, tests for occult blood in the stool, immunoglobulin, and complement levels are usually normal or negative. Circulating immunocomplexes may occasionally be found.[159]

Histopathologic examination of skin biopsy specimens demonstrates a small vessel leukocytoclastic vasculitis. Direct immunofluorescence shows deposition of C3 and fibrinogen in the vessel wall. IgM, IgG, IgA, and IgE deposition have also been noted in up to one third of cases.[159,161-163]

Differential Diagnosis

The differential diagnosis includes Henoch-Schönlein purpura, child abuse, meningococcemia and other infectious purpuras, erythema multiforme, Kawasaki disease, and Sweet syndrome.[155,160] Distinction from Henoch-Schönlein purpura may be impossible.[154] Perivascular deposits of IgA are not useful for differentiation because they may be present in both entities.

Course, Management, and Prognosis

The prognosis is excellent. The eruption resolves spontaneously without sequelae in 1 to 3 weeks. Treatment with corticosteroids is not necessary and may lead to complications and worsen the prognosis.[161] Exacerbations may be observed during the clinical evolution, with new crops of lesions and fever,[158,162] but true recurrences weeks or months after the first episode are rare.[154,160] There has been a single report of a fatal ileo-ileo intussusception in an infant with cutaneous lesions otherwise typical for AHE.[158]

THE PORPHYRIAS[164-168]

The porphyrias are a group of diseases characterized by abnormalities of porphyrin-heme metabolism. Each type results from deficient activity of one of the enzymes of the heme biosynthetic pathway, which leads to an accumulation of heme precursors. In infants, the enzymatic defects are always inherited. Porphyrias are classified as hepatic or erythropoietic according to the organ site in which the underlying heme synthetic defect is predominantly expressed (Table 17-2). Clinically, the porphyrias can be separated into those manifesting either cutaneous photosensitivity, neurovisceral symptoms, or both. Photosensitivity is maximum for ultraviolet wavelengths between 400 to 410 nm ("Soret band"), the spectrum of maximum absorption of porphyrins.

Photosensitivity in porphyrias may manifest as immediate phototoxicity with burning pain, edema, and erythema shortly after sun exposure, characteristic of erythropoietic types of porphyria, or as a more delayed photosensitivity manifesting as skin fragility, subepidermal blisters, milia, disorders of pigmentation, and sclerodermoid signs, characteristic of hepatic porphyrias.[168] The pathophysiologic

mechanisms involved in the cutaneous manifestations of the porphyrias are multiple.[165,166]

Congenital Erythropoietic Porphyria

Congenital erythropoietic porphyria (CEP), also called Günther disease, is a rare autosomal recessive disorder caused by deficient activity of uroporphyrinogen III (UROGEN III) synthase. This leads to excessive accumulation of isomer I porphyrins in bones, erythrocytes, skin, and teeth and excretion of large amounts of predominantly type I porphyrins in urine and feces.

Cutaneous Findings[164,165,169]
CEP presents with severe photosensitivity from birth or early infancy with formation of vesicles and bullae on areas exposed to sun, phototherapy devices, or even ambient lighting.[170] There is also marked skin fragility. As a result of the phototoxic injury and the increased skin fragility, there are severe mutilations mainly of fingers, hands, and face, particularly nose and ears, but also sun-protected areas. Hypertrichosis of the face and extremities, scarring alopecia of the scalp and eyebrows, and pigmentary changes (hyperpigmentation and hypopigmentation) are also common. Over time, severe facial mutilation results, with destruction of nasal and auricular cartilages, ectropion, and eclabium, as well as shortening and contraction of fingers.

Extracutaneous Findings
Accumulation of porphyrins in deciduous and permanent teeth produces red discoloration (erythrodontia) and reddish fluorescence on Wood's light examination. The urine is also reddish, which causes pink discoloration of the diapers, an early diagnostic sign. Ocular changes include ectropion, photophobia, and keratoconjunctivitis. Other manifestations include hemolytic anemia, osteodystrophy, splenomegaly, and porphyrin-rich gallstones.

Genetics
The gene for UROGEN III synthase is localized on chromosome 10. Several mutations have been identified,[171] and there is some correlation between the disease severity and genotypes.[172]

Laboratory Tests and Histopathology
Histologic examination of skin biopsy specimens from blisters reveals subepidermal cleavage (within the lamina lucida) with minimal inflammatory infiltrate. Perivascular accumulation of PAS-positive, diastase-resistant, homogeneous hyaline material (porphyrins) may be seen, which is best viewed with fluorescence microscopy. See

TABLE 17-2

Classification of the Porphyrias, Enzymatic Defect, Porphyrin Profile, and Age of Onset

Tissue origin	Type	Enzyme deficiency	Porphyrin profile				Age of onset
			Erythrocyte	Plasma	Urine	Stool	
Erythropoietic	Congenital erythropoietic porphyria (CEP)	Uroporphyrinogen III synthase	URO I, COPRO I, PROTO	URO I, COPRO I, PROTO	URO I> COPRO I	COPRO I	Birth, infancy
	Erythropoietic protoporphyria (EPP)	Ferrochelatase	PROTO	PROTO	Normal	PROTO	Infancy, early childhood
Hepatic	Acute intermittent porphyria (AIP)	Porphobilinogen deaminase	Normal	Normal	ALA, PBG	Normal	After puberty, no cutaneous manifestations
	Variegate porphyria (VP)	Protoporphyrinogen oxidase	Normal	COPRO, PROTO	COPRO> URO	PROTO> COPRO	Second decade, homozygous variant at birth, infancy, or early childhood
	Hereditary coproporphyria (HCP)	Coproporphyrinogen oxidase	Normal	COPRO	COPRO	COPRO	After puberty, homozygous variant (harderoporphyria) at birth, infancy, or early childhood
	Porphyria cutanea tarda (PCT)	Uroporphyrinogen decarboxylase	Normal	URO	URO I>III	ISOCOPRO	Third or fourth decade
	ALA dehydratase porphyria	ALA dehydratase	PROTO	ALA, COPRO, PROTO	ALA, COPRO, URO	COPRO, PROTO	Any age, no cutaneous manifestations
Hepatoerythropoietic	Hepatoerythropoietic porphyria (HEP)	Uroporphyrinogen decarboxylase	Zn-PROTO	URO	URO (I and III)	ISOCOPRO	Early infancy

ALA, 5-aminolevulinate; COPRO, coproporphyrin; ISOCOPRO, isocoproporphyrin; PBG, porphobilinogen; PROTO, protoporphyrin; URO, uroporphyrin.

Table 17-2 for porphyrin excretion profile. Measurement of URO III synthase activity may be made for genetic or scientific studies. Prenatal diagnosis from amniotic fluid is possible.[173]

Differential Diagnosis

Other photosensitivity diseases presenting early in life, such as xeroderma pigmentosum, or diseases manifesting with blisters, such as epidermolysis bullosa and bullous pemphigoid, should be considered. Determination of porphyrins is diagnostic and allows differentiation from other porphyrias presenting early in life with photosensitivity.

Prognosis

Clinical severity of CEP is highly variable, ranging from hydrops fetalis, hepatosplenomegaly, and severe anemia in utero to adult onset disease with only cutaneous manifestations.[174] In most cases, however, patients survive well into adulthood, although with severe mutilations or major disfigurement.

Treatment

Protection from sun exposure is essential. Chemical sunscreens do not achieve good protection against Soret band radiation, so protective clothing and physical sunblocks are necessary. Long-wavelength, UV-absorbing films are encouraged on car windows and windows at home. Repeated transfusions and hydroxyurea to suppress erythropoiesis,[177,178] splenectomy, activated charcoal,[179,180] and beta-carotene[181,182] have been helpful. Bone marrow transplantation offers the possibility of enzyme activity correction.[183,184] Replacement gene therapy has been accomplished in vitro.[185]

Erythropoietic Protoporphyria[164,166,186]

Erythropoietic protoporphyria (EPP) is the most common form of cutaneous porphyria apart from porphyria cutanea tarda (PCT). Clinical symptoms typically begin in infancy or early childhood, with a peak incidence between 2 to 4 years of age. EPP is usually inherited as an autosomal dominant condition with incomplete penetrance, but some families may have autosomal recessive inheritance.[187,188] EPP is caused by deficient activity of ferrochelatase, leading to accumulation of protoporphyrin in erythrocytes, plasma, and feces.

Cutaneous Manifestations

Clinical manifestations are those of an acute phototoxic reaction, which triggers an episode of crying within minutes of sunlight exposure due to burning pain or stinging sensations. Some patients are photosensitive to fluorescent lighting.[186] Erythema, edema, and urticarial lesions occur, but vesicles and bullae are rare (Fig. 17-17). Fine petechiae may occur on sun-exposed areas after prolonged sun exposure. Some patients have only subjective symptoms.[186] With chronic exposure, there is characteristic thickening and wrinkling of the knuckle pads, furrowing around the mouth (pseudorhagades), and shallow elliptical scars on the nose, cheeks, and forehead.

Hemolytic anemia is absent. Protoporphyrin-rich gallstones may develop in childhood. Fatal liver failure resulting from progressive accumulation of protoporphyrin in hepatocytes is a possible outcome in a minority of patients, altering the prognosis for an otherwise clinically benign disorder. Recessive inheritance may predispose to severe liver disease.[189]

Histopathologic examination of skin biopsy specimens of sun-exposed areas shows marked concentric deposits of a hyaline material around dermal blood vessels. This material is PAS positive and diastase resistant.

Diagnosis

The diagnosis of EPP is established by detecting elevated levels of protoporphyrin in erythrocytes, plasma, and feces. A rapid microfluorometric assay for free erythrocyte

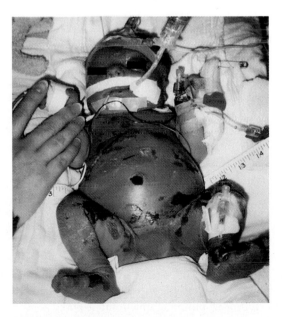

FIG. 17-17
Porphyria. (Courtesy Henry Lim and Tor Schwayder.)

protoporphyrin and examination of a blood smear for fluorescent erythrocytes may also be used as screening tests.[190] Differential diagnosis includes other types of porphyria, but causes of immediate photosensitivity such as PMLE or solar urticaria do not occur in infants.

The mainstay of treatment for erythropoietic protoporphyria is sun avoidance and oral administration of betacarotene to increase tolerance to sunlight exposure.[191] Cholestyramine, charcoal, and hematin have been used with clinical and biochemical improvement.[192] Avoidance of alcohol and drugs that interfere with hepatic excretory function is essential. Liver transplantation has been performed in a few patients with liver failure.[193]

Hepatoerythropoietic Porphyria

Hepatoerythropoietic porphyria (HEP), which is thought to represent the homozygous form of PCT,[194-197] is caused by a marked deficiency of uroporphyrinogen decarboxylase. Clinical manifestations begin in infancy or more commonly in early childhood and resemble both porphyria cutanea tarda and Günter disease. The disease usually presents with darkening of the urine and cutaneous photosensitivity of the delayed type with vesicles, skin fragility, milia, and scarring. With time, hypertrichosis, sclerodermoid changes, and mutilation similar to the manifestations of Günter disease become apparent.[198] Anemia, hepatosplenomegaly, and abnormalities of liver function of varying degrees may also occur. Treatment is directed to sun protection.

Other Porphyrias

Other porphyrias with onset of symptoms in infancy or early childhood include homozygous variants of coproporphyria (harderoporphyria) and variegate porphyria. In harderoporphyria, neonatal jaundice, hemolytic anemia, and hepatosplenomegaly dominate the clinical picture.[199-201] Blisters may occur during phototherapy for neonatal jaundice. Diagnosis depends on detecting very low coproporphyrinogen oxidase activity, elevated coproporphyrin in urine, markedly elevated harderoporphyrin and coproporphyrin in feces, and zinc protoporphyrin in erythrocytes.

Homozygous variegate porphyria may present shortly after birth with marked photosensitivity or, more commonly, in early childhood with erosions, blisters, and milia following minor trauma in sun-exposed areas.[202-205] Mental and growth retardation, seizures, nystagmus, and clinodactyly have been described.

TRANSIENT PORPHYRINEMIAS[206-208]

Transient increase of porphyrin levels has been described in neonates with hemolytic disease of the newborn. These infants develop erythema, violaceous discoloration, purpura, erosions, and blisters at areas exposed to phototherapy with sharp demarcation at photoprotected sites. Sensitivity to sunlight may occur.

Elevated levels of plasma porphyrins (mainly coproporphyrin) and/or erythrocyte protoporphyrin are found, which normalize spontaneously during the first few months. The cause of transient porphyrinemia is unclear. Many factors are likely involved, such as impaired liver and renal function, blood transfusions, and drugs.

PURPURA IN THE NEWBORN

Purpura in the neonate is almost always an emergency situation and should prompt the physician to begin an immediate search for an underlying disorder. Apart from trauma, purpura in the newborn may be due to coagulation defects, platelet abnormalities, or infections (Box 17-3). Extramedullary erythropoiesis also causes purpuric lesions by a different mechanism.

In the evaluation of a neonate with purpura it is important to obtain a maternal and familial history of bleeding diathesis and thromboembolic phenomena, drug intake, and symptoms of infectious diseases. A general physical examination and workup for sepsis is warranted. Laboratory studies should include hemoglobin and hematocrit values, platelet count, white blood count, coagulation studies, and TORCH serologies.

DERMAL ERYTHROPOIESIS (BLUEBERRY MUFFIN BABY)

Persistence of the erythropoietic activity of fetal dermal mesenchyme into the newborn period produces a characteristic purpuric eruption for which the term *blueberry muffin baby* was coined. The eruption, first observed in newborns with congenital rubella (Fig. 17-18), may be the result of other intrauterine infections (Fig. 17-19) and hematologic dyscrasias.[209-211] A blueberry muffin–like eruption may also represent metastatic infiltration of the dermis by congenital malignancies, without true extramedullary erythropoiesis.

Cutaneous Findings

The cutaneous lesions of blueberry muffin babies consist of dark blue or magenta, nonblanchable, round to oval papules ranging in size from 1 to 7 mm and have a gener-

BOX 17-3

Differential Diagnosis of Neonatal Purpura

1. Extramedullary erythropoiesis (blueberry muffin baby)
2. Coagulation defects
   Protein C and S deficiency (neonatal purpura fulminans)
   Hemorrhagic disease of the newborn
   Hereditary clotting factor deficiencies
3. Platelet abnormalities
   a. Immune platelet destruction
      Alloimmune neonatal thrombocytopenia
      Maternal autoimmune thrombocytopenia (ITP, lupus)
      Drug-related immune thrombocytopenia
   b. Primary platelet production/function defects
      Thrombocytopenia with absent radii syndrome
      Wiskott-Aldrich syndrome
      Fanconi anemia
      Congenital megakaryocytic thrombocytopenia
      X-linked recessive thrombocytopenia
      Other hereditary thrombocytopenias
      Giant platelet syndromes (Bernard-Soulier, May-Hegglin)
      Trisomy 13 or 18
      Alport syndrome variants
      Gray platelet syndrome
      Glanzmann thrombasthenia
      Hermansky-Pudlak syndrome
   c. Kasabach-Merritt syndrome*
4. Infections†
   Congenital (TORCH)
   Sepsis
   HIV
   Parvovirus B19
5. Trauma
6. Purpuric phototherapy-induced eruption

Modified from Baselga E, Drolet BA, Esterly NB. J Am Acad Dermatol 1997;37:673-705.
*Both thrombocytopenia and consumption coagulopathy are involved in the pathogenesis.
†Infection may cause purpura by several mechanisms.

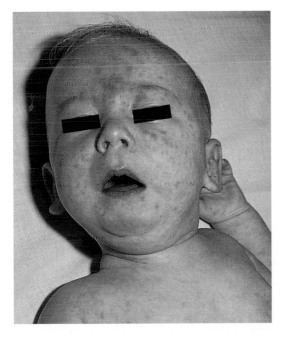

FIG. 17-18
Infant with congenital rubella and "blueberry muffin" lesions.

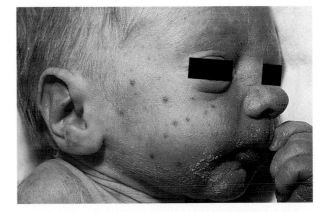

FIG. 17-19
"Blueberry muffin" lesions associated with cytomegalic inclusion disease.

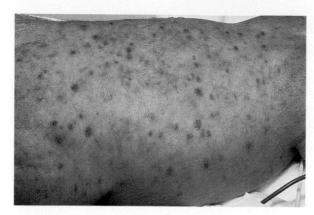

FIG. 17-20

Lesions of dermal erythropoiesis in an infant with Rh incompatibility due to RhoGAM failure.

alized distribution with accentuation on the head, neck, and trunk (Fig. 17-20). The papules are firm to palpation with an infiltrative quality that distinguishes them from petechiae and purpura, which often coexist in the same patient. These lesions evolve into dark purple to brown macules and spontaneously involute within 2 to 6 weeks.[155] Blueberry muffin lesions caused by infiltrative processes are usually larger, more nodular, less hemorrhagic, fewer in number, and firmer to palpation.

Extracutaneous Findings

Accompanying abnormalities vary with the underlying cause.

Etiology and Pathogenesis

In the prevaccination era, rubella was the most common cause of dermal erythropoiesis, but now congenital cytomegalovirus (CMV) infection is the major cause.[210,211] Dermal erythropoiesis has been associated with other intrauterine infections such as Coxsackie B-2[210] and parvovirus B19,[212] as well as hematologic dyscrasias such as Rh incompatibility,[213,214] maternal-fetal ABO incompatibility,[210] spherocytosis,[215] and the twin transfusion syndrome[210,216] (Box 17-4). In rare instances, it may occur in otherwise healthy newborns.[210,217]

Laboratory Tests and Histopathology

Histopathologic examination demonstrates poorly circumscribed collections of nucleated and nonnucleated red blood cells, predominantly confined to the reticular dermis and extending to the subcutaneous tissue.[209-211] Occasionally a few myeloid precursors may be interspersed.

Laboratory findings depend on the underlying cause. In the evaluation of a blueberry muffin baby the following tests are indicated: a peripheral blood count, hemoglobin level, TORCH serologies, viral cultures, and a Coombs' test. Skin biopsy is not always necessary for diagnosis but may be helpful if an infiltrative process is suspected.

Differential Diagnosis

The differential diagnosis includes other causes of neonatal purpura such as coagulation defects, platelet abnormalities, and infections.[155] Neoplastic diseases that produce infiltrative metastases in the neonatal period, such as neuroblastomas,[218-220] rhabdomyosarcomas,[221] myelogenous leukemias,[222-224] and Langerhans cell histiocytosis, especially the congenital self-healing reticulohistiocytosis variant (Hashimoto-Pritzker),[225-227] should be considered.

Course, Management, Treatment, and Prognosis

Lesions of true dermal erythropoiesis fade and resolve spontaneously in 3 to 6 weeks after birth. Treatment is directed at the underlying condition.

BOX 17-4

Differential Diagnosis of Blueberry Muffin Lesions

Dermal erythropoiesis
  Congenital infection
    Rubella
    Cytomegalovirus
    Parvovirus B19
    Coxsackievirus B2
  Hemolytic disease of the newborn
    Rh incompatibility
    Blood group incompatibility
  Hereditary spherocytosis
  Twin transfusion syndrome
Neoplastic-infiltrative diseases
  Neuroblastoma
  Rhabdomyosarcoma
  Langerhans cell histiocytosis
Congenital leukemia

Modified from Baselga E, Drolet BA, Esterly NB. J Am Acad Dermatol 1997;37:673-705.

PROTEINS C AND S DEFICIENCIES (NEONATAL PURPURA FULMINANS)

Neonatal purpura fulminans is a rare condition characterized by massive and progressive hemorrhagic necrosis of the skin accompanied by thrombosis of the cutaneous vasculature in the neonatal period.[228-233] Occasionally larger vessels and other organs are involved. The primary pathologic event is widespread thrombosis, which is responsible for a hematologic picture of disseminated intravascular coagulation (DIC). In neonates, purpura fulminans is usually the result of inherited thrombophilic disorders that are attributable to protein C deficiency, protein S deficiency, or resistance to activated protein C due to factor V mutations.

Cutaneous Findings

Neonatal purpura fulminans manifests 2 to 12 hours after birth. In rare instances, delayed onset of up to 6 to 10 months of age has been described.[234] Cutaneous lesions consist of extensive ecchymoses in a diffuse and often symmetric distribution that rapidly evolve into hemorrhagic bullae and purple-black necrotic skin lesions, which ultimately form a thick eschar (Fig. 17-21). The initial ecchymotic areas are sharply defined from the surrounding skin and usually have a red advancing inflammatory rim. They are most common at sites of trauma or pressure, the buttocks, extremities, trunk, and scalp. Mucous membranes may be involved rarely.[235] If treatment is instituted in the first 1 to 3 hours, before necrosis ensues, the initial lesions may be reversible.[229]

Extracutaneous Findings

Other organs may be affected by the microvascular thrombosis, most commonly the CNS and eye, but also the kidney and gastrointestinal tract. Cavernous sinus involvement, which may occur in utero, can result in hydrocephalus, seizures, intracerebral hemorrhage, and mental retardation.[232,236,237] Microphthalmia, cataracts, and blindness from vitreous or retinal hemorrhage may be seen.[231,232] Deep venous thrombosis and pulmonary embolism have also been described.[237]

Etiology and Pathogenesis

Purpura fulminans in the neonatal period is almost always caused by inherited thrombophilic states such as homozygous protein C and S deficiency or resistance to activated protein C. Severe bacterial infection associated with DIC can also induce purpura fulminans in the neonate, although it is more common in infancy or early child-

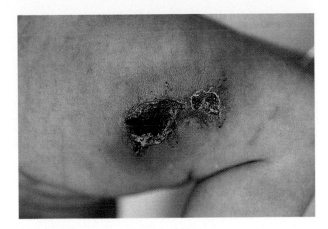

FIG. 17-21
Neonatal purpura fulminans caused by congenital coagulopathy.

hood.[238,239] Proteins C and S are vitamin K–dependent glycoproteins with antithrombotic properties.[240]

Protein C deficiency is an autosomal dominant disease with incomplete penetrance.[240] Homozygous or compound heterozygous patients have a severe clinical phenotype and usually present with neonatal purpura fulminans,* although they may be asymptomatic or present later in life with recurrent thrombosis.[244,245]

Protein S deficiency is also transmitted as an autosomal dominant trait with incomplete penetrance.[240] Homozygous patients may develop neonatal purpura fulminans, although the risk is lower than in patients with homozygous protein C deficiency.[230,246]

Neonatal purpura fulminans may also be caused by activated protein C resistance due to a mutation in the factor V gene.[235,247] Resistance to activated protein C may coexist with protein S and protein C deficiencies, becoming an additional genetic risk factor for purpura fulminans or thromboembolic complications and explaining in part the incomplete clinical penetrance of inherited thrombophilic disorders.

Laboratory Tests and Histopathology

Blood coagulation studies demonstrate evidence of DIC, including prolonged prothrombin and partial thromboplastin times, increased fibrin split products, decreased fibrinogen, and decreased platelets. Microangiopathic hemolytic anemia may occur.

---

*References 229, 231-233, 236, 241-243.

Biopsy of the early skin lesions demonstrates occlusion of dermal blood vessels by microthrombi. Hemorrhage and dermal necrosis are present in more advanced stages. Necrosis of the overlying epidermis with subepidermal hemorrhagic bullae occurs in later phases. Secondary fibrinoid necrosis of dermal vessel walls may be present in the necrotic areas, but primary vasculitis is absent.[229,248]

Definitive diagnosis of protein C and S deficiency is established by measurements of protein C and S levels.[240] Protein C deficiencies can be identified by immunoenzymatic assays measuring the actual concentration of the protein in plasma and two functional assays measuring the enzymatic activity and the anticoagulant activity. These tests distinguish two types of protein C deficiency. In type I deficiency, which is the most common, reduced synthesis of the normal protein leads to a low plasma concentration in all three assays. In type II disease, a qualitative deficiency, levels are normal but functional assays are abnormal. For protein S deficiency, functional and immunoenzymatic assays are available, and both the free form and the inactive form that circulates bound to C4b-binding protein have to be measured.[240] Type I deficiency is characterized by low total and free protein S, type II by normal free protein S and low activity, and type III by low free protein levels with normal total levels.

Interpreting the results of the assays may be difficult because protein C and S levels are physiologically reduced in the neonatal period and may be undetectable in sick newborns with liver disease, respiratory distress syndrome, DIC, or sepsis.[238,239,249-251] Therefore a complete sepsis workup is recommended in any case of neonatal purpura fulminans. Serial determination of protein levels in patients and other family members is necessary to exclude a transient deficiency and confirm true congenital deficiency.

Differential Diagnosis

The cutaneous lesions of purpura fulminans are very characteristic and rarely mistaken for any other condition. Other causes of purpuric eruptions in the newborn may be considered (see Box 17-3).

Course, Management, Treatment, and Prognosis

Without treatment, neonatal purpura fulminans is often fatal. If the diagnosis is suspected, therapy should be initiated immediately, without waiting for the results of protein C and S measurements. Prompt treatment may completely reverse early skin lesions. Initial therapy consists of the administration of fresh frozen plasma (10 to 15 ml/kg/12 hours) or prothrombin complex concentrate, sources of protein C, protein S, and activated protein C.[229,231] A protein C concentrate has been developed that has the advantage of avoiding blood volume overload and that does not carry the risk of transmission of viral diseases.[251-253] Protein S concentrate is not yet available for clinical use. Replacement therapy should be continued until all lesions have healed, usually after 4 to 8 weeks. Long-term treatment involves careful administration of oral anticoagulants, starting at very low doses and with protective replacement therapy to avoid coumarin-induced skin necrosis. Experience with long-term treatment with protein C infusions is limited. There is at least one case report of a successful liver transplant for homozygous protein C deficiency.[254]

PURPURIC PHOTOTHERAPY-INDUCED ERUPTION

This benign, transient purpura in transfused neonates who undergo phototherapy is characterized by raspberry-colored, nonblanching lesions at exposed sites, sparing sites that are protected from lights (e.g., leads and temperature probes).[206,208] The eruption develops after 1 to 4 days of phototherapy and clears spontaneously after discontinuation of light therapy. Histologically there is extravasation of red blood cells in the dermis without epidermal damage. The pathogenesis of this disease is unknown, although transient porphyrinemia has been detected in some patients.[206,208] The purpuric nature of the eruption and the absence of "sunburn cells" differentiate this eruption from "sunburn" due to exposure to UVA from fluorescent lamps.[255] Congenital erythropoietic porphyria and transient elevated porphyrin levels in neonates with hemolytic disease may also cause photosensitivity.[207] Drug-induced phototoxicity in neonates who have received photosensitizing chemicals such as fluorescein dye or furosemide must be considered.[256,257]

REFERENCES

1. Bressler GS, Jones RE. Erythema annulare centrifugum. J Am Acad Dermatol 1981;4:597-602.
2. Harrison PV. The annular erythemas. Int J Dermatol 1979; 18:282-290.
3. Toonstra J, deWit FE. "Persistent" annular erythema of infancy. Arch Dermatol 1984;120:1069-1072.
4. Peterson AO, Jarrat M. Annular erythema of infancy. Arch Dermatol 1981;117:145-148.
5. Cox NH, McQueen A, Evans TJ, et al. An annular erythema of infancy. Arch Dermatol 1987;123:510-513.

6. Hebert AA, Esterly NB. Annular erythema of infancy. Arch Dermatol 1981;117:145-148.

7. Gianotti F, Ermacora E. Erythema gyratum atrophicans transiens neonatale. Arch Dermatol 1975;111:615-616.

8. Tyring SK. Reactive erythemas: erythema annulare centrifugum and erythema gyratum repens. Clin Dermatol 1993;11:135-139.

9. Guillet MH, Dorval JC, Larregue M, et al. Erytheme annulaire centrifuge de Darier a debut neonatal avec 15 ans de suivi. Efficacite de l'interferon et role de cytokines. Ann Dermatol Venereol 1995;122:422-426.

10. Hammar H. Erythema annulare centrifugum coincident with Epstein-Barr virus infection in an infant. Acta Paediatr Scand 1974;63:788-792.

11. Fried R, Schonberg IL, Litt JZ. Erythema annulare centrifugum (Darier) in a newborn infant. J Pediatr 1957; 50:66-67.

12. Klaber R. Erythema gyratum perstans (Colcott Fox): a case report, with discussion on relations with erythema centrifugum annulare (Darier) and dermatitis herpetiformis. Br J Dermatol 1946;58:111-121.

13. Woerdeman MJ. Erythema gyratum perstans (Colcott Fox). Dermatologica 1964;128:392-393.

14. Vermeer DJH. Erythema gyratum perstans. Dermatologica 1968;136:449-450.

15. Larregue M, Beuve-Méry M, Dupuy JM, et al. Érythème annulaire centrifuge type Colcott-Fox (erythema gyratum perstans). Ann Dermatol Venereol 1977;104:217-223.

16. Schmid MH, Wollenberg A, Sander CA, et al. Erythema annulare centrifugum and intestinal Candida albicans infection—coincidence or connection? Acta Derm Venereol 1997;77:93-94.

17. Shelley WB. Erythema annulare centrifugum due to *Candida albicans*. Br J Dermatol 1965;77:383-384.

18. Hendricks AA, Lu C, Elfenbein GJ, et al. Erythema annulare centrifugum associated with ascariasis. Arch Dermatol 1981;117:582-585.

19. Ashurst PJ. Erythema annulare centrifugum due to hydroxychloroquine sulfate and chloroquine sulfate. Arch Dermatol 1967;95:37-39.

20. Shelley WB. Erythema annulare centrifugum: a case due to hypersensitivity to blue cheese *Penicillium*. Arch Dermatol Syph 1964;90:54-58.

21. Jillson OF. Allergic confirmation that some cases of erythema annulare centrifugum are dermatophytids. Arch Dermatol Syph 1954;70:355-359.

22. Beare JM, Froggatt P, Jones JH, et al. Familial annular erythema. An apparently new dominant mutation. Br J Dermatol 1966;78:60-68.

23. Watsky KL, Hansen T. Annular erythema in identical twins. Cutis 1989;44:139-140.

24. Kikuchi I, Ogata K, Inoue S. Pityrosporum infection in an infant with lesions resembling erythema annulare centrifugum. Arch Dermatol 1984;120:380-382.

25. Trevisan G, Stinco G, Cinco M. Neonatal skin lesions due to a spirochetal infection: a case of congenital Lyme borreliosis? Int J Dermatol 1997;36:677-680.

26. Silverman ED, Laxer RM. Neonatal lupus erythematosus. Rheum Dis Clin North Am 1997;23:599-618.

27. Lee LA. Neonatal lupus erythematosus. J Invest Dermatol 1993;100:9S-13S.

28. Watson RM, Lane AT, Barnett NK, et al. Neonatal lupus erythematosus: a clinical, serological, and immunogenetic study with review of the literature. Medicine 1984;63:362-378.

29. Weston WL, Morelli JG, Lee LA. The clinical spectrum of anti-Ro-positive cutaneous neonatal lupus erythematosus. J Am Acad Dermatol 1999 May;40(5 Pt 1):675-681.

30. Sheth AP, Esterly NB, Ratoosh SL, et al. U1RNP positive neonatal lupus erythematosus: association with anti-La antibodies? Br J Dermatol 1995;132:520-526.

31. Provost TT, Watson R, Gammon WR, et al. The neonatal lupus syndrome associated with U1RNP (mRNP) antibodies. N Engl J Med 1987;316:1135-1138.

32. Crowley E, Frieden IJ. Neonatal lupus erythematosus: an unusual congenital presentation with cutaneous atrophy, erosions, alopecia, and pancytopenia. Pediatr Dermatol 1998; 15:38-42.

33. Nitta Y. Lupus erythematosus profundus associated with neonatal lupus erythematosus. Br J Dermatol 1997;136: 112-114.

34. Thornton CM, Eichenfield LF, Shinall EA, et al. Cutaneous telangiectases in neonatal lupus erythematosus. J Am Acad Dermatol 1995;33:19-25.

35. Geggel RL, Tucker L, Szer I. Postnatal progression from second- to third-degree heart block in neonatal lupus syndrome. J Pediatr 1988;113:1049-1052.

36. Laxer RM, Roberts EA, Gross KR, et al. Liver disease in neonatal lupus erythematosus. J Pediatr 1990;116:238-242.

37. Watson R, Kang JE, May M, et al. Thrombocytopenia in the neonatal lupus syndrome. Arch Dermatol 1988;124:560-563.

38. Bourke JF, Burns DA. Neonatal lupus erythematosus with persistent telangiectasia and spastic paraparesis. Clin Exp Dermatol 1993;18:271-273.

39. Rider LG, Sherry DD, Glass ST. Neonatal lupus erythematosus simulating transient myasthenia gravis at presentation. J Pediatr 1991;118:417-419.

40. Contractor S, Hiatt M, Kosmin M, et al. Neonatal thrombosis with anticardiolipin antibody in baby and mother. Am J Perinatol 1992;9:409-410.

41. McCune AB, Weston WL, Lee LA. Maternal and fetal outcome in neonatal lupus erythematosus. Ann Intern Med 1987;106:518-523.

42. Press J, Uziel Y, Laxer RM, et al. Long-term outcome of mothers of children with complete congenital heart block. Am J Med 1996;100:328-332.

43. Silverman ED, Buyon J, Laxer RM, et al. Autoantibody response to the Ro/La particle may predict outcome in neonatal lupus erythematosus. Clin Exp Immunol 1995;100:499-505.

44. Ramsey-Goldman R, Hom D, Deng JS, et al. Anti-SSA antibodies and fetal outcome in maternal systemic lupus erythematosus. Arthritis Rheum 1986;29:1269-1273.

45. Ho YS, Esscher E, Anderson RH, et al. Anatomy of congenital complete heart block and relation to maternal anti-Ro antibodies. Am J Cardiol 1986;58:291-294.

46. Stephenson O, Cleland WP, Hallidie-Smith K. Congenital complete heart block and persistent ductus arteriosus associated with maternal systemic lupus erythematosus. Br Heart J 1981;46:104-106.

47. Lee LA, Coulter S, Erner S, et al. Cardiac immunoglobulin deposition in congenital heart block associated with maternal anti-Ro autoantibodies. Am J Med 1987;83:793-796.

48. Buyon JP, Swersky SH, Fox HE, et al. Intrauterine therapy for presumptive fetal myocarditis with acquired heart block due to systemic lupus erythematosus: experience in a mother with a predominance of SS-B (La) antibodies. Arthritis Rheum 1987;30:44-49.

49. Ishimaru S, Izaki S, Kitamura K, et al. Neonatal lupus erythematosus: dissolution of atrioventricular block after administration of corticosteroid to the pregnant mother. Dermatology 1994;189 Suppl 1:92-94.

50. Fox RJ Jr, McCuistion CH, Schoch EP Jr. Systemic lupus erythematosus: association with previous neonatal lupus erythematosus. Arch Dermatol 1979;115:340.

51. Wintroub BU, Stern R. Cutaneous drug reactions: pathogenesis and clinical classification. J Am Acad Dermatol 1985;13(2 Pt 1):167-179.

52. Sharma VK, Dhar S. Clinical pattern of cutaneous drug eruption among children and adolescents in north India. Pediatr Dermatol 1995;12:178-183.

53. Knowles S, Shapiro L, Shear NH. Serious dermatologic reactions in children. Curr Opin Pediatr 1997;9:388-395.

54. Kramer M, Hutchinson T, Flegel K, et al. Adverse drug reaction in general pediatric outpatients. J Pediatr 1985;106: 305-310.

55. Gourrier E, Karoubi P, el Hanache A, et al. Use of EMLA cream in a department of neonatology. Pain 1996;68 (2-3):431-434.

56. Calobrisi SD, Drolet BA, Esterly NB. Petechial eruption after the application of EMLA cream. Pediatrics 1998;101(3 Pt 1):471-473.

57. Lacouture PG, Epstein MF, Mitchell AA. Vancomycin-associated shock and rash in newborn infants. J Pediatr 1987; 111:615-616.

58. Odio C, Mohs E, Sklar FH, et al. Adverse reaction to vancomycin used as prophylaxis for CSF shunt procedures. Am J Dis Child 1984;138:17-19.

59. Schaad VB, McCracken GH, Nelson JD. Clinical pharmacology and efficacy of vancomycin in pediatric patients. J Pediatr 1980;96:119-126.

60. Prose NS, Mendez H, Menikoff H, et al. Pediatric human immunodeficiency virus infection and its cutaneous manifestations. Pediatr Dermatol 1987;4:267-274.

61. Salomon D, Saurat JH. Erythema multiforme major in a 2-month-old child with human immunodeficiency virus (HIV) infection. Br J Dermatol 1990;123:797-800.

62. Chanock SJ, Luginbuhl LM, McIntosh K, et al. Life-threatening reaction to trimethoprim/sulfamethoxazole in pediatric human immunodeficiency virus infection. Pediatrics 1994;93:519-521.

63. Cohen HA, Cohen Z, Frydman M. Fixed drug eruption of the scrotum due to hydroxyzine hydrochloride (Atarax). Cutis 1996;57:431-432.

64. Hebert AA, Sigman ES, Levy ML. Serum sickness–like reactions from cefaclor in children. J Am Acad Dermatol 1991; 25(5 Pt 1):805-808.

65. Vittorio C, Muglia J. Anticonvulsant hypersensitivity syndrome. Arch Intern Med 1995;155:2285-2290.

66. Konishi T, Naganuma Y, Hongo K, et al. Carbamazepine-induced skin rash in children with epilepsy. Eur J Pediatr 1993;152:605-608.

67. Mortureux P, Leaute-Labreze C, Legrain-Lifermann V, et al. Acute urticaria in infancy and early childhood: a prospective study. Arch Dermatol 1998;134:319-323.

68. Tamayo-Sanchez L, Ruiz-Maldonado R, Laterza A. Acute annular urticaria in infants and children. Pediatr Dermatol 1997;14:231-234.

69. Legrain V, Taieb A, Sage T, et al. Urticaria in infants: a study of forty patients. Pediatr Dermatol 1990;7:101-107.

70. Kauppinen K, Juntunen K, Lanki H. Urticaria in children: retrospective evaluation and follow-up. Allergy 1984;39: 469-472.

71. Beltrani VS. Urticaria and angioedema. Dermatol Clin 1996;14:171-198.

72. Ghosh S, Kanwar AJ, Kaur S. Urticaria in children. Pediatr Dermatol 1993;10:107-110.

73. Harris A, Twarog FJ, Geha RS. Chronic urticaria in childhood: natural course and etiology. Ann Allergy 1983;51: 161-165.

74. Carter EL, Garzon MC. Neonatal urticaria due to prostaglandin E1. Pediatr Dermatol 2000;17:58-61.

75. Massicot P, Billeau C, Fontan D, et al. Manifestations urticariennes chez le nourrison au cours de l'intolérance aux protéines du lait de vache. Ann Dermatol Venereol 1982; 109:237-246.

76. Hill DJ, Davidson GP, Cameron DS, et al. The spectrum of cow's milk allergy in childhood: clinical, gastroenterological, and immunological studies. Acta Paediatr Scand 1979; 68:847-852.

77. Jakobsson I, Lindberg T. A prospective study of cow's milk protein intolerance in Swedish infants. Acta Paediatr Scand 1979;68:853-859.

78. Ruiz-Maldonado R, Tamayo L, Ridaura C. Diffuse dermographic mastocytosis without visible skin lesions. Int J Dermatol 1975;14:126-128.

79. Tindall JP, Beeker SK, Rosse WF. Familial cold urticaria: a generalized reaction involving leukocytosis. Arch Intern Med 1969;124:129-134.

80. Zip CM, Ross JB, Greaves MW, et al. Familial cold urticaria. Clin Exp Dermatol 1993;18:338-341.

81. Doeglas HM, Bleumink E. Familial cold urticaria—clinical findings. Arch Dermatol 1974;110:382-388.

82. Ormerod AD, Smart L, Reid TS, et al. Familial cold urticaria: investigation of a family and response to stanozolol. Arch Dermatol 1993;129:343-346.

83. Muckle TJ. The Muckle-Wells syndrome. Br J Dermatol 1979;100:87-92.

84. Jedele KB, Michels VV. Familial dermographism. Am J Med Genet 1991;39(2):201-203.

85. Sahihi T, Esterly NB. Atypical diffuse cutaneous mastocytosis. Am J Dis Child 1972;124:133-135.

86. Epstein PA, Kidd KK. Dermodistortive urticaria. Am J Med Genet 1981;9:307-315.

87. Bonnetblanc JM, Andrieu-Pfahl F, Meraud JP, et al. Familial aquagenic urticaria. Dermatologica 1979;158:468-470.

88. Michaëlsson G, Ros AM. Familial localized heat urticaria of delayed type. Acta Derm Venereol 1971;51:279-283.

89. Prieur AM, Griscelli C, Lampert F, et al. A chronic, infantile, neurological, cutaneous, and articular (CINCA) syndrome: a specific entity analyzed in 30 patients. Scand J Rheumatol 1987;Suppl 66:57-68.

90. Torbiak RP, Dent PB, Cockshott WP. NOMID—a neonatal syndrome of multisystem inflammation. Skeletal Radiol 1989;18:359-364.

91. Huttenlocher A, Frieden IJ, Emery H. Neonatal onset multisystem inflammatory disease. J Rheumatol 1995;22:1171-1173.

92. Hassink SG, Goldsmith DP. Neonatal onset multisystem inflammatory disease. Arthritis Rheum 1983;26:668-673.

93. Prieur AM, Griscelli C. Arthropathy with rash, chronic meningitis, eye lesions, and mental retardation. J Pediatr 1981;99:79-83.

94. Miura M, Okabe T, Tsubata S, et al. Chronic infantile neurological cutaneous articular syndrome in a patient from Japan. Eur J Pediatr 1997;156:624-626.

95. Huff JC, Weston WL, Tonnesen MG. Erythema multiforme: A critical review of characteristics, diagnostic criteria, and causes. J Am Acad Dermatol 1983;8:763-775.

96. Roujeau JC. Stevens-Johnson syndrome and toxic epidermal necrolysis are severity variants of the same disease which differs from erythema multiforme. J Dermatol 1997;24:726-729.

97. Bastuji-Garin S, Rzany B, Stern RS, et al. Clinical classification of cases of toxic epidermal necrolysis, Stevens-Johnson syndrome, and erythema multiforme. Arch Dermatol 1993;129:92-96.

98. Dikland WJ, Oranje AP, Stolz E, et al. Erythema multiforme in childhood and early infancy. Pediatr Dermatol 1986,3:135-139.

99. Ginsburg CM. Stevens-Johnson syndrome in children. Pediatr Infect Dis 1982;1:155-158.

100. Ashkenazi S, Metzker A, Rachmel A, et al. Erythema multiforme as a single manifestation of cow's milk intolerance. Acta Paediatrica 1992;81:729-730.

101. Sakurai M. Erythema multiforme in children: unusual clinical features with seasonal occurrence. J Dermatol 1989;16:361-368.

102. Weston WL, Brice SL, Jester JD, et al. Herpes simplex virus in childhood erythema multiforme. Pediatrics 1992;89:32-34.

103. Roujeau JC, Kelly JP, Naldi L, et al. Medication use and the risk of Stevens-Johnson syndrome or toxic epidermal necrolysis. N Engl J Med 1995;333:1600-1607.

104. Ackerman AB, Ragaz A. Erythema multiforme. Am J Dermatopathol 1985;7:133-139.

105. Côté B, Wechsler HL, Bastuji-Garin S, et al. Clinicopathological correlations in erythema multiforme and Stevens-Johnson syndrome. Arch Dermatol 1995;131:1268-1272.

106. Anonymous. Corticosteroids for erythema multiforme? Pediatr Dermatol 1989;6:229-250.

107. Schofield JK, Tatnall FM, Leigh IM. Recurrent erythema multiforme: clinical features and treatment in a large series of patients. Br J Dermatol 1993;128:542-545.

108. Renfro L, Grant-Kels JM, Feder HM Jr, et al. Controversy: are systemic steroids indicated in the treatment of erythema multiforme? Pediatr Dermatol 1989;6:43-50.

109. Halebian PH, Madden MR, Finklestein JL, et al. Improved burn center survival of patients with toxic epidermal necrolysis managed without corticosteroids. Ann Surg 1986;204:503-512.

110. Fitzgerald RL, McBurney EI, Nesbitt LT Jr. Sweet's syndrome. Int J Dermatol 1996;35:9-15.

111. von den Driesch P. Sweet's syndrome (acute febrile neutrophilic dermatosis). J Am Acad Dermatol 1994;31:535-56;quiz 557-560.

112. Kemmett D, Hunter JA. Sweet's syndrome: a clinicopathologic review of twenty-nine cases. J Am Acad Dermatol 1990;23:503-507.

113. Sedel D, Huguet P, Lebbe C, et al. Sweet syndrome as the presenting manifestation of chronic granulomatous disease in an infant. Pediatr Dermatol 1994;11:237-240.

114. Dunn TR, Saperstein HW, Biederman A, et al. Sweet syndrome in a neonate with aseptic meningitis. Pediatr Dermatol 1992;9:288-292.

115. Collins P, Rogers S, Keenan P, et al. Acute febrile neutrophilic dermatosis in childhood (Sweet's syndrome). Br J Dermatol 1991;124:203-206.

116. Saxe N, Gordon W. Acute febrile neutrophilic dermatosis (Sweet's syndrome). S Afr Med J 1978;53:253-256.

117. Levin DL, Esterly NB, Herman JJ, et al. The Sweet syndrome in children. J Pediatr 1981;99:73-78.

118. Itami S, Nishioka K. Sweet's syndrome in infancy. Br J Dermatol 1980;103:449-451.

119. Hassouna L, Nabulsi Khalil M, Mroueh SM, et al. Multiple erythematous tender papules and nodules in an 11-month-old boy. Sweet syndrome (SS) (acute febrile neutrophilic dermatosis). Arch Dermatol 1996;132:1507-1510.

120. Hwang ST, Williams ML, McCalmont TH, et al. Sweet's syndrome leading to acquired cutis laxa (Marshall's syndrome) in an infant with alpha-1-antitrypsin deficiency. Arch Dermatol 1995;131:1175-1177.

121. Misery L, Blanc L, Perrot JL, et al. Syndrome de Sweet au cours d'une agranulocytose. Hypothese pathogenique. Ann Dermatol Venereol 1994;121:414-415.

122. Cohen PR, Kurzrock R. Sweet's syndrome and cancer. Clin Dermatol 1993,11:149-157.

123. Walker DC, Cohen PR. Trimethoprim-sulfamethoxazole-associated acute febrile neutrophilic dermatosis: case report and review of drug-induced Sweet's syndrome. J Am Acad Dermatol 1996;34(5 Pt 2):918-923.

124. Jain KK. Sweet's syndrome associated with granulocyte colony-stimulating factor. Cutis 1996;57:107-110.

125. Going JJ, Going SM, Myskow MW, et al. Sweet's syndrome: histological and immunohistological study of 15 cases. J Clin Pathol 1987;40:175-179.

126. Delaporte E, Gavoau DJ, Piette FA, et al. Acute febrile neutrophilic dermatosis (Sweet's syndrome). Arch Dermatol 1989;125:1101-1104.

127. Myatt AE, Baker DJ, Byfield DM. Sweet's syndrome: a report on the use of potassium iodide. Clin Exp Dermatol 1987;12:345-349.

128. Suehisa S, Tagami H, Inoue F, et al. Colchicine in the treatment of acute febrile dermatosis (Sweet's syndrome). Br J Dermatol 1983;108:99-101.

129. Aram H. Acute febrile neutrophilic dermatosis (Sweet's Syndrome): response to dapsone. Arch Dermatol 1984;120:245.

130. Kawasaki T, Kosaki F, Okawa S, et al. A new infantile acute febrile mucocutaneous lymph node syndrome (MLNS) prevailing in Japan. Pediatrics 1974;54:271-276.

131. Burns JC, Wiggins JW, Toews WH, et al. Clinical spectrum of Kawasaki disease in infants younger than 6 months of age. J Pediatr 1986;109:759-763.

132. Rosenfeld EA, Corydon KE, Shulman ST. Kawasaki disease in infants less than one year of age. J Pediatr 1995;126:524-529.

133. Fujita Y, Nakamura Y, Sakata J, et al. Kawasaki disease in families. Pediatrics 1989;84:666-669.

134. Yanagawa H, Nakamura Y, Yashiro M, et al. Update of the epidemiology of Kawasaki disease in Japan from the results of 1993-94 nationwide survey. J Epidemiol 1996;6:148-157.

135. Yanagawa H, Nakamura Y, Yashiro M, et al. Results of the nationwide epidemiologic survey of Kawasaki disease in 1995 and 1996 in Japan. Pediatrics 1998;102:E65.

136. Friter BS, Lucky AW. The perineal eruption of Kawasaki syndrome. Arch Dermatol 1988;124:1805-1810.

137. Kuniyuki S, Asada M. An ulcerated lesion at the BCG vaccination site during the course of Kawasaki disease. J Am Acad Dermatol 1997;37(2 Pt 2):303-304.

138. Dajani AS, Taubert KA, Gerber MA, et al. Diagnosis and therapy of Kawasaki disease in children. Circulation 1993;87:1776-1780.

139. Tomita S, Chung K, Mas M, et al. Peripheral gangrene associated with Kawasaki disease. Clin Infect Dis 1992;14:121-126.

140. Takahashi M. Kawasaki disease. Curr Opin Pediatr 1997;9:523-529.

141. Kikuta H, Sakiyama Y, Matsumoto S, et al. Detection of Epstein-Barr virus DNA in cardiac and aortic tissues from chronic, active Epstein-Barr virus infection associated with Kawasaki disease–like coronary aneurism artery. J Pediatr 1993;123:90-92.

142. Konishi N, Baba K, Abe J, et al. A case of Kawasaki disease with coronary artery aneurysms documenting *Yersinia pseudotuberculosis* infection. Acta Paediatrica 1997;86:661-664.

143. Hirao J, Hibi S, Andoh T, et al. High levels of circulating interleukin-4 and interleukin-10 in Kawasaki disease. Int Arch Allergy Immunol 1997;112:152-156.

144. Sato N, Sagawa K, Sasaguri Y, et al. Immunopathology and cytokine detection in the skin lesions of patients with Kawasaki disease. J Pediatr 1993;122:198-203.

145. Leung DY, Meissner HC, Fulton DR, et al. Toxic shock syndrome toxin-secreting *Staphylococcus aureus* in Kawasaki syndrome. Lancet 1993;342:1385-1388.

146. Fukushige J, Takahashi N, Ueda Y, et al. Incidence and clinical features of incomplete Kawasaki disease. Acta Paediatrica 1994;83:1057-1060.

147. Kato H, Sugimura T, Akagi T, et al. Long-term consequences of Kawasaki disease: a 10- to 21-year follow-up study of 594 patients. Circulation 1996;94:1379-1385.

148. Suzuki A, Yamagishi M, Kimura K, et al. Functional behavior and morphology of the coronary artery wall in patients with Kawasaki disease assessed by intravascular ultrasound. J Am Coll Cardiol 1996;27:291-296.

149. Nakamura Y, Yanagawa H, Kato H, et al. Mortality rates for patients with a history of Kawasaki disease in Japan. Kawasaki Disease Follow-up Group. J Pediatr 1996;128:75-81.

150. Dajani AS, Taubert KA, Takahashi M, et al. Guidelines for long-term management of patients with Kawasaki disease. Circulation 1994;89:916-922.

151. Newburger JW, Takahashi M, Burns JC, et al. The treatment of Kawasaki disease with intravenous gamma globulin. N Engl J Med 1986;315:341-347.

152. Wright DA, Newburger JW, Baker A, et al. Treatment of immune globulin–resistant Kawasaki disease with pulsed doses of corticosteroids. J Pediatr 1996;128:146-149.

153. Cunningham BB, Caro WA, Eramo LR. Neonatal acute hemorrhagic edema of childhood: case report and review of the English-language literature. Pediatr Dermatol 1996;13:39-44.

154. Legrain V, Lejean S, Taieb A, et al. Infantile acute hemorrhagic edema of the skin: study of ten cases. J Am Acad Dermatol 1991;24:17-22.

155. Baselga E, Drolet BA, Esterly NB. Purpura in infants and children. J Am Acad Dermatol 1997;37:673-705.

156. Gonggryp LA, Todd G. Acute hemorrhagic edema of childhood (AHE). Pediatr Dermatol 1998;15:91-96.

157. Ince E, Mumcu Y, Suskan E, et al. Infantile acute hemorrhagic edema: a variant of leukocytoclastic vasculitis. Pediatr Dermatol 1995;12:224-227.

158. Larregue M, Lorette G, Prigent F. Oedème aigu hémorragique du nourisson avec complication léthale digestive. Ann Dermatol Venereol 1980;197:901-905.

159. Saraçlar Y, Tinaztepe K, Adalioglu G, et al. Acute hemorrhagic edema of infancy (AHEI)—a variant of Henoch-Schönlein purpura or a distinct clinical entity? J Allergy Clin Immunol 1990;86(4 Pt 1):473-483.

160. Dubin BA, Bronson DM, Eng AM. Acute hemorrhagic edema of childhood: an unusual variant of leukocytoclastic vasculitis. J Am Acad Dermatol 1990;23(2 Pt 2):347-350.

161. Amitai Y, Gillis D, Wasserman D, et al. Henoch-Schönlein purpura in infants. Pediatrics 1993;92:865-867.

162. Lambert D, Laurent R, Bouilly D, et al. Oedème aigu hémorragique du nourisson: donnés immunologiques et ultrastructurales. Ann Dermatol Venereol 1979;106:975-987.

163. Saraçlar Y, Tinaztepe K. Infantile acute hemorrhagic edema of the skin. J Am Acad Dermatol 1992;26(2 Pt 1):275-276.

164. Poh-Fitzpatrick MB. Clinical features of the porphyrias. Clin Dermatol 1998;16:251-264.

165. Lim HW, Murphy GM. The porphyrias. Clin Dermatol 1996;14:375-387.

166. Bickers DR, Pathak MA, Lim HW. The porphyrias. In Freedberg IM, Eisen AZ, Wolff K, et al., eds. Fitzpatrick's dermatology in general medicine, 5th edition. New York: McGraw-Hill, 1999: pp 1766-1803.

167. Mascaro JM. Porphyrias in children. Pediatr Dermatol 1992;9:371-372.

168. Jensen JD, Resnick SD. Porphyria in childhood. Semin Dermatol 1995;14:33-39.

169. Fritsch C, Bolsen K, Ruzicka T, et al. Congenital erythropoietic porphyria. J Am Acad Dermatol 1997;36:594-610.

170. Huang JL, Zaider E, Roth P, et al. Congenital erythropoietic porphyria: clinical, biochemical, and enzymatic profile of a severely affected infant. J Am Acad Dermatol 1996;34(5 Pt 2):924-927.

171. Nordmann Y, de Verneuil H, Deybach JC, et al. Molecular genetics of porphyrias. Ann Med 1990;22:387-391.

172. Xu W, Warner CA, Desnick RJ. Congenital erythropoietic porphyria: identification and expression of 10 mutations in the uroporphyrinogen III synthase gene. J Clin Invest 1995;95:905-912.

173. Kaiser IH. Brown amniotic fluid in congenital erythropoietic porphyria. Obstet Gynecol 1980;56:383-384.
174. Horiguchi Y, Horio T, Yamamoto M, et al. Late onset erythropoietic porphyria. Br J Dermatol 1989;121:255-262.
175. Mathews-Roth MM. Treatment of the cutaneous porphyrias. Clin Dermatol 1998;16:295-298.
176. Mascaro JM. Management of the erythropoietic porphyrias. Photodermatol Photoimmunol Photomed 1998;14:44-45.
177. Guarini L, Piomelli S, Poh-Fitzpatrick MB. Hydroxyurea in congenital erythropoietic porphyria. N Engl J Med 1994;330(15):1091-1092.
178. Piomelli S, Poh-Fitzpatrick MB, Seaman C, et al. Complete suppression of the symptoms of congenital erythropoietic porphyria by long-term treatment with high-level transfusions. N Engl J Med 1986;314:1029-1031.
179. Minder EI, Schneider Yin X, Moll F. Lack of effect of oral charcoal in congenital erythropoietic porphyria. N Engl J Med 1994;330:1092-1094.
180. Pimstone NR, Gandhi SN, Mukerji SK. Therapeutic efficacy of oral charcoal in congenital erythropoietic porphyria. N Engl J Med 1987;316:390-393.
181. Maleville J, Babin JP, Mollard S, et al. Porphyrie erythropoietique congenitale de Gunther et carotenoides. Essai therapeutique de 4 ans. Ann Dermatol Venereol 1982;109:883-887.
182. Seip M, Thune PO, Eriksen L. Treatment of photosensitivity in congenital erythropoietic porphyria (CEP) with beta-carotene. Acta Derm Venereol 1974;54:239-240.
183. Thomas C, Ged C, Nordmann Y, et al. Correction of congenital erythropoietic porphyria by bone marrow transplantation. J Pediatr 1996;129:453-456.
184. Tezcan I, Xu W, Gurgey A, et al. Congenital erythropoietic porphyria successfully treated by allogeneic bone marrow transplantation. Blood 1998;92:4053-4058.
185. Moreau Gaudry F, Mazurier F, Bensidhoum M, et al. Metabolic correction of congenital erythropoietic porphyria by retrovirus-mediated gene transfer into Epstein-Barr virus-transformed B-cell lines. Blood 1995;85:1449-1453.
186. DeLeo VA, Poh-Fitzpatrick M, Mathews-Roth M, et al. Erythropoietic protoporphyria: 10 years' experience. Am J Med. 1976 Jan;60:8-22
187. Norris PG, Nunn AV, Hawk JL, Cox TM. Genetic heterogeneity in erythropoietic protoporphyria: a study of the enzymatic defect in nine affected families. J Invest Dermatol 1990;95:260-263.
188. Goerz G, Bunselmeyer S, Bolsen K, Schurer NY. Ferrochelatase activities in patients with erythropoietic protoporphyria and their families. Br J Dermatol 1996;134:880-885.
189. Sarkany RP, Alexander GJ, Cox TM: Recessive inheritance of erythropoietic protoporphyria with liver failure. Lancet 1994 4;343:1394-1396.
190. Poh-Fitzpatrick MB, Piomelli S, Young P, et al. Rapid quantitative assay for erythrocyte porphyrins. Arch Dermatol 1974;110:225-230.
191. Mathews-Roth MM. Treatment of the cutaneous porphyrias. Clin Dermatol 1998;16:295-298.
192. Bloomer JR. The liver in protoporphyria. Hepatology 1988;8:402-407.
193. Polson RJ, Lim CK, Rolles K, et al. The effect of liver transplantation in a 13-year-old boy with erythropoietic protoporphyria. Transplantation 1988;46:386-389.
194. Piñol-Aguade J, Herrero C, Almeida J, et al. Porphyrie hepato-erythroctaire, une nouvelle forme de porphyrie. Ann Dermatol Syph 1975;102:129-136.
195. Toback AC, Sassa S, Poh-Fitzpatrick MB, et al. Hepatoerythropoietic porphyria: clinical, biochemical, and enzymatic studies in a three generation family lineage. N Engl J Med 1987;316:645-650.
196. Lim HW, Poh-Fitzpatrick MB. Hepatoerythropoietic porphyria: A variant of childhood-onset porphyria cutanea tarda: porphyrin profiles and enzymatic studies of two cases in a family. J Am Acad Dermatol 1984;11:1103-1111.
197. Elder GH, Smith SG, Herrero C, et al. Hepatoerythropoietic porphyria: a new uroporphyrinogen decarboxylase defect or homozygous porphyria cutanea tarda? Lancet 1981;1:916-919.
198. Simon N, Berko NY, Schneider I. Hepato-erythropoietic porphyria presenting as scleroderma and acrosclerosis in a sibling pair. Br J Dermatol 1997;96:663-668.
199. Lamoril J, Martasek P, Deybach JC, et al. A molecular defect in coproporphyrinogen oxidase gene causing harderoporphyria, a variant form of hereditary coproporphyria. Hum Mol Genet 1995;4:275-278.
200. Nordmann Y, Grandchamp B, de Verneuil H, et al. Harderoporphyria: a variant hereditary coproporphyria. J Clin Invest 1983;72:1139-1149.
201. Doss M, von Tiepermann R, Kopp W. Harderoporphyrin coproporphyria. Lancet 1984;1:292-292.
202. Murphy GM, Hawk JLM, Magnus IA, et al. Homozygous variegate porphyria: two similar cases in unrelated families. J Roy Soc Med 1986;79:361-363.
203. Mustajoki P, Tenhunen R, Niemi KM, et al. Homozygous variegate porphyria: a severe skin disease of infancy. Clin Genet 1987;32:300-305.
204. Norris PG, Elder GH, Hawk JM. Homozygous variegate porphyria: a case report. Br J Dermatol 1990;122:253-257.
205. Korda V, Deybach JCH, Martasek P, et al. Homozygous variegate porphyria. Lancet 1984;1:851.
206. Paller AS, Eramo LR, Farrell EE, et al. Purpuric phototherapy-induced eruption in transfused neonates: relation to transient porphyrinemia. Pediatrics 1997;100(3 Pt 1):360-364.
207. Mallon E, Wojnarowska F, Hope P, et al. Neonatal bullous eruption as a result of transient porphyrinemia in a premature infant with hemolytic disease of the newborn. J Am Acad Dermatol 1995;33(2 Pt 2):333-336.
208. Crawford RI, Lawlor ER, Wadsworth LD, et al. Transient erythroporphyria in infancy. J Am Acad Dermatol 1996;35:833-834.
209. Klein HZ, Markarian M. Dermal erythropoiesis in congenital rubella: description of an infected newborn who had purpura associated with marked extramedullary erythropoiesis in the skin and elsewhere. Clin Pediatr 1969;8:604-607.
210. Bowden JB, Hebert AA, Rapini RP. Dermal hematopoiesis in neonates: report of five cases. J Am Acad Dermatol 1989;20:1104-1110.
211. Brough AJ, Jones D, Page RH, et al. Dermal erythropoiesis in neonatal infants: a manifestation of intrauterine viral disease. Pediatrics 1967;40:627-635.
212. Silver MM, Hellmann J, Zielenska M, et al. Anemia, blueberry-muffin rash, and hepatomegaly in a newborn infant. J Pediatr 1996;128:579-586.

213. Pizarro A, Elorza D, Gamallo C, et al. Neonatal dermal erythropoiesis associated with severe rhesus immunization: amelioration by high-dose intravenous immunoglobulin. Br J Dermatol 1995;133:334-336.

214. Hebert AA, Esterly NB, Gardner TH. Dermal erythropoiesis in Rh hemolytic disease of the newborn. J Pediatr 1985; 107:799-801.

215. Argyle JC, Zone JJ. Dermal erythropoiesis in a neonate. Arch Dermatol 1981;117:492-494.

216. Schwartz JL, Maniscalco WM, Lane AT, et al. Twin transfusion syndrome causing cutaneous erythropoiesis. Pediatrics 1984;74:527-529.

217. Hendricks WM, Hu CH. Blueberry muffin syndrome: cutaneous erythropoiesis and possible intrauterine viral infection. Cutis 1984;34:549-551.

218. Shown TE, Durfee MF. Blueberry muffin baby: neonatal neuroblastoma with subcutaneous metastases. J Urol 1970; 104:193-195.

219. Hawthorne HC, Nelson JS, Witzleben CL, et al. Blanching subcutaneous nodules in neonatal neuroblastoma. J Pediatr 1970;77:297-300.

220. van Erp IFR. Cutaneous metastasis in neuroblastoma. Dermatologica 1968;136:265-269.

221. Kitagawa N, Arata J, Ohtsuki Y, et al. Congenital alveolar rhabdomyosarcoma presenting as a blueberry muffin baby. J Dermatol 1989;16:409-411.

222. Meuleman V, Degreef H. Acute myelomonocytic leukemia with skin localizations. Dermatology 1995;190:346-348.

223. Gottesfeld E, Silverman RA, Coccia PF, et al. Transient blueberry muffin appearance of a newborn with congenital monoblastic leukemia. J Am Acad Dermatol 1989;21(2 Pt 2):347-351.

224. Resnik KS, Brod BB. Leukemia cutis in congenital leukemia: analysis and review of the world literature with report of an additional case. Arch Dermatol 1993;129:1301-1306.

225. Enjolras O, Leibowitch M, Bonacini F, et al. Histiocytoses langerhansiennes congenitales cutanees. A propos de 7 cas. Ann Dermatol Venereol 1992;119:111-117.

226. Enjolras O, Leibowitch M, Guillemette J, et al. "Blueberry muffin baby": hematopoiese extramedullaire neonatale? Leucemie monoblastique congenitale involutive? Ou histiocytose congenitale involutive? Ann Dermatol Venereol 1990;117:810-812.

227. Lerner LH, Bailey EM. A newborn with multiple hemorrhagic vesicles, lymphadenopathy, and respiratory distress. N Engl J Med 1996;24:1591-1597.

228. van der Horst RL. Purpura fulminans in a newborn baby. Arch Dis Child 1962;37:436-441.

229. Marlar RA, Neumann A. Neonatal purpura fulminans due to homozygous protein C or protein S deficiencies. Semin Thromb Hemost 1990;16:299-309.

230. Mahasandana C, Suvatte V, Chuansumrit A, et al. Homozygous protein S deficiency in an infant with purpura fulminans. J Pediatr 1990;117:750-753.

231. Marlar RA, Montgomery RR, Broekmans AW. Diagnosis and treatment of homozygous protein C deficiency. Report of the Working Party on Homozygous Protein C Deficiency of the Subcommittee on Protein C and Protein S, International Committee on Thrombosis and Haemostasis. J Pediatr 1989;114(4 Pt 1):528-534.

232. Marciniak E, Wilson HD, Marlar RA. Neonatal purpura fulminans: a genetic disorder related to the absence of protein C in blood. Blood 1985;65:15-20.

233. Auletta MJ, Headington JT. Purpura fulminans: a cutaneous manifestation of severe protein C deficiency. Arch Dermatol 1988;124:1387-1391.

234. Tuddenham EG, Takase T, Thomas AE, et al. Homozygous protein C deficiency with delayed onset of symptoms at 7 to 10 months. Thromb Res 1989;53:475-484.

235. Pipe SW, Schmaier AH, Nichols WC, et al. Neonatal purpura fulminans in association with factor V R506Q mutation. J Pediatr 1996;128:706-709.

236. Sills RH, Marlar RA, Montgomery RR, et al. Severe homozygous protein C deficiency. J Pediatr 1984;105:409-413.

237. Seligsohn U, Berger A, Abend M, et al. Homozygous protein C deficiency manifested by massive venous thrombosis in the newborn. N Engl J Med 1984;310:559-562.

238. Gürses N, Ozkan A. Neonatal and childhood purpura fulminans: review of seven cases. Cutis 1988;41:361-363.

239. Chuansumrit A, Hotrakitya S, Kruavit A. Severe acquired neonatal purpura fulminans. Clin Pediatr 1996;35:373-376.

240. Aiach M, Borgel D, Gaussem P, et al. Protein C and Protein S deficiencies. Semin Hematol 1997;34:205-217.

241. Auletta MJ, Headington JT. Purpura fulminans: a cutaneous manifestation of severe protein C deficiency. Arch Dermatol 1988;124:1387-1391.

242. Marlar RA, Mastovich S. Hereditary protein C deficiency: a review of the genetics, clinical presentation, diagnosis and treatment. Blood Coagul Fibrinolysis 1990;1:319-330.

243. Branson HE, Katz J, Marble R, et al. Inherited protein C deficiency and coumarin-responsive chronic relapsing purpura fulminans in a newborn infant. Lancet 1983;2:1165-1168.

244. Grundy CB, Melissari E, Lindo V, et al. Late-onset homozygous protein C deficiency. Lancet 1991;338:575-576.

245. Tripodi A, Franchi F, Krachmalnicoff A, et al. Asymptomatic homozygous protein C deficiency. Acta Haematol 1990;83: 152-155.

246. Gomez E, Ledford MR, Pegelow CH, et al. Homozygous protein S deficiency due to a one base pair deletion that leads to a stop codon in exon III of the protein S gene. Thromb Haemost 1994;71:723-726.

247. Dahlbäck B. Resistance to activated protein C as risk factor for thrombosis: molecular mechanisms, laboratory investigation, and clinical management. Semin Hematol 1997; 217-234.

248. Adcock DM, Hicks MJ. Dermatopathology of skin necrosis associated with purpura fulminans. Semin Thromb Hemost 1990;16:283-292.

249. Dominey A, Kettler A, Yiannias J, et al. Purpura fulminans and transient protein C and S deficiency. Arch Dermatol 1988;124:1442-1443.

250. Minutillo C, Pemberton PJ, Willoughby ML, et al. Neonatal purpura fulminans and transient protein C deficiency. Arch Dis Child 1990;65:561-562.

251. Gerson WT, Dickerman JD, Bovill EG, et al. Severe acquired protein C deficiency in purpura fulminans associated with disseminated intravascular coagulation: treatment with protein C concentrate. Pediatrics 1993;91:418-422.

252. Baliga V, Thwaites R, Tillyer ML, et al. Homozygous protein C deficiency—management with protein C concentrate. Eur J Pediatr 1995;154:534-538.

253. Dreyfus M, Magny JF, Bridey F, et al. Treatment of homozygous protein C deficiency and neonatal purpura fulminans with a purified protein C concentrate. N Engl J Med 1991; 325:1565-1568.

254. Casella JF, Lewis JH, Bontempo FA, et al. Successful treatment of homozygous protein C deficiency by hepatic transplantation. Lancet 1988;1:435-438.

255. Siegfried EC, Stone MS, Madison KC. Ultraviolet light burn: a cutaneous complication of visible light phototherapy of neonatal jaundice. Pediatr Dermatol 1992;9:278-282.

256. Burry JN, Lawrence JR. Phototoxic blisters from high furosemide dosage. Br J Dermatol 1976;94:495-499.

257. Kearns GL, Williams BJ, Timmons OD. Fluorescein phototoxicity in a premature infant. J Pediatr 1985;107:796-798.

18

Vascular Stains, Malformations, and Tumors

ODILE ENJOLRAS
MARIA C. GARZON

CLASSIFICATION OF VASCULAR BIRTHMARKS

In 1982, Mulliken and Glowacki[1] proposed a biologic classification of vascular birthmarks that subsequently has become widely accepted. It was modified slightly in 1996 by the International Society for the Study of Vascular Anomalies.[2] Two major groups of vascular birthmarks are recognized: *vascular malformations*, which are composed of dysplastic vessels, and *vascular tumors* that demonstrate cellular hyperplasia. Cellular markers, histologic appearance, and natural history demonstrate the biologic differences between malformations and vascular tumors.[3,4] This classification schema avoids confusing terminology such as *cavernous hemangioma*, which had been previously used to describe both tumors and malformations.[3]

Vascular malformations are subcategorized according to flow characteristics and predominant anomalous channels: slow flow (capillary [C], venous [V], lymphatic [L]) or fast flow (arterial = aneurysm [A] and arteriovenous fistula [AVF]). A number of complex-combined vascular malformations (M) exist: CVM, CLVM, LVM, AVM, CAVM, CLAVM, and so forth, some of them known by eponyms (e.g., Klippel-Trenaunay syndrome is a CVLM). Hemangioma is the most common vascular tumor of infancy; the others are rare, and some have only recently been characterized.

VASCULAR MALFORMATIONS

Capillary, venous, lymphatic, arterial, and arteriovenous malformations occur either alone or in combination. They are often localized and circumscribed lesions but can present in a segmental, systematized pattern or in a diffuse, dis-seminated form. Some are part of a more complex syndromic pathology. Vascular malformations are often erroneously referred to in the literature as *hemangioma* or *hemangiomatosis,* and this complicates analysis of the literature.

Capillary Malformations

Salmon Patch
A salmon patch is a midline capillary malformation (CM) that is also known as an "angel kiss" when it is located on the forehead and "stork bite" when on the nape. It is present in nearly half of all newborns and affects males and females equally.[5] It is most commonly located on the nape, as well as upper eyelids, glabella, nose, and upper lip[6] (Fig. 18-1).

If a salmon patch capillary malformation involves the upper eyelid and does not have a V-shaped patch in the middle of the forehead, it may be difficult to differentiate from a limited V1 port wine stain (the hallmark for the risk of Sturge-Weber syndrome) or a telangiectatic, ill-defined red stain that is a precursor mark for the development of an eyelid hemangioma. Salmon patches usually disappear within 1 or 2 years, but in some cases persist, particularly those at the nape.

Butterfly-Shaped Mark and Sacral Medial Telangiectatic Vascular Nevi
Localized in the midline sacral region, the butterfly-shaped mark has been described as a variant of the salmon patch without specific association, and some authors have asserted that evaluation of the spine seems unnecessary in these infants unless other signs are present.[7] Unlike the fa-

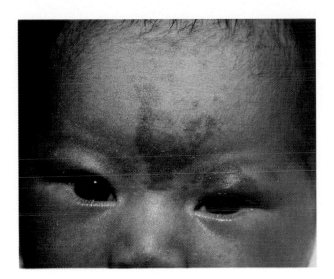

FIG. 18-1

Typical salmon patch on the mid-forehead and upper eyelid.

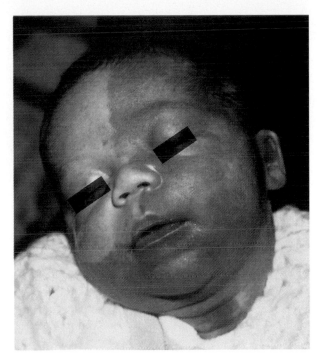

FIG. 18-2

Port wine stain involving left facial V1+V2+V3 and right V3 areas. The V1 involvement indicates a risk of Sturge-Weber syndrome, which this infant had.

cial salmon patch, this sacral stain tends to persist. A condition known as "sacral medial telangiectatic vascular nevi" is closely related; it is localized to the sacral midline or extends to the entire back or the buttocks. It is not reported to be associated with other local abnormalities or spinal dysraphism.[8] A more complete discussion of paraspinal skin abnormalities and their evaluation is found in Chapter 9.

Port Wine Stains

Port wine stains (PWS) are capillary malformations that are almost always evident at birth. They usually occur as sporadic lesions, but families with multiple PWS scattered over the body have demonstrated a possible autosomal dominant pattern of inheritance.

Cutaneous Findings. PWS are pink or red patches that arise at birth. They grow proportionate to the child's growth and persist throughout the patient's life if left untreated. They consist of ectatic dermal capillaries and may occur anywhere on the body (Fig. 18-2). PWS may appear to lighten over the first 6 to 12 months of life, but this should not be taken as a sign of involution. Skin changes commonly occur with age in facial PWS. The thickness increases over years, and the color changes from a pink-red to a crimson red or a deep purple hue. Nodular lesions

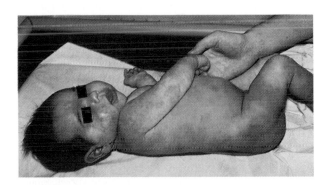

FIG. 18-3

Phakomatosis pigmentovascularis type IIA. Extensive port wine stain and dermal melanocytosis are admixed on the back of this infant, as well as elsewhere on her body.

may appear within them, requiring surgical intervention.[9] Other cutaneous lesions may coexist with PWS. PWS are sometimes contiguous to a nevus anemicus, and this may become more obvious in childhood. The association of PWS ("nevus flammeus") with pigmentary anomalies such as extensive mongolian spots (Fig. 18-3), nevus spilus, or nevoid hyperpigmentation are features of phakomatosis pigmentovascularis (see Chapter 20).

Extracutaneous Findings. Associated craniofacial abnormalities occur with some PWS.[10] Soft tissue and bony overgrowth underlying a facial PWS is common and develops throughout childhood. This occurs most frequently with V2 PWS. Asymmetric maxillary hypertrophy associated with distortion of the facial features requires orthodontic follow-up and treatment. Some patients require skeletal correction in late childhood. Gum hypertrophy may also appear in childhood. Two other well-documented extracutaneous associations, Sturge-Weber syndrome and Klippel-Trenaunay syndrome, are discussed later in this chapter. A capillary stain in the midline, in the lumbosacral area, dorsal or cervical region, or on the scalp, when associated with other midline developmental abnormalities, may be a marker for occult spinal or cranial dysraphism requiring early investigation (see Chapter 9).

Management and Treatment. The gradual thickening and nodularity provide a medical rationale for treatment of PWS during infancy and childhood.[9] The flashlamp-pumped pulsed dye laser is a well-established treatment for PWS and poses a very low risk of scarring. It causes less scarring than the argon laser, which was previously used to treat PWS, and also causes fewer pigmentary alterations than continuous-wave dye laser with the robotized scanner[11] and thus is more effective than either laser. Response to laser treatment varies by region.[12] Recent developments in laser technology may lead to more effective treatment of previously resistant lesions, but in large and confluent PWS, improvement rather than complete clearing is the most likely outcome. Controversy exists regarding the age at which treatment should begin. Some authors noted better therapeutic response with fewer treatments when treatment was begun in early infancy,[13] but others have found no evidence that treatment beginning early in childhood is more effective than treatment at older ages.[14] However, because of the increasing size of the stain over time due to the skin expanding with normal growth, we advise initiating laser treatment as early as possible in infancy, both to decrease stigmatization and to help prevent problematic skin thickening.

Telangiectasia

A number of telangiectatic nevi have been described. They are usually composed of small, punctate telangiectasias distributed either in a segmental, unilateral nevoid or a diffuse pattern. Most are poorly visible at birth; they extend before or at puberty. A pale halo of "anemic nevus" may surround small telangiectasia. Rendu-Osler-Weber disease, a familial disorder with various phenotypes corresponding to distinct genotypes, is characterized by skin and mucosal telangiectasias. Skin telangiectases are not visible during infancy, and mucosal and visceral hemorrhages from the telangiectasia do not occur until later in life.

Ataxia-telangiectasia (AT) is a rare autosomal recessive disease characterized by ataxia (due to progressive cerebellar degeneration), telangiectasia, immunodeficiency, cancer predisposition, sensitivity to ionizing radiation and radiomimetic drugs, and premature aging. Onset of telangiectasia in the newborn period is rare. In a group of 48 patients, the median age of onset of gait abnormalities was 15 months; it was 72 months for telangiectasia, but the median age of diagnosis of AT was 78 months, after the appearance of telangiectasia in two thirds of patients.[15] The mutated gene (ATM) was isolated in 1995, and more than 100 mutations have been documented in affected individuals.

Venous Malformations

Venous malformations (VMs) are slow-flow vascular malformations that are present at birth. They may involve skin, subcutaneous tissues, and mucosa. They are composed of ill-defined venous channels with irregularly attenuated walls dissecting the skin and surrounding normal follicles, nerves, or sweat glands.

Cutaneous Findings

At birth, the majority of VMs are subtle, bluish, ill-defined, compressible birthmarks, but a bulky venous mass develops in some patients during intrauterine life (Fig. 18-4). VMs are usually segmental or localized. Affected skin and mucous membranes are deep blue. The skin temperature

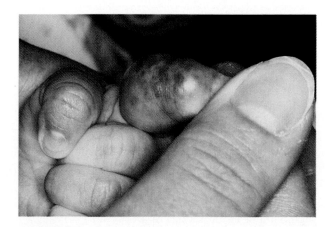

FIG. 18-4
Small venous malformation of the finger, with swelling and blue nodularity.

is normal, and a thrill or bruit is absent. Lesions swell when dependent or when the infant cries. Local venous thrombosis leads to the formation of round calcifications (phleboliths) that are visible on radiographs and are present at birth in rare cases. A majority of patients with extensive VMs have a chronic localized intravascular coagulopathy (LIC), which can manifest in newborns. This coagulopathy may lead to either thrombosis (with pain and phlebolith formation) or bleeding. It can persist throughout life. It differs from Kasabach-Merritt syndrome because the primary process is one of consumption of clotting factors, not platelet trapping.[16] Diffuse congenital genuine phlebectasia of Bockenheimer is a rare disorder; dilated blue linear veins visible on the entire skin surface (Fig. 18-5) increase with age.

Pathogenesis

VMs are sporadic in the majority of cases. However, familial VMs, inherited in an autosomal dominant fashion, have been described. Several genotypes for what appears to be the same phenotype have been elucidated, including VMCM1, a mutation on chromosome 9p[17]; this is an activating mutation in the kinase domain of the receptor tyrosine kinase Tie2, which has been found in two unrelated families.[18]

Diagnosis

The diagnosis is usually established on the basis of clinical features, but MRI and CT scans are useful for evaluating the extent of a VM. In the craniofacial area, as long as there is no major functional or cosmetic consequence, it is not necessary to image VMs in early infancy. Later on, imaging with MR (better than CT) is necessary before considering therapy. We advise examining the brain as well, since developmental venous anomalies (DVA) in the brain are more common in patients with craniofacial VMs than in the general population (25% vs. 0.5%).[19] DVA are uncommon trajectories of the brain venous drainage and pose no risk of cerebral hemorrhage.

Differential Diagnosis

Skin biopsy is rarely necessary to differentiate venous malformation from hemangioma or other well-vascularized growths. Extensive blue VMs in a leg or an arm and adjacent trunk must be differentiated from Klippel-Trenaunay syndrome (see later discussion). Sinus pericranii should be considered in the differential diagnosis of a VM located on the central forehead. It presents as a bluish, nonpulsating mass that is usually congenital and that expands when the patient is in a dependent position or with crying. Sinus pericranii represents a direct communication between superficial veins and intracranial venous sinuses through a bony defect. It is best imaged using CT bone windows.

Course

The clinical course and complications of venous malformations depend on anatomic location, with differing problems in the craniofacial area, trunk, and limbs.[16] The cheek and lip are common locations for superficial craniofacial VMs, and there is sometimes extension to the temporal and orbital areas. Swelling is noted with changes in position and activity. As the child grows older, the VM progressively molds the underlying developing bones and can result in deformities such as an open bite[20] or enlargement of the orbit. VMs located on the trunk and limbs may involve skin, skeletal muscles, joints, and bones.[16] During infancy and early childhood, the skin component of the VM expands and becomes deep blue. However, the deeper component may remain undiagnosed until it causes pain. Swelling, functional impairment, and limited joint motion occur when the child becomes older and more active, especially if playing sports. When this occurs, MRI can detect the deep component.

Treatment

Treatment of craniofacial VMs is instituted if there are significant functional impairments or disfigurement[20,21] but rarely is initiated in the first year of life. Therapy is aimed at preventing distortion of facial features, limiting bone deformity, gaping, shift of the dental midline, lip expansion, and lip commissural displacement. Small lesions can

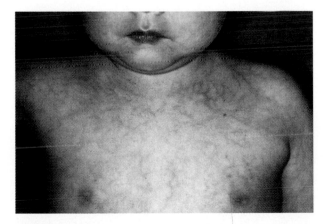

FIG. 18-5
Bockenheimer syndrome with an extensive network of dilated veins.

be treated using percutaneous sclerotherapy alone. Larger VMs are usually treated with percutaneous sclerotherapy combined with surgical excisions. Multiple treatments are often required over years. Deep laser surgery is occasionally helpful. Extensive pure VMs of the limb are usually managed in a conservative manner. Elastic stockings are encouraged from infancy. Compression increases comfort, limits swelling, and improves coagulopathy. Indications for treatment using sclerotherapy and surgery of limb VMs is limited in infancy, but well-localized lesions are sometimes excised.

Lymphatic Malformations

Lymphatic malformations (LMs) (known in much of the literature as "lymphangioma")[22] can be macrocystic microcystic, or combined.

Cutaneous Findings

Macrocystic LMs are usually visible at birth and are commonly diagnosed today by prenatal ultrasonographic investigation. They occur more commonly in the neck and axilla, where they are often referred to as *cystic hygroma* (Fig. 18-6). The detection of some huge LMs of the axilla

and thoracic area in utero may lead to discussion of terminating pregnancy, since the prognosis is poor. Microcystic LMs infiltrate diffusely throughout the dermis. Clear or hemorrhagic vesicles (so-called lymphangioma circumscriptum), which may intermittently leak lymphatic fluid, are visible on the surface of the lesion. This type of LM is rarely evident during the neonatal period and becomes apparent on skin and mucous membranes later in childhood. Combined microcystic-macrocystic LMs are more common in the head region, particularly the cheek and mouth (Fig. 18-7). Severe combined LMs may also occur on the trunk and limbs.

Extracutaneous Findings

Cervicofacial LMs or those involving the tongue and mouth interfere with normal development of the jaw.[23] Severe cervicofacial LMs, usually of combined microcystic-macrocystic type, that are not amenable to surgical resection and sclerotherapy can cause airway and esophageal obstruction, disfigurement, infection, and bleeding. Visceral LMs, intrathoracic or abdominal, are less common, representing about 8% of lesions.[22] A chronic coagulopathy is often associated with extensive LMs, and it may manifest even in infancy. LMs are more susceptible to bac-

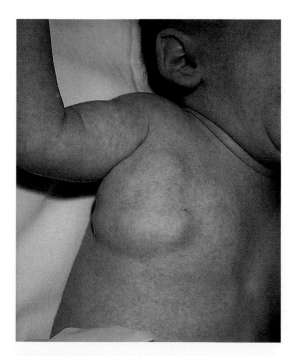

FIG. 18-6
Large thoracic lymphatic malformation ("cystic hygroma") at birth.

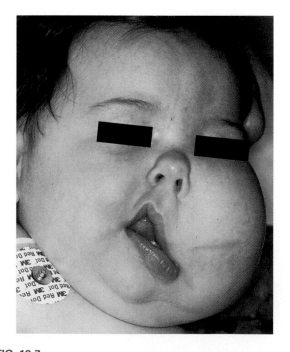

FIG. 18-7
Large lymphatic malformation of the face with both microcystic and macrocystic elements involving the skin and mucosa.

terial infections, and infection itself can worsen the malformation, particularly if the lower extremity is involved.

Pathogenesis

Severe hydrops fetalis and multiple cystic hygromas are the major cause of spontaneous abortion of fetuses with the 45,X genotype of Turner syndrome.[24] Controversy remains regarding the diagnostic and nosologic boundaries between microcystic and macrocystic LMs, diffuse lymphangiomatosis (both superficial and visceral), congenital diffuse lymphangioma of the leg,[25] transient localized lymphedema with puffiness of the dorsum of the feet (as seen in Turner and Noonan syndromes), and primary congenital lymphedema of limbs (Milroy-Meige-Nonne disease).

Diagnosis and Treatment

The diagnosis is established using either CT, MRI, or ultrasonography. Histologically, lymphatic vessels or cysts have thin walls, and lumens appear empty. Congenital macrocystic LMs can be treated after birth using fine-needle aspiration and sclerotherapy. A variety of sclerosing agents have been used, including Ethibloc, ethanol, killed bacteria–like OK-432, dextrose, sodium morrhuate, bleomycin, and doxycycline. Surgical resection is another therapeutic option for macrocystic LMs, as well as for microcystic types, but both techniques may result in recurrences and complications.[20,26-28]

Arteriovenous Malformations

Arteriovenous malformations (AVMs) are fast-flow anomalies that arise most commonly in the cephalic area. Forty percent are visible at birth.[29] In infants, AVMs have an ambiguous appearance and may mimic a port wine stain or an involuting hemangioma (Fig. 18-8). Redness with increased local warmth, atypical segmental distribution, and localized infiltration are specific signs of a high-flow lesion. A vascular mass, with tense draining veins, a thrill, and a bruit, is present in more active cases. The diagnosis is confirmed by color Doppler ultrasonographic examination. MR with MR angiography may also be helpful in delineating the extent of disease. Arteriography is not indicated in infants with quiescent AVMs.

AVMs are dangerous lesions and may severely worsen over time.[20] In some adults, an uncontrolled course may lead to death after a protracted course of disfigurement, pain, and hemorrhage. Among the main factors triggering this devastating evolution are puberty and trauma, which may be accidental or the result of ill-advised and partial treatment. Infants with superficial AVMs are rarely amen-

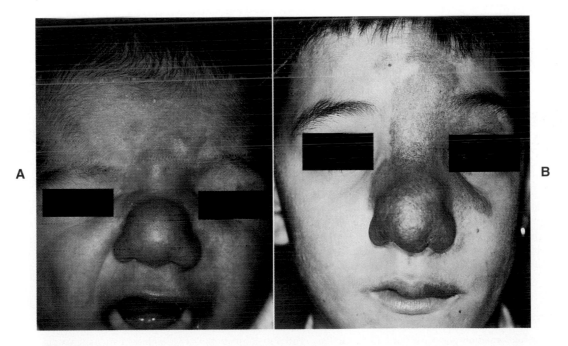

FIG. 18-8
A, Five-day-old neonate with midfacial quiescent arteriovenous malformation that subsequently worsened and proved to be part of a Bonnet-Dechaume-Blanc syndrome. B, Child at 8 years of age.

able to a satisfactory treatment. Laser treatment, cryosurgery, or partial excision may initiate AVM expansion and trigger growth. Severe congenital AVMs with associated high-output heart failure at birth a rare occurrence that requires endovascular embolization if pharmacologic treatment does not control cardiac complications.

Syndromes Associated with Vascular Malformations Detectable in the Neonate

Vascular malformations may be part of more complex dysmorphogenetic syndromes that may be diffuse or segmental (Table 18-1). Eponyms have been assigned to several of these syndromes. A number of these are diagnosed at birth, and the presence of vascular anomalies is a cardinal feature of these syndromes.[30] Their etiologies are unknown.

Cutis Marmorata Telangiectatica Congenita
Cutis marmorata telangiectatica congenita (CMTC) is a localized, segmental, or diffuse vascular anomaly that is vari-

ably associated with other defects. Most cases are sporadic. A female prevalence is reported.[31] At birth, a reticulate purple network is noted. The skin is streaked with linear and patchy vascular lesions intermingled with telangiectasia, often with focal areas of atrophy and in some cases ulceration (Fig. 18-9). These changes are often most prominent over the limb joints. This conspicuous atrophic reticulate pattern is clearly different from physiologic cutis marmorata, which is a normal physiologic finding in newborns. CMTC may be associated with port wine stains, which become more apparent after 1 year of age as the reticulate lesions of CMTC fade. CMTC may improve as the patient matures but rarely disappears completely. In some children, localized reticulate blue-red lesions persist throughout life in combination with atrophy, telangiectasia, and phlebectasia. Ulcerations may arise within CMTC during infancy and childhood, particularly in areas overlying the joints, and leave scaly scars.

In our experience, regional CMTC is far more common than the diffuse type but is probably less frequently re-

TABLE 18-1

Vascular Anomalies with Associated Extracutaneous Findings—Selected Syndromes

Syndrome	Cutaneous	Extracutaneous
Sturge-Weber	CM	Glaucoma, seizures
Klippel-Trenaunay	CVM, CLVM	Limb hypertrophy
Parkes-Weber	CAVM, CLAVM	Limb hypertrophy
Proteus	CM, LM, CLVM Epidermal nevi, thickened palms and soles	Hemihypertrophy, visceral lipomas, visceral vascular malformations, endocrine tumors
Servelle-Martorell	CVM	Limb undergrowth
Bannayan-Riley-Ruvalcaba	CM, LM, VM Lipomas, pigmented macules (genitalia)	Macrocephaly, mental retardation, visceral lipomas, intestinal polyposis
Beckwith-Wiedemann	CM	Macroglossia, macrosomia, renal disorders, embryonal tumors
Adams-Oliver	CMTC Aplasia cutis congenita	Cranium defects, limb anomalies
Blue rubber bleb nevus (Bean)	VM, LVM	Gastrointestinal, CNS vascular malformations
Wyburn-Mason	AVM	CNS AVM
Cobb	AVM	Spinal AVM
PHACE	Hemangioma	Posterior fossa, arterial, cardiac, ocular anomalies
Kasabach-Merritt	KHE, tufted angioma	Thrombocytopenic coagulopathy

CM, Capillary malformation/port wine stain; CVM, capillary venous malformation; CLVM, capillary lymphatic venous malformation; CAVM, capillary arteriovenous malformation; CLAVM, capillary lymphatic arteriovenous malformation; LM, lymphatic malformation; VM, venous malformation; CMTC, cutis marmorata telangiectatica congenita; AVM, arteriovenous malformation; KHE, kaposiform hemangioendothelioma.

ported in the literature. It generally involves one or more extremities, and such limb involvement can be ipsilateral or contralateral, often with corresponding trunk involvement. When only one limb is affected, a discrepancy in limb girth is common. The affected limb may have a thinner, pseudo-"athletic" appearance compared to the normal extremity as a result of less fat or diminished muscles and bones. Subsequent growth is usually proportionate to the original degree of limb asymmetry. Hypertrophy of the affected limb has been described but is less common in our experience.

Developmental defects are far more common in children affected with widespread CMTC than with more localized disease. Multiple associated abnormalities have been reported, including musculoskeletal anomalies, vascular abnormalities (arterial stenosis), cardiac defects, and the Adams-Oliver syndrome (see below). Less frequently reported anomalies include brain and spinal cord defects, glaucoma and other ocular anomalies, imperforate anus, abnormal genitalia, dystrophic teeth, congenital hypothyroidism, and stenosing tendinitis.[32-35]

CMTC can confused with a generalized reticulate capillary malformation (Fig. 18-10), but the latter lacks the patchy or linear atrophy and telangiectasia. This is a rare diffuse type of CM that in our experience is often associated with multiple visceral vascular anomalies (eye, kidney, and lungs) and may be associated with a risk of developing early ischemic brain symptoms (unpublished data). Extensive livedo, telangiectasia, and atrophic striae, which can be the sequelae of neonatal lupus during intrauterine life, should also be considered in the differential diagnosis of CMTC.[36]

The residual, persistent, reticulate vascular lesions of CMTC respond poorly to pulsed dye laser treatments and are associated with a greater risk of scarring than is usually associated with pulsed dye laser therapy. Associated port wine stains, however, may be more amenable to therapy. Management of extracutaneous associated abnormalities is directed at the specific anomaly. Those with a distribution similar to that of Sturge-Weber syndrome are at higher risk for CNS and ophthalmologic complications.

Sturge-Weber Syndrome

The classic triad in Sturge-Weber syndrome (SWS) includes the ipsilateral association of a facial port wine stain, which always involves V1 (although it may be more extensive) (see Fig. 18-2), eye abnormalities (choroidal vascular anomalies, increased ocular pressure, buphthalmos, and glaucoma in about 30% of patients with SWS), and leptomeningeal and brain abnormalities (leptomeningeal vascular malformation, calcifications, cerebral atrophy, enlarged choroid plexus, and developmental venous anomalies in the brain).

SWS occurs in 10% of neonates with either a V1 PWS alone or in combination with another facial, truncal, or limb PWS. Patients with V2 or V3 PWS alone and without involvement of the V1 skin are not at risk for SWS. However, individual anatomic variations in the distribution of V1 and V2 at the internal or external canthus of the eye may pose difficulties in evaluating whether V1, with its associated risk of SWS, is involved[37] (Fig. 18-11).

SWS can pose significant medical and ophthalmologic problems. Consequences of intracranial vascular anomalies include seizures, brain hypoxia, neuronal loss, dis-

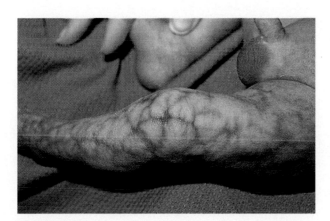

FIG. 18-9
Neonate with cutis marmorata telangiectatica congenita.

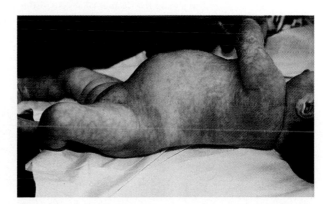

FIG. 18-10
This generalized reticulate capillary malformation is not true cutis marmorata telangiectatica congenita. This child had vascular renal anomalies, blindness, and brain ischemic attacks early in life.

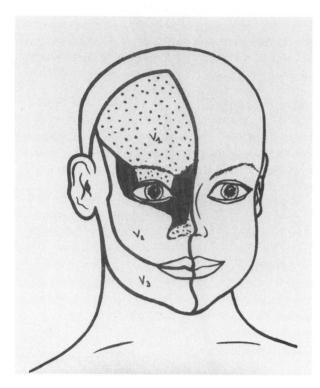

FIG. 18-11
Anatomic diagram of branches of the trigeminal nerve. The blackened area denotes the potential overlap of V1 and V2.

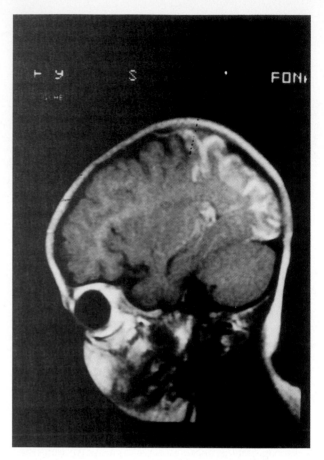

FIG. 18-12
Leptomeningeal lesion in Sturge-Weber syndrome well evidenced on T1-weighted MRI sequence with gadolinium enhancement.

turbed regional cerebral blood flow, and risk of contralateral hemiplegia. Developmental delay of cognitive skills may occur to varying degrees. Migraine headache is also common. Potential visual loss via acute or chronic glaucoma requires ongoing ophthalmologic follow-up.

The three mesectodermal tissues involved (the nasofrontal skin known as V1 skin, the ocular choroid, and the leptomeninges) have a common origin in the anterior neural primordium. A somatic mutation arising during development has been hypothesized.[20] The possibility of SWS should be considered in any infant with a PWS that includes the V1 distribution. Neuroimaging consisting of MRI with gadolinium enhancement (Fig. 18-12) or contrast-enhanced CT scans may be helpful in obtaining an early diagnosis. Nevertheless, the first evaluation in infants may not demonstrate typical neuroimaging changes (e.g., visualization of the pial angioma, calcifications of the lep-

tomeninges and of both the abnormal cortex and underlying white matter, and cerebral atrophy). Therefore subtle changes must be taken into account, such as an enlarged choroid plexus or a pattern of local accelerated myelination on MRI.[38] In most patients the first seizures in SWS occur before 2 years of age. The rapid cerebral impairment in these infants is stressed using functional neuroimaging tools. In the majority of infants studied the involved hemisphere is hyperperfused, as shown by SPECT, and hypermetabolizing, as shown by PET, before the first seizures develop. However, as soon as the seizures begin, hypoperfusion with decreased cerebral blood flow on SPECT and hypometabolism with decreased glucose utilization on PET in the damaged hemisphere are demonstrated.[39,40]

Careful clinical follow-up is recommended in newborns with an at-risk V1 PWS. Some pediatric neurologists believe that prophylactic antiseizure medication is war-

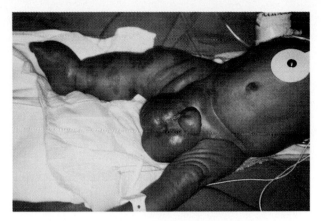

FIG. 18-13
Parkes-Weber syndrome in a newborn with evidence of a capillary lymphatic malformation, limb overgrowth, and arteriovenous fistulae (and cardiac failure) at birth.

ranted,[41] but this is controversial and currently represents a minority view. Therapeutic management of SWS is often characterized by a lifelong struggle to preserve vision, motor and psychomotor development, and cosmetic appearance and encompasses the following:

Regular ophthalmologic evaluation

Treatment of glaucoma when detected to prevent optic nerve damage and visual loss

Optimal control of epilepsy

Laser treatment of PWS

Control of maxilla overgrowth, open bite deformity, and gingival hyperplasia when present

The Sturge-Weber Foundation has been very active in supporting families and fundraising for SWS research (Box 18-1).

Klippel-Trenaunay, Parkes-Weber, and Servelle-Martorell Syndromes

These three syndromes are complex-combined vascular malformations of the limbs, visible at birth, with significant subsequent worsening. They are each different vascular anomalies and are not synonymous. Klippel-Trenaunay syndrome (KTS) is the association of capillary malformation (PWS) (some of which have lymphatic vessels intermingled), varicose veins, including persistent embryonic

veins, and overgrowth of the soft tissue and bone of the affected limb. This hypertrophy often increases progressively until the end of the growth of the child, but some affected individuals have PWS and soft tissue hypertrophy with proportionate growth, representing milder or different disease. Parkes-Weber syndrome (PaWS) is the association of limb overgrowth (length and girth), with capillary stains and multiple arteriovenous shunts (demonstrated on color Doppler ultrasonographic evaluation), and the variable presence of lymphedema at birth (Fig. 18-13). In rare instances PaWS may be complicated at birth by high-output cardiac failure requiring endovascular arterial embolization. Thus KTS is a slow-flow CVLM, whereas PaWS is a fast-flow CAVM, but both of these syndromes can result in gigantism of the affected limb. KTS may occur in association with SWS but not PaWS. Servelle-Martorell syndrome is the association of capillary stains and dysplastic veins, and unlike KTS, this slow-flow CVM also leads to discrepancy in limb length—a progressive *undergrowth* rather than overgrowth of the affected limb.

Diagnosis. These diagnoses are usually made clinically, but modern vascular imaging techniques help delineate the vascular defects. Doppler ultrasound evaluation is helpful, MRI may be helpful in more severe cases, but arteriography, phlebography, or lymphography is rarely needed during infancy and childhood.[42]

Treatment. Therapeutic management includes elastic stockings and close orthopedic follow-up of limb growth. If limb length discrepancy is significant after 1 year of age, radiographic studies may be appropriate, and a shoe lift or other orthopedic appliance may be used. Ultimately, surgical approaches to equalize limb lengths may be necessary, but these are not done during infancy. If capillary stains are extensive, they are often resistant to current laser technologies. Varicosities worsen over time, and later in life varicose veins in KTS, and AV fistulae in PaWS in selected patients, may require treatment. Long-term iatrogenic complications and a bad cosmetic outcome can result from overenthusiastic aggressive treatments early in life. Parents need educational information and support both in the newborn period and over time.[20,30,42] The Klippel-Trenaunay Association has a web page providing information to families: www.k-t.org.

Rarer Vascular Syndromes

Wyburn-Mason, Bonnet-Dechaume-Blanc, and Brégeat Syndromes

These syndromes are characterized by arteriovenous malformations occurring in the craniofacial area with a skin (midline or hemifacial), orbit, retina, and brain continuum of fast-flow vascular anomalies. In infancy, the cutaneous AVM commonly mimics a facial port wine stain, although it is either limited or not as clearly systematized as on the face. It is warm on palpation and is sometimes associated with an abnormally increased skin thickness at birth (see Fig. 18-8).

MR angiography and angio-CT scans are helpful noninvasive tools that may be used in infants for the detection of the enlarged tortuous vessels and AV shunting. These findings are more clearly delineated later in life with arteriography. Lesions slowly enlarge over years and may cause distortion of facial features, visual loss, and cerebral hemorrhage.

Cobb Syndrome

Cobb syndrome is the association of a dermatomal skin vascular malformation (trunk and arm or leg), a fast-flow intramedullary spinal AVM, and a vertebral vascular anomaly in the same segment. This metameric angiomatosis is the truncal counterpart of the syndromic cephalic AVMs. In infancy this syndrome may be undiagnosed because the cutaneous vascular signs are subtle or are misdiagnosed as skin capillary malformation. The diagnosis is often established later when an abnormal vertebra is incidentally imaged or if neurologic symptoms of spinal cord compression occur.

Maffucci Syndrome

Maffucci syndrome (MS) is a very rare sporadic syndrome, without sex prevalence, that begins in childhood and worsens during the patient's life. Congenital forms occur in only 17% of cases. MS is characterized by enchondromas of bones and skin lesions with a clinical aspect of venous malformations. Blue skin lesions are nodular, and they develop slowly and are rare in infancy. Although they have features of slow-flow venous anomalies on arteriography and MRI scans, histologic examination may reveal a spindle cell hemangioendothelioma, in addition to dysplastic venous channels.[4] Enchondromas, identical to those present in Ollier disease, involve both the metaphyses and diaphyses and may cause bony distortion and fragility. The hands and feet are involved in 90% of patients. Cranial and vertebral enchondromas have severe neurologic consequences. Enchondrosarcomas may develop.[43]

Blue Rubber Bleb Nevus Syndrome, or Bean Syndrome

The vascular anomalies associated with blue rubber bleb nevus syndrome (BRBNs) are small black-blue papules that can be present in infancy. Numerous lesions develop and are scattered over the skin.[44] Larger VM or LVM lesions coexist with smaller ones. BRBNs may be sporadic or inherited as an autosomal dominant trait. Early in life, before the occurrence of visceral hemorrhages, BRBNs presents with a similar appearance to the lesions observed in familial cutaneous and mucosal VMs. Evaluation includes gastrointestinal tract and bladder fibroscopic evaluation and neuroimaging of the brain and spinal cord, but it is not clear whether the evaluation should be carried out in an asymptomatic child. A coagulation disorder that sometimes manifests soon after birth with bleeding may occur in patients with BRBNs.

Gorham Syndrome

This sporadic syndrome of bony destruction is associated with a vascular lesion that is usually a lymphatic or capillary-venous-lymphatic malformation. The cause of the extensive bone destruction is not clearly understood. Lesions usually become obvious in childhood. If the thoracic cage is involved, pleural effusions may develop.

Hennekam Syndrome

An autosomal recessive disorder, Hennekam syndrome is the association of intestinal lymphangiectasia resulting in protein-losing enteropathy, lymphedema of the four limbs, abnormal facies, and mental retardation.[45] The expansion of the phenotype.[46] raises the question of more than one gene defect.

Aagenaes Syndrome (Hereditary Cholestasis with Lymphedema)

Aagenaes syndrome is an autosomal recessive disease occurring mostly in infants of Norwegian ancestry. Significant leg lymphedema due to lymph vessel hypoplasia that is congenital or develops later in life requires life-long treatment. Cholestasis and obstructive jaundice are present at birth and may improve in adulthood, but they may be lethal in childhood. Children have severe bleeding if vitamin K supplementation is not provided. They also complain of itching, and they have growth retardation.[47]

Beckwith-Wiedemann Syndrome
Beckwith-Wiedemann syndrome is associated with a capillary stain of the mid-forehead that is clinically identical to salmon patch but has a greater likelihood of persistence. Other common abnormalities include macroglossia and umbilical anomalies, usually omphalocele, and overgrowth of tissues and organs (liver, spleen, and kidney). There is a high risk of malignant embryonal tumors in infancy[48] and of nonmalignant renal diseases.[49] Other reported findings are a high body weight at birth, hemihypertrophy, and neonatal hypoglycemia. Intelligence is usually not impaired. Prenatal sonographic diagnosis is possible due to visceromegaly.

Proteus Syndrome
This sporadic syndrome, first described by Wiedemann,[50] is discussed in more detail in Chapter 24. It is characterized by asymmetric localized overgrowth of various body parts affecting soft tissues and bones. The syndrome is evident at birth.[51] It may become more complex over the years, or it may remain stable.

The most characteristic features are the asymmetric, disproportionate growth with regional gigantism and cutaneous manifestations, including cerebriform dermal thickening of soles and palms, epidermal nevi, lipomas, café au lait spots, and vascular malformations such as extensive capillary malformations, cystic lymphatic malformations, and limb gigantism with combined-complex capillary-venous-lymphatic anomalies (identical to Klippel-Trenaunay syndrome). Visceral benign tumors, mainly lipomas, but also tumors in the endocrine glands or CNS, and visceral vascular malformations are observed as well. Intelligence is normal in most patients, but learning disabilities are present in one third of patients.[52] Ophthalmologic and neurologic alterations or seizures have been reported.[52,53]

Some have suggested that Proteus syndrome is the result of a lethal postzygotic mutation surviving in a mosaic state. Surgical reconstruction is the primary method of rehabilitation for these children. Orthopedic management is essential because of discrepancy in limb and foot growth. Excision of lipomas or laser treatment of vascular lesions is sometimes indicated.

Riley-Smith, Bannayan-Zonana, and Ruvalcaba-Myhre-Smith Syndromes
These familial autosomal dominant disorders are now considered together because they share overlapping clinical features and may represent a continuum, the Bannayan-Riley-Ruvalcaba syndrome (BRRs).[54] BRRs is characterized by vascular anomalies and multiple other anomalies. The vascular lesions, many of which have not been well characterized, appear to represent several types of vascular anomalies, including capillary stains, venous malformations, and lymphatic malformations but are often referred to as "hemangiomas." Other features include the following:
- Macrocephaly with normal ventricular size
- Pseudopapilledema
- Localized superficial soft tissue and visceral overgrowths, mainly lipomas
- Mild to severe mental retardation
- Juvenile intestinal polyposis
- Pigmented macules arising on the genitalia[55]

The common feature of juvenile intestinal polyps in BRRs and Cowden disease may be explained by a common genetic defect (since both syndromes map to chromosome 10q23). Many of the features of BRRs are also seen in Proteus syndrome.

"Hemangiomatous" Branchial Clefts, Lip Pseudoclefts, Unusual Facies
Facial midline capillary malformation may occur in association with bony and facial abnormalities, including pseudocleft lip, cleft lip, cleft palate, unusual facies (hypoplastic nares, micrognathia, malformed ears, hypertelorism), and limb defects (hypomelia/phocomelia). When these features occur together, it is known as Roberts syndrome, pseudothalidomide syndrome, or SC phocomelia syndrome.[30] Marked growth retardation and sparse, silvery hair are also reported. The branchio-oculo-facial syndrome has a distinctive phenotype of ear, eye, mouth, and craniofacial anomalies and may include "hemangiomatous" aplastic skin overlying branchial or supraauricular defects.[56]

Adams-Oliver Syndrome
Adams-Oliver syndrome is characterized by CMTC occurring in association with scalp aplasia cutis congenita, cranium defects, and distal limb-reduction abnormalities varying from partial absence of toes or fingers to absence of a limb. Most cases are transmitted as an autosomal dominant trait[57] When the cranial bone defect exposes the dural membrane, necrosis, infection, and bleeding may be fatal.[58] The clinical spectrum of this disorder includes

palate and auricular malformations, microphthalmia, cardiac anomalies, spina bifida, and intracranial calcifications in a case without any proven intrauterine infection.[59]

Nova Syndrome

Nova syndrome is a familial disorder in which a congenital glabellar capillary stain occurs in association with neurologic malformations, including Dandy-Walker malformation, hydrocephalus, cerebellar vermis agenesis, and mega cisterna magna.[60]

VASCULAR TUMORS IN THE NEONATE

Hemangiomas of Infancy

Hemangioma of infancy (Table 18-2) is the most common vascular tumor encountered during the neonatal period. It is a benign proliferation of endothelial cells that undergoes a phase of rapid growth followed by spontaneous regression. Hemangiomas are noted in 1.0% to 2.6% of healthy infants in the immediate newborn period.[61] The majority of hemangiomas become apparent within the first few weeks of life, with a reported overall incidence of 10% to 13% at the first year. The incidence may vary among races. Some authors have noted hemangiomas to be less common in blacks, whereas other studies show a similar incidence within the first few days of life.[5,62] A study of Japanese infants revealed a slightly lower incidence of hemangioma than in white infants within the immediate neonatal period.[63] Hemangiomas are more common in females than in males with a ratio of 2:1 to 5:1.[30,64,65] They are also more common in premature infants, occurring in 22% to 30% of infants weighing less than 1000 g and in 15% of infants with birth weight between 1000 and 1500 g.[62,66] Infants weighing more than 1500 g show no significant increase when compared with term infants. A threefold increased incidence of hemangiomas has been noted in infants born to mothers who undergo chorionic villus sampling compared with those born to mothers who undergo amniocentesis.[67]

Superficial hemangiomas appear to be the most common type of hemangioma, occurring in approximately 50% to 60% of cases. Combined hemangiomas are estimated to occur in 25% to 35% of cases and deep hemangiomas in 15%.[30] Approximately 75% to 90% of infants present with a single hemangioma, but multiple lesions may appear in some infants. Some studies demonstrate a predilection for the head and neck area.[68] The majority of hemangiomas arise sporadically; however, a family history of hemangioma can be elicited in some patients. A recent study reported six families with autosomal dominant transmission of hemangiomas.[69]

Clinical Characteristics

Hemangioma Precursors. The medical literature frequently states that hemangiomas are rarely present at birth and develop within the first few weeks; however, a large series reviewing the natural history of hemangiomas has reported that 50% to 60% are present at birth.[65] The higher incidences reported reflect the recognition of precursor lesions. Telangiectasia surrounded by a halo of pallor, pale or erythematous patches, and bruiselike macules are the most commonly reported precursor lesions[63,70] (Figs. 18-14 and 18-15). It may be difficult to differentiate an erythematous patch precursor from a capillary malformation (although nascent hemangioma is more ill defined and telangiectatic). Follow-up physical examinations are essential to establish the correct diagnosis. Rarely a hemangioma on the perineum or lip may present in the neonate as ulceration without obvious hemangioma. In these cases the hemangioma becomes evident over the subsequent days to weeks. Furthermore, the area of ulceration may mimic bacterial or herpetic infection. Biopsies obtained from the border of the ulcers in these patients demonstrate increased vascularity in the dermis but are not clearly diagnostic of hemangioma.[71]

Congenital Hemangioma. Occasionally a fully developed hemangioma may be present at birth. The term *congenital hemangioma* is used to designate these tumors.[72,73] They are equally common in males and females. Three morphologic variations are described: a raised, violaceous tumor with large, radiating veins; a hemispheric tumor with overlying telangiectasia; and a firm, pink-violaceous tumor that is frequently located on the lower extremity, often with a pale halo (Fig. 18-16). Rarely the overlying skin may show hypertrichosis or milia that resolves in the first month of life.[2] Ulceration, necrosis, and hemorrhage

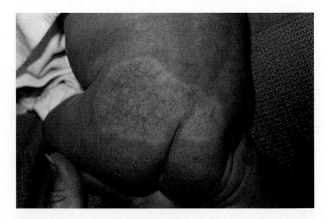

FIG. 18-14
A nascent hemangioma presenting as a vasoconstricted macule.

TABLE 18-2

Major Differences Between Hemangiomas and Vascular Malformations

	Hemangiomas	Vascular malformations (capillary, venous, lymphatic, arterial, and arteriovenous, pure or complex-combined)
Clinical	Variably visible at birth Subsequent rapid growth Slow, spontaneous involution	Usually visible at birth (AVMs may be quiescent) Growth proportionate to the skin's growth (or slow progression); present lifelong
Sex ratio	3:1 to 5:1 and 7:1 in severe cases	1:1
Pathology	Proliferating stage: hyperplasia of endothelial cells and SMC-actin+ cells Multilaminated basement membrane Higher mast cell content in involution	Flat endothelium Thin basement membrane Often irregularly attenuated walls (VM, LM)
Radiology	Fast-flow lesion on Doppler sonography Tumoral mass with flow voids on MR Lobular tumor on arteriogram	Slow flow (CM, LM, VM) or fast flow (AVM) on Doppler ultrasonography MR: Hypersignal on T2 when slow flow (LM, VM); flow voids on T1 and T2 when fast flow (AVM) Arteriography of AVM demonstrates AV shunting
Bone changes	Rarely mass effect with distortion but no invasion	*Slow-flow VM*: distortion of bones, thinning, underdevelopment *Slow-flow CM*: hypertrophy *Slow-flow LM*: distortion, hypertrophy, and invasion of bones *High-flow AVM*: destruction, rarely extensive lytic lesions *Combined malformations* (e.g., slow-flow [CVLM = Klippel-Trenaunay syndrome] or fast-flow [CAVM = Parkes-Weber syndrome]): overgrowth of limb bones, gigantism
Immunohistochemistry on tissue samples	*Proliferating hemangioma:* high expression of PCNA, type IV collagenase, VEGF, urokinase, and bFGF *Involuting hemangioma:* high TIMP-1, high bFGF	Lack expression of PCNA, type IV collagenase, urokinase, VEGF, and bFGF One familial (rare) form of VM linked to a mutated gene on 9p (VMCM1)
Hematology	No coagulopathy (Kasabach-Merritt syndrome is a complication of other vascular tumors of infancy, e.g., kaposiform hemangioendothelioma and tufted angioma, with a LM component)	Slow-flow VM or LM or LVM may have an associated LIC with risk of bleeding (DIC).

AVM, Arteriovenous malformation; *SMC,* smooth muscle cell; *VM,* venous malformation; *LM,* lymphatic malformation; *MR,* magnetic resonance imaging; *CM,* capillary malformation/port wine stain; *CLVM,* capillary lymphatic venous malformation; *CAVM,* capillary arteriovenous malformation; *PCNA,* proliferating cell nuclear antigen; *VEGF,* vascular endothelial growth factor; *bFGF,* basic fibroblast growth factor; *TIMP,* tissue inhibitor of metalloproteinase; *LIC,* localized intravascular coagulopathy; *DIC,* disseminated intravascular coagulation.

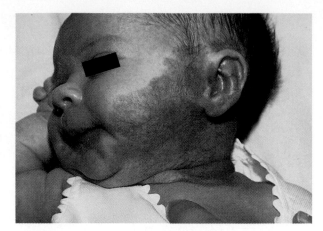

FIG. 18-15
Telangiectatic nascent hemangioma involving the "beard" area, neck, and extending intraorally, a distribution that carries a high risk of airway hemangioma. Despite high-dose corticosteroid therapy, this patient developed respiratory distress 2 weeks later and was found to have an extensive laryngeal hemangioma, which required excision and laryngoplasty using an ear cartilage graft.

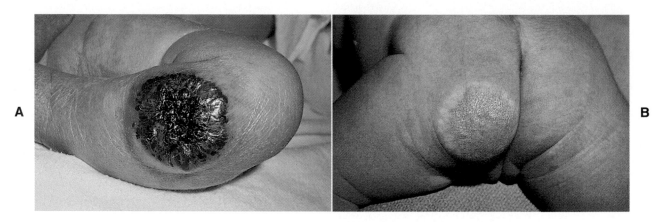

A   B

FIG. 18-16
Two examples of congenital hemangioma, a condition that usually involutes rapidly in the first year of life.

may complicate congenital hemangiomas. The congenital hemangioma may be noted on routine prenatal ultrasonographic evaluation. Those that are detected reveal prominent vascularity and high flow. The proliferating phase of congenital hemangiomas occurs in utero.[2] Congenital hemangiomas are usually diagnosed on physical examination. Radiologic evaluation, including Doppler ultrasonography and MRI, may assist in the diagnosis. A biopsy may be required to differentiate the tumor from other neoplasms, including fibrosarcomas and infantile myofibromatosis (see subsequent discussion).[72] The majority of reported cases of congenital hemangiomas demonstrated accelerated spontaneous involution[2,72,73] with regression by 14 months of age. In rare cases, ulceration and necrosis complicate the clinical course. Indications for treatment are similar to those for common post-

natal hemangiomas, including impairment of visual function and congestive heart failure.

Common Hemangioma. Hemangiomas can be classified into three types based on their clinical morphology: superficial hemangioma, combined hemangioma, and deep hemangioma. Superficial and combined hemangiomas are the most common types. Erythematous vascular plaques that are frequently bright red characterize superficial hemangiomas. The surface texture is finely lobulated.[74,75] These characteristics have led to the use of the term *strawberry hemangioma* (Fig. 18-17). Although the majority of superficial hemangiomas are small tumors, they can be more extensive (Fig. 18-18) and arise in localized or segmental pattern.[62] Multiple superficial hemangiomas may indicate visceral hemangiomatosis. Deep hemangiomas are not commonly noted in the neonatal

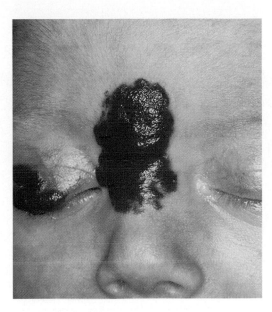

FIG. 18-17
A plaque-type superficial hemangioma.

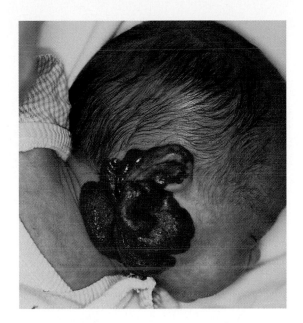

FIG. 18-18
Aggressive superficial growth of retro-auricular hemangioma in a premature infant.

period. They are characterized by the presence of a rather well-circumscribed, warm, subcutaneous mass that is caused by proliferation of the tumor in the deeper portion of the dermis or subcutis. The overlying skin may appear normal or have relatively inconspicuous superficial changes, such as telangiectasia or dilated veins, making it more difficult to diagnose. Larger, deep hemangiomas may be highly vascularized with "high-flow" arterial blood supplies during the proliferating phase. In some cases this may be detected on physical examination by the presence of a bruit. In these situations it is important to consider arteriovenous malformations in the differential diagnosis. Many hemangiomas exhibit characteristics of both deep and superficial hemangiomas and are called combined, or mixed, hemangiomas. These lesions frequently exhibit a configuration resembling a poached egg at the end of the proliferating phase, with a well-circumscribed superficial portion overlying a less well-defined deeper component.[74]

Extracutaneous Characteristics

Visceral Hemangiomas. Hemangiomas may arise in many organs; however, liver[75,76] and laryngeal involvement[77] are the most common. The liver may be affected with or without cutaneous involvement,[76] with solitary or multiple hemangiomas. Solitary hepatic lesions in the ab-

sence of cutaneous hemangiomas should be differentiated from a hepatic vascular malformation. Multiple hepatic hemangiomas are usually accompanied by cutaneous hemangiomas, with 83% showing more than five cutaneous lesions.

Extensive superficial hemangiomas located on the lower face and chin in a "beard distribution" correlate with symptomatic involvement of the airway,[77] upper airway, or subglottic area (see Fig. 18-15). There is a striking female predilection of 6-7:1 for "beard" and severe complicated hemangiomas.[77,78]

Multiple Neonatal Hemangiomas. Approximately 10% to 25% of infants with hemangiomas have multiple hemangiomas.[68] Numerous, small, superficial hemangiomas may herald visceral hemangiomatosis (Fig. 18-19). The term *benign neonatal hemangiomatosis* is used to describe infants with numerous cutaneous hemangiomas without clinically evident visceral lesions.[79] Diffuse neonatal hemangiomatosis describes infants with cutaneous and visceral hemangiomas.[80] Multiple hemangiomas appear early in the neonatal period, and girls are affected more commonly. Hepatic and cutaneous hemangiomas have been reported on prenatal sonographic evaluation at 32 weeks.[81] The cutaneous lesions may range in size from a few millimeters to more than several centimeters in diameter. There is no consensus regarding the number of cu-

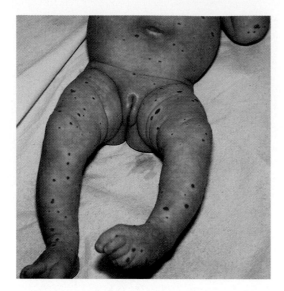

FIG. 18-19
Disseminated cutaneous (and liver) neonatal hemangiomatosis.

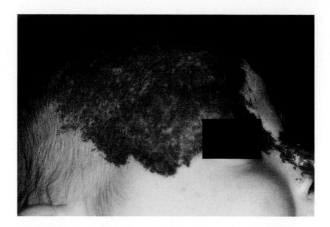

FIG. 18-20
Segmental distribution of a very flat hemangioma. Although located in V1 area, there is no risk of Sturge-Weber syndrome; this patient had intracranial arterial defects (PHACE syndrome).

taneous lesions required to suspect visceral involvement. Although the majority of children with diffuse neonatal hemangiomatosis have multiple skin lesions, visceral involvement may occur with few cutaneous lesions. Patients with diffuse neonatal hemangiomatosis and hepatic involvement demonstrate a high incidence of associated cardiac failure.[76] The gastrointestinal tract, lungs, and CNS are involved in over 50% of cases of diffuse neonatal hemangiomatosis.[75,79,80] The oral mucosa and eyes are also commonly affected. Patients with gastrointestinal hemangiomas most commonly present with bleeding.[82] Additional complications of diffuse neonatal hemangiomatosis include high-output congestive heart failure, visceral hemorrhage, hydrocephalus, and ocular abnormalities. Untreated patients have a high mortality rate. Mortality rates range between 29% and 81% with various treatment regimens.[75,76,83] Newborns with multiple cutaneous hemangiomas need to be monitored closely with serial physical examinations to assess for visceral involvement. Serial radiologic evaluation of the liver, including ultrasonography and CT or MRI, may be necessary to follow progression of visceral lesions. Not all patients with hepatic involvement require therapy, but close evaluation is essential, especially of very young infants, to determine which patients are at greater risk for complications associated with liver involvement.

Structural Malformations. Hemangiomas may rarely arise in association with structural malformations.[78,84-90] There is a striking female predilection in patients with he-

mangiomas and structural malformations that exceeds the 3:1 ratio reported for hemangiomas overall. Clinically, the hemangiomas are usually large, unilateral or bilateral, and may extend over a significant portion of the head and neck.

Central nervous system malformations, such as Dandy-Walker malformation, arachnoid cyst, enlarged fourth ventricle, enlarged cisterna magna, cerebellar or vermian hypoplasia, atrophy, and absent corpus callosum, may occur concomitantly with large facial hemangiomas.[88,90,91] Macrocephaly, ophthalmologic abnormalities, or psychomotor retardation may be a presenting sign of an underlying structural malformation.[90] Both extracranial and intracranial vascular anomalies may occur in association with facial hemangiomas (Fig. 18-20). These include anomalies of the brachiocephalic arteries and of the aortic arch, coarctation of the aorta, and cerebrovascular abnormalities (e.g., hypoplastic arteries, aneurysms, aberrant internal carotid artery, stenosis, occlusion of the internal carotid, posterior or anterior cerebral artery, persistent embryonic arteries, such as trigeminal artery, and so forth).[85,87,88,92] Patients with intracranial anomalous vessels may demonstrate progressive occlusive arterial changes and cerebral infarction.[89] Cardiac abnormalities include cortritriatum with partial anomalous pulmonary venous return, tricuspid and aortic atresia, patent ductus arteriosus, and ventricular septal defects.[85-88] Partial or

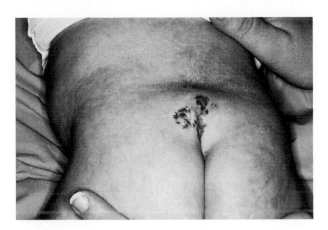

FIG. 18-21
Hemangioma in association with a cutaneous lipoma and spinal dysraphism.

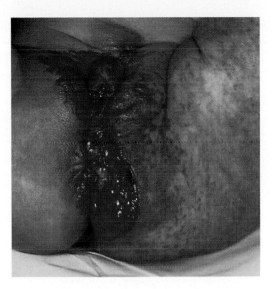

FIG. 18-22
This infant had perineal hemangioma as well as a telangiectatic hemangioma of the entire lower limb in association with abnormal external genitalia, exstrophy of the bladder, and umbilical malposition. Note the large ulceration, which is a common complication of perineal hemangiomas.

complete sternal agenesis and supraumbilical raphe may also occur in patients with large facial hemangiomas or multiple hemangiomas.[86,89,93,94] Recognition that structural anomalies and hemangiomas may coexist led to the proposal of the eponym PHACE syndrome to refer to the association of posterior fossa brain malformations, hemangiomas, arterial anomalies, coarctation of the aorta, cardiac defects, and eye abnormalities (e.g., microphthalmia, optic-nerve hypoplasia, cataracts, and increased retinal vascularity).[87] Hemangiomas arising over the lumbosacral area may be associated with malformations of the genitourinary, gastrointestinal, neurologic, and skeletal systems (Figs. 18-21 and 18-22). Imperforate anus, rectoscrotal fistula, renal anomalies, abnormal external genitalia, lipomyelomeningocele, tethered cord, and bony deformities of the sacrum have been reported.[79,95,96]

Pathogenesis
The pathogenesis of hemangiomas has not been clearly elucidated, and it remains poorly understood.[84,97] Preliminary investigations suggested that estrogens and their receptors play a role in the development and subsequent growth of hemangiomas. Mast cells are increased during the proliferating phase, and their number decreases in involuted hemangiomas; however, their role in pathogenesis is unclear.[98] Recent advances in the understanding of normal vascular development offer insight into the possible pathogenic mechanisms of this common spontaneously regressing vascular tumor.[97] During embryogenesis, the normal vascular system arises through a combination of two processes, vasculogenesis and angiogenesis. *Vasculogenesis* refers to the process by which new vessels arise by the de novo differentiation of early endothelial cells. *Angiogenesis* refers to the development of new capillary vessels from preexisting vasculature. Several factors are reported to play a role in angiogenesis, including vascular endothelial growth factor (VEGF) and basic fibroblast growth factor (bFGF).[97,99] VEGF and bFGF are overexpressed in proliferating hemangiomas. Patients with proliferating hemangiomas are noted to demonstrate increased levels of urinary bFGF, whereas those with vascular malformations do not.[97,99] Some authors have postulated that spontaneous involution of a hemangioma may be a result of apoptosis. Preliminary studies demonstrate increased apoptotic activity in involuting hemangioma compared with the common, noninvoluting, pyogenic granuloma.[100,101]

Diagnosis
Most hemangiomas can be diagnosed on the basis of their history and clinical appearance. The differential diagnosis includes other vascular and nonvascular tumors that are discussed in this chapter. In cases in which the history and physical examination are not helpful, further studies may

need to be conducted to confirm the diagnosis.[102] Doppler ultrasonography and MRI are most helpful in confirming the diagnosis of hemangioma. Doppler studies demonstrate the presence of a vascular lesion, but it may be difficult to differentiate a proliferating hemangioma from an arteriovenous malformation because both are high-flow lesions. Doppler ultrasonography is less helpful than MRI in delineating the extent of the hemangioma and its relationship to surrounding structures.[20] T1-weighted MRI sequences demonstrate flow voids as a result of high-flow vessels, but also delineate the solid tissue mass with an intermediate signal that enhances on T2. The presence of the solid tissue mass component of a hemangioma differentiates the hemangioma from an arteriovenous malformation. CT is less helpful than MRI for distinguishing a hemangioma from a vascular malformation but may define tissue involvement. Angiography is not needed to establish the diagnosis of hemangioma. It may be performed before embolization therapy. Measurement of urinary bFGF levels may be helpful for differentiating a proliferating hemangioma from a vascular malformation,[97-99] and it has proved to be valuable in following response to therapy.

A careful history and thorough physical examination should be performed in infants with multiple cutaneous hemangiomas to assess for visceral hemangiomatosis. Patients should be carefully evaluated for symptoms of liver involvement and signs of congestive heart failure. Further evaluation should be performed as indicated by the physical symptoms and location of hemangiomas. Patients may require ophthalmologic evaluation to assess for visual impairment in eyelid and orbital hemangiomas or rarely for ocular hemangiomatosis.

Histopathology

Rarely a biopsy may be necessary to rule out other neonatal tumors. Early in the proliferating stage the tumor consists predominantly of a mass of endothelial cells. Lumens become evident somewhat later in the proliferating phase, lined by normal-appearing endothelial cells. PAS stains reveal a thickened basement membrane. Mast cells are increased within proliferating hemangiomas when compared with normal tissue. As hemangiomas mature, the tumor shows lobules of endothelial channels separated by fibrous septae. Fibroblasts, smooth muscle cells, and fat cells are deposited around the vessels. Narrowed lumens, atrophy of the vessel walls, and ultimately obliteration of the vessel are noted in involuted hemangiomas.

Differential Diagnosis

Deep hemangiomas may be particularly difficult to differentiate from other tumors and malformations. Infantile myofibromatosis may mimic vascular tumors but is firmer to palpation and has distinct histopathologic features. Infantile fibrosarcoma, a rare tumor that is sometimes congenital, may resemble a deep hemangioma or lymphatic malformation.[103] Rhabdomyosarcoma is the most common sarcoma of early childhood and may present in newborns as a rapidly enlarging red cutaneous mass usually involving the head and neck that may be difficult to differentiate from a deep hemangioma. Other benign and malignant tumors that may resemble hemangiomas include adrenal carcinoma, spindle and epithelioid nevus, and neuroblastoma. Congenital Langerhans cell histiocytosis may mimic diffuse neonatal hemangiomatosis. Dermoid cysts are developmental anomalies that commonly arise on the head and neck. Periocular lesions are relatively common and may be difficult to distinguish from a periorbital deep hemangioma. Nasal glioma is a congenital lesion composed of extracranial brain tissue and meninges that usually arises in the glabellar area as a gray erythematous nodule. True encephalocele, meningocele, and teratoma may all be mistaken for deep hemangiomas.

Clinical Course

Several early studies have documented the natural history of hemangiomas. Three clinical phases are generally noted: proliferation, involution, and final involution. The proliferating phase occurs within the first several weeks to first year of life. Some studies indicate that superficial and combined hemangiomas proliferate for up to 9 months of life, whereas deep hemangiomas may have a longer period of growth. During the proliferating phase the hemangioma undergoes enlargement out of proportion to the growth of the infant. A superficial hemangioma is characteristically bright red during this phase. Both combined and deep hemangiomas may feel tense, and fluctuations in size and volume may be noted with crying or activity. The proliferating phase is followed by an involuting phase that may begin as early as within the first year of life. Change in the surface color and texture of a superficial hemangioma is often the earliest sign of spontaneous regression. The color changes from a bright crimson to a violaceous gray and is often accompanied by flattening of the surface texture. The superficial portion ultimately breaks up into smaller areas and then resolves. The deeper portion also regresses, but this is often not as apparent clinically. Parents may note less fluctuation in size during crying, and the tumor is less firm to touch.[62,74] Increased warmth slowly diminishes to normal temperature. Radial veins that are often quite prominent and may mimic a venous malformation are noted as the hemangioma involutes. Doppler studies indicate persistent high flow, and this assists in differentiating the involuting hemangioma from a venous malformation. During the later phase of involution, the surface is wrinkled, and the mass may develop a fibrofatty consistency. In some cases hemangiomas resolve completely, whereas in others they leave residua of variable cosmetic significance. Involuted hemangiomas often show residual telangiectasia, pallor or yellowish color, fibrofatty tissue deposition, and atrophy (Fig. 18-23). Several large studies have shown that the timing of involution is fairly consistent. Approximately 30% involute at 3 years, 50% at 5 years, 70% at 7 years, and over 90% by 10 to 12 years.[62,65,74]

Bleeding is a rare complication of superficial hemangiomas that are actively proliferating and usually can be controlled by firm pressure. Superficial ulceration is reported in less than 5% to 10% of hemangiomas during the proliferating phase. Ulceration is more common on the lip and perineum and may lead to secondary infection; moreover, it results in textural change or scarring of the skin surface.[65] Recurrent ulceration and infection may complicate hemangiomas located in the perineum, and conservative treatments routinely used to manage ulcerated hemangiomas may be ineffective. Lesions in this area need to be monitored closely for this potential complication.

In addition to perineal and lip hemangiomas, certain lesions arising on the head and neck require closer follow-up or intervention because of a greater likelihood of complications. Hemangiomas on the pinna may ulcerate and become secondarily infected, contributing to structural deformity. Hemangiomas obstructing the external auditory canal bilaterally may cause conductive hearing loss.[62] Growth of periorbital and lid hemangiomas may cause vi-

sual impairment by obstructing the visual axis, leading to amblyopia or deforming the young cornea, creating refractory errors. As many as 80% of patients with hemangiomas in this area have ocular complications.[104] Even small lesions may pose a threat to normal visual development. Astigmatism appears to be a relatively common ocular complication of periorbital hemangiomas.[105] Proliferation of retrobulbar lesions may lead to proptosis.[104] Strabismus may be associated. Mixed hemangiomas located on the nasal tip distort underlying cartilage. Plastic surgical repair is often necessary to correct the "cyrano-nose" deformity.

Large cervicofacial hemangiomas may impair vital functions, distort normal anatomy, or lead to congestive heart failure as they proliferate. Retrospective review of "alarming," life-threatening, or function-threatening hemangiomas (excluding vascular tumors complicated by Kasabach-Merritt syndrome) reveals several distinct characteristics. These problematic hemangiomas are more common in females than males and frequently arise on the head and neck. Alarming hemangiomas are more often identified at birth than uncomplicated hemangiomas, and rapid growth and proliferation are noted in the neonatal period in 80% of cases. In addition, although it is commonly recognized that multiple hemangiomas may be associated with visceral ones, large facial lesions may also signal visceral hemangiomatosis, including subglottic and gastrointestinal hemangiomas. Patients with large facial hemangiomas and visceral involvement have an increased incidence of congestive heart failure.[106] Congenital malformations also occur more commonly in these infants.[78,106] Thrombocytopenic consumptive coagulopathy

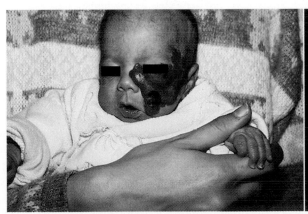 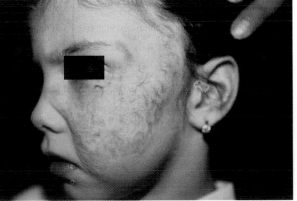

A   B

FIG. 18-23
A, Hemangioma growing rapidly with focal ulcerations in a premature infant girl weighing 2 kg. She had a dramatic response to corticosteroid treatment but did have some atrophic skin changes after involution (B).

(Kasabach-Merritt phenomenon) is described as a potential complication of large hemangiomas in the older literature. However, recent studies show that lesions that demonstrate this complication are not true hemangiomas but rather more aggressive vascular tumors, including Kaposiform hemangioendothelioma and tufted angioma (see subsequent discussion).

Management

Before the recognition that the majority of hemangiomas resolved spontaneously with few complications, x-ray therapy and surgery were the mainstay of treatment. Subsequently it was appreciated that allowing hemangiomas to regress spontaneously resulted in better cosmetic outcomes and fewer complications. In addition, long-term cutaneous and thyroid cancer, as well as increased risk of intracranial tumors, were reported after ionizing radiation treatment of hemangiomas in infants. More diverse management options[84] are currently available, but none is without potential side effects.[97]

Perhaps the greatest challenge in managing hemangiomas in infancy is the identification of lesions that will need intervention. It may be difficult to predict at the time of initial evaluation, and periodic assessment is necessary. There is no consensus regarding indications for treatment. The major goals of management are prevention and treatment of life-threatening or function-threatening complications caused by the growth of the hemangioma, prevention of permanent disfigurement left by residual skin changes after the hemangioma has regressed, avoidance of overly aggressive, potentially toxic or scarring procedures for hemangiomas that are likely to have a very good prognosis without active intervention, attention to the psychosocial needs of the patient and family, and treatment of ulcerated hemangiomas that may result in pain, infection, or permanent scarring.[107,108] Consequently, the following indications for treatment of hemangiomas have been proposed:

1. Life-threatening or function-threatening hemangiomas, including those causing impairment of vision, respiratory compromise, or congestive heart failure
2. Hemangiomas in certain anatomic locations (nose, lip, glabellar area, and ear) that may cause permanent deformity or scars
3. Large facial hemangiomas, particularly those with a large dermal component
4. Ulcerated hemangiomas

Other possible indications include smaller hemangiomas on the face or other exposed areas if the treatment method under consideration is unlikely to cause scarring

or significant side effects and pedunculated hemangiomas that are likely to leave significant fibrofatty residual lesions.[107,108]

Despite these recommended guidelines, determination of which hemangiomas should be treated and with what method may still be difficult. The potential benefits of any form of treatment should be carefully weighed against the risks associated with treatment. The long-term effects of newer treatment methods may not be known. It is important to consider not only anatomic location, but also the size and type of hemangioma (superficial, deep, or combined). It is extremely important to assess the phase of the hemangioma. Is it actively proliferating, is it stable, or is involution predominating? It is essential to have a candid discussion with the parents regarding the possible outcomes with and without therapy and the morbidity associated with treatments. The following sections describe some of the treatment methods that have been employed.

Active Nonintervention. The majority of hemangiomas are left to involute spontaneously. Parents may feel significant distress as they await spontaneous regression. A study of parents of children with facial hemangiomas measuring greater than 1 cm in diameter revealed that parents often report feelings of disbelief, fear, and mourning once the diagnosis is established. Some feel a degree of social stigmatization. Parent-child interactions may be adversely affected. Many report dissatisfaction with medical care, citing a lack of information, anticipatory guidance, and empathy.[109] In light of this experience, a careful discussion of the natural history of hemangiomas should be undertaken at the time of diagnosis, and it is often useful to discuss therapy of hemangiomas and why the patient would not be a candidate for such treatment. Frequent visits, measurements, and photographs during the proliferating phase are necessary. As the hemangioma begins to involute, regular visits and photography help to reassure parents that the hemangioma is indeed regressing. It may be appropriate to prepare parents for intrusive questions and advice they may receive.

Complications such as ulceration and infection should be treated promptly. Topical and oral antibiotics and biooclusive dressings are used as the initial treatment of ulcerated hemangiomas. Other forms of therapy include flashlamp-pumped pulsed dye laser and Nd:YAG laser (see Surgical Therapy section). Corticosteroids may be required.

Corticosteroid Therapy. Systemic corticosteroid has remained the mainstay of treatment for problematic hemangiomas since initial reports of efficacy in the 1960s. It is believed to act as an antiangiogenic agent. Prednisone or prednisolone at a dosage of 2 to 3 mg/kg/day is used during the proliferating phase to slow or halt growth of the hemangioma, with some authors advocating even higher doses.[84] Generally most patients receive 2 mg/kg/ day as a single morning dose. If a response is noted, patients are generally maintained on this regimen for 4 to 6 weeks. Thereafter the dose is slowly tapered over the following months. The duration of treatment depends on response to therapy and the amount of time the hemangioma remains in the proliferating period. Approximately 30% of patients respond to treatment within 2 to 3 weeks as evidenced by a cessation of growth and shrinkage of the mass (Fig. 18-24). Another 40% demonstrate cessation of growth without shrinkage in the size of the hemangioma, a finding that may be the result of either a corticosteroid effect or of spontaneous leveling off in the growth of the lesion. Approximately 30% fail to respond to therapy, even if prednisone dosages are increased.[78,106]

Before the initiation of corticosteroid therapy, parents should be counseled regarding potential side effects. Although the adverse effects of corticosteroids have been well documented in the literature for other systemic diseases, there is little information regarding side effects associated with the treatment of hemangiomas. Cushingoid facies, "personality changes," gastric irritation, and perineal and oral candidiasis are the most frequently reported short-term side effects.

Retardation of growth, including both height and weight, is also noted, with infants experiencing catch-up growth after cessation of therapy. Steroid myopathy is rare. Hypertension is a potential complication of higher dose therapy. In addition, patients should be cautioned about the risk of immunocompromise and susceptibility to infection, and live-virus vaccines should be avoided during corticosteroid treatment.

Intralesional corticosteroid treatment may be useful in the treatment of small, localized hemangiomas in problematic locations such as the lips, nasal tip, ear, or face. Long-acting triamcinolone acetonide, alone or in combination with the shorter-acting dexamethasone sodium phosphate, is the most frequently used agent.[20,110,111] Although no treatment protocols have been established and the frequency of injections is governed by clinical response, generally one to three treatments at 4- to 6-week intervals are needed. The dosage of triamcinolone should not exceed 3 to 5 mg/kg per treatment session. Intralesional injection of hemangiomas on the eyelid with long-acting corticosteroid preparations may be complicated by occlusion of the central retinal or ophthalmic arteries, which may cause blindness.[112] Other complications associated with intralesional treatment in this area include intraocular deposits, eyelid necrosis, and scleroderma-like linear atrophy of the skin. Therefore caution is advised when using these preparations in this location.[113]

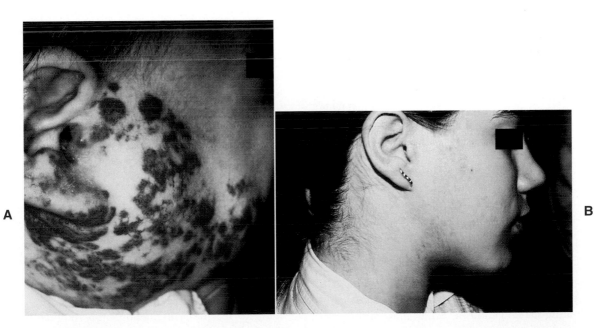

A   B

FIG. 18-24
Extensive hemangioma in infancy **(A)**, which responded to corticosteroid therapy, leaving virtually normal skin at 14 years **(B)**.

Interferon-alfa. Recombinant interferon-alfa has been successful in the treatment of life-threatening hemangiomas that have failed to respond to corticosteroid therapy.[114-117] Both interferon-alfa-2a and 2b have been used. The most common treatment regimen consists of a daily injection of 3 million U/m² as needed.[97] The response to therapy is variable, with some patients responding rapidly over the course of 3 to 6 months and others needing longer periods of treatment.[2] Side effects associated with treatment include fever, neutropenia, altered hepatic function chemistries, flulike complaints, and agitation. Spastic diplegia, a side effect reported in 5 of 26 infants receiving interferon-alfa-2a, is a particularly worrisome complication of treatment.[97,118] Although this has led some to recommend the use of the 2b preparation, this does not eliminate the risk cited by recent reports of spastic diplegia and neurotoxicity.[116,117] Therefore it is recommended that interferon-alfa be reserved for treatment of life-threatening hemangiomas that have failed corticosteroid therapy. Neurodevelopmental status should be assessed at baseline, during, and after treatment with interferon-alfa.[97,118]

Surgical Therapy. The flashlamp-pumped pulsed dye laser has been used to treat hemangiomas. Superficial lesions appear to respond best to this treatment.[119,120] Hemangiomas with a deeper dermal component may show lightening of the superficial erythematous portion, but treatment does not affect the deeper portion. Moreover, early laser treatment of a superficial hemangioma fails to prevent the growth of a deeper component. Multiple treatment sessions over several months may be needed to treat superficial hemangiomas. Treatment appears to be relatively well tolerated. Side effects include transient pigmentary alteration and atrophic scarring. The pulsed dye laser also is an effective treatment for residual telangiectasia in involuted hemangiomas, and it may be an effective treatment for ulcerated hemangiomas. Patients who failed to respond to treatment with topical agents respond with healing of the ulceration, and subjective reduction of pain may be noted after two or three treatments.[121] Other laser light sources including the argon and Nd:YAG lasers have been used to treat hemangiomas but may cause more significant scarring. Percutaneous treatment with a bare fiber Nd:YAG laser has been used to treat deep hemangiomas.[122] Experience with this technique is limited and is likely operator dependent. Contact cryotherapy has been used to treat small, early-proliferating hemangiomas.[123] Surgical excision is usually reserved for involuted hemangiomas to remove residual fibrofatty tissue and redundant skin. Early excision is generally not recommended, but possible indications include deep periorbital hemangiomas that fail to respond to pharmacologic therapy, or in which medical therapy is believed to pose a greater risk, and some cases of pedunculated hemangiomas that will ultimately result in prominent fibrofatty residual tissue. Excision may be considered during the preschool period for some patients with involuting hemangiomas in cosmetically significant areas such as the nasal tip. Arterial embolization has been employed to treat life-threatening hemangiomas with high output, that have failed medical therapy, improve the cardiovascular status by reducing the tumor volume.

Other Vascular Tumors

The diagnosis of the rare vascular tumors discussed in the following sections requires a skilled pathologist who is familiar with vascular lesions, since the criteria for their recognition are based primarily on histopathologic features and since the immunohistochemical markers that are used to help delineate one vascular growth from another are absent. Moreover, many of these entities have been described only recently, so they may be unfamiliar to some pathologists.[4]

Tufted Angioma

Tufted angioma (TA) was described by Wilson-Jones and Orkin.[124] It was long-known in the Japanese literature as *angioblastoma of Nakagawa*. The pathologic features are diagnostic. Most cases are acquired early in childhood and have a protracted course.[125] Rare congenital forms also exist.[125] Congenital TAs display various patterns at birth: large, plaquelike, infiltrated, inhomogeneous red lesions, some of them with lanugo or with a pale halo, or large, exophytic, firm, violaceous, cutaneous nodules (Fig. 18-25). A diagnostic biopsy is advised to rule out a congenital sarcoma. Histologically, both acquired and congenital TAs demonstrate vascular tufts of tightly packed capillaries, randomly dispersed throughout the dermis in a typical cannonball distribution, semilunar empty vascular spaces around the vascular tufts, and lymphatic-like spaces.[124] Congenital TAs must be differentiated from hemangiomas, the most common lobular capillary benign tumor of infancy. TAs may regress completely within a few years,[126] shrink, leaving a residuum, or persist unchanged, requiring further excisional treatment. A small number of congenital TAs develop Kasabach-Merritt phenomenon. After resolution of the coagulopathy, they may leave minor lesions with a fibrotic texture[128] or an extensive red stain with coalescent papules and tenderness.[128]

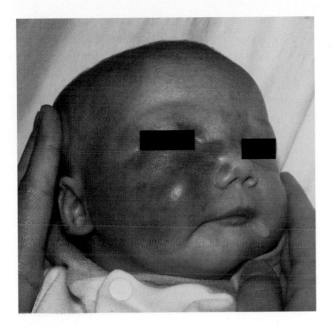

FIG. 18-25
This hemifacial congenital violaceous mass proved to be a tufted angioma, which involuted with corticosteroid treatment.

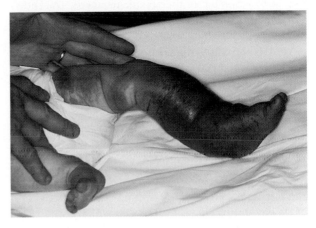

FIG. 18-26
Kasabach-Merritt phenomenon involving the leg. Note both the ecchymotic and inflammatory pattern of the skin.

Kaposiform Hemangioendothelioma

Kaposiform hemangioendothelioma is a rare vascular tumor that has been reported in association with Kasabach-Merritt syndrome (see following section) and with lymphangiomatosis.[129] Histologic examination reveals densely infiltrating nodules composed of spindled cells with minimal atypia and infrequent mitoses, lining slitlike or crescentic vessels containing hemosiderin. The proliferation is associated with lymphatic spaces. It is rarely recognized in neonates when, occurring without thrombocytopenia, it is probably misdiagnosed as "congenital hemangioma." It may involute spontaneously.

Kasabach-Merritt Syndrome

Since the first case report in 1940, the label *Kasabach-Merritt syndrome* (KMS) has been used for every infant with a vascular anomaly and thrombocytopenia, and the syndrome has been considered a complication of "hemangioma."[130] Several publications have now documented that this biologic phenomenon is not associated with a "true" hemangioma of infancy, but rather with other vascular tumors, especially kaposiform hemangioendothelioma (KHE) or tufted angioma (TA), which may occur in association with a lymphatic malformation.[131-135]

Cutaneous Findings. KMS is a rare and distinctive syndrome. Affected infants have a congenital tumor or a lesion soon after birth, with subsequent development of an inflammatory, bruising, reddish or purple mass, and purpura (Fig. 18-26). Before the development of thrombocytopenia and platelet trapping, the clinical appearance may be quite variable. Infants may have a yellowish, bluish, or red plaquelike lesion, often congenital, or no lesion at all; they may have a history of a congenital bulky tumor detected by prenatal ultrasonography and requiring a diagnostic biopsy in the neonate.[136]

Extracutaneous Findings. A severe thrombocytopenia is the hallmark of KMS. Consumption of fibrinogen and coagulation factors occurs to varying degrees, depending on the severity and phases of the disease. KMS has no anatomic site of predilection. It can be superficial or visceral. Visceral KMS—cervicothoracic, abdominal, pelvic, or intracranial—is always life threatening.

Course. Thrombocytopenia may persist for a few years but more commonly resolves with treatment by 12 to 18 months. Hemorrhage, infection, or iatrogenic complications may cause death. When the hematologic phenomenon is cured, the tumor shrinks but the patient has residual changes that are clearly different from those of an involuted hemangioma. These residua are more or less prominent and painful, persisting vascular tumors in a dormant stage. Their appearance varies from that of a pseudo–port wine stain, with infiltrated areas and papules, stainlike areas with halo, and nodular residua, to a poorly delineated, fibrotic-feeling plaque. Muscle and joint fibrosis remains in some cases.[137]

Treatment. KMS is a medical emergency. Infants with Kasabach-Merritt syndrome exhibit an inconsistent response to a number of therapeutic regimens. The choice of treatment is empiric. Both success and failure have been documented with various drugs prescribed alone or in combination, which increases the risk of toxicity. Currently the best therapeutic options appear to be corticosteroids, vincristine,[127] interferon-alfa, and ticlopidine plus aspirin. Surgical excision, arterial embolization, and radiotherapy may also benefit some patients.

Infantile Hemangiopericytoma (Versus Infantile Myofibromatosis)

Infantile hemangiopericytoma is considered a rare tumor and different from the more common adult type because of its benign prognosis.[138] The congenital form, more common in boys, is a red, partially necrotic tumor, with a branching vasculature, a multilobular pattern, a collagenous matrix, and mitotic figures. This is a controversial lesion,[4] now considered part of a continuum with solitary infantile myofibromatosis.[139] The latter presents as a congenital rubbery red or pink nodule, corresponding to a richly vascularized tumor and dense infiltration of plump, spindle-shaped cells. Solitary infantile myofibromatosis has a good outcome and involutes by massive apoptosis. A multinodular multisystemic form may be present in a neonate; this generalized form may have a bad outcome, being lethal soon after birth, although spontaneous resolution has also been reported.

Spindle Cell Hemangioendothelioma

Spindle cell hemangioendothelioma (SCHE) occurs at any age and site but seems more common in the limbs. It has a protracted course. Lesions are solitary or multiple. The nodular, dense, spindle cell proliferation is associated with "cavernous" vessels of attenuated, irregularly thickened walls. Lesions tend to multiply locally and to recur when excised. Among 78 cases,[140] 4 had Maffucci syndrome. No metastases were reported in this large series of SCHE, thereafter renamed *SC-hemangioma* (for solitary lesion) or *SC-hemangiomatosis* (for multiple skin lesions).[140]

Congenital Eccrine Angiomatous Hamartoma (Sudoriparous Angioma)

Congenital forms of this tumor present as a nodule or as a large, ill-defined angiomatous plaque with lanugo and sweating at the site of the lesion. They are usually located on the extremities or abdomen and may involute. It is not clear whether the rarely reported congenital cases[141,142] are identical to the slowly growing, persistent forms that are characterized by an acquired bluish or flesh-colored nodule or a bossed erythematous and pigmented firm nodule or plaque with excess hair, hyperhidrosis, and pain overlying a slow-flow vascular malformation. Diagnosis is established on the basis of the presence of characteristic histologic findings. Closely packed eccrine sweat glands are associated with dilated capillaries, a few dysplastic venous channels, and a dense collagenous matrix.

Congenital Cutaneous Plaquelike Glomus Tumors, Glomangiomas, and Familial Glomangiomatosis

Glomus tumors may be solitary or multiple. When present at birth, they are plaquelike, poorly demarcated, pink or bluish (or both) plaques or nodular lesions.[143] In our experience these tumors acquire a deep-blue hue and thicken during childhood. They are painful when palpated. Glomus tumors are composed of large tortuous channels with several rows of cuboid, proliferating glomus cells. They are treated by excision when possible. Congenital plaquelike glomangiomas may arise sporadically, or they occur in families with familial autosomal dominant glomangiomatosis. Affected members in a given family may have either small, blue vascular lesions scattered over the skin, the number of which increases with age, or congenital plaquelike lesions, with noticeable worsening during childhood.[144]

Pyogenic Granuloma[4]

A pyogenic granuloma is a red, rapidly growing, easily bleeding, papulonodular lesion that corresponds to dilated capillaries and a mucin-rich prominent stroma. It is quite common on the face in the malar area and frequent in young children. Rare multifocal forms have been observed in newborns. Destruction by electrocautery or laser is usually necessary.

REFERENCES

1. Mulliken JB, Glowacki J. Hemangiomas and vascular malformations in infants and children: a classification based on endothelial characteristics. Plast Reconstr Surg 1982;69: 412-420.
2. Enjolras O, Mulliken J. Vascular tumors and vascular malformations, new issues. Adv Dermatol 1998;13:375-423.
3. Takahashi K, Mulliken JB, Kozakewich H, et al. Cellular markers that distinguish the phases of hemangioma during infancy and childhood. J Clin Invest 1994;93:2357-2364.
4. Requena L, Sangueza OP. Cutaneous vascular proliferations. II. Hyperplasias and benign neoplasms. J Am Acad Dermatol 1997;37:887-920.
5. Pratt AG. Birthmarks in infants. Arch Dermatol Syph 1953; 67:302-305.

6. Leung AKC, Telmesani AMA. Salmon patches in Caucasian children. Pediatr Dermatol 1989;6:185-187.

7. Metzker A, Shamir R. Butterfly-shaped mark: a variant form of nevus flammeus simplex. Pediatrics 1990;85:1069-1071.

8. Patrizi A, Neri I, Orlandi C, et al. Sacral medial telangiectatic vascular nevus: a study of 43 children. Dermatology 1996; 192:301-306.

9. McClean K, Hanke CW. The medical necessity for treatment of port-wine stains. Dermatol Surg 1997;23:663-667.

10. Boyd JB, Mulliken JB, Kaban LB et al. Skeletal changes associated with vascular malformations. Plast Reconstr Surg 1984;74:789-795.

11. Dover JS, Geronemus R, Stern RS, et al. Dye laser treatment of port-wine stains: comparison of the continuous-wave dye laser with a robotized scanning device and the pulsed dye laser. J Am Acad Dermatol 1995;32:237-240.

12. Renfro L, Geronemus RG. Anatomical differences of port-wine stains in response to treatment with the pulsed dye laser. Arch Dermatol 1993;129:182-188.

13. Ashinoff R, Geronemus RG: Flashlamp-pumped pulsed dye laser for port-wine stains in infancy: earlier versus later treatment. J Am Acad Dermatol 1991;24:467-472.

14. Van Der Horst C, Koster P, De Borgie C, et al. Effect of the timing on the treatment of port-wine stains with the flash-lamp-pumped pulsed-dye laser. N Engl J Med 1998;338: 1028-1033.

15. Cabana M, Crawford TO, Winkelstein JA, et al. Consequences of the delayed diagnosis of ataxia-telangiectasia. Pediatrics 1998;102:98-100.

16. Enjolras O, Ciabrini D, Mazoyer E, et al. Extensive pure venous malformations in the upper and lower limbs: a review of 27 cases. J Am Acad Dermatol 1997;36:219-225

17. Boon LM, Mulliken JB, Vikkula M, et al. Assignment of a locus for dominantly inherited venous malformations to chromosome 9p. Hum Mol Genet 1994;3:1583-1587.

18. Vikkula M, Boon LM, Carraway KL, et al. Vascular dysmorphogenesis caused by an activating mutation in the receptor tyrosine kinase TIE2. Cell 1996;87:1181-1190.

19. Boukobza M, Enjolras O, Guichard JP, et al. Cerebral developmental venous anomaly associated with head and neck venous malformations. AJNR 1996;17:987-994.

20. Enjolras O, Mulliken JB. The current management of vascular birthmarks. Pediatr Dermatol 1993;10:311-333.

21. Burrows PE, Fellows KE. Techniques for management of pediatric vascular anomalies. In Cope C, ed. Current techniques in interventional radiology, Curr Med 1995;2:12-27.

22. Gimeno Aranguez M, Colomar Palmer P, Gonzalez Mediero I, et al. Aspectos clínicos y morfológicos de los linfangiomas infantiles, revisión de 145 casos. An Esp Pediatr 1996;45: 25-28.

23. Padwa BL, Hayward PG, Ferrero NF, et al. Cervicofacial lymphatic malformation, clinical course, surgical intervention, and pathogenesis of skeletal hypertrophy. Plast Reconstr Surg 1995;95:951-960.

24. Larralde M, Gardner SS, Torrado MV, et al. Lymphedema as a postulated cause of cutis verticis gyrata in Turner syndrome. Pediatr Dermatol 1998;15:18-22.

25. Piette F, Brevière GM, Catteau B, et al. Congenital diffuse elephantiasic lymphangioma. Ann Dermatol Venereol 1998;125(suppl 1):S167.

26. Enjolras O, Deffrennes D, Borsik M, et al. Les "tumeurs" vaculaires. Règles de prise en charge chirurgicale. Ann Chir Plast Esthét 1998;43:455-490.

27. Ogita S, Tsuto T, Deguchi E, et al. OK432 therapy for unresectable lymphangiomas in children. J Pediatr Surg 1991;26: 263-270.

28. Molitch HI, Unger EC, Witte CL, et al. Percutaneous sclerotherapy of lymphangiomas. Radiology 1995;194:343-347.

29. Enjolras O, Logeart I, Gelbert F, et al. Malformations artério-veineuses: à propos de 200 cas. Ann Dermatol Venereol 1999;127:17-22.

30. Esterly NB. Cutaneous hemangiomas, vascular stains and malformations, and associated syndromes. Curr Probl Dermatol 1995;3:69-107.

31. Picascia DD, Esterly NB. Cutis marmorata telangiectatica congenita: report of 22 cases. J Am Acad Dermatol 1989;20: 1098-1104.

32. Moroz PK. Cutis marmorata telangiectatica congenita: long-term follow-up, review of the literature, and report of a case in conjunction with congenital hypothyroidism. Pediatr Dermatol 1993;10:6-11.

33. Devillers ACA, de Waard-Van der Spek FB, Oranje AP. Cutis marmorata telangiectatica congenita: clinical features in 35 cases. Arch Dermatol 1999;135:34-38.

34. Kennedy C, Oranje AP, Keizer K, et al. Cutis marmorata telangiectatica congenita. Int J Dermatol 1992;31:249-252.

35. Gelmetti C, Schianchi R, Ermacora E. Cutis marmorata telangiectatica congenita: quatre nouveaux cas et revue de la littérature. Ann Dermatol Venereol 1987;114:1517-1528.

36. Carrascosa JM, Ribera M, Bielsa I, et al. Cutis marmorata telangiectatica congenita or neonatal lupus? Pediatr Dermatol 1996;13:230-232.

37. Enjolras O, Riché MC, Merland JJ. Facial port-wine stains and Sturge-Weber syndrome. Pediatrics 1985;76:48-51.

38. Adamsbaum C, Pinton F, Rolland Y, et al. Accelerated myelination in early Sturge-Weber syndrome: MRI-SPECT correlation. Pediatr Radiol 1996;26:759-762.

39. Pinton F, Chiron C, Enjolras O, et al. Early single photon emission computed tomography in Sturge-Weber syndrome. J Neurol Neurosurg Psychiatry 1997;63:616-621.

40. Chugani HT. The role of PET in childhood epilepsy. J Child Neurol 1994;9(suppl 1):82-88.

41. Salman MS. Is the prophylactic use of antiepileptic drugs in Sturge-Weber syndrome justified? Med Hypotheses 1998;51: 293-296.

42. Berry SA, Peterson C, Mize W, et al. Klippel-Trenaunay syndrome. Am J Med Genet 1998;79:319-326.

43. Ramina R, Coelho Neto M, Meneses MS, et al. Maffucci's syndrome associated with a cranial base chondrosarcoma: case report and literature review. Neurosurgery 1997;41: 269-272.

44. Radke M, Waldschmidt J, Stolpe HJ, et al. Blue rubber bleb nevus syndrome with predominant urinary bladder hemangiomatosis. Eur J Pediatr Surg 1993;3:313-316.

45. Hennekam RC, Geerdink RA, Hamel BC, et al. Autosomal recessive intestinal lymphangiectasia and lymphedema with facial anomalies and mental retardation. Am J Med Genet 1989;34:593-600.

46. Angle B, Hersch JH. Expansion of the phenotype of Hennekam syndrome: a case with new manifestations. Am J Med Genet 1997;71:211-214.

47. Aagenaes O. Hereditary cholestasis with lymphedema (Aagenaes syndrome, cholestasis-lymphedema syndrome). New cases and follow-up from infancy to adult age. Scand J Gastroenterol 1998;33:335-345.

48. Schneid H, Vasquez MP, Vacher C, et al. The Beckwith-Wiedemann syndrome phenotype and the risk of cancer. Med Pediatr Oncol 1997;28:411-415.

49. Choyke PL, Siegel MJ, Oz O, et al. Nonmalignant renal diseases in pediatric patients with Beckwith-Wiedemann syndrome. AJR 1998;171:733-737.

50. Wiedemann HR, Burgio GR, Aldendorff P, et al. The Proteus syndrome. Eur J Pediatr 1983;140:5-12.

51. Lacombe D, Taïeb A, Vergnes P, et al. Proteus syndrome in 7 patients: clinical and genetic considerations. Genet Counseling 1990;2:93-101.

52. Hotamisligil GS. Proteus syndrome and hamartoses with overgrowth. Dysmorphol Clin Genet 1990;4:87-102.

53. Barona-Mazuera MR, Hidalgo-Galvan LR, Orozco-Covarrubias ML, et al. Proteus syndrome: new findings in seven patients. Pediatr Dermatol 1997;14:1-5.

54. Cohen MM Jr. Bannayan-Riley-Ruvalcaba syndrome: renaming three formerly recognized syndromes as one etiologic entity. Am J Med Genet 1990;35:291.

55. Fargnoli MC, Orlow SJ, Semel-Concepcion J, et al. Clinicopathologic findings in the Bannayan-Riley-Ruvalcaba syndrome. Arch Dermatol 1996;132:1214-1218.

56. Lin AE, Gorlin RJ, Lurie IW, et al. Further delineation of the branchio-oculo-facial syndrome. Am J Med Genet 1995;56:42-59.

57. Martínez-Frías ML, Arroyo-Carrera I, Jiménez Munoz DN, et al. Síndrome de Adams-Oliver en nuestro medio: aspectos epidemiológicos. An Esp Pediatr 1996;45:57-61.

58. Dyall-Smith D, Ramsden A, Laurie S. Adams-Oliver syndrome: aplasia cutis congenita, terminal transverse limb defects, and cutis marmorata telangiectatica congenita. Australas J Dermatol 1994;35:19-22.

59. Romani J, Puig L, Aznar G, et al. Adams-Oliver syndrome with unusual central nervous system alterations. Pediatr Dermatol 1998;15:48-50.

60. Nova HR. Familial communicating hydrocephalus, posterior cerebellar agenesis, mega cisterna magna, and port wine nevi. J Neurosurg 1979;51:862-865.

61. Jacobs AH, Walton R. The incidence of birthmarks in neonate. Pediatrics 1976;58:218-222.

62. Mulliken JB. Diagnosis and natural history of hemangiomas. In Mulliken JB, Young AE, eds. Vascular birthmarks: hemangiomas and malformations. Philadelphia: WB Saunders, 1988: pp 41-62.

63. Hidano A, Nakajima S. Earliest features of the strawberry mark in the newborn. Br J Dermatol 1972;87:138-144.

64. Finn MC, Glowacki J, Mulliken JB. Congenital vascular lesions: clinical application of a new classification. J Pediatr Surg 1983;18:894-900.

65. Moroz B: Long-term follow-up of hemangiomas in children. In Williams HB, ed. Symposium on vascular malformations and melanotic lesions. St. Louis: CV Mosby, 1983: pp 162-171.

66. Amir J, Metzker A, Krikler R, et al. Strawberry hemangioma in preterm infants. Pediatr Dermatol 1986;3:331-332.

67. Burton BK, Schulz CJ, Angle B, et al. An increased incidence of haemangiomas in infants born following chorionic villus sampling (CVS). Prenatal Diagnosis 1995;15:209-214.

68. Achauer BM, Chang C, Vander VM. Management of hemangioma of infancy: review of 245 patients. Plast Reconstr Surg 1997;99:1301-1308.

69. Blei F, Walter J, Orlow SJ, et al. Familial segregation of hemangiomas and vascular malformations as an autosomal dominant trait. Arch Dermatol 1998;134:718-722.

70. Payne MM, Moyer F, Marcks KM, et al. The precursor to the hemangioma. Plast Reconstr Surg 1966;38:64-67.

71. Liang MG, Frieden IJ. Perineal and lip ulcerations as the presenting manifestation of hemangioma of infancy. Pediatrics 1997;99:256-259.

72. Boon LM, Enjolras O, Mulliken JB. Congenital hemangioma: evidence of accelerated involution. J Pediatr 1996;128:329-335.

73. Bonifazi E, Mileti F. Images in clinical medicine. Congenital hemangioma. N Engl J Med 1999;14:1080.

74. Lister WA. The natural history of strawberry nevi. Lancet 1938;1429-1434.

75. Golitz LE, Rudikoff J, O'Meara OP. Diffuse neonatal hemangiomatosis. Pediatr Dermatol 1986;3:145-152.

76. Boon LM, Burrows PE, Paltiel HJ, et al. Hepatic vascular anomalies in infancy: a twenty-seven-year experience. J Pediatr 1996;129:346-354.

77. Orlow SJ, Isakoff MS, Blei F. Increased risk of symptomatic hemangiomas of the airway in association with cutaneous hemangiomas in a "beard" distribution. J Pediatr 1997;131:643-646.

78. Enjolras O, Gelbert F. Superficial hemangiomas: associations and management. Pediatr Dermatol 1997;14:173-179.

79. Stern JK, Wolf JE, Jarratt M. Benign neonatal hemangiomatosis. J Am Acad Dermatol 1981;4:442-445.

80. Holden KR, Alexander F. Diffuse neonatal hemangiomatosis. Pediatrics 1970;46:411-421.

81. Sheu B, Shyu M, Ling Y, et al. Prenatal diagnosis and corticosteroid treatment of diffuse neonatal hemangiomatosis. J Ultrasound Med 1994;13:495-499.

82. Fishman SJ, Burrows PE, Mulliken JB. Gastrointestinal manifestations of vascular anomalies in childhood: varied etiologies require multiple therapeutic modalities. J Pediatr Surg 1998;33:1163-1167.

83. Berman B, Lim HWP. Concurrent cutaneous and hepatic hemangiomata in infancy: report of a case and review of the literature. J Dermatol Surg Oncol 1978;4:869-873.

84. Drolet BA, Esterly NB, Frieden IJ. Hemangiomas in children. N Engl J Med 1999;341:173- 181.

85. Burns AJ, Kaplan LC, Mulliken JB. Is there an association between hemangioma and syndromes with dysmorphic features? Pediatrics 1991;88:1257-1267.

86. Gorlin RJ, Kantaputra P, Aughton DJ, et al. Marked female predilection in some syndromes associated with facial hemangiomas. Am J Med Genet 1994;52:130-135.

87. Frieden IJ, Reese V, Cohen D. PHACE syndrome: the association of posterior fossa brain malformations, hemangiomas, arterial anomalies, coarctation of the aorta and cardiac defects, and eye abormalities. Arch Dermatol 1996;132:307-311.

88. Pascual-Castroviejo I, Viano J, Moreno F, et al. Hemangiomas of the head, neck, and chest with associated vascular and brain anomalies: a complex neurocutaneous syndrome. AJNR 1996;17:461-471.

89. Burrows PE, Robertson, RL, Mulliken JB, et al. Cerebral vasculopathy and neurologic sequelae in infants with cervicofacial hemangioma: report of eight patients. Radiology 1998;207:601-607.

90. Reese V, Frieden IJ, Paller AS, et al. Association of facial hemangiomas with Dandy-Walker and other posterior fossa malformations. J Pediatr 1993;122:379-384.

91. Geller JD, Topper SF, Hashimoto K, et al. Diffuse neonatal hemangiomatosis: a new constellation of findings. J Am Acad Dermatol 1991;24:816-818.

92. Vaillant L, Lorette G, Chantepie A, et al. Multiple cutaneous hemangiomas and coarctation of the aorta with right aotic arch. Pediatrics 1988;81:707-710.

93. Hersh JH, Waterfill D, Rutledge J, et al. Sternal malformation/vascular dysplasia association. Am J Med Genet 1985;21:177-186.

94. Blei F, Orlow SJ, Geronemus RG. Supraumbilical midabdominal raphe, sternal atresia, and hemangioma in an infant. Pediatr Dermatol 1993;10:71-76.

95. Goldberg NS, Hebert AA, Esterly NB. Sacral hemangiomas and multiple congenital abnormalities. Arch Dermatol 1986;122:684-687.

96. Albright AL, Gartner C, Wiener ES, et al. Lumbar cutaneous hemangiomas as indicators of tethered spinal cords. Pediatrics 1989;83:977-980.

97. Folkman J, Mulliken JB, Ezekowitz RAB. Angiogenesis and hemangiomas. In Oldham KT, Colombani PM, Foglia RP, eds. Surgery of infants and children: scientific principles and practice. Philadelphia: Lippincott-Raven, 1997: pp 569-580.

98. Glowacki J, Mulliken JB. Mast cells in hemangiomas and vascular malformations. Pediatrics 1982;70:48-51.

99. Folkman J. Clinical applications of research on angiogenesis. N Engl J Med 1995;333:1757-1763.

100. Iwata J, Sonobe H, Furihata M, et al. High frequency of apoptosis in infantile capillary haemangioma. J Pathol 1996;179:403-408.

101. Razon MJ, Kraling BM, Mulliken JB, Bischoff J. Increased apoptosis coincides with onset of involution in infantile hemangiomas. Microcirculation 1998;5:189-195.

102. Burrows PE, Laor T, Paltiel H, Robertson RL. Diagnostic imaging in the evaluation of vascular birthmarks. Dermatol Clin 1998;16:455-488.

103. Hayward PG, Orgill DP, Mulliken JB, et al. Congenital fibrosarcoma masquerading as lymphatic malformation: report of two cases. J Pediatr Surg 1995;30:84-88.

104. Haik BG, Jakobiec F, Ellsworth RM, et al. Capillary hemangioma of the lids and orbit: an analysis of the clinical features and therapeutic results in 101 cases. Ophthalmology 1979;86:760-789.

105. Robb R. Refractive errors associated with hemangiomas of the eyelids and orbit in infancy. Am J Ophthalmol 1977;83:52-58.

106. Enjolras O, Riche MC, Merland JJ, et al. Management of alarming hemangiomas in infancy: a review of 25 cases. Pediatrics 1990;85:491-498.

107. Frieden IJ, Eichenfield LF, Esterly NB, et al. Guidelines of care for hemangiomas of infancy. J Am Acad Dermatol 1997;37:631-637.

108. Frieden IJ. Which hemangiomas to treat-and how? Arch Dermatol 1997;133:1593-1595.

109. Tanner JL, Dechert MP, Frieden IJ. Growing up with a facial hemangioma: parent and child coping and adaptation. Pediatrics 1998;101:446-451.

110. Sloan GM, Reinisch JF, Nichter LS, et al. Intralesional corticosteroid therapy for infantile hemangiomas. Plast Reconstr Surg 1989;83:459-466.

111. Nelson LB, Melick JE, Harley R. Intralesional corticosteroid injections for infantile hemangiomas of the eyelid. Pediatrics 1984;74:241-245.

112. Schorr N, Seiff SR. Central retinal artery occlusion associated with periocular corticosteroid injection for juvenile hemangioma. Ophthalmol Surg 1986;17:229-231.

113. Egbert JE, Schwartz GS, Walsh AW. Diagnosis and treatment of an ophthalmic artery occlusion during an intralesional injection of corticosteroid into an eyelid capillary hemangioma. Am J Ophthalmol 1996;121:638-642.

114. Ezekowitz RAB, Mulliken JB, Folkman J. Interferon alfa-2a therapy for life-threatening hemangiomas of infancy. N Engl J Med 1992;326:1456-1463.

115. Tamayo L, Ortiz DM, Orozco-Covarrubias L, et al. Therapeutic efficacy of interferon alfa-2b in infants with life-threatening giant hemangiomas. Arch Dermatol 1997;133:1567-1571.

116. Chang E, Boyd A, Nelson CC, et al. Successful treatment of infantile hemangiomas with interferon alfa-2b. J Pediatr Hematol Oncol 1997;19:237-244.

117. Dubois J, Hershon L, Carmant L, et al. Toxicity profile of interferon alfa-2b in children: a prospective evaluation. J Pediatr 1999;135:782-785

118. Barlow CF, Priebe CJ, Mulliken JB, et al. Spastic diplegia as complication of interferon alfa-2a treatment of hemangiomas of infancy. J Pediatr 1998;132:527-530.

119. Garden JM, Bakus A, Paller A. Treatment of cutaneous hemangiomas by the flashlamp-pumped pulsed dye laser: prospective analysis. J Pediatr 1992;120:555-560.

120. Ashinoff R, Geronemus RG. Failure of the flashlamp-pumped pulsed dye laser to prevent progression to deep hemangioma. Pediatr Dermatol 1993;10:77-80.

121. Morelli JG, Tan OT, Yohn JJ, et al. Treatment of ulcerated hemangiomas in infancy. Arch Pediatr Adolesc Med 1994;148:1104-1105

122. Berlien HP, Müller G, Waldschmidt J. Lasers in pediatric surgery. Prog Pediatr Surg 1990;2:5-22.

123. Cremer HJ, Djawari D. Fruhtherapie der kutanen hamangiome mit der kontaktkryochirugie. Chir Praxis 1995;49:295-312.

124. Wilson-Jones E, Orkin M. Tufted angioma (angioblastoma): a benign progressive angioma not to be confused with Kaposi's sarcoma or low grade angiosarcoma. J Am Acad Dermatol 1989;20:214-225.

125. Catteau B, Enjolras O, Delaporte E, et al. Angiome en touffes sclérosant. A propos de 4 observations. Ann Dermatol Venereol 1998;125:682-687.

126. Lam WY, Mac-Moune Lai F, Look CN, et al. Tufted angioma with complete regression. J Cutan Pathol 1994;21:461-466.

127. Enjolras, M. Wassef, C. Dosquet, et al. Syndrome de Kasabach-Merritt sur angiome en touffes congénital. Ann Dermatol Venereol 1998;125:257-260.

128. Léauté-Labreze C, Bioulac-Sage P, Labbé L, et al. Tufted angioma with platelet trapping syndrome: response to aspirin. Arch Dermatol 1997;133:1077-1079.

129. Zukerberg LR, Nickoloff BJ, Weiss SW. Kaposiform hemangioendothelioma of infancy and childhood: an aggressive neoplasm associated with Kasabach-Merritt syndrome and lymphangiomatosis. Am J Surg Pathol 1993;17:321-328.

130. Kasabach HH, Merritt KK. Capillary hemangioma with extensive purpura, report of a case. Am J Dis Child 1940;59: 1063-1070.

131. Enjolras O, Wassef M, Mazoyer E, et al. Infants with Kasabach Merritt syndrome do not have "true" hemangioma. J Pediatr 1997;130:631-640.

132. Tsang WYW, Chan JKC. Kaposi-like hemangioendothelioma: a distinctive vascular neoplasm of the retroperineum. Am J Surg Pathol 1991;15:982-989.

133. Niedt GW, Greco MA, Wieczorek R, et al. Hemangioma with Kaposi's sarcoma–like features: report of two cases. Pediatr Pathol 1989;9:567-575.

134. Vin-Christian K, McCalmont TH, Frieden IJ. Kaposiform hemangioendothelioma, an aggressive locally invasive vascular tumor that can minic hemangioma of infancy. Arch Dermatol 1997;133:1573-1578.

135. Sarkar M, Mulliken JB, Kozakewich HPW, et al. Thrombocytopenic coagulopathy (Kasabach-Merritt phenomenon) is associated with kaposiform hemangioendothelioma and not with common infantile hemangioma. Plast Reconstr Surg 1997;100:1377-1386.

136. Raman S, Ramanujam T, Lim CT. Prenatal diagnosis of an extensive hemangioma of the fetal leg: a case report. J Obstet Gynecol Res 1996;22:375-378.

137. Enjolras O, Mulliken JB, Wassef M, et al. Residual lesions after Kasabach-Merritt phenomenon in 41 patients. J Am Acad Dermatol 2000;42:225-235.

138. Enzinger FM, Weiss SW. Infantile myofibromatosis. In Soft tissue tumors. St Louis: Mosby, 1995: pp 77-83.

139. Mentzel T, Calonje E, Nascimento AG, et al. Infantile hemangiopericytoma versus infantile myofibromatosis. Am J Surg Pathol 1994;18:922-930.

140. Perkins P, Weiss SW. Spindle cell hemangioendothelioma: an analysis of 78 cases with reassessment of its pathogenesis and biologic behavior. Am J Surg Pathol 1996;20:1196-204.

141. SanMartin O, Botella R, Alegre V, et al. Congenital eccrine angiomatous hamartoma. Am J Dermatopathol 1992;14: 161-164.

142. Michel JL, Secchi T, Balme B, et al. Hamartome angioeccrine congénital. Ann Dermatol Venereol 1997;124:623-625.

143. Landthaler M, Braun-Falco O, Exkert F, et al. Congenital multiple plaquelike glomus tumors. Arch Dermatol 1990; 126:1203-1207.

144. Glick SA, Markstein EA, Herreid P. Congenital glomangioma: case report and review of the world literature. Pediatr Dermatol 1995;12:242-244.

19

Hypopigmentation Disorders

SUSAN S. ELLIS
SUSAN BAYLISS MALLORY

A diverse group of diseases present with hypopigmentation in newborns or infants. Some, such as albinism, are genetic disorders due to abnormalities in melanin synthesis, which cause generalized hypopigmentation or depigmentation. Localized forms of hypopigmentation, such as nevus depigmentosus, are less dramatic, but more common. They may be present at birth, but because infants often have lighter skin color at birth than later in life, focal forms of hypopigmentation may be less obvious or even completely absent at birth, becoming manifest later in infancy or childhood. This chapter discusses a variety of clinical conditions causing hypopigmentation, many of which have a genetic or metabolic basis.

GENERALIZED DEPIGMENTATION

Albinism

Albinism refers to a group of genetic disorders involving abnormal melanin synthesis. Clinically, affected individuals have dilution or absence of ocular and cutaneous pigmentation. The skin of patients with albinism can vary from pink to light brown depending on ethnicity and the specific type of albinism. Photophobia, decreased visual acuity, and nystagmus are also constant findings. Typically, the affected individual is less pigmented than unaffected siblings. Albinism is found worldwide in all races with a 1:20,000 population incidence. African-Americans have a slightly higher prevalence rate than European Americans.[1]

Most types of oculocutaneous albinism (OCA) are autosomal recessive with a few reported families exhibiting autosomal dominant inheritance.[2] Affected infants are hypopigmented from birth.

Historically, albinism is divided into two clinical types based on the presence or absence of the tyrosinase enzyme. Tyrosinase is the major regulatory enzyme in the melanin biosynthetic pathway and is the rate limiting enzyme. It is the lack of or reduction of this enzyme that results in the characteristic color of the skin in albinism. In the past OCA has been classified by extracting tyrosine from hair bulb melanocytes and determining the presence or absence of this enzyme.[3] Recently, a more accurate classification has been achieved through molecular analysis by identifying specific genes involved.[4] Ten different variants of OCA have been described (Table 19-1).[1]

On a cellular level, the lack of pigment is caused by a decrease in the synthesis of normal melanin, although the melanocytes themselves are normal in structure and function.

Oculocutaneous Albinism–Type 1

Oculocutaneous albinism I (OCA-I), previously classified as tyrosinase-negative albinism, is one of the most common types of albinism and is caused by the loss of function of the tyrosinase gene. There are two subtypes of OCA-I: type IA and type IB. Type IB includes several disorders: OCA IB (yellow), OCA IB (minimal pigment), and OCA IB (temperature sensitive) (see Table 19-1). All of these subtypes are caused by defective tyrosinase activity.

Distinguishing OCA IA is the characteristic marked hypopigmentation of the skin and eyes at birth with white hair, milky white skin, and pale blue eyes (Figs. 19-1 and 19-2). In bright light, the entire iris can appear pink or red, which is caused by its translucency.[5] As the child matures, the irides may darken or become lightly pigmented with reduced translucency. With time, the skin may or may not

353

TABLE 19-1

Clinical Characteristics of Albinisms

	Type IA, tyrosine negative	Type IB, yellow	Type IB-MP, minimal pigment	Type IB-TS, temperature sensitive	Type II, tyrosine positive	Type II, Brown	Rufous Type III	HPS	CHS	Autosomal dominant
Skin color	White, pink as a baby	Milk-white	Milk-white	Milk-white	Creamy white	Light brown; only in Africans	Reddish brown	Creamy white	Creamy white to slate grey	Creamy white
Pigmented nevi and freckles	Absent	Present	Absent	Absent	Present	Absent	Present	Many in exposed sun areas	Present	Present
Skin neoplasia	++++	++++	++++	++++	++++	None	?	++ to ++++	Unknown	Unknown but expected to be low
Hair color	White throughout life; may become dirty white to light yellow	White at birth; turns yellow-blonde in first few years	White at birth; slight yellow tint with time	White at birth; after puberty: scalp and axillary hair white; arm + leg hair pigmented	White to yellow at birth; darkens with age	Medium brown	Ginger to red to mahogany	White to blonde to brown	Blonde to light brown; metallic silver-grey sheen	Blond to brown
Gene mutations	Tyrosinase gene (complete absence of tyrosinase activity)	Tyrosinase gene (decreased enzyme activity)	Tyrosinase gene is less active at higher temperatures	Tyrosinase gene	P gene (chromosome 15q)	TRP 1	Unknown	HPS	LYST	Unknown
Hair bulb melanosomes	Stages I & II	To stage III, pheomelanosomes	Late stage II, some with melanin	Stages I & II (scalp hair); stages II, III, IV (leg hair)	To stage III, eumelanosomes	Stage I to stage II, some lightly pigmented stage IV	Unknown	To stage III, phemelanosomes and eumelanosomes	Macromelanosomes and normal to stage IV	Stage I to early stage III; no structural abnormality

HPS, Hermansky-Pudlack syndrome; CHS, Chediak-Higashi syndrome.

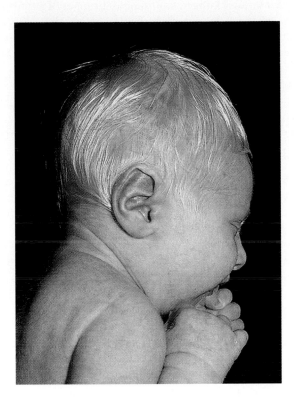

FIG. 19-1
Albinism. Note the snow-white hair at birth.

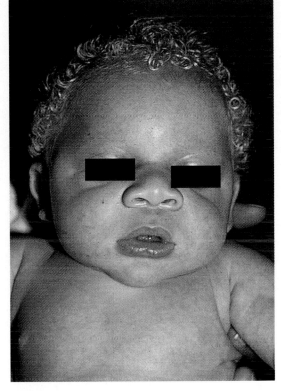

FIG. 19-2
Albinism. African-American infant with diffuse hair and skin hypopigmentation.

gain some pigment. Those who do develop color can also develop nevi, freckles, and lentigines with sun exposure. Severe photophobia results from a lack of fundal pigment. Associated ocular abnormalities include decreased visual acuity, nystagmus, and strabismus.[5]

Originally, the OCA IB phenotype was referred to as Yellow Mutant Albinism and was first described in an Amish family. Tyrosinase activity in their melanocytes is present but markedly reduced. Individuals with OCA IB form pheomelanin, resulting in some pigment production.[6] Affected individuals are described as having a similar appearance to those with OCA IA at birth but with time develop some pigment. Hair color can change from white to light blonde, and even progress to dark blonde or brown in adolescence. Irides can progressively darken to light tan or brown. With sun exposure, individuals with OCA IB may be able to tan, although it is more common to burn without tanning. Nevi and ephelides may develop.[5]

An interesting subtype of OCA IB is the temperature-sensitive phenotype in which the tyrosinase activity is seen mainly on the extremities. In these patients, the enzyme has no activity at 37° C, but some activity at 35° C. Indi-

viduals with this type of albinism are characterized with lightly pigmented hairs on the central body (axillae, pubic area) and darkly pigmented hair peripherally (legs, arms). The pattern is similar to that observed in Siamese cats.[6]

OCA I subtypes are caused by a loss of function of the melanocytic tyrosinase enzyme as a result of mutations in the tyrosinase gene found on chromosome 11. The OCA 1A phenotype is characterized by mutations that result in complete loss of tyrosinase activity, whereas OCA 1B is caused by mutations that result in reduced tyrosinase activity (5% to 10% of the normal level).

Oculocutaneous Albinism–Type II
Oculocutaneous albinism type II (OCA II), or tyrosinase-positive albinism, is characterized by the dilution of hair and iris pigment at birth and is most prevalent in African and African-American populations.[7] Affected individuals are able to make pigment but quantitatively less than normal. Comparison with a first-degree relative may be necessary to distinguish the degree of lightening.[6] Most individuals are born with creamy-colored skin, and white or light blonde hair. Depending on the individual's ethnic back-

ground, hair may also be golden blonde, reddish blonde, or brown. Pigmented birthmarks may also be present. With maturity, the amount of pigment in the skin, eyes, and hair tends to increase. In sun-exposed areas, nevi and freckles can develop. Photophobia and nystagmus are present but are generally not as severe as that seen in OCA IA.[4]

OCA II phenotype has been attributed to mutations of the P gene located on chromosome 15 (15q11.2-q12).[8] In the mouse, mutations of this gene have been shown to result in a decrease in eumelanin production.[9] It has been hypothesized that the P protein has a putative role as a tyrosinase transporter, but direct evidence for this theory is lacking.[10]

OCA II can be found in Prader-Willi syndrome and Angelman syndrome.[7] Prader-Willi involves loss of a gene on the paternally inherited copy of chromosome 15, whereas Angelman syndrome involves loss of the maternal allele.

Other Types of Albinism

Hermansky-Pudlak syndrome (HPS) is a type of OCA characterized by tyrosine-positive albinism, a bleeding disorder, and a lysosomal ceroid storage disease affecting the lungs and gut. The majority of individuals affected are of Puerto-Rican or Dutch descent. The bleeding diathesis is caused by the storage pool deficiency of platelets and results in epistaxis, gingival bleeding, or bleeding after surgical procedures such as tooth extractions. The ceroid material accumulation can result in pulmonary fibrosis, granulomatous colitis, cardiomyopathy, and renal failure. The defect has been mapped to chromosome 10q23.[11]

Diagnosis and Management. The diagnosis of albinism is usually made clinically. The hair bulb incubator test for tyrosinase activity has been used to differentiate between tyrosinase-positive and tyrosinase-negative albinism. In tyrosinase-negative albinism, there is the lack of pigment formation in hair bulbs when incubated with tyrosine, whereas in tyrosine-positive albinism, pigment is produced. Albinism can be determined prenatally using fetal cells obtained by fetal skin biopsy. Electron micrographic evaluation of fetal skin after 20 weeks gestation[12] shows melanin-containing melanosomes in OCA II, whereas OCA I has melanin-free melanosomes. Structurally, melanocytes are normal.[13] The melanosomes found in OCA II are in an arrested stage of development and fail to mature to stage IV melanosomes.

The importance of photoprotection should be stressed to reduce the risk of cutaneous malignancies, and daily sunscreen and protective clothing should be used. Ophthalmologic evaluation is also important. Because cutaneous squamous cell carcinomas have been known to develop in all types of OCA, yearly examination by a dermatologist is recommended.[6]

Cross-McKusick-Breen Syndrome

Cross-McKusick-Breen syndrome is a variant of albinism characterized by cutaneous hypopigmentation, silver-blonde hair, post-natal growth retardation, ocular, and neurological findings. The neurological findings may be manifest as mental retardation, spasticity, or athetoid movements.[14-16]

GENERALIZED PIGMENT DILUTION

Chediak-Higashi Syndrome

Chediak-Higashi syndrome (CHS) is an autosomal recessive disorder characterized by incomplete oculocutaneous albinism and recurrent bacterial infections. When compared with unaffected family members, the skin and the hair are both lighter in coloration. The hair often has a silvery tint (Fig. 19-3). Loss of iris pigmentation results in photophobia with an increased red reflex. Visual acuity is normal but strabismus and nystagmus are common.[17] The CHS gene is located on chromosome 1q.[18]

Multiple infections occur in early childhood but are not usually noted in the neonatal period. A previously affected sibling may warrant a high index of suspicion. Infectious episodes manifest as fever and most typically involve the

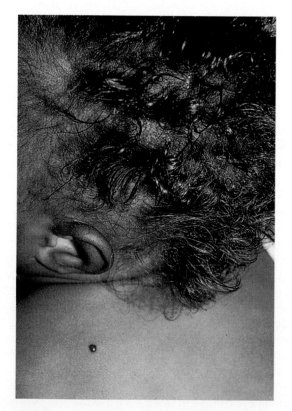

FIG. 19-3
Chediak-Higashi syndrome. The hair displays a silvery sheen.

skin, lungs, and upper respiratory tract. Common culprits include *Staphylococcus aureus, Streptococcus pyogenes,* and *Streptococcus pneumoniae.* Cutaneous involvement usually manifests as a pyoderma and there are a few reports of deeper involvement resembling pyoderma gangrenosum.[19]

Progressive neurologic deterioration with clumsiness, abnormal gait, paresthesias, and dysesthesias is often apparent later in childhood. Other neurologic abnormalities include peripheral and cranial neuropathies, spinocerebellar degeneration, ataxia, seizures, decreased deep tendon reflexes, cranial nerve palsies, and motor weakness.[20-25]

Natural killer cell function is drastically decreased. Diminished chemotaxis of granulocytes, monocytes, and lymphocytes has also been reported, as well as decreased antibody-dependent cytotoxicity and reduced suppressor T-cell function.[26-28] The resulting susceptibility to infections is caused by the combination of these factors.[29]

The diagnostic hallmark of CHS is the finding of giant lysosomal granules within leukocytes and other cells. In bone marrow myeloid cells, the giant granules appear prominent. In melanocytes, melanosomes fail to disperse melanin to adjacent keratinocytes, accounting for the decrease in pigmentation seen in the skin and hair.[30] On a cellular level, abnormal intracellular transport to and from the lysosomes has been detected.[31] Giant granules within the phagocytic cells cannot discharge their lysosomal and perioxidative enzymes into phagocytic vacuoles.[17,32] Prenatal diagnosis has been successfully performed using light microscopy by examining fetal hair shafts for characteristic clumping of melanosomes.[33]

Patients with CHS have an increased incidence of pyogenic infections and eventually develop an accelerated phase characterized by fever, hepatosplenomegaly, lymphadenopathy, pancytopenia, and bleeding.[21] Viral infections, particularly with the Epstein-Barr virus, have been implicated in causing the accelerated phase.[34,35]

Bone marrow transplantation (BMT) is the only definitive treatment for this disorder.[36] The natural killer cell defects and immunodeficiencies can be reversed, but the pigmentary dilution is not altered.[37] Without BMT, CHS is usually fatal during childhood,[21] although a few patients have survived for more than 20 years.[25,38,39] No patients with the accelerated phase have survived without BMT.[36,40]

Supportive treatments in early infancy include antibiotics for infections, and intravenous gamma globulin. Ascorbic acid has been shown to partially correct the granulocytic function in some patients.[26,27]

Phenylketonuria

Phenylketonuria (PKU) is an autosomal recessive disorder that results from the impaired conversion of phenylala-

nine to tyrosine, which is caused by the absence of hepatic phenylalanine hydroxylase (PAH) activity. The absence of this enzyme leads to a build-up of the amino acid phenylalanine and its by-products in the blood stream and spinal fluid.

If untreated, PKU results in mental retardation and oculocutaneous pigment diminution. Most affected individuals have blonde hair, blue eyes, fair skin, photosensitivity, a mousy body odor, and neurologic disturbances (seizures, psychosis, hyperreflexia).[41] The incidence in the United States is estimated at 1 in 10,000 among Caucasians.[42] It is most commonly observed in individuals of Scandinavian and northern European descent with males and females equally affected.

At birth, the infant appears normal but may have a musty odor secondary to urinary and sweat phenylacetic acid or phenylacetaldehyde. Caucasian children with PKU almost invariably have blonde hair, blue eyes, and fair skin. African-American and Asian children tend to be lighter in color than their parents and unaffected siblings. Hypotheses to account for the lighter skin color include a competitive inhibition of the binding of tyrosine to tyrosinase by excess phenylalanine or a decreased amount of tyrosine.[43]

In affected babies, serum phenylalanine levels begin to rise on the third or fourth day of life. Newborn screening with the Guthrie inhibition assay test was implemented in the United States beginning in 1963, testing all newborns for PKU. Prenatal diagnosis is also possible by performing amniocentesis or chorionic villus sampling with identification of the gene.[41]

With a low phenylalanine diet, the skin color, photosensitivity, odor, and eczema are reversible. Implementing a diet low in phenylalanine early in infancy can also dramatically reduce the mental retardation.[41] Although children with treated PKU typically have a lower IQ than the mean population, if the blood phenylalanine levels are maintained at reasonable levels in early childhood, affected individuals can be expected to have a normal to low-normal intelligence.[44]

Griscelli Syndrome

Griscelli syndrome was first described by both Griscelli[45] and Siccardi[46] in 1978. The syndrome is a rare autosomal recessive disorder and is characterized by pigmentary dilution, hepatosplenomegaly, lymphohistiocytosis, and a combined T- and B-cell immunodeficiency. Frequent pyogenic infections, acute febrile episodes, neutropenia, and thrombocytopenia usually begin between 4 months of age and 4 years. Fewer than 40 cases have been reported.[45-51]

In early childhood, the hair, eyebrows and eyelashes are silvery gray,[52] findings that may also be present in the neonatal period.[53] Cutaneous diminution of pigmentation has also been noted.[49,51]

Extracutaneous manifestations include pyogenic infections, episodic fevers, neutropenia, thrombocytopenia, and hepatosplenomegaly.[45,46] Neurologic findings include intracranial hypertension,[54] cerebellar signs, encephalopathy, hemiparesis, peripheral facial palsy, spasticity,[51] hypotonia,[49] seizures,[49,51] psychomotor retardation,[49,50,55] or progressive neurologic deterioration.[49-51,54]

Histologically, the hair shafts reveal uneven clumps of melanin, mainly in the medulla. Skin biopsy specimens reveal hyperpigmented oval melanocytes and poorly pigmented adjacent keratinocytes. On electron microscopic examination, epidermal melanocytes are found to contain perinuclear stage IV melanosomes. Adjacent keratinocytes contain only sparse melanosomes.[54]

Prenatal diagnosis of Griscelli syndrome has been accomplished by examination of hair from fetal scalp biopsies performed at 21 weeks' gestation, with confirmatory post-abortion examination of the fetus revealing silvery hair and identical microscopic findings.[33]

Differentiation from Chediak-Higashi syndrome can be made by pathognomonic light and electron microscopic features. Griscelli syndrome lacks the large cytoplasmic inclusions and granulocyte abnormalities that are characteristic of Chediak-Higashi syndrome. Both diseases, however, carry a poor prognosis without bone marrow transplantation.

Patients with Griscelli syndrome experience an accelerated phase similar to that of Chediak-Higashi syndrome.[54] Bone marrow transplant is most successful when done early in the course of disease.[54,56]

Recent studies link Griscelli syndrome to mutations of the gene encoding myosin V. These mutations result in a dilute or silvery hair color and neurological defects both in mice and humans with Griscelli syndrome.[57]

Elejalde Syndrome

Elejalde syndrome is an autosomal recessive disorder characterized by silvery hair, severe central nervous system (CNS) dysfunction, and abnormal intracytoplasmic inclusions in fibroblasts, histiocytes and lymphocytes.[58] Extracutaneous features include hypotonic facies, plagiocephaly, micrognathia, crowded teeth, narrow high palate, pectus excavatum, and cryptorchidism. Neurological abnormalities range from severe hypotonia, and the almost complete absence of movements to seizures and spasticity.[59,60]

Elejalde syndrome is thought to be the result of a distorted gene product responsible for early melanin formation. The resultant abnormal melanosomes are reflected by the silvery hair and defective CNS function.[59,60]

MOSAIC CONDITIONS

Mosaicism refers to the presence of two or more genetically distinct cell lines within an individual. These cell lines may be due to X-inactivation, as is normal in all human females, or from postzygotic somatic mutation. When mosaicism affects the skin, the affected skin may show patchy hypopigmentation or hyperpigmentation in a linear or segmental distribution (Figs. 19-4 and 19-5). (Pigmentary mosaicism associated with hyperpigmented disorders is discussed in Chapter 20, and other mosaic conditions in Chapter 24.) Segmental hypopigmented lesions may be seen as an isolated cutaneous skin condition or as part of a significant genetic disease. The presence of mosaicism can sometimes be documented by the karyotyping of lymphocytes from peripheral blood or by culturing fibroblasts from both involved and uninvolved skin, but in many cases chromosomal studies are normal, presumably because the defective gene is too small to detect with currently available techniques.

In 1901 Alfred Blaschko characterized the distribution of segmental and linear skin abnormalities by examining patients with linear lesions and formulating a patterned composite diagram. He described these patterns as V-shaped or fountainlike over the spine, S-shaped or whorled on the anterior and lateral aspects of the trunk, and linear over the extremities (see Chapter 3, p. 42.) These lines should not be confused with dermatomes, which are the segments of skin corresponding to sensory nerves.[61] Hypopigmentation that follows the lines of Blaschko and segmental patterns is thought to reflect cellular migration during embryogenesis, affecting pigmentation.[62] "Hypomelanosis of Ito," previously thought to be a distinct disease, appears to be a common cutaneous phenotype associated with mosaicism and several different chromosomal abnormalities, with systemic associations. This phenotype can be seen without associated extracutanous findings. In these cases, the skin findings are usually referred to as "nevoid hypopigmentation" or "nevus depigmentosus."[63]

Hypomelanosis of Ito

In 1952 a Japanese dermatologist named Minor Ito described a 21-year-old female with hypopigmented cutaneous whorls and streaks. Because the distribution of the hypopigmentation was analogous to that of the hyperpigmented streaks observed in incontinentia pigmenti, he called the disorder **incontinentia pigmenti achromians.** To avoid confusion of these two unrelated entities, the preferred terminology later became "hypomelanosis of Ito" (HI).[64] Hypomelanosis of Ito is a term used for a phenotype with linear streaks lighter than the patient's back-

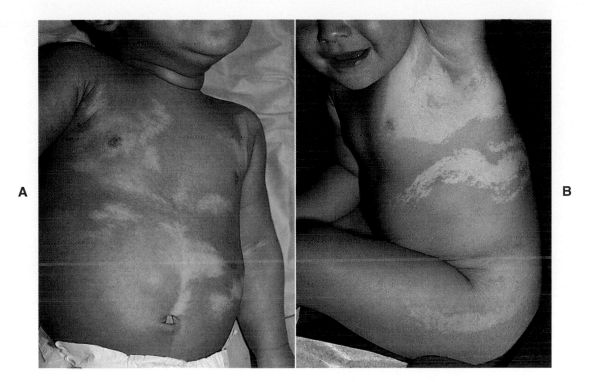

FIG. 19-4
Hypomelanosis of Ito. **A,** Segmental, streaky hypopigmentation. **B,** Hypopigmented macular lesions following Blaschko's lines are clearly seen.

ground skin color, extending around the trunk and down the long axes of the extremities in association with systemic findings.[65] The hypopigmented streaks follow the lines of Blaschko and are present at birth or become apparent during the first 2 years (see Fig. 19-4).[66] These markings tend to be stable, although there are cases reported in which the pigmentary changes become more or less pronounced over time.[67] In some cases, both hypopigmented and hyperpigmented streaks are evident. Wood's lamp examination may be useful to determine the extent of the lesions in lightly pigmented patients.

Hypopigmentation of the type seen with hypomelanosis of Ito may be seen without systemic associations, and many advocate that the name be used as a descriptive label, rather than a specific diagnosis.[68] Others will restrict the use of the diagnostic label to patients with systemic associations, advocating criteria for diagnosis (see Fig. 19-5).[69] Multiple chromosomal abnormalities have been associated with HI, and most cases are sporadic and have negligible recurrence risk.[64,70,71]

Extracutaneous findings are variable, and include the central nervous and musculoskeletal systems and/or ocular abnormalities. Defects of teeth, hair, nails, and sweat glands,[67] as well as aplasia cutis, fibromas,[70] and generalized or focal hypertrichosis, have been reported.[72] Additional abnormalities reported include limb-length discrepancies, facial hemiatrophy, scoliosis, sternal abnormalities, dysmorphic facies, and genitourinary and cardiac anomalies. Nearly all of the defects are detectable by a thorough physical examination and regular follow-up.

On histologic examination, the hypopigmented areas have either normal or reduced numbers of melanocytes, and those melanocytes that are present demonstrate a reduction in the number of melanosomes.[73] Infants should be observed for evidence of CNS involvement, reflected by developmental delay or seizures.[67] Most children with CNS involvement manifest with neurological abnormalities before 2 years of age. Differential diagnosis includes nevus depigmentosus (also known as nevus achromicus) and Goltz syndrome. Patients with Goltz syndrome have both increased and decreased pigmentation, as well as depressed areas of depigmentation following Blaschko's lines.

Cosmetic cover-up products such as Dermablend (Flori Roberts, Chicago, IL) or Covermark (Covermark Cosmet-

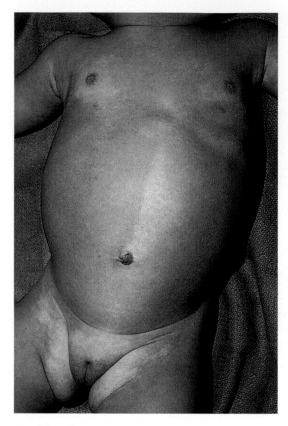

FIG. 19-5
Segmental hypopigmentation. This child was otherwise well.

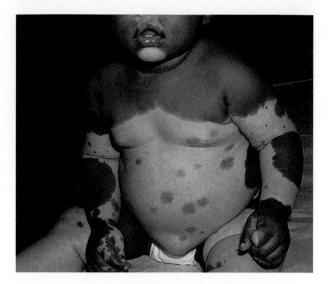

FIG. 19-6
Piebaldism.

ics, Rasbouck Heights, NJ) can be used to conceal the hypopigmented areas but is usually not needed. The use of sunscreens can prevent or lessen the accentuation of pigmentary differences.[67]

LOCALIZED AND SEGMENTAL HYPOPIGMENTED DISORDERS

Piebaldism

Piebaldism is an autosomal dominant disorder caused by defective cell proliferation and migration of melanocytes during embryogenesis. It is characterized by symmetric, well-demarcated patches of white skin and hair involving the frontal scalp, trunk, upper arms, and legs with normally pigmented skin on the hands and feet (Fig. 19-6). Normally pigmented patches or hyperpigmented spots can occur within the depigmented patches and are occasionally mistaken for café au lait macules.[63] Unlike vitiligo, patches of leukoderma in piebaldism are not pro-

gressive and are present at birth. Hyperpigmented areas can fluctuate in size. There are no extracutaneous findings in classic piebaldism.

Piebaldism is caused by different mutations in the c-KIT gene, which is necessary for melanocyte proliferation.[74] The c-KIT gene product is a member of the tyrosine kinase family of transmembrane receptors. Mutations in the c-KIT receptor results in decreased c-KIT-dependent signal transduction, abnormal distribution of melanoblasts during embryologic development, reduced proliferation of embryonic melanoblasts and in a decreased population of embryonic melanocytes in the dermis. c-KIT point mutations can be divided into four classes, each corresponding to a phenotype of differing severity.[75]

The clinical diagnosis of piebaldism can be confirmed by genetic analysis with the identification of the c-KIT mutation on chromosome 4q12. Disorders with similar clinical presentations are Waardenburg syndrome, nevus depigmentosus, and vitiligo. The latter can be differentiated from the others by progression of lesions and lack of presentation at birth.[76] Waardenburg syndrome is associated with depigmented patches in the skin and hair, deafness, heterochromic irides, and dystopia canthorum in classic cases. Piebaldism can be differentiated from other hypomelanotic lesions by determining the absence of melanocytic c-KIT protein with low to no expression of melanosomal markers. Nevus depigmentosus will show normal c-KIT and low melanosome expression.[76]

Melanocytes are absent from the depigmented areas of piebaldism but melanin and melanocytes are often in-

Types of Waardenburg Syndrome

Type I
Dystopia canthorum
White forelock (poliosis)
Synophrys (thickening of medial eyebrows)
Broad nasal root
Heterochromia irides
Hypoplasia of nasal alae
PAX 3 gene mutations (chromosome 2q35)

Type II
Sensorineural hearing loss
Heterochromia irides
Absence of dystopia canthorum
MITF mutations (chromosome 13q)

Type III (Waardenburg-Klein syndrome)
Features of type I
Musculoskeletal defects (limb abnormalities)
PAX3 gene mutations

Type IV (Waardenburg-Shah syndrome)
Extensive depigmentation
Hirschsprung disease
Endothelin receptor B gene mutations

creased at the margins and within the hyperpigmented or normally pigmented patches located within the areas of depigmentation. These melanocytes at these margins are atypical in morphology.[75]

Lesions of piebaldism generally grow proportionally with the individual and are usually stable. Photoprotection of the depigmented patches is important, beginning early in life to avoid skin cancers later in life.

Waardenburg Syndrome

Waardenburg syndrome is a disorder characterized by depigmented patches of the skin and hair and other associated findings.[77] Four types of Waardenburg syndrome have been described on clinical and genetic grounds (Box 19-1).[78,79] All types are inherited in an autosomal dominant fashion.

In *Type I Waardenburg syndrome* (WS1) dystopia canthorum, broad nasal root, medial hypertrichosis (synophrys), hypoplasia of the nasal alae, and deafness are present. The hearing loss is sensorineural, congenital, and in most cases, nonprogressive. The degree of deafness can

vary from mild to profound, and may be unilateral or bilateral. WS1 may also be associated with cleft lip and palate[80] and spina bifida.[81,82] It is considered to be the classic form and results from a mutation in the PAX 3 gene. The PAX3 gene product is a transcription factor critical for activating melanoblasts to proliferate or to begin migration from the neural crest.[75]

Waardenburg syndrome type II (WS2) lacks dystopia canthorum and is caused by the MITF gene. *Waardenburg syndrome type III* (WS3; Klein-Waardenburg syndrome) has features of type I and is associated with limb abnormalities[83] and is also caused by mutations in the PAX 3 gene. *Type IV Waardenburg syndrome* (WS4; Waardenburg-Shah syndrome) is a more severe phenotype that is associated with Hirschsprung disease (aganglionic megacolon)[84] and results from mutations in the endothelin B gene.

Through molecular genetic analysis, WS1 and WS3 have been shown to be allelic variants, whereas WS2 and WS4 are distinct entities.[75] Physical findings in neonates suggestive of Waardenburg syndrome warrant a hearing evaluation.

Nevus Depigmentosus

Nevus depigmentosus (nevus achromicus) is characterized by a well-circumscribed solitary hypopigmented patch, which may follow the lines of Blaschko, occur as a small isolated patch, or develop in a unilateral segmental distribution (Fig. 19-7).[85,86] The term *depigmentosus* is a misnomer because the lesions are actually hypopigmented. These lesions are usually present at birth or become evident shortly thereafter and remain stable over time.[85] Usual locations are on the trunk and proximal extremities. Males and females are affected equally.

Clinical examination is usually sufficient for establishing the diagnosis. In a lightly pigmented baby, Wood's lamp examination may make the lesion more evident. Rare associated findings include hemihypertrophy,[87] seizures and mental retardation.[88] Eleven percent of patients with a nevus depigmentosus can have systemic findings; this may reflect overlap with hypomelanosis of Ito.[63] On electron microscopic examination, a defect in transfer of pigment between the melanocyte and keratinocyte can be seen, resulting in a decreased number of melanosomes within the keratinocytes.[86]

Other entities with which nevus depigmentosus is sometimes confused include nevus anemicus, segmental vitiligo, hypopigmented lesions of tuberous sclerosis, and hypomelanosis of Ito. Stroking the lesion can differentiate nevus depigmentosus from nevus anemicus, since a normal erythematous flare will occur with nevus depigmentosus, but in nevus anemicus the surrounding skin will flare, and the actual lesion will remain unchanged.

Most patients do not require treatment. Camouflage makeup is useful if there is cosmetic concern. PUVA has been tried but has not shown to be beneficial.[87] Autologous grafting with noncultured melanocytes has been successful in two cases.[89]

Tuberous Sclerosis Complex

Tuberous sclerosis complex (TSC) (see also Chapter 24) is a term encompassing two autosomal dominant disorders with variable penetrance, characterized by cutaneous and neurologic abnormalities, as well as visceral hamartomas.[90] Estimates of prevalence range from 1:6,000[91] to 1:10,000, though some have quoted as low as 1:150,000.[92,93] Males and females are affected equally, and there is no racial predilection. Spontaneous mutations account for 50% to 75% of cases.[91,94,95] Criteria for diagnosis can be found in Box 19-2.

Cutaneous manifestations of TSC include hypopigmented macules, facial angiofibromas, forehead plaques, shagreen patch, ungual fibromas, and poliosis. Multiple hypopigmented macules are of concern for TSC, although three or less may be a variant of normal.[90] These macules can be one of the earliest indicators of the disease[96] and occur in 50% to 100% of patients with tuberous sclerosis.[97-102] The hypopigmented macules can be oval, lance-shaped, ash leaf–shaped, or confetti (Figs. 19-7, 19-8, and 19-9). The margins may be regular or irregular, and size ranges from one to several centimeters.[97,100] The macules are usually present at birth[97,100] but may appear later in childhood. Poliosis (white patches of the hair) can also be seen.[101]

It is rare for newborns to have other cutaneous signs of tuberous sclerosis. Shagreen patches (lumbosacral or forehead) may be present in infancy, but more commonly along with adenoma sebaceum around age 2 to 5 years. Periungual fibromas occur in adulthood.[101,102]

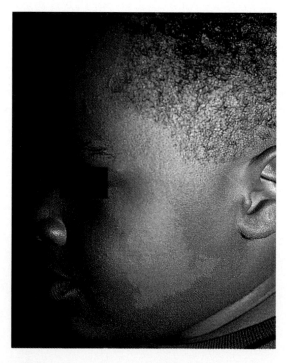

FIG. 19-7
Nevus depigmentosus. Sharply defined hypopigmented macular patch on the cheek that was present at birth.

BOX 19-2

Tuberous Sclerosis Complex Criteria

Major Features
Facial angiofibromas or forehead plaque
Nontraumatic ungual or periungual fibroma
Hypomelanotic macules (more than three)
Shagreen patch (connective tissue nevus)
Multiple retinal nodular hamartomas
Cortical tuber
Subependymal nodule
Subependymal giant cell astrocytoma
Cardiac rhabdomyoma, single or multiple
Lymphangiomyomatosis
Renal angiomyolipoma

Minor Features
Multiple randomly distributed pits in dental enamel
Hamartomatous rectal polyps
Bone cysts
Cerebral white matter radial migration lines
Gingival fibromas
Non-renal hamartoma
Retinal achromic patch
"Confetti" skin lesions
Multiple renal cysts
Definite TSC: either 2 major features or 1 major feature plus 2 minor features
Probable TSC: one major plus 1 minor feature
Possible TSC: either 1 major feature or 2 or more minor features

(From Roach ES, Gomez MR, Northrup H. J Child Neurol 1998;13:624-628.)

Electron microscopy of the hypopigmented macules reveals smaller organelles (Golgi apparatus, endoplasmic reticulum, free ribosomes, and mitochondria), as well as a reduction in the size and number of the melanosomes. The melanosomes exist mainly in the unmelanized stages.[86]

In children with light skin, hypopigmented macules may be better visualized with the aid of a Wood's lamp. Examination of the parents and other family members may be indicated, because this autosomal dominant disease can have marked variability.[103]

Lesions that should be distinguished from the cutaneous hypopigmented macules of TSC include nevus anemicus, pityriasis alba, postinflammatory hypopigmentation, tinea versicolor, vitiligo, and nevus depigmentosus.[90]

Nevus Anemicus

Nevus anemicus is a congenital vascular abnormality observed more frequently in females than in males. Unlike vascular malformations such as a port wine stain or nevus flammeus, which cause red or pink discolorations of the skin, nevus anemicus reflects an increased vascular reactivity to catecholamines resulting clinically in a circumscribed pale macule (Fig. 19-10).[104] Most instances of nevus anemicus are unilateral, located on the trunk, and asymptomatic.[105] Wood's lamp examination does not accentuate the lesion. Rubbing the lesion or temperature change causes erythema in the surrounding area but not

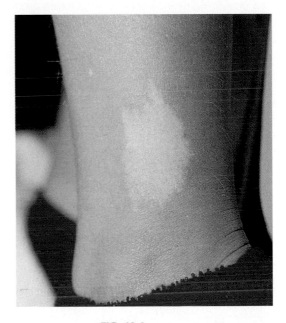

FIG. 19-9
Tuberous sclerosis.

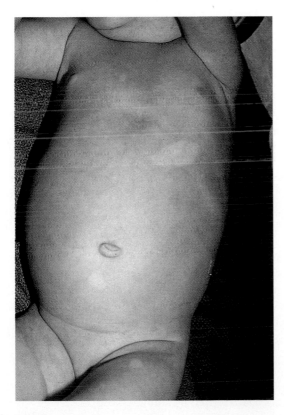

FIG. 19-8
Tuberous sclerosis. Hypopigmented macules in an infant with cardiac rhabdomyoma.

FIG. 19-10
Nevus anemicus.

within the lesion itself.[104] These physical maneuvers help to distinguish nevus anemicus from similar appearing entities such as vitiligo, nevus depigmentosus, tuberous sclerosis macules, and leprosy.

Histologic examination reveals normal vessels and normal skin.[106] With diascopic pressure, nevus anemicus becomes indistinguishable from the surrounding blanched skin.[104]

Treatment is cosmetic, and if so desired, the discoloration can be concealed with camouflage makeup. Patches remain stable in size and configuration throughout life.[107]

Postinflammatory Hypopigmentation

Postinflammatory hypopigmentation refers to the partial loss of cutaneous melanin in previously inflamed areas of skin. The clinical presentation appears as hypochromic macules or patches in the distribution of the inflammatory process and is more apparent in dark skin (Fig. 19-11). Because the hypopigmentation takes several weeks to develop, it is not usually seen in the neonate.

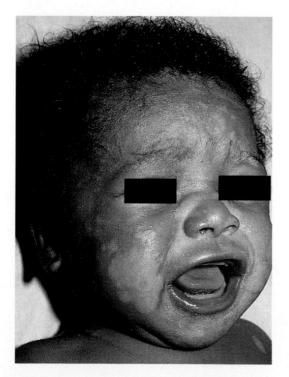

FIG. 19-11
Postinflammatory hypopigmentation secondary to seborrhea. Once the inflammation is gone, the hypopigmentation improves.

Pityriasis alba is a form of postinflammatory hypopigmentation commonly observed in children and adolescents but occasionally seen in the neonatal period. Most lesions occur on the sides of the face and present as ill-defined, hypopigmented, minimally scaly patches.[52]

Trauma and inflammation are thought to cause melanocyte dysfunction or complete loss, depending on the degree of insult. Infectious, allergic, immunologic, and papulosquamous conditions can result in postinflammatory hypopigmentation.

Wood's lamp examination will enhance the hypopigmented areas in light skin and helps to distinguish the presence of depigmentation versus hypopigmentation. Histology may help to establish the cause of hypopigmentation. In some cases, DOPA-stained sections or electron microscopic examination may be useful in evaluation of the process.[108] Treatment of the underlying cause of inflammation will improve the discoloration of the skin.

MISCELLAENOUS HYPOPIGMENTATION

Congenital Giant Halo Nevi

A halo nevus is a nevus, either junctional, compound, or intradermal, surrounded by a ring of depigmentation. Depigmented zones around nevi have also been reported with congenital nevi, Spitz nevi, blue nevi, and primary or metastatic melanomas.[109-111] In time, the nevus may eventually involute.

One hypothesis explains the appearance of a halo as an immune response to nevus antigens involving both specific antibodies and T cells. A cytotoxic cell-mediated immune response is thought to be responsible for causing the regression of nevi.[112] This theory of an immunologic mechanism is supported by the fact that a mononuclear cell infiltrate is seen surrounding the nevus cells. Furthermore, IgM and IgG antibodies directed against nevocellular antigens have been detected in the serum of some individuals. Unlike acquired halo nevi, congenital halo nevi may have an absence of inflammation and may not involute.[110,113]

Menkes Kinky Hair Syndrome

Menkes kinky hair syndrome is an X-linked recessive disorder characterized by abnormal copper storage. Lightly pigmented twisted hairs (pili torti) and a general decrease in skin pigmentation can be seen.

At birth, scalp hair may be sparse and lightly colored but otherwise normal. In the first months of life, the hair typically becomes fine, dull, lusterless, twisted, and more hypopigmented. The skin of affected infants is pale, and the cheeks are pudgy. The face lacks expression. Nail dystrophy and seborrheic dermatitis are also common.

The pathogenesis of Menkes kinky hair syndrome is an abnormal copper distribution within cells. The primary defect is thought to be a dysfunction of metallothienein, a copper binding protein important in cytoplasmic copper transport.[114,115] Copper accumulation in fibroblasts and macrophages, copper transport abnormalities, diminished intestinal absorption of copper, and cellular metabolism defects all result in a severe systemic copper deficiency responsible for the pathologic features.[116]

The twisted hairs result from a surplus of free sulfhydryl groups and a decrease in copper-dependent disulfide bonds. Depigmentation and hypopigmentation of hair and skin are caused by decreased tyrosinase, which is a copper-containing enzyme.[116]

The physiologic and phenotypic abnormalities of this syndrome can be traced to the defective functioning of several copper-dependent enzymes. Tyrosinase, lysyl oxidase, lactase, ascorbic acid oxidase, cytochrome oxidase, uricase, monoamine oxidase, and dopamine P-hydroxylase are all affected by the impaired copper metabolism.[117] The defective gene has been localized to chromosome Xp13.3 and is responsible for the absence of a copper transporting ATPase enzyme.[118] Constant findings in Menkes kinky hair syndrome are low ceruloplasmin and serum copper levels.

Histopathologically, hairs show features of pili torti, trichorrhexis nodosa, trichoclasis, and trichoptilosis. By hair analysis, low copper levels with an increase in free sulfhydryl content are observed.

Affected children may be mistaken for victims of child abuse because of bony changes such as the formation of spurs and fractures, subdural hematomas, and psychomotor retardation. Hair shaft abnormalities seen in this syndrome can also be observed in argininosuccinic aciduria, Bjornstad syndrome, and trichothiodystrophy. However, low copper and ceruloplasmin levels combined with bony abnormalities and clinical features are only found in Menkes kinky hair syndrome.[116]

No effective treatment has been found for this disease. Oral and parenteral copper and ceruloplasmin therapy have had varying results.[119] Copper histidine therapy[120] and oral D-penicillamine[121] have proven to be useful in some cases.

Severely affected individuals usually die before the age of 5 years. Mildly affected patients survive to adolescence.[122]

Ziprkowski-Margolis Syndrome

Ziprkowski-Margolis syndrome is characterized by cutaneous and hair hypomelanosis, localized hypermelanotic patches, heterochromia irides, congenital nerve deafness, and mutism. The syndrome was first described by Ziprkowski et al[123,124] and Margolis,[125] and was observed in an Israeli Jewish family of Sephardic origin.

At birth, the skin is white. With time, hypermelanotic macules begin to appear on the trunk and extremities, and more rarely, the scalp. The widespread and symmetric distribution of the macules gives the affected individual a leopard-like appearance. Scalp hair, eyelashes, eyebrows, and body hair are depigmented.

This disorder is seen in males and is on chromosome Xq26.3-q27.[126] Female carriers of the disease can demonstrate sensorineural hearing impairment.[127]

Skin biopsy of an affected child revealed weakly DOPA positive melanocytes in hypopigmented skin and strong DOPA positivity in the hyperpigmented macules. There was no increase or decrease in the number of melanocytes or abnormal distribution in either the hypopigmented or hyperpigmented skin.[124]

Alezzandrini Syndrome

In 1959 Casalo and Alezzandrini described a patient with the oculocutaneous findings of vitiligo, poliosis, and unilateral pigmentary retinitis with hypoacusis.[128] The findings of unilateral tapetoretinal degeneration with the ipsilateral appearance of facial vitiligo and poliosis, sometimes with accompanying perceptual deafness, have been known as Alezzandrini syndrome.[129,130]

Symptoms of visual loss begin in one eye between ages 12 to 30 years and are usually gradual in onset. Vitiligo and poliosis of the head ipsilateral to the retinal lesions tend to occur 3 to 13 years after visual decline.[129] This syndrome has not been reported in neonates.

REFERENCES

1. Sethi R, Schwartz RA, Janniger CK. Oculocutaneous albinism. Cutis 1996;57:397-400.
2. Frenk E, Calame A. [Familial oculo-cutaneous hypopigmentation of dominant transmission due to a disorder in melanocyte formation. Association of Prader-Willi syndrome with a chromosome abnormality in one of the subjects involved]. Schweiz Med Wochenschr 1977;107:1964-1968.

3. King RA, Olds DP. Hairbulb tyrosinase activity in oculocutaneous albinism: Suggestions for pathway control and block location. Am J Hum Genet 1985;20:49-55.

4. King RA. Albinism. In Nordlund JJ, Boissy RE, Hearing VJ, et al, eds. The pigmentary system. New York: Oxford University Press, 1998: pp 553-575.

5. King RA, Summers CG. Albinism. Dermatol Clin 1988;6: 217-227.

6. Bolognia JL. Disorders of hypopigmentation: Update on pathogenesis. Yale University/Glaxo Dermatology Lectureship Series in Dermatology, Glaxo: 1997.

7. Orlow SJ. Albinism: An update. Semin Cutan Med Surg 1997;16:24-29.

8. Ramsay M, Colman MA, Stevens G, et al. The tyrosine-positive oculocutaneous albinism locus maps to chromosome 15q11.2-q12. Am J Hum Genet 1992;51:879-884.

9. Tomita Y. The molecular genetics of albinism and piebaldism. Arch Dermatol 1994;130:355-358.

10. Gahl WA, Potterf B, Durham-Pierre D, et al. Melanosomal tyrosine transport in normal and pink-eyed dilution murine melanocytes. Pigment Cell Res 1995;8:229-233.

11. Fukai K, Oh J, Frenk E, et al. Linkage disequilibrium mapping of the gene for Hermansky-Pudlak syndrome to chromosome 10q23.1-q23.3. Hum Mol Genet 1995;4:1665-1669.

12. Eady RJ, Gunner DB, Garner A, et al. Prenatal diagnosis of oculocutaneous albinism by electron microscopy of fetal skin. J Invest Dermatol 1983;80:210-212.

13. Kugelman TP, Van Scott EJ. Tyrosinase activity in melanocytes of human albinos. J Invest Dermatol 1961;37: 73-76.

14. Courtens W, Broeckx W, Ledoux M, et al. Oculocerebral hypopigmentation syndrome (Cross syndrome) in a gypsy child. Acta Paediatr Scand 1989;78:806-810.

15. Cross HE, McKusick VA, Breen W. A new oculocerebral syndrome with hypopigmentation. J Pediatr 1967;70:398-406.

16. Fryns JP, Dereymaeker AM, Heremans G, et al. Oculocerebral syndrome with hypopigmentation (Cross syndrome): Report of two siblings born to consanguineous parents. Clin Genet 1988;34:81-84.

17. Dahl MV. Immunology. In Schachner LA, Hansen RC, eds. Pediatric dermatology. 2nd edition. New York: Churchill Livingstone, 1995: pp 71-119.

18. Barbosa MS, Nguyen QA, Tchernev VT, et al. Identification of the homologous beige and Chédiak-Higashi syndromes. Nature 1996;382:262-265.

19. Dahl MV. Immunology. In Schachner LA, Hansen RC, eds. Pediatric dermatology. 2nd edition. New York: Churchill Livingstone, 1995: pp 71-119.

20. Misra VP, King RM, Harding AE, et al. Peripheral neuropathy in the Chédiak-Higashi syndrome. Acta Neuropathol 1991; 81:354-358.

21. Blume RS, Wolff SM. The Chédiak-Higashi syndrome: Studies in four patients and review of the literature. Medicine 1972;51:247-280.

22. Sheramata W, Kott SH, Cyr DP. The Chédiak-Higashi-Steinbrinck Syndrome. Arch Neurol 1971;25:289-294.

23. Weary PE, Bender AS. Chédiak-Higashi syndrome with severe cutaneous involvement: Occurrence in two brothers 14 and 15 years of age. Arch Intern Med 1967;119:381-386.

24. Barak Y, Nir E. Chédiak-Higashi syndrome. Am J Pediatr Hematol Oncol 1987;9:42-55.

25. Pettit RE, Berdal KG. Chédiak-Higashi syndrome. Neurologic appearance. Arch Neurol 1984;41:1001-1002.

26. Boxer LA, Watanabe AM, Rister M, et al. Correction of leukocyte function in Chédiak-Higashi syndrome by ascorbate. N Engl J Med 1976;295:1041-1045.

27. Weening RS, Schoorel EP, Roos D, et al. Effect of ascorbate on abnormal neutrophil, platelet, and lymphocyte function in a patient with the Chédiak-Higashi syndrome. Blood 1981;57:856-865.

28. Roder JC, Haliotis T, Klein M, et al. A new immunodeficiency disorder in humans involving NK cells. Nature 1980; 284:553-555.

29. Nair MN, Gray RH, Boxer LA, et al. Deficiency of inducible suppressor cell activity in the Chédiak-Higashi syndrome. Am J Hematol 1987;26:56-66.

30. Amichai B, Zeharia A, Mimouni M, et al. Picture of the month. Arch Pediatr Adolesc Med 1997;151:425-426.

31. Brandt EJ, Elliot RW, Swank RT. Defective lysosomal enzyme secretion in kidneys of Chédiak-Higashi (beige) mice. J Cell Biol 1975;67:774-788.

32. Baetz K, Isaaz S, Griffiths GM. Loss of cytotoxic T lymphocyte function in Chédiak-Higashi syndrome arises from a secretory defect that prevents lytic granule exocytosis. J Immunol 1995;154:6122-6131.

33. Durandy A, Breton-Gorius J, Guy-Grand D, et al. Prenatal diagnosis of syndromes associating albinism and immune deficiencies (Chédiak-Higashi syndrome and variant). Prenatal Diagnosis 1993;13:13-20.

34. Rubin CM, Burke BA, McKenna RW, et al. The accelerated phase of Chédiak-Higashi syndrome. An expression of the virus-associated hemophagocytic syndrome? Cancer 1985; 56:524-530.

35. Kinugawa N. Epstein-Barr virus infection in Chédiak-Higashi syndrome mimicking acute lymphocytic leukemia. Am J Pediatr Hematol/Oncol 1990;12:182-186.

36. Haddad E, Le Deist F, Blanche S, et al. Treatment of Chédiak-Higashi syndrome by allogenic bone marrow transplantation: Report of ten cases. Blood 1995;85:3328-3333.

37. Griscelli C, Virelizier JL. Bone marrow transplantation in a patient with Chédiak-Higashi syndrome. Birth Defects 1983;19:333-334.

38. Price FV, Legro RS, Watt-Morse M, et al. Chédiak-Higashi syndrome in pregnancy. Obstet Gynecol 1992;79:804-806.

39. Uyama E, Hirano T, Ito K, et al. Adult Chédiak-Higashi syndrome presenting as parkinsonism and dementia. Acta Neurol Scand 1994;89:175-183.

40. Bejaoui M, Veber F, Girault D, et al. [The accelerated phase of Chediak-Higashi syndrome]. Arch Fr Pediatr 1989;46: 733-736.

41. Mineroff AD. Phenylketonuria. In Nordlund JJ, Boissy RE, Hearing VJ, et al, eds. The pigmentary system. New York: Oxford University Press, 1998: pp 590-591.

42. Lidsky AS, Robson KH, Thirumalachary C, et al. The PKU locus in man is on chromosome 12. Am J Hum Genet 1984; 36:527-533.

43. Rosenberg LE. Inherited disorders of amino acid metabolism and storage. In Isselbacher K, Braunwald E, Wilson J, et al, eds. Harrison's principles of internal medicine. 13th edition. New York: McGraw-Hill, 1994: pp 2117-2125.

44. Beasley MG, Costello PM, Smith I. Outcome of treatment in young adults with phenylketonuria detected by routine neonatal screening between 1964 and 1971. Q J Med 1994; 87:155-160.
45. Griscelli C, Durandy A, Guy-Grand D, et al. A syndrome associating partial albinism and immunodeficiency. Am J Med 1978;65:691-702.
46. Siccardi AG, Bianchi E, Calligari A, et al. A new familial defect in neutrophil bactericidal activity. Helv Paediatr Acta 1978;33:401-412.
47. Brambilla E, Dechelette E, Stoebner P. Partial albinism and immunodeficiency: Ultrastructural study of haemophago-cytosis and bone marrow erythroblasts in one case. Pathol Res Pract 1980;167:151-165.
48. Schneider LC, Berman RS, Shea CR, et al. Bone marrow transplantation (BMT) for the syndrome of pigmentary dilution and lymphohistiocytosis (Griscelli's syndrome). J Clin Immunol 1990;10:146-53.
49. Haraldsson A, Weemaes CR, Bakkeren JM, et al. Griscelli disease with cerebral involvement. Eur J Pediatr 1991;150:419-422.
50. Hurvitz H, Gillis R, Klaus S, et al. A kindred with Griscelli disease: spectrum of neurological involvement. Eur J Pediatr 1993;152:402-405.
51. Gogus S, Topcu M, Kucukali T, et al. Griscelli syndrome: Report of three cases. Pediatr Pathol Lab Med 1995;15:309-319.
52. Levine N. Pigmentary abnormalities. In Schachner LA, Hansen RC, eds. Pediatric dermatology. 2nd edition. New York: Churchill Livingstone, 1996: p 566.
53. Mancini AJ, Chan LS, Paller AS. Partial albinism with immunodeficiency: Griscelli syndrome: Report of a case and review of the literature. J Am Acad Dermatol 1998;38:295-300.
54. Klein C, Philippe N, Le Deist F, et al. Partial albinism with immunodeficiency (Griscelli syndrome). J Pediatr 1994;125:886-895.
55. Brismar J, Harfi HA. Partial albinism with immunodeficiency: A rare syndrome with prominent posterior fossa white matter changes. Am J Neuroradiol 1992;13:387-393.
56. Fischer A, Griscelli C, Friedrich W, et al. Bone marrow transplantation for immunodeficiencies and osteoporosis: European survey, 1968-1985. Lancet 1986;2:1080-1083.
57. Lambert J, Onderwater J, Vaner Haeghen Y, et al. Myosin V colocalizes with melanosomes and subcortical actin bundles not associated with stress fibers in human epidermal melanocytes. J Invest Dermatol 1998;111:835-840.
58. Elejalde BR, Holguin J, Valencia A, et al. Mutations affecting pigmentation in man: I. Neuroectodermal melanolysosomal disease. Am J Med Genet 1979;3:65-80.
59. Elejalde BR, De Elejalde MM. Neuroectodermal melanolysosomal disease. In Gomez MR, ed. Neurocutaneous diseases: A practical approach. Boston: Butterworths, 1987: pp 254-260.
60. Duran-McKinster C, Rodriguez-Jurado R, Ridaura C, et al. Elejalde Syndrome: A melanolysosomal neurocutaneous syndrome: Clinical and morphological findings in 7 patients. Arch Derm 1999;135:182-186.
61. Bolognia JL, Orlow SJ, Glick SA. Lines of Blaschko. J Am Acad Dermatol 1994;31:157-190.
62. Harre J, Millikan LE. Linear and whorled pigmentation. Intern J Dermatol 1994;33:529-537.
63. Nehal KS, PeBenito R, Orlow SJ. Analysis of 54 cases of hypopigmentation and hyperpigmentation along the lines of Blaschko. Arch Dermatol 1996;132:1167-1170.
64. Levine N. Pigmentary abnormalities. In Schachner LA, Hansen RC, eds. Pediatric dermatology. 2nd edition. New York: Churchill Livingstone, 1995: pp 539-582.
65. Ito M. Incontinentia pigmenti achromians: A singular case of nevus depigmentosus systematicus bilateralis. Tohoku J Exp Med 1952;55:57-59.
66. Ballmer-Weber BK, Inaebnit D, Brand CU, et al. Sporadic hypomelanosis of Ito with focal hypertrichosis in a 16-month-old girl. Dermatology 1996;193:63-64.
67. Loomis CA. Linear hypopigmentation and hyperpigmentation, including mosaicism. Semin Cutan Med Surg 1997;16:44-53.
68. Sybert VP. Hypomelanosis of Ito: A description, not a diagnosis. J Invest Dermatol 1994;103:141S-143S.
69. Ruiz-Maldonado R, Toussaint S, Tamayo L, et al. Hypomelanosis of Ito: Diagnostic criteria and report of 41 cases. Pediatr Dermatol 1992;9:1-10.
70. Sybert VP, Pagon RA, Donlan M, et al. Pigmentary abnormalities and mosaicism for chromosomal aberration: association with clinical features similar to hypomelanosis of Ito. J Pediatr 1990;116:581-586.
71. Vormittag W, Ensinger C, Raff M. Cytogenetic and dermatoglyphic findings in a familial case of hypomelanosis of Ito (incontinentia pigmenti achromians). Clin Genet 1992;41:309-314.
72. Takematsu H, Sato S, Igarashi M, et al. Incontinentia Pigmenti Achromians (Ito). Arch Dermatol 1983;119:391-395.
73. Montagna P, Procaccianti G, Galli G, et al. Familial hypomelanosis of Ito. Eur Neurol 1991;31:345-347.
74. Spritz RA, Ho L, Strunk KM. Inhibition of proliferation of human melanocytes by a KIT antisense oligodeoxynucleotide: Implications for human piebaldism and mouse dominant white spotting (W). J Invest Dermatol 1994;103:148-150.
75. Spritz RA. Piebaldism, Waardenburg syndrome, and related disorders of melanocyte development. Semin Cutan Med Surg 1997;16:15-23.
76. Dippel E, Haas N, Grabbe J, et al. Expression of c-kit receptor in hypomelanosis: A comparative study between piebaldism, naevus depigmentosis and vitiligo. Br J Dermatol 1995;132:182-189.
77. Read AP, Newton VE. Waardenburg syndrome. J Med Genet 1997;34:656-665.
78. Asher JH, Friedman TB. Mouse and hamster mutants as models for Waardenburg syndromes in humans. J Med Genet 1990;27:618-626.
79. Farrer LA, Arnos KS, Asher JH, et al. Locus heterogeneity for Waardenburg syndrome is predictive of clinical subtypes. Am J Hum Genet 1994;55:728-737.
80. Giacoia JP, Klein SW. Waardenburg's syndrome with bilateral cleft lip. Am J Dis Child 1969;117:344-348.
81. da Silva EO. Waardenburg I syndrome: A clinical and genetic study of two large Brazilian kindreds, and literature review. Am J Med Genet 1991;40:65-74.

82. Pantke OA, Cohen MM. The Waardenburg syndrome. Birth Defects 1971;7:147-152.

83. Klein PD. Albinisme partiel (leucisme) avec surdi-mutite, blepharophimosis et dysplasie myo-osteo-articulaire. Helv Paediatr Acta 1950;5:38-58.

84. Shah KN, Dalal SJ, Desai MP, et al: White forelock, pigmentary disorder of the irides, and long segment Hirschsprung disease: Possible variant of Waardenburg syndrome. J Pediatr 1981;99:432-435.

85. Bolognia JL, Pawelek JM. Biology of hypopigmentation. J Am Acad Dermatol 1988;19:217-255.

86. Jimbow K, Fitzpatrick TB, Szabo G, et al. Congenital circumscribed hypomelanosis: A characterization based on electron microscopic study of tuberous sclerosis, nevus depigmentosus, and piebaldism. J Invest Dermatol 1975;64: 50-62.

87. Berg M, Tarnowski W. Nevus pigmentosus. Arch Dermatol 1973;109:920-921.

88. Sugarman GI, Reed WB. Two unusual neurocutaneous disorders with facial cutaneous signs. Arch Neurol 1969;21: 242-247.

89. Gauthier Y, Surleve-Bazeille JE. Autologous grafting with noncultured melanocytes: A simplified method for treatment of depigmented lesions. J Am Acad Dermatol 1992; 26:191-194.

90. Vanderhooft SL, Francis JS, Pagon RA, et al. Prevalence of hypopigmented macules in a healthy population. J Pediatr 1996;129:355-361.

91. Hunt A, Lindenbaum RH. Tuberous sclerosis: A new estimate of prevalence within the Oxford region. J Med Genet 1984;21:272-277.

92. Stevenson AC, Fisher OD. Frequency of epiloia in northern Ireland. Br J Prev Soc Med 1956;10:134-135.

93. Zaremba J. Tuberous sclerosis: A clinical and genetical investigation. J Ment Defic Res 1968;12:63-80.

94. Zvulunov A, Esterly NB. Neurocutaneous syndromes associated with pigmentary skin lesions. J Am Acad Dermatol 1995;32:915-935.

95. Osborne JP, Fryer A, Webb D. Epidemiology of tuberous sclerosis. Ann N Y Acad Sci 1991;615:125-127.

96. Gold AP, Freeman JM. Depigmented nevi: The earliest sign of tuberous sclerosis. Pediatrics 1965;35:1003-1005.

97. Fitzpatrick TB, Szabo G, Hori Y, et al. White leaf-shaped macules: Earliest visible sign of tuberous sclerosis. Arch Derm 1968;98:1-6.

98. Harris R, Moynahan EJ. Tuberous sclerosis with vitiligo. Br J Dermatol 1966;78:419-420.

99. Hunt A. Tuberous sclerosis: A survey of 97 cases. II: Physical findings. Dev Med Child Neurol 1983;25:350-352.

100. Hurwitz S, Braverman IM. White spots in tuberous sclerosis. J Pediatr 1970;77:587-594.

101. Nickel WR, Reed WB. Tuberous sclerosis. Arch Dermatol 1962;85:89-106.

102. Roach ES, Delgado MR. Tuberous sclerosis. Dermatol Clin 1995;13:151-161.

103. Wagner AM, Hansen RC. Neonatal skin and skin disorders. In Schachner LA, Hansen RC, ed. Pediatric dermatology. 2nd edition. New York: Churchill Livingstone, 1995: pp.263-346.

104. Requena L, Sanqueza OP. Cutaneous vascular anomalies. Part I. Hamartomas, malformations, and dilatation of pre-existing vessels. J Am Acad Dermatol 1997;37:523-549.

105. Lacour JP. Hypopigmentation without hypomelanosis. In Nordlund JJ, Boissy RE, Hearing VJ, et al, eds. The pigmentary system. New York: Oxford University Press, 1998: pp 707-708.

106. Greaves MW, Birkett D, Johnson C. Nevus anemicus: A unique catecholamine-dependent nevus. Arch Dermatol 1970;102:172-176.

107. Hogan PA, Weston WL. Vascular reactions. In Schachner LA, Hansen RC, ed. Pediatric dermatology. 2nd edition. New York: Churchill Livingstone, 1995: pp 915-952.

108. Ruiz-Maldonado R, de la Luz Orozco-Covarrubias M. Post-inflammatory hypopigmentation and hyperpigmentation. Semin Cutan Med Surg 1997;16:36-43.

109. Brownstein MH, Kazam BB, Hashimoto K. Halo congenital nevus. Arch Dermatol Soc 1997;113:1572-1575.

110. Berger RS, Voorhees JJ. Multiple congenital giant nevocellular nevi with halos. Arch Dermatol 1971;104:515-521.

111. Ridley CM. Giant halo naevus with spontaneous resolution. Trans St. Johns Hosp Dermatol Soc 1974;60:54-58.

112. Zeff RA, Freitag A, Grin CM, et al. The immune response in halo nevi. J Am Acad Dermatol 1997;37:620-624.

113. Brownstein MH, Kazam BB, Hashimoto K. Halo congenital nevus. Arch Derm 1977;113:1572-1575.

114. Riordan JR, Jolicoeur-Paquet L. Metallothionein accumulation may account for intracellular copper retention in Menkes' disease. J Biol Chem 1982;257:4639-4645.

115. Yazaki M, Wada Y, Kojima Y, et al. Copper-binding proteins in the liver and kidney from the patients with Menkes' kinky hair disease. Tohoku J Exp Med 1983;139:97-102.

116. Ploysangam T. Menkes' kinky hair syndrome. In Nordlund JJ, Boissy RE, Hearing VJ, et al, eds. The pigmentary system. New York: Oxford University Press, 1998: pp 584-586.

117. Micali G, Bene-Bain MA, Guitart J, et al. Genodermatoses. In Schachner LA, Hansen RC, eds. Pediatric dermatology. 2nd edition. New York: Churchill Livingstone, 1995: pp 347-411.

118. Horn N, Stene J, Mollekaer AM, et al. Linkage studies in Menkes' disease. The Xg blood group system and C-banding of the X chromosome. Ann Hum Genet 1984;48:161-172.

119. Garnica AD. The failure of parenteral copper therapy in Menkes kinky hair syndrome. Eur J Pediatr 1984;142:98-102.

120. Sarkar B, Lingertat-Walsh K, Clarke JR. Copper-histidine therapy for Menkes disease. J Pediatr 1993;123:828-830.

121. Nadal D, Baerlocher K. Menkes' disease: long-term treatment with copper and D-penicillamine. Eur J Pediatr 1988; 147:621-625.

122. Gerdes AM, Tonnesen T, Pergament E, et al. Variability in clinical expression of Menkes syndrome. Eur J Pediatr 1988; 148:132-135.

123. Ziprkowski L, Adam A. Recessive total albinism and congenital deaf-mutism. Arch Dermatol 1964;89:151-155.

124. Ziprkowski L, Krakowski A, Adam A, et al. Partial albinism and deaf mutism due to a recessive sex-linked gene. Arch Dermatol 1962;86:530-539.

125. Margolis E. A new hereditary syndrome: Sex-linked deaf-mutism associated with total albinism. Acta Genet (Basel) 1962;12:12-19.

126. Shiloh Y, Litvak G, Ziv Y, et al. Genetic mapping of X-linked albinism-deafness syndrome (ADFN) to Xq26.3-q27.1. Am J Hum Genet 1990;47:20-27.

127. Fried K, Feinmesser M, Tsitsianov J. Hearing impairment in female carriers of the sex-linked syndrome of deafness with albinism. J Med Genet 1969;6:132-134.

128. Casala AM, Alezzandrini AA. Vitiligo y poliosis unilateral con retinitis pigmentaria e hipoacusia. Arch Arg Derm 1957; 9:449-456.

129. Hoffman MD, Dudley C. Suspected Alezzandriniís syndrome in a diabetic patient with unilateral retinal detachment and ipsilateral vitiligo and poliosis. J Am Acad Dermatol 1992;26:496-498.

130. Mosher DB, Fitzpatrick TB, Hori Y, et al: Disorders of pigmentation. In Fitzpatrick TB, Eisen AZ, Wolff K, et al, eds. Dermatology in general medicine. New York: McGraw-Hill, 1993: pp 903-995.

20

Hyperpigmentation Disorders

LAWRENCE F. EICHENFIELD
NEIL F. GIBBS

Hyperpigmented lesions are common at birth and in the first few weeks of life. Lesions range from small macules to large hyperpigmented plaques. Some, such as mongolian spots, are frequently seen in newborns and of little or no significance, whereas others may be signs of systemic diseases and genetic syndromes. An approach based on lesion morphology and location may be useful (Table 20-1). Excellent review articles discuss congenital and genetic hyperpigmentation in more detail, and may be helpful supplements to this chapter.[1,2]

LOCALIZED HYPERPIGMENTATION-FLAT LESIONS

Tan-Brown

Café au Lait Macules

Café au lait macules (CALMs) are usually round or oval flat lesions of light brown pigmentation with distinct margins ranging in size from a few millimeters to 15 to 20 cm in diameter, which can occur anywhere on the body (Figs. 20-1 and 20-2). They are seen in 0.3% to 18% of neonates with variation by ethnicity and race, and in 24% to 36% of older children.[3,4] Many or most are present at birth or develop in the first few months of life; they may increase in number and size with age.

Café au lait macules are most often unassociated with specific abnormalities, but can be markers for certain genetic diseases, most commonly neurofibromatosis type I (NF I).[5] Watson's syndrome presents with multiple café au lait macules, intertriginous freckling, short stature, pulmonary stenosis, and low intelligence, and is thought to be a subset, or allelic form of NF I. Large café au lait mac-

ules may be seen in McCune-Albright syndrome. Other syndromes in which café au lait macules appear to be strongly associated include neurofibromatosis type (NF-2) and ring chromosome syndrome.[2] Other conditions in which café au lait spots may be seen, though with less strong association, include tuberous sclerosis, Bloom syndrome, ataxia-telangiectasia syndrome, Silver-Russell syndrome, Jaffe-Campanacci syndrome, basal cell nevus syndrome, Gaucher disease, Turner syndrome, and Hunter syndrome.[6]

Diagnosis is based on the clinical appearance. The differential diagnosis of conditions associated with café au lait macules is extensive. In neonates, some flat congenital nevi may be indistinguishable from café au lait macules, although clinical differentiation is obvious with time. On biopsy, café au lait macules have increased epidermal melanin in both melanocytes and keratinocytes, without melanocytic proliferation, readily distinguishing them from melanocytic nevi. Giant pigment granules may be present, but these are nonspecific.[7]

The significance of café au lait macules is as a diagnostic aid to other disorders. Treatment is generally unnecessary. For disfiguring lesions, pigmented lesion lasers may be of value, although results are inconsistent, with complete clearance in some cases and rapid recurrence or no response in others.[8]

Neurofibromatosis

Neurofibromatosis refers to a group of disorders involving neuroectodermal and mesenchymal derivatives, characterized by café au lait spots and tumors of the nervous system. Neurofibromatosis type 1 is by far the most common, comprising 90% of all NF cases. Neurofibromatosis

TABLE 20-1

Diagnosis Using Lesion Morphology and Location

Description of lesions		Location	Possible diagnoses
Blue-gray/blue-black patches	Dermal melanocytosis	Torso	Mongolian spot
		Face	Nevus of Ota
		Shoulder/neck	Nevus of Ito
		Torso, in association with port wine stain	Phakomatosis pigmentovascularis
Labial macules	Involving mucosa	Perioral	Peutz-Jeghers syndrome
		More widespread facial	Carney syndrome
	More widespread, not involving mucosa	Face/trunk	LEOPARD syndrome
		Face	Carney syndrome
	Central face, not involving mucosa		Centrofacial lentiginosis
Brown sharply defined patches or plaques	Patch		Congenital nevus
			Café au lait macule
	Plaque		Congenital nevus
Small brown macules		Perioral/mucosal	Peutz-Jeghers syndrome
		Widespread, non mucosal	LEOPARD syndrome
			Generalized lentiginosis
			Inherited patterned lentiginosis
			Carney syndrome
		Central face/widespread Involves mucosa	Carney syndrome
		Axilliary/groin/neck only	Neurofibromatosis
		Central face only, not mucosa	Centrofacial lentiginosis
		Clustered in a defined body area or segment. Background skin color normal	Segmental lentiginosis Mosaicism
		Clustered in a defined body area or segment. Background skin color darker	Speckled lentiginous nevus Nevus spilus
		Single	Congenital nevus
Linear hyperpigmentation in swirled or Blaschko pattern		Flat	Linear and whorled nevoid hypermelanosis
			Epidermal nevus
			Incontinentia pigmenti
			Goltz syndrome
			Conradi-Hünermann syndrome
			Mosaicism
		Raised	Epidermal nevus
			Incontinentia pigmenti

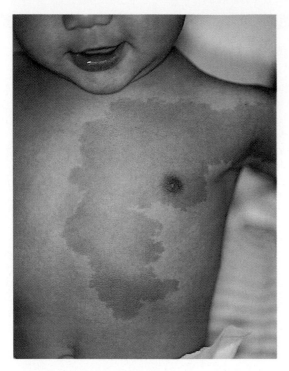

FIG. 20-1
Large café au lait macule. Child was otherwise well.

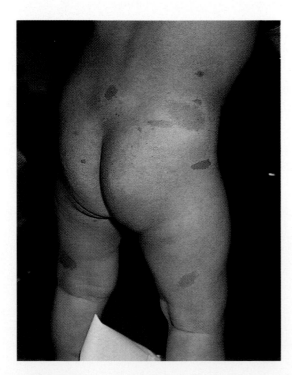

FIG. 20-2
Mulitple café au lait macules on a child with NF-1.

type 2 is a genetically distinct autosomal disorder, characterized by acoustic or central nervous system schwannomas. It may also present with CALMS, although these lesions tend to be fewer and paler than in NF-1. Segmental neurofibromatosis presents with localized CALMS, freckling, and/or neurofibromas, and is thought to be caused by mosaicism. Finally, some families appear to have autosomal dominant transmission of multiple CALMs, with or without axillary and inguinal freckling, and without systemic manifestations. A more extensive discussion of NF is found in Chapter 24.

Neonates with multiple café au lait macules should be carefully evaluated for stigmata of NF-1, including measuring and counting of lesions. Six or more CALMS greater than 5 mm in diameter in infants and children are presumptive evidence of NF-1. Axillary and/or inguinal freckling is only rarely present at birth and usually develops with time. Lisch nodules are extremely rare in neonates; their prevalence increases with age. A family history of NF or other syndromes should be sought, and parents examined when possible. Previously unrecognized findings in a parent may confirm the diagnosis. In one prospective study excluding those with segmental distribution, 75% of patients with 6 or more café au lait macules who were followed for 2 years, and 89% of patients followed for 3 or more years developed other signs of NF-1.[6] Manifestations of NF-1 may evolve over time, and neonates at risk or with presumptive evidence of disease should be monitored closely.[9]

McCune-Albright Syndrome

McCune-Albright syndrome refers to the triad of café au lait macules, polyostotic fibrous dysplasia, and endocrine dysfunction. Clinical findings are quite variable, and neonatal presentation may be limited to cutaneous findings. Café au lait macules in McCune-Albright syndrome are usually large, linear or segmental, unilateral or bilateral, and may have a jagged margin said to resemble the "coast of Maine" (Fig. 20-3). These skin lesions may be present at birth and can darken with time. The café au lait macules may follow Blaschko's lines in broader patterns. Bony lesions are usually on the same side as unilateral CALMS, consistent with the syndrome being a mosaic disorder.[10,11]

Extracutaneous findings include polyostotic fibrous dysplasia, where bone is replaced by fibrous tissue, resulting in asymmetry, bony growths and pathological fractures. These may be seen at birth, but more often develop in the first decade and frequently involve the face, hands, and legs. Multiple endocrine abnormalities have been reported, including precocious puberty, hyperthyroidism, Cushing's syndrome, hypersomatotropism, hyperprolactinemia, and hyperparathyroidism.[12-14]

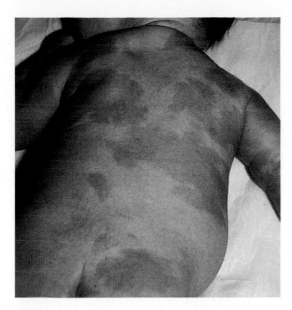

FIG. 20-3
Multiple patterned café au lait spots in a child with McCune-Albright syndrome.

McCune-Albright syndrome is more common in females than in males. It is believed to be to an autosomal dominant lethal mutation, which survives as a postzygotic mutation with resulting mosaicism.[15,16] Mutation of the GNAS1 gene that encodes for the α subunit of the guanine nucleotide binding protein causes loss of GTPase activity and increased stimulation of the adenylate cyclase system, resulting in proliferation and autonomous hyperfunction of hormonally responsive cells.[10,13,17]

Since the clinical expression may be variable and segmental, diagnosis may be difficult. Radiological studies may not reveal bony abnormalities in the neonatal period. McCune-Albright syndrome must be differentiated from NF 1. Café au lait macules of NF 1 tend to be smaller and have a more scattered distribution.[10,11] Histologic study of the café au lait macules does not help in differentiating McCune-Albright syndrome from the CALMS seen with other syndromes.[7,16]

Jaffe-Campanacci syndrome is evidenced by café au lait macules with a "coast of Maine" appearance, distributed unilaterally or diffusely, nonossifying fibromas (a condition distinct from polyostotic dysplasia), and multiple nevi.[1] The café au lait macules of McCune-Albright syndrome may also be confused with "segmental pigmentation disorder." In the hyperpigmented form of this condition, brown patches occur mainly on the trunk, sometimes in a dermatomal pattern. The size varies, but the lesions are usually larger than café au lait macules. Dif-

ferentiating clinical features include sharp delineation of the lesion at the midline with the lateral border less distinctly defined, and no endocrinologic or bony abnormalities as seen with McCune-Albright syndrome.[18]

McCune-Albright syndrome usually has a good prognosis. There is no specific treatment for the fibrous dysplasia, but care should be taken to avoid fractures. Close observation for endocrine abnormalities is appropriate. Referrals for orthopedic and endocrine evaluations are recommended.[13] Many patients develop normal reproductive function. Development of malignancy is rare, and life span is usually normal. Extensive osseous dysplasia in the early years portends a poor prognosis.[11]

Silver-Russell Syndrome

Silver-Russell patients have a low birth weight, skeletal asymmetry, and a triangular facies. Some have been noted to have café au lait macules and increased numbers of melanocytic nevi.[19]

Blue-Gray: Dermal Melanocytosis

Mongolian Spots

Mongolian spots are benign, brown, blue-gray, or blue-black patches that are usually located over the sacrum or lower back (see Chapter 7). They are present at birth or early infancy in over 80% of African-American and Asian babies, with lesser incidence in lighter skinned races.[3,20] Mongolian spots can range in size from a few millimeters to greater than 10 cm and can be single or multiple.[20] The sacrococcygeal area is most commonly affected, but lesions may occur on the buttock, dorsal trunk, and extremities (Fig. 20-4).[20,21] Lesion color stabilizes in infancy, with subsequent fading in the majority of lesions before adulthood. There are no known extracutaneous findings. Association of mongolian spots with port wine stains is seen with phakomatosis pigmentovascularis, and extensive mongolian spots may be seen with GM_1 gangliosidosis (see the following discussion).[1,22]

The etiology of dermal melanocytosis is thought to be due to arrested embryonal migration of melanocytes from neural crest to epidermis. Why the lesions almost always occur in the same areas is not well understood.[3] The blue color is characteristic of dermal melanin, as a result of the Tyndall effect.

Diagnosis is based on clinical morphology and location. Lesions are usually more blue in appearance than café au lait macules or congenital nevi. Biopsy will verify the dermal location of the melanocytes if the diagnosis is in question. Collections of greatly elongated, slender, spindle-shaped melanocytes are scattered be-

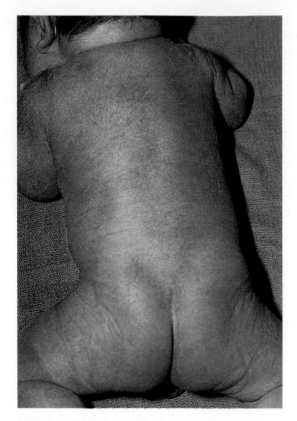

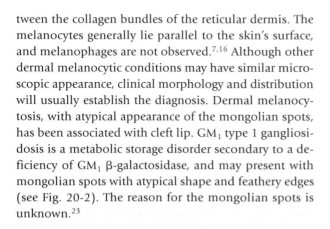

FIG. 20-4
Dermal melanocytosis/mongolian spot. Extensive involvement includes the trunk and lower extremity.

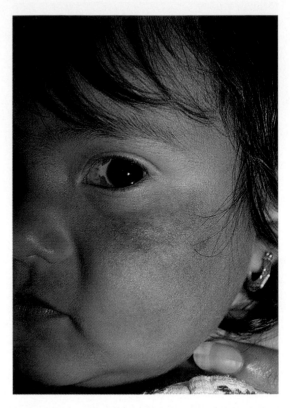

FIG. 20-5
Nevus of Ota. Periorbital blue-gray color associated with dermal melanocytosis.

tween the collagen bundles of the reticular dermis. The melanocytes generally lie parallel to the skin's surface, and melanophages are not observed.[7,16] Although other dermal melanocytic conditions may have similar microscopic appearance, clinical morphology and distribution will usually establish the diagnosis. Dermal melanocytosis, with atypical appearance of the mongolian spots, has been associated with cleft lip. GM_1 type 1 gangliosidosis is a metabolic storage disorder secondary to a deficiency of GM_1 β-galactosidase, and may present with mongolian spots with atypical shape and feathery edges (see Fig. 20-2). The reason for the mongolian spots is unknown.[23]

Nevus of Ota (Nevus Fuscoceruleus Ophthalmomaxillaris)

Periorbital dermal melanocytosis in the distribution of the first and second divisions of the trigeminal nerve is known as nevus of Ota. Lesions are present at birth in 50% of affected individuals, with a second peak onset during the

second decade of life.[24] Unilateral blue-gray lesions are typical. Pigmentation of the ipsilateral sclera is common (Fig. 20-5). Less commonly, the oral or nasal mucosa, retina, leptomeninges, or iris may be involved. Nevus of Ota is more common in Asians and the darker pigmented races and has female predominance.[24]

Malignant blue nevi and malignant melanoma can rarely occur with nevus of Ota. If ocular pigmentation is present, glaucoma may occur secondary to melanocytes in the ciliary body of the anterior chamber of the eye, impeding the normal flow of fluid.[24]

The etiology of nevus of Ota is presumed to be similar to that of mongolian spots, involving errors in melanocyte migration from the neural crest to the epidermis.[3,24,25]

The diagnosis is usually made clinically, based on appearance and location. Biopsy shows elongated dendritic melanocytes scattered among collagen bundles in the dermis. They are usually more numerous and superficial than in mongolian spots. At times, melanocytes surround the sheaths of adnexal structures.[7]

Unlike mongolian spots, nevus of Ota does not lighten or resolve with time, and may increase in size and color intensity.[24] If desired, treatment with pigmented lesion lasers (e.g., Alexandrite or Q-switched ruby) may lighten or clear the lesion. Alternatively, covering makeup can be used.[26,27] Regular ophthalmologic exams should be performed if ocular pigment is present.[1]

Nevus of Ito (Nevus Fuscoceruleus Acromiodeltoideus)

Nevus of Ito is a patchy blue-gray discoloration of skin on the shoulder, supraclavicular, neck, upper arm, scapular, and deltoid areas of the body (Fig. 20-6).[24] This condition has the same features as nevus of Ota, but its location approximates the distribution of the posterior supraclavicular and lateral brachial cutaneous nerves. It is generally a benign condition, but malignant melanoma/blue nevus can rarely develop.

The etiology is believed to be similar to mongolian spots and nevus of Ota (see previous discussion). The diagnosis is usually made clinically, based on appearance and location. Elongated dendritic melanocytes scattered among collagen bundles in the dermis are noted on biopsy. They are usually more numerous and superficial than in mongolian spots. At times, melanocytes surround the sheaths of adnexal structures.[7,24,28]

Unlike mongolian spots, nevus of Ito does not lighten or resolve with time, and may increase in size and intensity.[24] Treatment with one of the pigment lasers has shown the potential for good results, or a covering makeup can be used.[26,27]

Congenital Blue Nevus

A blue nevus is a hamartoma of dermal melanocytes. Congenital blue nevi are uncommon to rare. They may present in a similar fashion to large congenital melanocytic nevi, though with a blue-black color. Classically, two forms of blue nevi have been described: common and cellular. Common blue nevi, which are uncommon as congenital lesions, typically present as 2 to 10 mm, blue-black, smooth macules, or papules most frequently on the scalp or face (although they can occur anywhere), and are rarely associated with complications.[7,29] Typical cellular blue nevi are acquired, may range between 2 and 20 mm, may be single or multiple, and are most commonly present on the buttock and sacrococcygeal areas.[30,31] Cellular blue nevi may exhibit aggressive benign growth that may be confused with a malignant tumor, but may also undergo malignant change. Congenital blue nevi are usually of the cellular type; larger lesions of the head (usually >8 cm) may involve underlying muscle bone and

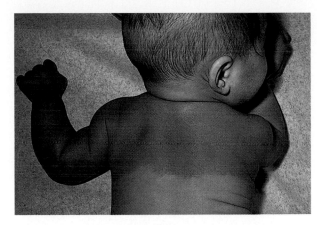

FIG. 20-6
Nevus of Ito.

dura.[7,30,31] Malignant melanoma may arise within giant congenital cellular blue nevi of the scalp, although incidence figures for this are unavailable due to the rarity of these lesions. Combined nevi, with features of melanocytic nevi and blue nevi, and blue nevi developing within lentiginous lesions (e.g., congenital unilateral speckled lentiginous blue nevi) or dermal melanocytosis, have been reported.[32] Familial multiple blue nevi may occur as part of Carney syndrome (a complex of myxomas, endocrine overactivity, and spotty pigmentation that includes epithelioid blue nevi), or without associated abnormalities.[33]

The etiology is unknown. Blue nevi may represent a defect in embryogenesis with abnormal migration of melanocytes from the neural crest to the epidermis.[3] The diagnosis is usually suggested by the blue-black clinical appearance; however, a biopsy may be needed. In the common form, dendritic melanocytes are found singly or in small aggregations in the reticular dermis, and may be clustered around adnexal structures, vessels, and nerves.[29,34] They resemble the cells in mongolian spot and in nevus of Ito, but their density is much greater. Melanophages are frequently observed. The cellular type has similar dendritic and spindled melanocytes, mixed in with cellular islands composed of closely aggregated, large, spindle-shaped cells with ovoid nuclei and abundant pale cytoplasm often containing little or no melanin.[30,31]

For both types of blue nevi, conservative surgical excision will usually suffice. The common type is rarely malignant, but is sometimes removed based on appearance and/or dark color. The aggressive cellular type may be associated with malignancy (malignant blue nevus), which some believe may actually represent malignant melanoma that arises from the blue nevus. This aggressive type may be difficult to remove completely and patients should have close follow-up.[30,31]

MOSAIC CONDITIONS AND WHORLED AND SEGMENTAL HYPERPIGMENTATION

Mosaic Conditions

A variety of hyperpigmented conditions may present in a segmental pattern or following lines of Blaschko (Box 20-1, also see Table 3-2). Many of these conditions are discussed in Chapter 24. Streaky, whorled macular hyperpigmentation is considered to be a physical representation of genomic mosaicism, and may be seen as an isolated cutaneous skin condition, or as part of a more significant genetic disease (Fig. 20-7). For example, the X-linked condition, incontinentia pigmenti, often displays hyperpigmented streaks following the lines of Blaschko. Incontinentia pigmenti is an X-linked dominant condition, with affected females being heterozygous for the mutation with inactivation of one of the X-chromosomes as predicted in the Lyon hypothesis. It is theorized that the pigmented whorls represent a clonal population of cells that arises during early development and progresses laterally, along the craniocaudal axis from the midline neuroectoderm. The peculiar but reproducible patterns reflect embryologic migration patterns, with linear appearance on the limbs, S-shapes on the chest, and V-shapes on the back. In addition to chromosome mosaicism, postzygotic somatic mu-

tations of other chromosomes can create populations of genetically differing cells. Segmental hyperpigmented (or hypopigmented) lesions in patients without specific syndromic diagnoses may be caused by functional cutaneous mosaicism, and careful physical examination and follow-up is reasonable to assess for systemic problems (Fig. 20-8). A number of other conditions listed in this chapter (e.g., McCune-Albright syndrome) are due to mosaicism, but have been described under the headings pertaining to their cutaneous manifestations.

Chimerism

Human chimerism is rare, but results from fusion of two or more genetically distinct zygotes. Chimerism may display pigmentation in a line of Blaschko distribution, checkerboard pattern, or asymmetric café au lait patches.

Linear and Whorled Nevoid Hypermelanosis

Linear and whorled nevoid hypermelanosis is a term used to describe asymmetric epidermal hypermelanosis in streaky or swirl-like patterns (Fig. 20-9). These pigmented areas follow lines of Blaschko, or occur in a segmental pattern. Linear and whorled hypermelanosis appears at birth or within a few weeks of age without a preceding inflammatory event. Pigmentation may become more evident over the first few years of life and then stabilizes, although fading with time has been observed in some individuals.[35-38]

Linear and whorled nevoid hypermelanosis is usually a benign condition. Patients with associated anomalies have been reported, although in most cases, chromoso-

---

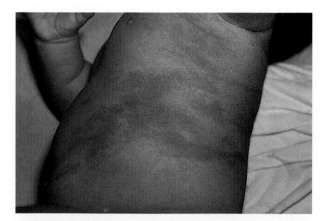

FIG. 20-7
Localized, whorled hyperpigmentation, considered a sign of cutaneous mosaicism. This child was clinically well.

mal analysis has not been performed to rule out other conditions that might exist as a result of mosaicism or chimerism as has been found in hypomelanosis of Ito.[35] The most likely etiological explanation is a developmental somatic mosaicism of neuroectodermal cells before migration from the neural crest, with the two skin colors representing two distinct populations of cells.[35,39]

Nevoid hypermelanosis is basically a diagnosis of exclusion. Biopsy specimens demonstrate diffuse increased pigmentation of the epidermal basal layer and a slight increase in the number of melanocytes without an increase in dermal melanophages or pigment incontinence.[7,35,36] It should be differentiated from other conditions with hyperpig-

mented lesions that follow Blaschko's lines, such as incontinentia pigmenti (third stage), linear epidermal nevus, nevoid hypermelanosis in human chimeras, Conradi-Hünermann syndrome, Goltz syndrome, and Naegeli-Franceschetti-Jadassohn syndrome.[37-39] These conditions may be excluded based on textural changes of the hyperpigmented areas and other clinical findings present. Diffuse hypopigmentation, seen with extensive hypomelanosis of Ito, may be difficult to distinguish from nevoid hypermelanosis, since it may be hard to determine the patient's natural color and if affected areas are pathologically lighter or darker.

No specific treatments have been described for linear and whorled hypermelanosis. Careful physical and developmental examinations are usually sufficient for detecting extracutaneous associations. If other anomalies exist, blood and skin fibroblast chromosomal analysis for mosaicism should be considered.[35,39]

Incontinentia Pigmenti

Incontinentia pigmenti is an X-linked dominant hereditary disorder, characterized by streaky, linear, or splash-like cuta-

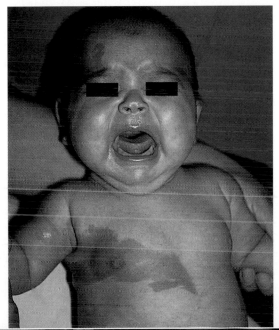
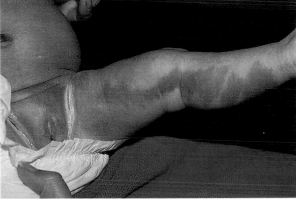

FIG. 20-8
Segmental hyperpigmentation affecting the right side of the face, chest, and left leg.

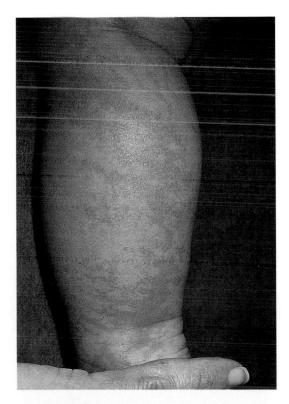

FIG. 20-9
Linear and whorled nevoid hypermelanosis.

neous lesions following the lines of Blaschko that are usually present at birth or shortly thereafter (see Chapter 24). Also known as Bloch-Sulzberger syndrome, it is found almost exclusively in females as a result of lethality in males. The gene responsible for the familial form (NEMO) has been mapped to Xq28, and a nonfamilial form to Xp11.21.[40]

There are four classic stages in the skin (see Chapter 24). Patients may demonstrate only some of the stages, and overlap or "skipping" of stages may occur. Neonates may be born with or develop the hyperpigmented lesions without signs of the preceding stages.[40,41] Stage 1 is an inflammatory vesicobullous stage with streaks of eosinophil-filled epidermal vesicles. It usually presents at birth or in the first few weeks of life, though later recurrences have been reported. A second stage with papules, pustules, verrucous, or lichenoid lesions usually appears within 2 to 6 weeks. These lesions may not correspond exactly to the same areas as stage 1, and usually resolve within weeks to months. A third stage of macular linear/whorled hyperpigmentation follows and gradually increases in intensity. There may be a fourth stage of hypopigmentation that replaces the hyperpigmentation.

Extracutaneous findings are common. Peripheral eosinophilia is often present during stage 1. Other organ system anomalies include defects of dentition (missing, pegged, and notched teeth), alopecia, ocular defects (retinal detachment, proliferative retinopathy, fibrovascular retrolental membrane, ciliary body atrophy, strabismus, cataracts, blindness, microphthalmia), central nervous system abnormalities (seizures, spastic paralysis, mental retardation), structural development problems, (dwarfism, club foot, spina bifida, hemiatrophy, congenital hip dysplasia), nail dystrophy, hemarthrosis, various internal malignancies, and immunological problems.[40,41]

Clinical diagnosis can usually be made by the distinctive skin changes. The skin biopsy results will be different for each stage.[7] The first stage is characterized by epidermal vesicles and spongiosis with eosinophils.[42] Scattered dyskeratotic cells and whorls of squamous cells with central keratinization are found between vesicles. The second stage shows acanthosis, irregular papillomatosis, hyperkeratosis, and more dyskeratotic cells and squamous whorls, usually with pigment dilution, vacuolar alteration, and degeneration of the basal layer. Mild inflammatory infiltrate with melanin within melanophages in the upper dermis ("incontinent pigment") is seen in the second and third stages of the disease. Further discussion of incontinentia pigmenti is found in Chapter 24.

Phakomatosis Pigmentovascularis

Phakomatosis pigmentovascularis is a term used to describe conditions involving the simultaneous occurrence of congenital cutaneous pigmented lesions, including dermal melanocytosis, nevus spilus, and linear and whorled nevoid hyperpigmentation in association with vascular malformations, particularly port wine stains.[22,43] A classification system with four types of phakomatosis pigmentovascularis has been proposed on the basis of the type of pigmented lesion, and each of these is subdivided on the basis of whether extracutaneous lesions are present (subtype 'b') or absent (subtype 'a') (Table 20-2).[1]

The most common by far is type II, the concordance of dermal melanocytosis with port wine stains (Fig. 20-10). Most of the coexistent extracutaneous abnormalities are those usually associated with each of the congenital birthmarks: Sturge-Weber syndrome with port wine stains in the trigeminal V1 distribution (and glaucoma, both with periorbital port wine stains and with nevus of Ota) and Klippel-Trenaunay syndrome with port wine stains on affected extremities. Reported extracutaneous anomalies include hypoplastic larynx and subglottic stenosis, multiple granular cell tumors, iris mammillations, scoliosis, anemia, malignant polyposis, mental disturbances, psychomotor retardation, epilepsy, intracranial calcifications, and cerebral atrophy.

Phakomatosis pigmentovascularis is a hereditary disorder believed to be explained by the "twin spot phenomenon" (see the following discussion). Proteus syndrome should be considered in the differential diagnosis of phakomatosis pigmentovascularis. Proteus syndrome may display coexisting epidermal and vascular nevi, though the presence of marked gigantism and asymmetry in Proteus syndrome usually helps to distinguish it. Laser treatments such as pulsed dye laser for the port wine stain

---

TABLE 20-2

Classification Schema of Phakomatosis Pigmentovascularis

Type	Vascular malformation	Pigmentary nevus
I	Port wine stain	Epidermal nevus
II	Port wine stain	Dermal melanocytosis (± nevus anemicus)
III	Port wine stain	Nevus spilus (± nevus anemicus)
IV	Port wine stain	Dermal melanocytosis and nevus spilus (± nevus anemicus)

and one of the pigmented lesion lasers for the melanocytosis may be helpful in decreasing disfigurement.[1]

Phakomatosis Pigmentokeratotica

Phakomatosis pigmentokeratotica (also known as phacomatosis pigmentokeratotica or melanocytic-epidermal twin nevus syndrome) is a term used for epidermal nevus of the nonepidermolytic type with contralateral segmental lentiginous or papular speckled melanocytic lesions. Its naming emphasizes its analogy to phakomatosis pigmentovascularis.[44] The epidermal nevi may be organoid or sebaceous, and follow Blaschko lines. Lentiginous elements may present in later life. Most reported cases have associated anomalies. These include neurologic abnormalities (seizures, retardation, hyperpathia, dysesthesia, hyperhidrosis), ophthalmologic abnormalities (including coloboma, lipodermoid of the conjunctiva, palpebral ptosis), and skeletal and limb defects (hemiatrophy, scoliosis, muscle weakness, gait disturbances). Basal cell epitheliomas may develop within sebaceous nevi, and ichthyosis-like hyperkeratosis has also been reported.[45] It has been sug

gested that the pathogenesis may involve the mechanism of "twin spotting," in which paired patches of genetically distinct clones exist in a background of normal cells. This may occur when an organism heterozygous for two different recessive mutations localized on the same chromosome undergoes somatic recombination, resulting in two homozygous daughter cells, which serve as stem cells for distinct clonal populations.[46]

Naegeli-Franceschetti-Jadassohn Syndrome

Naegeli-Franceschetti-Jadassohn syndrome is an autosomal dominantly inherited condition characterized by brown-gray reticulated hyperpigmentation beginning in early childhood, and a decreased ability to sweat. The pigmentation is more often on the abdomen, neck, and trunk, and less frequently on the flexures and face. Palmoplantar hyperkeratosis develops in late childhood.[47]

Striped Hyperpigmentation of the Torso
(see Chapter 7)

A case was described in an African-American neonate who had bands of horizontal pigmentation across the abdomen, which appeared after birth (Fig. 20-11). At birth, the baby's skin had some slight thickening and scaling

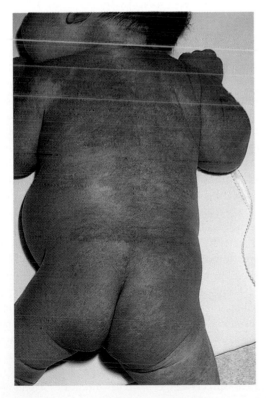

FIG. 20-10
Phakomatosis pigmentovascularis type II: Extensive dermal melanocytosis (mongolian spot) and port wine stain.

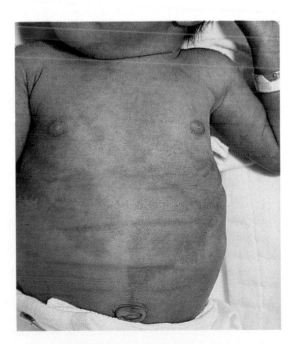

FIG. 20-11
Striped hyperpigmentation of the torso.

that decreased as the hyperpigmentation appeared. The dark stripes faded after a few months, and the skin became normal except for mild changes of ichthyosis vulgaris.[48] There were no known associations or signs of systemic disease. It was hypothesized that embryonal skin was unable to exfoliate normally, and that this was preceded by folding and fissuring of skin that promoted melanogenesis. Biopsy was not performed.

SPOTTY PIGMENTATION—DIFFUSE

Xeroderma Pigmentosum

Xeroderma pigmentosum is a severe, rare disease of autosomal recessive inheritance with clinical and cellular sensitivity to ultraviolet (UV) light, caused by decreased ability to repair DNA damage. Patients experience cutaneous and ocular photosensitivity and malignancies with pigment abnormalities.

The skin is normal at birth, but can start showing changes soon thereafter depending on the amount of UV exposure. An early sign may be acute sunburn reactions to minimal amounts of light, though not all patients have this. Subsequently, patients develop numerous pigmented macules (0.2 to 1 cm) on all sun-exposed areas. The number of macules correlates with sun exposure. Pigmented lesions may be brown, gray, or black, and may be so dense that they coalesce. Although they resemble freckles, they are actually solar lentigines, and do not fade with time.[49] Each macule is a clone of cells derived from a single mutated melanocyte.[50] Achromic spots, which may represent mutated melanocytes that have lost their ability to synthesize melanin, may also develop. After continued exposure, the skin enters a telangiectatic or atrophic stage. Skin malignancies may appear during the pigmented stage, but become more frequent in the atrophic stage. These include basal cell carcinomas, squamous cell carcinomas, and melanoma, as well as other rarer skin tumors.[50-52]

In approximately 20% of patients, there are neurological problems, including low intelligence, cerebral and cerebellar dysfunction, peripheral neuropathy, basal ganglia involvement, hyporeflexia, spasticity, sensory defects, and progressive dementia.[50,51] An increase in internal malignancies has been reported.

Xeroderma pigmentosum is found in all races worldwide, and is (so far) divided into 10 complementation groups (A, B, C, D, E, F, G, H, I, and Variant) based on in-vitro cell-fusion studies. Different races often have one dominant complementation group, and some groups consist of a single kindred. In groups A through I, the cause is a genetic mutation (different in each group) that impairs removal of pyrimidine dimers in DNA damaged by UV because of a defect in endonuclease activity. Functional endonuclease recognizes and removes damaged DNA regions so that other enzymes can initiate DNA repair (unscheduled DNA synthesis). In the Variant form, initiation of repair occurs normally, but a later step in postreplication repair is defective.[50,51]

There are no findings of xeroderma pigmentosum at birth, as there is only damage to the skin after exposure to UV light. A history of a young child developing erythema, lentigines, and increased pigmentation after UV exposure, particularly with conjunctivitis and photophobia, should prompt consideration of xeroderma pigmentosum. Other photosensitivity disorders, such as Cockayne syndrome (atrophy of the skin with telangiectasia) or trichothiodystrophy (brittle hair, ichthyosis, abnormal nails), should be easy to differentiate based on the clinical examination. Although erythropoietic protoporphyria has more burning pain and fewer skin findings, and erythropoietic porphyria (Günther) displays blistering, porphyrin screening is still recommended in suspected xeroderma pigmentosum cases. Hereditary polymorphous light eruption can cause similar symptoms, but without early malignancy. Peutz-Jeghers syndrome presents with the pigmented macules limited to the perioral skin and oral mucosa. Syndromes such as Rothmund-Thomson, Hartnup, or Bloom may display photosensitivity, but patients do not tend to have the hyperpigmented lesions of xeroderma pigmentosum.[53]

The histopathologic changes are nondiagnostic; lesional skin may show changes of severe photoaging, lentigines, or skin malignancy.[7] Specialized diagnostic tests may be performed from a specimen of nonlesional skin processed for cell culture. Select laboratories (such as the Armed Forces Institute of Pathology) can perform tests such as UV sensitivity or unscheduled DNA repair, which can confirm the diagnosis. Some centers can also perform similar testing for prenatal diagnosis on cultured cells from amniocentesis if there is a family history of xeroderma pigmentosum.[54]

The severity of xeroderma pigmentosum varies, depending on the particular defect and the amount of UV exposure. The most severely affected usually die of cancer before 10 years of age. Management involves genetic counseling, meticulous light avoidance, protective clothing, sunscreen, sunglasses, window coatings, long hairstyles, and methylcellulose eye drops for moist corneas. Skin examinations need to be frequent and thorough to catch premalignant/malignant changes early so they can be treated with cryosurgery, topical antimitotic agents such as 5-fluorouracil, or surgery. In some patients, high-dose oral isotretinoin can prevent new cancer formation, but is associated with side effects, especially in children.[55] Treatment with liposome-encapsulated endonuclease is under study, and may show promise for the future, as may advances in gene therapy.

Cutaneous Mastocytosis (Urticaria Pigmentosa)

Cutaneous mastocytosis, or urticaria pigmentosa (see Chapter 23), may develop in infancy or early childhood and is characterized by several to hundreds of brown, reddish-brown, or yellow macules, papules, and nodules composed of populations of cutaneous mast cells (see Figs. 23-6 and 23-7). Lesions can be single (solitary mastocytoma), multiple, or diffusely involve the skin surface. They are commonly on the trunk and extremities, but may be anywhere on the body, although infrequently on the scalp, palms, and soles, and are rarely on buccal, palatal, or pharyngeal mucosa or other mucous membranes. Lesions usually urticate in the characteristic manner when traumatized by friction (Darier's sign). In one study, 15% of patients had lesions at birth, and 64% of cases were apparent by age 6 months.[56]

The lesions tend to be larger on young children than adults, oval or round in shape, and usually between 1 and 10 mm in diameter. Vesicles or bullae may occur; recurrent blisters in the same anatomic location in the first few months of life should prompt consideration of mastocytosis.

The clinical appearance is often sufficient for diagnosis, especially if Darier's sign is present. Dermatographism of uninvolved skin occurs in 30% to 50% of all patients, due to an increase in mast cells throughout the dermis of normal skin, but in itself is not diagnostic.[56,57] Histopathologic examination demonstrates an infiltrate of mast cells in the upper third of the dermis, generally located around capillaries. In the larger papules, the cells may be packed into tumorlike aggregates.

Postinflammatory Hyperpigmentation

Postinflammatory hyperpigmentation refers to brown macules and patches in the skin, seen after an inflammatory condition. Lesions consistent with postinflammatory hyperpigmentation have been seen at birth, and certainly may develop within the first few weeks of life onward. Common factors inducing postinflammatory hyperpigmentation in hospitalized neonates include tape, adhesive monitor leads, and mechanical trauma, which may form distinct patterns. An indistinct pattern may form secondary to eczematous processes.

The dermal-epidermal junction and basal layer are disrupted due to epidermal injury (damaged epidermal keratinocytes and melanocytes). Melanin passes from its normal epidermal position into the dermis and is engulfed by macrophages to form melanophages.[58] This dermal melanin is slow to break down, causing delays in resolution of skin discoloration.

Diagnosis may be a process of exclusion. A clinical history of brown macules or patches that occur subsequent to inflammation in a corresponding pattern is suggestive. If the preceding inflammatory event was not noted, however, the appearance of the pigmentation often gives few clues to the nature of the cause. A Wood's light examination accentuates epidermal melanin and can be useful in delimiting the extent of pigment alteration. Biopsy is rarely indicated, but is characterized by melanophages in the superficial dermis along with a variably dense infiltrate of lymphohistiocytes around the superficial blood vessels and in dermal papillae. Necrotic keratinocytes and coarse collagen bundles are occasionally seen. There is increased pigment in the basal layer.[7,58]

The differential diagnosis of postinflammatory hyperpigmentation includes fixed drug eruption, which usually has more of a blue tint and appears after exposure to the causative drug. Postinflammatory hyperpigmentation may be seen as a sequela of transient neonatal pustular melanosis either at birth or after resolution of pustular lesions (see Chapter 7). Interestingly, biopsy does not show dermal melanophages.[58] **Striped hyperpigmentation of the torso** may also be a postinflammatory phenomenon.[48]

Prevention includes avoidance of frictional injury or inflammation. A low-potency topical steroid may help calm residual inflammation. Hyperpigmentation usually fades spontaneously with time.

Universal Melanosis

There are several progressive conditions in which the patient demonstrates patches of hyperpigmentation at birth or during infancy. In addition to the skin, including the palms and soles, they involve the oral mucosa, conjunctiva, and sclera. **Familial progressive hyperpigmentation** displays hyperpigmentation in varying-sized dots, whorls, streaks, and patches, not apparently following the lines of Blaschko,[59] whereas in **universal acquired melanosis (carbon baby),** the entire skin becomes deep black.[60] There are no known extracutaneous findings, and the etiologies are unknown.

Biopsy shows hyperpigmentation of the basal layer with pigment up to the stratum corneum. There are normal numbers of melanocytes, and some dermal melano-phages.[59,60] The clinical features, as well as the absence of significant melanin incontinence, should differentiate these conditions from incontinentia pigmenti, Naegeli-Franceschetti-Jadassohn syndrome, and linear and whorled nevoid hyperpigmentation.[59,60]

Poikiloderma

The term *poikiloderma* describes a tetrad of findings that characterize a number of photosensitivity syndromes that include the following:

- Telangiectasia (permanent dilatation of capillaries, venules, and arterioles in skin)
- Atrophy (cutaneous changes that result in thinning of epidermis, dermis, or both)
- Hyperpigmentation
- Hypopigmentation

Poikiloderma can be present at birth, beginning as diffuse erythema, evolving into a red-reticulated dermatosis. It generally appears first on the cheeks, then spreads to the buttocks, extensor surfaces of hands, forearms, and legs.[61]

Poikiloderma can be seen in a number of syndromes, including poikiloderma congenitale (Rothmund-Thomson syndrome), Bloom syndrome, Kindler syndrome, and dyskeratosis congenita. It may be a later finding in conditions such as xeroderma pigmentosum, connective tissue disorders, Cockayne syndrome, and Fanconi anemia.[61]

The pathogenesis and etiology are unknown. It is a finding in a number of disorders with differing causes, and is exacerbated by light exposure.

Diagnosis is made by the clinical appearance of the reticulated eruption. Biopsy results will differ depending on the severity. Abnormal findings include varying degrees of epidermal thinning with hyperkeratosis, dilated vessels, hydropic degeneration of the basal layer, variable numbers of pigment-laden melanophages, and a bandlike or perivascular lymphocytic infiltrate in the dermis.[7,61] Prognosis depends on the particular condition. Early recognition of the correct diagnosis, careful monitoring of the patient for associated abnormalities, and sun protection are all critical.[61]

Metabolic Causes

Addison Disease and Adrenocortical-Unresponsiveness Syndrome

Addison disease is caused by deficiency of adrenocortical hormones. Changes in pigmentation, including diffuse tan, brown, or bronze darkening of all skin surfaces, especially exposed areas, and blue-black patches on mucous membranes. Associated signs and symptoms such as weakness, weight loss, and hypotension may be present. Hyponatremia, hyperkalemia, hypoglycemia, and eosinophilia accompany these changes. The prohormone proopiomelanocortin is secreted and cleaved, producing excessive ACTH and β-MSH (melanocyte-stimulating hormone). The increased level of β-MSH stimulates production of melanin.[62,63]

Congenital insensitivity to functionally normal ACTH secretion has been termed *ACTH-insensitivity syndrome,* or adrenocortical-unresponsiveness syndrome.[64,65] Diffuse hyperpigmentation in the neonatal period may herald this condition before clinical hypoadrenalism. The histologic findings are nondiagnostic, and include increased amounts of melanin in the basal keratinocytes and often in the keratinocytes in the upper spinous layer. The number of melanocytes is not increased.[7]

LENTIGINES

Spotty Pigmentation–Diffuse, With Lentigines

LEOPARD Syndrome (Multiple Lentigines Syndrome, Moynahan Syndrome)

LEOPARD is an acronym for the following:

Lentigines
Electrocardiographic conduction defects
Ocular hypertelorism
Pulmonary stenosis
Abnormalities of genitalia
Retardation of growth, and
sensorineural **D**eafness.

It is a syndrome of probable autosomal dominant inheritance with variable expressivity involving multiple organ systems.[66] The lentigines may be present at birth, increasing in number until puberty, and are most numerous on the face, neck, upper trunk, upper arms, and diffusely elsewhere, but spare the mucous membranes.[66]

A variety of extracutaneous abnormalities with variable expressivity have been associated.[66-69] Cardiac abnormalities include conduction defects and pulmonary or subaortic stenosis. Genital anomalies include gonadal hypoplasia, hypospadias, undescended testes, hypoplastic testes/ovaries, and delayed puberty. Short stature, pectus excavatum, kyphosis, ocular hypertelorism, mandibular prognathism, and other craniofacial defects constitute the skeletal abnormalities. Neurological findings include sensorineural deafness, mental retardation, seizures, abnormal nerve conduction, oculomotor defects, and an abnormal electroencephalogram (EEG).

The pathogenesis and etiology are unknown. Since most of the extracutaneous findings do not occur until puberty, a firm diagnosis before that may not be possible. The family history may be useful.[66] In the neonatal period, evaluation of a suspected case should include complete physical examination for associated extracutaneous findings, electrocardiogram (ECG), hearing evaluation, and other studies as directed by symptomatology. Patients with suspected LEOPARD syndrome should have chest x-rays and ECGs periodically throughout childhood.[66,67]

On biopsy, the pigmented lesions are typical for lentigines, showing elongation of the rete ridges, increase in concentration in melanocytes in the basal layer, an increase in the amount of melanin in both the melanocytes and the basal keratinocytes, and the presence of melanophages in the upper dermis.[7,66,68]

Differential diagnosis includes generalized lentiginosis and inherited patterned lentiginosis, Carney/NAME/LAMB syndrome (see the following discussion), and Peutz-Jeghers syndrome (see the following discussion). Xeroderma pigmentosa patients can have widespread lentigines, but these are related to UV exposure and would not be present at birth. Associated abnormalities should be managed, and genetic counseling should be provided. There are reports of treatment of lentigines by cryotherapy and other surgical means.[70]

Carney/NAME/LAMB Syndrome

Several previously described syndromes have recently been consolidated under the classification of Carney syndrome, since it is now believed that they represent various manifestations of the same complex. These include the **NAME** syndrome (Nevi, Atrial myxoma, Myxoid neurofibromata, Ephelides) and the **LAMB** syndrome (Lentigines, Atrial myxoma, Myxoid tumors, and Blue nevi).[33] Spotty pigmentation, mainly lentigines, is seen in the majority of patients (65%), but blue and junctional nevi may also occur.[33] The lentigines may be present at birth, have the highest concentration in the central face, and in contrast to LEOPARD syndrome, may involve the mucosa. They can also involve the neck, trunk, extremities, and genitalia. Cutaneous myxomas, nontender dermal nodules, usually do not develop until the second decade of life, and typically are on the head and neck.[71,72] Psammomatous melanotic schwannomas may occur subcutaneously, but are usually in the nerve roots or GI tract, and do not appear until the third decade of life. This is an autosomal dominant-inherited disorder of suspected neuroectodermal origin. The defective gene has been mapped to chromosome 2p.[73] Candidate genes include those involved in tumor suppression and control of the cell cycle, as well as those with specific effects on the function and growth of mesenchymal cells and melanocytes.

The diagnosis of Carney requires two or more of the following findings[1,33]:

- Spotty skin pigmentation (lentigines, blue nevi)
- Cutaneous myxomas
- Myxoid mammary fibroadenomas
- Primary pigmented nodular adrenocortical disease
- Testicular Sertoli cell tumors
- Pituitary adenomas with acromegaly or gigantism
- Cardiac myxomas
- Psammomatous melanotic schwannomas

Biopsy reveals findings typical of lentigines (as described in LEOPARD syndrome).[7] This condition needs to be differentiated from LEOPARD and Peutz-Jeghers syndromes. Neurofibromatosis is distinguished by freckling restricted to the axillary/groin/neck areas.[9] If a neonate has skin findings suggestive of Carney syndrome, electrocardiogram, echocardiography, and biopsy of a suspected blue nevus should be considered.[33]

Localized, Spotty Pigmentation

Zosteriform Lentiginous Nevus

Zosteriform lentiginous nevus is morphologically similar to nevus spilus, but in a larger dermatomal or segmental distribution. Clinical and semantic overlap exists with unilateral lentiginosis, segmental lentiginosis, lentiginous mosaicism, and speckled giant café au lait macule.[74,75] Onset is generally at birth or in early childhood, though lesions may continue to evolve into adulthood. Lesions usually respect the midline. Histologic examination shows a lentigines pattern or increased basilar melanocytes. They may have nests of melanocytes at the dermal-epidermal junction, which has also been termed a "jentigo" pattern. Axillary lesions may suggest the diagnosis of neurofibromatosis, though the unilateral or segmental cut-off and histology displaying increased number of melanocytes allow differentiation. Segmental lentiginosis is considered by many to be a distinct condition (see the following discussion).[76] Extracutaneous findings have been reported primarily in patients with segmental lentiginosis. Rare cases of melanoma arising within zosteriform lentiginous nevi have been reported.[77] Observation of lesions is reasonable due to the apparently rarity of malignancy, though excision might be considered if marked atypical nevus elements are present on biopsy. Cryotherapy and various lasers may be of benefit in some patients.

Centrofacial Lentiginosis

These patients develop lentigines over the nose and cheeks in early childhood. The mucosa is spared, and there may be associated extracutaneous abnormalities. Neonatal presentation has not been reported.[78]

Segmental Lentiginosis (Partial Unilateral Lentiginosis, Lentiginous Mosaicism)

This rare pigmentary disorder consists of clustered lentigines in a segmental pattern. Lentigines may be present at birth or manifest in early childhood. Individual lesions are small, well-circumscribed, hyperpigmented macules grouped on a background of normal-appearing skin. This is in contrast to speckled (zosteriform) lentiginous nevus, which has similar macules on a slightly hyperpigmented background.[74,75,79] Associated ipsilateral cerebrovascular hypertrophy and proliferation, and prominent neuropsychiatric findings with ipsilateral pes cavus have been reported.[80] There is speculation that affected individuals are mosaics of one of the more generalized lentigines syndromes.

Biopsy of lesions demonstrates findings typical of lentigo, including elongation of the rete ridges, an increase in the concentration of melanocytes in the basal layer, an increase in the amount of melanin in both the melanocytes and the basal keratinocytes, and the presence of melanophages in the upper dermis.[80] In a few cases the histological picture has appeared to represent a combination of lentigo and junctional nevus patterns.[74]

It may be difficult to distinguish segmental lentiginosis from zosteriform lentiginous nevus, agminated Spitz nevi, and segmental NF. Signs and symptoms that might indicate an alternative diagnosis should be looked for. Examination of the skin with Wood's light, and skin biopsy may be indicated.[1] Cryotherapy and pigment lasers may be useful in removing the lentigines, if desired.[8] Prognosis depends on the specific systemic abnormalities.

Peutz-Jeghers Syndrome

Peutz-Jeghers syndrome is an autosomal dominant-inherited disorder with variable expressivity, characterized by mucocutaneous pigmentation and GI polyps. The lesions are dark-brown to black, 1 to 5 mm, irregular macules that primarily involve the lips and buccal mucosa, but may also involve the palate, gingiva, face, fingers, elbows, palms, toes, and rarely even the periumbilical, perianal, or labial areas (Fig. 20-12).[81,82] There may be pigmented bands in the nail plates.[1] Hyperpigmented macules may be present at birth, but often develop later.

Later in life these patients develop hamartomatous polyps in the jejunum, ileum, colon, rectum, stomach,

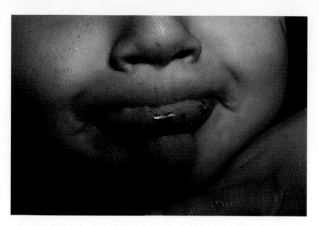

FIG. 20-12
Peutz-Jehger syndrome. Hyperpigmented labial macules.

and duodenum, resulting in crampy pain, intussusception, and rectal bleeding. There can also be adenomatous polyps, and there is a slightly increased risk of gastrointestinal (GI) and other cancers, such as breast, cervix, uterus, lung, and testes in later life.[81,82]

A mutation has been identified in the gene for serine threonine kinase 11 (STK 11) on the short arm of chromosome 19. The disease manifestations are triggered by the loss of the functional copy of this gene in somatic cells. The mechanism by which this gene controls cellular differentiation is unknown.[83]

The histopathology of the pigmented lesions is typical for lentigines, that is, elongation of the rete ridges, increase in concentration of melanocytes in the basal layer, an increase in the amount of melanin in both the melanocytes and the basal keratinocytes, and the presence of melanophages in the upper dermis.[7] Abdominal pain, melena, or intussusception may be the presenting sign in older patients.[81,82] Facial lentigines may also be seen during the neonatal period in LEOPARD syndrome, NAME/LAMB/ Carney syndrome, and generalized lentiginosis. Labial melanosis may occur secondary to photo or sun damage, but would not involve the oral mucosa, nor be seen during the neonatal period.

Hematocrits and stool guaiacs should be performed at regular intervals in later childhood. Most of the GI polyps are not premalignant, but may cause symptoms requiring surgical intervention for relief. Referral to gastroenterology is prudent, as well as serial examination for malignancy of the GI tract and other associated organs. The cutaneous macules may fade after puberty, but the mucosal ones do not.[81,82] The macules may respond to treatment with liquid nitrogen or a pigment laser.

Bannayan-Riley-Ruvalcaba Syndrome

Bannayan-Riley-Ruvalcaba syndrome, a unifying term proposed to reflect overlap among three previously described conditions (Bannayan-Zonana, Riley-Smith, and Ruvalcaba-Myhre-Smith syndromes), is a condition with phenotypic variability with the common clinical features of macrocephaly with normal ventricular size, multiple subcutaneous and/or visceral lipomas, and vascular malformations, intestinal hamartomatous polyps, and lentigines of the penis and vulva.[84-86]

Pigmented macules, 2 to 6 mm in diameter, consistent with lentigines, occur on the glans and shaft of the penis. Lesions may be present at birth, or develop postnatally through adolescence.[85,87] Vulvar lesions have been reported in affected females. Café au lait macules, single or multiple, may be observed. Other reported mucocutaneous findings include multiple subcutaneous lipomas, vascular malformations (termed *hemangiomas* in several reported cases), facial papules displaying features of trichilemmomas and verrucae, oral and perianal papillomas, acrochordons, acral keratoses, and acanthosis nigricans.

Macrocephaly (and macrosomia) is usually noted at birth or in early infancy. Central nervous system manifestations include hypotonia, developmental delay, mental retardation, seizures, arteriovenous malformations, meningiomas, and pseudopapilledema. Skeletal features include pectus excavatum, scoliosis and kyphoscoliosis, accelerated growth of digits, and high arched palate. Hamartomatous polyps of the GI tract are seen in almost half of the patients, but are not clinically significant in neonates. Lipid storage myopathy may present with increased limb size.[88] Ocular abnormalities include prominent Schwalbe lines and corneal nerves, strabismus, and amblyopia. Thyroiditis, adenomatous goiter, and thyroid carcinoma have been reported.

Autosomal dominant inheritance is observed, with sporadic occurrences and phenotypic variability. Germ-line mutations in PTEN, a tyrosine phosphatase and putative tumor suppressor gene, have been demonstrated in some families with Bannayan-Riley-Ruvalcaba syndrome, correlating with chromatin loss on chromosome 10q23.[25,89] Allelism with Cowden disease has been proposed. However, PTEN germ-line mutations were absent in several patients with sporadic Bannayan-Riley-Ruvalcaba syndrome.[90] Lipid-storage myopathy in a patient with Bannayan-Riley-Ruvalcaba syndrome has been attributed to long-chain L-3 hydroxyacyl-Coenzyme A dehydrogenase (L-CHAD) deficiency.[88]

Biopsy of the hyperpigmented penile macules display lentiginous hyperplasia of the epidermis with increased pigment in the basal layer and slight increase in the melanocyte number. Cowden disease (multiple hamartoma syndrome) has many features in common, and may be allelic or have common genetic expression with Bannayan-Riley-Ruvalcaba syndrome, but it does not have neonatal manifestations. Lentiginosis with intestinal polyposis is seen with Peutz-Jeghers syndrome and Cronkhite-Canada syndrome, though the distribution of lentigines is different. Proteus syndrome (skull exostoses, epidermal nevi, pigmentary changes along Blaschko's lines, and palmoplantar masses) should be easily distinguishable. Recognition of the disease and specialty referral for management of systemic associations is appropriate.

PIGMENTARY VARIATIONS

Dyschromatosis

The dyschromatoses are a group of disorders characterized by both macular hyperpigmentation and hypopigmentation without atrophy or telangiectasia as seen in poikiloderma. Cases are extremely rare, and have been reported most commonly from Japan.[91] **Dyschromatosis universalis hereditaria** presents with generalized well-demarcated brown macules with various-sized hypopigmented macules. Cases have been reported with sparing of the face, hands, and feet, and generalized leukomelanoderma and leukotrichia have been observed.[92] Rare cases of universal dyschromia have been reported with small stature, high-tone deafness, idiopathic torsion dystonia, X-linked ocular albinism, photosensitivity, and neurosensory hearing loss.[93-95] Tissue histopathology shows increased epidermal melanin in the hyperpigmented areas without increased melanocyte number. Achromic skin shows an absence of melanin despite intact melanocytes, suggesting a disorder of melanosome production and distribution.[96] **Dyschromatosis symmetrica hereditaria** (reticulate acropigmentation of Dohi) presents with dyschromia restricted to sun-exposed skin, with distribution usually on the dorsal aspects of the extremities and face.[97] Findings generally develop after infancy. There is uncertainty if this condition is functionally related to the universal type.

Pigmentary Demarcation Lines

Pigmentary demarcation lines have been described and categorized into five types. They are most commonly seen in black and Asian individuals.[98,99] Type A (anterobrachial demarcation) is a line extending from the presternal area to the antecubital fossa on the dorsal-ventral surface of the upper arms. It is seen in 16% to 26% of blacks and 6% of Japanese adults. Type B is on the lower extremities in the posterior-medial position, and is seen in 40% of black adults. Type C is paired hypopigmented lines in a vertical direction from the clavicular area to the inferior sternal border. Type D is a hyperpigmented line on the midback, occurring rarely in Asians. Type E is periareolar hypopigmentation, seen in 69% of black children and often becoming less noticeable with age.

MELANOCYTIC NEVI

Congenital melanocytic nevi (CMN) are proliferations of nested melanocytes in the skin present at birth or appearing in the first few months of life. Various classification schemes exist, and although not based on biologic principles, congenital nevi are usually categorized based on the size of the largest lesional diameter.[100,101] Several definitions have been used to define large congenital nevi, with the most common being a size of 20 cm or greater in adolescents or adults. Small congenital nevi are lesions 1 to 1.5 cm or less in size (Fig. 20-13), and intermediate sized lesions range

from 1 to 1.5 cm up to 20 cm (Fig. 20-14). Size assessments are generally based on adult size, and since lesions grow proportionate with the individual, lesions approximately 9 cm in diameter on the head or 6 cm on the body in a neonate may be considered large congenital melanocytic nevi (LCMN), or giant. Other names for LCMN include "garment," "bathing trunk," or "giant hairy nevi."

The nevi are tan, brown to dark brown macules, papules, or plaques at birth. Color is quite variable, with some lesions having black or purple foci, whereas others are light tan, mimicking café au lait spots. They may have a smooth, nodular, verrucous, or rough cobblestone-like texture. Lesions may or may not have hair. The presence or absence of hair does not indicate malignant potential. The hairs may vary from light vellus to long, coarse, and darkly pigmented terminal hair. Scalp lesions may be cerebriform, similar to cutis verticis gyrata.

Small and Intermediate Congenital Nevi

Small nevi are seen in 1% to 2% of newborns, intermediate-sized lesions in 0.6%, and LCMN in no more than 0.02%.[102-104] The risk of malignant melanoma arising within small and intermediate congenital melanocytic nevi is quite small, though prospective data are limited. Estimates range greatly, with several studies suggesting that there may not be a clinically significant increased risk for melanoma arising in banal-appearing, medium-sized CMN or small congenital nevi, while rare cases of prepubertal melanoma have been reported in intermediate-sized lesions.[105-107] Based on histologic retrospective findings of contiguous dermal nevi suggestive of congenital

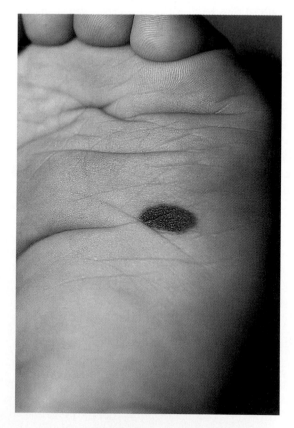

FIG. 20-13
Small congenital nevus.

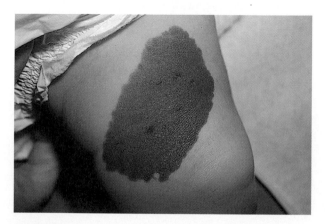

FIG. 20-14
Intermediate-sized congenital melanocytic nevus with irregular hyperpigmentation.

nevi in continuity with melanomas, rates of melanoma arising in small CMN range from 2.6% to 8.1%.[108,109] Although it does appear that there is some risk for melanoma developing within both small and intermediate CMN, neonatal risk is minimal, and the extent of lifetime risk is uncertain and low. Factors other than size that may confer added risk of malignant transformation are unknown (e.g., family history, sun exposure).

A number of congenital disorders include increased numbers of small congenital and acquired nevi as a clinical feature.[110] In many cases a critical reading of the literature raises the issue of whether the lesions described are truly melanocytic nevi or rather other melanocytic proliferations such as lentigines, or freckles, and whether the nevi are truly an associated finding or merely a chance occurrence.

Differential diagnosis includes smooth muscle hamartoma, urticaria pigmentosa, nevus spilus, and in early life, café au lait spots. The histologic appearance may be the same as acquired nevi or may show features diagnostic of congenital nevi.[108,111] Lesions may be junctional, compound, or intradermal, superficial, or deep. Features considered useful in differentiating congenital lesions from acquired nevi include presence of melanocytes around and within hair follicles, sweat ducts, eccrine glands, vessel walls and perineurium of nerves, extension between collagen bundles in rows, or extension into deep reticular dermis or subcutis.[112] However, these features may be seen in acquired lesions, and it is unknown if the features defining "nevi with histologic pattern of the congenital type" are of any significance as risk markers for melanoma.[34]

Management of small and intermediate congenital nevi is controversial, secondary to limited studies on the natural history.[113,114] Most small and intermediate CMN may be managed during childhood by observation alone, commonly with photographic documentation. However, management may be individualized, with factors in decision making about surgical excision including the appearance of the lesion (color, presence of papules or nodules), location of the lesion, ease of excision (easily performed under local anesthesia versus staged excisions under general anesthesia), and expected cosmetic result. Laser treatment (e.g., Q-switched laser) has been advocated for small congenital nevi, but often yields only temporary improvement without completely removing the melanocytes.[115]

Large Congenital Melanocytic Nevi

LCMN are most common on the posterior trunk, but may also be seen on the anterior and lateral trunk, head and neck, or extremities (Fig. 20-15).[116,117] Multiple small satellite CMN are seen in the majority of patients with LCMN and often continue to develop over time.[117,118] Dermatomal distribution of congenital nevi has been reported rarely.[119] LCMN may have multiple pink to purple areas that may mimic melanoma, or be mistaken for open neural tube defects or hemangiomas.[53] Erosions may be present at birth or in early infancy, and may represent benign superficial epidermal breakdown or melanoma (Fig. 20-16).[120] Intradermal nevi may develop within giant nevi as slow-growing, firm, asymptomatic nodules.

Large congenital nevi of the scalp and dorsal axis have been associated with neurocutaneous melanosis (NCM), also known as leptomeningeal melanosis (LMM) (see the following section). Limb hypoplasia with reduction in subcutaneous fat may be seen underlying giant congenital melanocytic nevi.[121] Large CMN in the lumbosacral area may be associated with spinal dysraphism, including myelomeningocele.[122,123] Malignant tumors reported to arise within LCMN other than melanoma include rhabdomyosarcoma, liposarcoma, neuroblastoma, prim-

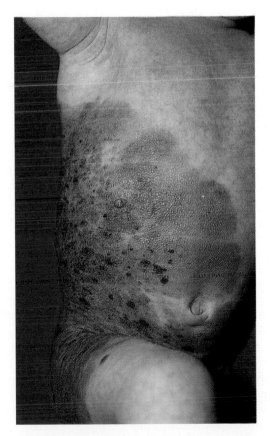

FIG. 20-15
Large congenital melanocytic nevus.

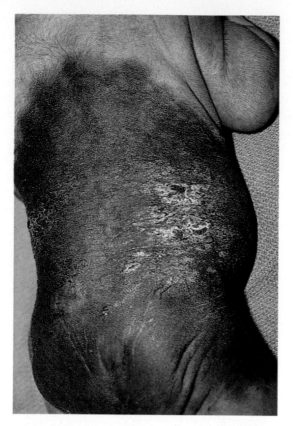

FIG. 20-16
Erosions within large congenital melanocytic nevus. Biopsy displayed features of a normal nevus of the congenital type.

itive neuroectodermal tumors, and mixed malignant neoplasms.[121,124,125]

Other reported associated malformations with LCMN include vascular malformations, supernumerary nipples, ear deformities, preauricular appendages, cryptorchidism, and clubfeet.[1] Large CMN (>10 cm) are reported in 2% of patients with neurofibromatosis type 1, a frequency greater than that of the general population. Care should be taken to distinguish pachydermatous overgrowth within LCMN from plexiform neurofibromas, since they are distinct entities.[119]

Cutaneous melanoma may arise from LCMN from both epidermal and nonepidermal sites.[126] The lifetime risk of melanoma associated with LCMN is difficult to determine precisely. Methodological problems in study design and hampering study comparisons include differing size definitions, histologic overdiagnosis of melanoma in the newborn period, varying ages of entry of patients into studies, and failure to consider the impact of surgical ex-

cision or partial excision. Most investigators, however, estimate the lifetime risk of melanoma in a patient with LCMN to be approximately 6% to 8%.[116,117,121,126-128] Onset of melanomas in utero has been reported. Approximately half of melanomas associated with LCMN may occur by 3 to 5 years of age, and the greatest risk for malignant transformation appears to be in the prepubertal years.[117] LCMN on the extremities appear to have a markedly lower risk of melanoma than those in an axial location. No cases of melanoma have been reported as having arisen from satellite nevi. Melanomas associated with LCMN appear to have a poorer prognosis than de novo melanomas, with earlier development of metastatic disease.[129]

Congenital nevi are proliferations of melanocytes and may be considered as hamartomas or benign neoplasms of melanocytic cells. Lesions that are clinically and histologically consistent with congenital nevi may appear weeks or months after birth, and it is believed that these lesions were present in the skin but inapparent. Some have used the term *tardive congenital nevi* for these lesions. The mechanisms of malignant transformation of CMN are uncertain. Congenital nevi may have higher numbers of estrogen and progesterone binding cells as compared with acquired melanocytic nevi, similar to malignant melanoma and dysplastic nevi.[130] Chromosomal abnormalities have been documented in some lesions; whereas LCMN are genetically polyclonal, melanomas arising within LCMN are monoclonal neoplasms.[131] DNA content of melanocyte nuclei has shown more aneuploidy relative to acquired nevi.[132]

Most CMN will grow proportionately with the anatomic site, though certain studies have found that some smaller lesions do not appear to grow with time, and that some will have disproportionately rapid expansion.[133-135] CMNs may evolve with change in texture and color. Some LCMN may decrease in pigment after birth, whereas other lesions may darken with age focally or generally.[117,136] Papules and nodules may develop with time, most commonly in the first 2 years of life. Histologically, these lesions may be benign intradermal nevi, atypical melanocytic nevi with dysplasia, or unusual dysplastic or hamartoma-like lesions, including neurocristic dysplastic, neural crest hamartomas, spindle cell tumors, and neurofibromas.[117] Melanomas may present with similar nodules, though rapid growth, ulceration, and regional lymph node enlargement are more suggestive of melanoma.

Differential diagnosis is as listed previously for small and intermediate sized congenital nevi. Melanoma arising within LCMN must be considered when there are lesional changes in color or the development of papules, nodules, or erosions though all of these may simply indicate normal maturation of the lesion. Early lesions may appear identical to café au lait macules, though speckled pigmentation or a papular component may differentiate CMN.

A biopsy should be diagnostic, displaying a benign proliferation of melanocytes in a nested pattern, which may extend from the superficial epidermis through the subcutaneous fat. Congenital nevi may have melanocytes that are fully intraepidermal in location (junctional melanocytic nevi), though more commonly melanocytes will be present in the reticular dermis and below. Dermal congenital nevi without an epidermal component may also be seen.[137] Common features in larger lesions include melanocytes around or within epithelial structures of adnexa (including hair follicles and eccrine ducts), nonepithelial adnexa (hair erectile muscle, smooth muscle, and nerve fascicles) and around venules.[138-140] Larger CMN display melanocytes situated in the lower two thirds of the reticular dermis, and in subcutaneous fat, and may extend into fascia, skeletal muscles, and occasionally lymph nodes. However, histologic features of small congenital nevi may not display similar patterns of melanocyte distribution.[111]

Differentiation from other pigmented lesions may be aided by use of staining techniques with antibodies to S100 protein and myelin basic protein: melanocytes are S100 positive; myelin basic protein is negative.[133] Melanocytic dysplasia and cytologic atypia are not common features of CMN in early infancy and childhood. Distinguishing abnormal histologic features from normal in large congenital nevi may be difficult, and expert dermatopathology consultation may be appropriate.

The management of large CMN should be individualized, with consideration of the risk of melanoma, risks and functional impact of surgery, disfigurement from the lesion or surgical intervention, and ease of observation of lesional changes. While data are insufficient to recommend prophylactic excision of all congenital nevi, many specialists recommend partial or complete excision of large CMN.[114,126] Surgical excision is often complex, requiring multiple surgeries, tissue expansion or grafting, and artificial skin replacement, and may not be technically feasible. Other surgical options that more superficially treat LCMN include curettage, which may be more effective in the first few weeks of life, dermabrasion, laser surgery (including carbon dioxide, ruby, and Q-switched lasers), cryosurgery, and electrocautery.[141-143] Spontaneous resolution of giant congenital melanotic nevi may occur due to vigorous host response against aberrant clone of melanocytes, which may suggest a possible therapeutic

option for those whose congenital nevi are not amenable to surgery.[144]

Neurocutaneous Melanosis

Neurocutaneous melanosis (NCM), also known as neurocutaneous melanocytosis or leptomeningeal melanosis, is a rare condition characterized by benign or malignant melanocytic infiltration of the leptomeninges associated with large or multiple (greater than 3) congenital melanocytic nevi.[145]

CMN on the posterior midline trunk, most commonly in the lumbosacral area, or on the head and neck are seen in virtually all patients with NCM. The appearance and histopathologic features of cutaneous lesions are not distinguishable from CMN not associated with NCM.

Macrocephaly may be seen in infants due to hydrocephalus with or without increased intracranial pressure, which may develop secondary to obstructed CSF flow, excess absorption due to subarachnoid infiltration by pigmented cells, or associated Dandy-Walker syndrome.[146] Leptomeningeal melanoma develops in 40% to 62% of symptomatic patients, often within the first few years of life, though delayed presentations after puberty are reported. Asymptomatic children with LCMN of the scalp, neck, and posterior midline trunk have distinctive MRI findings suggestive of leptomeningeal melanosis.[147] While the course of these children is unknown, it may be that the findings correlate to the biology of cutaneous congenital nevi; lesions may be present that are melanocytic hamartomas, with some small risk of symptomatic or malignant change. Interestingly children with neurologic alterations without evidence of NCM on CT or MRI scans have also been reported.[148]

The pathogenesis is considered to be due to an error in the morphogenesis of embryonal neuroectoderm, though the mechanisms are unknown. Diagnosis of leptomeningeal melanosis may be made with magnetic resonance imaging (MRI) with gadolinium, with hyperintense regions on T1-weighted images (T1-shortening) seen most commonly in the cerebellar hemispheres and anterior temporal lobes. A normal MRI does not fully rule out neurocutaneous melanosis, and cytologic examination of cerebrospinal fluid may be necessary. Differential diagnosis includes melanoma, including prenatal metastases.[146]

The prognosis of symptomatic NCM is poor, with death occurring within 3 years in more than half of patients, and in 70% within 10 years. Not all patients die from melanoma, as structural damage from benign lesions may be severe enough to cause death. Neurosurgical consultation is appropriate, though procedures may be palliative.

Spontaneous resolution of nodules presumed to be NCM has been reported, and the natural history of asymptomatic leptomeningeal melanosis is not fully known.

Congenital Malignant Melanoma

Congenital melanoma may present in neonates secondary to maternal melanoma, in association with a giant congenital melanocytic nevus, arising from leptomeningeal melanocytosis and de novo. Darkly pigmented, rapidly growing nodules, with or without ulceration may be the initial signs of malignant melanoma arising in each of the above settings. Prenatal metastatic disease has been reported. Care should be taken to have pathologic specimens examined by an experienced dermatopathologist, as misdiagnosis of benign congenital melanocytic nevi as melanoma is not uncommon. Congenital melanoma is discussed in more detail in Chapter 23.

Nevus Spilus (Speckled Lentiginous Nevus)

Nevus spilus, or speckled lentiginous nevus, is a circumscribed patch of hyperpigmentation with smaller, darker pigmented macules or papules within the patch. It is seen in 1.7 of 1000 newborns, though prevalence in white schoolchildren and adults has ranged from 1.3% to 2%.[4,24] There is no sex predilection. Solitary, non-hairy, flat, light to medium brown patches of pigmentation are generally present at birth. These are dotted by smaller dark brown to black freckle-like areas of pigmentation that may not appear until later in childhood. Acquired lesions are not uncommon (Fig. 20-17). Size is quite varied, from 1 cm to greater than 20 cm. Extensive lesions, including segmental (zosteriform lentinginous nevus), unilateral or generalized lesions, have been reported. Nevus spilus lesions that involve upper and lower eyelids have been reported, termed divided nevi, and are presumed to develop prior to eyelid separation at 12 to 14 weeks' gestational age.[149] Speckled areas, generally 2 to 4 mm in size, may continue to develop in childhood. Nevus spilus may be seen in association with vascular malformations in phakomatosis pigmentovascularis type III and IV.

Histologic features are increased epidermal hyperpigmentation often with macromelanosomes, or epidermal melanocytes with or without nest formation.[79] Some authors restrict the use of the term nevus spilus to lesions without increased melanocytes, though this is not a consistent semantic distinction. Speckled areas correspond to junctional or dermal melanocytes. Blue nevi or spindle and epithelioid nevi have been described as variants of speckles.

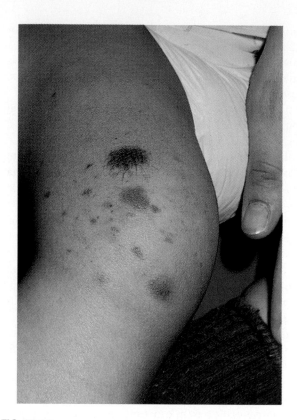

FIG. 20-17
Nevus spilus, with even-colored hyperpigmented background and brown, frecklelike pigmented areas within it.

Differential diagnosis includes café au lait spots, congenital melanocytic nevi, and Becker nevi. Rare cases of malignant melanoma arising from nevus spilus have been reported, though this has not been documented in the neonatal period. Observation for distinct pigmentary changes is reasonable, with excision considered only if histologic atypia is seen. Successful laser treatment with pigmented specific lesion lasers has been reported.[150]

Spindle and Epithelioid Cell Nevi (Spitz Nevi)

Spitz nevi, also known as spindle and epithelioid nevi, or in the past as benign juvenile melanoma, are variants of melanocytic nevi with spindle and epithelioid histologic appearance. Sophie Spitz first described these lesions in 1948.[151] Spitz nevi are commonly found in the first or second decade of life, and appear as hairless, red or brownish-red, smooth or verrucous, dome-shaped papules, 2 to 15 mm in size.

Congenital Spitz nevi may be present at birth or develop within the first few months of life. Typically they present as an area of hyperpigmentation, usually described as a café au lait spot with subsequent development of multiple agminated Spitz nevi.[152-154] Other presentations include isolated Spitz nevi present at birth, or developing within a compound nevus or congenital speckled lentiginous nevus.[155,156] There are no associated extracutaneous findings.

Histologic examination reveals collections of melanocytes with irregular cytoplasmic and nuclear shapes, in a spindle and epithelioid pattern. Surface telangiectasia may be prominent in lesions with reddish color resembling vascular tumors. Spindle and epithelioid nevi should be differentiated from intradermal melanocytic nevi, pyogenic granulomas, juvenile xanthogranulomas, mastocytomas, and malignant melanoma. Spitz nevi with atypical pathologic features should be evaluated by experienced dermatopathologists to rule out malignant melanoma. If atypia is confirmed, conservative reexcision is recommended.

Spitz nevi are benign melanocytic neoplasms, but can in some cases be difficult to distinguish histologically from melanoma. Although there is apparently no malignant potential, regional lymph node involvement has been reported.[153] Routine excision is advocated by many, due to concern over misdiagnosis of melanomas as Spitz nevi and uncertainty about the natural history of the tumors. Without excision, lesions may remain stable for years, evolve into compound nevi, flatten over time, or involute spontaneously.

REFERENCES

1. Salmon J, Frieden IJ. Congenital and genetic disorders of hyperpigmentation. Curr Prob Dermatol 1995;7:143-198.
2. Landau M, Krafchik B. The diagnostic value of café au lait macules. J Amer Acad Dermatol 1999;40:877-890.
3. Jacobs A. Birthmarks. Pediatr Ann 1976;5:743-758.
4. McLean DI, Gallagher RP. "Sunburn" freckles, café au lait macules, and other pigmented lesions of schoolchildren: The Vancouver Mole Study. J Am Acad Dermatol 1995;32:565-570.
5. Crowe FW, Schull WJ. Diagnostic importance of cafe-au-lait spots in neurofibromatosis. Arch Intern Med 1993;91:758-766.
6. Korf BR. Diagnostic outcome in children with multiple cafe au lait spots. Pediatrics 1992;90:924-927.
7. Elder D. Lever's histopathology of the skin. Philadelphia: Lippincott-Raven, 1997:pp 970, 980.
8. Shimbashi T, Kamide R, Hashimoto T. Long-term follow-up in treatment of solar lentigo and café au lait macules with Q-switched ruby laser. Aesthetic Plast Surg 1997;21:445-448.
9. Riccardi VM. Neurofibromatosis: Clinical heterogeneity. Curr Probl Cancer 1982;7:1-34.
10. Levine MA. The McCune-Albright syndrome. The whys and wherefores of abnormal signal transduction. N Engl J Med 1991;325:1738-1740.
11. Roth JG, Esterly NB. McCune-Albright syndrome with multiple bilateral cafe au lait spots. Pediatr Dermatol 1991;8:35-39.
12. Yoshimoto M, Nakayama M, Baba T, et al. A case of neonatal McCune-Albright syndrome with Cushing syndrome and hyperthyroidism. Acta Paediatr Scand 1991;80:984-987.
13. Shenker A, Weinstein LS, Moran A, et al. Severe endocrine and nonendocrine manifestations of the McCune-Albright syndrome associated with activating mutations of stimulatory G protein GS. J Pediatr 1993;123:509-518.
14. Aarskog D, Tveteraas E. McCune-Albright's syndrome following adrenalectomy for Cushing's syndrome in infancy. J Pediatr 1968;73:89-96.
15. Happle R. The McCune-Albright syndrome: A lethal gene surviving by mosaicism. Clin Genet 1986;29:321-324.
16. Rieger E, Kofler R, Borkenstein M, et al. Melanotic macules following Blaschko's lines in McCune-Albright syndrome. Br J Dermatol 1994;130:215-220.
17. Olsen BR. "A rare disorder, yes; an unimportant one, never." J Clin Invest 1998;101:1545-1546.
18. Metzker A, Morag C, Weitz R. Segmental pigmentation disorder. Acta Derm Venereol 1983;63:167-169.
19. Duncan PA, Hall JG, Shapiro LR, et al. Three-generation dominant transmission of the Silver-Russell syndrome. Am J Med Genet 1990;35:245-250.
20. Cordova A. The Mongolian spot: A study of ethnic differences and a literature review. Clin Pediatr 1981;20:714-719.
21. Jacobs A. The incidence of birthmarks in the neonate. Pediatrics 1976;58:218-222.
22. Ruiz-Maldonado R, Tamayo L, Laterza AM, et al. Phacomatosis pigmentovascularis: A new syndrome? Report of four cases. Pediatr Dermatol 1987;4:189-196.
23. Tang TT, Esterly NB, Lubinsky MS, et al. GM$_1$-gangliosidosis type 1 involving the cutaneous vascular endothelial cells in a black infant with multiple ectopic Mongolian spots. Acta Derm Venereol 1993;73:412-415.
24. Kopf AW, Bart RS. Malignant blue (Ota's?) nevus. J Dermatol Surg Oncol 1982;8:442-445.
25. Zigman AF, Lavine JE, Jones MC, et al. Localization of the Bannayan-Riley-Ruvalcaba syndrome gene to chromosome 10q23. Gastroenterology 1997;113:1433-1437.
26. Shimbashi T, Hyakusoku H, Okinaga M. Treatment of nevus of Ota by Q-switched ruby laser. Aesthetic Plast Surg 1997;21:118-121.
27. Raulin C, Schonermark MP, Greve B, Werner S. Q-switched ruby laser treatment of tattoos and benign pigmented skin lesions: A critical review. Ann Plast Surg 1998;41:555-565.
28. Okawa Y, Yokota R, Yamauchi A. On the extracellular sheath of dermal melanocytes in nevus fusco- ceruleus acromiodeltoideus (Ito) and Mongolian spot. An ultrastructural study. J Invest Dermatol 1979;73:224-230.
29. Radentz WH, Vogel P. Congenital common blue nevus. Arch Dermatol 1990;126:124-125.
30. Kawasaki T, Tsuboi R, Ueki R, et al. Congenital giant common blue nevus. J Am Acad Dermatol 1993;28:653-654.
31. Marano SR, Brooks RA, Spetzler RF, et al. Giant congenital cellular blue nevus of the scalp of a newborn with an underlying skull defect and invasion of the dura mater. Neurosurgery 1986;18:85-89.

32. Hofmann U, Wagner N, Grimm T, et al. [Linear and whorled nevoid hypermelanosis. Case report and review of the literature]. Hautarzt 1998;49:408-412.

33. Carney JA, Gordon H, Carpenter PC, et al. The complex of myxomas, spotty pigmentation, and endocrine overactivity. Medicine (Baltimore) 1985;64:270-283.

34. Elder D, Elenitsas R. Benign pigmented lesions and malignant melanoma. In Elder D, et al, eds. Lever's histopathology of the skin. Philadelphia: Raven Publishers, 1997:pp 626-630.

35. Van Gysel D, Oranje AP, Stroink H, et al. Phakomatosis pigmentovascularis. Pediatr Dermatol 1996;13:33-35.

36. Happle R, Hoffmann R, Restano L, et al. Phacomatosis pigmentokeratotica: A melanocytic-epidermal twin nevus syndrome. Am J Med Genet 1996;65:363-365.

37. Tadini G, Restano L, Gonzales-Perez R, et al. Phacomatosis pigmentokeratotica: Report of new cases and further delineation of the syndrome. Arch Dermatol 1998;134:333-337.

38. Koopman R. Concept of twin spotting. Am J Med Genet 1999;85:355-358.

39. Kalter DC, Griffiths WA, Atherton DJ. Linear and whorled nevoid hypermelanosis. J Am Acad Dermatol 1988;19:1037-1044.

40. Alvarez J, Peteiro C, Toribio J. Linear and whorled nevoid hypermelanosis. Pediatr Dermatol 1993;10:156-158.

41. Quecedo E, Febrer I, Aliaga A. Linear and whorled nevoid hypermelanosis. A spectrum of pigmentary disorders. Pediatr Dermatol 1997;14:247-248.

42. Akiyama M, Aranami A, Sasaki Y, et al. Familial linear and whorled nevoid hypermelanosis. J Am Acad Dermatol 1994;30:831-833.

43. Kubota Y, Shimura Y, Shimada S, et al. Linear and whorled nevoid hypermelanosis in a child with chromosomal mosaicism. Int J Dermatol 1992;31:345-347.

44. Roberts JL, Morrow B, Vega-Rich C, et al. Incontinentia pigmenti in a newborn male infant with DNA confirmation. Am J Med Genet 1998;75:159-163.

45. Wagner A. Distinguishing vesicular and pustular disorders in the neonate. Curr Opin Pediatr 1997;9:396-405.

46. Thyresson NH, Goldberg NC, Tye MJ, et al. Localization of eosinophil granule major basic protein in incontinentia pigmenti. Pediatr Dermatol 1991;8:102-106.

47. Itin PH, Lautenschlager S, Meyer R, et al. Natural history of the Naegeli-Franceschetti-Jadassohn syndrome and further delineation of its clinical manifestations. J Am Acad Dermatol 1993;28:942-950.

48. Gibbs RC. Unusual striped hyperpigmentation of the torso. A sequel of abnormalities of epitrichial exfoliation. Arch Dermatol 1967;95:385-386.

49. Kraemer KH. Xeroderma pigmentosum knockout mice: an immunologic tale. J Invest Dermatol 1996;107:291-292.

50. Robbins JH. Xeroderma pigmentosum. Defective DNA repair causes skin cancer and neurodegeneration. JAMA 1988;260:384-388.

51. Kraemer KH, Lee MM, Scotto J. Xeroderma pigmentosum. Cutaneous, ocular, and neurologic abnormalities in 830 published cases. Arch Dermatol 1987;123:241-250.

52. Masinjila H, Arnbjornsson E. Two children with xeroderma pigmentosum developing two different types of malignancies simultaneously. Pediatr Surg Int 1998;13:299-300.

53. Sybert V. Genetic skin disorders. New York: Oxford University Press, 1997.

54. Ramsay CA, Coltart TM, Blunt S, et al. Prenatal diagnosis of xeroderma pigmentosum. Report of the first successful case. Lancet 1974;2:1109-1112.

55. Kraemer KH, DiGiovanna JJ, Moshell AN, et al. Prevention of skin cancer in xeroderma pigmentosum with the use of oral isotretinoin. N Engl J Med 1988;318:1633-1637.

56. Soter NA. The skin in mastocytosis. J Invest Dermatol 1991;96:32S-39S.

57. Lazarus GS, Guzzo C, Lavker RM, et al. Urticaria pigmentosum: Nature's experiment in mast cell biology. J Dermatol Sci 1991;2:395-401.

58. Epstein JH. Postinflammatory hyperpigmentation. Clin Dermatol 1989;7:55-65.

59. Chernosky M, Anderson DE, Chang JP, et al. Familial progressive hyperpigmentation. Arch Dermatol 1971;103:581-598.

60. Ruiz-Maldonado R, Tamayo L, Fernandez-Diez J. Universal acquired melanosis. The carbon baby. Arch Dermatol 1978;114:775-778.

61. Collins P, Barnes L, McCabe M. Poikiloderma congenitale: Case report and review of the literature. Pediatr Dermatol 1991;8:58-60.

62. Williams G, Dluhy RG. Diseases of the adrenal cortex. In Fauci AS, et al, eds. Harrison's principles of internal medicine. New York: McGraw-Hill, 1998: pp 2051-2054.

63. Mulligan TM, Sowers JR. Hyperpigmentation, vitiligo, and Addison's disease. Cutis 1985;36:317-318, 322.

64. Migeon C, Kenny EM, Kowarski A, et al. The syndrome of congenital adrenocortical unresponsiveness to ACTH. Report of six cases. Pediatr Res 1968;2:501-513.

65. Moshang T Jr, Rosenfield RL, Bongiovanni AM, et al. Familial glucocorticoid insufficiency. J Pediatr 1973;82:821-826.

66. Gorlin RJ, Anderson RC, Moller JH. The Leopard (multiple lentigines) syndrome revisited. Birth Defects Orig Artic Ser 1971;7:110-115.

67. Lassonde M, Trudeau JG, Girard C. Generalized lentigines associated with multiple congenital defects (leopard syndrome). Can Med Assoc J 1970;103:293-294.

68. Nordlund JJ, Lerner AB, Braverman IM, et al. The multiple lentigines syndrome. Arch Dermatol 1973;107:259-261.

69. Arnsmeier SL, Paller AS. Pigmentary anomalies in the multiple lentigines syndrome: Is it distinct from LEOPARD syndrome? Pediatr Dermatol 1996;13:100-104.

70. Rosenblum GA. Cryotherapy of lentiginous mosaicism. Cutis 1985;35:543-544.

71. Atherton DJ, Pitcher DW, Wells RS, et al. A syndrome of various cutaneous pigmented lesions, myxoid neurofibromata and atrial myxoma: The NAME syndrome. Br J Dermatol 1980;103:421-429.

72. Rhodes A, Silverman RA, Harrist TJ, et al. The "LAMB" syndrome. J Am Acad Dermatol 1984;10:72-82.

73. Stratakis C, Carney JA, Lin J, et al. Carney complex, a familial multiple neoplasia and lentiginosis syndrome. J Clin Invest 1996;97:699-705.

74. Marchesi L, Naldi L, Di Landro A, et al. Segmental lentiginosis with "jentigo" histologic pattern. Am J Dermatopathol 1992;14:323-327.

75. Altman DA, Banse L. Zosteriform speckled lentiginous nevus. J Am Acad Dermatol 1992;27:106-108.

76. Trattner A, Metzker A. Unilateral dermatomal pigmentary dermatosis: A variant dyschromatosis? J Am Acad Dermatol 1993;29:1060.

77. Bolognia JL. Fatal melanoma arising in a zosteriform speckled lentiginous nevus. Arch Dermatol 1991;127:1240-1241.
78. Dociu I, Galaction-Nitelea O, Sirjita N, et al. Centrofacial lentiginosis. A survey of 40 cases. Br J Dermatol 1976; 94:39-43.
79. Stewart DM, Altman J, Mehregan AH. Speckled lentiginous nevus. Arch Dermatol 1978;114:895-896.
80. Trattner A, Metzker A. Partial unilateral lentiginosis. J Am Acad Dermatol 1993;29:693-695.
81. Tovar JA, Eizaguirre I, Albert A, et al. Peutz-Jeghers syndrome in children: Report of two cases and review of the literature. J Pediatr Surg 1983;18:1-6.
82. Fernandez SM, Martinez Soto MI, Fernandez Lorenzo JR, et al. Peutz-Jehgers syndrome in a neonate. J of Ped 1995; 126:965-967.
83. Jenne DE, Reimann H, Nezu J, et al. Peutz-Jeghers syndrome is caused by mutations in a novel serine threonine kinase. Nat Genet 1998;18:38-43.
84. Cohen JM. Bannayan-Riley-Ruvalcaba syndrome: Renaming three formerly recognized syndromes as one etiologic entity. Am J Med Genet 1990;35:291.
85. Fargnoli M, Orlow SJ, Semel-Concepcion J, et al. Clinicopathologic findings in the Bannayan-Riley-Ruvalcaba syndrome. Arch Dermatol 1996;132:1214-1218.
86. Gorlin R, Cohen MM Jr, Condon LM, et al. Bannayan-Riley-Ruvalcaba syndrome. Am J Med Genet 1992;44:301-314.
87. Gretzula JC, Hevia O, Schachner LS, et al. Myhre-Smith-Ruvalcaba Syndrome. Pediatr Dermatol 1988;5:28-32.
88. Fryburg JS, Pelegano JP, Bennett MJ, et al. Long-chain 3-hydoxylacyl-coenzymeA dehydrogenase (L-CHAD) defiency in a patient with Bannayan-Riley-Ruvalcaba syndrome. Am J Med Genetics 1994;52:97-102.
89. Arch E, Goodman BK, Van Wesep RA, et al. Deletion of PTEN in a patient with Bannayan-Riley-Ruvalcaba Syndrome suggests allelism with Cowden disease. Am J Med Genet 1997;275:1943-1947.
90. Carethers J, Furnari FB, Zigman AF, et al. Absence of PTEN/MMAC1 germ line mutations in sporadic Bannayan-Riley-Ruvalcaba Syndrome. Cancer Res 1998;58:2724-2726.
91. Urabe K, Hori Y. Dyschromatosis. Semin Cutan Med Surg 1997;16:81-85.
92. Schoenlaub P, Leroy JP, Dupre D, et al. [Universal dyschromatosis: a familial case]. Ann Dermatol Venereol 1998;125:700-704.
93. Yang JH, Wong CK. Dyschromatosis universalis with X-linked ocular albinism. Clin Exp Dermatol 1991;16:436-440.
94. Shono S, Toda K. Universal dyschromatosis associated with photosensitivity and neurosensory hearing defect. Arch Dermatol 1990;126:1659-1660.
95. Rycroft RJ, Calnan CD, Wells RS. Universal dyschromatosis, small stature and high-tone deafness. Clin Exp Dermatol 1977;2:45-48.
96. Kim NS, Im S, Kim SC. Dyschromatosis universalis hereditaria: An electron microscopic examination. J Dermatol 1997;24:161-164.
97. Oyama M, Shimizu H, Ohata Y, et al. Dyschromatosis symmetrica hereditaria (reticulate acropigmentation of Dohl): Report of a Japanese family with the condition and a literature review of 185 cases. Br J Dermatol 1999;140:491-496.
98. Grimes PE, Stockton T. Pigmentary disorders in blacks. Dermatol Clin 1988;6:271-281.
99. Selmanowitz VJ, Krivo JM. Pigmentary demarcation lines. Comparison of Negroes with Japanese. Br J Dermatol 1975; 93:371-377.
100. Gari LM, Rivers JK, Kopf AW. Melanomas arising in large congenital nevocytic nevi: A prospective study. Pediatr Dermatol 1988;5:151-158.
101. Kopf AW, Bart RS, Hennessey P. Congenital nevocytic nevi and malignant melanomas. J Am Acad Dermatol 1979;1:123-130.
102. Castilla EE, da Graca Dutra M, Orioli-Parreiras IM. Epidemiology of congenital pigmented naevi: I. Incidence rates and relative frequencies. Br J Dermatol 1981;104:307-315.
103. Kroon S, Clemmensen OJ, Hastrup N. Incidence of congenital melanocytic nevi in newborn babies in Denmark. J Am Acad Dermatol 1987;17:422-426.
104. Walton RG, Jacobs AH, Cox AJ. Pigmented lesions in newborn infants. Br J Dermatol 1976;95:389-396.
105. Sahin S, Levin L, Kopf AW, et al. Risk of melanoma in medium-sized congenital melanocytic nevi: A follow-up study. J Am Acad Dermatol 1998;39:428-433.
106. Swerdlow AJ EJ, Qiao Z. The risk of melanoma in patients with congenital nevi: A cohort study. J Am Acad Dermatol 1995;32:595-599.
107. DaRaeve L, Danau W, DeBacker A, et al. Prepubertal melanoma in a medium-sized congenital naevus. Eur J Pediatr 1993;152:734-736.
108. Rhodes AR, Sober AJ, Day CL, et al. The malignant potential of small congenital nevocellular nevi. An estimate of association based on a histologic study of 234 primary cutaneous melanomas. J Am Acad Dermatol 1982;6:230-241.
109. Illig L, Weidner F, Hundeiker M, et al. Congenital nevi less than or equal to 10 cm as precursors to melanoma. 52 cases, a review, and a new conception. Arch Dermatol 1985;121:1274-1281.
110. Marghoob AA, Orlow SJ, Kopf AW. Syndromes associated with melanocytic nevi. J Am Acad Dermatol 1993;29:373-390.
111. Everett MA. Histopathology of congenital pigmented nevi. Am J Dermatopathol 1989;11:11-12.
112. Caputo R, Ackerman AB, Sison-Torre EQ. Congenital melanocytic nevi in pediatric dermatology and dermatopathology. Philadelphia: Lea & Febiger, 1990: pp 331.
113. Williams ML, Pennella R. Melanoma, melanocytic nevi, and other melanoma risk factors in children. J Pediatr 1994;124:833-845.
114. Sweren R. Management of congenital nevocytic nevi: A survery of current practices. J Am Acad Dermatol 1984;11:629-633.
115. Chamlin SL, Williams ML. Moles and melanoma. Curr Opin Pediatr 1998;10:398-404.
116. Gari LM, Rivers JK, Kopf AW. Melanomas arising in large congenital nevocytic nevi: A prosepective study. Pediatr Dermatol 1988;5:151-158.
117. Egan CL, Oliveria SA, Elenitsas R, et al. Cutaneous melanoma risk and phenotypic changes in large congenital nevi: a follow-up study of 46 patients. J Am Acad Dermatol 1998;39:923-932.
118. Castilla EE, da Graca Dutra M, Orioli-Parreiras IM. Epidemiology of congenital pigmented naevi: II. Risk factors. Br J Dermatol 1981;104:421-427.

119. Giam YC, Williams ML, Leboit PE, et al. Neonatal erosions and ulcerations in giant congenital melanocytic nevi. Pediatr Dermatol 1999;16:354-358.

120. Ruiz-Maldonado R, Tamayo L, Laterza AM, et al. Giant pigmented nevi: Clinical, histopathologic, and therapeutic considerations. J Pediatr 1992;120:906-911.

121. Arons MS, Hurwitz S. Congenital nevocellular nevus: A review of the treatment controversy and a report of 46 cases. Plast Reconstr Surg 1983;72:355-365.

122. James HE. Intrinsically derived deformational defects secondary to spinal dysraphism. Semin Perinatol 1983;7:253-256.

123. Hendrickson MR, Ross JC. Neoplasms arising in congenital giant nevi: Morphologic study of seven cases and a review of the literature. Am J Surg Pathol 1981;5:109-135.

124. Zuniga S, Las Heras J, Benveniste S. Rhabdomyosarcoma arising in a congenital giant nevus associated with neurocutaneous melanosis in a a neonate. J Ped Surg 1987;22:1036-1038.

125. Reed W, Becker SW Sr, Becker SW Jr, et al. Giant pigmented nevi, melanoma, and leptomeningeal melanocytosis. Arch Dermato 1965;91:100-119.

126. Rhodes A, Wood WC, Sober AJ, et al. Nonepidermal origin of malignant melanoma associated with a giant congenital nevocellular nevus. Plast Reconst Surg 1981;67:782-790.

127. Marghoob AA, Schoenbach SP, Kopf AW, et al. Large congenital melanocytic nevi and the risk for the development of malignant melanoma. A prospective study. Arch Dermatol 1996;132:170-175.

128. DeDavid M, Orlow SJ, Provost N, et al. A study of large congenital melanocytic nevi and associated malignant melanomas: Review of cases in the New York University Registry and the world literature. J Am Acad Dermatol 1997;36:409-416.

129. Quaba AA, Wallace AF. The incidence of malignant melanoma (0 to 15 years of age) arising in "large" congenital nevocellular nevi. Plast Reconstr Surg 1986;78:174-181.

130. Ellis DL, Wheeland RG, Solomon H. Estrogen and progesterone receptors in congenital melanocytic nevi. J Am Acad Dermatol 1985;12:235-244.

131. Harada M, Suzuki M, Ikeda T, et al. Clonality in nevocellular nevus and melanoma: an expression-based clonality analysis at the X-linked genes by polymerase chain reaction. J Invest Dermatol 1997;109:656-660.

132. Stenzinger W, Suter L, Schumann J. DNA aneuploidy in congenital melanocytic nevi: suggestive evidence for premalignant changes. J Invest Dermatol 1984;82:569-572.

133. Nickoloff BJ, Walton R, Pregerson-Rodan K, et al. Immunohistologic patterns of congenital nevocellular nevi. Arch Dermatol 1986;122:1263-1268.

134. Rhodes A. Congenital Nevomelanoctyic nevi: Histologic patterns in the first year of life and evolution during childhood. Arch Dermatol 1986;122:1257-1262.

135. Rhodes A, Albert LS, Weinstock MA. Congenital nevomelanocytic nevi: proportionate area expansion during infancy and early childhood. J Am Acad Dermatol 1996;34: 51-62.

136. Ruiz-Maldonado R, Tamayo L, Laterza AM, et al . Giant pigmented nevi: clinical, histopathologic, and therapeutic considerations. J Pediatr 1992;120: 906-911.

137. Zitelli JA, Grant MG, Abell E, et al. Histologic patterns of congenital nevocytic nevi and implications for treatment. J Am Acad Dermatol 1984;11:402-409.

138. Nickoloff B, Walton R, Pregerson-Rodan K, et al. Immunohistologic patterns of congenital nevocellular nevi. Arch Dermatol 1986;26:173-183.

139. Mark GJ, Mihm MC, Liteplo MG, et al. Congenital melanocytic nevi of the small and garment type. Clinical, histologic, and ultrastructural studies. Hum Pathol 1973;4:395-418.

140. Rhodes A, Silverman RA, Harrist TJ, et al. A histologi comparison of congenital and acquired nevomelanocytic nevi. Arch Dermatol 1985;121:1266-1273.

141. Casanova D, Bardot J, Aubert JP, et al. Management of nevus spilus. Pediatr Dermatol 1996;13:233-238.

142. Grevelink JM, van Leeuwen RL, Anderson RR, et al. Clinical and histological responses of congenital melanocytic nevi after single treatment with Q-switched lasers. Arch Dermatol 1997;133:349-353.

143. Rompel R, Moser M, Petres J. Dermabrasion of congenital nevocellular nevi: experience in 215 patients. Dermatology 1997;194:261-267.

144. Hogan DJ, Murphy F, Bremner RM. Spontaneous resolution of a giant congenital melanocytic nevus. Pediatr Dermatol 1988;5:170-172.

145. Kadonaga JN, Frieden IJ. Neurocutaneous melanosis: Definition and review of the literature. J Am Acad Dermatol 1991;24:747-755.

146. Schneiderman H, Wu AY, Campbell WA, et al. Congenital melanoma with multiple prenatal metastases. Cancer 1987;60:1371-1377.

147. Frieden IJ, Williams ML, Barkovich AJ. Giant congenital melanocytic nevi: Brain magnetic resonance findings in neurologically asymptomatic children. J Am Acad Dermatol 1994;31:423-429.

148. Ruiz-Maldonado R, del Rosario Barona-Mazuera M, Hidalgo-Galvan LR, et al. Giant congenital melanocytic nevi, neurocutaneous melanosis and neurological alterations. Dermatology 1997;195:125-128.

149. Sato S, Kato H, Hidano A. Divided nevus spilus and divided form of spotted grouped pigmented nevus. J Cutan Pathol 1979;6:507-512.

150. Nelson JS, Applebaum J. Treatment of superficial cutaneous pigmented lesions by melanin-specific selective photothermolysis using the Q-switched ruby laser. Ann Plast Surg 1992;29:231-237.

151. Spitz S. Melanomas of childhood. 1948 [classical article]. CA Cancer J Clin 1991;41:40-51.

152. Hamm H, Happle R, Brocker EB. Multiple agminate Spitz naevi: Review of the literature and report of a case with distinctive immunohistological features. Br J Dermatol 1987;117:511-522.

153. Renfro L, Grant-Kels JM, Brown SA. Multiple agminate Spitz nevi. Pediatr Dermatol 1989;6:114-117.

154. Prose NS, Heilman E, Felman YM, et al. Multiple benign juvenile melanoma. J Am Acad Dermatol 1983;9:236-242.

155. Betti R, Inselvini E, Palvarini M, et al. Agminated intradermal Spitz nevi arising on an unusual speckled lentiginous nevus with localized lentiginosis: a continuum? Am J Dermatopathol 1997;19:524-527.

156. Aloi F, Tomasini C, Pippione M. Agminated Spitz nevi occurring within a congenital speckled lentiginous nevus. Am J Dermatopathol 1995;17:594-598.

21

Lumps, Bumps, and Hamartomas

JULIE S. PRENDIVILLE

LUMPS AND BUMPS

A wide variety of conditions affecting the skin and subcutaneous tissues present as papulonodular lesions, or "lumps and bumps." Benign and malignant neoplasms, hamartomas, and inflammatory and infectious disorders, as well as a number of infiltrative diseases, could be included in this category. Some of these conditions are discussed in detail in other chapters. This section deals with a group of nonmalignant disorders that present as discrete, circumscribed skin lesions in the newborn and young infant.

Fibromatoses

The fibromatoses represent a diverse collection of mesenchymal tumors that are characterized by fibroblastic-myofibroblastic proliferation.[1] They are locally invasive neoplasms that do not metastasize but may recur following surgical excision. They vary in clinical behavior from benign lesions that regress spontaneously to aggressive life-threatening tumors. They can be solitary or multifocal, and may exhibit skin, soft tissue, bone, or visceral involvement. Most of these tumors are sporadic but some occur in a familial setting.

The fibromatoses are classified as juvenile or adult in type (Box 21-1).[1] The juvenile fibromatoses are a unique group of fibroblastic-myofibroblastic proliferations that present at birth or in the first years of life (Table 21-1). They account for approximately 12% of pediatric soft tissue tumors.[1] Adult-type fibromatoses are occasionally observed in infancy and childhood.[1] The fibromatoses have also been subdivided according to the site of fibrous tissue overgrowth into superficial or fascial fibromatoses, and deep or musculoaponeurotic (desmoid-type) fibromatoses.[2]

Infantile Myofibromatosis

The term *infantile myofibromatosis* was introduced by Chung and Enzinger in 1981 to designate a disorder previously described under numerous synonyms, including congenital multiple fibromatosis, diffuse congenital fibromatosis, multiple congenital mesenchymal tumors,

---

BOX 21-1

Fibromatoses of the Skin and Soft Tissues

Juvenile Fibromatoses
Infantile myofibromatosis
Infantile desmoid-type fibromatosis
Fibromatosis colli
Infantile digital fibromatosis
Fibrous hamartoma of infancy
Gingival fibromatosis
Juvenile hyaline fibromatosis
Infantile systemic fibromatosis

Adult-Type Fibromatoses
Superficial
Dupuytren-type fibromatosis
- Palmar
- Plantar
Knuckle pads

Deep
Desmoid fibromatosis
- Intraabdominal
- Abdominal
- Extraabdominal

TABLE 21-1

Juvenile Fibromatoses

	Location	Inheritance	Associated features	Course	Treatment
Infantile myofibromatosis	Solitary, multicentric or generalized	Sporadic, autosomal dominant, "?" autosomal recessive	Lytic bone lesions, visceral involvement	Spontaneous regression of bone and skin lesions; visceral lesions may be fatal	Await spontaneous regression, local excision if necessary; "?" chemotherapy or radiation for visceral lesions
Infantile desmoid-type fibromatosis	Any site	Usually sporadic, autosomal dominant	Other congenital anomalies	Locally invasive; does not metastasize; recurs after excision	Local excision with wide margins; "?" chemotherapy for non-resectable lesions
Fibromatosis colli	Neck	Rarely familial	None	Spontaneous regression	Physiotherapy
Infantile digital fibromatosis	Fingers and toes	Sporadic	None	Spontaneous regression reported; may recur	Await spontaneous regression; local excision if necessary
Fibrous hamartoma of infancy	Axillae, shoulders, chest wall	Sporadic	None	Does not regress	Local excision
Gingival fibromatosis	Gums	Autosomal dominant, recessive	Generalized hypertrichosis	May interfere with ability to eat, speak	Surgical debulking
Juvenile hyaline fibromatosis	Nodules on face and elsewhere	Autosomal recessive	Gingival hypertrophy, joint contractures	Chronic physical and cosmetic disability, overlaps with ISH	Supportive care, surgical excision of nodules if necessary
Infantile systemic hyalinosis (ISH)	Generalized thickening of skin	Autosomal recessive	Painful joint contractures, protein-losing enteropathy	Usually fatal within first few years of life	Supportive care

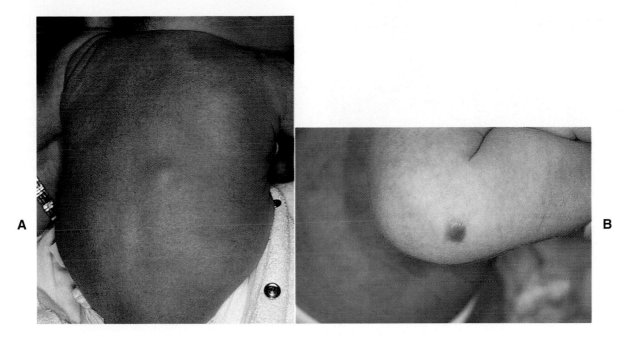

FIG. 21-1
A, Flesh-colored nodule in infantile myofibromatosis. B, Cutaneous myofibroma with a vascular appearance.

and multiple vascular leiomyomas of the newborn.[3] There are three clinical patterns of presentation: *solitary* infantile myofibroma; *multicentric* infantile myofibromatosis, with multiple lesions in the skin, soft tissues, and bone; and *generalized* infantile myofibromatosis, in which there is also visceral involvement.[1]

Cutaneous Findings. Over 80% of myofibromas present in the first two years of life, and 60% are apparent at birth or shortly thereafter.[3] Lesions may be superficial or deep, involving the skin, subcutaneous tissues, and muscle. They appear clinically as discrete, rubbery firm to hard nodules measuring from 0.5 to 7 cm in diameter (Fig. 21-1, A). Cutaneous myofibromas may be skin-colored or have a prominent vascular appearance, resembling hemangioma (Fig. 21-1, B). Sites of predilection for solitary lesions are the head, neck, trunk, and upper extremities. In the multicentric and generalized forms, there are multiple and widespread myofibromas, numbering from a few to over 100 lesions (Fig. 21-2).[4] Skin and soft tissue lesions are asymptomatic and usually cause little morbidity. Rarely, a myofibroma presents with surface ulceration or an atrophic morphology (Fig. 21-3).[5] Joint contractures have been observed with extensive limb lesions.[6]

Extracutaneous Findings. In the multicentric form of the disease, myofibromas in the skin and soft tissues are

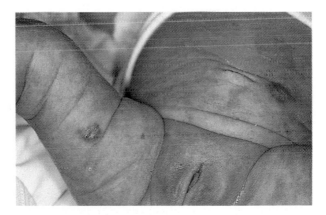

FIG. 21-2
Multicentric cutaneous myofibromas in an infant with extensive bone lesions. This case was familial with autosomal dominant transmission.

associated with multiple lytic bone lesions. These may be extensive and can involve any bone.[4] Progression in size and number has been observed during infancy.[4] The bone tumors eventually stabilize, and spontaneous healing occurs with complete regression during the first few years

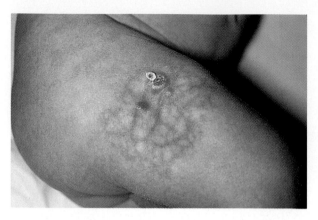

FIG. 21-3
Infantile myofibroma presenting as a congenital area of atrophy and telangiectasia with central red nodules, one of which was ulcerated.

of life. Development of sclerotic borders around lytic areas may be an early sign of regression.[4] In most cases there are no clinical signs or symptoms of bone disease. Pathologic fractures occur rarely and usually heal without residual deformity.[4] Vertebral body collapse has been described with residual loss of vertebral height in early childhood.[4] There are reports of fatal spinal cord compression resulting from extension into the spinal canal.[7]

The much rarer generalized form of infantile myofibromatosis is characterized by involvement of visceral organs in addition to skin, soft tissue, and bone tumors. The gastrointestinal tract, heart, and lungs are most frequently affected. Involvement of the central nervous system is rare. Myofibromatosis in visceral organs is locally invasive and may severely compromise organ function. Cardiopulmonary, gastrointestinal, and hepatobiliary complications can be fatal, particularly in the newborn period or early infancy.[8]

Multiple skin and soft-tissue tumors in the absence of bone or visceral involvement may occasionally occur.[1] Conversely, bone involvement has been observed in association with a single soft-tissue lesion,[8] and uncommonly in the absence of skin lesions.[4]

Etiology and Pathogenesis. The pathogenesis is unknown. Most cases are sporadic. There are a few reports of familial occurrence for which both autosomal dominant and recessive inheritance has been postulated.[9]

Diagnosis. Myofibromatosis may be suspected by the presence of firm, cutaneous and subcutaneous nodules. A biopsy is required to confirm the diagnosis. All three forms of infantile myofibromatosis show interlacing fas-

cicles of spindle-shaped fibroblasts.[1] Central vascular areas resembling hemangiopericytoma are variably present. Focal necrosis, calcification, hyalinization, macrophages containing hemosiderin, and chronic inflammation may be seen.[1] A giant cell variant containing multiple multinucleated giant cells has also been described. There is positive immunoreactivity for vimentin and actin consistent with the presumed myofibroblastic derivation of the tumor; desmin staining is variable. Electron microscopy shows cells with features of both fibroblasts and smooth muscle cells.

Infants with cutaneous myofibromas should be evaluated for bone and visceral involvement, particularly when there are multiple lesions. Recommended initial investigations include a skeletal survey, chest x-ray, echocardiogram, and abdominal imaging studies.[8]

Differential Diagnosis. Infantile myofibromatosis can be distinguished from other pediatric soft-tissue tumors by histopathologic examination of biopsy material. These include other forms of fibromatosis, as well as congenital fibrosarcoma, leiomyoma and leiomyosarcoma, neurofibroma, metastatic neuroblastoma, hemangioma, hemangiopericytoma, chondromatosis, and nodular fasciitis.[1]

Treatment and Prognosis. The prognosis for infantile myofibromatosis is good in the absence of visceral involvement. Lesions in the skin and soft tissues show spontaneous involution during the first few years of life, sometimes leaving residual areas of skin atrophy or hyperpigmentation. Bone lesions also regress spontaneously, usually without significant disability or residual radiologic change.[4] They do not interfere with enchondral bone growth.[4] The prognosis is grave for newborns with visceral disease in whom a mortality rate of 76% has been documented.[8]

Surgical excision may be necessary to obtain tissue for diagnosis. Otherwise, excision should be limited to lesions that result in functional impairment or severe cosmetic disability.[6,8] The benefit of chemotherapy or radiation therapy for symptomatic, recurrent, and nonresectable disease has not been established.

Infantile Desmoid-Type Fibromatosis

Although desmoid fibromatosis has traditionally been considered a deep fibromatosis of adulthood, with abdominal, intraabdominal, and extraabdominal variants, a specific juvenile subset has become increasingly recognized.[1] Description of this entity under a variety of synonyms, including aggressive fibromatosis of infancy, musculoaponeurotic fibromatosis, desmoma, and fibrosarcoma grade 1-desmoid type, among others, has led to confusion in the literature.[10] Up to 30% of juvenile desmoid tumors

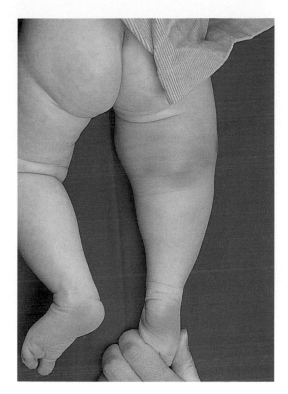

FIG. 21-4
Desmoid fibromatosis: firm mass on the thigh of an infant, diagnosed as "aggressive fibromatosis of infancy."

present in the first year of life, and congenital cases have been reported.[1,11]

Clinical Findings. Infantile desmoid-like fibromatosis involves deep tissues and is generally extraabdominal.[1] The usual clinical presentation is a slowly growing, nontender subcutaneous mass that has been present for weeks or months (Fig. 21-4). Sites of predilection in children are the head and neck, extremities, shoulder girdle, trunk, and hip regions. The abdomen, retroperitoneum, spermatic cord, and breast may also be involved. Rarely, there are multiple lesions. The tumor tends to be very locally aggressive with infiltration of adjacent skeletal muscles, tendons, or periosteum, and erosion of bone.

Approximately 12% of pediatric patients with desmoid fibromatosis have other congenital abnormalities.[1] Adult-type intraabdominal desmoid tumors are associated with Gardner syndrome and with familial polyposis coli.[1,12]

Etiology and Pathogenesis. The finding of minor radiologic bone abnormalities in 80% of patients with desmoids and 48% of their relatives suggests an autosomal dominant mode of inheritance.[1] Antecedent trauma, including surgery or irradiation, is reported in 12% to 63% of patients with all forms of desmoid tumor.[1] It is postulated that desmoid tumors are associated with a familial defect in the regulation of connective tissue and may be precipitated by multiple factors.[1,12]

Diagnosis. The tumor is composed of bundles of slender, uniform spindle cells surrounded by variable amounts of collagen. Cleft or slit-like blood vessels are variable in number and more abundant at the periphery. The fibrous proliferation may be indistinguishable from scar tissue except that it infiltrates skeletal muscle and tendons.[1] Cellularity is variable. Some childhood lesions have an increased number of mitoses and greater cellularity.[1] Immunohistochemical and ultrastructural studies show that the lesion is composed of fibroblasts and myofibroblasts.

Differential Diagnosis. Myofibromatosis and other juvenile fibromatoses should be considered in the differential diagnosis. Keloid scars are more superficial than desmoid tumors. Cellular variants can be difficult to differentiate histologically from fibrosarcoma.

Treatment and Prognosis. The treatment of choice is local excision with wide margins if possible.[11-13] The recurrence rate varies from 30% to 80%.[1] Higher recurrence rates are associated with a young age at diagnosis, intralesional or marginal excision, mesenteric location, and associated Gardner syndrome. Microscopic features of high vascularity, myxoid foci, and abundant immature myofibroblasts are associated with a higher recurrence rate.[1] Treatment with combination chemotherapy and radiotherapy, or with tamoxifen and nonsteroidal antiinflammatory agents, has been advocated for nonresectable lesions.[14,15] Mortality from locally aggressive desmoids is less than 10%.[1]

Fibromatosis Colli

Fibromatosis colli, or congenital muscular torticollis, is a congenital fibromatosis of the sternocleidomastoid muscle. It occurs in up to 0.4% of live newborns.[1] Males are affected more than females. It does not involve the skin.

Clinical Findings. A hard, nontender, lobulated subcutaneous mass is palpable in the lower third of the sternocleidomastoid muscle. The trapezoid muscle is sometimes involved. Following an initial rapid period of growth, the tumor stabilizes in size. Torticollis and facial asymmetry are variable and may be transient. There is a right-sided predominance, and 2% to 3% of cases are bilateral.[1]

Etiology and Pathogenesis. The pathogenesis is unknown. Birth trauma has been implicated, since 86% of cases have a history of complicated delivery; whether this is a cause or effect of the tumor is not clear. Familial cases are rare.[1]

Diagnosis. Histologically, bands of fibroblasts with abundant collagen are intermingled with residual angulated skeletal muscle fibers. The diagnosis may be established by fine needle aspiration, which shows benign spindle cells and degenerating skeletal muscle fibers. Magnetic resonance imaging may also be useful.[16]

Differential Diagnosis. A combination of the typical location of the lesion in the neck and the characteristic histology is diagnostic. The clinical differential diagnosis includes lymphangioma, hemangioma, and malignant neoplasms. The histopathologic features may resemble those of a desmoid tumor.[1]

Treatment and Prognosis. The majority of lesions regress within the first year of life. Most resolve completely, but minor residual asymmetry or tightening of the sternocleidomastoid muscle is seen in 25% of cases.[1] Only 9% have persistence of the tumor and torticollis. Physiotherapy is the treatment of choice. Surgery is rarely necessary unless the diagnosis is in doubt or the mass fails to resolve.

Infantile Digital Fibromatosis

Infantile digital fibromatosis is a recurring myofibroblastic proliferation of the fingers and toes. Synonyms for this tumor include digital fibrous tumor of Reye, digital fibrous swelling, recurring digital fibrous tumor of childhood, and inclusion body fibromatosis.[1]

Cutaneous Findings. Almost all lesions are diagnosed in infancy, and one third are present at birth. Both sexes are affected equally. The typical lesion is an asymptomatic firm, smooth, pink nodule located on the lateral or dorsal aspect of the digit, measuring less than 3 cm in diameter (Fig. 21-5). Lesions are more common on the fingers than

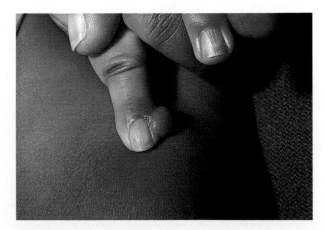

FIG. 21-5
Infantile digital fibroma presenting as a smooth, pink nodule.

on the toes. The thumbs and great toes are spared. There is often deformity of the affected digit. There may be single or multiple nodules. Rarely, more than one digit is involved or extradigital lesions are seen.[17]

Extracutaneous Findings. Periosteal attachment is not unusual, but underlying bone erosion is rare.

Etiology and Pathogenesis. The pathogenesis is not known. Defective actin filament organization in myofibroblasts has been hypothesized.[1]

Diagnosis. Whorls and inderdigitating sheets of uniform fibroblasts in a densely collagenous stroma are seen in the dermis or subcutis.[1] A unique feature is the presence of distinctive, eosinophilic, perinuclear cytoplasmic inclusions surrounded by a clear halo that stain red with a trichrome stain. Electron microscopy shows abundant cytoplasmic filaments that form whorled bodies; these are the ultrastructural correlate of the cytoplasmic inclusions. Immunostaining is positive for desmin, actin, vimentin, and keratin.

Differential Diagnosis. The digital location and the characteristic histology distinguish this lesion from other fibromatoses and pediatric soft-tissue tumors.

Treatment and Prognosis. The local recurrence rate is 60% to 90% following surgical excision. Many tumors regress spontaneously within a few years.[17] The indications for surgical excision are controversial.[1,17] Conservative management without surgery is appropriate unless there is functional impairment.

Fibrous Hamartoma of Infancy

Fibrous hamartoma of infancy is a benign fibrous tumor that develops during the first 2 years of life.[18] Up to 20% are present at birth.[1] Occasional cases have been described in children between 2 and 10 years. Males are affected more frequently than females.

Cutaneous Findings. Fibrous hamartoma presents as a subcutaneous lesion located around the axillae, shoulders, and upper chest wall.[19] It may involve other sites such as the inguinal region, extremities, and head and neck. It is usually a solitary nodule, measuring 2 to 5 cm in diameter, that feels lumpy to palpation. Occasionally, these lesions are multifocal. There are no symptoms.

Extracutaneous Findings. There are no systemic associations.

Etiology and Pathogenesis. Fibrous hamartoma of infancy is believed to represent a hamartomatous process rather than a true neoplasm. It is not familial.

Diagnosis. The hamartoma is located in the subcutaneous and musculoaponeurotic tissues.[18,19] Histopathologic examination reveals three characteristic elements: a fibrous component consisting of well defined fascicles of fibroblasts or disorderly fibroblasts in a collagenous stroma; mature adipose tissue; and myxoid mesenchymal tissue in a basophilic matrix. Electronmicroscopy reveals the presence of both fibroblasts and myofibroblasts, primitive mesenchymal cells, small blood vessels, and mature adipocytes.[1]

Differential Diagnosis. The clinical differential diagnosis of fibrous hamartoma of infancy includes cystic hygroma, hemangioma, and other soft-tissue tumors.[19] Identification of the three histologic components of this lesion distinguishes it from other fibroblastic proliferations.

Treatment and Prognosis. There is no tendency to spontaneous regression. The treatment of choice is surgical excision. The recurrence rate is less than 15%.[1]

Gingival Fibromatosis

This is a rare familial disorder that manifests at the time of eruption of the deciduous or permanent teeth.[1]

Cutaneous Findings. There is slowly progressive gingival enlargement that may cover the crowns of the teeth and result in difficulty in eating or speaking. It is associated with generalized hypertrichosis.

Extracutaneous Findings. Rarely there is associated mental retardation and epilepsy.

Etiology and Pathogenesis. Inheritance is autosomal dominant. Autosomal recessive and sporadic cases are also reported.[20] The pathogenesis is unknown.

Diagnosis. Mucosal biopsy shows coarse, interlacing, collagen bundles with sparse fibroblasts and myofibroblasts. There may be calcification, ossification, abundant amorphous extracellular material, and cellular fibroblastic proliferation.[1]

Differential Diagnosis. The differential diagnosis includes phenytoin usage, chronic gingivitis, cherubism, and juvenile hyaline fibromatosis.

Treatment and Prognosis. Treatment options include repeated surgical debulking of the gums or dental extraction.

Adult-Type Fibromatoses

The superficial fibromatoses of adulthood are the most common type of fibromatosis in the general population but are rare in infants and children. Fibromatosis may involve the palm (Dupuytren contracture), the plantar surface of the foot (Ledderhose disease), or the penis (Peyronie disease). Dupuytren-type fibromatosis of the palms and soles may be seen in childhood, and is occasionally congenital (Fig. 21-6).[1] Surgical excision is only necessary for diagnosis or release of contractures. Knuckle pads are seen in older children and adolescents but not in infants.

Leiomyoma

Leiomyoma is a benign tumor of smooth muscle. Cutaneous leiomyoma may arise from the arrector pili muscle in hair follicles, the dartos muscle of the scrotum and labia majora, the erectile muscle of the nipple, and the muscular wall of veins (angioleiomyoma). Leiomyomas are uncommon in children and are extremely rare in the newborn period.[21,22]

Cutaneous Findings. Cutaneous leiomyomas appear as discrete papules or nodules with a pink or brown discoloration of the overlying skin. They are usually solitary but may be multiple. Rarely, a leiomyoma may present as a pedunculated mass at birth or as a papular plaque in early infancy.[22,23] Leiomyomas are often painful, particularly on exposure to cold.

Extracutaneous Findings. Most cutaneous leiomyomas are not associated with visceral disease. The multiple leiomyomas of the esophagus and tracheobronchial tree in Alport syndrome may be associated with female genital leiomyomas in older children and adults.[21] Leiomyomas that occur in immunocompromised children only rarely involve the skin or soft tissues.[24]

Etiology and Pathogenesis. Multiple cutaneous leiomyomas may be inherited as an autosomal dominant trait, but the etiology of other forms is unknown.

Diagnosis. The diagnosis is made by skin biopsy, which demonstrates whorls and bundles of well-differentiated spindle cells with cigar-shaped nuclei in the dermis. There is a variable collagenous component. The smooth muscle stains red with the Masson trichrome stain. Immunochemistry is positive for muscle-specific actin and desmin reactivity.

Differential Diagnosis. Leiomyoma must be distinguished from the fibroblastic and myofibroblastic prolif-

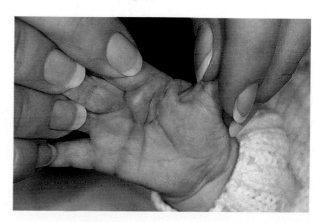

FIG. 21-6
Congenital fibromatosis of the palm.

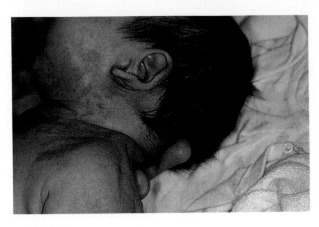

FIG. 21-7
Congenital area of hyperpigmentation overlying a plexiform neurofibroma in NF1.

erations of infancy and childhood, as well as from other spindle cell tumors such as neurofibroma and leiomyosarcoma. Immunohistochemistry may be helpful as myofibroblastic tumors express smooth muscle actin more than muscle-specific actin or desmin.[21] The circumscribed spindle cell appearance of leiomyoma differs from the smooth muscle bundles of congenital smooth muscle hamartoma.

Treatment and Prognosis. Excision is curative for solitary lesions.

Neurofibromas and Other Neural Tumors

Cutaneous neurofibromas in infants and young children are almost invariably associated with neurofibromatosis type 1 (NF1). These benign tumors consist of Schwann cells, nerve fibers, and fibroblasts, and may be cutaneous, subcutaneous, or plexiform. Cutaneous and subcutaneous neurofibromas are rarely seen at birth but may sometimes appear within the first year of life. Plexiform neurofibromas are often present at birth and are considered pathognomonic of neurofibromatosis. There may be a large area of hyperpigmentation overlying the plexiform neurofibroma that predates the characteristic "bag of worms" consistency of the tumor (Fig. 21-7). These lesions enlarge with time and can cause considerable cosmetic disfigurement, particularly on the face and around the eye. A plexiform neurofibroma in the neck may compromise airway function, and large lesions over the back are very often associated with underlying spinal involvement.

Pacinian neurofibromas, or nerve-sheath myxomas, are uncommon tumors with components that resemble Vater-Pacini corpuscles.[25] Multiple hairy pacinian neurofibro-

mas have been reported in children without neurofibromatosis type 1 and may be congenital.[25] Underlying skeletal anomalies may be associated with pacinian neurofibromas in a sacrococcygeal location.

In neurilemmomatosis, a syndrome reported in Japanese children, multiple cutaneous neurilemmomas derived from Schwann cells are present at birth or develop during childhood.[26] These lesions are a marker for development of central nervous system tumors in later childhood and adult life. Cutaneous schwannomas associated with neurofibromatosis type 2 (NF2) may also rarely present in early life.[27] The gene locus for neurilemmomatosis has recently been reported to lie within the NF2 gene region suggesting that these two disorders may be the same disease.[28]

Non-Langerhans' Cell Histiocytoses

The non-Langerhans' cell histiocytoses encompass a diverse group of disorders in which there is proliferation of mononuclear phagocytes other than Langerhans cells. Two variants, juvenile xanthogranuloma and benign cephalic histiocytosis, occur primarily in infants and young children. Other benign histiocytoses such as papular xanthoma, xanthoma disseminatum, and generalized eruptive xanthoma may rarely present in childhood, but are extremely unusual in infancy.[29,30]

Juvenile Xanthogranuloma

Juvenile xanthogranuloma is a benign, self-healing, non-Langerhans' cell histiocytosis characterized by solitary or multiple yellow-red papules and nodules in the skin and occasionally in other organs.[31] Although adults may be affected, it is predominantly a disorder of infancy and early childhood. There is an increased frequency of juvenile xanthogranuloma in children with neurofibromatosis type 1, juvenile myeloid leukemia, and urticaria pigmentosa.[32,33]

Cutaneous Findings. The typical juvenile xanthogranuloma is an asymptomatic, firm, well-demarcated papule or nodule that measures from 1 mm to 2 cm in diameter. Early lesions are pink or red in color, later changing to a distinctive yellow or orange/brown (Fig. 21-8). There may be overlying telangiectasia with a purpuric appearance, and occasionally surface ulceration and bleeding with associated pruritus and discomfort. Solitary lesions with a hyperkeratotic surface, pedunculated, or plaque-like morphology are also reported.[31] As many as 17% of juvenile xanthogranulomas are present at birth, and 70% develop within the first year of life.[31] The majority are solitary lesions. Multiple lesions may be few or number in the hundreds (Fig. 21-9). They can be located

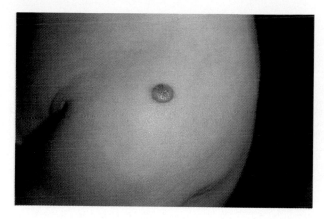

FIG. 21-8
Juvenile xanthogranuloma.

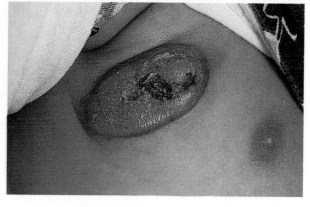

FIG. 21-10
Giant juvenile xanthogranuloma with ulceration.

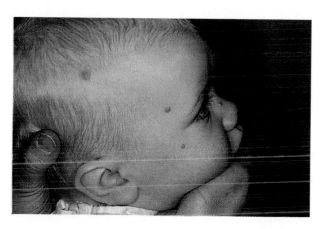

FIG. 21-9
Multiple juvenile xanthogranulomas.

at virtually any body site but are most common on the head, neck, and upper trunk.

Juvenile xanthogranulomas may be classified as micronodular, measuring 2 to 5 mm, or macronodular, measuring 0.5 to 2 cm in diameter. An unusual variant is the giant juvenile xanthogranuloma, which measures from 2 to 10 cm in diameter (Fig. 21-10).[34] These lesions are congenital or appear in early infancy and may have a greater propensity to ulcerate. Rarely, numerous micronodular lesions may present as a generalized lichenoid eruption.[35]

Extracutaneous Findings. Extracutaneous juvenile xanthogranuloma is rare, and less than 50% of these patients have associated cutaneous lesions.[36] The most frequent extracutaneous sites are the eye and orbit, central nervous system, liver/spleen, lung, oropharynx, and mus-

cle. In contrast to cutaneous lesions, a systemic juvenile xanthogranuloma may produce symptoms related to a mass effect or infiltration of the involved organ. The incidence of ocular disease in patients with cutaneous lesions is 0.3% to 0.4%.[37] Eye lesions manifest as an asymptomatic mass on the iris, unilateral glaucoma, spontaneous hyphema, or color change of the iris. Risk factors for eye involvement include multiple lesions, age less than 2 years, and recently diagnosed disease.[37]

Juvenile xanthogranulomas are seen with increased frequency in patients with neurofibromatosis type 1 and juvenile chronic myeloid leukemia. A triple association between juvenile chronic myeloid leukemia, juvenile xanthogranulomas, and neurofibromatosis type 1 is described (Fig. 21-11).[32] Urticaria pigmentosa and juvenile xanthogranuloma have also been associated.[33]

Etiology. The etiology of juvenile xanthogranuloma is unknown. It is believed to be a reactive rather than a neoplastic process.

Diagnosis. The typical histologic appearance consists of a dense dermal infiltrate of foamy histiocytes with Touton giant cells. There is an admixture of other cell types, including lymphocytes, eosinophils, neutrophils, and foreign body giant cells, as well as infrequent mitoses. In early lesions there may be few or absent foam cells or Touton giant cells, with a variable number of spindle cells and numerous mitotic figures.[38,39] Immunohistochemistry shows negative staining for S-100 and MAC 387, and positive staining for HAM56, HHF35, KP1, and vimentin. There are no Birbeck granules visible on ultrastructural examination.

Differential Diagnosis. Distinction of a small juvenile xanthogranuloma from clinically similar lesions such as

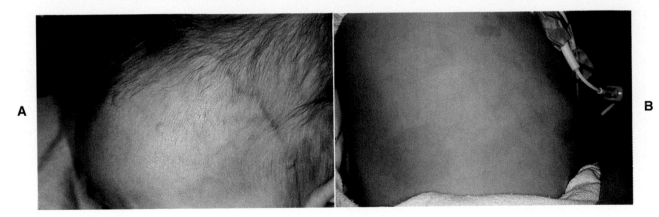

FIG. 21-11
A, Multiple juvenile xanthogranulomas and **B,** café au lait macules in an child with juvenile chronic myeloid leukemia.

xanthoma, mastocytoma, Spitz nevus, and a number of other benign skin tumors may require a skin biopsy. Giant lesions may be mistaken for a hemangioma or malignant tumor. Early lesions that lack the characteristic lipid-laden histiocytes and Touton giant cells may resemble Langerhans' cell histiocytosis on histologic examination.[38,39] The absence of Birbeck granules and negative staining for S-100 is characteristic of juvenile xanthogranuloma.

Treatment and Prognosis. Most cutaneous lesions resolve spontaneously over months or years and do not require treatment. Ulcerating, symptomatic, or large unsightly lesions may require surgical excision. Most lesions resolve completely, but some leave a residual area of hyperpigmentation or skin atrophy resembling anetoderma. Ocular and systemic lesions can be more problematic. Treatment options include observation, corticosteroids, surgical excision, radiation therapy, and chemotherapy.[31]

Benign Cephalic Histiocytosis

Benign cephalic histiocytosis is a non-Langerhans' cell histiocytosis characterized clinically by multiple brownish-yellow macules and papules on the face and adjacent areas. Some authors believe that benign cephalic histiocytosis is a localized variant of micronodular juvenile xanthogranuloma.[40]

Cutaneous Findings. Lesions first appear between the ages of 2 months and 2 years.[41] The face is the site of predilection, but the scalp, neck, and ears can also be involved. A few lesions may be scattered over the shoulders and upper arms.[42] Typical lesions are slightly raised, asymptomatic papules measuring 2 to 3 mm in diameter. They vary from erythematous to light-brown or yellowish

in color. The mucous membranes are not involved. There are no extracutaneous findings.

Diagnosis. Histologically, a monomorphous histiocytic infiltrate is located in the upper and mid-dermis. There may be a few lymphocytes and eosinophils also. Unlike juvenile xanthogranuloma, there are no foamy histiocytes or Touton giant cells. Staining for S-100 protein is negative. Electron microscopy reveals coated vesicles and comma- or worm-shaped bodies. Birbeck granules are absent.

Differential Diagnosis. The differential diagnosis includes juvenile xanthogranuloma, Langerhans' cell histiocytosis, and cutaneous mastocytosis. The lesions of mastocytosis have a similar color but urticate when rubbed (Darier's sign) and have a distinctive histology. Benign cephalic histiocytosis can be distinguished from Langerhans' cell histiocytosis by immunohistochemical stains and the absence of Birbeck granules on electron microscopy.

Treatment and Prognosis. There is no effective treatment. The skin lesions regress spontaneously over months to years. There may be residual hyperpigmentation and anetoderma-like atrophy.

Calcifying Disorders of the Skin

Calcium deposition in the skin, or *calcinosis cutis,* is found in a diverse group of disorders. It is termed *dystrophic calcification* when calcium is deposited in abnormal or injured tissue in patients with no abnormality of calcium or phosphate metabolism. *Metastatic calcification* develops in normal tissues as a result of abnormal calcium and phosphorus metabolism. *Idiopathic calcification* occurs in the absence of any discernible tissue injury or metabolic abnormality. *Iatrogenic calcification* may develop as a complication of calcium infusions or application of calcium containing paste to abraded skin. Cutaneous ossification, in which normal bone is formed in the dermis and subcutaneous soft tissues, is termed *osteoma cutis*.

Dystrophic Calcification

Dystrophic calcification arises at sites of skin trauma or in association with inflammatory lesions, connective tissue disorders, skin tumors, and cysts. Calcinosis cutis on the heels is a not uncommon sequela of drawing blood by heel sticks during the neonatal period.[43,44] It presents some months later as one or more white papules or nodules and usually resolves spontaneously by 18 to 30 months of age. Calcification may also occur in association with subcutaneous fat necrosis of the newborn.[45,46] Calcium deposition has been observed histologically both in the septa and within the fat lobules.[45,47] Widespread subcutaneous calcification may develop in cases of subcutaneous fat necrosis complicating hypothermic cardiac surgery.[16,47,48] Although hypercalcemia is a known complication of subcutaneous fat necrosis, the majority of reported cases of soft-tissue calcification have occurred in normocalcemic patients. Conversely, most infants with subcutaneous fat necrosis and hypercalcemia do not show evidence of calcium deposition in biopsies taken from affected sites.[16]

Dystrophic calcification has been reported in the skin lesions of a newborn infant with intrauterine-acquired herpes simplex infection.[49] The calcification was present at birth and appeared to have developed in utero. A lethal disorder characterized by extensive congenital skin necrosis and follicular calcification has been described in three newborn females.[50] Dystrophic calcification may also occur as a complication of intralesional corticosteroid injection of infantile periocular hemangiomas.[51]

Metastatic Calcification

Metastatic calcification occurs when calcium salts are precipitated in normal tissues as a result of high serum calcium or phosphate levels. The calcium deposits usually consist of hydroxyapatite crystals. This is associated primarily with chronic renal insufficiency in which ulceration of the skin may be caused by calcification of blood vessels, leading to ischemic skin necrosis, or by painful disseminated calcification of the dermis and subcutaneous tissues (calciphylaxis).[52] Chronic renal failure is also associated with benign nodular calcification. Calcium deposits in the skin may develop as a result of hypervitaminosis D, milk-alkali syndrome, and other causes of hypercalcemia and hyperphosphatemia.

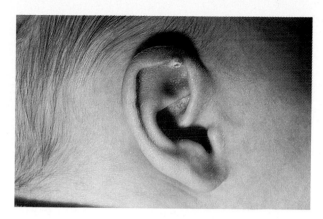

FIG. 21-12
Calcified ear nodule, also known as nodular calcification of Winer.

Metastatic calcinosis in the skin is rarely seen in infancy and childhood.[53] In contrast, the cutaneous bone formation, or osteoma cutis, associated with Albright hereditary osteodystrophy frequently appears first in infancy or childhood and may present in the neonatal period. This metabolic disorder is discussed in the following section.

Idiopathic Calcification

Idiopathic calcification can be congenital or acquired. Congenital calcified nodules occur most frequently on the ear, but may be seen elsewhere on the face and limbs. These lesions are variously described as *congenital calcified nodule of the ear, subepidermal calcified nodule,* or *solitary congenital nodular calcification of Winer*.[54,55,56] Other types of idiopathic calcinosis cutis, such as idiopathic calcification of the scrotum and the milia-like lesions associated with Down syndrome, present later in childhood or adolescence and are not seen in the newborn. There are rare reports of juxtaarticular *tumoral calcinosis* in infancy.[57-60]

Calcified Ear Nodule

A solitary calcified nodule on the pinna or earlobe is the most common presentation of idiopathic calcinosis in the newborn (Fig. 21-12). These nodules may occur elsewhere on the face or limbs, and occasionally there is more than one nodule. Auricular lesions developing after birth have also been described. There is a male preponderance.

Cutaneous Findings. The nodule is firm and measures 3 to 10 mm in diameter. The surface may be warty in appearance or smooth and dome-shaped. The color is chalky white or yellow. Surface ulceration and discharge of calcified material may occur spontaneously or as a result of trauma. There are usually no associated symptoms.

Extracutaneous Findings. Serum calcium and phosphate levels are normal. There are no systemic abnormalities.

Etiology and Pathogenesis. The pathogenesis of these lesions is not clear. Most authors believe that they represent dystrophic calcification following dermal damage from some unknown source. Proposed hypotheses include derivation from milia, syringomas, other sweat gland hamartomas, nevi, trauma, and degranulation of mast cells with secondary calcification.[55,56]

Diagnosis. The diagnosis is often made on the clinical appearance. Histologically, amorphous, and/or globular masses of calcified material are seen in the papillary dermis and may extend to the reticular dermis. Foreign body giant cells may be observed in association with the calcified masses. The overlying epidermis shows a warty architecture with variable amounts of pseudoepitheliomatous hyperplasia. Ulceration and transepidermal elimination of calcium may occur.

Differential Diagnosis. Clinically, calcified nodules may be misdiagnosed as viral warts, molluscum contagiosum, pilomatricomas, syringomas, and congenital inclusion cysts.

Treatment and Prognosis. If treatment is necessary, the nodule can be removed by curettage or excision. Calcified nodules sometimes recur following curettage or shave excision. Intralesional injection of triamcinolone at the time of shave excision has been suggested for recurrent lesions.[54]

Tumoral Calcinosis

Tumoral calcinosis is characterized by painless, calcified soft-tissue nodules located close to large joints in otherwise healthy children and adults.[57-60] It occurs most frequently in patients of African heritage. There have been five reported cases in infancy, the youngest of whom was 3 weeks old.[59]

Cutaneous Findings. Tumoral calcinosis presents as progressively growing, lobulated masses in a juxtaarticular location. The hip joints, shoulders, and elbows are most frequently affected in older children and adults. A predilection for the anterior aspect of the knee has been noted in three infants.[59] Involvement of the buttock, axilla, and supraclavicular region has also been observed in infancy.[58,60] Lesions may be multifocal and, occasionally, bilateral. Rarely, ulceration of the overlying skin with discharge of a chalky white substance may occur.[58] Large lesions may interfere with joint or muscle function.

Extracutaneous Findings. About one third of patients with tumoral calcinosis have idiopathic hyperphos-

phatemia. Transient and marginally elevated serum phosphate levels were found in one affected infant.[60] Serum calcium levels are normal.

Etiology and Pathogenesis. The etiology is unknown. Both abnormal phosphate metabolism and trauma have been proposed as possible causes. An inborn error of phosphate metabolism has been postulated because of reports in the literature of tumoral calcinosis in multiple family members. A mechanical pathogenesis is based on the observation that lesions occur in areas of chronic mechanical trauma, particularly in Africans who carry heavy loads and sleep on hard floors.

Diagnosis. Radiographs show discrete, sometimes lobulated, calcified areas. There is no joint involvement, and the underlying bones appear normal. Excisional biopsy specimens usually show a well-encapsulated calcified mass, but there may be invasion of the surrounding musculature. Histologic examination reveals calcification, central necrosis, a chronic inflammatory cell infiltrate including multinucleate giant cells, and fibrosis.[57,60]

Treatment. Excision is the treatment of choice. There may be recurrence after excision. Spontaneous resolution was observed in one infant after incisional biopsy of a supraclavicular mass.[60]

Iatrogenic Calcification

Iatrogenic calcinosis cutis (see Chapter 8) may result from intravenous infusion of calcium gluconate, with or without extravasation of the solution into the tissues. In addition to cutaneous calcification, there may be an intense inflammatory response and occasionally soft-tissue necrosis.[61]

Iatrogenic calcification has also been described following electrode placement for electroencephalography, electromyography, and brain stem auditory evoked potentials when calcium containing electrode paste was applied to abraded skin.[62] Treatment is generally symptomatic, and spontaneous resolution occurs over several months.

Osteoma Cutis

Heterotopic ossification of the skin, or osteoma cutis, is classified as primary and secondary. In primary osteoma cutis there is no preexisting skin pathology. In secondary osteoma cutis, bone formation develops within scars, inflammatory lesions, skin tumors, hamartomas, or cysts.

Primary osteoma cutis may present in infancy as a manifestation of Albright hereditary osteodystrophy (AHO),[63] or as an idiopathic disorder. Idiopathic variants have been described as progressive osseous heteroplasia,[64] congenital platelike osteoma cutis,[65] and familial ectopic ossification or hereditary osteoma cutis.[66]

Albright Hereditary Osteodystrophy

Albright hereditary osteodystrophy (AHO) is a genetic disorder that manifests clinically as pseudohypoparathyroidism (PHP) or pseudopseudohypoparathyroidism (PPHP). Both variants of the disorder have a similar phenotype. PHP is characterized by a lack of end-organ responsiveness to parathormone and variable degrees of hypocalcemia and hyperphosphatemia. In PPHP, serum calcium and phosphate levels are normal. PHP and PPHP may occur in the same kindred and PPHP may progress to PHP in a single individual.[63]

Cutaneous Findings. Osteoma cutis is present in up to 42% of patients with PHP and PPHP. Lesions are usually first noted in infancy or childhood. They may be located anywhere on the body and have a predilection for sites of friction or mild trauma. The characteristic lesions are blue-tinged, stony-hard papules, nodules, or plaques that range in size from pinpoint to 5 cm in diameter. Early lesions may present as barely discernible blue macules (Fig. 21-13). Rarely, more extensive cutaneous ossification may occur (Fig. 21-14). Ulceration occurs occasionally.

Extracutaneous Findings. The characteristic phenotype of AHO includes short stature, round face, obesity, and brachydactyly, in particular a shortened fourth metacarpal. Other manifestations include dental defects, short broad nails, cataracts, calcification of the basal ganglia, and mental retardation. These findings are easier to discern in late childhood and adulthood and are not usually manifest in infancy. Hypocalcemia may cause seizures and tetany. Some patients with PHP have evidence of other endocrine abnormalities such as hypogonadism or hypothyroidism.

Etiology and Pathogenesis. The metabolic changes in PHP result from a failure of receptors in renal and skeletal target tissues to respond to PTH. This resistance to the action of PTH is variable in PHP and apparently absent in PPHP. The mechanism of end-organ resistance to PTH is not fully understood. In some cases (PHP type 1a), it is associated with reduced expression or function of a guanine nucleotide stimulatory protein (G$_s$-alpha) that is required for activation of adenylate cyclase by the hormone-bound receptor.[67] Inheritance of AHO was originally believed to be X-linked dominant, but autosomal dominant inheritance is now considered more likely. The gene for G$_s$ alpha is located on chromosome 20q13. A second candidate gene is the vasoactive intestinal peptide receptor (RDCI), which has been mapped to 2q37.[68]

Diagnosis. Skin biopsy shows bone formation in the dermis and subcutis. Osteoblasts, osteocytes, and osteoclasts are present within the spicules of bone. When ossification is severe and progressive, a proliferation of spindle cells, resembling fibroblasts, may be prominent.

In PHP there is hypocalcemia, hyperphosphatemia, and an elevated serum PTH. In PPHP, there is no discernible abnormality of calcium and phosphate metabolism. Urinary excretion of cAMP in response to intravenous infusion of PTH is impaired in most cases of PHP but is normal in PPHP.

Radiologic abnormalities include ossification of the skin and subcutaneous tissues; shortening of the metacarpal, metatarsal, and phalangeal bones, notably the distal phalanx of the thumb and the fourth metacarpal; and cone epiphyses. Occasionally, there may be radiographic evidence of hyperparathyroidism or osteomalacia.

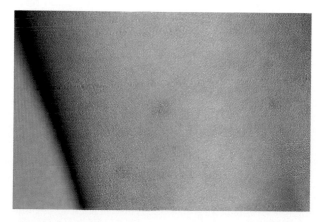

FIG. 21-13
Violaceous macules and papules of osteoma cutis in an infant with osteoma cutis with Albright hereditary osteodystrophy.

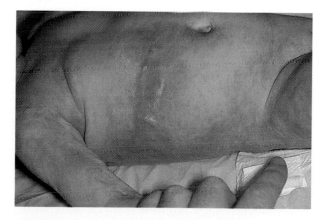

FIG. 21-14
Progressive osseous heteroplasia in an infant with familial Albright hereditary osteodystrophy at 1 year of age.

Differential Diagnosis. Hypocalcemia, hyperphosphatemia, and elevated levels of circulating PTH in the absence of renal disease, steatorrhea, or generalized osteomalacia are characteristic of PHP. A diagnosis of PPHP may be difficult to establish in infancy, particularly when there is no family history of AHO. The differential diagnosis includes idiopathic variants of osteoma cutis that present in this age group, such as progressive osseous heteroplasia, congenital plate-like osteoma cutis, and familial osteoma cutis in families with no evidence of AHO.[66]

Treatment and Prognosis. Treatment of PHP is directed towards controlling hypocalcemia by careful administration and monitoring of calcium and vitamin D. Normocalcemic patients must be monitored closely and evaluated regularly for development of cataracts or hypocalcemia. Mental retardation may be causally related to poorly controlled or undetected hypocalcemia. Patients should also be screened for hypothyroidism. There is no effective treatment for osteoma cutis. Surgical excision may be considered for individual lesions that cause pain or cosmetic disfigurement.

Congenital Plate-Like Osteoma Cutis

Congenital plate-like cutaneous osteoma is a rare entity that occurs in infants with no abnormality of calcium or phosphate metabolism. Lesions present at birth or in the first year of life as a large, asymptomatic, skin-colored plaque, varying in size from 1 to 15 cm.[65] There are no predisposing events such as trauma or infection to explain the heterotopic ossification. The scalp is the site of predilection, but lesions may also be found on the limbs or trunk. There are no associated abnormalities. Radiographs reveal calcified sheets or nodules in the subcutaneous soft tissues. Histology shows mature spongy bone in the dermis and subcutis. There may be gradual progression of the lesion with time and clinical overlap with progressive osseous heteroplasia. It is proposed that the term *congenital plate-like osteoma cutis* should be reserved for nonprogressive, superficial lesions to distinguish this disorder from progressive osseous heteroplasia in which ossification extends deeper into muscle and is relentlessly progressive.[52] Treatment is by excision, if necessary and feasible. Recurrence after excision has been reported.

Progressive Osseous Heteroplasia

Progressive osseous heteroplasia (POH) is a recently described entity that is characterized by progressive heterotopic ossification of the skin and deeper soft tissues, including muscle.[64,69,70,71] It presents at birth or in early infancy with focal areas of dermal ossification that resemble rice grains and have a gritty consistency.[64] These enlarge and coalesce to form large nodules and plaques. Extension to the deeper tissues and muscle often results in ankylosis of affected joints and growth retardation of involved limbs. There have been case reports of ossification limited to one half of the body or to a single limb.[70] Histologic examination reveals mainly intramembranous ossification similar to that seen in AHO, although foci of enchondral bone formation with cartilage are sometimes present. There is a female predominance. Most reported cases are sporadic, although familial cases showing autosomal dominant inheritance have been observed with smaller, more trivial lesions occurring in other affected family members.[69] POH is not typically associated with endocrine dysfunction. However, although the lesions in Albright hereditary osteodystrophy (AHO) are usually more superficial and limited to the dermis and subcutis, the clinical phenotype of POH has been observed in association with AHO (see Fig. 21-14).[72] The relationship between these disorders and other congenital and familial forms of osteoma cutis awaits better understanding of the pathogenesis of heterotopic ossification and the underlying genetic defects.

HAMARTOMAS

A *hamartoma* is a developmental abnormality of the skin in which there is an excess of one or more mature or nearly mature tissue structures normally found at that site.[73] The term *nevus* is often used synonymously, although not all "nevi" are hamartomas (e.g., nevus anemicus, nevus depigmentosus). Whether a lesion is designated a hamartoma or a nevus largely depends on tradition.[74] An *organoid nevus* or *organoid hamartoma* refers to a malformation that consists of more than one type of tissue structure, and where identification of a single tissue of origin is not possible.[74]

Most hamartomas are isolated, sporadic malformations. They can be single or multiple, localized or extensive, and may be distributed in a linear or whorled pattern corresponding to the lines of Blaschko. Some arise from a post-zygotic mutation in the embryo that leads to somatic mosaicism.[75] Others are manifestations of well-defined genetic disorders such as tuberous sclerosis. Epidermal hamartomas may be associated with underlying abnormalities in the central nervous system, skeleton, or other organs. Rarely, a post-zygotic mutation that involves the germ line results in transmission of generalized skin disease to subsequent offspring.[75,76]

Nevus Sebaceus

The nevus sebaceus (of Jadassohn) is an organoid hamartoma of appendageal structures that is usually evident at birth.[77] It occurs where pilosebaceous and apocrine structures are prominent and is considered to be a variant of epidermal nevus on the head and neck.[74,77] A nevus sebaceus is seen in 0.3% of newborns.[78]

Cutaneous Findings. The typical nevus sebaceus is a pink-yellow or yellow-orange plaque with a pebbly or velvety surface that is located on the scalp or face (Fig. 21-15). It varies in size from one to several centimeters and can be round, oval, or linear in shape. Lesions on the scalp present as a congenital area of circumscribed alopecia (Fig. 21-16). There may be evolution from a slightly raised plaque at birth to a flat, almost macular lesion in infancy and childhood. A verrucous or cobblestone appearance develops in adolescence when the sebaceous and apocrine glands enlarge and proliferate.[73] Some lesions present with an atypical papillomatous or cerebriform morphology (Fig. 21-17). There can be some overlap between the morphology of a sebaceus nevus and an epidermal verrucous nevus on the head and neck. Both types of nevus may coexist at different sites when extensive lesions are present.

Extracutaneous Findings. The nevus sebaceus is usually an isolated lesion with no extracutaneous findings. Rarely, it is associated with other developmental abnormalities in a variable malformation syndrome known as

the "Schimmelpenning-Feuerstein-Mims syndrome," "linear nevus sebaceus syndrome" or "epidermal nevus syndrome."[24,77,79] The nevus sebaceus can be of any size or shape but is often extensive or linear, with a distribution following the lines of Blaschko. Extracutaneous manifestations include mental retardation, seizures, coloboma of the eyelid, lipodermoids of the conjunctiva, choristomas, and other ophthalmologic and central nervous system abnormalities.[74,77,79,80] Skeletal, cardiac and genitourinary

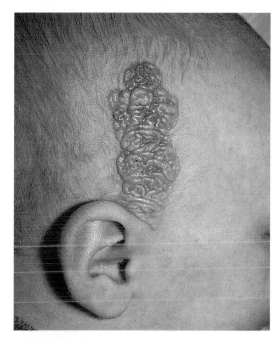

FIG. 21-16
Nevus sebaceus on the scalp with overlying alopecia.

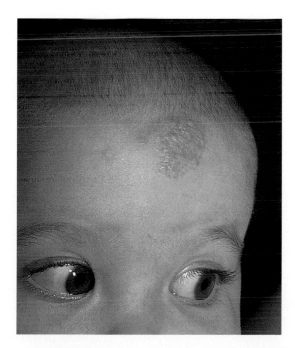

FIG. 21-15
Nevus sebaceus on the forehead of a newborn.

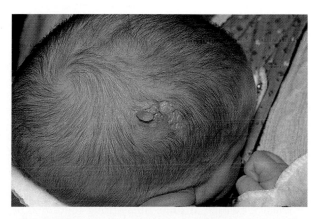

FIG. 21-17
Nevus sebaceus with pedunculated, cerebriform appearance.

abnormalities, and vitamin D–resistant rickets are also reported.[74,77,81,82]

Etiology and Pathogenesis. The pathogenesis of this hamartoma is not known. There is no racial or gender predilection. There have been rare reports of familial lesions.[83,84] The linear nevus sebaceus (or epidermal nevus) syndrome occurs sporadically, and an autosomal lethal mutation that survives by mosaicism has been postulated.[85]

Diagnosis. The diagnosis is usually made on clinical grounds except in atypical cases. In infancy and childhood, the characteristic histologic changes of nevus sebaceus are less developed than in adolescence and adulthood. Mature lesions show numerous sebaceous and apocrine glands in the dermis with overlying epidermal hyperplasia. In infants, the histologic findings are more subtle with rudimentary hair follicles and immature glandular structures. It can sometimes be difficult to distinguish a linear nevus sebaceus from a verrucous epidermal nevus histologically, as well as clinically, during childhood.

Differential Diagnosis. The differential diagnosis of a circumscribed area of alopecia on the scalp at birth includes aplasia cutis congenita and neural tube closure defects such as meningocele, encephalocele, and rests of heterotopic meningeal or brain tissue in the skin (see Chapter 9). Aplasia cutis congenita can be distinguished by the presence of atrophy and scarring, and in some cases ulceration of the skin at birth. Neural tube defects are located in or close to the midline at the vertex, nasal bridge, or lower occipital scalp. Both aplasia cutis congenita and neural tube closure defects may show a collarette of dark terminal hair in the newborn.[86]

Treatment and Prognosis. The nevus sebaceus has a propensity to develop neoplastic growths, most of which are benign appendageal tumors such as syringocystadenoma papilliferum, trichilemmoma, trichoblastoma, and apocrine cystadenoma. Malignant tumors include basal cell epithelioma, squamous cell carcinoma, and tubular apocrine carcinoma.[87] These tumors are localized to the skin lesion and rarely metastasize, although they may be locally invasive.[88] The lifetime risk of developing a superimposed malignant tumor is uncertain, and very high figures may be subject to ascertainment bias.[87,88] Neoplastic change in a nevus sebaceus is unusual in childhood. Changes that should lead one to suspect a neoplastic growth include surface ulceration or development of a nodule within the lesion.

Elective excision at some time during childhood or adolescence is recommended both for cosmetic reasons and because of the risk of developing a superimposed adnexal tumor in adult life.

As the lifetime risk of aggressive malignant transformation is low, observation may be preferable to surgery for lesions that are extensive or difficult to excise with a good cosmetic result, particularly on the face.

Epidermal Nevus

The term *epidermal nevus* is used to encompass a group of hamartomas of ectodermal origin in which there is clinical and histologic overlap. These include the linear verrucous epidermal nevus, inflammatory linear verrucous epidermal nevus (ILVEN), nevus sebaceus, and nevus comedonicus. Other hamartomas that may be considered epidermal nevi are syringocystadenoma papilliferum, linear porokeratosis, and porokeratotic eccrine and ostial dermal duct tumor. Epidermal nevi also occur as a component of the Proteus syndrome and CHILD (congenital hemidysplasia with ichthyosiform nevus and limb defects) syndrome.[85] When applied without qualification, the term *epidermal nevus* usually refers to a linear verrucous epidermal nevus. Epidermal nevi affect about 1 in 1000 people.[75]

Cutaneous Findings. The verrucous epidermal nevus presents at birth or during early childhood and may continue to extend for a variable period of time.[77] Rarely, new lesions become apparent in adolescence or adult life. Lesions vary in extent from a small cluster or linear arrangement of pigmented, warty papules to widespread linear and swirled areas of pigmentation following the lines of Blaschko (Fig. 21-18). A linear epidermal nevus may involve an entire limb, half of the body in a unilateral distribution, or both sides of the trunk, limbs, and face in a symmetric pattern with demarcation at the midline. Extensive bilateral lesions have been referred to historically as "systematized epidermal nevus" or "ichthyosis hystrix," and unilateral lesions as "nevus unius lateris."

Epidermal nevi may have a macerated appearance at birth because of prolonged contact with amniotic fluid (Fig. 21-19). During childhood, the degree of verrucosity varies from subtle, almost flat pigmentation to a grossly elevated, warty appearance.[77] There is a tendency to become more verrucous with age, particularly during puberty. Epidermal nevi involving the head and neck often exhibit the morphology of a nevus sebaceus. Scalp lesions may also be associated with woolly hair nevus, and occasional epidermal nevi have overlying hypertrichosis.[89,90] A linear lesion that impinges on the nail matrix may cause dystrophy of the involved nail.

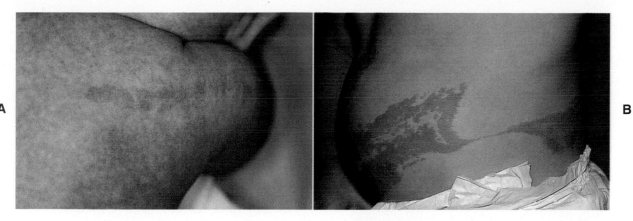

FIG. 21-18
Linear epidermal nevus following the lines of Blaschko on **A**, a shoulder and arm and **B**, the trunk.

The linear inflammatory verrucous epidermal nevus (ILVEN) is a verrucous, erythematous lesion that can occur at any site, but is most often seen on the limbs or perineum in girls (Fig. 21-20). It is extremely pruritic and may simulate linear psoriasis or linear lichen planus. It is rarely present at birth, but may appear in the first months of life.

Extracutaneous Findings. The majority of epidermal nevi are isolated lesions with no evidence of extracutaneous disease. Multiple associated anomalies are seen in the "epidermal nevus syndrome."[74,77] Manifestations of this variable syndrome include developmental abnormalities of the central nervous system, skeleton, eye, and heart, as well as tumors of the genitourinary tract, precocious puberty, and vitamin D–resistant rickets.[90-94]

In the Proteus syndrome, epidermal nevi occur in association with limb overgrowth, lipomatous lesions, cerebriform malformations of the feet, and cutaneous vascular anomalies.[85] The CHILD syndrome is characterized by verrucous lesions corresponding to the lines of Blaschko in conjunction with limb reduction defects.[85]

Diagnosis. The most common histologic pattern is that of a benign papilloma, with acanthosis, elongation of rete ridges, hyperkeratosis, and papillomatosis. This histologic appearance may be shared by viral warts, seborrheic keratosis, or acanthosis nigricans. Histology of lesions from the scalp may reveal features of a nevus sebaceus, especially after puberty. A subset of epidermal nevi shows the histologic features of epidermolytic hyperkeratosis, characterized by perinuclear vacuolization of keratinocytes and increased numbers of enlarged keratohyalin granules with overlying hyperkeratosis. In a less

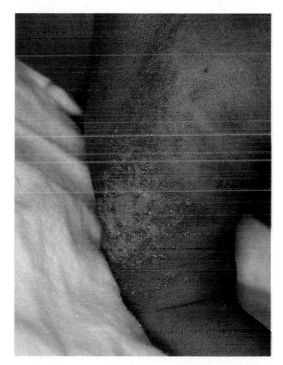

FIG. 21-19
Epidermal nevus on the leg shortly after delivery.

common variant, there is acantholytic hyperkeratosis similar to that seen in Darier's disease.[95]

Etiology and Pathogenesis. The distribution of lesions following the lines of Blaschko suggests somatic mosaicism. Chromosomal mosaicism has been demonstrated

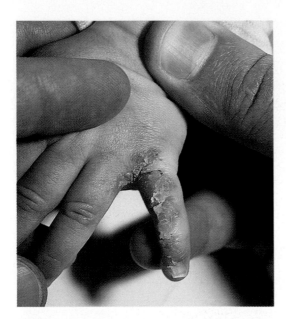

FIG. 21-20
Inflammatory linear epidermal nevus (ILVEN) on dorsal hand and finger.

in two patients with linear verrucous epidermal nevi.[96] The concept of mosaicism is supported by observation of lesions with the histology of epidermolytic hyperkeratosis in the parents of children with bullous ichthyosiform erythroderma.[75,76] The same keratin 10 gene mutation was identified in lesional skin from parents with epidermal nevi, and in their offspring with generalized skin disease.[75] This phenomenon has not been observed with other epidermal nevi, suggesting that the genetic defects in these cases may be lethal if inherited.[85] Epidermal nevi are now thought to represent a phenotypic expression of several genetic defects due to post-zygotic mutations, rather than a single disease. Whether the basic pathogenetic defect of nonepidermolytic lesions lies in the dermal fibroblast or in the keratinocyte is not known.

Differential Diagnosis. The differential diagnosis of a localized cluster of lesions includes viral warts, which do not commonly have a linear arrangement and spontaneously regress with time. Linear lesions at birth may be confused with the verrucous stage of incontinentia pigmenti. Linear epidermal nevi that develop during infancy and childhood differ in morphology, if not in distribution, from lichen striatus, a self-limiting disorder with an inflammatory, papular appearance and lichenoid histology. The differential diagnosis of ILVEN includes lichen simplex chronicus, linear psoriasis, and linear lichen planus, none of which is seen in the newborn period.

The CHILD syndrome and Proteus syndrome have distinctive clinical features. Happle considers these two entities to be well-defined epidermal nevus syndromes.[85] In *phakomatosis pigmentokeratotica* (PPK), the coexistence of an epidermal nevus of the nonepidermolytic type and a melanocytic speckled lentiginous nevus is frequently associated with neurologic and musculoskeletal anomalies (see Chapter 20).

Treatment and Prognosis. Unlike nevus sebaceus, the linear verrucous epidermal nevus is rarely associated with development of superimposed benign or malignant tumors in adult life. Patients with epidermal nevi should be evaluated clinically and followed for developmental anomalies and other manifestations of the epidermal nevus syndrome.[77] When histologic examination shows epidermolytic hyperkeratosis, the patient should receive counseling about the possible risk of genetic transmission. The risk of transmission is not known.

Treatment may be requested for cosmetically disfiguring lesions but is generally undertaken later in life. Excision of small lesions or localized areas of larger lesions may be feasible. Treatment of extensive lesions is difficult. Various destructive modalities, including CO_2 laser ablation, dermabrasion, or liquid nitrogen cryotherapy, have been attempted, but there is frequent recurrence.[97] The same is true for pharmacologic treatments such as topical or oral retinoids and 5-fluorouracil.[98]

Nevus Comedonicus

A nevus comedonicus is a developmental abnormality of the pilosebaceous unit that appears as a grouped or linear arrangement of small or large comedones. Lesions present at birth or during infancy in the majority of cases. Nevus comedonicus is considered a rare type of epidermal nevus.

Cutaneous Findings. Groups of enlarged follicular openings containing pigmented, comedone-like keratin plugs may be localized or extensive (Fig. 21-21, *A* and *B*). Most nevi are unilateral and located on the face or upper trunk. They frequently have a linear arrangement. Extensive lesions are distributed along the lines of Blaschko and are limited at the midline.[99,100] There may be associated white papules representing milia, closed comedones, or deeper follicular cystic structures. Later in childhood or adolescence, these lesions may develop painful, inflammatory cystic nodules and acneiform scarring (Fig. 21-21, *C*).[101] Coexistence of a nevus comedonicus and a verrucous epidermal nevus is reported[102]; comedone-like structures may also be seen within verrucous epidermal nevi.[77]

Extracutaneous Findings. In most cases there are no extracutaneous manifestations. Rarely, a nevus comedonicus is associated with central nervous system, skele-

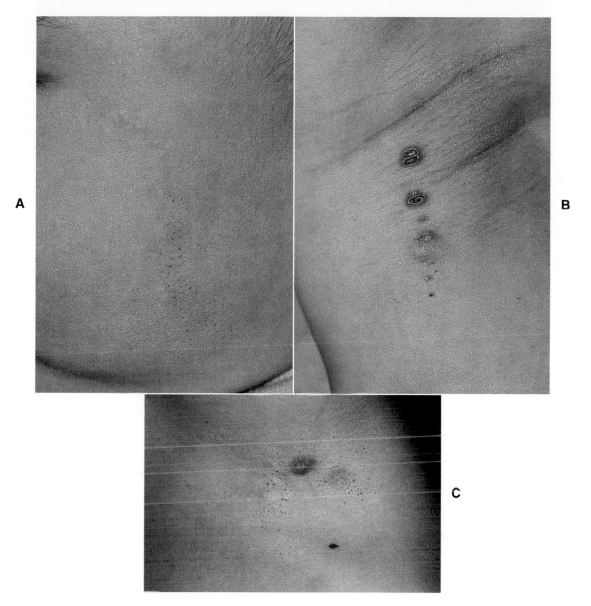

FIG. 21-21

Nevus comedonicus. **A,** Open and closed comedones in a linear arrangement on the face of an infant; **B,** large pigmented follicular keratin plugs and a deep follicular cyst; **C,** comedones, inflammatory and noninflammatory cysts in an adolescent.

tal, and ocular abnormalities.[101] In these cases, unilateral cataract and skeletal abnormalities are found on the same side of the body as the nevus.[101] The nevus comedonicus syndrome is considered a variant or subtype of the epidermal nevus syndrome.[85,101]

Etiology and Pathogenesis. Nevus comedonicus is a sporadic disorder and is not inherited. The pathogenesis is believed to involve somatic mosaicism.[85,100]

Diagnosis. The diagnosis is made on the clinical ap-

pearance of the lesion. Histopathologic examination reveals hyperkeratosis and acanthosis of the epidermis with widely dilated, keratin-filled, cystic structures. Epidermolytic hyperkeratosis may be observed in the keratinocytes of the follicular epithelial wall.[99,101]

Differential Diagnosis. The localized appearance of the lesion is very characteristic and unlikely to be mistaken for comedonal acne unless bilateral.[100] Porokeratotic eccrine ostial and dermal duct nevus presents with comedo-like lesions on the palms and soles and has distinctive histologic features. Inflammatory cysts may closely resemble cystic acne.

Treatment and Prognosis. Recurrent inflammation and scarring can cause cosmetic disfigurement. Treatment is difficult. Excision of smaller lesions is curative.[103] Inflammatory acneiform cysts may recur if excision is incomplete. Pharmacologic agents such as oral or topical retinoids are of minimal benefit. Topical and systemic antibiotics have been used to treat inflammatory lesions with variable success.[100]

Porokeratotic Eccrine and Ostial Dermal Duct Nevus

The porokeratotic eccrine and ostial dermal duct nevus is a congenital hamartoma of the eccrine ducts. Although usually present at birth, lesions may first appear in later childhood or adult life.

Cutaneous and Extracutaneous Findings. This hamartoma is characterized clinically by grouped comedo-like keratotic papules or pits on a palm or sole.[104] Occasionally lesions may be more widespread with a linear distribution.[105] Keratotic papules and plaques that are located in sites other than the palms and soles resemble linear verrucous epidermal nevi.[105-107] There are no symptoms. There may be associated anhidrosis. There are no recognized systemic manifestations.

Etiology and Pathogenesis. The pathogenesis is believed to represent a circumscribed disorder of keratinization localized to the acrosyringium.[105]

Diagnosis. Histologically, there are epidermal invaginations with parakeratotic plugs emerging from dilated eccrine ostia and surrounded by parakeratotic columns of cornoid lamellae.[106] The eccrine origin of the lesion is confirmed by positive staining for carcinoembryonic antigen (CEA).[105]

Differential Diagnosis. The clinical differential diagnosis includes linear porokeratosis, nevus comedonicus, and linear verrucous nevus. Histologically, punctate porokeratosis and linear porokeratosis of Mibelli can be distinguished by the lack of epidermal invaginations.

Treatment and Prognosis. Benefit from treatment with the UltraPulse CO_2 laser has been reported, although recurrence was noted.[105]

Congenital Smooth Muscle Hamartoma

Congenital smooth muscle hamartoma is a benign cutaneous developmental anomaly characterized by an excess of arrector pili muscle within the reticular dermis.[108] It is usually evident at birth or shortly thereafter. The estimated prevalence is 1 in 2600 live births with a slight male predominance.[109] Rarely, extensive involvement may be associated with the phenotype of the Michelin tire baby.[110-112]

Cutaneous Findings. The typical congenital smooth muscle hamartoma presents as a lightly pigmented plaque or patch with overlying hypertrichosis (Fig. 21-22). The trunk, in particular the lumbosacral area, is the site of predilection but lesions may also occur on the proximal limbs. Perifollicular papules are sometimes evident.[113] The overlying hair is vellus in type. Hypertrichosis is not invariable, and the hamartoma may present as a plaque of perifollicular papules with little or no increase in hair growth (Fig. 21-23).[114] Transient elevation or a rippling

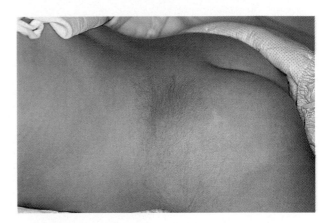

FIG. 21-22
Congenital smooth muscle hamartoma with overlying hypertrichosis.

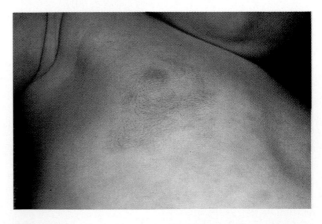

FIG. 21-23
Plaque of congenital smooth muscle hamartoma with minimal hypertrichosis.

movement of the lesion due to contraction of the muscle bundles can sometimes be elicited by rubbing or stroking the surface. Rarely, a congenital smooth muscle hamartoma has a linear configuration or presents with multiple lesions.[115,116]

Extracutaneous Findings. There are no systemic findings with localized lesions. There may be associated mental retardation, seizures, and other developmental abnormalities in children with extensive smooth muscle hamartoma as a manifestation of the Michelin tire baby syndrome.[112] Unilateral hypoplasia of the breast and other cutaneous, muscular, or skeletal defects may be associated with smooth muscle hamartoma in the Becker nevus syndrome.[117]

Etiology and Pathogenesis. Congenital smooth muscle hamartoma is believed to represent aberrant development of pilar smooth muscle during fetal life. It has been suggested that the hamartoma involves other structures such as neural tissue and hair.[113] The hypertrichosis appears to result from increased hair length and diameter rather than an increase in hair density.[114]

Diagnosis. Light microscopic examination of a skin biopsy specimen will establish the diagnosis if the clinical appearance is atypical. Numerous well-defined and variably oriented bundles of smooth muscle are seen within the reticular dermis. They may or may not be associated with follicular structures. Increased epidermal pigmentation may be observed.

Differential Diagnosis. The differential diagnosis of congenital smooth muscle hamartoma includes Becker nevus, nevus pilosus, leiomyoma, connective tissue nevus, solitary mastocytoma, plexiform neurofibroma, and congenital hairy melanocytic nevus. Smooth muscle may be observed in the dermis in Becker nevus and a continuum between the two conditions has been proposed.[113] Unlike Becker nevus, the congenital smooth muscle hamartoma is always present at birth, does not show prominent epidermal changes, and may demonstrate abnormally whorled myofilaments on electron microscopy.[114]

A nevus pilosus, or hairy patch, shows no alteration in skin texture or pigmentation, and the hair is usually terminal in type. A congenital pigmented hairy nevus is more deeply pigmented, and the overlying hypertrichosis is composed of terminal hair. Leiomyoma is a circumscribed spindle-cell tumor. Connective tissue nevi and mastocytoma may be distinguished by skin biopsy.[114]

Prognosis. This hamartoma has no malignant potential, and the prognosis is excellent. There is a tendency for the pigmentation and hair growth to become less noticeable with age.[109] Treatment is unnecessary unless there are cosmetic concerns in later life.

Congenital Becker Nevus and Becker Nevus Syndrome

Becker nevus is an organoid hamartoma characterized by a circumscribed area of hyperpigmentation and hypertrichosis. It is commonly located over the shoulder, chest, or scapula and has a predilection for males. Although usually acquired in adolescence, a number of congenital cases of Becker nevus have been described.[117-120] Histopathologic examination reveals acanthosis and hyperpigmentation of the basal layer of the epidermis, as well as a variable dermal component consisting of smooth muscle bundles that resemble congenital smooth muscle hamartoma.

The Becker nevus syndrome refers to an association with unilateral hypoplasia of the female breast and ipsilateral skeletal defects such as hypoplasia of the shoulder girdle or arm. Other reported anomalies include supernumerary nipples, scoliosis, spina bifida occulta, congenital adrenal hyperplasia, and accessory scrotum.[117,119,121] The syndrome is twice as common in females, possibly because ipsilateral hypoplasia of the breast is easily recognized and reported.[117] A postzygotic mutation that gives rise to mosaicism may explain the location of the nevus and associated anomalies in a similar body region.[117] Although both the isolated nevus and the Becker nevus syndrome are generally sporadic, there have been a few reports of familial aggregation.[117,118]

Michelin Tire Baby

The "Michelin tire baby" is characterized by numerous transverse skin folds on all four limbs. These circumferential ringed creases may be associated with an underlying diffuse nevus lipomatosus or a smooth muscle hamartoma.[111] There have been two reports of autosomal dominant transmission.[112] There may be an association with other congenital defects, such as mental retardation, microcephaly, hemiplegia, hemihypertrophy, and chromosomal defects, suggesting a contiguous gene syndrome.[112] When the syndrome is associated with an underlying smooth muscle hamartoma, there is often diffuse hyperpigmentation and hypertrichosis. In one such patient, there were also moderate joint hyperextensibility and perifollicular papules.[111] No treatment is available. The skin folds usually diminish slowly as the child grows.

Nevus Lipomatosus

Nevus lipomatosus cutaneous superficialis is a hamartoma composed of mature fat. Clinically, these lesions present at birth or later in childhood as an asymptomatic, soft or rubbery plaque with a polypoid or cerebriform appearance.[122] A linear arrangement of flesh-colored to yellow lesions in a zosteriform pattern is the most common presentation (Fig. 21-24). They are frequently observed in the lumbosacral or perineal areas but can be located elsewhere. Histologic specimens show mature unencapsulated adipose tissue infiltrating between collagen bundles in the superficial and deep dermis. Similar features may be observed in the lipomatous lesions of encephalocraniocutaneous lipomatosis, focal dermal hypoplasia, or benign fat herniations on the feet of infants. Although asymptomatic, they may require excision for cosmetic reasons.

Connective Tissue Nevus

A connective tissue nevus is characterized by excessive deposition of one or both of the collagen or elastin components of dermal connective tissue. These hamartomas may occur sporadically or as a familial disorder with autosomal dominant transmission.[123] Connective tissue nevi are also seen as a manifestation of genetic syndromes, notably the "shagreen patch" or collagenoma in tuberous sclerosis, and the multiple elastic tissue nevi of Buschke-Ollendorff syndrome.[124] A connective tissue nevus may be present at birth, but most become evident during childhood or adolescence.

Cutaneous Findings. Connective tissue nevi present clinically as asymptomatic, firm, skin-colored to yellowish nodules or plaques located on the trunk or limbs (Fig. 21-25). The surface of the lesion may be smooth or have a "cobblestone," "leather-grain," or "peau d'orange" appearance. They may be solitary or multiple. A linear or "zosteriform" morphology is sometimes observed.

Extracutaneous Findings. Osteopoikilosis is seen in association with elastic tissue nevi in the Buschke-Ollendorff syndrome.[124] The skin lesions in this condition may rarely be present at birth, but the distinctive bone changes are not reported in infancy. The collagenoma or "shagreen patch" of tuberous sclerosis develops in later childhood, although other stigmata of the disease may be present at birth or in early infancy. Cardiomyopathy may occur in association with the multiple lesions of familial cutaneous collagenoma and with collagenomas and hypogonadism.[123] Multiple collagenomas in Down syndrome have been reported in adolescence.[125] A cerebriform collagenoma on the sole of the foot may be an isolated phenomenon or a component of Proteus syndrome.[126]

Etiology and Pathogenesis. The pathogenesis is unknown. In familial cutaneous collagenoma, the skin lesions are inherited as an autosomal dominant trait. Tuberous sclerosis and Buschke-Ollendorff syndrome are also inherited by autosomal dominant transmission. Somatic mosaicism may be postulated for sporadic lesions, particularly those with a linear distribution.

Diagnosis. Histologic examination of connective tissue nevi shows an excess of collagen or elastic tissue in the dermis. This may not be apparent unless a specimen of normal adjacent skin is obtained for comparison. Thus biopsies of connective tissue nevi are often reported as "normal skin." Special elastic stains are necessary to demonstrate the increased numbers of elastic fibers in elastic tissue nevi.

Differential Diagnosis. The differential diagnosis includes other cutaneous hamartomas such as neurofibromas, leiomyomas, smooth muscle hamartoma, nevus lipomatosus, and epidermal nevus. These entities may be

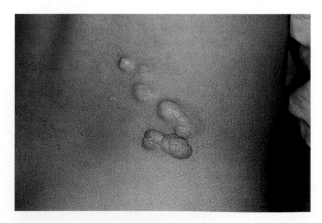

FIG. 21-24
Nevus lipomatosus with soft polypoid nodules on the lower back.

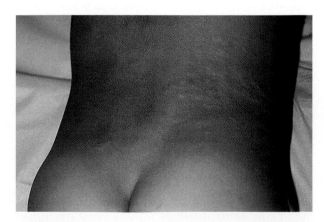

FIG. 21-25
Flesh-colored nodules of connective tissue nevi on the back.

distinguished by histopathologic examination of a skin biopsy.

Treatment and Prognosis. Connective tissue nevi are permanent lesions. They grow in proportion to the child's growth. There is no malignant potential and most lesions do not require treatment. Surgical excision may occasionally be indicated for cosmetic reasons.

REFERENCES

1. Coffin CM. Fibromyoblastic-myofibroblastic tumors. In Coffin CM, Dehner LP, O'Shea PA. Pediatric soft tissue tumors: A clinical, pathological, and therapeutic approach. Philadelphia: Williams & Wilkins, 1997: pp 133-178.
2. Enzinger FM, Weiss SW. Fibromatoses. In Soft tissue tumors. 2nd edition. St Louis: Mosby, 1988: pp 171-178.
3. Chung EB, Enzinger FM. Infantile myofibromatosis. Cancer 1981;48:1807-1818.
4. Brill PW, Yandow DR, Langer LO, et al. Pediatr Radiol 1982;12:269-278.
5. Parker RK, Mallory SB, Baker GF. Infantile myofibromatosis. Pediatr Dermatol 1991;8:129-132.
6. Goldberg NS, Bauer BS, Kraus H, et al. Infantile myofibromatosis: A review of clinicopathology with perspectives on new treatment choices. Pediatr Dermatol 1988;5:37-46.
7. Wada H, Akiyama H, Seki H, et al. Spinal canal involvement in infantile myofibromatosis: Case report and review of the literature. J Pediatr Hematol Oncol 1998;20:353-356.
8. Wiswell TE, Sakas EL, Stephenson SR, et al. Infantile myofibromatosis. Pediatrics 1985;76:981-984.
9. Bracko M, Cindro L, Golouh R. Familial occurrence of infantile myofibromatosis. Cancer 1992;69:1294-1299.
10. Keltz M, DiCostanzo D, Desai P, et al. Infantile (Desmoid-type) fibromatosis. Pediatr Dermatol 1995;12:149-151.
11. Martinez-Lage JF, Acosta J, Sola J, et al. Congenital desmoid tumor of the scalp: A histologically benign lesion with aggressive clinical behavior. Child's Nerv Sys 1996;12:409-412.
12. Pereyo NG, Heimer WL. Extraabdominal desmoid tumor. J Am Acad Dermatol 1996;34:352-356.
13. Faulkner LB, Hajdu SI, Kher U, et al. Pediatric desmoid tumor: Retrospective analysis of 63 cases. J Clin Oncol 1995;13:2813-2818.
14. Skapek SX, Hawk BJ, Hoffer FA, et al. Combination chemotherapy using vinblastine and methotrexate for the treatment of progressive desmoid tumor in children. J Clin Oncol 1998;16:3021-3027.
15. Lackner H, Urban C, Kerbl R, et al. Noncytotoxic drug therapy in children with unresectable desmoid tumors. Cancer 1997;80:334-340.
16. Eich GF, Hoeffel JC, Tschappeler H, et al. Fibrous tumors in children: imaging features of a heterogeneous group of disorders. Pediatric Radiology 1998;28:500-509.
17. Ishii N, Matsui K, Ichiyama S, et al. A case of infantile digital fibromatosis showing spontaneous regression. Br J Dermatol 1989;121:129-133.
18. Paller AS, Gonzalez-Crussi, Sherman JO. Fibrous hamartoma of infancy. Arch Dermatol 1989;125:88-91.
19. Sotelo-Avila C, Bale PM. Subdermal fibrous hamartoma of infancy: Pathology of 40 cases and differential diagnosis. Pediatr Pathol 1994;14:39-52.
20. Tagaki M, Yamamoto H, Mega H, et al. Heterogeneity in the gingival fibromatoses. Cancer 1991;68:2202-2212.
21. O'Shea PA. Myogenic tumors of soft tissue. In Coffin CM, Dehner LP, O'Shea PA. Pediatric soft tissue tumors: a clinical, pathological, and therapeutic approach. Philadelphia: Williams & Wilkins, 1997: pp 214-253.
22. Lupton GP, Naik DG, Rodman OG. An unusual congenital leiomyoma. Pediatr Dermatol 1986;3:158-160.
23. Henderson CA, Ruban A, Porter DL. Multiple leiomyomata presenting in a child. Pediatr Dermatol 1997;14:287-289.
24. Yang SS, Williams RJ, Bear BJ, et al. Leiomyoma of the hand in a child who has the human immunodeficiency virus: A case report. J Bone Joint Surg Am 1996;78-A:1904-1906.
25. McCormack K, Kaplan D, Murray JC, et al. Multiple hairy pacinian neurofibromas (nerve-sheath myxomas). J Am Acad Dermatol 1988;18:416-419.
26. Murato Y, Kumano K, Ugai K, et al. Neurilemmomatosis. Br J Dermatol 1991;125:466-468.
27. Mautner VF, Lindenau M, Baser ME, et al. Skin abnormalities in neurofibromatosis 2. Arch Dermatol 1997;133:1539-1543.
28. Iyengar V, Golomb CA, Schachner L. Neurilemmomatosis, NF2 and juvenile xanthogranuloma. J Am Acad Dermatol 1998;39:831-834.
29. Caputo R, Ermacora E, Gelmetti C, et al. Generalized eruptive histiocytoma in children. J Am Acad Dermatol 1987;17:449-454.
30. Jang KA, Lee HJ, Choi JH, et al. Generalized eruptive histiocytoma of childhood. Br J Dermatol 1999;140:174-176.
31. Hernandez-Martin A, Baselga E, Drolet BA, et al. Juvenile xanthogranuloma. J Am Acad Dermatol 1997;36:355-367.
32. Zvulunov A, Barak Y, Metzker A. Juvenile xanthogranuloma, neurofibromatosis, and juvenile chronic myelogenous leukemia. Arch Dermatol 1995;131:904-908.
33. Mann RE, Friedman KJ, Milgraum SS. Urticaria pigmentosa and juvenile xanthogranuloma: Case report and brief review of the literature. Pediatr Dermatol 1996;13:122-126.
34. Resnick SD, Woosly J, Azizkhan RG. Giant juvenile xanthogranuloma: Exophytic and endophytic variants. Pediatr Dermatol 1990;7:185-188.
35. Kolde G, Bonsmann G. Generalized lichenoid juvenile xanthogranuloma. Br J Dermatol 1992;126:66-70.
36. Freyer DR, Kennedy R, Bostrom BC, et al. Juvenile xanthogranuloma: Forms of systemic disease and their clinical implications. J Pediatr 1996;129:227-237.
37. Chang MW, Frieden IJ, Good W. The risk of intraocular juvenile xanthogranuloma: Survey of current practices and assessment of risk. J Am Acad Dermatol 1996;34:445-449.
38. Shapiro PE, Silvers DN, Treiber RK, et al. Juvenile xanthogranulomas with inconspicuous or absent foam cells and giant cells. J Am Acad Dermatol 1991;24:1005-1009.
39. Newman CC, Raimer SS, Sanchez RL. Nonlipidized juvenile xanthogranuloma: A histologic and immunohistochemical study. Pediatr Dermatol 1997;14:98-102.
40. Zelger BG, Zelger B, Steiner H, et al. Solitary giant xanthogranuloma and benign cephalic histiocytosis—variants of juvenile xanthogranuloma. Br J Dermatol 1995;133:598-604.
41. Godfrey KM, James MP. Benign cephalic histiocytosis: a case report. Br J Dermatol 1990;123:245-248.
42. Gianotti F, Caputo R. Histiocytic syndromes: a review. J Am Acad Dermatol 1985;13:383-404.

43. Sell EJ, Hansen RC, Struck-Pierce S. Calcified nodules of the heel: A complication of neonatal intensive care. J Pediatr 1985;96:473-475.

44. Leung A. Calcification following heel sticks. J Pediatr 1985; 106:168.

45. Fretzin DF, Arias AM. Sclerema neonatorum and subcutaneous fat necrosis of the newborn. Pediatr Dermatol 1987; 4:112-122.

46. Glover MT, Catterall MD, Atherton DJ. Subcutaneous fat necrosis in two infants after hypothermic cardiac surgery. Pediatr Dermatol 1991;8:210-212.

47. Chuang SD, Chiu HC, Chang CC. Subcutaneous fat necrosis of the newborn complicating hypothermic cardiac surgery. Br J Dermatol 1995;132:805-810.

48. Duhn R, Schoen E, Sui M. Subcutaneous fat necrosis with extensive calcification after hypothermia in two newborn infants. Pediatrics 1968;41:661-664.

49. Beers BB, Flowers FP, Sherertz EF, et al. Dystrophic calcinosis cutis secondary to intrauterine herpes simplex. Pediatr Dermatol 1986;3:208-211.

50. Ruiz-Maldonado R, Duran-McKinster C, Carrasco-Daza D, et al. Intrauterine epidermal necrosis: report of three cases. J Am Acad Dermatol 1998;38:712-715.

51. Carruthers J, Jevon G, Prendiville J. Localized dystrophic periocular calcification: A complication of intralesional corticosteroid therapy for infantile periocular hemangiomas. Pediatr Dermatol 1998;15:23-26.

52. Walsh JS, Fairley JA. Calcifying disorders of the skin. J Am Acad Dermatol 1995;33:693-706.

53. Zouboulis CC, Blume-Peytavi U, Lennert T, et al. Fulminant metastatic calcinosis with cutaneous necrosis in a child with end-stage renal disease and tertiary hyperparathyroidism. Br J Dermatol 1996;135:617-622.

54. Plott T, Wiss K, Raimer SS, et al. Recurrent subepidermal calcified nodule of the nose. Pediatr Dermatol 1988;5:107-111.

55. Evans MJ, Blessing K, Gray ES. Subepidermal calcified nodule in children: A clinicopathologic study of 21 cases. Pediatr Dermatol 1995;12:307-310.

56. Azon-Masoliver A, Ferrando J, Navarra E, et al. Solitary congenital nodular calcification of Winer located on the ear: report of two cases. Pediatr Dermatol 1989;6:191-193.

57. Bostrum B. Tumoral calcinosis in an infant. Am J Dis Child 1981;135:246-247.

58. Heydemann JS, McCarthy RE. Tumoral calcinosis in a child. J Pediatr Orthop 1988;8:474-477.

59. Greenberg SB. Tumoral calcinosis in an infant. Pediatr Radiol 1990;20:206-207.

60. Niall DM, Fogarty EE, Dowling FE, et al. Spontaneous regression of tumoral calcinosis in an infant: A case report. J Pediatr Surg 1998;33:1429-1431.

61. Sahn EE, Smith DJ. Annular dystrophic calcinosis cutis in an infant. J Am Acad Dermatol 1992;6:1015-1017.

62. Puig L, Rocamora V, Romani J, et al. Calcinosis cutis following calcium chloride electrode paste application for auditory-brainstem evoked potentials recording. Pediatr Dermatol 1998;15:27-30.

63. Prendiville JS, Lucky AW, Mallory SB, et al. Osteoma cutis as a presenting sign of pseudohypoparathyroidism. Pediatr Dermatol 1992;9:11-18.

64. Miller ES, Esterly NB, Fairley JA. Progressive osseous heteroplasia. Arch Dermatol 1996;132:787-791.

65. Sanmartin O, Alegre V, Martinez-Aparicio A, et al. Congenital platelike osteoma cutis: Case report and review of the literature. Pediatr Dermatol 1993;10:182-186.

66. Gardner RJM, Yun K, Craw SM. Familial ectopic ossification. J Med Genet 1988;25:113-117.

67. Patten JL, Johns JR, Valle D, et al. Mutation in the gene encoding the stimulatory G protein of adenylate cyclase in Albright's hereditary osteodystrophy. N Engl J Med 1990;322: 1412-1419.

68. Power MM, James RS, Barber JC, et al. RDCI, the vasoactive intestinal peptide receptor: A candidate gene for the features of Albright hereditary osteodystrophy associated with deletion of 2q37. J Med Genet 1997;34:287-290.

69. Kaplan KS, Craver R, MacEwan GD, et al. Progressive osseous heteroplasia: A distinct developmental disorder of heterotopic ossification. J Bone Joint Surg 1994;76-A425-436.

70. Schmidt AH, Vincent KA, Aiona MD. Hemimelic progressive osseous heteroplasia. J Bone Joint Surg 1994;76-A:907-912.

71. Athanasou NA, Benson MK, Brenton DP, et al. Progressive osseous heteroplasia: A case report. Bone 1994;15:471-475.

72. Kaplan FS. Skin and bones. Arch Dermatol 1996;132:815-818.

73. Poomeechaiwong S, Golitz LE. Hamartomas. Adv Dermatol 1990;5:257-288.

74. Solomon LM, Esterly NB. Epidermal and other congenital organoid nevi. Curr Probl Pediatr 1975;6:1-55.

75. Paller AS, Syder AJ, Chan Y-M, et al. Genetic and clinical mosaicism in a type of epidermal nevus. N Engl J Med 1994;331:1408-1415

76. Nazarro V, Ermacora E, Santucci B, et al. Epidermolytic hyperkeratosis: Generalized form in children from parents with systematized linear form. Br J Dermatol 1990;122:417-422.

77. Rogers M, McCrossin I, Commens C. Epidermal nevi and the epidermal nevus syndrome. J Am Acad Dermatol 1989; 20:476-488.

78. Alper J, Holmes LB, Mihm MC. Birthmarks with serious medical significance: Nevocellular nevi, sebaceous nevi, and multiple cafe au lait spots. J Pediatr 1979;95:696-700.

79. Baker RS, Ross PA, Baumann RJ. Neurologic complications of the epidermal nevus syndrome. Arch Neurol 1987; 44:227-232.

80. Palazzi P, Artese O, Paolini A, et al. Linear sebaceous nevus syndrome: Report of a patient with unusual associated abnormalities. Pediatr Dermatol 1996;13:22-24.

81. Goldblum JR, Headington JT. Hypophosphatemic vitamin D-resistant rickets and multiple spindle and epithelioid nevi associated with linear nevus sebaceus syndrome. J Am Acad Dermatol 1993;29:109-111.

82. Oranje AP, Przyrembel H, Meradji M, et al. Solomon's epidermal nevus syndrome (Type: linear sebaceus nevus) and hypophosphatemic vitamin D-resistant rickets. Arch Dermatol 1994;130:1167-1171.

83. Benedetto L, Sood U, Blumenthal N, et al. Familial nevus sebaceus. J Am Acad Dermatol 1990;23:130-132.

84. Sahl WJ. Familial nevus sebaceus of Jadassohn: occurrence in three generations. J Am Acad Dermatol 1990;22:853-854.

85. Happle R. How many epidermal nevus syndromes exist? A clinicogenetic classification. J Am Acad Dermatol 1991;25: 550-556.

86. Drolet BA, Prendiville J, Golden J, et al. Membranous aplasia cutis with hair collars: Congenital absence of the skin or neuroectodermal defect. Arch Dermatol 1997;133:1551-1554.

87. Wilson-Jones E, Heyl T. Naevus sebaceus: A report of 140 cases with special report of the development of secondary malignant tumours. Br J Dermatol 1970;82:99-117.

88. Domingo J, Helwig EB. Malignant neoplasms associated with nevus sebaceus of Jadassohn. J Am Acad Dermatol 1979;1:545-556.

89. Tay Y-K, Weston WL, Ganong CA, et al. Epidermal nevus syndrome: association with central precocious puberty and woolly hair nevus. J Am Acad Dermatol 1996;35:839-842.

90. Allison MA, Dunn CL, Pedersen RC. Epidermal nevus syndrome: A neurologic variant with hemimeganencephaly, facial hemihypertrophy and gyral malformation. Pediatr Dermatol 1998;15:59-61.

91. Grebe TA, Rinsen ME, Richter SF, et al. Further delineation of the epidermal nevus syndrome: Two cases with new findings and literature review. Am J Med Genet 1993;47:24-30.

92. Ivker R, Resnick SD, Skidmore RA. Hypophosphatemic vitamin D-resistant rickets, precocious puberty, and the epidermal nevus syndrome. Arch Dermatol 1997;133:1557-1561.

93. Moss C, Parkin JM, Comaish JS. Precocious puberty in a boy with a widespread linear epidermal nevus. Br J Dermatol 1991;125:178-182.

94. Rongioletti F, Rebora A. Epidermal nevus with transitional cell carcinomas in the urinary tract. J Am Acad Dermatol 1991;25:856-858.

95. Munro CS, Cox NH. An acantholytic dyskeratotic epidermal naevus with other features of Darier's disease on the same side of the body. Br J Dermatol 1992;127:168-171.

96. Stosiek N, Ulmer R, von den Driesch P, et al. Chromosomal mosaicism in two patients with epidermal verrucous nevus: demonstration of chromosomal breakpoint. J Am Acad Dermatol 1994;30:622-625.

97. Wagner A. Lumps and bumps in childhood. Curr Probl Dermatol 1996;8:137-188.

98. Nelson BR, Kolansky G, Gillard M, et al. Management of linear verrucous epidermal nevus with topical 5-fluorouracil and tretinoin. J Am Acad Dermatol 1994;30:287.

99. Cestari T, Rubim M, Valentini BC. Nevus comedonicus: case report and brief review of the literature. Pediatr Dermatol 1991;8:300-305.

100. Vassiloudes PE, Morelli JP, Weston WL. Inflammatory nevus comedonicus in children. J Am Acad Dermatol 1998;38:834-836.

101. Patrizi A, Neri I, Fiorentini C, et al. Nevus comedonicus syndrome: a new pediatric case. Pediatr Dermatol 1998;15:304-306.

102. Kim SC, Kang WH. Nevus comedonicus associated with epidermal nevus. J Am Acad Dermatol 1989;21:1085-1088.

103. Marcus J, Esterly NB, Bauer BS. Tissue expansion in a patient with extensive nevus comedonicus. Ann Plast Surg 1992;29:362-366.

104. Abell E, Read SI. Porokeratotic eccrine ostial and dermal duct naevus. Br J Dermatol 1980;103:435-441.

105. Leung CS, Tang WYM, Lam WY, et al. Porokeratotic eccrine ostial and dermal duct naevus. Br J Dermatol 1998;138:684-688.

106. Fernandez-Redondo V, Toribi J. Porokeratotic eccrine ostial and dermal duct nevus. J Cutan Pathol 1988;15:393-395.

107. Aloi F, Pippione M. Porokeratotic eccrine ostial and dermal duct nevus. Arch Dermatol 1986;122:892-895.

108. Prendiville JS, Esterly NB. Congenital smooth muscle hamartoma. J Pediatr 1987;110:742-744.

109. Zvulunov A, Rotem A, Merlob P, et al. Congenital smooth muscle hamartoma: Prevalence, clinical findings, and follow-up in 15 patients. AJDC 1990;144:782-784.

110. Sato M, Ishiwawa O, Miyachi Y, et al. Michelin tyre syndrome: A congenital disorder of elastic fibre formation. Br J Dermatol 1997;136:583-586.

111. Oku T, Iwasaki K, Fujita H. Folded skin with an underlying cutaneous smooth muscle hamartoma. Br J Dermatol 1993;129:606-608.

112. Schnur RE, Herzberg AJ, Spinner N, et al. Variability in the Michelin tire syndrome: A child with multiple anomalies, smooth muscle hamartoma, and familial paracentric inversion of chromosome 7q.102. J Am Acad Dermatol 1993;28:364-370.

113. Johnson MD, Jacobs AH. Congenital smooth muscle hamartoma. Arch Dermatol 1989;125:820-822.

114. Gagne EJ, Su WPD. Congenital smooth muscle hamartoma of the skin. Pediatr Dermatol 1993;10:142-145.

115. Grau-Massanes M, Raimer S, Colome-Grimmer M, et al. Congenital smooth muscle hamartoma presenting as a linear atrophic plaque: Case report and review of the literature. Pediatr Dermatol 1996;13:222-225.

116. Guillot B, Huet P, Joujoux JM, et al. Multiple congenital smooth muscle hamartomas. Ann Dermatol Venereol 1998;125:118-120.

117. Happle R, Koopman RJJ. Becker nevus syndrome. Am J Med Genet 1997;68:357-361.

118. Book SE, Glass AT, Laude TA. Congenital Becker's nevus with a familial association. Pediatr Dermatol 1997;14:373-375.

119. Lambert JR, Willems P, Abs R, et al. Becker's nevus associated with chromosomal mosaicism and congenital adrenal hyperplasia. J Am Acad Dermatol 1994;30:655-657.

120. Ferreira MJ, Bajanca R, Fiadeiro T. Congenital melanosis and hypertrichosis in a bilateral distribution. Pediatr Dermatol 1998;15:290-292.

121. Urbani CE, Betti R. Supernumerary nipple in association with Becker nevus vs. Becker nevus syndrome: A semantic problem only. Am J Med Genet 1998;77:76-77.

122. Wilson-Jones E, Marks R, Pongsehirun D. Naevus superficialis lipomatosus. Br J Dermatol 1975;93:121-133.

123. Uitto J, Santa Cruz DJ, Eisen AZ. Connective tissue nevi of the skin: Clinical, genetic and histopathologic classification of hamartomas of the collagen, elastin, and proteoglycan type. J Am Acad Dermatol 1980;3:441-461.

124. Verbov J, Graham R. Buschke-Ollendorff syndrome-disseminated dermatofibrosis with osteopoikilosis. Clin Exp Dermatol 1986;11:17-26.

125. Smith JB, Hogan DJ, Glass LF, et al. Multiple collagenomas in a patient with Down syndrome. J Am Acad Dermatol 1995;33:835-837.

126. Botella-Estrada R, Alegre V, Sanmartin O, et al. Isolated plantar cerebriform collagenoma. Arch Dermatol 1991;127:1589-1590.

22

Disorders of the Subcutaneous Tissue

BERNARD A. COHEN

The subcutaneous fat cushions the overlying skin, insulates and provides energy storage, and protects underlying soft tissue and bony structures. Although not fully functional at birth, a well-developed fatty layer is present in the neonate even in the premature infant.[1] Disorders of the fat can interfere with normal function and may have systemic implications.

The nomenclature and classification of subcutaneous fat disorders of the newborn are inconsistent and confusing. However, a number of entities have been recognized because of distinctive clinical patterns, histopathology, biochemical markers, inheritance, and course. The clinician must distinguish disorders that are innocent and self-limiting from those that are associated with significant morbidity or underlying systemic disease.

SUBCUTANEOUS FAT NECROSIS OF THE NEWBORN

Subcutaneous fat necrosis of the newborn (SCFN) is an uncommon disorder that occurs primarily in full-term and post-mature infants during the first few weeks of life. Although lesions can develop in infants with a normal delivery and neonatal course, SCFN has been associated with perinatal complications, including asphyxia, hypothermia, seizures, preeclampsia, meconium aspiration, and intrapartum medication.[2,3] Extensive subcutaneous fat necrosis has also been reported following induced hypothermia used in cardiac surgery.[4]

Although the first reports of SCFN appeared during the early nineteenth century, many investigators continued to use the terms scleroderma or scleredema to describe SCFN, as well as a number of diverse disorders of the subcutaneous tissue associated with the development of distinct nodules or widespread induration. Over a century later, the term subcutaneous fat necrosis was first applied to this clinically benign condition with histologic characteristics of fat necrosis.[3]

Cutaneous Findings

Affected infants typically present with one or several indurated, variably circumscribed, violaceous or red plaques or subcutaneous nodules from 1 to several cm in diameter on the buttocks, thighs, trunk, face, and/or arms (Figs. 22-1 and 22-2). In some cases, the nodules may be subtle, not associated with overlying color change, and only appreciated by careful palpation of the underlying fat. Rarely, large plaques may cover extensive areas of the trunk or extremities. However, lesions are usually freely movable over subjacent muscles and fascia. Although SCFN may be tender, affected infants are afebrile and usually asymptomatic.

Most SCFN regresses spontaneously without scarring in several weeks to several months. Rarely nodules persist for over 6 months.[5] Occasionally fluctuance and abscesslike changes occur, resulting in spontaneous drainage and scar formation. Variable amounts of calcification develop, which can be appreciated radiographically.[6]

Etiology and Pathogenesis

Some investigators have proposed that SCFN results from hypoxic injury to fat caused by local trauma, particularly in the child with perinatal complications.[7,8] This is supported by the observation that fat necrosis occurs commonly over bony prominences. Others have suggested that the susceptibility to SCFN results from an increased proportion of the saturated fats palmitic and stearic acid relative to the monounsaturated fat oleic acid in neonatal sub-

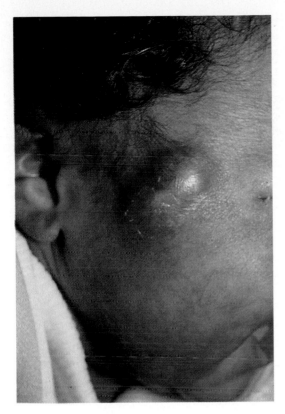

FIG. 22-1
Fat necrosis of the temple secondary to forceps injury.

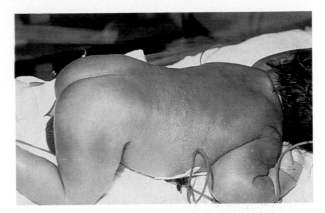

FIG. 22-2
Extensive fat necrosis involving the back, upper arm, and thigh. This infant also had transient thrombocytopenia.

cutaneous tissue.[5,7,9] Saturated fatty acids have a higher melting point than unsaturated fats, which may predispose newborn fat to crystallization at higher ambient temperatures than fat in older children and adults. Consequently, even in the setting of mild hypothermia, crystallization of fat may occur with subsequent fat necrosis. Finally, an underlying defect in neonatal fat composition or metabolism, possibly related to immaturity, in the setting of perinatal stress may lead to fat necrosis.

Diagnosis
When subcutaneous nodules develop in an otherwise healthy newborn, the diagnosis of SCFN can be confirmed by the characteristic histopathologic findings of patchy areas of necrosis and crystallization of fat. The involved fat lobules contain pathognomonic needle-shaped clefts surrounded by a mixed inflammatory infiltrate composed of lymphocytes, histiocytes, fibroblasts, and foreign body giant cells.[3]

Although laboratory tests are usually normal, hypercalcemia is occasionally noted from 1 to 4 months after the appearance of skin lesions.[5,7-9] Rarely hypercalcemia is severe and has been implicated in the deaths of three infants.

Nephrocalcinosis, vomiting, failure to thrive, poor weight gain, irritability, and seizures can complicate hypercalcemia. Although the exact cause of hypercalcemia is unknown, several explanations, including elevated parathyroid hormone levels, prostaglandin E2 release, calcium release from necrotic fat, and elevated levels of vitamin D, have been proposed. Calcitriol produced by macrophages in the inflammatory infiltrate of SCFN with increased calcium absorption in the gastrointestinal tract is the favored explanation.[2,3,7-9]

Soft-tissue calcification may occur in the absence of hypercalcemia and can be detected radiographically. Tests of parathyroid function, vitamin D metabolites, and urinary prostaglandins may be useful in the evaluation of infants with hypercalcemia. Thrombocytopenia has also been reported in several children, but the implications are unknown.

Differential Diagnosis
The subcutaneous nodules following the abrupt withdrawal of systemic steroids can be difficult to distinguish from SCFN. However, they usually occur on the cheeks, arms, and trunk 1 to 2 weeks after discontinuation of steroids. SCFN can be distinguished from sclerema neonatorum, lipogranulomatosus, infectious panniculitis, and nodular panniculitis by the general well-being of the infant with SCFN and characteristic clinical and histopathologic features. Infants with sclerema neonatorum present with diffuse skin stiffness and severe multisystem disease. Deep soft-tissue infections in neonates are usually associated with fever and other signs of sepsis. When hypercalcemia and/or soft tissue calcification is present, primary hyperparathyroidism, osteoma cutis, and calcification associated with Albright osteodystrophy should be excluded.

Management

In most infants with SCFN treatment is limited to parental reassurance and supportive measures.[2,7-9] Hypercalcemia, if present, may have clinical signs such as poor growth or irritability, or may be entirely asymptomatic. Monitoring of serum calcium levels for several months should be considered, especially with large areas of cutaneous involvement or if symptoms are present. Treatment of hypercalcemia may require intravenous saline, calcium-wasting diuretics, and rarely intravenous corticosteroids. Etidronate therapy has also been reported to be successful in controlling severe hypercalcemia in SCFN.[9] Ulcerated lesions, which rarely occur in otherwise healthy infants, usually respond to topical antibiotics and biooclusive dressings.

SCLEREMA NEONATORUM

Sclerema neonatorum is a rare clinical finding rather than a distinct disorder that affects debilitated term and premature infants during the first 1 to 2 weeks of life.[3] It occasionally occurs in older infants up to 4 months of age with severe underlying disease.

Cutaneous Findings

Diffuse hardening of the skin usually appears suddenly on the third or fourth day of life, starting over the lower extremities, especially the calves, spreading to the thighs, buttocks, and cheeks, and eventually the trunk.[3,10-12] Sclerema eventually involves most of the skin, particularly in premature infants, with the exception of the palms, soles, and genitals. The skin feels cold, smooth, hard, and bound down. The joints are immobile, and the face appears masklike.

Extracutaneous Findings

Affected infants are usually poorly nourished, dehydrated, hypotensive, hypothermic, and septic. Necrotizing enterocolitis, pneumonia, intracranial hemorrhage, hypoglycemia, and electrolyte disturbances are also often associated with sclerema.[3,10-14]

In most cases, sclerema is limited to the subcutaneous fat. However, in two infants autopsy revealed identical changes in the visceral fat.[15]

Etiology and Pathogenesis

The development of sclerema is probably a result of dysfunction of the neonatal enzymatic system involved in the conversion of saturated palmitic and stearic acids to unsaturated oleic acid. Immaturity of the neonatal lipoenzymes is further compromised by hypothermia, infection, shock, dehydration, and surgical and environmental stresses. The relative abundance of saturated fatty acids and depletion of unsaturated fatty acid allows for fat solidification to occur more readily, with the subsequent development of sclerema.[3]

Diagnosis

On gross pathologic examination, the subcutaneous tissue of affected infants is markedly thickened, firm, and lardlike with fibrous bands noted to extend from the fat into the lower dermis. Microscopically, early lesions demonstrate distinctive lipid crystals within fat cells, forming rosettes of fine needlelike clefts.[3] Although there is usually no inflammatory reaction to fat necrosis, occasionally some giant cells are present. Older lesions often show thickened septae and rarely calcification.

Other laboratory findings in neonates with sclerema are nonspecific and usually reflect the underlying systemic medical problems. Thrombocytopenia, neutropenia, active bleeding, and worsening acidosis carry a poor prognosis.[3,13,14]

Differential Diagnosis

The lack of inflammation and extensive involvement of the subcutis help to distinguish sclerema from SCFN and cold panniculitis, in which the lesions are localized and associated with exuberant granulomatous inflammation. Diffuse edema resulting from hemolytic anemia, renal, and/or cardiac dysfunction manifests as pitting edema, unlike sclerema. Congenital lymphedema or Milroy's disease is nonpitting and often widespread. However, in lymphedema the infant is otherwise healthy, and a skin biopsy reveals normal fat and dilated lymphatics. Erysipelas or lymphangitis is red, tender, and more localized than sclerema. Diffuse sclerodermatous changes associated with systemic sclerosis, which is extremely rare in the newborn, can also mimic sclerema. However, histology demonstrates characteristic hypertrophy and sclerosis of collagen, which eventually replaces the fat in scleroderma.

Treatment

Attention to the maintenance of a neutral-thermal environment, electrolyte and water balance, adequate hydration and ventilation, and aggressive treatment of shock and infection in the modern nursery intensive care unit undoubtedly account for the extremely low incidence of sclerema today. Although most infants with sclerema succumb to sepsis and shock, reversal of the underlying systemic disease can result in recovery.

The role of systemic steroids in the management of infants with sclerema is controversial. Several investigators have reported a favorable outcome when exchange transfusion was combined with conventional therapy.[14]

PANNICULITIS CAUSED BY PHYSICAL AGENTS

Although physical agents may contribute to the development of SCFNN and sclerema neonatorum, a number of environmental factors can cause direct injury to the fat. Cold, heat, mechanical trauma, and chemical injury can lead to the formation of nodules in the fat. The overlying epidermis is usually unaffected in cold and mechanical trauma, whereas bullae, erosions, and ulcerations from epidermal and dermal necrosis characterize heat and chemical insults.

Cold Panniculitis

The development of panniculitis following exposure to subfreezing temperatures was first noted over 50 years ago by Haxthausen, who described four young children and an adolescent with facial plaques.[16,17] In his paper he referred to several earlier reports of hardening of the fat associated with cold exposure and application of ice directly to the skin.[18,19] Similar cases have been reported following the use of ice to induce hypothermia before cardiac surgery,[18] and the application of ice bags to the face for management of supraventricular tachycardia.[19,20] Widespread fat necrosis has also been described following the use of ice to induce hypothermia before cardiac surgery. Popsicle panniculitis is a term coined by Epstein in 1970, to refer to a specific subset of cold panniculitis triggered by infants sucking on flavored ice.[21] Although lesions may develop in older children and adults, most cases occur in infants under a year.

Cutaneous Findings
Symmetric, tender, indurated nodules and plaques 1 to 3 cm in diameter typically appear on the cheeks of infants 1 to 2 days after cold exposure.[16,17,20-22] The overlying skin appears red to violaceous (Fig. 22-3), and the infants are otherwise well. In a study by Rotman, the application of an ice cube to the volar aspect of the forearm of an 8-month-old girl resulted in mild transient erythema for 15 minutes.[17] A red plaque developed 12 to 18 hours later and resolved 13 days later. Lesions usually soften, flatten, and heal over 2 to 3 weeks, leaving postinflammatory pigmentary changes particularly in darkly pigmented individuals.

Etiology and Pathogenesis
As in subcutaneous fat necrosis of the newborn and sclerema neonatorum, exposure to low ambient temperatures is thought to result in crystallization of subcutaneous tissue in infants, which is relatively high in saturated fats compared with older children and adults. Applying ice to the skin for 50 seconds results in nodules in all newborns,

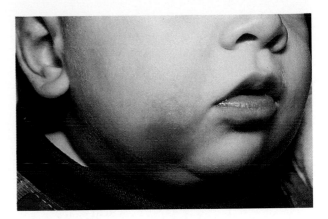

FIG. 22-3
Erythematous nodule of panniculitis resulting from cold exposure (popsicle).

but only in 40% of 6 month olds, and only occasionally in 9 month olds.[21] In 1966 Duncan described a child in whom nodules followed the application of ice for several minutes at 6 months of age, and 8 minutes at 18 months of age.[23] When the child was 22 months old, ice applied for 15 minutes did not trigger panniculitis. The resistance to cold injury correlates with the relative increase in unsaturated fats in the subcutaneous tissue of older infants and children.

Diagnosis
The development of subcutaneous nodules in any neonate or young infant exposed to ice or subfreezing temperatures in the preceding 1 to 3 days should suggest the diagnosis of cold panniculitis. Histologic changes evolve over several days.[23] The earliest changes 24 hours after cold injury include an infiltrate of macrophages and lymphocytes at the dermal-epidermal junction extending into the dermis and fat. At 48 hours the inflammation is more intense and fat necrosis is present. Lipid from ruptured fat cells forms large cystic structures surrounded by histiocytes, neutrophils, and lymphocytes. These changes become more pronounced over the next few days and subside completely in 2 weeks.

Other laboratory studies, including blood counts, cold agglutinins, cryoglobulins, and general chemistry studies, are usually normal.

Differential Diagnosis
The history of cold exposure in an otherwise healthy infant will help to distinguish cold panniculitis from other causes of subcutaneous nodules. Clinical lesions of SCFN

can overlap with cold panniculitis. Although a skin biopsy is not usually necessary to distinguish these two disorders, the distribution of nodules and histological changes are usually distinctive. Cellulitis should also be considered in any child with tender red facial nodules. However, the lack of progression of lesions or fever in a healthy appearing infant is against the diagnosis of infection.

Post-steroid panniculitis can be clinically indistinguishable from cold panniculitis.[24] Subcutaneous nodules or plaques appear on the cheeks of infants within 2 weeks of rapidly discontinuing high-dose systemic steroids after a prolonged course. A biopsy reveals granulomatous inflammation in the fat lobules and needle-shaped clefts within histiocytes identical to those of SCFNN. However, in a child with the typical history a biopsy is unnecessary, and nodules resolve over a period of months without treatment.

Treatment and Course

Although skin lesions are self-limiting and no treatment is recommended, early recognition of cold panniculitis is important to prevent unnecessary parental anxiety or laboratory studies. Nodules heal in 1 to 3 weeks without scarring.

Mechanical Trauma

Cutaneous Findings

Firm, subcutaneous nodules may follow blunt trauma to the skin especially in areas prone to trauma where the fat is in close proximity to the underlying bone.[25] This occurs most commonly on the cheeks in children between 6 and 12 years old. However, nodules can also develop in infants and over other bony prominences after accidental or deliberate injury.

Diganosis

Traumatic fat injury should be considered in any child with subcutaneous nodules over injury-prone areas. Skin biopsies will demonstrate fat necrosis with granulomatous inflammation. However, a biopsy is usually not necessary.

Treatment and Course

Nodules slowly resolve over 6 to 12 months without treatment. In some patients localized lipoatrophy can lead to a depression with normal overlying epidermis and dermis.

Injection-Site Granuloma

Cutaneous Findings

Firm, tender, subcutaneous nodules commonly appear 1 to 2 days after vaccinations in the buttocks or thighs in infants and in the deltoid area in older children and adults.[26] Although lesions occasionally result from direct trauma to the subcutaneous tissue when the needle is accidentally placed in the fat, some patients develop aluminum granulomas when an aluminum-adsorbed vaccine is used.

Diagnosis

The diagnosis is apparent when one or several nodules develop in a vaccination injection site. Skin biopsies demonstrate characteristic findings, including lymphoid follicles with germinal centers and dense surrounding infiltrate of lymphocytes, histiocytes, plasma cells, and eosinophils. Staining for aluminum is also positive, confirming the diagnosis.[26]

Differential Diagnosis

Other foreign material injected into the skin can produce panniculitis with resultant nodule formation and fat necrosis. This can occur with certain medications and intravenous fluid extravasation.[27] Munchhausen syndrome by proxy should be considered when recurrent panniculitis with associated cellulitis and/or ulceration occurs in an otherwise healthy infant without a clear diagnosis.

Treatment and Course

Injection-site granulomas usually resolve without scarring within 2 weeks. Occasionally liponecrosis leads to ulceration and/or lipoatrophy with persistent dimpling of the skin.

INFECTIOUS PANNICULITIS

Although this entity usually occurs in immunocompromised adults, there are rare reports of affected children in the pediatric and infectious disease literature.[28,29] In infants, infectious panniculitis can occur as an extension of primary cutaneous infection or direct hematogenous dissemination to fat.

Cutaneous Findings

Septic emboli produce tender red subcutaneous nodules that are usually confined to one area, such as a portion of an extremity, but widespread dissemination can occur (Fig. 22-4).

In primary cutaneous infection, superficial tissue destruction by the invading organism and ischemia from invasion of local blood vessels and lymphatics leads to necrosis and ulceration of the skin and deeper soft-tissue structures.

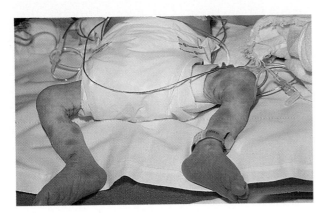

FIG. 22-4
Multiple nodules of panniculitis in an infant with *E. coli* sepsis.

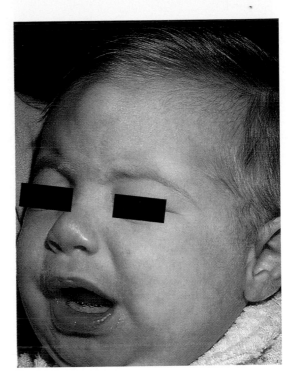

FIG. 22-5
Lipoma of the forehead in a young infant.

Extracutaneous Findings

Infected children are febrile, irritable, and appear ill. There may be other signs of systemic infection or sepsis. Although infectious panniculitis is more common in immunocompromised individuals, it has been reported in immunocompetent children.[28]

Etiology and Pathogenesis

Infectious panniculitis has been associated with gram-positive (*Staphylococcus aureus*, *Staphylococcus epidermidis*, *Streptococcal* species) and gram negative (*Pseudomonas* species, *Klebsiella* species, *Fusobacterium*, *Fusarium*) bacteria, fungi (*Candida* species, *Nocardia* species), and atypical mycobacteria.

Diagnosis

Skin biopsies from subcutaneous nodules reveal a mixed septal-lobular panniculitis with infiltration by neutrophils.[28,29] Special stains demonstrate organisms scattered throughout fat lobules. Blood cultures and cultures of other body fluids may also be positive.

Differential Diagnosis

Other conditions to be considered in the setting of possible panniculitis associated with fever include erythema nodosum, Henoch-Schonlein purpura (HSP), and cellulitis. The most difficult of these to exclude is erythema nodosum, an immunologically mediated phenomenon commonly associated with streptococcal and other infections. In erythema nodosum, the panniculitis occurs primarily in the fat septae, and the infecting organisms are not found in the skin nodules. HSP is not usually associated with fever, and skin biopsy shows leukocytoclastic vasculitis.

Treatment and Course

Treatment should be directed against the specific organism. Skin biopsy for pathology and cultures, blood cultures, and other appropriate cultures will hopefully identify a specific organism and direct antibiotic and/or antifungal therapy.

TUMORS OF FAT

Tumors of fat include a number of neoplasms and hamartomatous malformations. A specific diagnosis is important to distinguish between those disorders with isolated cutaneous findings and those with systemic implications.

Lipoma

Cutaneous Findings

Although lipomas represent the most common tumor of the mesenchyme in adults, they are rare in infants. Lipomas are soft, rounded or lobulated, mobile, slightly compressible, subcutaneous tumors with smooth margins (Fig. 22-5). Lumbosacral lipomas are usually congenital and occur in conjunction with intraspinal lipomas and anomalies of the spine (Fig. 22-6).[30-33] They are often softer and less discrete than lipomas found in other sites.

Extracutaneous Findings

In 1967 Lassman and James described 26 cases of lumbosacral lipomas associated with laminar defects on x-ray and spinal anomalies at surgery.[30] The recognition of lipomas as markers of underlying spinal dysraphism has been reemphasized by a number of investigators.[30-33] Conversely, most cases of intraspinal lipomas are associated with congenital lumbosacral cutaneous markers, including lipoma, myelocele closure scar, hairy patch, vascular lesions and dimpling.[32] (See also Chapter 9.)

Diagnosis

The presence of a soft, spongy congenital mass in the lumbosacral area is characteristic, and requires a radioimaging evaluation to exclude anomalies of the underlying cord and bony spine. Histologic findings are typical of lipomas in other sites and show mature adipocytes within a thin connective tissue capsule.

Treatment, Course, and Management

Although the need for surgical management of intraspinal lipomas associated with lumbosacral lipomas is controversial, it should be recognized that the development of neurologic impairment can be delayed for years.[30-33] Unfortunately, many patients present in later childhood and adolescence with neurologic defects in the lower extremities, including weakness and foot deformities. Consequently, immediate neurosurgical evaluation and long-term neurologic follow-up is required.

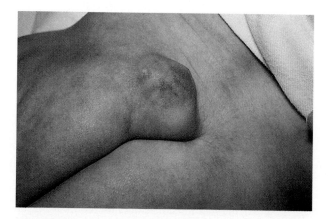

FIG. 22-6
Lumbosacral lipoma associated with lipoma of the cord. Note the deviation of the gluteal cleft.

Nevus Lipomatosus Cutaneous Superficialis

Nevus lipomatosus cutaneous superficialis (NLCS) is a malformation of the subcutaneous tissue consisting of multiple or solitary papules usually occurring on the lower trunk, buttocks, or upper thighs.[34-37] Based on the paucity of reports, NLCS is either rare or underdiagnosed. In 1921 Hoffmann and Zurhelle described the original case of a 25-year-old man with multiple papules on the left buttock.[37] In 1975 Jones and Marks summarized the findings of an additional 40 cases subsequently reported in the literature and 20 of their own patients. A number of other reports have expanded our understanding of the clinical expression and pathogenesis of NLCS.

Cutaneous Findings

Most patients report that lesions were present at birth or appeared in the first two decades of life.[34-37] NLCS typically presents as multiple, soft, skin-colored to yellowish lobules that may coalesce into plaques with a cerebriform surface. Unilateral involvement of the buttock is most common, but plaques may extend to the adjacent skin of the upper thigh or lower back. Lesions may be confined to the upper thigh, lower back, hip, or abdomen. Usually lesions do not cross the midline, but bilateral involvement of opposing surfaces of the buttocks has been reported. Once formed, papules usually remain stable. However, new lobules may develop slowly for decades.

Solitary nevi have been described at various sites, including the scalp, ear, and neck, but these lesions probably represent fibromas or polypoid fibrolipomas rather than true NLCS.

Extracutaneous Findings

NLCS is not usually associated with extracutaneous findings.[34-37] Cases reported with bony, dental, and other anomalies probably represent focal dermal hypoplasia (Goltz syndrome), which can be confused clinically and histologically with NLCS. However, there are several reports of NLCS associated with pigment anomalies, including café au lait spots and hypopigmented macules.

Etiology and Pathogenesis

Although the origin of NLCS is not clear, electron microscopic studies support the hypothesis of several investigators that the hamartomatous lesion arises from pluripotential vascular elements in the dermis.[35] The presence of varying amounts of other connective tissue components also suggests a relationship with connective tissue nevi.

Diagnosis

Although the clinical appearance of NLCS varies, the presence of typical nodules and plaques in the pelvic girdle region should suggest the diagnosis. Histopathology shows some hyperkeratosis and acanthosis of the epidermis and a marked increase in mature fat cells throughout the dermis.[35,37] Adipocytes are most prominent in the reticular dermis, where they are arranged in clusters and interspersed by broad, interwoven, collagen bundles. However, they may extend into the papillary dermis, and the distinction between the dermis and subcutaneous fat may be poorly defined. Although the remainder of the dermis often appears normal, other connective tissue anomalies, including thickening of collagen and elastic fibers, and increased numbers of fibroblasts and blood vessels with a perivascular mononuclear infiltrate may also develop.

Differential Diagnosis

The varying clinical findings explain the wide range of clinical diagnoses suspected before skin biopsy. These include pigmented nevi, supernumerary nipples, lipomas, neurofibromas, connective tissue nevi, sebaceous nevi, epidermal nevi, and warts.

Encephalocraniocutaneous lipomatosis and congenital diffuse lipomatosis (Michelin tire baby) may represent distinctive variants of NLCS (see the following discussion).

Treatment, Course, and Management

Although new lobules may develop in adolescence and adult life, NLCS is usually static and not associated with pain, pruritus, or other symptoms. Consequently, treatment is not necessary, but surgical excision particularly for small lesions, gives a good cosmetic result.

Encephalocraniocutaneous Lipomatosis

In encephalocraniocutaneous lipomatosis (ECL), unilateral cerebral malformations are associated with ipsilateral scalp, face, and eye lesions.[38] Since the first description of this congenital neurocutaneous disorder in 1970 by Haberland and Perou,[39] 12 cases with similar clinical and histologic findings have been reported.[40-42]

Cutaneous Findings

Soft, spongy, hairless, pink to yellowish tumors characteristically involve the scalp often in a linear configuration but may extend to the legs and paravertebral area.[38-42] Although lesions are usually unilateral, bilateral involvement has been reported. Papular and polypoid nodules,

often contiguous to the scalp lesions, are constant features on the face of affected infants. Atrophic hairless patches may also be present on the scalp and face.[38]

Extracutaneous Findings

Characteristic papules and nodules on the bulbar conjunctivae show histologic features of desmoid tumors.[38] Anomalies of the hyaloid vessel system, lens, and cornea are also common.

Cerebral defects are usually ipsilateral to the main cutaneous scalp lesions and include ventricular dilatation and cerebral atrophy.[38] Other anomalies, including arachnoidal cyst, pontocerebellar lipoma, porencephaly, agenesis of the corpus callosum, and paramedullary lipomas have also been described.

Etiology and Pathogenesis

There is no evidence of genetic transmission or chromosomal aberration, and all cases have been sporadic. Happle proposed that ECL might be caused by a lethal autosomal mutation that survives in the mosaic state.[43]

Diagnosis

Biopsies of the cutaneous nodules show normal epidermis overlying a dermis with irregularly shaped collagen fibers that extend into the subcutis and form large fibrous septae associated with increased amounts of fat.[38-42] These histologic features typical of fibrolipoma seen in children with characteristic cutaneous, ocular, and cerebral features should suggest the diagnosis of ECL.

Differential Diagnosis

The clinical features of ECL may overlap with focal dermal hypoplasia (Goltz syndrome), oculoauricular vertebral dysplasia (Goldenhar syndrome), Schimmelpenning syndrome, oculocerebrocutaneous (Dellman) syndrome, Proteus syndrome, and the epidermal nevus syndrome. However, careful analysis of clinical and histologic features will help to distinguish these neurocutaneous genodermatoses.

Treatment and Course

Care of affected children is determined by neurologic symptoms, which range from normal to global neurodevelopmental retardation, unilateral spasticity, and mental retardation.[38] Seizures are variable and may develop later in childhood. Moreover, the severity of neurologic symptoms does not seem to correlate with the extent of cutaneous involvement. Ocular and cutaneous lesions appear to be static and amenable to surgical repair.

Congenital Diffuse Lipomatosis

Congenital diffuse lipomatosis (Michelin tire baby) was initially referred to by Ross in 1969, who described a child with ringed creases of the skin reminiscent of the mascot of the French tire manufacturer, Michelin.[44] Since then a number of cases of this rare hamartomatous disorder have been reported demonstrating the variability of clinical and histologic findings.[44-48]

Cutaneous Findings

Symmetric ringed creases of the extremities may be associated with hirsutism of the arms, legs, shoulders, and buttocks (Fig. 22-7).[44-48] The palmar and plantar skin may also demonstrate excessive folding. Although scalp hair is usually normal, long curled eyelashes and thick eyebrows are typical.

Extracutaneous Findings

Although affected children may be otherwise normal, a number of anomalies have been reported.[44-48] Facial dysmorphisms have included epicanthal folds, hypertelorism, antimongoloid slant to the eyes, flat nasal bridge, and low-set ears. Variable oral anomalies, including cleft lip and palate, high-arched palate, dental hypoplasia, and micrognathia, are common. Orthopedic defects such as rocker-bottom feet, metatarsus abductus, coxa valga, genu valgus, overlapping of toes, and pectus excavatum may require surgical intervention. Psychomotor delay and the development of seizures are also variable.

Etiology and Pathogenesis

Although no specific chromosomal abnormality has been identified in congenital diffuse lipomatosis, autosomal dominant inheritance has been noted in two families in which the cutaneous findings occurred as isolated defects.[47] In two other patients with multiple associated anomalies, unrelated cytogenetic defects were found.[45] Further studies may help to detect a Michelin tire baby gene, although this syndrome may represent disparate disorders with similar phenotypic expression.

Diagnosis

Skin biopsies from the extremities of affected children have shown changes in the dermis consistent with nevus lipomatosus cutaneous superficialis or smooth muscle hamartoma.[45,46] A recent report in which histopathology showed fragmented elastic fibers and decreased deposition of elastin on electron microscopy suggests that some cases may result from a primary defect in elastic fibers.[46]

Differential Diagnosis

Although congenital diffuse lipomatosis may be confused histologically with localized smooth muscle hamartoma, Becker's nevus, and nevus lipomatosis cutaneous superficialis, the diffuse, symmetric, and dramatic cutaneous findings are distinctive.

Treatment, Course, and Management

Management of affected individuals depends on the presence of associated anomalies. Clinicians should look carefully for oral and orthopedic anomalies, which may require early surgical intervention. Neurodevelopmental parameters will also require long-term follow-up.

Congenital Pedal Nodules

Congenital nodules of the plantar surface of the feet have been described under a variety of names, including congenital pedal papules, congenital piezogenic-like papules, plantar fibromatosus of the heel, "podalic papules of the newborn," and precalcaneous fibrolipomatous hamartoma.[49-51]

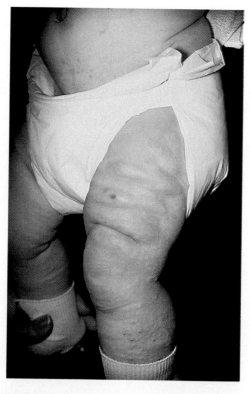

FIG. 22-7
Multiple ringed creases of congenital diffuse lipomatosis. (From Novice FM, Collison DW, Burgdorf WHC, Esterly NB. Handbook of genetic skin disorders. Philadelphia: WB Saunders, 1994.)

Cutaneous Findings

Pedal nodules are asymptomatic, symmetric, flesh-colored nodules of the medial plantar surface of the feet, generally 0.5 to 1.5 cm in size (Fig. 22-8). The nodules are ill defined and may go unnoticed by parents. Lesions undergo minimal change over time, though proportionate growth may be seen.

Etiology and Pathogenesis

The pathogenesis is uncertain. Possible etiologies include a hamartomatous condition or a developmental defect in the plantar aponeurosis. Histopathology displays increased mature adipocytes in the mid and deep dermis within fibrous sheaths.

Diagnosis and Differential Diagnosis

The diagnosis is a clinical one. Differential diagnosis includes piezogenic papules seen on the lateral surface of the feet in older children, fibrous hamartoma of infancy, and aponeurotic fibroma.

Treatment and Course

Although the natural history is not fully known, lesions seem to persist over time. Treatment is unnecessary.

Lipoblastoma and Lipoblastomatosis

Lipoblastoma is a term first used by Jaffe in 1926, to describe recurrent fatty tumors of the groin in infants and young children.[52] Van Meurs subsequently wrote of his experience with an infant with a lipomatous tumor in the right axilla that required four surgeries over a 2-year period before she was free of recurrence.[53] Histologic changes from biopsies over the 2-year period in Van Meurs case demonstrated maturation from a tumor comprised primarily of lipoblasts to a mature lipoma. In 1973 Chung and Enzinger reported a large series of lipomatous tumors in infancy and proposed that the term *lipoblastoma* be used to describe the well-encapsulated variant and *lipoblastomatosis* be reserved for unencapsulated infiltrating lesions.[54]

Cutaneous Findings

Clinically, the tumors are soft, subcutaneous or deep, soft-tissue masses ranging in size from 1 to 12 cm in diameter.[55,56] Although cases have been diagnosed in children as old as 10 years of age, most appear before 3 years of age, and congenital tumors are common. The most common location is the extremities (Fig. 22-9) followed by the trunk and face. However, unusual sites, including the parotid gland, mediastinum, and tonsils, have been reported.

Etiology and Pathogenesis

Although the cause of lipoblastoma is unknown, electronmicroscopic findings suggest a close resemblance to

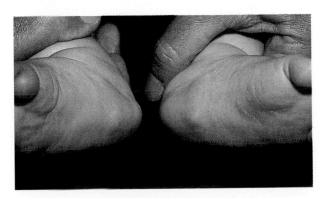

FIG. 22-8
Congenital pedal papules.

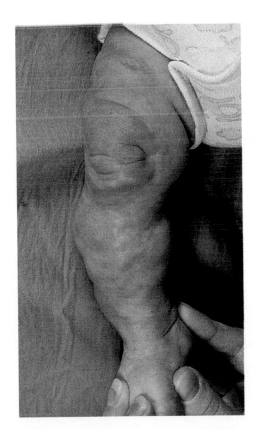

FIG. 22-9
Lipoblastomatosis involving the entire leg and foot, present from birth.

human fetal adipose tissue.[57] Some investigators propose that lipomatoblastoma results from the continued proliferation of fetal lipoblasts in the postnatal period. This is supported by observations of histologic maturation of adipose cells in recurrent tumors.

Diagnosis

Histologically lipoblastoma is encapsulated or well circumscribed, whereas in lipoblastomatosis, the tumor infiltrates surrounding normal structures.[54-56] The diagnostic feature is the presence of lobules of mature and immature fat cells, primitive mesenchymal cells, and lipoblasts with varying degrees of differentiation. The lobules are separated by fibrous septae containing small blood vessels, hyaline collagen, and fibroblasts. There is no evidence of atypia, and mitotic figures are rare.

Differential Diagnosis

Lipoblastomatosis should be differentiated from liposarcoma, an exceedingly rare tumor in children under 10 years of age.[56] Although histologic distinction is occasionally difficult, the lack of cytologic atypia and mitotic figures and the presence of a uniform growth pattern and extensive lobulation favor lipoblastoma.

Treatment and Course

Encapsulated tumors represent the majority of lesions and generally respond well to simple excision. However, in some series lipoblastomatosis accounts for nearly a third of the cases. Metastases do not occur, but recurrences are common. Although extensive infiltration into local muscle and fascial structures precludes complete excision, in most cases maturation of recurrent tumor results in a favorable outcome.

LIPODYSTROPHIES

The lipodystrophies are a rare group of disorders characterized by complete or partial loss of fat. The congenital variants are inherited in an autosomal recessive pattern and express variable abnormalities in carbohydrate and lipid metabolism and insulin resistance.

Leprechaunism

Donohue and Uchida were the first to describe this rare syndrome when they reported their observations on two sisters of consanguineous parents with intrauterine growth retardation, gnomelike facies, and severe endocrine dysfunction evidenced by emaciation, enlargement of the breasts and clitoris, and histologic changes in the ovaries,

pancreas, and breasts.[58,59] Leprechaunism was the term applied to the elfinlike facial features and poor growth characteristic of this disorder.

The incidence of this autosomal recessive disorder has been estimated at 1 in 4 million live births and the prevalence of the carrier state as at least 1 in 1000 individuals.[60]

Cutaneous Findings

In a review of 31 patients with Leprechaunism reported since the original description by Donohue in 1948, Elsas summarized the clinical findings, including severe growth retardation; elfinlike face with large protuberant low-set ears; depressed nasal bridge with a broad nasal tip and flared nares; thick lips; distended abdomen; relatively large hands, feet, nipples, and genitalia; and abnormal skin with hyperpigmentation, café au lait spots, hypertrichosis, acanthosis nigricans, pachyderma, and decreased subcutaneous fat (Fig. 22-10).[61-63] The virtual absence of fat gives a cachectic appearance with wrinkled skin hanging loosely over the skeletal frame.

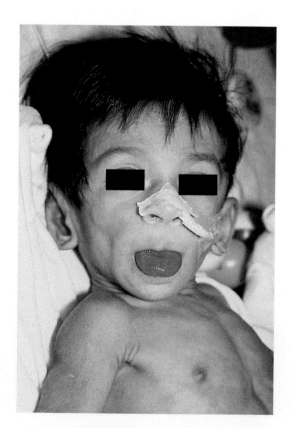

FIG. 22-10
Infant with Leprechaunism.

Etiology and Pathogenesis

Initially Leprechaunism was identified as a primary endocrinologic disorder because of the associated cystic changes of the gonads and hyperplasia of the islet cells of the pancreas. In the 1970s and 1980s laboratory advances led to the identification of severe insulin resistance resulting from a genetic defect of the insulin receptor system in infants with Leprechaunism.[61,62] Using molecular genetic techniques, the first defect in the insulin receptor gene was discovered in a child with Leprechaunism in 1988.[64] Subsequently, multiple mutations have been described indicating that there is great genetic heterogeneity in this disorder. Overactivation of insulin-like growth factor 1 by high levels of insulin and lack of functional insulin receptors in a number of organ systems lead to growth failure, lipodystrophy, and other cutaneous findings.

Diagnosis

The diagnosis can be made by DNA analysis of fibroblasts grown in culture from skin biopsies of affected infants. Specific mutations in the insulin receptor gene can be identified. Prenatal diagnosis is possible by similar evaluation of chorionic villus biopsy specimens.

Differential Diagnosis

Leprechaunism shares many features with congenital total lipoatrophy, including insulin resistance, absence of subcutaneous fat, acanthosis nigricans, and hyperpigmentation. However, the elfin facies, wrinkled skin, and other cutaneous markers are distinctive.

Treatment and Course

Post-natal growth is invariably poor, and affected children are severely motor and mentally retarded. Infants rarely survive beyond the first few months of life unless they have some residual insulin receptor function.

Congenital Generalized Lipodystrophy (Seip-Berardinelli Syndrome)

Congenital generalized lipodystrophy (CGL) was first described by Berardinelli in 1954, and in greater detail by Seip in 1959.[65,66] In 1996 Seip published a follow-up study of the original patients and summarized the findings from over 90 cases reported in the literature.[67]

Cutaneous Findings

Complete absence of subcutaneous fat and marked muscular hypertrophy are evident at birth and persist through adolescence. The skin tends to become coarse, particularly in boys, and patients often develop warty fibromas on the upper half of the body.[65,67] Acanthosis nigricans develops to a variable degree in early childhood but disappears in adolescence. Excessive, curly scalp hair and hypertrichosis are also common.

Extracutaneous Features

An anabolic state develops with increased height velocity, advanced bone and dental age, muscular hypertrophy, masculine body build, acromegaloid stigmata, organomegaly, and enlarged genitals.[65-67] Growth velocity is already advanced at birth and continues throughout childhood. The absence of facial fat pads and enlarged muscles gives adolescent girls a female body builder look.

Patients tend to be hypermetabolic with a voracious appetite, increased energy consumption, and associated hyperhidrosis and decreased heat tolerance. Cardiac muscle hypertrophy is also present at birth and may result in progressive hypertrophic cardiomyopathy with decrease in cardiac function. Most patients with CGL demonstrate mild to moderate developmental delay and mental retardation.

Etiology and Pathogenesis

Although the cause is unknown, clinical and biochemical findings point to a mutation in a gene controlling the transport and storage of glucose and fatty acids in subcutaneous tissue.[67] Recent studies suggest that the primary cause may be a defect in the insulin receptor or post-receptor mechanisms.

Diagnosis

This is a well-characterized disorder inherited in an autosomal recessive pattern with clinical and metabolic features that allow for diagnosis at birth. However, CGD syndrome is genetically heterogeneous, allowing for some variation in phenotypic expression.

Metabolic features include insulin resistance, hyperinsulinemia, hypertriglyceridemia, and nonketotic diabetes. Skin biopsies demonstrate a marked decrease in adipocyte size and number.[67] Unlike the subcutaneous fat, glycogen and triglycerides are abundant in the liver, where variable amounts of connective tissue with liver cirrhosis have been noted. Hypertriglyceridemia varies from patient to patient, but tends to increase at puberty and with increased dietary fat consumption. In childhood, glucose and insulin levels tend to be normal except with large glucose challenges. However, at or shortly after puberty, glucose metabolism deteriorates with the development of clinical diabetes with hyperinsulinemia, elevated serum glucose, and glycosuria.

Differential Diagnosis

CGL can be distinguished from other lipodystrophies by the characteristic clinical and metabolic findings.

Treatment and Course

Treatment is complex and should emphasize dietary measures to control energy consumption, hyperglycemia, and hypertriglyceridemia.[67] Appetite suppressants have been used with some success. Therapy is further complicated by moderate to severe mental retardation in most individuals with CGL. Despite therapy, many patients die in childhood of liver cirrhosis or associated complications and/or cardiomyopathy.

Carbohydrate-Deficient Glycoprotein Syndrome

Although carbohydrate-deficient glycoprotein syndrome (CDGS) represents a heterogeneous group of disorders, they share clinical features resulting from a defect in the synthesis of N-linked oligosaccharides.[68,69] This entity was first recognized by Jaeken in 1980, who reported monozygotic twins with psychomotor retardation, increased CSF protein, delayed nerve conduction velocity, thyroxine-binding deficiency, and increased serum arylsulfatase A activity.[70] Carbohydrate analysis of a number of subsequent patients resulted in identification of the common defect in N-linked glycoproteins.

Cutaneous Findings

Dysmorphic features typical of CDGS appear in infancy, including inverted nipples and an abnormal distribution of fat over the suprapubic region and labia majora.[68,69] Peculiar fat pads, which tend to disappear in later childhood, are noted on the superior lateral portion of the buttocks. Lipoatrophy can be marked on the rest of the buttocks, and lipoatrophic streaks often extend down the legs. Variable facial dysmorphisms include a high nasal bridge, prominent jaw, and large pinnae.

Extracutaneous Findings

Neurologic features of CDGS include hypotonia, hyporeflexia, and alternating esotropia.[67] Infants often suck poorly and present with feeding difficulties. Even when nutritional intake is good, lipoatrophy gives many children an emaciated appearance. Although most children are full-term and appropriate weight for gestational age,

developmental delay and failure to thrive usually occur by 3 months of age.

Significant coagulopathy may result in strokelike episodes, and hepatomegaly with hepatic dysfunction is common. Renal cysts, pericardial effusions, pericardial tamponade, and hypertrophic obstructive cardiomyopathy have been reported.

Although the central nervous system involvement tends to be static, musculoskeletal complications, including muscular atrophy, contractures, and spinal deformities, progress in later childhood and adulthood. In girls, defective peptide hormone glycosylation results in hypogonadotrophic hypogonadism with failure to undergo pubertal sexual development. Males are virilized at puberty, but may exhibit decreased testicular volume. Other endocrinologic findings result from hyperglycemia-induced growth hormone release, hyperprolactinemia, and insulin resistance.

Etiology and Pathogenesis

A recessive mode of inheritance is supported by several cases. Recent genetic studies have demonstrated linkage to a locus on chromosome 16 p.[67,71] Although a common clinical phenotype is recognized, at least four different defects in N-linked oligosaccharide synthesis have been identified, and more types are expected to emerge. In subtypes 1 and 2, specific enzymatic deficiencies have been identified.

Diagnosis

Typical clinical features seen in association with the presence of abnormally glycosylated serum proteins, typically transferrin detected by cathodal migration on serum isoelectric focusing, may allow for diagnosis in the neonatal period. Other serum glycoproteins also show abnormal bands on isoelectric focusing.

Prenatal diagnosis of CDGS type 1A by lysosomal enzyme analysis of amniotic fluid and genetic linkage analysis of cultured amniocytes was recently reported.[71]

Differential Diagnosis

Although other lipodystrophies should be considered, the clinical features are usually distinctive. When dysmorphic features are subtle, biochemical studies are required to distinguish CDGS from related disorders.

Treatment and Course

Supportive treatment is necessary to avoid complications from the central nervous system, as well as ophthalmologic and hematologic manifestations of CDGS. Mannose has been used to deal with some of the acute crises of infancy, including intractable seizures, severe coagulopathy, and pericardial effusions, but does not change the dismal prognosis.

FARBER LIPOGRANULOMATOSIS

Farber disease is a rare autosomal recessive disorder of lipid metabolism that usually presents with a fatal course in early infancy.[72,73] Although skin, joint, and laryngeal symptoms associated with neurodegeneration are characteristic, some patients may present with later onset of primarily neurologic findings.

Clinical Findings

Tender, red, subcutaneous nodules and swelling appear during the first few weeks of life over joints and areas of trauma, particularly the wrists and ankles. Granulomatous infiltration of the larynx results in a weak, hoarse cry.[72-73] Infants are usually irritable, and psychomotor retardation is severe. Reticuloendothelial involvement may produce generalized lymphadenopathy and marked hepatosplenomegaly.

Etiology and Pathogenesis

In Farber disease, ceramide, a normal intermediate in the metabolism of gangliosides and structurally important sphingolipids and glycolipids, accumulates as a result of a deficiency of lysosomal acid ceramidase.[72] Variable storage of ceramide occurs in visceral organs and brain white matter.

Diagnosis

The biochemical defect can be demonstrated in kidney, liver, cultured fibroblasts, and leukocytes.[72,73] Prenatal diagnosis is also possible by amniocentesis and chorionic villus sampling.

Differential Diagnosis

In the young infant, the diagnosis can usually be made clinically when the classic findings are present. However, when various aspects are missing, Farber disease can be confused with juvenile rheumatoid arthritis, multicentric reticulohistiocytosis, and juvenile hyaline fibromatosis.[73] Ceramide levels are normal in all of these conditions.

Treatment and Course

The clinical course is usually characterized by recurrent fever and pulmonary infiltrates, with death occurring by 2 years of age. Rarely patients present with later onset of neurologic disease followed by extraneuronal granulomas in skin and viscera. Some patients with little or no involvement of the central nervous system develop normally and survive longer.

REFERENCES

1. Holbrook KA. Structure and function of the developing human skin. In Goldsmith LE, ed. *Physiology, biochemistry and molecular biology of the skin.* 2nd edition. vol 1. New York: Oxford University Press, 1991: p 63.
2. Scales JW, Krowchuk DP, Schwartz RP, et al. An infant with firm fixed plaques. Arch Dermatol 1998;134:425-426.
3. Fretzin DF, Arias AM. Sclerema neonatorum and subcutaneous fat necrosis of the newborn. Pediatr Dermatol 1987;4: 112-122.
4. Rosbotham JL, Johnson A, Haque KN, et al. Painful subcutaneous fat necrosis of the newborn associated with intrapartum use of a calcium channel blocker. Clin Exp Dermatol 1998;23:19-21.
5. Silverman AK, Michels EH, Rasmussen JE. Subcutaneous fat necrosis in an infant occurring after hypothermic cardiac surgery. J Am Acad Dermatol 1986;15:331-336.
6. Duhn R, Schoen E, Sui M. Subcutaneous fat necrosis with extensive calcification after hypothermia in two newborn infants. Pediatrics 1968; 41:661-664.
7. Hicks MJ, Levy ML, Alexander J, et al. Subcutaneous fat necrosis of the newborn and hypercalcemia: A case report and review of the literature. Pediatr Dermatol 1993;10:271-276.
8. Fernandez-Lopez E, Garcia-Dorado J, de Unamuno P, et al. Subcutaneous fat necrosis of the newborn and idiopathic hypercalcemia. Dermatology 1990;180:250-254.
9. Rice AM, Rivkees SA. Etidronate therapy for hypercalcemia in subcutaneous fat necrosis of the newborn. J Pediatr 1999; 134:349-351.
10. Kellum RE, Ray TL, Brown CR. Sclerema neonatorum. Arch Dermatol 1968;97:372-376.
11. Horsfield MB, Yardley H. Sclerema neonatorum. J Invest Dermatol 1965;44:326-332.
12. Warwick WJ, Ruttenberg HD, Quie PG. Sclerema neonatorum, a sign, not a disease. JAMA 1963;184:680.
13. Gupta AK, Shashi S Mohon M, et al. Epidemiology of *Pseudomonas aeruginosa* infection in a nursery intensive care unit. J Trop Pediatr 1993;39:32-36.
14. Gupta P, Murali MV, Furidi MM, et al. Clinical profile of Klebsiella septicemia in neonates. Indian J Pediatr 1993;60: 568-572.
15. Zeck P, Madden EM. Sclerema neonatorum of both internal and external adipose tissue. Arch Pathol 1946;41:166.
16. Haxthausen H. Adiponecrosis e frigore. Br J Dermatol 1941; 53:83.
17. Rotman H. Cold panniculitis in children. Arch Dermatol 1966;94:720-721.
18. Collins HA, Stahlman M, Scott HW Jr. The occurrence of subcutaneous fat necrosis in an infant following induced hypothermia used as an adjuvant in cardiac surgery. Ann Surg 1953;138:880-885.
19. Mimouni F, Merlob P, Metzker A, et al. Supraventricular tachycardia: The icebag technique may be harmful in newborn infants. J Pediatr 1983;103:337.

20. Ter Poorten JC, Hebert AA, Ilkiw R. Cold panniculitis in a neonate. J Am Acad Dermatol 1995;33:383-385.
21. Epstein EH Jr, Oren ME. Popsicle panniculitis. N Eng J Med 1970;282:966-967.
22. Lowe IB Jr. Cold panniculitis in children. Am J Dis Child 11968;115:709-713.
23. Duncan WC, Freeman RG, Heaton CL. Cold panniculitis. Arch Dermatol 1966;94:722-724.
24. Silverman RA, Newman AJ, LeVine MJ, et al. Poststeroid panniculitis: A case report. Pediatr Dermatol 1988;5:92-93.
25. Buswell WA. Traumatic fat necrosis of the face in children. Br J Plast Surg 1979;32:127-128.
26. Fawcett HA, smith NP. Injection-site granuloma due to aluminum. Arch Dermatol 1984;120:1318-1322.
27. Forstrom L, Winkelmann RK. Factitial panniculitis. Arch Dermatol 1974;110:747-750.
28. Pao W, Duncan KO, Bolognia JL, et al. Numerous eruptive lesions of panniculitis associated with Group A Streptococcus bacteremia in an immunocompetent child. Clin Infect Dis 1998;27:430-433.
29. Patterson J, Brown PO, Broecker LR. Infection-induced panniculitis. J Cutan Pathol 1989;161:183-193.
30. Lassman LP, James CC. Lumbosacral lipomas: critical survey of 26 cases submitted to laminectomy. J Neurol Neurosurg Psychiatry 1967;30:174-181.
31. Harrist TJ, Gary DL, Kleinman GM, et al. Unusual sacrococcygeal embryologic malformation with cutaneous manifestation. Arch Dermatol 1982;118:643-648.
32. Goldberg NS, Hebert AA, Esterly NB. Sacral lipomas: The need for neurologic and radiologic evaluation. Arch Dermatol 1987;123:711-712.
33. Lhowe D, Ehrlich MC, Chapman PH, et al. Congenital intraspinal lipomas: Clinical presentation and response to therapy. J Pediatr Orthopaedics 1987;7:531-537.
34. Park HJ, Park CJ, Yi TY, et al. Nevus lipomatosus cutaneous superficialis. Int J Dermatol 1997;36:435-437.
35. Raymond JL, Stoebner P, Amblard P. Nevus lipomatosus cutaneous superficialis, an electron microscopic study of 4 cases. J Cutan Pathol 1980;7:295-301.
36. Orteau CH, Hughes JR. Nevus lipomatosus cutaneous superficialis: Overlap with connective tissue naevi (Letter). Acta Derm Venereol 1996;76:243-245.
37. Jones EW, Marks R, Pongsehirun D. Nevus superficialis lipomatosus, a clinicopathological report of 20 cases. Br J Dermatol 1975;93:121-133.
38. Grimalt R, Ermacora E, Mistura L, et al. Encephalocraniocutaneous lipomatosis: Case report and review of the literature. Pediatr Dermatol 1993;10:164-168.
39. Haberland C, Perou M. Encephalocraniocutaneous lipomatosis. A new example of ectodermal dysgenesis. Arch Neurol 1970;22:144-155.
40. Fishman MA, Chang CS, Miller JE. Encephalocraniocutaneous lipomatosis. Pediatrics 1978;61:580-582.
41. Miyao M, Saito T, Yamamoto Y, Kamoshita S. Encephalocraniocutaneous lipomatosis: A recently described neurocutaneous syndrome. Childs Brain 1984;11:280-284.
42. Fishman MA. Encephalocraniocutaneous lipomatosis. J Child Neurol 1987;2:186-193.
43. Happle R. How many epidermal nevus syndromes exist? J Am Acad Dermatol 1991;25:550-556.
44. Ross CM. Generalized folded skin with an underlying lipomatous nevus. Arch Dermatol 1969;100:320-323.
45. Schnur RE, Herzberg AJ, Spinner N, et al. Variability in the Michelin tire syndrome, a child with multiple anomalies, smooth muscle hamartoma and familial paracentric inversion of chromosome 7q. J Am Acad Dermatol 1993;28:364-370.
46. Sato M, Ishikawa O, Miyachi Y, et al. Michelin tyre syndrome: A congenital disorder of elastic fibre formation? Br J Dermatol 1997;136:583-586.
47. Kunze J, Riehm H. A new genetic disorder: Autosomal dominant multiple benign ring-shaped skin creases. Eur J Pediatr 1982;138:301-313.
48. Gardner EW, Miller HM, Lowney ED. Folded skin associated with underlying nevus lipomatous. Arch Dermatol 1979;115:978-979.
49. Eichenfield LF, Cunningham BC, Friedlander SF. Congenital piezogenic-like papules. Ann Dermatol 1998;125(S1):182.
50. Larralde De Luna M, Ruiz Leon J, Cabrerea HN. [Pedal papules in newborn infants]. [Spanish] Med Cutan Ibero Lat Am 1987;15:135-139.
51. Larregue M, Varbres P, Echard P, et al. Precalcaneal congenital fibrolipomatous hamartoma. Vth Int Congress Pediatric Dermatology, September, 1996.
52. Jaffe RH. Recurrent lipomatous tumors of the groin: Liposarcoma and lipoma pseudomyxomatodes. Arch Pathol 1926;1:381-387.
53. Van Meurs DP. The transformation of an embryonic lipoma to common lipoma. Br J Surg 1947;34:282-284.
54. Chung EF, Enzinger FM. Benign lipoblastomatosis: an analysis of 35 cases. Cancer 1973;32:482-492.
55. Mahour GH, Bryan BJ, Isaacs H. Lipoblastoma and lipoblastomatosis—a report of six cases. Surgery 1988;104:577-579.
56. Mentzel T, Calonje E, Fletcher CD. Lipoblastoma and lipoblastomatosis: A clinicopathological study of 14 cases. Histopathology 1993;23:527-533.
57. Gaffney EF, Vellios F, Hiliary K, et al. Lipoblastoma ultrastructure of two cases and relationship to human fetal white adipose tissue. Pediatr Pathol 1986;5:207-216.
58. Donohue WL, Uchida IA. Leprechaunism: A euphemism for a rare familial disorder. J Pediatr 1954;45:505-519.
59. Donohue WL. Dysendocrinism. J Pediatr 1948;32:739-748.
60. Taylor SI. Lilly lecture: Molecular mechanism of insulin resistance. Diabetes 1992;41:1473-1490.
61. Elsas LJ, Endo F, Strumlauf E, et al. Leprechaunism: An inherited defect in high-affinity insulin receptor. Am J Human Genet 1985;37:73-88.
62. Kosztolanyi F. Leprechaunism/Donohue syndrome/insulin receptor gene mutations: A syndrome delineation story from clinicopathological description to molecular understanding. Eur J Pediatr 1997;156:253-255.
63. Ozbey H, Ozbey N, Tunnessen W. Picture of the month: Leprechaunism. Arch Pediatr Adolesc Med 1998;1998;152:1031-1032.
64. Kadowaki T, Bevins CL, Cama A. Two mutant alleles of the insulin receptor gene in a patient with extreme insulin resistance. Science 1998;240:787-790.
65. Berardinelli W. An undiagnosed endocrinometabolic syndrome: Report of 2 cases. J Clin Endocrin 1954;14:193-204.

66. Seip M. Lipodystrophy and gigantism with associated endocrine manifestations: A new diencephalic syndrome? Acta Pediatr Scand 1959;48:555-574.

67. Seip M, Trugstad O. Generalized lipodystrophy, congenital and acquired (lipoatrophy). Acta Pediatr 1996; Suppl 413: 2-28.

68. Jaeken J, Stibler H, Hagberg B. The carbohydrate-deficient glycoprotein syndrome. Acta Paediatr Scand 1991;375:5S-71S.

69. Krasnewich D, Gahl WA. Carbohydrate-deficient glycoprotein syndrome. Adv Pediatr 1997;44:109-139.

70. Jaeken J, Vanderschueren-Lodewyckx M, Casaer P. Familial psychomotor retardation with markedly fluctuative serum prolactin, FSH and GH levels, partial TBG deficiency, increased CSF protein: a new syndrome? Pediatr Res 1980; 14:129.

71. Charlwood J, Clayton P, Keir G, et al. Prenatal diagnosis of the carbohydrate-deficient glycoprotein syndrome type 1A (CDG1A) by a combination of enzymology and genetic linkage analysis after amniocentesis or chorionic villus sampling. Prenat Diagn 1998;18:693-699.

72. Rutledge P. Gangliodoses and related lipid storage diseases. In Rimoin DL, Connor JM, Pyeritz RE, eds. *Emery and Rimoin's principles and practice of medical genetics, 3rd edition.* New York: Churchill Livingstone, 1996: p 2113-2114.

73. Antonarakis SE, Valle D, Hugo M, et al. Phenotypic variability in siblings with Farber disease. J Pediatr 1984;104:406-409.

23

Neoplastic and Infiltrative Diseases

NEIL S. PROSE
RICHARD J. ANTAYA

Skin disorders characterized by infiltrative lesions can be present at birth or develop during the first few months of life. Some represent frank neoplasms, both benign and malignant, whereas others are the result of metabolic errors. In most instances, diagnosis is facilitated by skin biopsy in which certain cell types can be identified by special stains and immunologic markers. Others require special enzyme assays for definitive diagnosis.

LEUKEMIA

Congenital leukemia is a rare hematologic disorder. Of the two distinct types, acute nonlymphocytic leukemia is far more common than the lymphocytic variety. To differentiate congenital leukemia from the several infectious and proliferative disorders that can easily mimic this condition, the following diagnostic criteria are employed:

1. The presence of immature white cells in the blood
2. Infiltration of these cells into extrahematopoietic tissues
3. The absence of diseases that can cause leukemoid reactions (such as erythroblastosis fetalis and a variety of congenital infections)
4. The absence of chromosomal disorders that are associated with "unstable" hematopoiesis (such as trisomy 21)[1,2]

Cutaneous Findings
The cutaneous manifestations of congenital leukemia consist of petechiae, ecchymoses, and skin nodules. The firm nodules are usually 1 to 2.5 cm in diameter and blue to purple in color (Fig. 23-1). They are often widely spread over the skin surface, although congenital leukemia may present as a single cutaneous lesion. Congenital monoblastic leukemia may be manifested by "blueberry muffin" lesions,[3] and Darier's sign has been observed.[4] The clinical signs and symptoms include hepatosplenomegaly, pallor, lethargy, and respiratory distress. Lymphadenopathy occurs in some infants.

Diagnosis
Biopsy of a cutaneous lesion reveals a dense pleomorphic mononuclear cell infiltrate in the dermis and subcutaneous fat. Atypical mitotic figures may be present. The diagnosis of congenital leukemia can usually be confirmed by a complete blood count, bone marrow aspirate, and radiographs of the skull and long bones. In every case, cytogenetic studies must be performed to exclude the possibility of transient myeloproliferative disorder, which is usually associated with trisomy 21.[5]

Treatment and Course
Although a few cases of temporary and permanent spontaneous remission have been reported, congenital leukemia, when untreated, is almost always a lethal neoplastic disorder. Treatment alternatives include chemotherapy and bone marrow transplant.

LANGERHANS' CELL HISTIOCYTOSIS

Langerhans' cell histiocytosis (LCH), a rare proliferative disorder, may be present at birth or may develop during the first few months of life. The spectrum of clinical presentations, and the clinical course, is extremely varied and ranges from the simple presence of one or several nodules or crusted papules to severe, progressive multisystem disease.

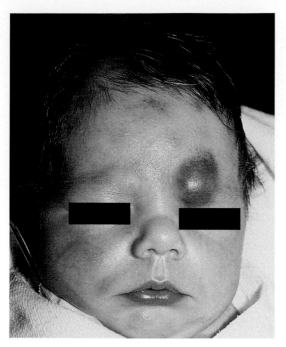

FIG. 23-1
The large nodule above the eye of this neonate represented a manifestation of congenital leukemia resulting from acute lymphocytic leukemia.

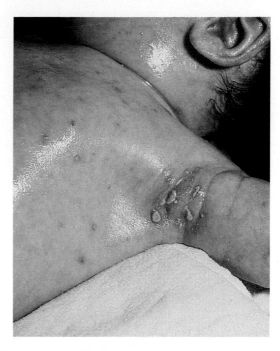

FIG. 23-2
Multiple pustules and erosions are evident in this young infant with Langerhans' cell histiocytosis and multisystem involvement.

Cutaneous Findings

The most frequent cutaneous presentation consists of multiple widespread vesiculopustules with umbilication and hemorrhagic crust.[6-10] Nodules and petechiae, which may involve the palms and soles, are also observed. Over time, eczematous lesions in the scalp and diaper area may develop (Fig. 23-2). Gingival and palatal lesions consist of ulcerations, areas of necrosis, and nodular infiltrates. Premature exfoliation and eruption of teeth, and destruction of alveolar bone are characteristic.

In 1973 Hashimoto and Pritzker described a disorder characterized by congenital papulonodular and papulovesicular skin lesions composed of S-100 positive histiocytes and eosinophils in children who did not develop other organ system involvement (Figs. 23-3 and 23-4).[11] The lesions in these patients seemed to resolve spontaneously, without sequellae.[12-14] However, the progression to severe LCH has now been reported in children who initially met the clinical criteria of "congenital self-healing histiocytosis."[15] Therefore Hashimoto-Pritzker disease should probably be considered a mild form of LCH, and patients who present with only papular or nodular skin lesions should also be closely monitored for the later development of visceral disease.

Extracutaneous Findings

The majority of infants with all forms of congenital or neonatal Langerhans' cell histiocytosis will show evidence of multisystem disease.[16,17] Single or multifocal bone lesions are particularly common, and intercranial disease may result in exopthalmos and diabetes insipidus. Lymph node involvement is seen in a significant percentage of patients. Invasion of the liver, spleen, lung, bone marrow, gastrointestinal tract (GI), and central nervous system (CNS) may occur and may result in symptomatology and even organ failure.

Diagnosis

Biopsy of a cutaneous lesion reveals a diffuse infiltration of histiocytes with abundant eosinophilic cytoplasm and eccentric, indented nuclei. In some cases, the nuclei may appear pleomorphic or atypical. Cells are S-100 and CD-1a positive, and electron microscopy reveals the presence of Langerhans' granules in a significant percentage of histiocytes.

Preliminary laboratory evaluation of the patient with biopsy-proven skin lesions must include a complete blood count (CBC), serum electrolytes, urine specific gravity, and assessment of liver function. Examination

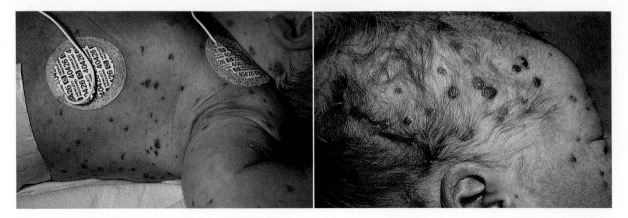

FIG. 23-3
Multiple crusted papules are typical of the "self-healing" variant of congenital Langerhans' cell histiocytosis.

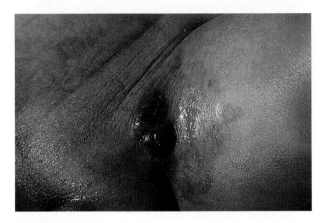

FIG. 23-4
A congenital nodule in the inguinal area was found on biopsy to be congenital Langerhans' cell histiocytosis. It resolved without further sequellae.

of the bone marrow may show the presence of increased histiocytes. Skeletal survey, chest radiographs, and magnetic resonance imaging (MRI) may be used to determine the extent of bone, pulmonary, liver, spleen, and CNS involvement.

Differential Diagnosis

Congenital Langerhans' cell histiocytosis must be differentiated from other neoplastic disorders, such as leukemia and lymphoma; from congenital infections, especially herpes simplex; and from those viral disorders associated with blueberry muffin lesions.

Treatment and Course

Congenital Langerhans' cell histiocytosis with organ involvement is most often a rapidly fatal disease. Treatment consists of chemotherapy, but in general, presentation at a young age is a particularly poor prognostic factor.[9]

FAMILIAL HEMOPHAGOCYTIC LYMPHOHISTIOCYTOSIS

Familial hemophagocytic lymphohistiocytosis (FHL) is an autosomal recessive disorder that most often presents during the first year of life.[18] Some children have been noted to have an evanescent macular and papular skin eruption, sometimes associated with episodes of fever. Most patients have pronounced hepatosplenomegaly, and many develop symptoms related to CNS involvement. Diagnosis is made by the detection of a nonmalignant mixed lymphohistiocytic proliferation in the reticuloendothelial system, with evidence of hemophagocytosis. Without treatment, FLH is usually rapidly fatal. Chemotherapy and bone marrow transplant are the preferred therapies.

FIBROSARCOMA

Congenital/infantile fibrosarcoma is a rare tumor that occurs most frequently on the extremities. Lesions are seen less commonly on the head, neck, and trunk and may also occur in the retroperitoneum.[19] The tumor may be present at birth, or may develop during early infancy.

Cutaneous Findings

Fibrosarcoma most often presents as a soft-tissue mass, sometimes with rapid growth. The overlying skin may be

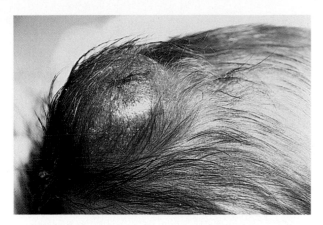

FIG. 23-5
Infantile fibrosarcoma of the scalp in a 15-day-old boy.

tense, shiny, and erythematous, and ulceration may occur (Fig. 23-5).[20]

Diagnosis
MRI is useful in defining the extent of the lesion, but diagnosis is based on histology. Histologic examination reveals a highly cellular fibroblastic proliferation, with sizeable vascular clefts and occasional myxoid degeneration and hemorrhagic necrosis.[21]

Differential Diagnosis
Clinically, infantile fibrosarcomas are easily confused with either hemangiomas or vascular/lymphatic malformations.[22,23] The differential diagnosis also includes rhabdomyosarcoma and infantile myofibromatosis.

Treatment and Course
Most authors suggest that the risk of metastasis, especially in cutaneous lesions, is considerably lower in infants (approximately 8%) than in older patients.[24] Treatment consists of wide local excision. Chemotherapy has been used in some patients to reduce the lesion mass preoperatively, and for lesions that are not resectable. Close follow-up, to monitor for the presence of local recurrence and metastatic disease, is mandatory.

DERMATOFIBROSARCOMA PROTUBERANS

Dermatofibrosarcoma protuberans (DFSP) is a fibrohistiocytic tumor with low metastatic potential and a high incidence of local recurrence. Congenital DFSP is rare, but several cases have been reported.[25,26] Another condition,

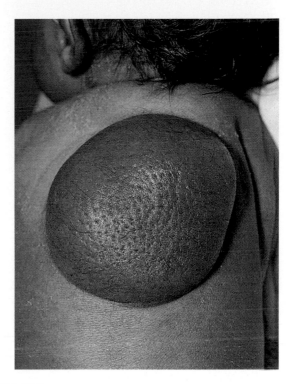

FIG. 23-6
Giant cell fibroblastoma, considered a variant of dermatofibrosarcoma protuberans.

so-called giant cell fibroblastoma, can also present in early infancy and is now considered to be a variant of DFSP (Fig. 23-6).

Cutaneous Findings
Characteristically, DFSP begins as an atrophic plaque, surrounded by an area of bluish discoloration. Over time, as the cellular proliferation extends into the deep dermis and subcutaneous tissues, nodules develop on the plaque surface (Fig. 23-7). Similar to the lesions seen in older patients, congenital DFSP occurs most commonly on the trunk and proximal extremities.

Diagnosis
Histologically, DFSP is characterized by the presence of spindle cells in a well-defined and uniform storiform pattern. Focal myxoid change and scarring may occur. Tumor cells express vimentin, but are negative for S-100 protein, epithelial membrane antigen, and smooth muscle actin.[27]

Differential Diagnosis
Clinically, the differential diagnosis of congenital DFSP includes fibrous hamartoma of infancy, infantile myofi-

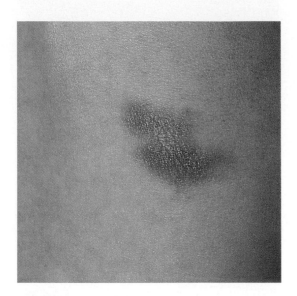

FIG. 23-7
Nodular, plaque-type dermatofibrosarcoma protuberans.

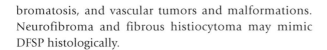

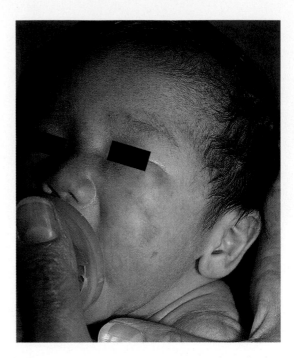

FIG. 23-8
Congenital neuroblastoma: blue nodules on the face. (Courtesy of Bari Cunningham, MD.)

bromatosis, and vascular tumors and malformations. Neurofibroma and fibrous histiocytoma may mimic DFSP histologically.

Treatment
Because of the high risk of recurrence, adequate surgical margins must be obtained. Mohs micrographic surgery is an alternative approach in some patients.[28]

NEUROBLASTOMA

Cutaneous Findings
Neuroblastoma is among the most common solid tumors of early childhood, and presentation at birth or in early infancy may occur. Cutaneous metastases present as bluish, firm papules and nodules on the trunk and extremities (Fig. 23-8). Several authors have reported that these lesions may blanch after palpation, and that the blanching persists for 30 to 60 minutes.[29,30] This phenomenon has been related to the localized release of catecholamines. Periorbital ecchymoses, secondary to orbital metastases, may also occur.

Extracutaneous Findings
Metastatic disease, characterized by fever, hepatomegaly, and failure to thrive, is often present at the time of diag-

nosis. The primary lesion is usually located in the upper abdomen, arising within the adrenal gland, and may be detected as an enlarging mass.

Diagnosis
Diagnosis of the cutaneous lesions is based on histologic examination. The dermal or subcutaneous infiltrate consists of small cells with scant cytoplasm and heterochromatic nuclei. Pseudorosettes and mature ganglion cells are present in differentiated lesions. Immunoperoxidase staining may establish the presence of neuron-specific proteins.

Although most cases of neuroblastoma are sporadic, autosomal dominant inheritance may occur. Concordance in monozygotic twins has also been reported.[31] The location and extent of the primary lesion is most often established by computed tomography (CT) or MRI. Increased urinary catecholamines are present in the majority of patients.

Differential Diagnosis
Clinically and histologically, the lesions of neuroblastoma must be differentiated from leukemia and lymphoma. In addition, the blueberry-muffin appearance of some lesions may mimic congenital rubella or cytomegalovirus infection.

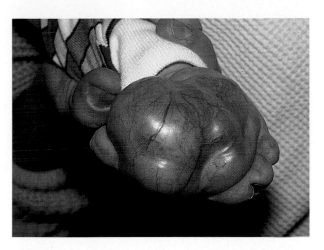

FIG. 23-9
Rhabdomyosarcoma: firm, vascular appearing tumor of the hand.

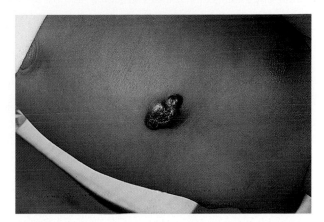

FIG. 23-10
Congenital malignant melanoma, arising de novo on normal skin.

Treatment and Course

The prognosis of neuroblastoma depends on the age of the patient and the extent of the disease (Stages I to IV-s). The survival rate at 2 years in children who are diagnosed under the age of 1 year exceeds 80%. In some patients, especially with Stage IV-s, spontaneous differentiation to neural ganglion cells, and regression without treatment have been reported. The choice of treatment depends on staging and patient age, and consists of various combinations of surgery, radiation therapy, and chemotherapy.[37]

RHABDOMYOSARCOMA

Rhabdomyosarcoma presents most commonly as a tumor of the head and neck. Other locations include the genitourinary tract, extremities, and trunk (Fig. 23-9). Two percent of cases are present at birth. An association between rhabdomyosarcoma and both neurofibromatosis type 1 and major congenital abnormalities has been observed.[33]

Cutaneous origin of rhabdomyosarcoma is rare. Most commonly, extension of the tumor into the dermis results in the evolution of a nodule or plaque.[34] Facial lesions are most common, and these must be differentiated clinically from dermoid cysts, hemangiomas, and inflammatory disorders. Histologically, there is a dermal infiltrate of small blue cells with occasional differentiation toward rhabdomyoblasts. The presence of desmin staining with immunoperoxidase may help to differentiate these lesions from neuroblastoma and lymphoma.

Treatment is based on the extent of local, regional, and distant disease, and consists of combinations of surgery,

radiation, and chemotherapy. Combined modality therapy results in a long-term survival of greater than 50%.[35]

CONGENITAL MELANOMA

Congenital malignant melanoma may develop in several different clinical situations[36,37]:

1. *Congenital malignant melanoma arising de novo.* Malignant melanoma may present at birth as a nodular, darkly pigmented, and rapidly growing skin lesion, sometimes with ulceration.[38,39] In these neonates, there is no clinical or histologic evidence of an underlying congenital melanocytic nevus, and there is no maternal history of melanoma (Fig. 23-10).
2. *Congenital malignant melanoma arising in a giant congenital melanocytic nevus.* In these patients, ulcerated and nonulcerated nodules may be present in the congenital melanocytic nevus and on adjoining skin. The presence of prenatal metastatic disease has been noted to occur in some children.[40,41]
3. *Congenital malignant melanoma arising from leptomeningeal melanocytosis.* Children with leptomeningeal melanocytosis may have a high lifetime incidence of metastatic malignant melanoma. Rarely, these metastatic cutaneous lesions may be present at birth.
4. *Congenital malignant melanoma secondary to maternal melanoma.* Transplacental transmission from a mother with metastatic disease may occur.[42] Typically, the skin lesions are multiple pigmented macules, papules and nodules, and multiorgan involvement may occur.

The diagnosis of malignant melanoma is made by excisional biopsy of the suspicious skin lesion, and the cellular and architectural features are similar to those seen in melanoma in older patients. However, a wide variety of benign and malignant tumors, with small round cell, spindled, neural, and epitheloid components, have been observed within congenital melanocytic nevi.[39] In addition, histologic changes within a benign, congenital melanocytic nevus may include displaced large melanocytes within the epidermis, and heterogeneous patterns of melanocytic hyperplasia.[40] In some cases, findings of this type have led to the incorrect diagnosis of malignant melanoma. Biopsies of congenital melanocytic nevi, especially in the neonate, must therefore be interpreted with caution.[43-45]

The evaluation of children with all forms of melanoma must include a complete evaluation for local and distant lymph node involvement. Metastases are most frequently seen in the CNS, bones, lungs, and liver.

Treatment is based on lesion thickness and the stage of the disease. Therapeutic options include lymph-node dissection of enlarged draining regional nodes and chemotherapy for metastatic disease.[41] Lesions arising de novo have an unpredictable prognosis, and long-term survival has been reported in children who developed both local recurrences and metastatic lesions. Melanomas arising in congenital melanocytic nevi appear to have a significantly worse prognosis. Congenital malignant melanoma secondary to maternal melanoma is usually fatal, but spontaneous regression has been reported to occur.[42]

CONGENITAL TERATOMA

Congenital teratomas most frequently present as masses in the cervical region or nasopharynx.[46] These benign tumors, which are derived from elements of all three germinal layers, result in significant morbidity and mortality because of their location, size, and tendency to cause airway obstruction. The differential diagnosis includes dermoids and lymphatic or vascular malformations. Treatment consists of complete surgical excision.

MASTOCYTOSIS

Mastocytosis refers to a spectrum of conditions characterized by the infiltration of benign mast cells in the skin or other organs. Fifty-five percent of cases develop during the first 2 years, and an additional 10% develop before age 15 years.[47] Both sexes are affected equally. Mastocytoma, urticaria pigmentosa (UP), and diffuse cutaneous mastocytosis (DCM) are most likely to affect neonates and infants (see the following discussion). Mastocytoma is the most

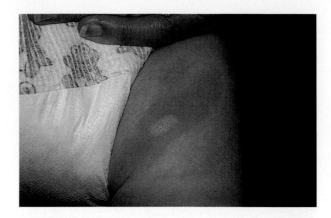

FIG. 23-11
Mastocytoma on the leg of a young infant with a centrally urticated plaque with surrounding flare, demonstrating a positive Darier's sign.

common clinical manifestation of mastocytosis. UP is less common, and DCM, the most severe form, is rare. Most cases are sporadic; however, there have been several reports of UP affecting multiple family members, and some believe diffuse cutaneous mastocytosis can be inherited in an autosomal dominant fashion.[47-49]

Mastocytoma

Mastocytoma most often appears in the first 3 months of life. It presents as one or several, isolated, skin-colored to light brown, 1 to 5 cm, oval to round macules or slightly elevated nodules or plaques (Fig. 23-11). Some lesions have a pink or yellow hue. Any cutaneous surface may be affected, and the trunk, upper extremities and neck are favored locations. Most new lesions appear within 2 months of the initial lesion, but individual lesions may enlarge for several months.

Urticaria Pigmentosa

Urticaria pigmentosa generally develops between 3 and 9 months of life. The lesions appear as multiple, reddish-brown, hyperpigmented macules, papules and nodules (Fig. 23-12) that have a tendency to coalesce into plaques and often exhibit increased skin markings. Early lesions of UP may mimic recurrent urticaria until pigmentation becomes apparent. Any cutaneous surface may be affected, including mucous membranes, but most are on the trunk. Additional lesions of UP may develop for several months after the initial diagnosis is made.

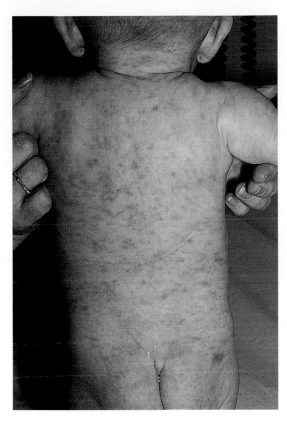

FIG. 23-12
Multiple lesions of urticaria pigmentosa in a 1-month-old infant.

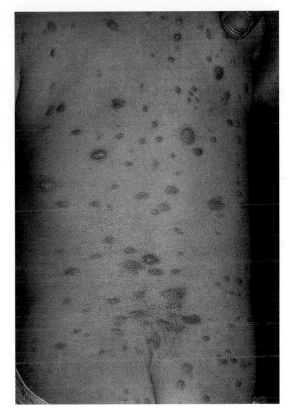

FIG. 23-13
Focal blister formation in an infant with diffuse cutaneous mastocytosis.

Diffuse Cutaneous Mastocytosis

Diffuse cutaneous mastocytosis (DCM) is characterized by widespread infiltration of mast cells throughout the skin (Fig. 23-13). It presents in the first 3 years of life, and is characterized by generalized thickening and palpable edema of the skin. The skin may be normal in color or display a reddish-yellow hue. The first sign of DCM most often is hemorrhagic bullae and erosions, sometimes following minor trauma. Severe dermatographism with resultant bullae and flushing may also occur.

With mastocytosis most patients exhibit Darier's sign, which is the development of an urticarial wheal and flare after firm stroking of lesional skin. This cutaneous finding represents the response to physical disruption of mast cells' granular contents, particularly histamine. Rarely, flushing and hypotension have resulted from stroking of a large lesion, or from surgery. Darier's sign is a common finding in UP. Dermatographism, the formation of linear urticarial plaques following scratching of uninvolved skin, is also seen. However, this nonspecific finding occurs in up to 5% of the normal population. A variety of physical stimulants and drugs can evoke mast cell degranulation, resulting in urtication, bulla formation, or systemic manifestations (flushing, hypotension, or shock) (Box 23-1).

Many patients have no symptoms, but when present, the major presenting symptom is pruritus. It may be periodic or unremitting. Excoriations may be observed. In children less than 2 years of age vesicles and bullae occur, and are seen in all three forms of cutaneous mastocytosis. The tendency to blister diminishes over 1 to 3 years. In one series, generalized flushing was observed in 65% of patients with all forms of the disease.[50]

Hepatosplenomegaly, lymphadenopathy, or skeletal lesions caused by mast cell hyperplasia occur infrequently in infants with DCM or UP.[51] Associated systemic findings in infants with these forms of the disease include diarrhea, vomiting, abdominal pain, bone pain, headache, hypotension, and rarely shock. Prolonged bleeding in the skin and GI tract may occur, and is more frequent in infants with DCM. In these children, heparin from mast cells acts as a local anticoagulant. Elevated levels of circulating histamine, which stimulates gastric acid secretion, may result in gastric ulceration and gastrointestinal hemorrhage.[52] Children with DCM have the highest incidence of visceral mast cell disease and associated systemic manifestations. UP in infants is rarely (less than 3%) associated with visceral involvement, and visceral involvement does not appear to occur in children with cutaneous mastocytomas. The incidence of allergic disease is not increased in children with mastocytosis.

The cause of mastocytosis is unknown. A mutation in the *c-kit* protooncogene has been identified in some patients with mastocytosis. *C-kit* codes for a receptor for stem cell factor, and is expressed on mast cells, melanocytes, and hematopoietic stem cells. This mutation may contribute to the characteristic proliferation of mast cells, the hyperpigmentation of the skin seen in cutaneous mastocytosis, or the myeloproliferative diseases observed in some patients with mastocytosis.[53] The clinical presentation and characteristic cutaneous lesions usually allow for easy diagnosis. Skin biopsy should be performed when the diagnosis is unclear or when bullae are the main feature. Histopathologic sections may demonstrate variable degrees of mast cell infiltration around blood vessels and within skin appendages. Bullae, when present, are subepidermal.

Determination of plasma histamine levels may be useful in infants at high risk of GI bleeding, as in DCM.[52] Clinical evidence of extracutaneous mastocytosis should guide any additional diagnostic studies (ultrasound, bone and liver-spleen scans, GI endoscopy, skeletal survey, and bone marrow evaluation).[54] The usefulness of studies performed empirically is limited, and they do not appear to provide any prognostic information.[47]

Mastocytomas should be differentiated from xanthomas, juvenile xanthogranulomas, and congenital nevi. Where bullae are prominent, biopsy is often indicated to differentiate mastocytosis from the immunobullous diseases, staphylococcal scalded skin syndrome, and epidermolysis bullosa.

The course of most cases of pediatric mastocytosis is benign and the prognosis generally favorable. Solitary mastocytomas have not been reported to progress to systemic involvement.[54] Greater than 50% of childhood cases of urticaria pigmentosa resolve by adolescence, and the remaining cases experience a marked reduction in cutaneous symptoms.[50,55] Fifteen to thirty percent of patients whose disease persists into adulthood develop systemic involvement, which is similar to the rate observed in adult-onset disease.[50]

Treatment is aimed at decreasing pruritus and, in some children, minimizing blister formation. The regular use of H_1 antihistamines such as hydroxyzine is effective in treating pruritus, bullae, flushing, and abdominal pain. The addition of H_2 blockers and oral cromolyn sodium may be effective for patients with gastrointestinal signs or symptoms.[57-58]

Solitary mastocytomas may be treated with a short course of a super-potent topical steroid, and very problematic lesions may be excised. Rare instances of circulatory collapse as a result of systemic histamine release should be treated with careful fluid management and intravenous epinephrine.[59] A self-injectable epinephrine device may be prescribed for children with a history of such episodes.[47] PUVA therapy is effective for severe UP and DCM.[60] Parents should be provided with a list of substances that stimulate mast cell activity, and therefore should be avoided (see Box 23-1).

JUVENILE HYALINE FIBROMATOSIS

Juvenile hyaline fibromatosis (JHF) is a rare, progressive, autosomal recessive disease. It first manifests from birth through the first several years of life with papulonodular skin lesions, joint contractures, skeletal and soft-tissue lesions, gingival hyperplasia, and stunted growth.

Cutaneous Findings

There are several distinct, characteristic skin lesions observed in JHF. Small, pearly white papules are found predominately on the face and neck. Translucent appearing, larger papules and nodules are found around the nose, behind the ears, and on the tips of digits. These have a gelatinous consistency. Subcutaneous nodules are seen widely distributed over the trunk, extremities, and scalp, and may exhibit variable consistency. Papillomatous perianal lesions, resembling condylomata, have been observed in some patients.[61]

Extracutaneous Findings

The most consistent and earliest extracutaneous manifestation of JHF is joint flexion contractures, especially of the knees and elbows. Many patients become severely disabled by these progressively severe contractures. Gingival hyperplasia is seen in nearly all patients, and the majority have osteolytic bone lesions and osteoporosis.[62] JHF generally does not involve the viscera; however, there is considerable clinical and histologic overlap with a more severe and uniformly fatal condition, infantile systemic hyalinosis (ISH). Some believe JHF and ISH to represent different points on the same clinical spectrum.[61]

Etiology and Pathogenesis

The etiology is unknown. Recent evidence suggests a possible malfunction in the synthesis of collagen types I and III, with altered proportions of cutaneous glycosaminoglycans and collagens I, III, and VI.[63,64]

On routine histology, the dermal papules show thinning of the epidermis and a dermis occupied by abundant, amorphous, PAS-positive, diastase resistant material containing wavy filamentous elements. Cells with oval or spindle-shaped nuclei are embedded in this stroma, imparting a chondroid appearance. These fibroblastic cells often display PAS-positive cytoplasmic vacuoles. Ultrastructurally, the fibroblastic stromal cells display a hyperplastic and dilated rough endoplasmic reticulum with collections of smooth surfaced cisternae, filled with tangled microfilaments.[61] Osteoporosis and osteolytic bone lesions are observed on radiographic examination of most patients. Routine laboratory evaluations are normal.

Differential Diagnosis

The differential diagnosis should first include Winchester syndrome, a rare autosomal recessive condition that has many overlapping features with JHF, including joint con-

tractures, dwarfism, hypertrophic lips and gingivae, severe osteoporosis, thickened leathery skin, and corneal opacities.[65] Lipoid proteinosis may be distinguished from JHF by distinctly different histology, a characteristic hoarse cry, and a more benign clinical course.

Treatment and Course

The course is progressive. Excluding those most severely affected with hyalin material in the viscera, most patients appear to survive into adulthood with severe physical deformities from joint contractures, delayed motor development, and skin nodules that recur after surgical excision. Treatment, which is unsatisfactory, includes excision of skin lesions and systemic corticosteroids for joint symptoms.

FARBER DISEASE

Farber disease, or Farber lipogranulomatosis, is a rare, progressive, autosomal recessive mucolipidosis. The disorder primarily involves the musculoskeletal, respiratory, integumentary, and nervous systems of affected infants, and onset occurs in the first year of life.[66]

Cutaneous Findings

The characteristic cutaneous features include multiple subcutaneous nodules, flesh-colored papules, and periarticular tumors or nodules. Coarse facial features and xanthoma-like papules on the face and hands have also been reported.[67]

Extracutaneous Findings

Painful, deforming joint swelling with restriction of movement, particularly of distal interphalangeal and metacarpal joints, is characteristic. Infants frequently exhibit marked failure to thrive, recurrent infections, a hoarse cry attributed to laryngomalacia, dyspnea,[68] noisy breathing, and hyperirritability. Impairment of cognitive development, seizures, hepatosplenomegaly, macroglossia, recurrent fevers, and hyporeflexia are variably present.

Etiology and Pathogenesis

Farber lipogranulomatosis is caused by a deficiency of the lysosomal acid ceramidase with resultant progressive accumulation of ceramide in tissues. The characteristic clinical presentation and the detection of low levels of acid ceramidase are diagnostic for Farber disease. Light microscopic examination of skin and other affected tissues is nonspecific, demonstrating foam cells and a granulomatous infiltrate. Several characteristic structures are observed ultramicroscopically, probably resulting from the accumulation of ceramide in cells. Curvilinear tubular bodies, comma-shaped, tubular structures consisting of two single membranes separated by a clear space, are observed in dermal fibroblasts among other affected cells. Banana bodies, variably membrane-bound structures that have a spindle and usually curved shape, are found predominantly in Schwann cells of peripheral nerves.[67]

Diagnosis

Radiologic examination reveals diffuse osteopenia, underdevelopment of terminal phalanges, and reduced long bone diameters.[68] The diagnosis should be confirmed by detection of deficient lysosomal acid ceramidase activity in leukocytes, fibroblasts, or other tissues.

Differential Diagnosis

The differential diagnosis includes metabolic storage diseases, particularly other mucolipidoses. Some cases have been misdiagnosed as juvenile rheumatoid arthritis because of the severe joint involvement seen early in the course.

Treatment and Course

Most patients die in the first decade of life. There is no specific medical therapy. Various treatments, including corticosteroids and radiotherapy, have been attempted and are ineffective.[68] The potassium-titanyl-phosphate (KTP) laser has been used for treatment of severe oral lesions.[69]

Because transmission is autosomal recessive, genetic counseling is mandatory. Prenatal diagnosis, performed by assaying acid ceramidase levels in skin cells cultured from amniotic fluid, is now possible.[70]

I-CELL DISEASE

I-cell disease, or mucolipidosis II, is a severe autosomal recessive form of lysosomal storage disease. The skeletal and central nervous systems are most severely affected, but characteristic skin changes also occur. I-cell disease exhibits signs and symptoms of both the mucopolysaccharidoses and sphingolipidoses. The inclusion cell, or I-cell, refers to the presence of cytoplasmic inclusions associated with lysosomes. Onset occurs at birth, and disease progression results in death during the first decade.

Cutaneous Findings

The most notable cutaneous findings are the facial features: small orbits and prominent eyes, puffy and swollen eyelids with a prominent venous pattern, and fullness of the lower face with rounded cheeks. Many small telangiectases impart a ruddy appearance to the cheeks. Patients often exhibit a fish mouth appearance in profile resulting from prominent maxillary bones. The neck is short, and the skin has a thickened and rigid texture, particularly of the neck and ears. Gingival hypertrophy is progressive and severe.

Extracutaneous Findings

Neonates commonly exhibit intrauterine growth retardation, with birth weights often below 2500 g. Linear growth is below normal and ceases at 1 year of age. Orthopedic problems, such as club foot, diaphyseal bending of long bones, and hip dislocation, may be presenting features. Inguinal hernias, especially in boys, may be noted at birth, and patients of both sexes have frequent upper respiratory tract infections. All patients experience severe psychomotor retardation, and the majority neither walk unaided nor develop more than primitive language skills. There is progressive stiffness of all joints, first apparent in the shoulders, with decreased mobility by 2 years of age.[71]

The long bones of affected infants younger than 6 months display periosteal cloaking, possibly from repeated new bone formation. Also observed are cone-shaped phalanges and abnormalities of the skull and pelvis.[72]

I-cell disease is caused by an underlying defect in N-acetyl-glucosamine-1-phosphotransferase, an enzyme involved in the synthesis of a mannose-6-phosphate marker of hydrolases normally found in lysosomes. Because newly synthesized lysosomal enzymes are not marked correctly, the mannose-6-phosphate receptor–dependent transport fails, and the enzymes are secreted out of cells, instead of being targeted to lysosomes. This results in failed lysosomal degradation of macromolecules, simulating a catabolic enzyme defect.[73] Fibroblast lysosomal enzymes are deficient in patients with I-cell disease, whereas the serum levels of the same enzymes are elevated.[74] The finding that some tissues have normal levels of lysosomal enzymes suggests that there may be an alternative method for targeting lysosomal hydrolases in these tissues.[75] The defective phosphotransferase gene has been mapped to chromosome 4q.[76]

Diagnosis

The diagnosis of I-cell disease is suggested by detection of an increase in the activity of several hydrolases in plasma. It is confirmed by dermal fibroblast cultures, which show the characteristic cytoplasmic inclusions (I-cells) in the cultured cells. These cytoplasmic inclusions stain positively for PAS and Sudan black, but almost negatively for Alcian blue, suggesting the inclusion bodies represent an abnormal accumulation of glycolipid.[72] Reduced activity of lysosomal hydrolases in the fibroblasts provides additional confirmation of the diagnosis.

Differential Diagnosis

I-cell disease shares most of the clinical features of Hurler syndrome, including coarse facial features, severe psychomotor retardation, and skeletal dysplasia. However, patients with I-cell disease do not exhibit mucopolysaccharides in their urine. Gingival hypertrophy and vacuolated peripheral blood lymphocytes, characteristic of I-cell disease, are not present in Hurler disease.

Treatment and Course

Death in early childhood is usually secondary to lower respiratory tract infection or congestive heart failure. No specific treatment exists. Because of the recessive inheritance pattern, genetic counseling should be offered. Successful prenatal diagnosis has been accomplished by demonstration of elevated enzyme levels in amniotic fluid in conjunction with enzyme assays from cultured amniotic fluid cells.[77]

MUCOPOLYSACCHARIDOSES

The mucopolysaccharidoses (MPSs) are a heterogeneous group of rare lysosomal storage disorders that display several variable clinical features, including coarse facies, skeletal abnormalities, mental retardation, corneal clouding, and hepatosplenomegaly. The degree of progression varies among the diseases, as does the constellation of clinical and laboratory findings. Each disease results from the deficiency of one specific lysosomal enzyme, but all are characterized by accumulation of mucopolysaccharides (glycosaminoglycans) in lysosomes and excessive amounts of mucopolysaccharides in the urine.[78] Sanfilippo syndrome is the most common, and has an incidence of about 1:25,000. This is contrasted with Sly syndrome, of which only 40 cases have been reported worldwide.[79]

Cutaneous Findings

The most characteristic cutaneous feature, manifest in all types of MPS, is coarse, thickened skin. This cutaneous alteration, along with underlying craniofacial abnormalities combine to impart coarse facial features. Patients have a thick nose with a depressed nasal bridge, thick tongue and lips, short neck, and macrocephaly. The severity of the facial abnormalities is variable, and the most striking features are observed in Hurler and Hunter syndromes. Coarse facies may not be present in young infants.[80] Patients also display variable degrees of coarse hair and generalized hirsutism.

Aside from Sanfilippo syndrome, which presents with synophrys, Hunter syndrome is the only MPS that regularly presents with specific cutaneous findings. Children with Hunter syndrome may develop firm, discrete or coalescing, ivory-colored papules on the arms or symmetrically distributed between the angles of the scapulae and the posterior axillary lines. Recently, this same finding was described in a patient with Hurler-Scheie syndrome.[81]

Extracutaneous Findings

Infants may appear normal at birth, but usually develop characteristic findings in the first few years of life. Each disease has its own array of clinical findings; however, the most important extracutaneous features are mental retardation, deafness, hyperactivity/behavior problems, stiff joints, skeletal dysplasia, kyphoscoliosis, corneal clouding, valvular and coronary heart disease, hepatosplenomegaly, noisy breathing, and lower respiratory tract infections. Table 23-1 lists the cardinal characteristics and pertinent negative findings for each disorder.

The skeletal abnormalities in the MPSs are referred to as dysostosis multiplex and comprise the following elements: large, thickened skull with premature closure of lambdoid and sagittal sutures, shallow orbits, enlarged J-shaped sella, and anterior hypoplasia of the lumbar vertebrae. In addition, the long bones display enlarged diaphyses, irregular metaphyses, and poor development of the epiphyseal centers.

Etiology and Pathogenesis

Each type of MPS is caused by a deficiency of a specific lysosomal enzyme responsible for the degradation of mucopolysaccharides. This deficiency results in excessive accumulation of the mucopolysaccharides, dermatan sulfate, heparan sulfate, and keratan sulfate throughout the body. The deficient enzyme has been elucidated for each disease, and the genetic locus has been mapped for several.[82] All have an autosomal recessive inheritance except for Hunter syndrome, which is X-linked recessive. Excluding an increased incidence of Hunter syndrome in the Jewish population in Israel and Morquio syndrome in French-Canadians, MPSs appear to affect all ethnic groups equally.

Diagnosis

The testing of urine for glycosaminoglycans is the basis for screening patients suspected of having MPS. If screening tests are positive for glycosaminoglycans, a quantitative analysis should be performed to confirm the presence of MPS. The type and quantity of urinary glycosaminoglycans combined with the child's clinical presentation are

TABLE 23-1

Classification and Features of the Mucopolysaccharidoses*

Eponym	MPS number	Main clinical features (and pertinent negatives)	Urinary mucopolysaccharide
Hurler	I-H	IH, UH, HSM, SS, JS, URI, MR, HL, HD, DM, CC, Hc	DS, HS
Hurler-Scheie	I-H/S	HL, JS, CC, HD, Mg, *no MR*	DS, HS
Scheie	I-S	JS, HD, CC, *no MR, no SS*	DS, HS
Hunter (severe)	II-A	SP, IH, UH, HSM, SS, JS, URI, MR, HL, DM, RD, Hc, *no CC*	DS, HS
Hunter (mild)	II-B	SP, HL, JS, HD, mild CC, *no MR*	DS, HS
Sanfilippo	III A-D	MR (onset 3-4 yrs), mild HSM, mild DM, synophrys	HS†
Morquio (classic)	IV-A	SD, SS, CC, *no MR*	KS
Maroteaux-Lamy	VI	IH, UH, SS, JS, URI, HD, HSM, HLHc, DM, CC, *no MR*	DS
Sly	VII	IH, UH, HSM, SS, JS, URI, MR, HL, HD, Hc, DM, CC‡	DS, HS

*Some subtypes omitted.
†May be missed due to small amount.
‡Large variability of phenotypes observed.
CC, Corneal clouding; DM, dysostosis multiplex; DS, dermatan sulfate; Hc, hydrocephalus; HD, heart disease; HL, hearing loss; HS, heparan sulfate; HSM, hepatosplenomegaly; IH, inguinal hernia; JS, joint stiffness; KS, keratan sulfate; Mg, micrognathism; MR, mental retardation; RD, retinal degeneration; SD, spondyloepiphyseal dysplasia; SP, skin papules; SS, short stature; UH, umbilical hernia; URI, upper respiratory tract infections.

used to determine the most appropriate enzyme assay to establish definitively the specific type of MPS.[78]

The enzymatic diagnosis should be determined on all patients in whom MPS is suspected. Lysosomal enzyme analysis may be carried out using serum, leukocytes, or cultured cells. In all the MPSs, histopathologic examination of skin with alcian blue, colloidal iron, or Giemsa stain reveals metachromatic granules in fibroblasts, and occasionally in keratinocytes and in the secretory and ductal cells of eccrine glands. In addition, the cutaneous papules, mostly seen in Hunter syndrome, exhibit extracellular dermal deposits of metachromatic material.[82]

Differential Diagnosis

The mucolipidoses are the most important group of diseases to be differentiated from the MPSs. I-cell disease (mucolipidosis II) shares most of the clinical features of Hurler syndrome, but patients with I-cell disease do not exhibit urine mucopolysaccharides or acceleration of skeletal growth around 1 year of age.

Treatment, Course, and Management

The natural course of the more severe forms is progressive, and death resulting from respiratory or cardiac complica-

tions often occurs during the second decade. Some types, such as Scheie syndrome, have a normal life expectancy. Bone marrow transplantation lessens the severity and slows the progression of most cases.[79,83]

Management revolves around supportive care. Physical therapy and nighttime splinting may prevent contractures. Special education and frequent audiologic evaluation should be instituted. Many patients benefit from hearing aids. Echocardiograms are recommended to evaluate for valvular abnormalities. Surgical interventions, including corneal transplants for cloudy corneas, cardiac valve replacement, ventriculoperitoneal shunts for communicating hydrocephalus, tracheostomies for obstructive sleep apnea, and occasionally herniorrhaphies, may be helpful. Patients may possess atlantoaxial joint instability, and injury to the head or spine may result in paralysis. Because of this potentially devastating complication, all patients at risk should undergo careful evaluation, and spinal fusion is recommended for those who are severely affected.

Prenatal diagnosis is performed by enzyme assays of cultured amniotic cells, or of cells obtained in chorionic villus sampling.[84] Experimental gene therapy employing animal models is showing promising results for several of the MPSs.[85]

REFERENCES

1. Francis JS, Sybert VP, Benjamin, DR. Congenital monocytic leukemia: Report of a case with cutaneous involvement, and review of the literature. Pediatr Dermatol 1989;6:306-311.

2. Resnik KS, Brod BB: Leukemia cutis in congenital leukemia. Arch Dermatol 1993;129:1301-1306.

3. Gottesfeld E, Silverman A, Coccia PF, et al. Transient blueberry muffin appearance of a newborn with congenital monoblastic leukemia. J Am Acad Dermatol 1989;21:347-351.

4. Yen A, Sanchez R, Oblender M, et al. Leukemia cutis: Darier's sign in a neonate with acute lymphoblastic leukemia. J Am Acad Dermatol 1996;34:375-378.

5. Bhatt S, Schreck R, Graham JM, et al. Transient leukemia with trisomy 21: Description of a case and review of the literature. Am J Genet 1995;58:310-314.

6. Stiakaki E, Giannakopoulou C, Kouvidi E, et al. Congenital systemic Langerhans cell histiocytosis (Report of two cases). Haematologia 1997;28(4):215-222.

7. Esterly NB, Maurer HS, Gonzalez-Crussi F. Histiocytosis X: A seven-year experience at a children's hospital. J Am Acad Dermatol 1985;13:481-496.

8. Enjolras O, Leibowitch M, Bocanini F, et al. Congenital cutaneous Langerhans' cell histiocytosis; a seven cases report. Ann Dermatol Venerol 1992;119:111-117.

9. The French Langerhans' Cell Histiocytosis Study Group. A multicentre retrospective survey of Langerhans' cell histiocytosis: 348 cases observed between 1983 and 1993. Arch Dis Child 1996;75:17-24.

10. Munn S, Chu AC. Langerhans cell histiocytosis of the skin. Hematol Oncol Clin North Am 1998;12:269-286.

11. Hashimoto K, Pritzker MS. Electron microscopic study of reticulohistiocytoma; an unusual case of congenital, self-healing reticulohistiocytosis. Arch Dermatol 1973;107:263-270.

12. Herman LE, Rothman KF, Harawi S, et al. Congenital self-healing reticulohistiocytosis. Arch Dermatol 1990;126:210-212.

13. Hashimoto K, Takahashi S, Lee RG, et al. Congenital self-healing reticulohistiocytosis. J Am Acad Dermatol 1984;11:447-454.

14. Kapila PK, Grant-Kels JM, Allred C, et al. Congenital, spontaneously regressing histiocytosis: Case report and review of the literature Pediatr Dermatol 1985;2(4):312-317.

15. Longaker MA, Frieden IJ, LeBoit PE, et al. Congenital "self-healing" Langerhans cell histiocytosis: the need for long term follow-up. J Am Acad Dermatol 1994;31:910-916.

16. Arico M, Egeler RM. Clinical aspects of Langerhans cell histiocytosis. Hem Oncol Clin North Am 1998;12:247-258.

17. Schmitz L, Favara BE. Nosology and pathology of Langerhans cell histiocytosis. Hem Oncol Clin North Am 1998;12:221-247.

18. Henter, J-I, Arico M, Elinder G, et al. Familail hemophagocytic lymphohistiiocytosis. Hematol Oncol Clin North Am 1998,12:417-433.

19. Soule EH, Pritchard DJ. Fibrosarcoma in infants and children. Cancer 1977;40:1711-1721.

20. Balsaver AM, Butler JJ, Martin RG. Congenital fibrosarcoma. Cancer 1967;20:1607-1616.

21. Chung EB, Enzinger FM. Infantile fibrosarcoma. Cancer 1976;38:729-739.

22. Hayward PG, Orgill DP, Mulliken JB, et al. Congenital fibrosarcoma masquerading as lymphatic malformation: Report of two cases. J Pediatr Surg 1995;30:84-88.

23. Boon LM, Fishman SJ, Lund DP, et al. Congenital fibrosarcoma masquerading as congenital hemangioma: Report of two cases. J Pediatr Surg 1995;30(9):1378-1381.

24. Neifeld JP, Berg JW, Godwin D, et al. A retrospective epidemiologic study of pediatric fibrosarcomas. J Pediatr Surg 1978;13(6D):735-739.

25. Kahn TA, Liranzo MO, Vidimos AT, et al. Pathological case of the month. Arch Pediatr Adolesc Med 1996;150:549-550.

26. Annessi G, Cimitan A, Girolomoni G, et al. Congenital dermatofibrosarcoma protuberans. Pediatr Dermatol 1993;10:40-42.

27. McKee PH, Fletcher CD. Dermatofibrosarcoma protuberans presenting in infancy and childhood. J Cutan Pathol 1991;18:241-246.

28. Hobbs ER, Wheeland RG, Bailin PL, et al. Treatment of dermatofibrosarcoma protuberans with Mohs micrographic surgery. Ann Surg 1988;207:102-107.

29. Hawthorne HC, Nelson JS, Witzleben CL, et al. Blanching subcutaneous nodules in neonatal neuroblastoma. J Pediatr 1970;77:297-300.

30. Lucky AW, McGuire J, Komp DM. Infantile neuroblastoma presenting with cutaneous blanching nodules. J Am Acad Dermatol 1982;6:389-391.

31. Boyd TK, Schofield DE. Monozygotic twins concordant for congenital neuroblastoma: Case report and review of the literature. Pediatr Pathol of Lab Med 1995;15:931-940.

32. Brodeur GM, Pritchard J, Berthold F. Revisions of the international criteria of neuroblastoma diagnosis. J Clin Oncol 1993;11:1466-1477.

33. Yang P, Grufferman S, Khoury MJ, et al. Association of childhood rhabdomyosarcoma with neurofibromatosis type I and birth defects. Gen Epidem 1995;12:467-474.

34. Wiss K, Solomon A, Ralmer S, et al. Rhabdomyosarcoma presenting as a cutaneous nodule. Arch Dermatol 1988;124:1687.

35. Maurer HM, Gehan EA, Hayes DM, et al. The intergroup rhabdomyosarcoma Study-II. Cancer 1993;71:1904-1922.

36. Ceballos PI, Ruiz-Maldonado R, Mihm MC. Melanoma in children. N Engl J Med 1995;332:656-662.

37. Trozak DJ, Rowland WD, Hu F. Metastatic malignant melanoma in prepubertal children. Pediatr Clinician 1973; 191-204.

38. Prose NS, Laude TA, Heilman ER, et al. Congenital malignant melanoma. Pediatrics 1987;79:967-970.

39. Ruiz-Maldonado R, Orozco-Covarrubias L. Malignant melanoma in children. Arch Dermatol 1997;133:363-371.

40. Naraysingh V, Busby GO. Congenital malignant melanoma. J Pediatr Surg 1986;21:81-82.

41. Schneiderman H, Wu AY, Campbell WA. Congenital melanoma with multiple prenatal metastases. Cancer 1987; 60:1371-1377.

42. Cavell B. Transplacental metastasis of malignant melanoma. Acta Pediatr suppl. 1963;146:37-40.

43. Hendrickson MR, Ross JC. Neoplasms arsing in giant congenital nevi. Morphlogic study of seven cases and a review of the literature. Am J Surg Pathol 1981;5:109-135.

44. Silvers DN, Helwig EB. Melanocytic nevi in neonates. J Am Acad Dermatol 1981;4:166-175.

45. Ceballos PI, Ruiz-Maldonado R, Mihm MC. Melanoma in children. N Engl J Med 1995;332:656-662.

46. April MM, Ward RF, Garelick JM. Diagnosis, management, and follow-up of congenital head and neck teratomas. Laryngoscope 1998;108:1398-1401.

47. Kettelhut BV, Metcalfe OD. Pediatric mastocytosis. J Invest Dermatol 1991;96:15s-18s.

48. Stein DH. Mastocytosis: a review. Pediatr Dermatol 1986;3: 365-375.

49. Boyano T, Carrascosa T, Val J, et al. Urticaria pigmentosa in monozygotic twins. Arch Dermatol 1990;126:1375-1376.

50. Caplan RM. The natural course of urticaria pigmentosa. Arch Dermatol 1963;87:146-157.

51. Lucaya J, Perez-Candela V, Celestina A, et al. Mastocytosis with skeletal and gastrointestinal involvement in infancy. Two case reports and a review of the literature. Radiology 1979;131:363-366.

52. Kettelhut BV, Metcalfe DD. Plasma histamine concentration in the evaluation of pediatric mastocytosis. J Pediatr 1987; 111:419-421.

53. Shah PY, Sharma V, Worobec AS, et al. Congenital bullous mastocytosis with myeloproliferative disorder and c-kit mutation. J Am Acad Dermatol 1998;39:119-121.

54. Kettelhut BV, Metcalfe DD. Pediatric mastocytosis. Ann Allergy 1994;73:197-202.

55. Azana MJ, Torrelo A, Mediero IG, et al. Urticaria pigmentosa: A review of 67 pediatric cases. Pediatr Dermatol 1994;11: 102-106.

56. Robinson HM, Kile RL, Hitch JM, et al. Bullous urticaria pigmentosa. Arch Dermatol 1962;85:86-96.

57. Kettelhut BV, Berkebile C, Bradley D, et al. A double-blind placebo controlled, crossover trial of ketotifen versus hydroxyzine in the treatment of pediatric mastocytosis. J Allergy Clin Immunol 1989;83:866-870.

58. Horan RF, Sheffer AL, Austen KF. Cromolyn sodium in the management of systemic mastocytosis. J Allergy Clin Immunol 1990;85:852-855.

59. Turk J, Oates JA, Roberts LJ. Intervention with epinephrine in hypotension associated with mastocytosis. J Allergy Clin Immunol 1983;71:189-192.

60. Smith ML, Orton PW, Chu H, et al. Photochemotherapy of dominant, diffuse, cutaneous mastocytosis. Pediatr Dermatol 1990;7:251-255.

61. Kan AE, Rogers M. Juvenile Hyalin fibromatosis: An expanded clinicopathologic spectrum. Pediatr Dermatol 1989;6:68-75.

62. Fayad MN, Yacoub A, Salman S, et al. Juvenile hyaline fibromatosis: Two new patients and review of the literature. Am J Med Genet 1987;26:123-131.

63. Breir F, Fang-Kircher S, Wolff K, et al. Juvenile hyaline fibromatosis: Impaired collagen metabolism in human skin fibroblasts. Arch Dis Child 1997;77:436-440.

64. Katagiri K, Takasaki S, Fujiwara S, et al. Purification and structural analysis of extracellular matrix of a skin tumor from a patient with juvenile hyaline fibromatosis. J Dermatol Sci 1996;13:37-48.

65. Winchester P, Grossman H, Lim WN, et al. A new acid mucopolysaccharidosis with skeletal deformities simulating rheumatoid arthritis. AJR 1969;106:121-128.

66. Farber S. A lipid metabolic disorder-disseminated "lipogranulomatosis" a syndrome with similarity to, and important difference from, Niemann-Pick and Hand-Schuller-Christian disease. Am J Dis Child 1952;84:499-500.

67. Abenoza P, Sibley RK. Farber's disease: A fine structural study. Ultrastruct Pathol 1987;11:397-403.

68. Jameson RA, Holt PJ, Keen JH. Farber's disease (lysosomal acid ceramidase deficiency). Ann Rheum Dis 1987;46:559-561.

69. Haraoka G, Muraoka M, Yoshioka N, et al. First case of surgical treatment of Farber's disease. Ann Plast Surg 1997;39: 405-410.

70. Fensome AH, Benson PF, Neville BR, et al. Prenatal diagnosis of Farber's disease. Lancet 1979;2:990-992.

71. Leroy JG, Martin JJ. Mucolipidosis II (I-cell disease): Present status of knowledge. Birth Defects Orig Artic Ser 1975;11: 283-293.

72. Terashima Y, Tsuda K, Isomura S, et al. I-cell disease: Report of three cases. Am J Dis Child 1975;129:1083-1090.

73. McDowell G, Gahl WA. Inherited disorders of glycoprotein synthesis: Cell biological insights. Proc Soc Exp Biol Med 1997;215:145-157.

74. Leroy JG, Demars RI. Mutant enzymatic and cytological phenotypes in cultured human fibroblasts. Science 1967;157: 804-806.

75. von Figura K, Haslik A, Pohlmann R, et al. Mutations affecting transport and stability of lysosomal enzymes. Enzyme 1987;38(1-4):144-153.

76. Mueller OT, Wasmuth JJ, Murray JC, et al. Chromosomal assignment of N-acetylglucosaminylphosphotransferase, the lysosomal hydrolase targeting enzyme deficient in mucolipidosis II and III. Cytogenet Cell Genet 1987;69.

77. Aula P, Rapola J, Autio S, et al. Prenatal diagnosis and fetal pathology of I-cell disease (mucolipidosis type II). J Pediatr 1975;87:221-226.

78. Muenzer J. Mucopolysaccharidoses. Adv Pediatr 1986;33: 269-302.

79. Matsuyama T, Sly WS, Kondo N, et al. Treatment of MPS VII (Sly syndrome) by allogeneic BMT in a female with homozygous A619V mutation. Bone Marrow Transplant 1998; 21:629-634.

80. Hirschhorn K, Willner J. Disorders of metabolism. In Spitz JL, ed. Genodermatoses a full-color clinical guide to genetic skin disorders. Baltimore: Williams & Wilkins, 1996.

81. Schiro JA, Mallory SB, Demmer L, et al. Grouped papules in Hurler-Scheie syndrome. J Am Acad Dermatol 1996;35:868-870.

82. Maize J, Metcalf J. Metabolic diseases of the skin. In Elder D, Elenitsas R, Jaworsky C, et al, eds. Lever's Histopathology of the skin, 8th edition. Philadelphia: Lippincott-Raven, 1997: p 393.

83. Vellodi A, Young EP, Cooper A, et al. Bone marrow transplantation for mucopolysaccharidosis type I: Experience of two British centres. Arch Dis Child 1997;76:92-99.

84. Fensom AH, Benson PF. Recent advances in the prenatal diagnosis of the mucopolysaccharidoses. Prenat Diagn 1994; 14:1-12.

85. Huang MM, Wong A, Yu X, et al. Retrovirus-mediated transfer of human alpha-L-iduronidase cDNA into human hematopoietic progenitor cells leads to correction in trans of Hurler fibroblasts. Gene Ther 1997;4:1150-1159.

24

Selected Hereditary Diseases

VIRGINIA P. SYBERT

The understanding of disease inheritance is rapidly evolving. This chapter discusses selected hereditary diseases with significant cutaneous manifestations, including neurocutaneous syndromes, disorders of laxity and redundant skin, mosaic disorders, photosensitivity disorders, and some metabolic diseases. A multitude of other inherited disorders are discussed in other chapters of the book. Several textbook and websites discuss genetic diseases in a comprehensive fashion. The reader is referred Sybert VP *Genetic Skin Disorders.* New York. Oxford University Press, 1997, for a more expanded discussion of genetic disease with cutaneous findings and to OMIM, On-line Mendelian Inheritance in Man (http://www3.ncbi.nlm.nih.gov/omim/).

NEUROCUTANEOUS SYNDROMES

Many disorders share neurologic and dermatologic findings. Disorders for which the major diagnostic features occur in the skin and in which the neurologic abnormalities figure significantly are referred to as neurocutaneous syndromes. A variety of conditions are included in this category. Each textbook and review offers different listings of included disorders. The most universally accepted conditions under this heading are neurofibromatosis, tuberous sclerosis, and Sturge-Weber syndrome (see Chapter 18). This text includes familial dysautonomia (Riley-Day syndrome), although it is not traditionally characterized as such.

Neurofibromatosis 1

Neurofibromatosis 1 (NF1) is the most common of the neurocutaneous disorders, occurring in 1/3000 to 1/4000

newborns. Of these infants, half are born to an affected parent. The other half are the first in the family to be affected (sporadic), the disorder resulting from a new dominant mutation in the NF1 gene that occurred either in the maternal or paternal gamete. NF1 occurs with equal frequency among racial groups. There is no difference in severity of expression between males and females.

This autosomal dominant disorder enjoys a multiplicity of complications, all of which occur in tissues that derive from the cells of the embryonic neural crest. It is marked by clinical variability, both within and between families.

Some of the features of NF1 are congenital. Others develop during infancy and childhood or occur throughout adult life.

Consensus criteria for the diagnosis of NF1 were developed at an NIH conference (Box 24-1).[1] The purpose of the criteria was to allow for uniform designation of individuals as affected or unaffected, primarily to aid in the search for the NF gene by linkage studies. These criteria have limited diagnostic utility in young children. Except for café au lait spots, most features are not present early. In one follow-up study of 41 children, between 1 month and 14 years of age, who presented initially with 6 or more café au lait spots greater than 5 mm in diameter without other signs of NF1, 24 developed other features of the condition over the course of the next 2 to 10 years. An additional six were diagnosed as having segmental NF1.[2] Fois et al[3] reevaluated 21 children who had only café au lait spots at the time of first assessment. Nine subsequently developed other features of NF1. These studies likely underestimate the number of children with multiple café au lait spots who will subsequently show other signs of NF1, because the follow-up times are not

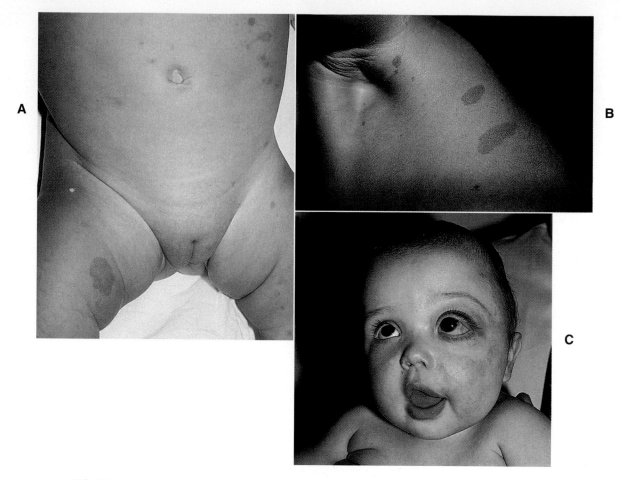

FIG. 24-1
A, Multiple café au lait spots in a child with neurofibromatosis. **B,** Axillary freckling and multiple café au lait spots. **C,** Plexiform neurofibroma of the left orbit.

BOX 24-1

NIH Consensus Criteria for NF1

Diagnosis Requires Two Criteria
- ≥6 café au lait macules, ≥5mm diameter in children, ≥15mm in adults
- ≥2 neurofibromas of any type or 1 plexiform neurofibroma
- Axillary/inguinal freckling
- Optic glioma
- ≥2 Lisch nodules
- Distinctive osseous changes (e.g., sphenoid wing dysplasia or pseudoarthrosis)
- First-degree relative with NF1

---

very long and many subjects have not yet gone through puberty.

Café au lait spots[4] are flat, light to dark brown macules and patches with sharply defined, although not necessarily smooth, borders (Fig. 24-1, *A*). They are the major sign of NF1 evident in children under 5 years of age.[5,6] They may be present at birth. Café au lait spots appear on any skin surface except the palms, soles, and scalp.[7] Although Riccardi[7] states emphatically that "by the first birthday café au lait spots will be obvious if they are to appear at all . . ." in fact they may not be evident in sufficient numbers to reach the diagnostic criterion until several years of life.[8] The spots continue to appear throughout childhood and darken with tanning. In very fair-skinned individuals, use of the Wood's lamp may be helpful to identify all café au lait spots.

All infants or children with six or more café au lait spots greater than 5 mm in diameter and no other signs of NF1 should be followed through puberty as if they have NF1, at which time the question of diagnosis can be re-opened. It is not uncommon for children of African or Hispanic ancestry to have several café au lait spots, and these are not cause for concern. However, in all racial groups, six or more café au lait spots of sufficient size are equally suggestive of NF1.

There are no histologic or ultrastructural characteristics of the café au lait spots in NF1 that distinguish them from café au lait spots resulting from other causes. Any café au lait spot may contain giant pigment granules (macromelanosomes) demonstrable by electron microscopic examination.

The terms *axillary* and *inguinal freckling* (Fig. 24-1, *B*) refer to the presence of small, usually a few millimeters in diameter, hyperpigmented macules that appear in the groin, armpits, and inframammary region in individuals with NF1. These usually do not appear until late toddler/childhood years or beyond. Similar freckling on the neck and on the trunk is also common in individuals with NF1, but because these areas are sun-exposed, their occurrence in these locations is a less reliable diagnostic feature. The "freckles" of NF are qualitatively different from solar ephelides, with more distinct borders and less of a reddish tint (personal observation). Wood's lamp examination may also be necessary to detect axillary and inguinal freckling.

Peripheral neurofibromas are uncommon in childhood NF1 (Fig. 24-1, *C*). North[9] found neurofibromas in only 14% of children less than 10 years of age, in 44% of adolescents 10 to 15 years of age, and in 85% of adults by age 30. No child under 10 years of age had more than five neurofibromas. Leppig and colleagues[10] have suggested that a subset of children with large deletions of the NF1 gene typically present early in childhood with multiple neurofibromas.

Plexiform neurofibromas of the face, neck, or mediastinum are an uncommon feature of NF1 (occurring in approximately 1% or less of patients). These neurofibromas present at birth or soon thereafter.[8] Often initially appreciated only as mild asymmetric fullness of the face, these lesions can grow rapidly. There may be an orange-hued, coarsely textured quality to the skin overlying some plexiform neurofibromas. Increased hair growth over these areas has also been described. If a plexiform neurofibroma is suspected, neuroradiologic imaging is warranted. These growths present difficult management problems, since they interdigitate with and surround normal structures. Plexiform neurofibromas can occur at other sites throughout life. These are also relatively uncommon.

Optic gliomas are astrocytomas that develop anywhere along the optic pathway. Present in about 15% of individuals with NF1, they are symptomatic in less than 5%. These tumors can grow and result in visual loss and may lead to blindness. This is a complication of early childhood. Optic gliomas do not appear to proliferate significantly after the age of 5 or 6 years. The best method for initial examination for, and monitoring of, optic gliomas is debated. Routine MRI imaging is encouraged by Riccardi[7] to be performed within the first year of life and repeated at least once thereafter. Others prefer regular ophthalmologic evaluation at initial presentation and yearly thereafter during the first decade. This evaluation is to include visual fields and/or visual evoked responses.[11] Treatment for symptomatic optic gliomas is problematic, and there is no one preferred approach.

Lisch nodules are pigmented iris hamartomas that are a major diagnostic feature of NF1, but are rarely present in infants. They are similar to café au lait spots in that while they have diagnostic utility, they result in no functional disability. They are bilateral and multiple. They are best seen on slit lamp examination and can be confused with iris nevi by the nonexpert. The proportion of individuals with NF1 with Lisch nodules increases from 20% in the first 5 years of life to 95% of adults.

Congenital glaucoma is an unusual (less than 0.05%), but recognized complication of NF1. It may be presaged by the presence of a neurofibroma of the overlying eyelid.

Congenital pseudoarthrosis is a major diagnostic criterion of NF1, occurring in 3% or fewer of newborns and infants with the condition. It is usually unilateral, isolated, and most commonly involves the tibia, although other tubular bones can be affected. At birth, minor bowing of the foreleg may be the only sign. This can progress, ultimately resulting in severe deformity and fracture. Other structural alterations of the skeleton include vertebral scalloping, sphenoid wing dysplasia, and lytic lesions. These alterations are usually asymptomatic. Scoliosis is a feature common in later childhood, rare before the age of 6 years. Macrocephaly (relative and absolute) appears to be frequent in NF1, but is not a diagnostic feature. Although learning disabilities are a common finding in NF1, frank mental retardation is less so. Estimates of mental retardation in NF1 range from 3% to 30%, the lower figures representing population-based prevalence with presumably lower bias of ascertainment. Mental handicaps usually are not evident in the newborn. More subtle learning disabilities may not be appreciated until the school years.

NF1 results from mutations in a gene that resides on the long arm of chromosome 17 (17q22.2). Its product, neurofibromin, appears to function as a negative feedback control for cell proliferation.[11] Commercially available molecular testing has a sensitivity of approximately 70%. The diagnosis of NF1 remains primarily clinical.

Neurofibromatosis 1 should be suspected in any infant with the following signs:

- Multiple café au lait spots
- Pseudoarthrosis
- Congenital glaucoma
- A plexiform neurofibroma

In the absence of a positive family history, it is unusual to make the diagnosis of NF1 in infants less than 6 months of age.

There are many other conditions in which café au lait spots may be found (see chapter 20). None is easily confused with neurofibromatosis with the exception of autosomal dominant multiple café au lait spots. This condition is very rare. The gene for it has not yet been identified. It is the diagnosis of choice in any adult with café au lait spots only and no other features of neurofibromatosis.

Occasionally infants and children present with a single or multiple giant café au lait spot(s). Giant café au lait spots may be an isolated finding of no diagnostic importance or can be a feature of McCune-Albright syndrome (polyostotic fibrous dysplasia), chromosomal mosaicism, and neurofibromatosis 1, or segmental NF. It may not be possible in early infancy to distinguish these entities clinically. If other malformations are present or developmental delay is suspected, chromosome testing may be warranted to rule out chromosome mosaicism. In general, a wait and watch approach is best.

Tuberous Sclerosis

There are two autosomal dominant genetic disorders encompassed by the term *tuberous sclerosis complex* (TSC). Tuberous sclerosis complex 1 (TSC1) is due to mutations in the gene (TSC1) that produces the protein hamartin, on chromosome 9, located at 9q34.3.[12] Tuberous sclerosis complex 2 (TSC2) is caused by mutations in the TSC2 gene, coding for the protein tuberin on chromosome 16 at 16p13.3.[13] For the most part, the two disorders are clinically indistinguishable.

Consensus-based diagnostic criteria for these autosomal dominant disorders have been attempted[14,15] but are not universally accepted (Boxes 24-2, *A* and 24-2, *B*). They are not as easily utilized as the diagnostic criteria for NF1.

Tuberous sclerosis is much less common than neurofibromatosis, with an incidence rate of 1/6000 to 1/10,000. The cutaneous features of tuberous sclerosis are often not the first feature to be recognized.

BOX 24-2, A

Tuberous Sclerosis Complex Criteria (From Roach et al)

Major Features
Facial angiofibromas or forehead plaque
Nontraumatic ungual or periungual fibroma
Hypomelanotic macules (more than three)
Shagreen patch (connective tissue nevus)
Multiple retinal nodular hamartomas
Cortical tuber
Subependymal nodule
Subependymal giant cell astrocytoma
Cardiac rhabdomyoma, single or multiple
Lymphangiomyomatosis
Renal angiomyolipoma

Minor Features
Multiple randomly distributed pits in dental enamel
Hamartomatous rectal polyps
Bone cysts
Cerebral white matter radial migration lines
Gingival fibromas
Nonrenal hamartoma
Retinal achromic patch
"Confetti" skin lesions
Multiple renal cysts

Definite TSC: either 2 major features or 1 major feature plus 2 minor features
Probable TSC: 1 major plus 1 minor feature
Possible TSC: either 1 major feature or 2 or more minor features

---

The infant with tuberous sclerosis complex may present with seizures, most often infantile spasms or generalized tonic clonic seizures. Epilepsy occurs in upwards of 60% to 80%[16,17] of patients with TSC. Of infants with infantile spasms, it is estimated that 4% to 50% have tuberous sclerosis.[18,19] Presumably this wide range reflects bias of ascertainment. Mental retardation is a major deleterious consequence of TSC, occurring in 38% to 50% have patients.[17,20] The risk for mental retardation is greater in those individuals who have had early onset of seizures (less than 2 years of age) and greatest in those with early onset of infantile spasms. Mental retardation in children with TSC without epilepsy is rare. A recent study has suggested that mental retardation is more common in TSC2 than in TSC1, but this observation remains to be validated.[21]

BOX 24-2, B

Tuberous Sclerosis Complex Criteria (From Ruiz Maldonado et al)

Major Features

Hypomelanotic macules
Facial angiofibromas
Periungal fibromas
Shagreen patches
Retinal hamartomas
Cortical tuber
Subependymal glial nodule
Renal cysts or angiomyolipomas
First-degree relative with TSC

Minor Features

Infantile spasms
Seizures
Intracranial calcification
Mental retardation
Gingival fibromas
Dental enamel pits
Multicystic kidneys
Cardiac rhabdomyoma
Radiologic lung changes
Patch of depigmented hair

Definitive diagnosis requires 1 major and 1 minor feature
A probable diagnosis can be made with 1 major diagnostic feature*

*Author's note: This is obviously untrue. A positive family history alone would be inadequate for probable diagnosis.

Other findings in the newborn and infant suggestive of the diagnosis of tuberous sclerosis are cardiac rhabdomyomas and renal cysts. Cardiac rhabdomyomas have been detected by fetal sonography of fetuses with TSC. Rhabdomyomas are hamartomas that can occur anywhere in the heart. In TSC they are often multiple and are found in 30% to 50% of affected infants. Conversely, it is estimated that 80% to 90% of infants with cardiac rhabdomyomas have TSC.[22,23] These growths can interfere with cardiac output when they obstruct outflow, can cause arrhythmia, or can be asymptomatic. The growths often regress after birth. They do not require surgical intervention if asymptomatic.[23]

Renal cysts and angiomyolipomas are found in two thirds of patients with tuberous sclerosis complex,[24] their frequency increasing with age. One quarter of infants and children less than 5 years of age with TSC, adequately studied, have been found to have renal cysts; 8% were found to have renal angiomyolipomas. Similar to cardiac rhabdomyomas, renal cysts have been detected in utero in TSC. A number of infants with TSC2 and severe polycystic kidney disease have been found to have deletions of both the TSC2 and the neighboring PKD1 genes[25]; however, renal involvement in TSC is not limited to this contiguous gene syndrome.

The cutaneous features of tuberous sclerosis include hypomelanotic lesions (Figs. 24-2, *A* and *B*), angiofibromas, collagenomas (shagreen patches) (Figs. 24-2, *C*), periungual fibromas, forehead fibrous plaques, gingival fibromas, and soft cutaneous fibromas (molluscum fibrosum pendulum). In infancy, only the hypomelanotic lesions are likely to be found. Shagreen patches can be present at birth or early on, but tend to erupt in mid to late childhood, as do the angiofibromas, fibrous forehead plaques, and gingival fibromas. Periungual fibromas rarely appear before puberty.

The classic hypomelanotic lesion of TSC is the ash leaf macule or patch, an oval area with decrease in, but not absence of, pigment (see Fig. 24-2, *A*). These can also be more irregular in outline and shape. They may be very small and guttate, or confetti-like (see Fig. 24-2, *B*). They are found in almost 90% of patients with TSC. Although they may be present at birth, often only evident on Wood's lamp examination, the lesions are usually not noticed until several months to year(s) of life as normal pigment develops and the contrast between the color of the macules and the normal skin becomes greater. Some authors maintain that all ash leaf spots are congenital, but spots have been documented to develop over several months to years in patients who have been thoroughly and completely examined with a Wood's lamp[26] (personal observation). They may disappear in adult life. They can also occur on the scalp with lightening of the hair in the patch.

A single, hypopigmented macule in an infant is not cause for concern.[27] Multiple lesions should raise the question of TSC. It is more common that the neurologic, cardiac, or renal features of TSC will raise the question of the diagnosis in the newborn, at which time a complete skin examination will be performed. A complete skin examination under both ambient and Wood's lamp illumination should be performed in every infant with infantile spasms, cardiac rhabdomyomas, or renal cysts. Although there are specific electron microscopic features of the hypopigmented lesions of TSC (decrease in number, size, melanization, and transfer of melanosomes, along with stubby melanocytic dendrites), skin biopsy is not necessary for confirmation of the diagnosis. In the infant with a hypopigmented patch distributed along the

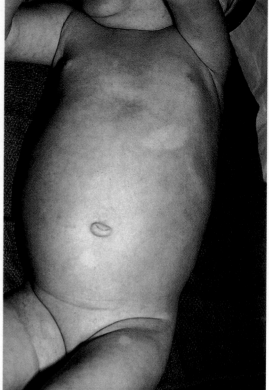

FIG. 24-2
A, Typical hypopigmented ash leaf spots of tuberous sclerosis. **B**, Confetti hypopigmentation in tuberous sclerosis. **C**, Shagreen patch in TSC. (**B** and **C**, From Sybert VP. Genetic skin disorders. New York: Oxford University Press, 1997.)

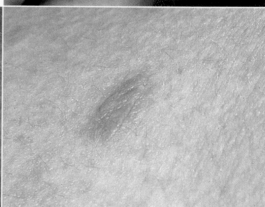

lines of Blaschko and no other features of TSC, the diagnosis of nevus depigmentosus rather than TSC may be more likely. Jimbow[28] states that histologic differences can distinguish between the two. This author is less certain that in hands other than Jimbow's, such diagnostic accuracy is possible.

Angiofibromas generally do not appear until 4 years of age or older. They are not pathognomonic for TSC. They have been described in MEN1[29] and as an isolated autosomal dominant disorder.

Even more than one periungual fibroma, long thought to be pathognomonic for TSC, can occur in an otherwise healthy adult. Isolated shagreen patches or connective tissue nevi are also lesions that can occur outside the setting of TSC. In the absence of a positive family history or other obvious cutaneous signs of TSC, a complete work-up for TSC (MRI/CT, renal ultrasound, cardiac ultrasound, dilated eye examination) may not always be indicated. The clinician can exercise judgment, considering the age of the patient, familial concern, and reproductive implications. Currently, molecular testing for TSC1 and TSC2 is not readily available commercially.

Although the genes for both TSC1 and TSC2 have been identified and their gene products are now known, their function has yet to be fully determined.

Riley-Day Syndrome

Riley-Day syndrome (familial dysautonomia, hereditary sensory, and autonomic neuropathy III) is an autosomal recessive condition seen almost exclusively in Ashkenazi Jews.[30] Although affected individuals are usually not diagnosed until several years of age, generalized signs appear within the newborn period in over 80% of patients.[31] These features include breech birth in one quarter, intrauterine growth retardation, hypotonia, respiratory insufficiency, and poor feeding with swallowing difficulty and aspiration. Unexplained episodes of fever and failure to thrive, aspiration pneumonia, and repeated episodes of vomiting are typical. The diagnostic significance of absence of tearing, a cardinal feature of Riley-Day syndrome, is usually not appreciated in young infants, since overflow tearing does not develop until 2 to 3 months of age in normal infants. Affected babies often have blotching and mottling of the skin. This usually appears after a month of age and within the first year or so, as do bouts of hyperexia. Emotional excitement often precipitates the appearance of the red blotches. Deep tendon reflexes are in variably absent.

In older children, excessive drooling and sweating, often in response to inappropriate stimuli, occur, as do orthostatic hypotension and labile hypertension. In familial dysautonomia, the indifference or insensitivity to pain results in progressive self-mutilation, biting of the tongue, loss of teeth, burns, and ulcers. Mechanically induced ulceration of the tongue in teething infants has been reported. There is absence of fungiform papillae on the tongue and a decrease in the ability to taste. Other complications tend to occur in later childhood and adult life. Survival is decreased, and almost one fifth of affected infants die in infancy or childhood.

Faced with an infant with unexplainable hyperpyrexia, sweating abnormalities, and failure to thrive, the primary differential diagnosis is hypohidrotic ectodermal dysplasia versus Riley-Day syndrome. Injection of histamine (1:10,000) does not elicit a flare response in Riley-Day syndrome. The flare response can be used to discriminate between the two conditions, as can the presence of teeth on a panorex examination of the jaw.

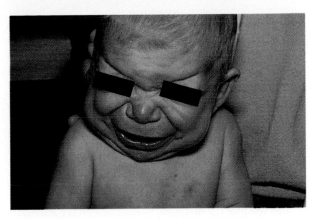

FIG. 24-3
Infant with cutis laxa. Droopy appearing face.

The gene for Riley-Day syndrome has been mapped to 9q31, but has not been identified. Prenatal diagnosis using linked markers has been successfully performed.[32] The basic defect in Riley-Day syndrome is also unknown. There appears to be a decrease in survival of sensory, sympathetic, and some parasympathetic nerves.

The astute physician, aware of the feature of random blotching and mottling of the skin, may be able to make the diagnosis of Riley-Day syndrome in an infant whose multiplicity of problems have failed to lead to the correct diagnosis.

DISORDERS WITH SKIN LAXITY AND REDUNDANT SKIN

Soft, hyperelastic skin, lax skin, or redundant skin, with or without bruising, fragility, or abnormal healing, is seen in a variety of related and distinct inherited disorders. Most are clinically evident in the infant and young child, although a correct diagnosis is often not recognized until later childhood.

Cutis Laxa

Cutis laxa is a term applied to a group of three genetic conditions in which the skin is loose and nonelastic, drooping rather than stretching. Autosomal dominant, autosomal recessive, and X-linked forms have been identified. All three conditions can present in the newborn period with skin changes and abdominal and inguinal hernias (Fig. 24-3). The autosomal dominant form of cutis

laxa tends to be the mildest with the fewest internal manifestations and with skin laxity more likely to develop in
later childhood or even adult life.[33] In the autosomal recessive form, flaccid skin is often evident at birth. Di-
aphragmatic hernias have also been reported. Early onset
emphysema is typical of autosomal recessive cutis laxa.

The X-linked form of cutis laxa is also called occipital
horn disease and Ehlers-Danlos IX. It is caused by mutations in the MNK gene, which result in a defect in copper
transport and a secondary deficiency of copper dependent
enzymes.[34] Allelic mutations (different mutated versions
of the same gene) cause Menkes syndrome. In addition to
shared features of cutis laxa, X-linked cutis laxa is marked
by bladder and gastrointestinal diverticuli. Mild intellectual handicap is common. The development of occipital
horns, bony excrescences on the occiput, occurs over time.
Among the other skeletal changes seen, the one most
likely to be found in the newborn and young infant is
congenital dislocation of the hip.

There are histopathologic distinctions between the
X-linked and autosomal forms of cutis laxa. In the former, there are abnormally large collagen fibrils with normal elastic fibers. In the latter, the elastin is decreased.
The dense amorphous component is abnormal. There are
occasional collagen "flowers" and variation in collagen
fibril diameter. There is no way to reliably distinguish
histologically between the autosomal dominant and autosomal recessive forms of cutis laxa. The basic defect in
autosomal recessive cutis laxa is not known. Heterozygous mutations in the elastin gene (ELN) have been
identified in some individuals with autosomal dominant
cutis laxa.[35] Other mutations in this gene also cause
Williams syndrome and familial supravalvular aortic
stenonsis.

Treatment for cutis laxa is limited. Plastic surgery to repair drooping skin can give only temporary relief. Surgical
intervention may be required for other complications.

Other conditions that can present with lax skin in the
newborn period include Costello syndrome, SCARF syndrome, de Barsy syndrome, and the neonatal Marfan syndrome. Prenatal exposure to maternal ingestion of penicillamine can cause cutis laxa in the newborn.[36]

Ehlers-Danlos Syndromes

The severity of skin involvement in the disorders that
share the eponym Ehlers-Danlos syndrome (EDS) varies,
as do the associated features. Type III EDS is characterized
by marked joint hypermobility and few or no cutaneous
abnormalities. Types VIIA and VIIB EDS have minimal
skin involvement. These are not discussed here. Type IX

EDS is better designated as occipital horn disease or
X-linked cutis laxa (vide supra).

Babies with EDS types I and II have very soft, velvety,
extensible skin that feels almost like pudding. It bruises
impressively. The skin is fragile, splitting with minimal
trauma. Wounds are slow to heal, quick to dehisce, and
often resolve with cigarette paper atrophic scars. The forehead is a favorite site for scarring during the toddler years
as a result of frequent falls. Pregnancies of infants with
EDS I or II can have premature rupture of membranes, and
preterm delivery is common. Joint hypermobility is
marked. Developmental milestones may be delayed because of joint instability. The difference between EDS I and
EDS II is in degree, and it may not be readily obvious in
the neonatal or infancy period how severely affected the
child will be. With age, molluscoid pseudotumors develop
in areas of repeated trauma; spheroids, firm subcutaneous
nodules, develop over bony prominences, and hemosiderin deposition from repeated bruising is typical. These
are changes of later childhood and adult life.

The diagnosis is often not made in sporadic cases of
these autosomal dominant conditions until after repeated
visits to the physician for wounds and referral for concerns
regarding child abuse. Delaying removal of sutures, liberal
use of Steri-Strips, and protection may help decrease the
scarring. There is no information regarding the efficacy of
cyanoacrylates in wound management. However, their
limited effectiveness in wounds subjected to stretch (e.g.,
over knees and elbows) suggests they might not be useful
in EDS. Conservative orthopedic management may help
decrease the development of osteoarthritis in later life.

Light microscopic features are not diagnostic. Large irregular collagen fibrils are the typical ultrastructural features of EDS I and EDS II. One cannot distinguish between
types I and II histologically.

Linkage to COL5A1, the alpha 1 chain of type V collagen,[37] and mutations in COL5A2, the alpha 2 chain of
type V collagen,[38] have been demonstrated in EDS I and
EDS II. There are likely to be other causal genes as well.

Ehlers-Danlos IV, also known as the arterial or Sack-
Barabas type, is also autosomal dominant and is due to
mutations in type III collagen. In EDS IV, rather than being extensible and doughy, the skin is thin and translucent
with a visible prominent vascular pattern (Fig. 24-4).
Bruising is common, but the skin is not fragile and healing
is usually normal. None of these features is likely to be appreciated in a newborn or young infant unless the disorder is already known to be in the family. There is a typical
facial appearance in EDS IV, with thin nose, thin lips, and
prominent eyes. In adulthood, elastosis perforans serpiginosa may develop, as does hemosiderin deposition re-

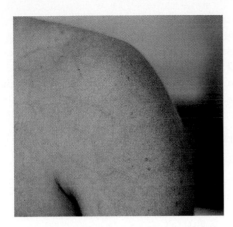

FIG. 24-4
Prominent visible venous pattern in EDS IV. (From Sybert VP: Genetic skin disorders. New York: Oxford University Press, 1997.)

sulting from bruising. The internal complications of EDS IV are dire and common. Rupture of viscera and major vessels is almost invariable. Rupture of the uterus in pregnant women with EDS IV is not uncommon. The mean age of death (albeit probably lowered by bias of ascertainment of more severe cases) in EDS IV is between 35 and 40 years of age.[39] Histology at the light level shows thinning of the dermis. On electron microscopy, collagen fiber diameter can vary, and some patients show storage of type III collagen in fibroblasts.

EDS VI[40] is extremely rare, has dermatologic features similar to, but milder than EDS I and EDS IV, and associated problems of hypotonia, joint laxity, and severe scoliosis, which may even be present at birth. EDS VI is also referred to as the ocular form, since the globe is fragile. Glaucoma, retinal detachment, and ocular rupture have occurred. Arterial rupture has also been reported. This condition appears to be autosomal recessive and heterogeneous. Individuals with EDS VIA have lysyl hydroxylase deficiency; those with VIB do not. Again, both small and large collagen fibrils are seen with electron microscopic evaluation of the dermis.

Dermatosparaxis, a recently described addition to the Ehlers-Danlos family, is also called EDS VIIC.[41] Infants with dermatosparaxis have soft, doughy skin that ruptures readily with minimal trauma. Inguinal tears have occurred at birth, and the face appears puffy and the skin sagging. Healing appears to be normal as is the appearance of the scars, in contrast to EDS I. Premature rupture of membranes, ligamentous laxity, blue sclerae, umbilical hernia, and micrognathia are features common to the handful of infants reported with this autosomal recessive disorder. It

appears to be caused by alterations in the activity of type I pro collagen-N-proteinase. The collagen bundles of the dermis appear ribbonlike and look like hieroglyphics on cross-section with electron microscopy.

The periodontal form of EDS, EDS VIII,[42] is also very rare. The skin findings are similar to EDS II. In addition, excessive wrinkling of the palms and soles and marked atrophy and hyperpigmentation of the skin develop over time. Joint laxity is usually mild. Periodontitis is a feature that typically develops in the early teens, but may be seen in younger children. In the one patient with this condition that this author has seen, she was struck by the nature of his skin and joint findings. These were clearly not normal, and yet not severe enough to be compatible with a diagnosis of EDS I or II. When this child subsequently developed gum disease, the diagnosis of EDS VIII became obvious. This condition is also autosomal dominant, and the basic defect is unknown.

Marfan Syndrome

Marfan syndrome is an autosomal dominant disorder rarely diagnosed in the newborn. Its cardinal features are arachnodactyly, tall, disproportionate stature with relatively long extremities, progressive aortic root dilatation that leads to aortic dissection, and dislocated lenses. Cutaneous features are usually minor. Progressive striae are seen in almost two thirds of patients. There may be mild thinning of the skin and mild distensibility. Despite its mention as a feature of Marfan syndrome in many reviews, elastosis perforans serpiginosa has been documented in only one patient.[43]

The infantile form of Marfan syndrome is quite rare and distinctive.[44] In addition to the typical skeletal disproportion and arachnodactyly, the majority of newborns with infantile Marfan syndrome have congenital contractures or arthrogryposis. About a third have hyperextensible joints. Congenital scoliosis has been described in approximately a fifth of infants with this condition. Two fifths of these babies have had congenital dislocation of the lenses, and four fifths have had aortic root dilatation evident before 3 months of life. Progressive cardiac disease is the rule. The babies' faces are characterized by a "worried look" with megalocornea (in over one third), frontal bossing, and deep-set eyes. There are usually no distinctive skin findings in this age group.

Other diagnostic considerations in the newborn include Beals contractural arachnodactyly.

Mutations in the fibrillin gene, FBN1, on chromosome 15 have been found in classic and neonatal Marfan syndrome. Most mutations are private; that is, most families have distinct mutations, and there is no evidence for a hot spot or site of frequent mutation.[45] Alterations at the beginning of the longest calcium binding EGF-like motif of the fibrillin gene were found in three infants with neonatal Marfan syndrome, suggesting that mutations in this region may give rise to a more severe phenotype.[46]

There is no information regarding the response of the striae distensae, caused by Marfan syndrome, to standard therapies.

Costello Syndrome

Costello syndrome is an extremely rare disorder. Newborns with Costello syndrome are often large for gestational age. Pregnancies have been complicated by polyhydramnios. At birth, these babies have loose, redundant skin at the neck, the backs of the hands, and the tops of the feet. The palms and soles are thickened with deep creases without hyperkeratosis. Poor feeding is typical. These babies go from being large for gestational age to having failure to thrive. The degree of ensuing growth retardation exceeds that as a result of poor nutrition alone.

Over time, acanthosis nigricans develops at the neck and in the folds. Dark, olive complexion has been noted in the majority of patients. Nasal and perioral papillomas develop in childhood and may occur elsewhere on the body. Acrochordons have been noted in some patients. The hair is usually sparse and curly and the nails may be brittle with koilonychia.[47,48]

Mental retardation, varying in severity, is a universal feature. In general, joints are hyperextensible, although tightening of the Achilles tendon has been reported. Congenital clubfeet are common. Facial features are described as coarse with full lips, depressed nasal bridge, and low-set ears with thick lobes. The neck is short, and the voice is hoarse. These features usually develop after a year or two of life. Cardiac involvement is common. Arrhythmias, hypertrophic cardiomyopathy, and structural cardiac malformations have been described in half of the reported patients.[49]

Histopathologic features are inconstant and described only for a few patients. The basic defect is unknown. Inheritance is possibly autosomal recessive with occurrence reported in two sibling pairs. Most cases have been sporadic, suggesting that mutation for an autosomal dominant disorder might be a cause.

Lipoid proteinosis shares coarse features, hoarse voice, and facial papules with Costello syndrome, but lacks redundant skin, abnormal hair, and facies. Patients with the cutis laxa syndromes do not have the palmar and plantar findings, or the facial papules of Costello syndrome. Lep-

rechaunism is marked by similar laxity of skin and acanthosis nigricans, but lacks the facial features and papillomas. There is some overlap with the noncutaneous features of Noonan syndrome and cardiofaciocutaneous syndrome. These conditions do not have the skin findings of Costello syndrome.[50]

de Barsy Syndrome

Infants with de Barsy syndrome[51] have very lax, wrinkled skin. They have a "progeroid" facial appearance with thin hair, thin skin, pinched midface, and lack of subcutaneous tissue. These features are present at birth and nonprogressive. The underlying vascular pattern of the skin is readily apparent, probably resulting from the thinness of the dermis. These babies have intrauterine growth retardation and poor growth postnatally. The hands are typically held in fists, whereas other joints are lax. These children are severely mentally retarded and develop progressive choreoathetosis. Eye findings have included cataracts, strabismus, and myopia.

In some case reports, a decrease in elastic fibers was seen by light microscopy. Ultrastructural studies have shown variability in the size of collagen bundles and a decrease in the amorphous component of elastin with an increase in the microfibrillar component.

The mode of inheritance of de Barsy syndrome is uncertain.

Infants with cutis laxa do not have the same progeroid appearance. Infants with progeria develop their features progressively; those with de Barsy present at birth. Weidemann-Rautenstrauch syndrome is clinically very similar to de Barsy syndrome. However, infants with this neonatal progeria syndrome do not develop choreoathetosis.

Turner Syndrome

Females with gonadal dysgenesis and sex chromosome aneuploidy, Turner syndrome, have a number of skin findings. In utero lymphedema is typical, and the presence of bilateral cystic hygromas detected by fetal ultrasonography often leads to prenatal diagnosis of this chromosome disorder. The lymphedema gradually resolves, leaving residual nuchal webbing, and puffy hands and feet at birth. Approximately one third of patients with Turner syndrome are diagnosed at birth because of edema. It is present but overlooked in another third. A number of newborns with Turner syndrome have had cutis verticis gyrata, areas of fixed folds of skin noted at birth.[52] These are presumably caused by in utero entrapment and fixation of edematous skin. The puffiness of the hands and feet gradually resolve, in the hands faster than in the feet. The puffiness persists in a minority of patients. In some, it recurs in the feet and/or legs in childhood or later.

The toenails are often tiny, very deep set, and grow out vertically (Fig. 24-5). The fingernails can be hyperconvex and deep set or flat.

Girls with Turner syndrome often have many typical acquired nevi. They commonly occur on the face and arms. It is not so much that these nevi appear unusual, as it is that they are so numerous. These nevi often have fine hairs in them. Dysplastic nevi and an increased risk for malignant melanoma are not features of Turner syndrome.

Adults with Turner syndrome often appear younger than their stated age because of their short stature. We have seen what appears to be a premature wrinkling of the skin in a significant proportion of adult patients whom we have followed for many years. In their late thirties and early forties, many of these women experience a fairly rapid, fine, generalized wrinkling, especially of the face. It looks similar to the fine wrinkled skin seen in longtime smokers. It has occurred in patients who have been on adequate estrogen and progesterone replacement. The cause has not been actively sought.

Vitiligo and alopecia areata may occur more commonly in Turner syndrome than in the general pediatric population, but the absolute risk is still low. A subset of patients with Turner syndrome who are mosaic for their chromosome alterations present with hyperpigmentation or hypopigmentation along the lines of Blaschko. These features should always prompt karyotyping of blood and then skin if necessary.

Hypertrophic scars and keloid formation may be more likely to occur in girls with Turner syndrome. However, this risk may be more apparent than real, as it may be a consequence of the surgeries these patients tend to undergo, reduction of nuchal webbing, and cardiac repair. These involve scarring in areas of the body with a baseline increased likelihood of keloid formation and/or hypertrophic scarring.

The extracutaneous features of Turner syndrome are legion. The major clinical findings are short stature and gonadal dysgenesis. Any newborn with lymphedema should be karyotyped.[53]

Noonan Syndrome

Noonan syndrome is an autosomal dominant disorder that shares the features of congenital edema and short stature with the Turner syndrome. Nuchal webbing is also seen. There are typical facies with ptosis, downslanting palpebral fissures, and high palate. The classic cardiac lesion in Noonan syndrome is pulmonic stenosis, in contrast to bicuspid aortic valve and coarctation of the aorta in Turner syndrome.

The neonate with Noonan syndrome is unlikely to have dermatologic manifestations other than nuchal webbing that lead to diagnosis. In older children, keratosis pilaris atrophicans faciei (ulerythema ophryogenes) has been noted. Infants with cardiofaciocutaneous syndrome have, in addition to the usual features of Noonan syndrome, curly hair with a high frontal and temporal hairline. They almost invariably have ulerythema ophryogenes.[54] Koilonychia is also seen.

Some children with neurofibromatosis have facial features of Noonan syndrome, and some children with features of Noonan syndrome have multiple café au lait spots. The relationship between the two disorders remains uncertain, but a designation of Noonan/NF exists. Watson syndrome is a term also applied to this combination of features, and it appears to be allelic to NF1.

Cutis Verticis Gyrata

Cutis verticis gyrata refers to the presence of fixed, furrowed folds of skin. It is a feature that can be primary or secondary, present at birth or acquired.

The skin in cutis verticis gyrata is usually normal in color. The scalp is the most commonly involved area, and there may be an absence of hair when it occurs in the hair-bearing areas. The forehead and neck (and scrotum in males) can also be involved.

Primary cutis verticis gyrata can occur in isolation or in association with mental retardation. Occurrence at birth does not automatically confer a risk for mental retardation; cutis verticis gyrata more often develops later in those

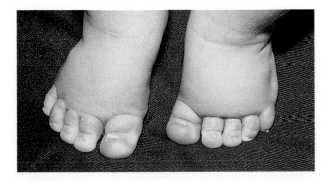

FIG. 24-5
Residual puffiness of the feet in Turner syndrome, with tiny imbedded toenails.

children in whom it is associated with mental retardation. Familial occurrence is rare.

Fixed folds of apparently normal skin have been reported in association with Turner syndrome and with Noonan syndrome, perhaps as a result of unusual pinching of edematous, redundant skin.[52,55] Pachydermoperiostosis[56] is a possibly autosomal dominant disorder in which progressive cutis verticis gyrata, clubbing of the nails, and periostosis of the long bones occur.

Beare-Stevenson Syndrome

Beare-Stevenson syndrome is a rare condition, known to be autosomal dominant by molecular analysis.[57] All cases have been sporadic. Infants with Beare-Stevenson present with extensive cutis verticis gyrata on the face and extremities, and extensive acanthosis nigricans-like changes. They have craniofacial dyostosis, large umbilical stumps, genital abnormalities, and anal anomalies. Natal teeth, accessory nipples, and pyloric stenosis have also been described. This is a striking disorder unlikely to be confused with any other condition in which cutis verticis gyrata or acanthosis nigricans occurs. Mutations in fibroblast growth factor receptor 2 (FGFR2) have been found in some but not all affected infants, and genetic heterogeneity is likely.

The histologic findings in cutis verticis gyrata are inconstant and not diagnostic. Excision of involved skin is the only treatment.

MOSAIC DISORDERS

There are a number of genodermatoses that are tolerated only in the mosaic state. They are lethal when expressed in all the cells of the body. The mosaicism can be real, as a result of the presence of distinct cell lines, or functional, resulting from X inactivation.

Mosaicism

Mosaicism is defined as the presence in a single organism, in this instance, human, of two or more genetically or chromosomally different cell lines. The cell lines may be normal, as in a chimera, or abnormal, as in a girl with 45,X/46,X,i(Xq) Turner syndrome. All human females are functionally mosaic for genes located on the inactivated segments of the X chromosome. Each female has a mixture of two cell lines, one in which the paternal X has been inactivated and no longer is transcribed, and the other in which the maternally derived X is quiescent. In contrast to heterozygosity for autosomal genes, in which each cell expresses the products of both the alleles, cells from females

heterozygous for a mutation in a gene on the portions of the X chromosome that undergo inactivation express product from one or the other allele, but not both.

In the skin, mosaicism appears to be expressed in specific patterns. Female carriers of X-linked disorders such as incontinentia pigmenti express pigment changes along the lines of Blaschko. Children mosaic for chromosomal aneuploidy have hyperpigmentation or hypopigmentation along the lines of Blaschko. Other disorders for which mosaicism has been invoked as an explanation demonstrate pigment change along these same lines, or in a phylloid (Happle) pattern, or a segmental checkerboard pattern. Presumably, all these cutaneous designs represent the endpoint of the orderly migration of cells during embryogenesis and the commitment of specific cells to specific regions occurring at the time of expression of the gene/gene products affected.

Incontinentia Pigmenti

Incontinentia pigmenti (IP)[58] is an X-linked dominant disorder with striking cutaneous features.

In the newborn period, affected infants develop small, clustered blisters on an erythematous base, scattered over the body surface along the lines of Blaschko (Fig. 24-6, A). The scalp can be involved. This stage resolves, usually by 6 months of age, and is followed by the second phase, characterized by warty, hyperkeratotic lesions, also on a red base (Fig. 24-6, B and C). In turn, these lesions crust over and disappear, to be replaced by swirly hyperpigmentation (Fig. 24-6, D). The lesions of more than one stage can be present at a given time, and one or more stages may be skipped in a particular individual. All three stages are distributed along the lines of Blaschko, but may not overlap in the areas involved. The fourth stage of incontinentia pigmenti develops very slowly. The hyperpigmentation may fade during childhood, to be replaced by hypopigmentation and loss of hair and sweat glands (Fig. 24-6, E). The face is usually not involved in any of the stages.

Congenital scarring alopecia and nail dystrophy can be seen. Missing teeth and peg-shaped teeth are common. There is variability in the manifestations in other organ systems. The most important and worrisome ocular finding is retinal vascular proliferation, which can result in retinal detachment and vision loss.[59] Any baby with the diagnosis of IP needs to be followed early and closely by an ophthalmologist skilled in evaluation of and management of retinal vascular abnormalities. It appears that the risk for eye involvement is before 1 year of age.

Mental retardation, seizures, spastic diplegia, hemiplegia, and quadriplegia are additional features in approximately 20% of patients. In our experience, those infants

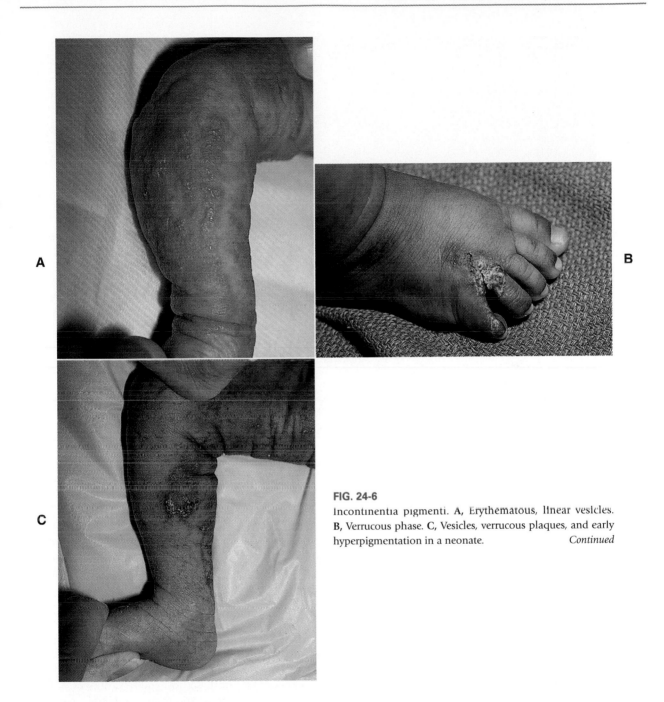

FIG. 24-6
Incontinentia pigmenti. **A,** Erythematous, linear vesicles. **B,** Verrucous phase. **C,** Vesicles, verrucous plaques, and early hyperpigmentation in a neonate.   *Continued*

with eye involvement are more likely to also have neurologic problems.

A host of other malformations have been described in patients with IP, since a poorly characterized immune defect is observed in some patients. Whether they are coincidental or related remains an open question.

IP results from mutations in the gene NEMO (NF-kappa B essential modulator),[60] located on the long arm of the X chromosome at Xq28. This mutation is believed to be lethal in the hemizygous male; very few males with IP have been reported. A woman with IP has a 1 in 3 chance of having an affected daughter, a 1 in 3 chance of having an unaffected daughter, and a 1 in 3 chance of having an unaffected son among pregnancies carried to term. Males who inherit the gene for IP presumably are aborted spontaneously, since the gene is lethal during embryogenesis if expressed in all cells.

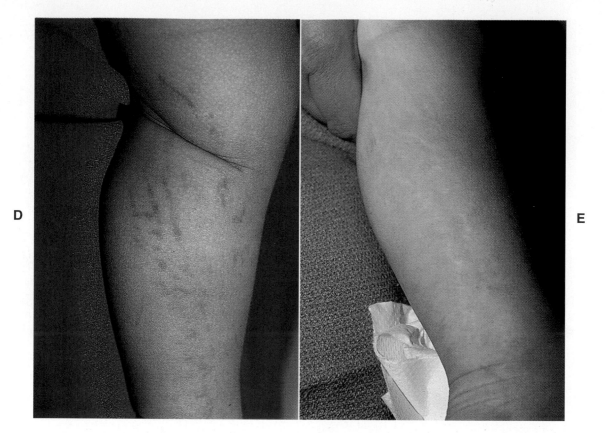

FIG. 24-6, cont'd
D, Hyperpigmentation of phase 3. E, Striate hypopigmentation.

The histopathology of IP is specific to each stage. The blisters show intercellular edema and intraepidermal vesicles filled with eosinophils, along with dyskeratotic keratinocytes. There can be a peripheral eosinophilia or leukocytosis as well. The warty lesions show hyperkeratosis, papillomatosis, and mild dyskeratosis. In the areas of increased pigment, basal cells are degenerated and there are pigment-laden melanophages in the dermis.

In the newborn period, IP must be differentiated from infectious causes of blistering, including bacteria and herpes simplex virus, and from the epidermolysis bullosa syndromes. This is usually straightforward. It is wise to treat the neonate appropriately for possible infection while awaiting the results of the Tzanck preparation or fluorescent antibody test for herpes simplex or a skin biopsy if indicated. The warty phase of IP is unique, and the diagnosis is unlikely to present difficulty, although a linear epidermal nevus might cause some confusion, which a biopsy will resolve.

Linear and whorled nevoid hypermelanosis can appear identical to stage 3 of IP. History should help distinguish between the two conditions. Occasionally, a biopsy may be necessary, since stage 3 IP has occurred as late as 15 months

of age without any antecedent skin changes. There has been some attempt to classify IP into IP1 and IP2. IP1 refers to a handful of patients with hyperpigmentation distributed along the lines of Blaschko who have been found to have X:autosome translocations, involving a breakpoint on the short arm of the X. These individuals do not have IP—their pigment abnormalities are presumed to be on the same basis as that for other children with a hypomelanosis of Ito phenotype (i.e., chromosomal mosaicism). The terms IP1 and IP2 should be abandoned.[61]

Skin changes of IP do not require treatment. Management of other malformations and problems needs to be individualized. Every infant needs a baseline eye examination by an ophthalmologist and anticipatory evaluation for the possibility of neurologic deficits by the primary care provider.

Focal Dermal Hypoplasia of Goltz

Newborns with this X-linked dominant disorder present with linear, streaky cutaneous atrophy, in which telangiectases predominate (Fig. 24-7, *A*). There is cribiform scar-

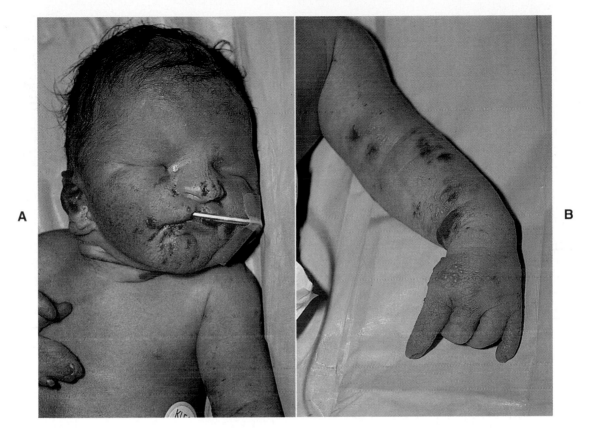

FIG. 24-7
A, Streaky areas of atrophy in focal dermal hypoplasia of Goltz syndrome. Note syndactyly. **B,** Linear fat herniation with vesiculation.

ring with pinpoint porelike depressions. Focal areas of dermal hypotrophy and atrophy are typical, and the subcutaneous fat can herniate up against the epidermis, resulting in visible yellowish excrescences (Fig. 24-7, *B*). The lines of Blaschko define the distribution of these skin changes.[62]

Over time, fleshy and vascular papillomas can develop, most frequently on mucosal, perioral, perigenital, and intertriginous areas. Nail dystrophy is common and variable. Patchy alopecia, sparse or brittle hair, aplasia cutis congenita, hyperhidrosis, and hyperkeratotic papules on the palms and soles have also been described in some patients.

Similar to incontinentia pigmenti, FDH can affect the eyes and teeth.[63] The eye abnormalities range from strabismus to microphthalmia. Teeth may be missing or malformed. The skeleton is also affected. Striated osteopathy (vertical streaking of no known clinical significance) is a characteristic finding in older patients. Cutaneous or bony syndactyly is common. Short stature, asymmetry and numerous other bony alterations have been described in a minority of patients. Mental retardation occurs in approximately 15% of affected individuals, and there can be accompanying microcephaly.

The diagnosis of focal dermal hypoplasia of Goltz (FDH) is made on the basis of the skin changes. Associated malformations need not be present.

FDH is presumed lethal in hemizygous males. The few affected males who have been described are believed to have resulted from post-zygotic mutations in the gene. The gene has not been mapped or identified.

The diagnosis of FDH is clinical with histologic corroboration. There is diminution to absence of the dermal collagen, and adipose cells extend up to the epidermis. When collagen bundles are present, they appear thinned and fragmented. There is no specific treatment. The differential diagnosis is fairly limited. FDH does not have the blisters of IP, or the hyperpigmentation. The cribiform atrophic lesions of FDH resemble those of X-linked dominant chondrodysplasia punctata, but there is no epiphyseal stippling.

Proteus Syndrome

Proteus syndrome is a fascinating disorder that is likely to prove heterogeneous in cause. Affected newborns have a variety of hamartomas and malformations, hence the name honoring the shape-changing Greek god. Overgrowth of soft tissues resulting from lipomatosis, asymmetric bone growth, hemihypertrophy, and macrodactyly are typical and variable (Fig. 24-8).[64] These changes can present at birth or develop over time. There is a very striking cerebriform hyperplasia of the feet seen in many children with Proteus syndrome. Hyperpigmentation in patchy, linear, or diffuse patterns has been described, as have been connective tissue, epidermal and organoid nevi. Lymphangiomas and angiomas can occur anywhere on the body at any time. They may progressively enlarge, stabilize, or regress. Extraosseous calcification in the soft tissues of the overgrown digits is common.

Asymmetric bony overgrowth is a typical feature and can involve any long bone. Benign bony tumors are also described. Ophthalmologic findings[65] are frequent and range from minimal strabismus to epibulbar harmartomatous masses. Intelligence can be normal or compromised severely. Cystic malformations of the lung have been reported in a few affected children.

The histopathologic features of Proteus are typical of the suspected hamartoma—lipomas, angiomas, and angiolipomas.

The cause of Proteus syndrome is unknown. It has been suggested[66] that it represents a post-zygotic mutation for a dominant gene that would be lethal in the heterozygous state, but is tolerated to some degree when not present in all tissues. There have been no recurrences in families.

Treatment of Proteus syndrome is often difficult. Surgical extirpation of rapidly growing lesions may not be effective. Orthopedic, ophthalmologic, neurologic, and pediatric care needs to be individualized. The condition can be relatively static, or there may be progressive debilitating overgrowth of skin lesions and bones.[67]

There are other disorders that share asymmetric hypertrophy with Proteus syndrome. The most likely to be considered in the differential diagnosis include Maffucci syndrome (in which lipomas do not occur); neurofibromatosis (café au lait spots have been described in Proteus syndrome, but axillary freckling and neurofibromas have not); Klippel-Trenaunay-Weber (the majority of soft tissue growths in Proteus are lipomas, although vascular tumors can occur); and Bannayan-Riley-Ruvalcaba syndrome. This last condition is clinically very similar. Affected males often have pigmented penile macules. Cerebriform plantar nevi are said not to occur. Bannayan-Riley-Ruvalcaba syndrome appears to be caused by mutations in PTEN1, allelic with Cowden syndrome.[68] Careful observation coupled with appropriate biopsies should help correctly distinguish among these conditions.[69]

Microphthalmia/Linear Skin Defects

Microphthalmia, dermal aplasia, and sclerocornea are the major features of MIDAS or MLS (microphthalmia and linear skin defects). This appears to be an X-linked dominant disorder and is extremely rare. Affected female infants show atrophic linear scars on the face and neck[70] (Fig. 24-9). The skin shows striking, irregular, linear, red

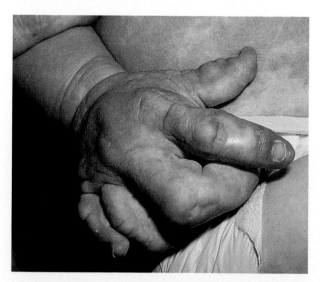

FIG. 24-8
Proteus syndrome. Hemihypertrophy and lipomatosis.

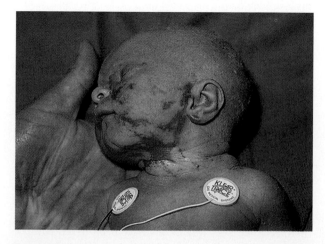

FIG. 24-9
Microphthalmia/linear skin defects. Atrophic linear scars on the face and neck.

areas of atrophic skin similar in appearance to fresh lesions of aplasia cutis congenita. In contrast to focal dermal hypoplasia of Goltz, fat herniation does not occur.

Eye defects are usually bilateral and include microphthalmia, corneal opacities, and orbital cysts. Among the less than 15 cases reported to date, a variety of other malformations have occurred. Survival can be compromised by congenital heart disease and neurologic abnormalities.[71] The disorder is clinically distinctive.

PHOTOSENSITIVITY DISORDERS AND MISCELLANEOUS METABOLIC DISORDERS

Although some inherited skin disorders are exacerbated by sun exposure, few do so in the neonate or young infant. Congenital erythropoietic porphyria (Gunther disease) is discussed in Chapter 10, Hartnup disorder in Chapter 14, and xeroderma pigmentosum in Chapter 20.

Bloom Syndrome

Bloom syndrome[72] is an autosomal recessive condition that is most frequent among Ashkenazi Jews. Infants with this disorder develop facial telangiectases and erythema in a butterfly distribution after exposure to sunlight. Progressive atrophy and actinic pigmentary changes ensue. The forearms and hands may become involved. Café au lait spots may be more common in these children. Acanthosis nigricans has occasionally been noted, usually in older children.

The major nondermatologic features of Bloom syndrome include immunodeficiency manifested primarily by severe recurrent pneumonia. Malignancies have been reported in over one half of patients with Bloom syndrome. There is a wide variety in the types of cancers that occur. Skin cancers often occur, but surprisingly, primarily in non–sun-exposed areas.

Fertility appears to be decreased among females. Males with Bloom syndrome do not produce sperm. Growth failure is universal and of prenatal onset. Death before age 40 is the rule.[73] The histologic features of the facial rash are nonspecific.

The gene for Bloom syndrome, BLM, maps to 15q26.1 and encodes a DNA helicase.[74] Chromosome studies show increased sister chromatid exchanges and an increase in chromosome breakage.

The differential diagnosis of Bloom syndrome includes all disorders with facial telangiectases. Lupus erythematosus is rare in infants and young children and is not associated with growth failure. The face of Rothmund-Thomson syndrome is different, as are the associated malformations. Children with polymorphic light eruption and congenital erythropoietic porphyria usually present later with their skin changes, and prenatal growth failure does not occur. Infants with xeroderma pigmentosa may show similar skin findings if exposed to sufficient sunlight early on, although telangiectases are not as prominent a feature as they are in Bloom syndrome.

Rothmund-Thomson Syndrome

Infants with Rothmund-Thomson syndrome[75] are usually identified as abnormal at birth because of associated limb defects that include radial ray deficiency and absent patellae. They develop progressive facial telangiectases with atrophy and hypopigmentation early in infancy. Occasionally blisters may occur. Involvement of the arms, legs, and buttocks is gradual. The trunk and flexures are spared. Later in life, hyperkeratoses and frank photosensitivity develop in about one third of patients. Nail dystrophy is reported in one quarter and is variable. In adults, squamous cell carcinoma has occurred.

Other skeletal features include short stature in over one half of patients and osteoporosis. There is an increased risk for osteogenic sarcoma. Approximately one quarter of affected individuals have hypogonadism and infertility. Juvenile cataracts develop in about 50%.

Histopathologic features include epidermal atrophy, a perivascular lymphocytic infiltrate, telangiectases, and fragmented elastin fibers. These features are not diagnostic. The basic defect in this autosomal recessive disorder remains unknown.

The poikiloderma that accompanies the telangiectases of Rothmund-Thomson syndrome distinguish it from the Fanconi, Bloom, and ataxia telangiectasia syndromes. Kindler syndrome is marked by bullae, a minor finding in Rothmund-Thomson syndrome.

Farber Disease

Farber disease, or lipogranulomatosis,[76] is an autosomal recessive disorder of acid ceramidase deficiency. Affected infants are typically mentally retarded and slowly develop failure to thrive. There is a gradual appearance of flesh-colored nodules over joints, on the scalp, and in the larynx. The trunk is usually spared. There is progressive loss of range of motion in the joints and ensuing disuse atrophy. Internal organ involvement is widespread. Death usually occurs by 3 years of age.

The nodules lie deep within the dermis and are composed of foamy histiocytes. A lymphoplasmacytic infiltrate occurs, and capillaries are dilated. On electron microscopy, the foamy cells in the peripheral and central nervous system show inclusions described as "banana bodies" or "zebralike bodies."

Systemic hyalinosis is marked by failure to thrive, progressive stiffening, and diffuse nodules. Affected infants have normal acid ceramidase activity, differentiating this condition from Farber disease.

ECTODERMAL DYSPLASIA SYNDROMES

There are over a hundred syndromes whose primary features involve alterations in two or more of the structures that derive from the embryonic ectoderm. These are referred to as ectodermal dysplasias.[76] Most are rare. Some are associated with major findings in other organs and are therefore not generally classified as an ectodermal dysplasia.

Among those syndromes characterized by developmental defects in hair, teeth, nails, sweat glands, and lens of the eye, the following are the relatively more common, although in absolute terms, still infrequent or rare.

AEC Syndrome

The upper and lower eyelids of the newborn with autosomal dominant ankyloblepharon filiforme adnatum–ectodermal dysplasia–cleft palate syndrome (AEC, Hay-Wells syndrome)[78] have fine strands of skin between them (Fig. 24-10, A). Ankyloblepharon are pieces of tissue that can be thick or thin, may tear spontaneously, or require surgical lysis. They are a cardinal feature of this condition, but are not mandatory for diagnosis. The rest of the skin is red and fissured with a collodion membrane appearance,

resembling the skin in bullous congenital ichthyosiform erythroderma (Chapters 10 and 16) with peeling, erythema, and erosions (Fig. 24-10, B). This sheds over the first few weeks. The underlying skin is dry and thin. Recurrent scalp infections, erosions, and granulation tissue plague two thirds to three quarters of older infants, children, and adults with this condition.[79]

The hair is sparse and coarse. Sweating is usually not significantly affected. Nail dystrophy is variable. The nails can be thickened and malformed, thin or absent.

Cleft palate, the third major sign of AEC syndrome, occurs in 80% of affected newborns. The lip may or may not be involved. The reported hypodontia associated with the condition may reflect the degree of severity of the clefting, rather than a primary ectodermal defect.

A few males with AEC have had hypospadias. External ear malformations are described in some patients. Supernumerary nipples and ectopic breast tissue occur in a minority of cases. There may be tear duct abnormalities and recurrent lid inflammation.

The gene for AEC and its product remain to be identified. There are no diagnostic histopathologic features. Other diagnoses to be considered when presented with an infant with cleft palate and a collodion membrane include EEC syndrome, distinguished by its limb involvement and Rapp-Hodgkin syndrome. Chronic involvement of the scalp is less typical of Rapp-Hodgkin ectodermal dysplasia. Both conditions are autosomal dominant, and there is considerable overlap between them. When ankyloblepharon are present, the diagnosis of AEC syndrome is self-evident.

Treatment is limited to surgical management of eyelid involvement and oral facial clefting. Use of light emol-

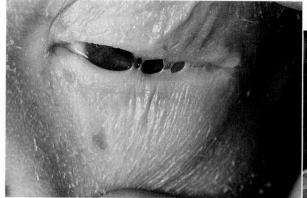
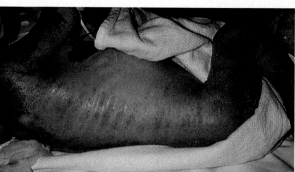

FIG. 24-10
Fine strands of tissue between eyelids in AEC syndrome. **B,** Cracking erosions of skin of body in AEC. (**A,** From Sybert VP. Genetic skin disorders. New York: Oxford University Press, 1997. **B,** From Vanderhooft SL, Stephan MJ, Sybert VP. *Pediatr Derm* 1993;10:334-340.)

lients may speed the shedding of the dry, cracking neonatal skin. Careful handling of the scalp and prompt attention to folliculitis may decrease long-term complications.

Hidrotic Ectodermal Dysplasia

Clouston syndrome, named after the Canadian physician who first described it in a French-Canadian kindred, is an autosomal dominant form of hidrotic or "sweating" ectodermal dysplasia.[80] Affected newborns may have milky white–appearing nails and dry skin or may show no clinical signs. The diagnosis may not be recognized until abnormal hair growth is detected or progressive nail dystrophy develops. Although it is a relatively common form of ectodermal dysplasia, it is not a diagnosis likely to be made in the newborn period in the absence of a positive family history.

Hypohidrotic Ectodermal Dysplasia

Hypohidrotic ectodermal dysplasia (HED) (Christ-Siemens-Touraine syndrome)[81] is an X-linked recessive form of ectodermal dysplasia and is the most common of this group of disorders. Affected male infants often present with a collodion membrane at birth,[82] which may be misconstrued as a marker of congenital ichthyosis or of postmaturity. The classic facial features of periorbital hyperpigmentation and wrinkling, saddle nose, and hypoplastic gum ridges with everted lips may not be appreciated (Fig. 24-11). It is, more often, repeated bouts of unexplained fevers that bring the infant with HED to medical attention. The fevers occur when the ambient temperature rises to a

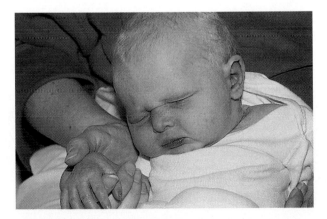

FIG. 24-11
Two-week-old with HED syndrome. Periorbital hyperpigmentation is evident. (From Sybert VP. Genetic skin disorders. New York: Oxford University Press, 1997.)

degree requiring sweating for cooling. Since these infants produce little to no sweat, they cannot make the appropriate physiologic response to an increase in the environmental temperature and their core temperature rises. Diminished or absent sweat pores can be appreciated both clinically and histologically.

In the toddler years, the sparse fine blond hairs and variable hypodontia of this condition become evident. Atopic disease is common in these infants and children. The nails are normal.

Gastroesophageal reflux occurs frequently, and failure to thrive may be significant. Nasal secretions are thick; recurrent upper respiratory tract infection is common. Cerumen may be tenacious and impacted.

The gene for HED resides at Xq12-q13.1 and is homologous to the Tabby gene in the mouse. It has been identified and sequenced.

Female carriers with the gene for HED may show no signs, display some features, or be as severely affected as males.[83] The degree to which the disorder is manifested in a carrier female depends on the random event of X inactivation.

The diagnosis of HED in an affected male born to a family known to be at risk is readily made by the mother or grandmother who immediately recognizes the facial features. The diagnosis in an infant not known to be at risk is usually made after an exhaustive search for other causes of fever of unknown origin in the infant. An examination for sweating or sweat pores and a panorex film of the jaw will confirm the suspicion of HED. There may be an autosomal recessive form of HED that needs to be considered when evaluating a severely affected female infant. X-linkage is the much more likely mode of inheritance, even in a fully manifesting female.

Treatment consists of control of the environment to keep the temperature normal and restorative dental work starting as early as age 2.5 to 3 years. Management of otolaryngologic complications and for atopic disease needs to be individualized.

EEC Syndrome

EEC syndrome (ectrodactyly-ectodermal dysplasia-clefting) is a rare autosomal dominant condition. Limb abnormalities that serve to distinguish this disorder from other ectodermal dysplasias occur in 80% to 100% of affected individuals. The feet are more often involved than the hands. There is deficiency of the medial ray of the limbs, resulting in a lobster claw deformity of varying degree. Cleft palate, with or without cleft lip, occurs in 70% to 100% of patients. Genitourinary malformations and hydronephrosis have been found in one third of persons with EEC. Malformed tear ducts, photophobia, blepharitis, and tearing abnormalities are typical.[84]

The dermatologic manifestations of EEC are mild and minor. The scalp hair is fine, sparse, and usually blond. Nails overlying abnormal phalanges are invariably abnormal. Those overlying uninvolved fingers may be dystrophic or pitted as well. Dry skin is an occasional complaint.

The diagnosis of EEC is self-evident when all three features are present. In the absence of limb defects, other ectodermal dysplasias associated with oral facial clefting need to be considered. A gene for ectrodactyly has been mapped to 7q21.3 – q22.1. Whether this gene is responsible for EEC syndrome is unknown. Some families with EEC have shown linkage to this region. In others, linkage to the pericentric region of chromosome 19 has been demonstrated. In yet another set of families, mutations in p63 have been found.[85] Treatment for EEC is surgical and orthodontic for the clefting. Orthopedic management of limb defects is individualized. The skin does not usually require specific therapy.

Absence of Dermatoglyphics

Isolated absence of dermatoglyphics is an interesting anomaly and exceedingly rare. Affected individuals have no fingertip ridge patterns, no palmar-plantar sweating, and thin, ridged nails. There may be two subtypes, one with palmar plantar thickening and the other with congenital blistering of the hands and feet. The former is also marked by camptodactyly.[86] Both appear to be autosomal dominant and of limited medical consequence, responsive to no specific therapy, and for which the basic defects are unknown. Males with HED may also have effaced fingerprints. The other clinical features of HED readily distinguish it from absence of dermatoglyphics.

ACKNOWLEDGMENTS

This work was supported in part by a grant from the National Institute of Health (NIH POI AM2155).

REFERENCES

1. NIH-CDC. Neurofibromatosis Conference Statement. Arch Neurol 1988;45:575-578.
2. Korf B. Diagnostic outcome in children with multiple cafe-au-lait spots. Pediatrics 1992;90:924-927.
3. Fois A, Calistri L, Balestri P, et al. Relationship between cafe-au-lait spots as the only symptom (sic) and peripheral neurofibromatosis (NF1): A follow-up study. Eur J Pediatr 1993; 152:500-504.
4. Chauffard A. Dermo-fibromatose pigmentaire (ou neuro-fibromatose generalise) mort par adenomes capsules surrenales et du pancreas. Bull Mem Soc Med Hop Paris 1896;13: 777-784.
5. Obringer A, Meadows A, Zackai E. The diagnosis of neurofibromatosis-1 in the child under the age of 6 years. Am J Dis Child 1989;14:717-719.
6. Whitehouse D. Diagnostic value of the cafe-au-lait spot in children. Arch Dis Childh 1966;41:316-319.
7. Riccardi V. Neurofibromatosis: Phenotype, natural history and pathogenesis. 2nd edition. Baltimore: Johns Hopkins University Press, 1992.
8. Huson S, Harper P, Compston D, et al. Von Recklinghausen neurofibromatosis. A clinical and population study in southeast Wales. Brain 1988;111:1355-1381.
9. North K. NF type 1 in childhood. In International review of child neurology series. London: MacKeith Press, 1997.
10. Leppig K, Kaplan P, Viskochil D, et al. Familial neurofibromatosis 1 microdeletions: Cosegregation with distinct facial phenotype and early onset of neurofibromata. Am J Med Genet 1997;73:197-204.
11. Gutmann D, Aylsworth A, Carey J, et al. The diagnostic evaluation and multidisciplinary management of neurofibromatosis 1 and neurofibromatosis 2. JAMA 1997;278:51-57.
12. Tuberous Sclerosis Consortium. Identification of the tuberous sclerosis gene TSC1 on chromosome 9q34. Science 1997;277:805-808.
13. The European Chromosome 16 Tuberous Sclerosis Consortium. Identification and characterisation of the tuberous sclerosis gene on chromosome 16. Cell 1993;75:1305-1315.
14. Roach E, Smith M, Northrup H, et al. Tuberous sclerosis complex consensus conference; revised clinical diagnostic criteria. J Child Neurol 1998;13:624-628.
15. Ruiz Maldonado, R Tamayo L. Neurocutaneous syndromes. In Harper J, ed. Inherited skin disorders: The genodermatoses. Boston: Butterworth-Heinemann, 1996.
16. Webb D, Fryer A, Osborne J. Morbidity associated with tuberous sclerosis: A population study. Dev Med Child Neurol 1996;38:146-155.
17. Gomez M. Tuberous sclerosis. 2nd edition. New York: Raven Press, 1988.
18. Sidenvall R, Eeg-Olofsson O. Epidemiology of infantile spasms in Sweden. Epilepsia 1995;36:572-574.
19. Webb D, Osborne J. Tuberous sclerosis. Arch Dis Child 1995;72:471-474.
20. Webb D, Fryer A, Osborne J. On the incidence of fits and mental retardation in tuberous sclerosis. J Med Genet 1991;28:395-397.
21. Jones A, Daniells C, Snell R, et al. Molecular genetic and phenotypic analysis reveals differences between TSC1 and TSC2 associated with familial and sporadic tuberous sclerosis. Hum Mol Genet 1997;6:2155-2161.
22. Webb D, Thomas R, Osborne J. Cardiac rhabdomyomas and their association with tuberous sclerosis. Arch Dis Child 1993;68:367-370.
23. Bosi G, Lintermans J, Pellgrino P, et al. The natural history of cardiac rhabdomyomas with and without tuberous sclerosis. Arch Paediatr 1996;85:928-931.
24. Cook J, Oliver K, Mueller R, et al. A cross sectional study of renal involvement in tuberous sclerosis. J Med Genet 1996; 33:480-484.

25. Brook-Carter P, Peral B, Ward C. Deletion of the TSC2 and PKD1 genes associated with severe infantile polycystic kidney disease—a contiguous gene syndrome. Nat Genet 1994; 8:328-332.

26. Ramenghi LA, Verrotti A, Domizio S, et al. Neonatal diagnosis of tuberous sclerosis. Childs Nerv Syst 1996;12:121-123.

27. Vanderhooft S, Francis J, Pagon R, et al. Prevalence of hypopigmented macules in a healthy population. J Pediatr 1996;129:355-361.

28. Jimbow K. Tuberous sclerosis and guttate leukodermas. Sem Cutan Med Surg 1997;16:30-35.

29. Darling T, Skarulis M, Steinberg S, et al. Multiple facial angiofibromas and collagenomas in patients with multiple endocrine neoplasia type 1. Arch Dermatol 1997;133:853-857.

30. Levine S, Manniello R, Farrell P. Familial dysautonomia: unusual presentation in an infant of non-Jewish ancestry. J Pediatr 1977;90:79-81.

31. Axelrod F, Porges R, Sein M. Neonatal recognition of familial dysautonomia. J Pediatr 1987;110:946-948.

32. Eng C, Slaugenhaupt S, Blumenfeld A, et al. Prenatal diagnosis of familial dysautonomia by analysis of linked CA-repeat polymorphisms on chromosome 9q31-q33. Am J Med Genet 1995;59:349-355.

33. Damkier A, Brandup F, Starklint H. Cutis laxa: autosomal dominant inheritance in five generations. Clin Genet 1991; 39:321-329.

34. Peltonen L, Kuivaniemi H, Palotic A, et al. Alterations in copper and collagen metabolism in the Menkes syndrome and a new subtype of the Ehlers-Danlos syndrome. Biochemistry 1983;22:6156-6163.

35. Zhang M-C, He L, Giro M, et al. Cutis laxa arising from frameshift mutations in axon 30 of the elastin gene (ELN). J Biol Chem 1999;274:981-986.

36. Harpey JP, Jaudon MC, Clavel JP, et al. Cutis laxa and low serum zinc after antenatal exposure to penicillamine. Lancet 1983;2:838.

37. Burrows N, Nicholls A, Yates J, et al. Genetic linkage to the collagen alpha 1 (V) gene (COL5A1) in two British Ehlers-Danlos syndrome families with variable type I and II phenotypes. Clin Exp Dermatol 1997;22:174-176.

38. Michalickova K, Susic M, Willing M, et al. Mutations of the alpha1(V) chain of type V collagen impair matrix assembly and produce Ehlers-Danlos syndrome type I. Hum Mol Genet 1998;7:249-255.

39. Wenstrup R, Murad S, Pinnell S. Ehlers-Danlos syndrome type VI: clinical manifestation of collagen lysyl hydroxylase deficiency. J Pediatr 1989;115:405-409.

40. Pepin M, Schwarze U, Superti-Furga A, Byers PH. Clinical and genetic features of Ehlers-Danlos syndrome type IV, the vascular type. N Engl J Med 2000;342:673-680.

41. Smith L, Wertelicki W, Milstone L, et al. Human dermatosparaxis: a form of Ehlers-Danlos syndrome that results from failure to remove the amino-terminal propeptide of type I pro collagen. Am J Hum Genet 1997;51:235-244.

42. Nelson D, King R. Ehlers-Danlos syndrome type VIII. J Am Acad Dermatol 1981;5:297-303.

43. Cohen P, Schneiderman P. Clinical manifestations of the Marfan syndrome. Int J Dermatol 1989;28:291-299.

44. Morse R, Rockenmacher S, Pyeritz R, et al. Diagnosis and management of infantile Marfan syndrome. Pediatrics 1990; 86:888-895.

45. Adès L, Haan E, Colley A, et al. Characterisation of four novel fibrillin-1 (FBN1) mutations in Marfan syndrome. J Med Genet 1996;33:665-671.

46. Kainulainen K, Karttunen L, Puhakka L, et al. Mutations in the fibrillin gene responsible for dominant ectopia lentis and neonatal Marfan syndrome. Nat Genet 1994;6:64-69.

47. Costello J. A new syndrome-mental subnormality and nasal papillomata. Aust Paediatr J 1977;13:114-118.

48. Zampino G, Mastroiacovo P, Ricci R, et al. Costello syndrome: further clinical delineation, natural history, and nosology. Am J Med Genet 1993;47:176-183.

49. Siwik E, Zahka K. Cardiac disease in Costello syndrome. Pediatrics 1998;101:706-709.

50. Philip N, Sigaudy S. Costello syndrome. J Med Genet 1998; 35:238-240.

51. de Barsy A, Moens E, Dierckx L. Dwarfism, oligophrenia, and degeneration of the elastic tissue in skin and cornea a new syndrome? Helv Paediatr Acta 1966;23:305-313.

52. Larralde M, Gardner S, Torrado M, et al. Lymphedema as a postulated cause of cutis verticis gyrata in Turner syndrome. Pediatr Dermatol 1998;15:18-22.

53. Sybert V. Turner syndrome in a life span perspective: Research and clinical aspects. in 4th International Symposium on Turner Syndrome. 1995. Gothenburg, Sweden: Elsevier.

54. Sybert VP. Genetic skin disorders. New York: Oxford University Press, 1997.

55. Lacombe D, Taieb A, Masson P, et al. Neonatal Noonan syndrome with a molluscoid cutaneous excess over the scalp. Genet Counsel 1991;2:249-253.

56. Rimoin D. Pachydermoperiostosis (idiopathic clubbing and periostosis). Genetic and physiologic considerations. N Engl J Med 1965;272:923-931.

57. Przylepa K, Paznekas W, Zhang M, et al. Fibroblast growth factor receptor 2 mutations in Beare-Stevenson cutis gyrata syndrome. Nat Genet 1996;13:492-494.

58. Carney RJ. Incontinentia pigmenti: a world of statistical analysis. Arch Dermatol 1976;112:535-542.

59. Watzke R, Stevens T, Carney RJ. Retinal vascular changes of incontinentia pigmenti. Arch Ophthalmol 1976;94:743-746.

60. Smahi A, Courtois G, Vabres P, et al. Genomic rearrangement in NEMO impairs NF-KappaB activation and is a cause of incontinentia pigment. Nature 2000;405:466-472.

61. Sybert V. Incontinentia pigmenti nomenclature. Am J Hum Genet 1994;55:209-211.

62. Goltz R, Henderson R, Hitch J, et al. Focal dermal hypoplasia syndrome. A review of the literature and report of two cases. Arch Dermatol 1970;101:1-11.

63. Hall E, Terezhalmy G. Focal dermal hypoplasia syndrome. Case report and literature review. J Am Acad Dermatol 1983; 9:443-451.

64. Biesecker LG, Peters KF, Darling TN, et al. Clinical differentiation between Proteus syndrome and hemihyperplasia: description of a distinct form of hemihyperplasia. *Am J Med Genet* 1998;79:311-318.

65. Burke J, Bowell R, O'Doherty N. Proteus syndrome: ocular complications. J Pediatr Ophthalmol Strabismus 1988;25: 99-102.

66. Happle R. Cutaneous manifestation of lethal genes. Hum Genet 1986;72:280.

67. Clark R, Donnai D, Rogers J, et al. Proteus syndrome: an expanded phenotype. Am J Med Genet 1987;27:99-117.

68. Marsh D, Coulon V, Lunetta K, et al. Mutation spectrum and genotype-phenotype analyses in Cowden disease and Bannayan-Zonana syndrome, two hamartoma syndromes with germline PTEN mutation. Hum Mol Genet 1998;7: 507-515.

69. Viljoen D, Nelson N, de Jong G, et al. Proteus syndrome in Southern Africa: Natural history and clinical manifestations in six individuals. Am J Med Genet 1987;27:87-97.

70. Al-Gazali L, Mueller R, Caine A, et al. Two 46,XX,t(X;Y) females with linear skin defects and congenital microphthalmia: a new syndrome at Xp22.3. J Med Genet 1990;27: 59-63.

71. Happle R, Daniels O, Koopman RJ. MIDAS syndrome (microphthalmia, dermal aplasia, and Sclerocornea): An X-linked phenotype distinct from Goltz syndrome. Am J Med Genet 1993;47:710-713.

72. Bloom D. The syndrome of congenital telangiectatic erythema and stunted growth. J Pediatr 1966;68:103-113.

73. German J, Passarge E. Report from the registry for 1987. Clin Genet 1989;35:57-69.

74. Ellis N, German J. Molecular genetics of Bloom's syndrome. Hum Mol Genet 1996;5:1457-1463.

75. Vennos E, Collins M, James W. Rothmund-Thomson syndrome: review of the world literature. J Am Acad Dermatol 1992;27:750-762.

76. Zappatini-Tommasi L, Dumontel C, et al. Farber disease: An ultrastructural study. Virchows Arch A Pathol Anat Histopathol 1992;420:281-290.

77. Freiere-Maia N, Pinheiro M. Ectodermal dysplasias: A clinical and genetic study. New York: AR Liss, 1984.

78. Hay R, Wells R. The syndrome of ankyloblepharon, ectodermal defects and cleft lip and palate: An autosomal dominant condition. Br J Dermatol 1976;94:277-289.

79. Vanderhooft S, Stephan M, Sybert V. Severe skin erosions and scalp infections in AEC syndrome. Pediatr Dermatol 1993; 10:334-340.

80. Clouston H. A hereditary ectodermal dysplasia. Can Med Assoc J 1929;21:18-31.

81. Clarke A, Phillips D, Brown R, et al. Clinical aspects of X-linked hypohidrotic ectodermal dysplasia. Arch Dis Child 1987;62:989-996.

82. Executive and Scientific Advisory Boards of the National Foundation of Ectodermal Dysplasias. Scaling skin in the neonate: A clue to the early diagnosis of X-linked hypohidrotic ectodermal dysplasia (Christ-Siemens-Touraine syndrome). J Pediatr 1989;114:600-602.

83. Sybert V. Hypohidrotic ectodermal dysplasia: Argument against an autosomal recessive form clinically indistinguishable from X-linked hypohidrotic ectodermal dysplasia (Christ-Siemens-Touraine syndrome). Pediatr Dermatol 1989;6:76-81.

84. Rodini E, Richieri-Costa A. EED syndrome: Report on 20 new patients, clinical and genetic considerations. Am J Med Genet 1990;37:42-53.

85. Celli J, Duijf P, Hamel BCJ, et al. Heterozygous germline mutations in the p53 homolog p63 are the cause of EEC syndrome. Cell 1999;99:143-153.

86. Cirillo-Hyland V, Zackai E, Honig P, et al. Re-evaluation of a kindred with congenital absence of dermal ridges, syndactyly, and facial milia. J Am Acad Dermatol 1995;32:315-318.

25

Neonatal Mucous Membrane Disorders

DENISE W. METRY
ADELAIDE A. HEBERT

Examination of the mucous membranes is an important, yet often overlooked, part of the neonatal evaluation. In this chapter we discuss abnormal cutaneous findings of the oral, genital, and ocular systems. Many of these abnormalities provide important clues to the diagnosis of underlying disease and/or developmental syndromes in the newborn infant.

DISORDERS OF THE ORAL MUCOUS MEMBRANES (Table 25-1)

Bohn's Nodules

Bohn's nodules are multiple, small cystic structures found along the lingual gum margins and lateral palate (Fig. 25-1). These lesions are commonly found in up to 85% of newborn infants. Bohn's nodules most likely develop from epithelial remnants of salivary gland tissue or from remnants of the dental lamina. However, some authors refute this idea because mucinous glands are rarely found on the lateral edge of the gingival margins. Therapy for Bohn's nodules is unnecessary, since spontaneous involution or shedding is the rule.[1-3]

Congenital Epulis

The congenital epulis is a rare, benign tumor of the newborn. Clinically, the lesion is a solitary soft nodule, from 1 to several mm in diameter, which is often pedunculated. The epulis forms over the gingival margin, most frequently along the anterior maxillary ridge or the incisor-canine.[4,5] Lesions are nine times more frequent in female newborns.

Fetal-ovarian estrogen levels were originally thought to account for this predominance, but this concept has been challenged.[6]

Histologic examination shows tightly packed granular cells surrounded by a prominent fibrovascular network. The absence of pseudoepitheliomatous hyperplasia and neural elements differentiates the epulis from a granular cell myoblastoma.

Lesions may regress spontaneously over time. However, difficulties with feeding and respiration can occur with large or multiple lesions. Simple excision is curative; recurrences have not been reported.

Congenital Ranula

The congenital ranula is a very rare type of mucocele that results from an obstructed, imperforate, or atretic sublingual or submandibular salivary gland duct. Lesions are found specifically on the anterior floor of the mouth, lateral to the lingual frenulum. The overlying mucosa may be normal in color or have a translucent blue hue.

Ranulae may resemble mucous retention cysts, dermoid cysts, or cystic hygromas. Differentiation of a ranula from a mucous retention cyst can be confirmed only by histopathologic examination. Although the mucous retention cyst is a true cyst lined by epithelium, the ranula is a pseudocyst.

Ranulae may rupture spontaneously during feeding and sucking; however, obstructed ducts should be treated early with marsupialization. In some cases, failure to operate may lead to sialadenitis. If surgery is warranted, the risk of recurrence postoperatively is minimal.[7]

TABLE 25-1

Benign Papular Lesions of the Tongue/Oral Mucosa

Lesion	Morphology	Most common location
Bohn's nodules	Multiple, small cysts	Gingival margin, lateral palate
Congenital epulis	Pedunculated, soft nodule from 1 mm to several cm in diameter	Gingival margin
Congenital ranula	Translucent, firm papule or nodule	Anterior floor of mouth, lateral to lingual frenulum
Epstein's pearls	Multiple, tiny (< few mm) cysts	Median palatal raphe
Eruption cysts	Circumscribed, fluctuant swelling; may have bluish-red to black surface if hemorrhage has occurred	Alveolar ridge of mandible or maxilla
Granular cell tumor	Small (<3 cm in diameter), firm, flesh-colored nodule	Tongue
Hemangiomas	Red to blue, soft to semi-firm nodule	Lips, buccal mucosa, palate
Lymphangiomas	Translucent papules or nodule	Tongue
Neurofibromas	Soft, flesh-colored nodule	Tongue
Venous malformations	Bluish, compressible nodule; often intermittently painful	Oropharynx
White sponge nevus	White plaque with thick, folded surface	Buccal mucosa

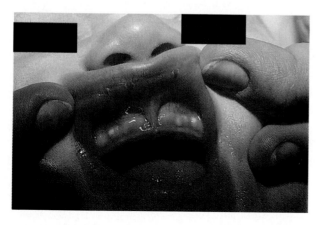

FIG. 25-1
Bohn's nodules along the upper alveolar ridge.

Granular Cell Tumor

The granular cell tumor, first described in 1926, was originally thought to arise from skeletal muscle and was hence named a granular cell myoblastoma.[8] However, recent immunohistochemical testing suggests a neural origin.[9] Intraoral granular cell tumors most commonly occur on the tongue, but may also affect the lips and gingiva. The lesion is typically a solitary, small (less than 3 cm), firm, asymptomatic nodule, with a smooth, nonulcerated sur-

face. The differential diagnosis includes other benign neural neoplasms (neuromas, neurofibromas), and vascular tumors (hemangiomas, venous malformations).[10-12]

Histologically, large, eosinophilic granular cells are arranged in clusters and fascicles. Pseudoepitheliomatous hyperplasia of the overlying epithelium may be present, mimicking squamous cell carcinoma.[13] Although the majority of granular cell tumors are entirely benign, these tumors can be locally invasive and metastases have been rarely reported. Surgical excision is recommended and curative. Recurrences are uncommon.[14]

Epstein's Pearls

Epstein's pearls are benign cystic lesions that occur along the median palatal raphe, most commonly at the junction of the hard and soft palate (Fig. 25-2). Lesions are multiple and small, ranging in size from less than a millimeter to several millimeters in diameter. The overall appearance is similar to the Bohn's nodule, but the location and etiology make this a distinct entity. Epstein's pearls are common, occurring in 60% to 85% of newborn infants. Japanese newborns are most commonly affected (up to 92%), followed by Caucasians and African-Americans.[1,15,16]

Epstein's pearls are epidermal inclusion cysts formed during the fusion of the soft and hard palates, and contain desquamated keratin within their lumens. They are considered the counterpart of milia, which are commonly

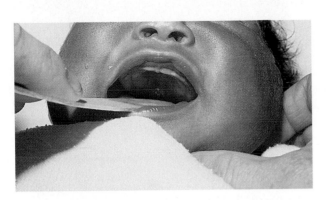

FIG. 25-2
Epstein's pearls of the hard palate.

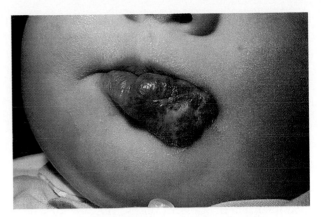

FIG. 25-4
Hemangioma of the lower lip.

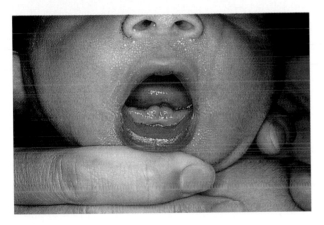

FIG. 25-3
Eruption cysts on the lower alveolar ridge of an infant.

seen on the faces of neonates. No therapy is indicated, since most lesions spontaneously rupture within the first few weeks to months of life.[1,15]

Eruption Cysts

An eruption cyst (or eruption hematoma) is a circumscribed fluctuant swelling that develops over the site of an erupting tooth (Fig. 25-3). Lesions in the newborn may occur secondary to natal or neonatal teeth, but these cysts are more commonly associated with the eruption of deciduous, or permanent teeth. Eruption cysts most commonly develop on the alveolar ridge of the maxilla or mandible. Size varies with the type of tooth overlaid, but most lesions are approximately 0.6 cm in diameter. The surface of the cyst may appear flesh-colored or have a bluish-red to blue-black color if the cyst cavity contains

blood. Although removal of the tissue overlying the tooth may aid in its eruption, most eruption cysts resolve spontaneously within several weeks without treatment.[17]

Hemangiomas

Hemangiomas of the oral mucosa in newborns most commonly develop over the lips, buccal mucosa, or palate (Fig. 25-4). Superficial lesions are red to blue nodules, which are soft or semifirm to palpation. In contrast, deep-seated hemangiomas are firmer, flesh-colored nodules with poorly defined borders. Although biopsy is seldom warranted, histology demonstrates numerous, dilated vascular spaces.[4]

Hemangiomas of the oral cavity are prone to trauma, which can lead to ulceration, hemorrhage, or infection. Lesions in a cervicofacial, or "beard" distribution (preauricular skin, chin, anterior neck, or lower lip) have a 63% association with the development of airway hemangiomas. Such infants are at greatest risk between 2 and 6 weeks of life and should be followed closely for the development of stridor or other signs of airway compromise.[18]

Hemangiomas involute spontaneously over time, but lesions of the tongue or lip may do so more slowly, and lip lesions in particular may leave permanent soft-tissue damage. Therapeutic intervention is required only if the function of the oral cavity and/or airway becomes compromised. Treatment modalities in such cases include systemic or intralesional steroids, alpha or beta interferon, cryosurgery, laser therapy, or intravascular embolization (see Chapter 18).[19]

Lymphangiomas (Lymphatic Malformations)

Lymphangiomas are benign malformations of lymphatic vessels, and are much less common than hemangiomas.

The majority of lymphangiomas are detected at birth or within the first 2 years of life. No apparent sexual predilection or hereditary predisposition exists. Unlike hemangiomas, lymphangiomas rarely undergo any significant degree of involution.[20-22]

Most lymphangiomas are found in the head and neck region. Lesions may be single or multiple and most often present as translucent papules or nodules. The most common location for intraoral lymphangiomas is the tongue, although lesions can also develop over the lips, buccal mucosa, palate, or alveolar ridges. Tongue lymphangiomas most commonly affect the dorsal anterior two thirds and may result in macroglossia. Consequently, abnormal bone development, drooling, and difficulties with feeding and speech may occur. Airflow obstruction is fortunately rare if the nasopharyngeal airway is patent.[21,23]

Histologically, lymphangiomas consist of multiple lymphatic channels lined by single or multiple layers of endothelial cells. Treatment is based on lesion size and location. As spontaneous regression is rare, surgery remains the mainstay of therapy. However, post-surgical recurrences are common.[20,21] The neodymium-YAG laser has recently been employed, and long-term studies will determine its effectiveness. Injection of cystic areas with sclerosing agents such as alcohol or sotraderol is also effective in some cases. Systemic steroids have been used acutely to decrease edema, but have no role in the chronic management of these lesions.[16]

Cystic hygromas are a subset of lymphangiomas that develop when the jugular lymph sac fails to communicate with the thoracic duct or the internal jugular vein. Typically, lesions present at birth or shortly thereafter as smooth, firm, fluctuant nodules, which transilluminate. Cystic hygromas are predominantly found in the posterior triangle of the neck, and often involve the floor of the mouth and submandibular space. Enlargement may result in life-threatening respiratory distress (Fig. 25-5). Treatment consists of surgical reduction or complete removal if possible.[24-26]

Neurofibromas

A neurofibroma is a tumor of neural origin, which may occur as an isolated finding or in association with the syndrome of neurofibromatosis. Neurofibromatosis may be difficult to diagnose in the newborn period, when many of the features of the syndrome are not yet evident.

Neurofibromas may be found on the skin or within the oral cavity, although intraoral lesions are exceedingly rare in the newborn. The most common intraoral location is the tongue, though tumors have also been observed over the buccal mucosa and palate. Oral lesions are typically asymptomatic, slow growing, soft nodules, of the same

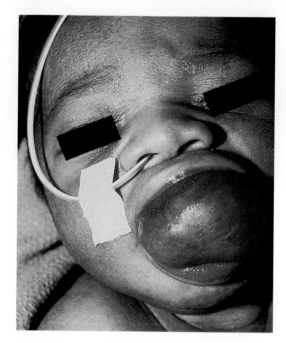

FIG. 25-5
Large, oral cystic hygromas (lymphangioma) may result in life-threatening respiratory distress.

color as the surrounding mucosa. Neurofibromas range in size from a few millimeters to a few centimeters in diameter. Histologically, the tumor is unencapsulated and composed of Schwann cells, perineural cells, and fibroblasts. Neurofibromas are benign and can be electively surgically excised with little risk of recurrence.[27,28]

Venous Malformations

Venous malformations (VM) are slow-flow vascular malformations usually present at birth. Lesions most commonly involve the face and oropharynx but may occur in any anatomic location. Though usually solitary, lesions may be multiple, especially when associated with the Maffuci or blue rubber bleb nevus syndromes. VMs are bluish, compressible nodules, which are often intermittently painful. Lesions may result in skeletal alterations, such as facial asymmetry, dental malalignment, and bony hypertrophy.

The best means of establishing the diagnosis of a VM and determining the extent of tissue involvement is with magnetic resonance imaging. In addition, the presence of phleboliths is highly characteristic of the diagnosis. Extensive lesions may be complicated by a localized, intravascular coagulopathy, characterized by a slightly low platelet count, low fibrinogen, increased D-dimers, and normal prothrombin and partial thromboplastin times.

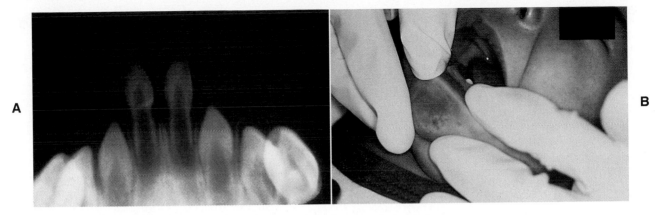

FIG. 25-6
A, Radiograph of natal teeth. B, Natal teeth on the lower alveolar ridge of an infant.

Treatment of venous malformations is rarely necessary within the first year of life. However, VMs may slowly increase in size. Intervention may eventually be required for those lesions resulting in persistent pain, functional impairment, or cosmetic disfigurement.[29]

White Sponge Nevus (of Cannon)

White sponge nevus is a rare, benign condition inherited as an autosomal dominant trait. Typical lesions are asymptomatic white plaques in which the oral mucosa appears thickened and folded with a spongy texture. The most common location for a white sponge nevus is on the buccal mucosa, often in a bilateral distribution. Extraoral lesions such as labial, nasal, vaginal, esophageal, and anal mucosa are uncommon and usually do not occur in the absence of oral involvement. The white sponge nevus is most often present at birth or discovered during early childhood.[30]

The clinical differential diagnosis of white sponge nevus includes candidiasis, leukoderma, leukoplakia, lichen planus, and local irritation. It is sometimes seen in association with pachyonychia congenita. However, the clinical and histologic findings are usually characteristic enough to differentiate this condition from other white mucosal lesions.[31] The histopathology of a white sponge nevus shows epithelial thickening with hyperkeratosis and acanthosis. The suprabasal cells exhibit intracellular edema with pyknotic nuclei and compact aggregates of keratin intermediate filaments within the upper spinous layer.[32]

Natal Teeth

Natal teeth are defined as teeth present at birth. *Natal* teeth are to be differentiated from *neonatal* teeth, which erupt during the first month of life. The reported incidence of both natal and neonatal teeth varies widely but is decidedly rare. Both may occur in either premature or term infants. However, natal teeth occur three times more often than neonatal teeth and are twice as common in females. Two thirds of natal teeth occur in pairs. The most common location for natal teeth is at the sites of the central mandibular incisors (85%), followed by the maxillary incisors (11%) (Fig. 25-6).[33-35]

Although the exact etiology for natal teeth remains unknown, it appears that the primary tooth bud develops in a more superficial location than normal, and therefore erupts prematurely.[36] Many syndromes have been associated with natal teeth (Table 25-2), and newborns with this finding should be examined carefully. Other reported associations include congenital syphilis, endocrine disturbances, febrile systemic illness, hypovitaminosis, and pyelitis during pregnancy.[4]

Natal teeth usually represent deciduous rather than supernumerary teeth, which can be distinguished by radiography. Supernumerary teeth are extraneous teeth, which should be extracted, since they may interfere with normal tooth eruption. The lower central incisors are normally the first teeth in the oral cavity to erupt. The condition of Riga-Fede describes a traumatic ulcerative lesion of the tongue or frenulum, produced when an infant rakes the tongue over the primary lower incisors, which may be mobile and/or have poorly formed crowns (Fig. 25-7). This condition may be related to pain insensitivity, and has been associated with familial dysautonomia.[4,37]

Treatment of natal teeth is dependent on morphology, amount of root development, and mobility. If the tooth is only minimally loose, it will tend to stabilize over time and can be left in place. Problematic teeth should be extracted to prevent trauma or aspiration.[38,39]

TABLE 25-2

Syndromes Associated With Natal Teeth

Syndrome	Associated anomalies	Inheritance/chromosomal abnormality/prevalence
Ellis-van Creveld (chondroectodermal dysplasia)	Bilateral postaxial polydactyly of hands, chondrodysplasia of long bones resulting in acromesolic dwarfism, ectodermal dysplasia affecting nails/teeth, congenital heart malformation	Autosomal-recessive Not known $7/1 \times 10^6$
Hallermann-Streiff	Dyscephaly, hypotrichosis, micro-ophthalmia, cataracts, beaked nose, micrognathia, proportionate short stature	Sporadic Not known 150 cases to date
Pachyonychia congenita (Jadassohn-Lewandowsky or Jackson-Lawler)	Dystrophic nails, palmoplantar keratosis, hyperhidrosis, follicular keratosis, oral leukokeratosis, cutaneous cysts	Autosomal–dominant Not known $0.07/1 \times 10^6$ 9:5 male to female
Pallister-Hall (hypothalamic hamartoblastoma)	Hypothalamic hamartoblastoma, craniofacial abnormalities, postaxial polydactyly, cardiac and renal defects	Sporadic Not known 13 cases to date 8:5 male to female
Weidemann-Rautenstrauch	Endocrine dysfunction, aged facies, frontal and biparietal bossing, small facial bones, sparse scalp hair, prominent scalp veins, small beaked nose, low-set ears	Autosomal-recessive Not known 1 case to date
Natal teeth, patent ductus arteriosus, intestinal pseudoobstruction	Dilatation/hypermobility of small bowel, short or microcolon without obstruction, incomplete rotation of midgut, patent ductus arteriosus	X-linked recessive Not known 2 cases to date, brothers

From Hebert AA, Berg JH. Mucous membrane disorders. In Schachner LA, Hansen RC, eds. Pediatric dermatology, 2nd edition. New York: Churchill Livingstone, 1995.

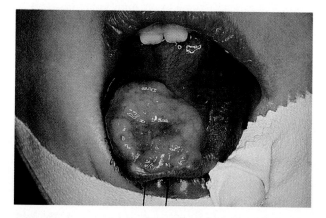

FIG. 25-7
Traumatic ulcerative granuloma lesion of the tongue in Riga-Fede syndrome.

Sucking Calluses

Sucking calluses (or sucking pads) develop on the lips or buccal mucosa as solitary, oval thickenings (Fig. 25-8). When these lesions are congenital, they are indicative of vigorous sucking in utero. Presentation after birth is more common in breast fed, black infants. Histology reveals a thickened epidermis secondary to intracellular edema and hyperkeratosis. Sucking calluses involute spontaneously within a few days or weeks after birth or on cessation of breast-feeding.[3,15]

Congenital Fistulae of the Lower Lip

Congenital fistulae of the lower lip (or lip pits) are rare developmental anomalies. The estimated frequency of lower lip pits in the Caucasian population is uncommon, with approximately one in 100,000 persons affected; the frequency in the black population is rare. Clinically, bilateral indentations are seen on the vermilion portion of the

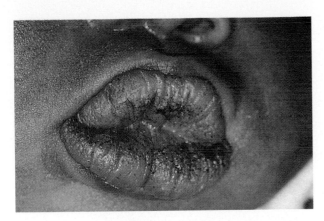

FIG. 25-8
Sucking calluses of the lips.

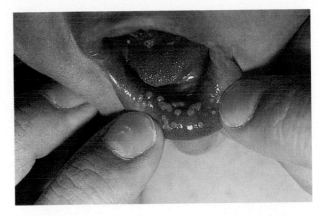

FIG. 25-9
Sebaceous hyperplasia (Fordyce spots) involving the lower gingiva.

lower lip. The pits are usually 1 cm apart and equidistant from the midline. The defect results from incomplete closure of the furrows on the fetal mandibular process. The pits range in depth from a few millimeters to 25 mm; longer fistulae can transverse the orbicularis oris muscle. The proximal opening of the fistula at the lip may extrude saliva, either spontaneously or during mastication. Histologically, the fistula lumen is lined by stratified squamous epithelium, similar to lip mucosa. At the distal end of the fistula, scattered acini of mucinous glands with tubular ducts are present. True salivary glands are not seen.[16,40]

Congenital fistulae are inherited as an autosomal dominant trait with an estimated penetrance of 80% to 100%. The presence of a single fistula is considered an incomplete expression of the trait and not a separate entity. The evaluation of a patient with lower lip pits should include a search for other possible anomalies. Lip pits are strongly associated with the formation of cleft lip and/or palate. This association approaches 80% and is now referred to as the Van de Woude syndrome. Newborn infants with single lip pits are at equal risk to those with double pits for associated clefting. Congenital fistulae of the lip are only treated to correct visible deformity or to eradicate significant aberrant salivation.[16,40-42]

Sebaceous Hyperplasia of the Lip (Fordyce Spots or Granules)

Fordyce spots represent collections of normal sebaceous glands within the oral cavity. Lesions appear as white to yellow macules and papules visible through the transparent oral mucosa. The papules measure 1 to 3 mm in size and may be clustered (Fig. 25-9). Plaques form when large numbers of sebaceous glands coalesce. Sebaceous hyperplasia is most commonly seen on the upper lip but may also be evident on the buccal mucosa, tongue, gingiva, or palate. No treatment is warranted, as these lesions are asymptomatic, resolve spontaneously, and are of no medical consequence.[16]

Annulus Migrans (Geographic Tongue)

Annulus migrans (or geographic tongue) is a common condition that may present as early as 2 weeks of life. Characteristically, multiple erythematous patches surrounded by white, polycyclic borders are seen over the dorsum of the tongue. The lesions are often migratory and transient in nature. The etiology of annulus migrans is most likely reactive in nature; reported associated disorders have included psoriasis (especially pustular), Reiter's syndrome, atopic and seborrheic dermatitis, and spasmodic bronchitis of childhood. Histologically, geographic tongue is indistinguishable from pustular psoriasis or Reiter's syndrome. Therapy of this benign condition is generally unsuccessful and unwarranted.[16]

Macroglossia

Macroglossia is defined as a resting tongue that protrudes beyond the teeth or gum line (Fig. 25-10). When this finding is present in a newborn, a thorough evaluation should be performed to rule out genetic, metabolic, or other possibly contributing factors. True macroglossia may be "primary," whereby the tongue is enlarged due to hyperplasia or hypertrophy of normal lingual structures, or, more commonly, "secondary" to an underlying process, as with a lymphangioma or in amyloidosis (Box 25-1).

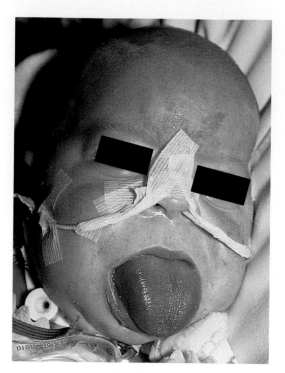

FIG. 25-10
Macroglossia in an infant with Beckwith-Weidemann syndrome.

True macroglossia must be distinguished from *pseudomacroglossia*. In pseudomacroglossia, the tongue size is normal, but functionally enlarged as a result of a small or inferiorly displaced mandible. This situation occurs in the Pierre-Robin syndrome, and is also seen in some newborns ultimately diagnosed with cerebral palsy.

An enlarged tongue may affect feeding, speech, and respiration. In later infancy, macroglossia may also cause malocclusion as a result of increased pressure on the teeth.

Surgical trimming or reduction of the tongue is often effective in reducing tissue bulk. However, therapeutic intervention, when feasible, should be aimed at treating any underlying cause.[16]

Macular Pigmentation

Macular pigmentation of the oral mucosa is a normal variant found in darker-skinned persons. Several patterns of pigmentation may occur. Most commonly, a pigmented band is present at the junction of the free and attached alveolar mucosa. Patchy pigmentation may also be evident over the buccal mucosa, on the lips, and on the floor of the mouth (Fig. 25-11). When the tongue is involved, which is rare, the pigment is localized to the filiform papillae. The increased pigmentation occurs as a result of an increase in melanocytic activity rather than an increase in the number of melanocytes. No therapy is necessary.[43]

Linugal Melanotic Macule

Congenital lingual melanotic macules have been observed as solitary or multiple, well-circumscribed, brown lesions present on the dorsal surface of the tongue at birth that grow proportionately to the tongue (personal observation). Histological features are those of increased basal pigmentation with minimal melanocytic hyperplasia and mild pigment incontinence. It is distinct from macular pigmentation, and appears to be a benign process.

Acatalasemia

Acatalasemia is a genetically heterogeneous disease characterized by an inherited absence of the enzyme catalase. Affected infants are unable to degrade endogenous or exoge-

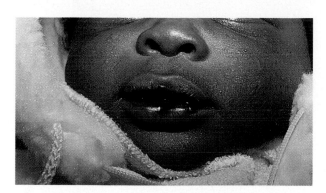

FIG. 25-11
Macular hyperpigmentation involving the lower lip.

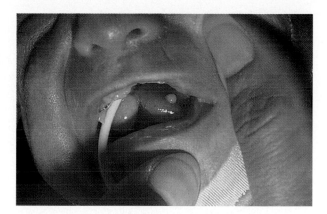

FIG. 25-12
Lobulated tongue of a female infant with oral-facial-digital I syndrome.

nous hydrogen peroxide, which accumulates, resulting in oxidation deprivation. The soft tissues of the mouth and nasal mucosa are preferentially affected, leading to ulceration, necrosis, and gangrene in severe cases. The physical examination is otherwise normal. The diagnosis is confirmed by the absence of blood catalase. Therapy consists of meticulous oral hygiene, early removal of diseased teeth and tonsils, and the administration of systemic antibiotics as necessary to control bacterial proliferation.[16,44]

Oral-Facial-Digital Syndrome, Type I

Oral-facial-digital (OFD) syndrome is a rare and complex condition. Seven types of OFD are currently recognized. Oral abnormalities are the most consistent and characteristic findings of type I OFD. Features may include multiple hyperplastic frenulae between the buccal mucosa and alveolar ridge, cleft lip or palate, a lobated or bifid tongue with small hamartomas (Fig. 25-12), dental caries, and/or anomalous anterior teeth. Distinguishing facial features are frontal bossing, hypoplasia of the malar bones and alar cartilages, a broad nasal root, and milia of the ears. Skeletal findings include asymmetric shortening of digits, clinodactyly and brachydactyly of the hands, and unilateral polydactyly of the feet. Infants may also have a dry, rough scalp with significant alopecia.

Newborns with OFD type I may also have internal manifestations, the most common of which are multiple renal, hepatic, or pancreatic cysts. Significant CNS abnormalities, especially agenesis or absence of the corpus callosum, also occur. The overall prognosis is poor; one third of affected patients die within the first year of life. Therapy must be individualized based on the presence of vis-

ceral anomalies. Surgical intervention may be necessary to ensure proper feeding and oral communication.[16,45,46]

Oral and Genital Ulcerations with Immunodeficiency

The presentation of oral and genital ulcers in a newborn may be a sign of underlying congenital immunodeficiency (Fig. 25-13). In particular, ulcers in these locations appear to be a distinctive marker, and often are the presenting feature of severe combined immunodeficiency disease with T- and B-cell lymphopenia (T-B-SCID) in Athabascan-speaking American Indian infants.[47] In this population, ulcers are typically punched-out and deep, though without invasion to underlying structures, and do not result in functional sequelae or significant scarring. This is to be distinguished from the condition *neonatal noma*, which is a rare condition of preterm infants in developing countries. Neonatal noma causes aggressive, orofacial tissue gangrene, accompanied by a high mortality rate, and is most commonly associated with *Pseudomonas aueruginosa* sepsis.[48,49] In contrast, the ulcers found in American Indian children with T-B-SCID are most likely a result of T-cell immunodeficiency combined with a genetic predisposition. In such children, treatment of the underlying condition with bone marrow transplantation results in ulcer resolution. Early recognition and diagnosis can lead to prompt intervention and prevention of complications.[47]

Ectopic Thyroid Tissue

Ectopic thyroid tissue is defined by the development of thyroid tissue outside of the usual pretracheal position

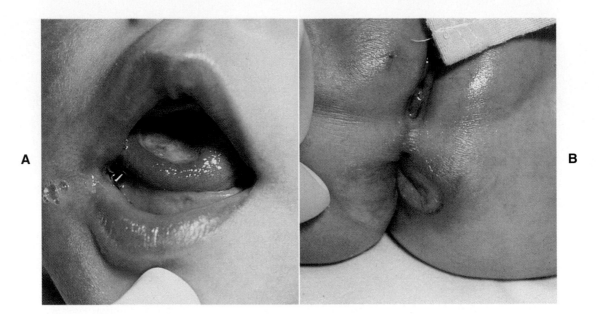

FIG. 25-13

A, Oral ulceration associated with immunodeficiency. **B,** Genital ulceration associated with immunodeficiency. (From Kwong PC, O'Marcaigh AS, Howard R, et al. Arch Dermatol 1999;135:927-931.)

(inferior to the thyroid cartilage). This abnormality results from an arrest or irregularity in thyroid descent during embryologic development. Ectopic thyroid tissue, also referred to as a thyroglossal duct cyst, may be classified as lingual, sublingual, pretracheal, or substernal. Lingual is the most common type, representing over 90% of cases. A lingual thyroglossal duct cyst presents as a painless, nodular mass in the cervical midline or at the base of the tongue between the circumvallate papillae and epiglottis. Lesions may be present at birth or develop in early infancy. However, most become evident during the first or second decade of life, at which time associated symptoms may occur.[50-53]

Thyroglossal duct cysts are a rare but serious cause of airway obstruction in newborns and infants; mortality rates of up to 43% have been reported. Though usually asymptomatic, lesions may be associated with cough, dysphagia, hemorrhage, or pain. If a cutaneous tract is present, mucous drainage can occur.

Ectopic thyroid tissue occurs in less than 1 in 100,000 to 300,000 persons. The incidence is much more common among patients with thyroid disease.[51,54] The extraglandular tissue secretes chemically normal thyroid hormone, but in quantities sometimes insufficient to meet metabolic needs. Hypothyroidism occurs in up to one third of patients; thus a serum TSH, T4 andT3 level should be performed in all suspected cases.[52] If the quan-

tity of thyroid hormone is insufficient, a compensatory increase of TSH from the anterior pituitary will lead to hypertrophy of the thyroid tissue. Thyroid hormone supplementation is indicated if clinical hypothyroidism develops, or to reduce the size of an enlarged thyroid tissue mass. Some authors suggest thyroid hormone supplementation on discovery of a thyroglossal duct cyst to prevent such complications.[52,55-58]

Surgical treatment may be necessary, particularly in cases where hemorrhage or failure of medical measures occurs. A thyroid scan preoperatively can assist in localizing the ectopic thyroid tissue. If the duct cannot be adequately excised due to size, marsupialization may be attempted.[53]

DISORDERS OF THE GENITAL MUCOUS MEMBRANES

Labial Adhesions

Labial adhesions are exceedingly rare during the newborn period. The rarity of this finding has been attributed to the presence of maternal estrogens at birth. Infants between the ages of 13 and 23 months are most commonly affected, with an incidence of 3.3%. Clinically a thin membrane extends between the labia, which may partially or completely conceal the vaginal opening. Recommended treatments include A and D ointment for asymptomatic

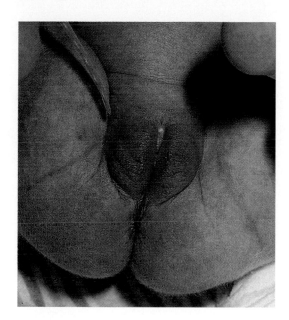

FIG. 25-14
Perianal pyramidal protrusion in a female infant.

cases, and topical estrogen cream or ointment if urinary or vaginal drainage is impaired.[59,60]

Perianal Pyramidal Protrusion

Perianal pyramidal protrusion is an increasingly recognized entity characteristically located on the perineal median raphe, anterior to the anus. Clinically the lesion is pyramidal in shape, with a smooth, red- or rose-colored surface (Fig. 25-14). The average age at presentation is 14.1 months, and 94% occur in females. Histologic examination shows epidermal acanthosis, marked edema in the upper dermis, and a mild dermal inflammatory infiltrate.[61] The pathogenesis is unknown but some cases have been related to constipation and lichen sclerosus et atrophicus.[62,63] This condition is not associated with child abuse. Differential diagnosis includes genital warts, granulomatous lesions of inflammatory bowel disease, rectal prolapse, hemorrhoids, acrochordons, and perineal midline malformation. Though most lesions show spontaneous reduction without any specific treatment, treating associated constipation may hasten resolution.[61]

Pyoderma Gangrenosum

Pyoderma gangrenosum (PG) is an ulcerative skin disorder most commonly seen on the lower legs of adults. In adults, PG is often associated with an underlying systemic disease, especially ulcerative colitis, Crohn's disease, or leukemia. The condition is rare in children (4% of cases), and rarer still in infants less than 2 years of age. Diagnosis in infancy is challenging due to the atypical location of lesions (perianal or genital) and the lack of associated systemic illness. Differential diagnosis in infancy includes ecthyma gangrenosum caused by *Pseudomonas* infection, herpes simplex infection, and severe diaper dermatitis. Successful treatment has been reported with systemic, topical, and intralesional corticosteroids.[64]

Urethral Retention Cyst

The urethral retention cyst is an inclusion cyst that forms at the urethral opening of male newborns. This lesion is simply a milium, which develops either as a result of friction or from remnants of epithelial tissue trapped along a line of skin fusion. No therapy is necessary, as the white, firm, smooth-surfaced papule will spontaneously rupture and be shed during the first weeks of life. These cysts are not likely to cause urinary retention or symptoms.[65]

DISORDERS OF THE OCULAR MUCOUS MEMBRANES

Behçet's Disease

Behçet's disease is a complex, multisystem disease characterized clinically by the presence of oral aphthae and at least two of the following: genital aphthae, synovitis, cutaneous pustular vasculitis, posterior uveitis, or meningoencephalitis.

Although uncommon, pediatric Behçet's disease does occur. Neonatal cases have been described in which affected mothers had oral and genital ulcerations during pregnancy.[66] A case of transient neonatal Behçet's disease with life-threatening complications has been reported.[67] In comparison with adults, oral and genital ulcers are less common in children with Behçet's disease. Uveitis, however, is more common. As in adults, ocular lesions in children pose a serious threat because they may lead to blindness.[68]

Colobomata

The term *coloboma* describes a defect such as a notch, gap, fissure, or hole due to the loss of ocular tissue or an ocular structure. Colobomata may occur as an isolated anomaly, but are most frequently associated with chromosomal defects, especially trisomies 13 and 18, often in association with significant central nervous system abnormalities.[69]

Infants with the CHARGE syndrome (congenital heart disease, choanal atresia, growth and/or mental retardation, genital hypoplasia, ear anomalies and/or deafness) have a 79% incidence of colobomata.[70] Colobomata may occasionally be associated with an impaired vision. Retinal colobomas are also a regular feature of the CHIME syndrome (see Chapter 16).

Congenital Obstruction of the Nasolacrimal Duct

Congenital obstruction of the nasolacrimal duct is the most common abnormality of the lacrimal system in children. Up to 6% of newborn infants are affected. Symptoms typically begin shortly after birth and are variable. Many infants will have only a wet-looking eye or overflow tearing, but most will have recurrent infections manifested by reflux or mucopurulent material from the lacrimal sac. The majority of nasolacrimal duct obstructions clear spontaneously. Simple medical management with antibiotics and massage may hasten resolution. When spontaneous resolution does not occur, ophthalmologic probing and/or irrigation may be required.[71]

Glaucoma

Glaucoma is defined as abnormal elevation of intraocular pressure, which may cause damage to the eye and changes in visual function. In infants, the principal signs of glaucoma are tearing, conjunctival hyperemia, photophobia, blepharospasm, corneal clouding, and an enlargement of the cornea and globe, referred to as *buphthalmos* (Fig. 25-15). Glaucoma in infants is usually due to a developmental disorder in which residual mesodermal tissue impedes the drainage of aqueous humor from the anterior chamber. This *primary* or *simple congenital* glaucoma is probably a multifactorial, recessively inherited condition. Other major causes of glaucoma in children are trauma, intraocular hemorrhage, ocular inflammatory disease, and intraocular tumors.

Infantile glaucoma has been associated with a variety of other ocular conditions as well as a number of systemic disorders. Those systemic disorders relevant to the dermatologist include the Sturge-Weber syndrome, neurofibromatosis, the congenital infection (TORCH) syndromes, and juvenile xanthogranulomas.

Ocular manifestations of the Sturge-Weber syndrome include a port wine stain (nevus flammeus) involving the eyelids; dilatation and tortuosity of the conjunctival, scleral, and retinal vessels; angiomatous lesions of the uveal

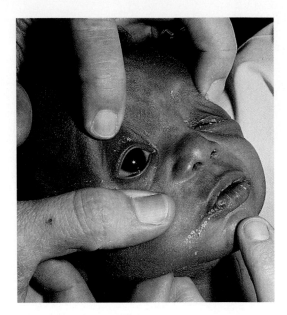

FIG. 25-15
Corneal clouding characteristic of congenital glaucoma.

tract; and glaucoma.[69] Childhood glaucoma occurs in 45% of children if both the ophthalmic and maxillary divisions of the trigeminal are involved.[72] In some children signs of glaucoma may develop later in infancy, and long-term monitoring of children at risk is advised.

Ocular manifestations associated with neurofibromatosis include plexiform neurofibromas of the eyelid (often presenting with ptosis), optic gliomas or meningiomas, pulsatile exophthalmos secondary to bony defects of the orbital wall, and Lisch nodules (yellowish-brown hamartomas of the iris). Glaucoma, most frequently unilateral, is uncommon. The mechanism of glaucoma development in neurofibromatosis is often unclear but may be associated with developmental abnormalities of the orbital tissue, plexiform neurofibromas of the eyelid, or neurofibromas of the uvea.

Children with the congenital infection (TORCH) syndromes may develop glaucoma in infancy or later in life. This occurs as a result of intraocular inflammation, except in the case of congenital rubella, in which anomalies of the optic angle have been found.

The most frequent systemic complication found in infants with multiple juvenile xanthogranulomas other than neurofibromatosis type I, is involvement of the iris and epibulbar area with this histiocytic tumor. Complications include glaucoma, hemorrhage, and blindness.[69,72]

Mucocele of the Lacrimal Sac

The mucocele of the lacrimal sac is a rare anomaly. It presents at birth or shortly thereafter as a bluish, cystic swelling located just below the medial canthus. The lesion is typically about 1 cm in diameter and may be confused with a hemangioma because of its color. Blockage of both the proximal and distal ends of the lacrimal drainage system leads to the accumulation of mucus within the lacrimal sac. The natural course is variable. In some cases the blockage may spontaneously open, but many lesions become infected and/or inflamed with erythema, edema, and surrounding cellulitis. Treatment includes gentle application of warm compresses and systemic antibiotics if infection is suspected. Mucoceles unresponsive to conservative treatment may require ophthalmologic probing.[71]

Seborrheic Blepharitis

Seborrheic blepharitis is an inflammatory condition of the eyelid margin. In infants, seborrheic blepharitis usually occurs in association with dermatitis of the scalp (termed *cradle cap*) or diaper area and is most commonly seen between the second and tenth weeks of life. The lid margins are typically erythematous and scaly with accumulation of debris at the base of the lashes. The severity of the blepharitis usually correlates with degree of dermatitis and rarely may cause a superficial, marginal keratitis.

Treatment consists of warm water compresses and gentle cleansing using a dilute amount of an isotonic (baby) shampoo. If necessary, a soft-bristled toothbrush can be used to mechanically remove the scale. A low-potency, nonfluorinated corticosteroid (hydrocortisone) or sulfacetamide ointment may then be gently massaged into the lid margin. These procedures should be repeated daily until the blepharitis has subsided.[73]

REFERENCES

1. Hurwitz S. Miscellaneous cutaneous disorders. In Clinical pediatric dermatology, 2nd edition. Philadelphia: WB Saunders, 1993: p 13.
2. Oski FA, ed. Dental problems. In Principles and practice of pediatrics. 2nd edition. Philadelphia: Lippincott, 1994: p 862.
3. Wagner AM, Hansen RC. Neonatal skin and skin disorders. In Schachner LA, Hansen RC, eds. Pediatric dermatology, 2nd edition. New York: Churchill Livingstone, 1995: pp 273-275.
4. Dilley DC, Siegel MA, Budnick S. Diagnosing and treating common oral pathologies. Pediatr Clin Noth Am 1991;38: 1227-1264.
5. Zuker RM, Buenechea R. Congenital epulis: Review of the literature and case report. J Oral Maxillofac Surg 1993;51:1040-1043.
6. Al-Qattan MM, Clarke HM. Congenital epulis: evidence against the intrauterine estrogen stimulus theory. Ann Plast Surg 1994;33:320-321.
7. Steelman R, Weisse M, Ramadan H. Congenital ranula. Clin Pediatr 1998;37:205-206.
8. Buley ID, Gatter KC, Kelly PM, et al. Granular cell tumors revisited. An immunohistochemical and ultrastructural study. Histopathology 1988;12: 263.
9. Junquera LM, deVincente JC, Vega JA, et al. Granular-cell tumours: an immunohistochemical study. Br J Oral Maxillofac Surg 1997;35:180-184.
10. Noonan JD, Horton CE, Old WL, Stokes TL. Granular cell myoblastoma of the head and neck. Am J Surg 1979;138: 611-614.
11. Peterson LJ. Granular-cell tumor: review of the literature and report of a case. Oral Surg 1974;37:728-735.
12. Robinson HBG, Miller AS, eds. Colby, Kerr and Robinson's color atlas of pathology. St Louis: Lippincott, 1990: p 149.
13. Reed RJ, Argenyi Z. Tumors of neural tissue. In Elder D, Elenitsas R, Jaworsky C, Johnson B, eds. Lever's histopathology of the skin, 8th edition. Philadelphia: Lippincott-Raven, 1997; 36:994.
14. Kershisnik M, et al. Granular cell tumors. Ann Otol Rhinol Laryngol 1994;103:416-419.
15. Weston WL, ed. Neonatal dermatology. In Color textbook of pediatric dermatology. St Louis: Mosby, 1991: pp 224 and 227.
16. Hebert AA, Berg JH. Mucous membrane disorders. In Schachner LA, Hansen RC, eds. Pediatric dermatology, 2nd edition. New York: Churchill Livingstone, 1995: pp 469-537.
17. Peters R, Schock RK. Oral cysts in newborn infants. Oral Surg 1971;7:10-14.
18. Orlow SJ, Isakoff MS, Blei F. Increased risk of symptomatic hemangiomas of the airway in association with cutaneous hemangiomas in a "beard" distribution. J Pediatr 1997;131: 643-646.
19. Frieden IJ. Which hemangiomas to treat—and how? Arch Dermatol 1997;133:1593-1595.
20. Eisen D, Lynch D: Developmental disorders. In The mouth: Diagnosis and treatment. St Louis: Mosby, 1998: p 48.
21. Shafer WG, Hine MK, Levy BM, eds. Benign and malignant tumors of the oral cavity. In A textbook of oral pathology, 4th edition. Philadelphia: WB Saunders, 1983: p 159-160.
22. Stal S, Hamilton S, Spira M. Hemangiomas, lymphangiomas, and vascular malformations of the head and neck. Otolaryngol Clin North Am 1986;19:769-884.
23. Levin SL, Jorgeson RJ, Jarvey BA. Lymphangiomas of the alveolar ridges in neonates. Pediatrics 1976;58:881-884.
24. Birrel JF, ed. Cysts, tumors, and miscellaneous conditions. In Paediatric otolaryngology. Chicago: Year Book, 1978: p 38.
25. Bordley JE, et al: Neck. In Ear, nose, and throat disorders in children. New York: Raven Press, 1986: p 392.
26. Hebert AA, Lopez MC: Oral lesions in pediatric patients. In Advances in dermatology, vol 12. St Louis: Mosby, 1997: p 181.
27. Chrysomali E, Papanicolaou SI, Dekker NP, Regezi JA. Benign neural tumors of the oral cavity. Oral Surg Oral Med Oral Pathol Oral Radiol Endod 1997;84:381-390.
28. Geist JR, Gander DL, Stefanac SJ. Oral manifestation of neurofibromatosis type I and II. Oral Surg Oral Med Oral Pathol 1992;73:376-382.

29. Grevelink SV, Mulliken JB. Vascular anomalies. In Freedberg IM, et al, eds. Fitzpatrick's dermatology in general medicine, 5th edition. New York: McGraw-Hill, 1999: pp 1175-1194.

30. Krajewska IA, Moore L, Brown LH. White sponge nevus presenting in the esophagus—case report and literature review. Pathology 1992; 24:112-115.

31. Eisen D, Lynch D: Genodermatoses. In The mouth: diagnosis and treatment. St Louis; Mosby, 1998: pp 193-194.

32. Miller CS, Craig RM. White corrugated mucosa. JADA 1988; 117:345-347.

33. Bodenhoff J. Dentitio connatalis et neonatalis. Odont Tidskr 1959;67:645-695.

34. Kates GA, Needleman HL, Holmes LB. Natal and neonatal teeth: a clinical study. JADA 1984;109:441-443.

35. Zhu J, King D. Natal and neonatal teeth. J Dent Child 1995; 3:123-128.

36. Nelson WE, ed. Disorders of the teeth associated with other conditions. In Nelson's textbook of pediatrics. Philadelphia: WB Saunders, 1996: p 1039.

37. Eichenfield LF, Honig PJ, Nelson L. Traumatic granuloma of the tongue (Riga-Fede disease): Association with familial dysautonomia. J Pediatr 1990,116:742-744.

38. Cohen RL. Clinical perspectives on premature tooth eruption and cyst formation in neonates. Pediatr Dermatol 1984;1: 301-306.

39. Shafer WG, Hine MK, Levy BM, eds. Developmental disturbance of oral and paraoral structures. In A textbook of oral pathology, 4th edition. Philadelphia: WB Saunders, 1983: p 64.

40. Iregbulem LM. Congenital lower lip sinuses in Nigerian children. Br J Plast Surg 1997;50:649-650.

41. Mohrenschlager M, Kohler LD, Vogt HJ, Ring J. Congenital lower lip pits—a very rare syndrome? Report of two cases and review of the literature. Cutis 1998;61:127-128.

42. Velez A, Gorslay M, Buchner A, et al. Congenital lower lip pits (Van der Woude Syndrome). J Am Acad Dermatol 1995;3: 520-521.

43. Amir E, et al. Physiologic pigmentation of the oral mucosa in Israeli children. Oral Surg Med Oral Pathol 1991;71:396-398.

44. Ogata M. Acatalasemia. Hum Genet 1991;86:331-340.

45. Larralde de Luna M, Raspa ML, Ibargoyen J. Oral-facial-digital type I syndrome of Papillon-Leage and Psaume. Pediatr Dermatol 1992;9:52-56.

46. Patrizi A, Orlandi C, Neri I, et al. What syndrome is this? Oral-Facial-Digital Type I. Pediatr Dermatol 1999;16:329-331.

47. Kwong PC, O'Marcaigh AS, Howard R, et al. Oral and genital ulceration: a unique presentation of immunodeficiency in Athabascan-speaking American Indian children with severe combined immunodeficiency. Arch Dermatol 1999; 135:927-31.

48. Ghosal SP, Gupta PC, Muhherjee AK. Noma neonatorum: Its aetiopathogenesis. Lancet 1978;2:289-290.

49. Juster-Reicher A, Mogilner BM, Levi G, et al. Neonatal noma. Am J Perinatol 1993;10:409-411.

50. Damiano A, Glickman AB, Rubin JS, Cohen AF. Ectopic thyroid tissue presenting as a midline neck mass. Int J Pediatr Otorhinolaryngol 1996;34:141-148.

51. Krishnamurthy GT, Bajd WH. Lingual thyroid associated with Zenker's and vallecular diverticula: report of a case and review of the literature. Arch Otolaryngol 1972;96:171-175.

52. Leung AK, Wong AL, Robson WL. Ectopic thyroid gland simulating a thyroglossal duct cyst: a case report. Can J Surg 1995;38:87-89.

53. Fanaroff AA, Martin RJ, eds. The respiratory system. In Neonatal-perinatal medicine: diseases of the fetus and infant. vol 2. St Louis: Mosby, 1997: p 1068.

54. Temmel AF, Baumgartner WD, Steiner E, et al. Ectopic thyroid gland simulating a submandibular tumor. Am J Otolaryngol 1998;19:342-344.

55. Neinas, FW, Gorman CA, Devine KD, Woolner LB. Lingual thyroid: clinical characteristics of 15 cases. Ann Int Med 1973;79:205-210.

56. Hulse JA, Grant DB, Clayton BE, et al. Population screening for congenital hypothyroidism. Br Med J 1980;280:675-678.

57. Jones JA. Lingual thyroid. Br J Oral Maxillofac Surg 1986; 24:58-62.

58. Kansal P, Sakati N, Rifai A, Woodhouse N. Lingual thyroid: diagnosis and treatment. Arch Intern Med 1987;147:2046-2048.

59. Leung AK, Robson WL, Tay-Uyboco J. The incidence of labial fusion in children. J Paediatr Child Health 1993;29:235-236.

60. Starr NB. Labial adhesions in childhood. J Paediatr Child Health 1996;10:26-27.

61. Kayashima K, Kitoh M, Ono T. Infantile perianal pyramidal protrusion. Arch Dermatol 1996;132:1481-1484.

62. Merigou D, Labreze C, Lamireau T, et al. Infantile perianal pyramidal protrusion: A marker of constipation? Pediatr Dermatol 1998;15:143-144.

63. Cruces MJ, DeLaTorre C, Losada A, et al. Infantile pyramidal protrusion as a manifestation of lichen sclerosus et atrophicus. Arch Dermatol 1998;134:1118-1120.

64. Graham JA, Hansen KK, Rabinowitz LG, Esterly NB. Pyoderma gangrenosum in infants and children. Pediatr Dermatol 1994;11:10-17.

65. Yaffe D, Zissin R. Cowper's glands duct: radiographic findings. Urol Radiol 1991;13:123-125.

66. Fain O, Mathieu E, Lachassinne E, et al. Neonatal Behçet's disease. Am J Med 1995;98:310-311.

67. Stark AC, Bhakta B, Chamberlain MA, et al. Life threatening transient neonatal Behçet's disease. J Rheumatol 1997;36: 700-702.

68. Kaklamani V, Vaiopoulos G, Kaklamanis PG. Behçet's Disease. Sem Arth Rheum 1998;27:197-217.

69. Martyn LJ, DiGeorge A. Pediatric ophthalmology. Pediatr Clin North Am 1987;34;1530-1536.

70. Tellier AL, Cormier-Daire V, Abadie V, et al. CHARGE syndrome: Report of 47 cases and review. Am J Med Genet 1998;76:402-409.

71. Calhoun JH. Problems of the lacrimal system in children. Pediatr Clin North Am 1987;34:1457-1465.

72. Stevenson RF, Thomson HG, Marin JD: Unrecognized ocular problems associated with port-wine stain of the face in children. Can Med Assoc J 1974;111:953-954.

73. Hurwitz S: Eczematous eruptions in childhood. In Clinical pediatric dermatology, 2nd edition. Philadelphia: WB Saunders, 1993: p 62.

26

Hair Disorders

MAUREEN ROGERS

This chapter covers neonatal hair patterns, genetic hair shaft abnormalities, and the conditions in which hypotrichosis or hypertrichosis are present in the neonatal period. There are many syndromes in which hypotrichosis or atrichia occur, and those in which it is a prominent feature are discussed. Localized alopecia can occur physiologically, with trauma, and as a nevoid disorder, alone or associated with other nevi. Diffuse hypertrichosis can occur alone or as part of various syndromes. Localized hypertrichosis may occur with other nevi, but also may be a marker for serious neural tube closure defects.

SCALP HAIR WHORLS

Ninety-five to ninety-eight percent of normal Caucasian infants have a single hair whorl in the parietal area,[1,2] usually clockwise but inconsistent in position. The remainder have a double parietal whorl. Only 10% of African-American individuals with short curly hair have a parietal whorl.[2] A mild frontal upsweep or "cowlick" is present in 7% of normal infants.[1] Hair patterns may be very abnormal in infants with structural abnormalities of the brain, demonstrating a striking frontal upsweep and absent or aberrant parietal whorls.[1] Multiple parietal whorls occur with increased frequency in developmentally delayed children and their presence in the neonate may be an early dysmorphic sign.[3]

THE HAIRLINE

The frontal hairline of neonates is lower than in older children, a feature most striking in racial groups in which there is profuse hair at birth. These terminal hairs on the brow are gradually replaced by vellus hairs over the first 12 months of life. Displacement of the hairline may be a

dysmorphic feature. A low frontal hairline is a feature of several syndromes, including Costello, Cornelia de Lange (Brachmann–de Lange), Coffin Siris, Fanconi, and fetal hydantoin syndromes. The syndromes in which a low posterior hairline occurs include Noonan, Turner, Kabuki, Cornelia de Lange, and fetal hydantoin syndromes.

HETEROCHROMIA OF SCALP HAIR

This may be noted at birth as a result of several clinical situations.[4] In piebaldism there is a white forelock, which will be obvious in a dark-haired neonate. A congenital melanocytic nevus may present as a tuft of dark hair, which is often also longer than the surrounding normal hair. In hereditary, usually autosomal dominant, heterochromia there may be, for example, a tuft of red hair in a dark-haired neonate or a dark tuft in a fair individual. There has been a recent report of a diffuse heterochromia of scalp hair, present from birth, with black and red hairs evenly distributed over the scalp.[4]

HAIR SHAFT ABNORMALITIES

These conditions have been reviewed in detail by Whiting,[5] Price,[6] and Rogers.[7,8]

Monilethrix

Monilethrix is an autosomal dominant condition producing a beaded appearance of the hair.[5-8] On microscopy, spindle-shaped "nodes" separated by constricted internodes are seen (Fig. 26-1). The nodes have the diameter of normal hair and may be medullated, whereas the internodes are narrower and usually non-medullated and are the sites of fracture.

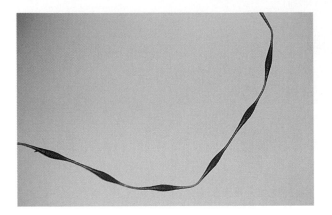

FIG. 26-1
Monilethrix: microscopic appearance.

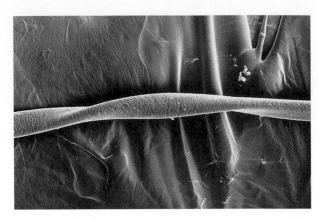

FIG. 26-3
Pili torti: electron microscopic appearance.

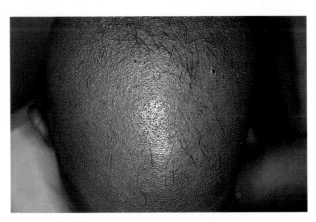

FIG. 26-2
Monilethrix: follicular plugging and short, broken hairs.

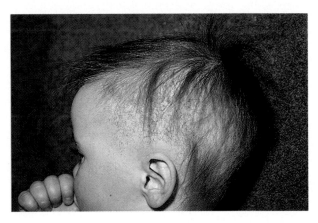

FIG. 26-4
Pili torti in Menkes syndrome.

Recently the condition has been mapped to the type II hair cortex keratin gene cluster.[9,10] However, the exclusion of these candidate genes in one family suggests the possibility of genetic heterogeneity.[11] The hair is usually normal at birth but is replaced within weeks by affected hairs that are dry, dull and brittle, breaking spontaneously, leaving a stublelike appearance (Fig. 26-2). The hairs may break almost flush with the scalp or may attain lengths of 0.5 to 2.5 cm, or occasionally longer. Follicular keratosis is commonly associated and may involve the scalp, face and limbs.

Pili Torti

This is characterized by groups of three or four regularly spaced twists of the hair shaft on its own axis (Fig. 26-3).[6-8] Microscopically, twists are seen, each 0.4 to 0.9 mm in width, occurring usually in groups of 3 or more at irregular intervals. Twists are almost always through 180 degrees, although some are through 90 or 360 degrees. The hair shaft is somewhat flattened. Pili torti may occur as an isolated phenomenon with the onset at birth or in the early months of life. The hair is usually fairer than expected and is spangled, dry, and brittle, breaking at different lengths (Fig. 26-4). It may stand out from the scalp and tends to be short, especially in areas subject to trauma.

Pili torti occurs as a feature of other defined syndromes, some of which are identifiable in the neonatal period. Menkes syndrome is an X-linked recessive condition due to mutations in a gene encoding for a protein believed to be a copper-transporting P-type ATP-ase,[12] and the multiple abnormalities are due to decreased bioavailability of copper with resultant functional deficiencies of copper-dependent

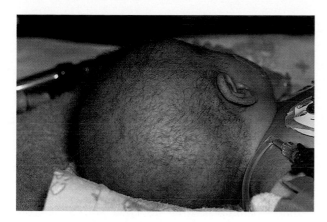

FIG. 26-5
Pili torti in Crandall syndrome.

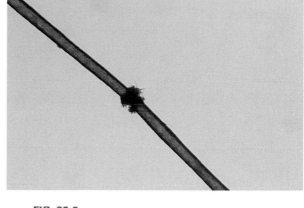

FIG. 26-6
Trichorrhexis nodosa: light microscopic appearance.

enzymes. In the early months of life, scalp and eyebrow hair becomes kinky, coarse, and sparse. Lax, pale skin, hypotonia, and early neurodegenerative changes may already be seen in the neonatal period. In Bazex syndrome, inherited as an X-linked dominant trait,[13] congenital hypotrichosis with pili torti is associated with follicular atrophoderma and multiple facia milia, both of which may also be present from birth. These patients have an increased susceptibility to development of basal cell carcinomas. In Crandall syndrome, congenital hypotrichosis with pili torti is associated with sensorineural deafness and hypopituitarism (Fig 26-5).[14] Pili torti may occur also in Rapp-Hodgkin syndrome, although pili canaliculi is the more characteristic finding.

Trichorrhexis Nodosa

The term *trichorrhexis nodosa* refers to the light microscopic appearance of a fracture with splaying out and release of individual cortical cells from the main body of the hair shaft, producing an appearance suggestive of the ends of two brushes pushed together (Fig. 26-6).[5-8] When the break occurs, the brushlike end is clearly seen. Electron microscopy shows the disrupted cuticle and splaying of cortical cells. The defect renders the hair very fragile, and it breaks readily with trauma or sometimes probably spontaneously. In congenital trichorrhexis nodosa, the hair is usually normal at birth but is replaced within a few months with abnormal, fragile hair.

Trichothiodystrophy

The term *trichothiodystrophy* refers to the sulfur-deficient brittle hair that is a marker for a neuroectodermal symptom complex occurring in a group of autosomal recessive

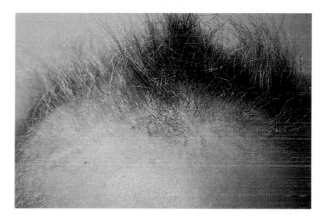

FIG. 26-7
Short, broken, dull hair in trichothiodystrophy.

genetic disorders.[15] Named syndromes that fit into this spectrum include Tay syndrome, Pollitt syndrome, Sabinas brittle hair syndrome, and Marinesco Sjögren syndrome. The words describing the various clinical features of the condition have lead to other mnemonic names, including BIDS, IBIDS, and PIBIDS.[16] The major clinical features seen in this group of conditions are brittle hair, ichthyosis, short stature, decreased fertility, intellectual impairment, photosensitivity with a DNA repair defect (due to mutations in the XPD ECCR2 DNA repair/transcription gene),[17,18] and osteosclerosis. Features that may be evident in the neonatal period are intrauterine growth retardation, severe infections, congenital cataracts, nail dystrophy, facial dysmorphism, a collodion baby phenotype, and the characteristic fragile, dull, short, disordered hair involving scalp hair, eyebrows, and eyelashes (Fig. 26-7).[19,20]

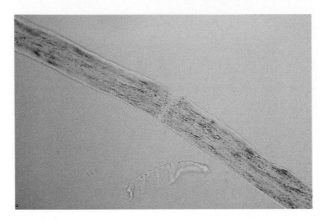

FIG. 26-8
Trichoschisis in trichothiodystrophy: light microscopic appearance.

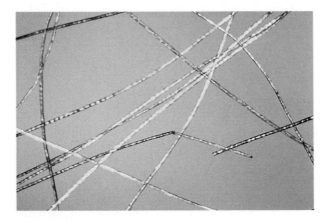

FIG. 26-9
"Tiger tail" appearance of light and dark bands on polarizing microscopy of hair in trichothiodystrophy.

On light microscopy, the hair has a wavy, irregular outline and a flattened shaft in which twists like a folded ribbon occur. Two types of fracture are seen—an atypical trichorrhexis nodosa and trichoschisis, a clean, transverse fracture (Fig. 26-8). Using crossed polarizers, light and dark bands are seen when the hair is aligned in one of the polarizer directions, the so-called tiger-tail appearance (Fig. 26-9). This may be absent at birth and is not fully developed until 3 months of age.[21] Scanning electron microscopy shows irregular ridging and fluting and a disordered, reduced or absent cuticle scale pattern.

Woolly Hair

This is tight, curly hair, differing considerably from other areas of scalp hair and that of family members. It is usu-

ally abnormal from birth. Fragility of the hair is rarely significant in this condition. A wide variety of changes are described in shaft cross-sectional shape, follicle morphology and cuticular appearance on scanning electron microscopy. The pathogenesis is unclear and may vary case to case. There are three main groups, two diffuse and inherited, one autosomal recessive, and one autosomal dominant and one localized and sporadic, the woolly hair nevus. The condition is important to define early because there are many associations. Diffuse woolly hair has been associated with ocular abnormalities, some present at birth,[22] keratosis pilaris atrophicans,[23] Noonan syndrome,[23] palmoplantar keratoderma, and cardiac conduction defects,[24] giant axonal neuropathy,[25] and primary osteoma cutis.[26] Woolly hair nevus has been associated with ocular abnormalities[22] and epidermal nevi, usually away from the site of the woolly hair nevus and sometimes quite extensive.[27]

Uncombable Hair

This is a condition defined by its clinical features.[6-8] Synonyms are spun glass hair, pili canaliculi, and pili trianguli et canaliculi. In the classical clinical form, the hair is a light silvery-blond, paler than expected. It is frizzy, stands away from the scalp and cannot be combed flat. It is often "spangled" or glistening. It is usually normal in length, quantity and tensile strength. The onset may be with the first terminal growth or later. Eyebrows, lashes, and body hair are normal. There are reports suggesting both dominant and recessive inheritance patterns. Scanning electron microscopy best demonstrates the characteristic shallow grooving or flattening of the surface.[28] These areas are often discontinuous and change orientation many times along the length of the hair, occurring on different faces of the hair at different points. Cross-sectional microscopy shows triangular, reniform, and other unusual shapes. It is now clear that longitudinal grooving of hair shafts and/or irregular cross-section is not specific for the clinical entity of uncombable hair. It has been demonstrated in a variety of other syndromes with congenital onset, including progeria, Marie Unna hypotrichosis,[29] Rapp-Hodgkin syndrome,[30] oral-facial digital syndrome type I,[31] ectrodactyly ectodermal dysplasia and clefting syndrome,[31] and hypohidrotic ectodermal dysplasia.[31] The classical clinical appearance of spun glass or uncombable hair would seem to depend on the proportion of abnormal hairs. The typical spangled appearance is usually found in patients with no other abnormalities, but has been seen in patients with Rapp-Hodgkin syndrome[30] and in hypohidrotic ectodermal dysplasia.[32]

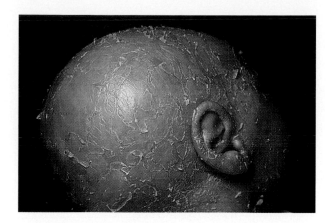

FIG. 26-10
Absence of scalp hair and erythroderma in a neonate with Netherton syndrome.

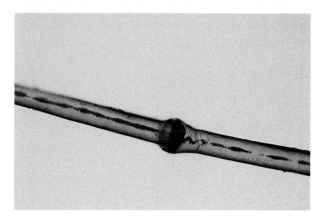

FIG. 26-11
Trichorrhexis invaginata in Netherton syndrome; light microscopic appearance.

Pili Annulati

This hair shaft abnormality, which may be present at birth, does not render the hair fragile. The hair looks pleasantly shiny, and on close observation, alternating bright and dark bands are seen. There are usually no associated abnormalities. The condition may be sporadic or inherited, usually as a dominant characteristic. The bright areas are due to light scattered from clusters of air filled cavities within the cortex, and in a hair mount, viewed with transmitted light, the light areas appear as dark patches. Scanning electron microscopy shows longitudinal wrinkling and folding in bands corresponding to the abnormal areas, possibly due to the evaporation of air in the spaces when the hair is coated in the vacuum. Transmission electron microscopy demonstrates multiple holes within the cortex.

Trichorrhexis Invaginata

This is the characteristic hair shaft abnormality of **Netherton syndrome,** and although the severity varies considerably, the clinical and microscopic findings are present from birth. In the severely affected neonate, the hair may be extremely sparse or even absent altogether (Fig. 26-10). What hair is present is short and dull and breaks easily. The changes may affect eyebrows, eyelashes, and general body hair as well.

Microscopically, a ball and socket configuration with various patterns is seen (Fig. 26-11). The classical "bamboo hair" occurs when the soft abnormal hair shaft wraps around a firmer distal shaft, producing the appearance of a shallow invagination of the distal into the proximal shaft. There is a tuliplike form with a deeper invagination and longer sides of the "cup."[6] Circumferential strictures

may be found, representing the earliest stage of the invagination. The term *golf-tee hair* has been given to the expanded proximal end of an invaginate node after a break has occurred.[33] Thin vellus hairs may show multiple invaginations, the so-called "canestick hairs."[34] A helical pattern of twisting with obliquely running parallel invaginations has recently been described.[35]

DIFFUSE ALOPECIA OR HYPOTRICHOSIS (Box 26-1)

Hypotrichosis With Hair Shaft Abnormalities

As discussed in the previous section, many hair shaft abnormalities present in the neonatal period or in early infancy with significant hypotrichosis.

Isolated Congenital Alopecia or Hypotrichosis Without Other Defects

There appear to be several distinct genotypes within this group, with recessive, dominant, and X-linked inheritance patterns being represented.[36-40] Those with recessive inheritance are in general the most severe and of congenital onset. In some pedigrees, there is total absence of hair (congenital atrichia, atrichia congenita) and on biopsy no hair follicles are found. In others, the hair is present but extremely sparse (congenital hypotrichosis), with biopsy demonstrating a few scattered, miniaturized follicles occurring in decreased numbers. In most cases, the condition involves eyebrow, eyelash, and general body hair as well. In one family with recessive inheritance the gene has been mapped to chromosome 8p.[40]

Diffuse Alopecia or Hypotrichosis

Hypotrichosis with major hair shaft abnormalities
Congenital alopecia or hypotrichosis without
    other defects
    Atrichia congenita
    Congenital hypotrichosis
Marie Unna hypotrichosis
Atrichia with papular lesions
Congenital hypotrichosis and milia
Hypotrichosis in ectodermal dysplasias
    Hidrotic ectodermal dysplasia
    Hypohidrotic ectodermal dysplasia
    Ankyloblepharon ectodermal dysplasia and cleft-
        ing syndrome and Rapp-Hodgkin syndrome
    Bazex-Dupre-Christol syndrome
    Congenital atrichia with nail dystrophy, abnor-
        mal facies and retarded psychomotor
        development
Hypotrichosis with ichthyoses
    Ichthyoses presenting as the collodion baby
        phenotype
    Congenital ichthyosis, follicular atrophoderma,
        hypotrichosis and hypohidrosis
    Ichthyosis follicularis, congenital atrichia and
        photophobia
    Keratitis, ichthyosis and deafness syndrome
Hypotrichosis with premature aging syndromes
Hypotrichosis with immunodeficiency syndromes

Marie Unna Hypotrichosis

The hair in this autosomal dominant condition is usually sparse or absent at birth,[41] but it is not until early childhood that the characteristic coarse, wiry hair appears, showing longitudinal ridging and irregularly distributed twisting on scanning electron microscopy. Histopathology demonstrates multiple small hair follicles appearing to bud from scalp epidermis and from the outer root sheath of the few normal follicles present.[42]

Atrichia With Papular Lesions

This is a distinctive association of congenital atrichia and tiny, white papules.[43-45] Atrichia of the scalp may be present from birth or appear in early childhood. In most cases, fetal hair is shed in the first 3 months of life and never replaced;[46] eyebrows and eyelashes may or may not be involved. The papular lesions, which occur diffusely but predominate on the face and scalp, are not present in the

neonatal period. A recent histopathologic study[45] showed the papules to represent keratin-filled follicular cysts in contact with the overlying epidermis. The bald scalp showed tubular epithelial structures devoid of hair bulbs, but demonstrating sebaceous and outer root sheath differentiation, extending from the epidermis to the deep dermis, resembling epidermoid cysts. Recent work has demonstrated molecular homologies between the mutated gene in these patients and the mouse hairless gene.[47,48] In the mice carrying this mutation, a very similar clinical picture occurs with hair shed at about two weeks of age and not replaced, and cystic structures developing in the superficial and deep dermis.[48]

Congenital Hypotrichosis and Milia

In this condition, which bears some clinical similarity to atrichia with papular lesions, there is hypotrichosis with sparse, coarse hair and multiple milia are present at birth on the face and sometimes also the limbs and trunk. Study of a large pedigree suggests X-linked dominant inheritance.[49]

Hypotrichosis With Ectodermal Dysplasias

Hypotrichosis is an important feature in many syndromes but becomes obvious only after the neonatal period. A selection of conditions in which there may be congenital severe hypotrichosis or atrichia will be considered here.

Hidrotic Ectodermal Dysplasia

Hypotrichosis of a variable and sometimes very severe degree of scalp hair, eyebrows, eyelashes, and body hair is usually present at birth.[50,51] Any hair present is fine and fragile. Later significant features are leukoplakia, nail dystrophy, and palmoplantar keratoderma.

Hypohidrotic Ectodermal Dysplasia

Marked hypotrichosis of all hair-bearing areas may be evident in the neonatal period; hair that is present is fine and fair and often shows pili canaliculi on microscopy. Other features that may be evident in the neonatal period include impaired heat regulation, diffuse scaling of skin, hypoplastic or absent nipples, and the typical facies with a depressed nasal bridge and prominent brow.[52]

Ankyloblepharon, Ectodermal Dysplasia and Clefting Syndrome (AEC, Hay-Wells) and Rapp-Hodgkin Syndrome

At birth in the ankyloblepharon, ectodermal dysplasia, and clefting syndrome (AEC, Hay-Wells) the scalp is usually red and scaly with extensive erosions and crusts and there is a severe hypotrichosis.[53] Other neonatal features include a generalized erythroderma with or without erosive lesions, ankyloblepharon filiforme, lacrimal duct atresia, cleft palate and lip, and hypoplastic nails. It seems very likely that Rapp-Hodgkin syndrome[54,55] and AEC syndromes are variable expressions of the same entity with reported cases of Rapp-Hodgkin syndrome sharing all the features of AEC apart from the ankyloblepharon.[56]

Bazex-Dupre-Christol Syndrome
The main features of this probable X-linked dominant condition are congenital hypotrichosis, milia with onset in the first 3 months of life, later appearance of follicular atrophoderma as the milia are shed, and early development of basal cell carcinomas.[13] Microscopic hair shaft examination may show trichorrhexis nodosa and an irregular twisting.

Congenital Atrichia With Nail Dystrophy, Abnormal Facies, and Retarded Psychomotor Development
In this condition, after the shedding in the first weeks of life of an initial sparse cover of hair, there is almost total alopecia with only tiny vellus hairs being evident; scalp biopsy demonstrates atrophy of hair follicles with rudimentary hair shafts.[57] Nail dystrophy and an abnormal facies with a broad nasal bridge, hypertelorism, a broad nose, and a long philtrum are other congenital features.

Hypotrichosis With Ichthyoses

Ichthyoses Presenting as the Collodion Baby Phenotype
The hair is often either absent or shed in the early weeks of life with the collodion scale in this group of conditions, which includes autosomal recessive and autosomal dominant forms of lamellar ichthyosis (Fig. 26-12), congenital ichthyosiform erythroderma and lamellar ichthyosis of the newborn (self-healing collodion baby).

Congenital Ichthyosis, Follicular Atrophoderma, Hypotrichosis and Hypohidrosis
This combination of traits has been described as a new autosomal recessive genodermatosis.[58] Hypotrichosis of scalp, eyebrows, and eyelashes is evident in the neonatal period, and the ichthyosis and follicular atrophoderma are both also congenital.

Ichthyosis Follicularis, Congenital Atrichia and Photophobia
From birth these individuals demonstrate keratotic follicular papules, atrichia, or severe hypotrichosis and photophobia.[59,60] The reports in some cases of other features such as periorificial erosions and plaques, nail dystrophy,

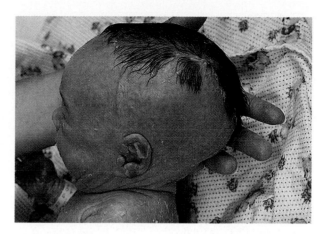

FIG. 26-12
Alopecia in neonate with lamellar ichthyosis.

gingival erythema, and recurrent infections suggest that this condition and hereditary mucoepithelial dysplasia, which demonstrates the same congenital features,[61] may be the same condition.[62]

Keratitis, Ichthyosis and Deafness Syndrome
Severe hypotrichosis of scalp, eyebrows, and eyelashes may be evident at birth. Other congenital features include spiny follicular plugs, perioral furrowing, reticulate hyperkeratosis of the palms and soles, widespread thickened erythematous plaques, and hearing loss.[63]

Hypotrichosis With Premature Aging Syndromes

Although the onset of obvious hypotrichosis is often delayed until several years of age in these conditions, in some cases of Hutchison-Gilford progeria, Cockayne syndrome, and Rothmund Thomson syndrome, sparse hair is evident in early infancy. A severe neonatal progeroid syndrome has been described, which may be a separate entity, in which sparse anterior scalp hair, thin eyebrows, and absent eyelashes were evident at birth, along with redundant skin, absent subcutaneous fat, and prominent blood vessels.[64]

Hypotrichosis With Immunodeficiency Syndromes

In cartilage hair hypoplasia syndrome, sparsity of scalp, eyebrow, and eyelash hair is often evident in the neonatal period together with short limbs and prenatal growth failure.[65] Alopecia is also often a striking feature of a heterogeneous group of congenital immunodeficiency conditions presenting with erythroderma, failure to thrive, and diarrhea in early infancy, which includes Omenn syndrome and severe combined immunodeficiency-associated congenital graft-versus-host disease.[66-68]

LOCALIZED ALOPECIA (Box 26-2)

Trauma

Alopecia in the neonatal period may occur in areas of scalp damaged by instrumentation such as forceps, scalp monitors, and vacuum extractor, and also over cephalohematomas (see Chapter 8).

Neonatal Occipital Alopecia

A well-defined patch of alopecia commonly develops in the occipital area in the early months of life (Fig. 26-13). This has been attributed entirely to rubbing the back of the head on the bedding surface. It is explained more fully by an understanding of the patterns of hair cycle evolution in fetal and early neonatal life.[69] By 20 weeks' gestation there are well-developed hair follicles containing anagen hairs all over the scalp. Although the hair roots enter catagen and then telogen in a progressive manner from frontal to parietal areas at 26 to 28 weeks' gestation, the roots in the occipital area remain in anagen until around the time of birth when they abruptly enter telogen. These hairs inevitably fall 8 to 12 weeks later. Often there are considerable numbers of hairs in the parietal area still in telogen at birth, and a more extensive post-natal alopecia can occur, leaving hair only on the vertex. In children with a dark complexion there is a delay in onset of the changes, most roots are still in anagen at birth, and the mean diameter of the hairs is greater than in fair-complexioned neonates.[70] For these reasons the hair is often prolific at a time when the fair neonates are developing significant alopecia.

Triangular Alopecia

This noncicatricial circumscribed area of hypotrichosis is triangular or lance-shaped[71] and is positioned in the frontotemporal area, with the base facing the temporal edge of the hairline but sometimes separated from it by a small fringe of normal hair. In a recent study of 6200 randomly selected individuals, the condition was identified in 7 cases (0.11%).[72] Triangular alopecia is unilateral in 80% of cases. It is a hypotrichosis rather than a true alopecia because vellus hairs are present in the affected area.[71] Occasionally a few terminal hairs are retained.[71,73] It is possible that it represents a mosaic disorder. Histopathologic examination of transverse sections of a biopsy specimen demonstrates that the majority of follicles are vellus; a normal number of follicles is present, but the follicular size is abnormal for the scalp.[71] The condition certainly may be congenital and may be noted in the neonatal period in infants with abundant scalp hair, in whom it is often erroneously ascribed to forceps trauma. Whether it is always congenital is disputed.[71]

BOX 26-2

Localized Alopecia

Trauma
Neonatal occipital alopecia
Triangular alopecia
With other nevoid conditions
    Aplastic nevus
    Sebaceous nevus
    Congenital melanocytic nevus
    Meningocele, encephalocele, heterotopic
        meningeal and brain tissue
    Aplasia cutis
Alopecia areata
Localized alopecia as part of syndromes
    Hallermann-Streiff syndrome
    X-linked dominant conditions

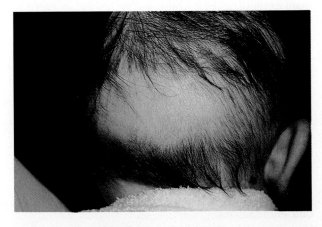

FIG. 26-13
Neonatal occipital alopecia.

Localized Alopecia Associated With Other Nevoid Conditions

Aplastic Nevus (Minus Nevus)
This is a nevoid condition in which there is a complete absence of skin appendages in an area of otherwise normal skin.[74]

Sebaceous Nevus
These nevi are characteristically hairless. Sometimes the nevus is so flat and subtle that it is only recognized as such later, and the presentation is as a patch of congenital alopecia.

Congenital Melanocytic Nevus
These lesions are usually associated with hypertrichosis, but large, folded lesions on the scalp causing a cutis verticis gyrata appearance may have sparse covering hair.

Cranial Meningoceles, Encephaloceles and Heterotopic Meningeal or Brain Tissue
These present characteristically as tumors or cysts that are either hairless or have sparse overlying hair. There is often a surrounding collar of long hair (see the following discussion).

Alopecia Areata

This condition is very rarely encountered in early infancy, and until recently the earliest documented case had its onset at 2 weeks of age.[75] De Viragh et al[76] have now reported a case in which a patch of alopecia was present at birth in a premature infant. A biopsy specimen obtained at 14 months of age showed the typical histology of alopecia areata with miniaturized anagen follicles with a dense peribulbar lymphocytic infiltrate. The condition subsequently appeared to respond to topical corticosteroid and minoxidil 2% solution.

Localized Alopecia Associated With Syndromes

Hallermann Streiff Syndrome
The hair may be normal at birth, but in some cases the typical alopecia, located in the frontal and parietal areas over the cranial sutures, may be evident in early months together with atrophic facial skin and multiple craniofacial and ocular abnormalities.[77]

X-linked Dominant Conditions
Several rare syndromes, caused by X-linked dominant genes that interfere with hair growth, produce a mosaic pattern of alopecia in affected females as a result of functional X-chromosome mosaicism.[78] The hemizygous males with these conditions rarely survive. The conditions include incontinentia pigmenti, focal dermal hypoplasia (Goltz syndrome), X-linked dominant chondrodysplasia punctata, oral-facial digital syndrome, and CHILD syndrome. The alopecia in these conditions has a patchy distribution, sometimes obviously linear or spiral as it follows the lines of Blaschko.[78]

DIFFUSE HYPERTRICHOSIS (Box 26-3)

Primary Hypertrichosis

There is much confusion about congenital hypertrichosis occurring alone or with only occasional associations, because of the wide variety of designations given and the poor clinical descriptions in the early literature. Baumeister et al[79] have attempted to clarify the classification, but confusion persists. However several individual entities can probably be separated out.

BOX 26-3

Diffuse Hypertrichosis

Primary hypertrichosis
    Hypertrichosis lanuginosa
    Ambras syndrome
    Prepubertal hypertrichosis
    X-linked hypertrichosis
Hypertrichosis as part of other genetically determined disorders
    Hypertrichosis with gingival fibromatosis
    Hypertrichosis with osteochondrodysplasia
    Hypertrichosis, pigmentary retinopathy and facial anomalies
    Coffin-Siris syndrome
    Cornelia de Lange syndrome
    Leprechaunism
    Seip-Berardinelli syndrome (congenital generalized lipodystrophy)
    Rubinstein-Taybi syndrome
    Barber-Say syndrome
Drug-induced hypertrichosis
    Fetal alcohol syndrome
    Maternal minoxidil
    Diazoxide

Hypertrichosis Lanuginosa

This rare condition is characterized by retention of lanugo hair, and the infant is born with a coat of profuse, long, fair, silky, fine hair affecting all the usual hair bearing areas of skin.[80-83] It may reach 10 cm in length and blends with the terminal hair of scalp and eyebrows (Fig. 26-14). There may be accentuation in certain areas, particularly over the spine and on the pinnae. Profuse growth in the ear may lead to infection and reduced hearing and need to be cleared. Matted hair in the diaper area is particularly troublesome, and shaving of this and other areas may be indicated.[84] The outcome is variable, with many authors reporting improvement,[83,84] whereas others report persistence or even worsening. At puberty there may be no conversion to terminal hair in secondary sexual hair areas with long, fine, lanugo hairs growing in beard, pubic, and axillary areas. Although about one third of cases are sporadic, autosomal dominant inheritance is well-established;[80,81] a single family with possible autosomal recessive inheritance is reported.[82] Most patients are free of other abnormalities, but congenital glaucoma[83] and dental abnormalities,[81,84] including neonatal teeth,[84] have been observed.

Prepubertal Hypertrichosis

A series is reported of otherwise healthy children, with no clinical evidence of endocrinopathy, but generalized hyper-

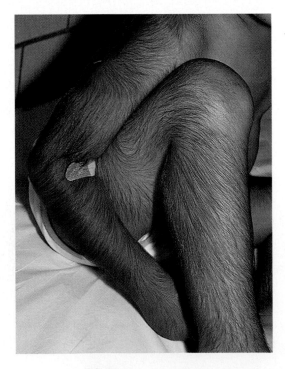

FIG. 26-14
Hypertrichosis lanuginosa

trichosis present from birth and increasing in severity in early childhood. There is terminal hair growth on the temples, spreading across the brow and merging with bushy eyebrows and also profusely on the back and proximal limbs.[85] The pattern does not resemble hirsutism. There was a patterning of the hair growth on the back with an inverted fir tree distribution centering on the spine. It is not clear whether this represents an abnormality or whether it is an extreme form of the normal range of hair growth, resembling as it does the patterns of hair growth seen regularly in some racial groups.[85] However, a recent study has demonstrated elevated plasma dihydrotestosterone levels in several patients, suggesting that an endocrine abnormality may indeed be the basis for this condition.[86]

X-Linked Dominant Hypertrichosis

A pedigree has been reported with probable X-linked dominant inheritance in whose affected members there was generalized terminal hair hypertrichosis present at birth.[87] The involvement was most severe over the face, pubic area, back, and upper chest. There may be an improvement on the trunk and limbs after puberty. This condition has recently been mapped to chromosome Xq24-q27.1.[88]

Ambras Syndrome

Baumeister et al[89] have delineated what they regard as a unique form of diffuse congenital hypertrichosis, which has been previously reported under a variety of names, and have demonstrated a balanced structural chromosomal aberration in a patient with this condition. It has been designated Ambras syndrome in reference to the first documented case. The hair, which may demonstrate pigmentation and medullation, is said to be vellus rather than lanugo hair, which is nonpigmented and nonmedullated. The hypertrichosis is most marked on face, ears, and shoulders and persists through life. A number of dysmorphic facial features have occurred in these patients.

Hypertrichosis as Part of Other Genetically Determined Disorders

Many syndromes have hypertrichosis as a feature, and in some of these it is present in the neonatal period. A selection of these conditions is considered here.

Hypertrichosis With Gingival Fibromatosis

Congenital hypertrichosis may occur in patients with the inherited condition of gingival fibromatosis,[90] but it is usually relatively mild. However, several patients have been reported with severe hypertrichosis in association with gingival fibromatosis and epilepsy.[91] Most cases are familial, and while some heterogeneity is postulated, the inheritance is usually autosomal dominant. The gingival fibromatosis in this condition usually presents in the second decade but has been reported in infancy. The hypertrichosis is congenital, and the hair varies from fine to coarse and is pigmented. The face, arms, and lumbosacral area are affected most severely. It is possible, however, that these conditions are within a single spectrum.[90] Further overlap is suggested with the Laband syndrome of gingival hyperplasia, dysplasia of the terminal phalanges, hepatosplenomegaly, and facial dysmorphism, with the recent report of marked congenital hypertrichosis as an additional feature in one patient.[92]

Hypertrichosis With Osteochondrodysplasia

This is a rare autosomal recessive syndrome in which congenital macrosomia and cardiomegaly, which may be present at birth, are additional features.[93-95] The hypertrichosis is diffuse. The hair may be fine initially but after several months becomes thicker and more profuse. The radiologic changes include the following:

- A wide posterior cranial fossa
- Verticalized base of the cranium
- Narrow thorax
- Broad ribs
- Coxa valga
- Short distal phalanx of the thumb
- Short and broad distal phalanx of the first toe
- Generalized osteopenia
- Bands of growth arrest
- Delayed bone age[95]

Hypertrichosis, Pigmentary Retinopathy, and Facial Anomalies

An apparently distinct form of congenital hypertrichosis has been reported in one male patient.[96] At birth, long, fine, dark hair covered the shoulders, back, buttocks, and limbs; the chest and abdomen were relatively spared. A biopsy from an arm showed a smooth muscle proliferation suggestive of smooth muscle hamartoma. Associated findings were pigmentary retinopathy and dysmorphic facial features. The finding of hypopigmented and hyperpigmented streaks following Blaschko's lines on the limbs suggested mosaicism, but this could not be confirmed on chromosomal studies of lymphocytes and skin fibroblasts.

Coffin-Siris Syndrome

Hypertrichosis is a feature in many cases,[97,98] particularly of face and back; there is a low frontal hairline, bushy eyebrows, and long eyelashes, but often sparse scalp hair. Also evident in the neonatal period are absence or hypoplasia of the nails and distal phalanges of the fifth fingers and toes, microcephaly, facial dysmorphism, and low birth weight. Growth failure and mental retardation become evident later.

Cornelia de Lange Syndrome

There is a mild generalized hypertrichosis with low frontal and occipital hairlines, thick eyebrows, synophrys, and long, upturned lashes (Fig. 26-15). The hair on the lateral elbows and sacral area may be very long and fine. Other features notable in the neonatal period include congenital livedo, low birth weight, feeding difficulties, increased susceptibility to infection, and an unusual low-pitched growling cry. There is a distinctive facies with hypertelorism, an anti-Mongoloid slant of the palpebral fissures, long philtrum, and thin lips. Other features in occasional cases include micromelia and phocomelia, cryptorchidism, and hypospadias.

Leprechaunism

These infants have coarse, curly scalp hair, and 75% of cases have extensive body and facial hypertrichosis.[99] There

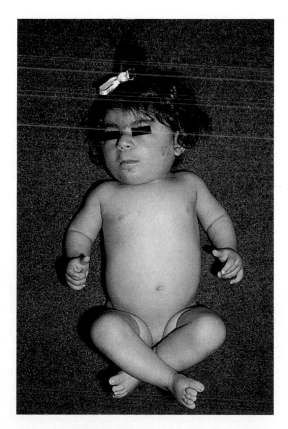

FIG. 26-15
Cornelia de Lange syndrome.

is low birth weight, wrinkled loose skin with decreased or absence of subcutaneous fat, acanthosis nigricans, periorificial rugosity of skin, thick lips, gingival hypertrophy, large low-set ears, and hypertrophic external genitalia.

Seip-Berardinelli Syndrome (Congenital Generalized Lipodystrophy)

Hypertrichosis of the face, neck, and limbs may be present at birth. There is thick, curly scalp hair with a low frontal hairline. Other features that may be evident in the neonatal period include deficiency of subcutaneous fat, acanthosis nigricans, organomegaly, and hypertrophy of genitalia.

Rubenstein-Taybi Syndrome

In Rubenstein Taybi syndrome[100,101] hypertrichosis of trunk, limbs, and face occurs in two thirds of cases. The eyebrows are highly arched and the eyelashes unusually long. Other features evident in the neonatal period include capillary vascular malformations, beaked nose, hypertelorism, high arched palate, cryptorchidism, broad thumbs and great toes, and sometimes broad terminal phalanges of other digits.

Barber-Say Syndrome

In this rare syndrome, extensive generalized hypertrichosis, most marked over the back, is associated with redundant atrophic skin, telecanthus, ectropion, macrostomia, a broad bulbous nose, and abnormal pinnae.[102]

Drug-Induced Neonatal Hypertrichosis

Fetal Alcohol Syndrome

Neonatal hypertrichosis is an occasional feature of this condition.[103] The infant is small and microcephalic with dysmorphic facial features, including short palpebral fissures, microphthalmia, midfacial hypoplasia, and a long philtrum.

Maternal Minoxidil

Maternal use of minoxidil during pregnancy has been associated with a striking hypertrichosis of the back and extremities in the neonate, accompanied by multiple dysmorphic facial features, uneven fat distribution, omphalocele, and cardiac anomalies.[104]

Diazoxide

Diazoxide is commenced in babies with hyperinsulinemia as soon as the diagnosis is established, usually in the first week of life; hypertrichosis of brow, limbs, and back becomes obvious in the first 4 weeks of treatment and is dose dependent.

LOCALIZED CONGENITAL HYPERTRICHOSIS

Localized hypertrichosis may occur in association with certain nevi or developmental abnormalities (Box 26-4).

Congenital Melanocytic Nevus

Congenital melanocytic nevi may be covered with dense, dark terminal hair at birth over part or all of their surface (Fig. 26-16). In areas other than the scalp, the degree of hairiness is usually proportional to the degree of elevation of the lesion. On the scalp, however, even very flat lesions often have a dense covering of hair that is longer, darker, and coarser than the surrounding scalp hair.

BOX 26-4

Localized Hypertrichosis

Congenital melanocytic nevus
Congenital smooth muscle hamartoma
Hypertrichosis over plexiform neurofibroma
Hypertrichosis with spinal fusion abnormalities
Familial cervical hypertrichosis with kyphoscoliosis
Associated with cranial meningoceles, encephaloceles, and heterotopic meningeal or brain tissue
Nevoid hypertrichosis
Hemihypertrophy with hypertrichosis
Scrotal hair
Anterior cervical hypertrichosis

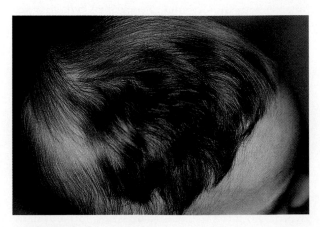

FIG. 26-16
Long, dark hair on congenital melanocytic nevus of scalp.

Congenital Smooth Muscle Hamartoma

These nevi present most commonly as congenital, slightly elevated, pebbly, firm plaques of background skin color, or slightly pigmented with local hypertrichosis.[105] Most occur on the trunk or the proximal extremities, but other areas, including the scalp,[106] may be affected. A pseudo-Darier sign of transient piloerection or elevation of the lesion after it is rubbed is a characteristic feature. Extensive hypertrichosis overlying diffuse, widespread, smooth muscle hamartomas has been reported.[107,108] Histopathologic examination demonstrates a proliferation of variably oriented smooth muscle bundles, often associated with hair follicles. There may also be epidermal changes of acanthosis and papillomatosis as seen in Becker nevus. Becker nevus usually presents in late childhood or adolescence as a patch of thickened, pigmented, hypertrichotic skin, but congenital cases have been reported, although usually lacking hypertrichosis in the neonatal period.[109] An unusual presentation with congenital bilaterally symmetric lesions, hypertrichotic at birth, has been reported.[110] Some believe that congenital smooth muscle hamartoma and Becker nevus are in a spectrum,[105] whereas others feel they are distinct entities.[111]

Plexiform Neurofibroma

The skin over these lesions is often notable for a patch of hyperpigmentation with an irregular border and hypertrichosis of varying degree.[112] A prominent paraspinal hair whorl may also occur at the site of a deep mediastinal plexiform neurofibroma.[113] A similar paraspinal whorl has been described in a patient with a posterior mediastinal ganglioneuroma.[114]

Hypertrichosis With Spinal Fusion Abnormalities

These occur mainly in the lumbosacral area but can occur elsewhere in the spine. A tuft of long, silky hair often marks the abnormal area, with or without other cutaneous markers such as dimple, sinus tract, aplasia cutis, capillary malformation, hemangioma, lipoma, or pigmented nevus.[115,116] These cutaneous lesions may be found in the presence of clinical spina bifida with myelomeningocele, but are particularly helpful as markers for occult spinal dysraphism.

Familial Cervical Hypertrichosis With Kyphoscoliosis

A family has been reported with congenital localized hypertrichosis of the cervical area overlying a kyphoscoliosis without other spinal or cutaneous abnormalities.[117] The inheritance pattern was autosomal dominant.

Hypertrichosis With Cranial Meningoceles, Encephaloceles, and Heterotopic Meningeal or Brain Tissue

These conditions are described in detail in Chapter 9. They are often marked by a peripheral collar of hair (Fig. 26-17), a tuft of hair nearby, or overlying hair.[118-121] For scalp lesions the hair is longer, thicker, and often darker than the surrounding normal hair. With lesions away from the scalp, the presence of hair may be an indication that one is dealing with a neural lesion (Figs. 26-18 and 26-19).

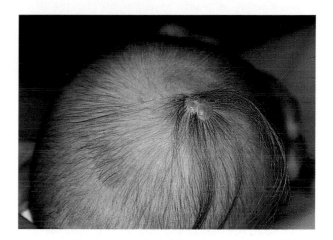

FIG. 26-17
Heterotopic brain tissue on scalp with hair collar.

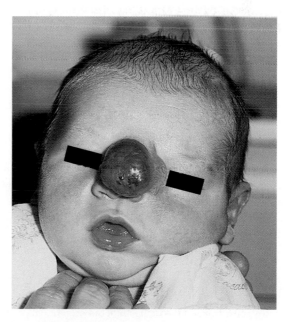

FIG. 26-18
Encephalocele with surrounding hypertrichosis.

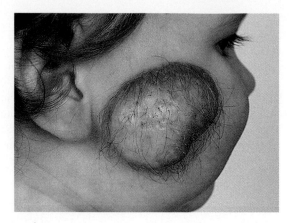

FIG. 26-19
Heterotopic brain tissue on the cheek with prominent follicle orifices and superimposed hypertrichosis.

Prominent hair follicle orifices may also be a feature. It is now clear that the membranous form of aplasia cutis, which may also demonstrate a hair collar, is a forme fruste of a neural tube closure defect and in the same spectrum as cranial meningoceles, encephaloceles, and heterotopic brain tissue.[122] A patient has been reported with a congenital patch of hypertrichosis over the lumbar area, well away from the spine, overlying what was demonstrated histologically to be meningeal tissue; in this case, displacement of meningeal cells along nerves during embryogenesis is postulated as the mechanism rather than entrapment of meningeal membranes at the time of closure of the neural tube.[123,124]

Nevoid Hypertrichosis

Several patients have been reported with single or multiple localized patches of terminal hair growing from skin of normal color and texture.[125,126] In one case, underlying lipoatrophy was found in some patches.[125] Additional abnormalities in one patient included areas of lipoatrophy and streaky depigmentation away from the areas of hypertrichosis, developmental delay and seizures, congenital lung cyst, congenital malrotation of the gut, and multiple skeletal, dental, and ocular abnormalities.[126] This constellation of findings did not fit into any recognized syndrome.

Hemihypertrophy With Hypertrichosis

Hemihypertrophy is a rare congenital disorder in which the whole body is enlarged or, less commonly part of one side of the body. Serious associated malformations include Wilms tumor and tumors of the brain and adrenals. The skin is often normal, but cutaneous abnormalities reported include pigmentation, telangiectasia, abnormal nail growth, and hypertrichosis, which can be very striking.[127]

Scrotal Hair

Several infant boys have been reported who developed scrotal hair within the first 3 months of life in the absence of clinical or biochemical evidence of excessive androgen production.[128,129] The condition was nonprogressive, and the hair usually disappeared by the age of 18 months.[128]

Anterior Cervical Hypertrichosis

A congenital patch of hypertrichosis localized to the front of the neck has been described as an isolated phenomenon[130] and in association with peripheral sensory and motor neuropathy,[131] and sometimes retinal abnormalities.[132]

Hairy Cutaneous Malformations of Palms and Soles

There have been reports of the familial occurrence of hair growth on circumscribed areas of the palms and soles.[133] In one family, the skin in the area showed exaggerated skin markings in a geometric pattern. The condition was present at birth and persisted through life. Histopathology demonstrated the presence of ectopic hair follicles and some increase in the amount of elastic fibers in the dermis.

REFERENCES

1. Smith DW, Gong BT. Scalp hair patterning as a clue to early fetal brain development. J Pediatr 1973;83:374-380.
2. Wunderlich RC, Heerema NA. Hair crown patterns of human newborns. Clin Pediatr 1975;14:1045-1049.
3. Tirosh E, Jaffe M, Dar H. The clinical significance of multiple hair whorls and their association with unusual dermatoglyphics and dysmorphic features in mentally retarded Israeli children. Eur J Pediatr 1987;146:568-570.
4. Lee WS, Lee IW, Ahn SK. Diffuse heterochromia of scalp hair. J Am Acad Dermatol 1996;35:823-825.
5. Whiting D. Structural abnormalities of the hair shaft. J Am Acad Dermatol 1987;16:1-25.
6. Price VH. Structural abnormalities of the hair shaft. In Orfanos C, Happle R, eds. Hair and hair diseases. Berlin: Springer Verlag, 1990: pp 363-422.
7. Rogers M. Hair shaft abnormalities: Part I. Aust J Dermatol 1995;36:179-186.
8. Rogers M. Hair shaft abnormalities: Part II. Aust J Dermatol 1996;37:1-11.
9. Winter H, Rogers MA, Langbein L, et al. Mutations in the hair cortex keratin hHb6 cause the inherited hair disease monilethrix. Nat Genet 1997;16:372-374.

10. Winter H, Rogers MA, Gebhardt M, et al. A new mutation in the type II hair cortex keratin hHb1 involved in the inherited hair disorder monilethrix. Hum Genet 1997;101:165-169.
11. Richard G, Itin P, Lin JP, et al. Evidence for genetic heterogeneity in monilethrix. J Invest Dermatol 1996;107:812-814.
12. Chelly J, Tumer Z, Tonnesen T, et al. Isolation of a candidate gene for Menkes disease that encodes a potential heavy metal binding protein. Nat Genet 1993;3:14-19.
13. Goetyn M, Geerts M-L, Kint A, et al. The Bazex-Dupre-Christol syndrome. Arch Dermatol 1994;130:337-342.
14. Crandall B, Samec L, Sparkes RS, et al. A familial syndrome of deafness, alopecia and hypogonadism. J Pediatr 1973;82:461-465.
15. Price VH, Odom RB, Ward WH, et al. Trichothiodystrophy. Sulfur-deficient brittle hair as a marker for neuroectodermal symptom complex. Arch Dermatol 1980;116:1375-1384.
16. Itin PH, Pittelkow MR. Trichothiodystrophy: review of sulfur-deficient brittle hair syndromes and association with the ectodermal dysplasias. J Am Acad Dermatol 1990;22:705-717.
17. Taylor EM, Broughton BC, Botta E, et al. Xeroderma pigmentosum and trichothiodystrophy are associated with different mutations in the XPD(ERCC2) repair/transcription gene. Proc Nat Acad Sci USA 1997;94:8658-8663.
18. Weeda G, Eveno E, Donker I, et al. A mutation in the XPB/ERCC3 DNA repair transcription gene, associated with trichothiodystrophy. Am J Hum Genet 1997;60:320-329.
19. Petrin JH, Meckler KA, Sybert VP. A new variant of trichothiodystrophy with recurrent infections, failure to thrive and death. Pediatr Dermatol 1998;15: 31-34.
20. Tolmie JL, de Berker D, Dawber R, et al. Syndromes associated with trichothiodystrophy. Clin Dysmorphol 1994;3:1-14.
21. Brusasco A. The typical "tiger-tail" pattern of the hair shaft in trichothiodystrophy may not be evident at birth. Arch Dermatol 1997;133:249.
22. Taylor A. Hereditary woolly hair with ocular involvement. Br J Dermatol 1990;123:523-526.
23. Neild VS, Pegum JS, Wells RS. The association of keratosis pilaris atrophicans and woolly hair, with or without Noonan's syndrome. Br J Dermatol 1984;110:357-362.
24. Tosti A, Misciali C, Barbareschi M, et al. Woolly hair, palmoplantar keratoderma and cardiac abnormalities: report of a family. Arch Dermatol 1994;130:522-524.
25. Ouvrier RA. Giant axonal neuropathy. Brain Develop 1989;11:207-214.
26. Ruggieri M, Pavone V, Smilari P, et al. Primary osteoma cutis—multiple cafe-au-lait spots and woolly hair abnormality. Pediatr Radiol 1995;25:34-36.
27. Wright S, Lemoine NR, Leigh IM. Woolly hair naevi with systematized linear epidermal nevus. Clin Exp Dermatol 1986;11:179-182.
28. Matis WL, Baden H, Green R, et al. Un-combable hair syndrome. Pediatr Dermatol 1987;4:215-219.
29. Marren P, Wilson C, Dawber RPR, et al. Hereditary hypotrichosis (Marie-Unna type) and juvenile macular degeneration. Clin Exp Dermatol 1992;17:189-191.
30. Camacho F, Ferrando J, Pichardo AR, et al. Rapp-Hodgkin syndrome with pili canaliculi. Pediatr Dermatol 1993;10:54-57.
31. Micali GM, Cook B, Blekys I, et al. Structural hair abnormalities in ectodermal dysplasia. Pediatr Dermatol 1990;7:27-32.
32. Shelley WB, Shelley ED. Uncombable hair syndrome: Observations on response to biotin and occurrence in siblings with ectodermal dysplasia. J Am Acad Dermatol 1985;13:97-102.
33. de Berker D, Paige D, Harper, J et al. Golf tee hairs: A new sign in Netherton syndrome. Br J Dermatol 1992; 127 (suppl 40):30.
34. Menne T, Weisman K. Canestick lesions of vellus hair in Netherton's syndrome. Arch Dermatol 1985;121:451.
35. Lurie R, Ben-Zion G. Helical hairs: A new hair anomaly in a patient with Netherton's syndrome. Cutis 1995;55:349-352.
36. Baden HP, Kubilus J. Analysis of hair from alopecia congenita. J Am Acad Dermatol 1980;3:623-626.
37. Ahmad M, Abbas H, Haque S. Alopecia universalis as a single abnormality in an inbred Pakistani kindred. Am J Med Genet 1993;46:369-371.
38. Pinheiro M, Freire-Maia N. Atrichias and hypotrichoses; a brief review with description of a recessive atrichia in two brothers. Hum Hered 1985;35:53-55.
39. Kenue RK, al-Dhafri KS. Isolated congenital atrichia in an Omani kindred. Dermatology 1994;188:72-75.
40. Nothen MM, Cichon S, Vogt IR, et al. A gene for congenital alopecia maps to chromosome 8p21-22. Am J Hum Genet 1998;62:386-390.
41. Peachey RDG, Wells RS. Hereditary hypotrichosis (Marie Unna type). Trans St John's Hosp Dermatol Soc 1971;57:157-166.
42. Mallon E, Dawber RPR, Dover R, et al. Marie-Unna hypotrichosis - histopathology findings and pathogenesis. Brit J Dermatol 1995;133(suppl 45):55.
43. Lowenthal LJA, Prakken JR. Atrichia with papular lesions. Dermatologica 1961;122:85-89.
44. Delprat A, Bonafe JL, Lugardon Y. Atrichie congenitale avec kystes. Ann Dermatol Venereol 1994;121:802-804.
45. Misciali C, Tosti A, Fanti PA, et al. Atrichia and papular lesions. Report of a case. Dermatology 1992;185:284-288.
46. Miller L, Loffreda M, Lyle S, et al. Atrichia with papules. Presented at the Second Intercontinental Hair Research Societies' Meeting, Washington, DC, November 6, 1998.
47. Ahmad W, Haque M, Brancolini V, et al. Alopecia universalis associated with a mutation in the human hairless gene. Science 1998;279:720-724.
48. Sundberg JP, Price VH, King LE. The "hairless" gene in mouse and man. Arch Dermatol 1999;135:718-720.
49. Rapelanoro R, Taieb A, Lacombe D. Congenital hypotrichosis and milia: Report of a large family suggesting X-linked dominant inheritance. Am J Med Genet 1994;52:487-490.
50. McNaughton PZ, Pierson DL, Rodman OG. Hidrotic ectodermal dysplasia in a black mother and daughter. Arch Dermatol 1976;112:1448-1450.
51. Rajagopalan K, Tay CH. Hidrotic ectodermal dysplasia: Study of a large Chinese pedigree. Arch Dermatol 1977;113:481-485.
52. Clarke A, Phillips DIM, Brown R, et al. Clinical aspects of X-linked hypohidrotic ectodermal dysplasia. Arch Dis Child 1987;62:989-996.

53. Vanderhooft SL, Stephan MJ, Sybert VP. Severe skin erosions and scalp infections in AEC syndrome. Pediatr Dermatol 1993;10:334-340.

54. Felding IB, Bjorklund LJ. Rapp-Hodgkin ectodermal dysplasia. Pediatr Dermatol 1990;7:126-131.

55. Camacho F, Ferrando J, Pichardo AR, et al. Rapp-Hodgkin syndrome with pili canaliculi. Pediatr Dermatol 1993; 10:54-57.

56. Cambiaghi S, Tadini G, Barbareschi M, et al. Rapp-Hodgkin syndrome and AEC syndrome: Are they the same entity? Brit J Dermatol 1994;130:97-101.

57. Vogt BR, Traupe H, Hamm H. Congenital atrichia with nail dystrophy, abnormal facies and retarded psychomotor development in two siblings: A new autosomal recessive syndrome? Pediatr Dermatol 1988;5:236-242.

58. Lestringant GG, Kuster W, Frossard PM, et al. Congenital ichthyosis, follicular atrophoderma, hypotrichosis and hypohidrosis. Am J Med Genet 1998;75:186-189.

59. Eramo LR, Esterly NB, Zieserl EJ. Ichthyosis follicularis with alopecia and photophobia. Arch Dermatol 1985;121:1167-1174.

60. Rothe MJ, Weiss DS, Dubner BH. Ichthyosis follicularis in two girls: an autosomal dominant disorder. Pediatr Dermatol 1990;7:287-292.

61. Rogers M, Kourt G, Cameron A. Hereditary mucoepithelial dysplasia. Pediatr Dermatol 1994;11:133-138.

62. Rothe MJ, Lucky AW. Are ichthyosis follicularis and hereditary mucoepithelial dystrophy related diseases? Pediatr Dermatol 1995;12:195.

63. Harms M, Gilardi S, Levy PM, et al. KID syndrome (keratitis, ichthyosis and deafness) and chronic mucocutaneous candidiasis: Case report and review of the literature. Pediatr Dermatol 1984;2:1-7.

64. Megarbane A, Loiselet J. Clinical manifestations of a severe neonatal progeroid syndrome. Clin Genet 1997;51:200-204.

65. Makitie O, Sulisalo T, de la Chapelle A, et al. Cartilage-hair hypoplasia. J Med Genet 1995;32:39-43.

66. Glover MT, Atherton DJ, Levinsky RJ. Syndrome of erythroderma, failure to thrive and diarrhea in infancy: A manifestation of immunodeficiency. Pediatr 1988;81:66-72.

67. Ricci, G, Patrizi A, Specchia F. Omenn syndrome. Pediatr Dermatol 1997;14:49-52.

68. Farrell A, Scerri L, Stevens A, et al. Acute graft-versus-host disease with unusual cutaneous intracellular vacuolation in an infant with severe combined immunodeficiency. Pediatr Dermatol 1995;12:311-313.

69. Barman JM, Pecoraro V, Astore I, et al. The first stage in the natural history of the human scalp hair cycle. J Invest Dermatol 1967;48:138-142.

70. Pecoraro V, Astore I, Barman J. Cycle of the scalp hair of the new-born child. J Invest Dermatol 1964;43:145-147.

71. Trakimas C, Sperling LC, Skelton HG, et al. Clinical and histologic findings in temporal triangular alopecia. J Am Acad Dermatol 1994;31:205-209.

72. Garcia-Hernandez MJ, Rodriguez-Pichardo A, Camacho F. Congenital triangular alopecia. Pediatr Dermatol 1995;12:301-303.

73. Tosti A. Congenital triangular alopecia. J Am Acad Dermatol 1987;16:991-993.

74. Schoenfeld RJ, Mehregan AH. Aplastic nevus—the 'minus nevus'. Cutis 1973;12:386-389.

75. Bentivoglio GC. Un caso di alopecia areata primitiva in un lattante. Pediatria 1926;34:952-960.

76. de Viragh PA, Giannada B, Levy ML. Congenital alopecia areata. Dermatology 1997;195:96-98.

77. Cohen JJ. Hallermann-Streiff syndrome: A review. Am J Med Genet 1991;41:488-489.

78. Happle R. Genetic defects involving the hair. In Orfanos CE, Happle R, eds. Hair and hair diseases, Berlin: Springer-Verlag, 1989; p 345.

79. Baumeister FAM, Schwartz HP, Stengel-Rutkowski S. childhood hypertrichosis: Diagnosis and management. Arch Dis Child 1995;72:457-459.

80. Felgenhauer WR. Hypertrichosis lanuginosa universalis. J Genet Hum 1969;17:1-44.

81. Freire-Maia M, Felizali J, de Figueiredo AC, et al. Hypertrichosis lanuginosa in a mother and son. Clin Genet 1976; 10:303-306.

82. Janssen TAE, de Lange C. Hypertrichosis (trichostasis) lanuginosa. Ned Tijdschr Geneesk 1946;90:198.

83. Judge MR, Rice NSC, Christopher A, et al. Congenital hypertrichosis lanuginosa and congenital glaucoma. Br J Dermatol 1991;124:495-497.

84. Partridge JW. Congenital hypertrichosis lanuginosa: Neonatal shaving. Arch Dis Child 1987;62:623-625.

85. Barth JH, Wilkinson JD, Dawber RPR. Prepubertal hypertrichosis: Normal or abnormal? Arch Dis Child 1988;63:666-668.

86. Balducci R, Toscano V. Bioactive and peripheral androgens in prepubertal simple hypertrichosis. Clin Endocrinol 1990; 33:407-414.

87. Macias-Flores MA, Garcia-Cruz D, Rivera H, et al. A new form of hypertrichosis inherited as an X-linked dominant trait. Hum Genet 1984;66:66-70.

88. Figuera LE, Pandolfo M, Dunne PW, et al. Mapping of the congenital generalized hypertrichosis locus to chromosome Xq24-q27.1. Nat Genet 1995;10:202-207.

89. Baumeister FAM, Egger J, Schildhaure MT, et al. Ambras syndrome: Delineation of a unique hypertrichosis universalis congenita and association with a balanced pericentric inversion (8)(p11.2;q22). Clin Genet 1993;44:121-128.

90. Lee IJ, Im SB, Kim D-K. Hypertrichosis universalis congenita: A separate entity, or the same disease as gingival fibromatosis. Pediatr Dermatol 1993;10:263-266.

91. Witkop CJ. Heterogeneity in gingival fibromatosis. Birth Defects: Original Article Series VII 1971;7:210-221.

92. Lacombe D, Bioulac-Sage P, Sibout M, et al. Congenital marked hypertrichosis and Laband syndrome in a child: Overlap between the gingival fibromatosis-hypertrichosis and Laband syndromes. Genet Couns 1994;5:251-256.

93. Cantu JM, Garcia-Cruz D, Sanchez-Corona J, et al. A distinct osteochondrodysplasia with hypertrichosis. Hum Genet 1982;60:36-41.

94. Nevin NC, Mulholland HC, Thomas P. Congenital hypertrichosis, cardiomegaly and mild osteochondrodysplasia. Am J Med Genet 1996;66:33-38.

95. Garcia-Cruz D, Sanchez-Corona J, Nazara Z, et al. Congenital hypertrichosis, osteochondrodysplasia and cardiomegaly: Further delineation of a new genetic syndrome. Am J Med Genet 1997;69:138-151.

96. Pivnick EK, Wilroy RS, Martens PR, et al. Hypertrichosis, pigmentatary retinopathy and facial anomalies: A new syndrome? Am J Med Genet 1996;62:386-390.

97. Tunnessen WW, McMillan JA, Levin MB. The Coffin-Siris syndrome. Am J Dis Child 1978;132:393-395.

98. Levy P, Baraitser M. Coffin-Siris syndrome. J Med Genet 1991;28:338-341.

99. Roth SI, Schedewie HK, Herzberg VK, et al. Cutaneous manifestations of leprechaunism. Arch Dermatol 1981;117:531-535.

100. Selmanowitz VJ, Stiller MJ. Rubinstein-Taybi syndrome. Arch Dermatol 1981;117:504-506.

101. Cambiaghi S, Ermacora E, Brusasco A, et al. Multiple pilomatricomas in Rubinstein-Taybi syndrome. Pediatr Dermatol 1994;11:21-25.

102. Santana SM, Alvarez FP, Frias JL, et al. Hypertrichosis, atrophic skin, ectropion and macrostomia (Barber-Say) syndrome: Report of a new case. Am J Med Genet 1993;47:20-23.

103. Hanson JW, Jones KL, Smith DW. Fetal alcohol syndrome: experience with 41 patients. JAMA 1976;235:1458-1460.

104. Kaler SG, Patrinos ME, Lambert GH, et al. Hypertrichosis and congenital anomalies associated with maternal use of Minoxidil. Pediatrics 1987;79;434-436.

105. Johnson MD, Jacobs AJ. Congenital smooth muscle hamartoma. Arch Dermatol 1989;125:820-822.

106. Knable A, Treadwell P. Pigmented plaque with hypertrichosis on the scalp of an infant. Pediatr Dermatol 1996;13 431-433.

107. Glover MT, Malone M, Atherton DJ. Michelin-tire baby syndrome resulting from diffuse smooth muscle hamartoma. Pediatr Dermatol 1989;6:329-331.

108. Larregue M, Vabre P, Cavaroc Y, et al. Hamartome diffus des muscles arrecteurs et hypertrichose lanugineuse congénitale. Ann Dermatol Venereol (Paris) 1991;118:796-798.

109. Book SE, Glass AT, Laude TA. Congenital Becker's nevus with a familial association. Pediatr Dermatol 1997;14:373-375.

110. Ferreira MJ, Bajanca R, Fiadeiro T. Congenital melanosis and hypertrichosis in a bilateral distribution. Pediatr Dermatol 1998;15:290-292.

111. Gagne EJ, Su WPD. Congenital smooth muscle hamartoma of the skin. Pediatr Dermatol 1993;10:142-145.

112. Ettl A, Marinkovic M, Koornneef L. Localized hypertrichosis associated with periorbital neurofibroma; clinical findings and differential diagnosis. Ophthalmol 1996;103:942-948.

113. Pivnik EK, Lobe TE, Fitch SJ, et al. Hair whorl as an indicator of a mediastinal plexiform neurofibroma. Pediatr Dermatol 1997;14:196-198.

114. Flannery DB, Howell CG. Confirmation of the Riccardi sign. Proc Greenwood Genet Centre 1986;6:161.

115. Tavafoghi V, Ghandchi A, Hambrick GW, et al. Cutaneous signs of spinal dysraphism. Arch Dermatol 1978;114:573-577.

116. Davis DA, Cohen PR, George RE. Cutaneous stigmata of occult spinal dysraphism. J Am Acad Dermatol 1994;31:892-896.

117. Reed OM, Mellette JR, Fitzpatrick JE. Familial cervical hypertrichosis with underlying kyphoscoliosis. J Am Acad Dermatol 1989;20:1069-1072.

118. Commens C, Rogers M. Heterotropic brain tissue presenting as bald cysts with a collar of hypertrophic hair. Arch Dermatol 1989;125:1253-1256.

119. Stone MS, Walker PS, Kennard CD. Rudimentary meningocele presenting with a scalp hair tuft. Arch Dermatol 1994;130:775-777.

120. Khallouf R, Fetissof F, Machet MC. Sequestrated meningocele of the scalp: Diagnostic value of hair abnormalities. Pediatr Dermatol 1994;11:315-318.

121. Drolet BA, Clowry L, McTigue K, et al. The hair collar sign: Marker for spinal dysraphism. Pediatrics 1995;96:309-313.

122. Drolet B, Prendiville J, Golden J, et al. 'Membranous aplasia cutis' with hair collars. Arch Dermatol 1995;131:1427-1431.

123. Penas PF, Jones-Caballero M, Amigo A, et al. Cutaneous meningioma underlying congenital localized hypertrichosis. J Am Acad Dermatol 1994;30:363-366.

124. Penas PF, Jones-Caballero M, Garcia-Diez A. Cutaneous heterotopic meningeal nodules. Arch Dermatol 1995;131:731.

125. Cox NH, McClure JP, Hardie RA. Naevoid hypertrichosis—report of a patient with multiple lesions. Clin Exp Dermatol 1989;14:62-64.

126. Rogers M. Naevoid hypertrichosis. Clin Exp Dermatol 1981:16:74.

127. Hurwitz S, Klaus SN. Congenital hemihypertrophy with hypertrichosis. Arch Dermatol 1971;103:98-100.

128. Diamond FB, Shulman DI, Root AW. Scrotal hair in infancy. J Pediatr 1989;114:999-1001.

129. Slyper AH, Esterly NB. Nonprogressive scrotal hair growth in two infants. Pediatr Dermatol 1993;10:34-35.

130. Braddock SR, Jones KL, Bird LM, et al. Anterior cervical hypertrichosis. A dominantly inherited isolated defect. Am J Med Genet 1995;55:498-499.

131. Trattner A, Hodak E, Sagie-Lerman T, et al. Familial congenital anterior cervical hypertrichosis associated with peripheral sensory and motor neuropathy—A new syndrome? J Am Acad Dermatol 1991;25:767-770.

132. Garty BZ, Snir M, Kremer I, et al. Retinal changes in familial peripheral sensory and motor neuropathy associated with anterior cervical hypertrichosis. J Pediatr Ophthalmol and Strabismus 1997;34:309-312.

133. Jackson CE, Callies QC, Krull EA, et al. Hairy cutaneous malformations of the palms and soles. Arch Dermatol 1975;111:1146-1149.

27

Nail Defects

ROBERT A. SILVERMAN

Nails are specialized cutaneous appendages, are composed of hard keratins similar to those found in hair, and are unique to primates. In humans, nails function as a stabilizing unit to aid in tactile sensation, grasping, and scratching. Well-manicured or adorned nails in adolescents and adults may be perceived as an attribute of social acceptability and serve as a source of personal satisfaction. Although abnormalities of the nails are rare, they may affect an individual's self-esteem and their relationships with others. Abnormal nails in a neonate may be indicative of a more widespread inherited or sporadic syndrome, or they may be a localized congenital malformation. In either case, parents of a newborn may be concerned about their infant's nails, seemingly out of proportion to the magnitude of any other problems that may be present. Investigation and consultations to uncover any associated illness and to allay any untoward parental anxiety are warranted.

The nail unit is composed of a rectangular nail plate bordered by proximal and lateral nail folds[1] (Fig. 27-1). The cuticle attaches the proximal nail fold to the nail plate. This acellular membrane is tightly adherent and prevents invasion of microorganisms from reaching the underlying matrix. The lunula (half moon) represents the distal portion of the nail's proliferative matrix. The ventral side of the nail plate has longitudinal ridges that orient the direction of growth from the root over a complementary grooved nail bed. At birth, the dorsal surface of the nail displays unique, somewhat oblique ridges as well. These ridges become parallel and disappear slowly, and over time the surface becomes smooth. The distal free edge of the plate separates from the bed at the hyponychium. The shape of the nail plate is convex. It is normally thickest at its proximal portion and thins distally.

The size of the nail plate is determined by the size and growth of the underlying distal phalanx. Since embryologic development occurs in a cephalocaudal direction, it is not surprising that at birth, especially in premature infants, toenails may be smaller than fingernails. In premature infants less than 32 weeks' gestation, nail plates may not extend beyond the distal groove of the hyponychium. In postmature infants, such as macrosomic infants or infants of diabetic mothers, the nail plate may extend well beyond the hyponychium. In adults, it is estimated that fingernails grow 0.1 mm/day and toenails grow 1 mm/month. Similar data in newborns and infants are not available. Box 27-1 lists pathologic factors that affect nail growth.

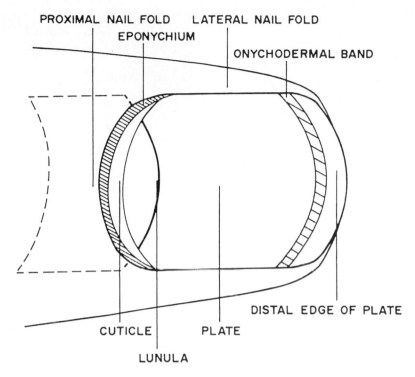

PROXIMAL NAIL FOLD   LATERAL NAIL FOLD

EPONYCHIUM

ONYCHODERMAL BAND

DISTAL EDGE OF PLATE

CUTICLE   PLATE

LUNULA

FIG. 27-1
Dorsal view of the nail unit. (From Scher & Daniel: Nails: therapy diagnosis, surgery, 2nd edition. New York: WB Saunders, 1997.)

The anatomic structure of the nail unit is affected by many disease states. Conditions may be primary or secondary, localized or generalized, congenital or acquired, inherited, associated with syndromes, known genetic defects or drug exposures, and infectious or systemic disease. Nail morphogenesis begins during the ninth week of gestation and is completed by the end of the second trimester (see Chapter 1).

BEAU'S LINES

Beau's lines are transverse grooves, or moatlike depressions, that extend across the nail plate from one lateral nail fold to the other.[2,3] This deformity is a manifestation of nail matrix arrest and is first observed adjacent to the proximal nail fold. Beau's lines slowly move toward the distal free edge of the nail plate as nail growth resumes. If the rate of nail growth is known, one can estimate the date of nail matrix arrest by measuring the distance between the proximal nail fold and the Beau's line. Causes of Beau's lines include high fevers caused by infection, severe cutaneous inflammatory diseases such as Stevens-Johnson syndrome or Kawasaki disease, a reaction to medications, and acrodermatitis enteropathica. Beau's

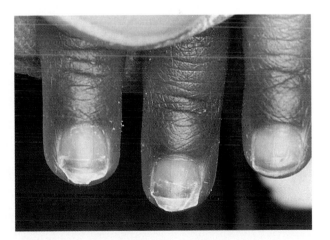

FIG. 27-2
Beau's lines are transverse grooves of the nail plate that represent a brief reduction of growth from the nail matrix.

lines may occur in infants, 4 to 10 weeks of age, as a result of the stress of delivery. They have also been reported at birth as a result of intrauterine stress in a premature infant[4] (Fig. 27-2). Although Beau's lines should develop on all fingernails and toenails, they are usually most prominent on the thumbs and great toe nails because of their slower rate of growth.

Onychomadesis refers to proximal separation of the nail plate from the nail bed. Latent onychomadesis occurs when the nail separates sometime after a profound interruption in nail growth. Causes are similar to those that produce Beau's lines and may occur during the neonatal period as well.

ALTERATIONS IN NAIL SHAPE

It is not uncommon for newborns to have variations of the normal convex curvature of the nail. *Koilonychia* refers to nails that exhibit a concave, or spoon, shape.[5] This may be a normal variant in newborns, especially when it involves the great toe nails. It is widely accepted that koilonychia in infants and toddlers may be indicative of iron deficiency. According to some investigators, koilonychia may precede clinical or laboratory evidence of anemia.[6] However, well-controlled studies of iron deficiency in large numbers of infants with and without koilonychia have not been reported, and improvement of nail shape with administration of iron has not been documented. As the child grows, koilonychia gradually improves. Familial koilonychia has rarely been reported.[7] It has also been described with other ectodermal defects such as monilethrix, palmoplantar keratoderma, and steatocystoma multiplex, as well as Turner syndrome.[8]

Other deformities in nail shape include pincer nails, claw nails, and racquet nails. Pincer nails are characterized by a transverse overcurvature of the nail plates.[9] The condition is usually acquired, but some cases may result from an inherited developmental anomaly. If the convex overcurvature is prominent, nails may appear similar to those in patients with pachyonychia congenita and occasionally may be quite painful. Congenital clawlike nails have also been reported.[10] The nail plates have a dorsal convexity and then curve downward to resemble onychogryphosis. This is usually noted on the second to fourth toes and may be associated with a cleft hand. Hypoplasia of the distal phalanx with absence of the ossification center is observed on radiographs of the affected digits.[11] Correction of the deformity is desirable because of the tendency toward recurrent bleeding and ulceration of the tip of the toe. Racquet nails occur when the width of the nail plate exceeds its length, also referred to as *brachyonychia*. It may be a sign of foreshortening of the terminal phalanx and may be associated with other congenital anomalies.[12]

Clubbing is a curved or beaklike deformity of the nail unit that accompanies hypertrophy and hyperplasia of the

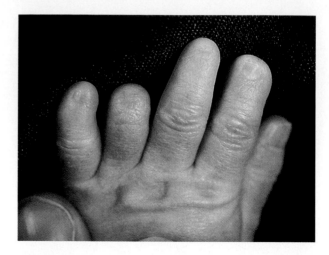

FIG. 27-3
Anonychia with absence of the distal phalanx and foreshortening of the digit.

fibrovascular support stroma of the distal phalanx. It is an acquired sign of both systemic and hereditary diseases.[13] In neonates or infants, clubbing may be an early manifestation of cyanotic congenital heart disease, bronchopulmonary diseases, or HIV disease.[14,15]

ALTERATIONS IN NAIL SIZE

Anonychia refers to the absence of nails. The most widely known association is with nail-patella syndrome (see subsequent discussion). Isolated congenital anonychia has been reported in families with both autosomal recessive[16,17] and autosomal dominant inheritance (OMIM 206800).* Rudimentary nail units may be evident, but the underlying phalangeal structure is normal. Anonychia and hypoplasia of the nails may be observed with absence of the distal phalanges and foreshortening of the affected digits (Fig. 27-3). Anonychia has been reported with limb defects (OMIM 106990),[18] ectrodactyly,[19] flexural pigmentation (OMIM 106750),[20] isolated to the thumbnails (OMIM 188200),[21] and with sensorineural hearing loss (OMIM 124480, 220500).[22] These latter cases have been termed *DOOR syndrome* (deafness, onycho-osteodystrophy, and retardation). Elevated urinary amino acids have been detected in some patients with DOOR syndrome.[23]

---

*OMIM: Online Mendelian Inheritance in Man (www.ncbi.nlm.nih.gov/Omim/).

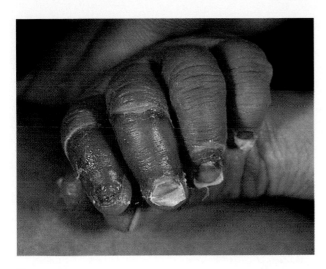

FIG. 27-4
Anonychia of the index finger in a case of junctional epidermolysis bullosa.

Anonychia of the fifth fingers and toenails is characteristic of Coffin-Siris syndrome (OMIM 135900).[24] Other features include growth and mental retardation, generalized hypertrichosis and scalp hypotrichosis, lax joints, and abnormal facies.

Infants with junctional and dystrophic forms of epidermolysis bullosa (EB) frequently have anonychia at birth[25] (Fig. 27-4). Onycholysis (separation of the nail plate from the nail bed) and onychomadesis precede nail loss. One or more fingernails are usually affected. The periungual tissues and nail beds are frequently swollen and inflamed. Granulation tissue develops quickly. Meticulous hygiene, application of topical antibiotics, and wound care with synthetic dressings may optimize regrowth if possible. It is the author's opinion that in utero sucking of the fingers results in most of the nail disease in EB present at birth.

MICRONYCHIA

Small nails may be localized to one or a few digits or involve all of the nail fields. Conditions associated with micronychia are listed in Table 27-1.[26 30] Current theory suggests that at least some forms of micronychia, such as in fetal alcohol syndrome and anticonvulsant exposure, are due to inhibition of retinoic acid synthesis during early embryologic development.[31,32] Selected specific causes of micronychia are discussed in subsequent sections.

TABLE 27-1

Micronychias

Disorder	Clinical manifestations
Nail-patella syndrome	Small or absent patellas, iliac horns, triangular lunulas
Congenital onychodysplasia	
Ectodermal dysplasias	Variable sweating, hair and tooth abnormalities
Fetal Teratogens	
Alcohol	Microcephaly, short palpebral fissures, maxillary hypoplasia
Hydantoins (and other anticonvulsants)	Short stature, retardation, hypertelorism, depressed nasal bridge, cardiac anomalies, mucosal changes
Polychlorinated biphenyls	Natal teeth, pigment anomalies, mucosal changes
Warfarin	Nasal hypoplasia, stippled epiphyses
Coffin-Siris syndrome	Hypoplasia of the fifth digit, lax joints, blepharoptosis
Dyskeratosis congenita	Hyperpigmentation and hypopigmentation, Fanconi-like anemia, blepharitis, leukoplakia, XLR* (OMIM30500)
Chromosome Abnormalities	
Trisomies	3q, 8, 13, 18
Turner syndrome	XO, webbed neck, nevi, lymphedema, coarctation of the aorta
Noonan syndrome	XY male with a Turner phenotype and pulmonic stenosis
Amniotic bands	Hypoplasia of the distal phalanx associated with aplasia cutis

*X-linked recessive inheritance.

NAIL-PATELLA SYNDROME (OMIM 161200)

Nail-patella syndrome, also known as hereditary osteo-onychodysplasia (HOOD), is an autosomal dominant genodermatosis associated with chronic renal disease and debilitating osteoarthritis. This disorder has a high degree of penetrance and widely variable expressivity.[33] During the neonatal period, nail disease is usually the only manifestation. However, there are rare reports of infants with proteinuria, signifying the early onset of renal pathology.[34]

Ungual manifestations are most prominent on the ulnar sides of the thumbs and index fingers, and to a lesser degree on other digits. They include micronychia, hemionychia, and occasionally anonychia. If present, a triangularly shaped lunula with a distal apex is nearly pathognomonic for the condition.[35] The nail plates may be thin and display koilonychia, resulting in frequent chipping and splitting later in childhood.

Skeletal deformities are not visible until ossification centers develop. Parents may be screened for small, easily subluxed patellas, characteristic posterior iliac horns, hypoplasia of the proximal radius and ulna, scoliosis, and thickened scapulas. Generally, patients with nail-patella syndrome are not identified until early adulthood, when knee dislocation, pain, and gait disturbances bring them to medical attention.[36]

Renal disease that presents as asymptomatic proteinuria is the most serious manifestation of nail-patella syndrome. It is usually not apparent until adulthood, but a newborn and a 2-year-old child with nephrosis have been reported.[37] Renal biopsies have uncovered glomerulonephritis secondary to glomerular basement membrane zone thickening from collagen fibril deposition. These findings have even been noted in a spontaneously aborted 18-week-old fetus.[38,39]

Other manifestations include heterochromic irides, colobomas, microcorneas, glaucoma,[40] popliteal pterygia, and mild mental deficiency. It has been suggested that these, as well as other findings such as colon cancer, in specific kindreds may be a result of contiguous gene defects, translocations, or other genetic aberrations.[41] Complications from cerebral and large vessel dilation have also been reported.[42] These are also caused by collagenous basal lamina reduplication.

The gene for nail-patella syndrome has been mapped to the region of 9q34. It is linked to the ABO blood group and had been believed to be an abnormality in COL5A1, which is necessary for the production of collagen type V, an important component in the glomerular and other

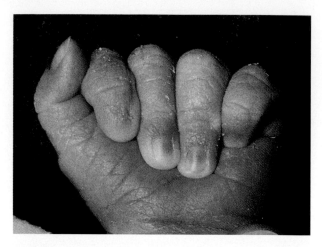

FIG. 27-5
Absence or hypoplasia of the nail unit of the index fingers is characteristic of congenital onychodysplasia of the index fingers.

basement membrane zones.[43] However, recent evidence suggests that a LIM-homeodomain protein, Lmx1b, coded for at the same site, is probably the major factor in this disorder.[44] This protein plays a central role in dorsal/ventral patterning of the vertebrate limb, and targeted disruption of Lmx1b results in skeletal defects, including hypoplastic nails, absent patellae, and renal dysplasia.

CONGENITAL ONYCHODYSPLASIA OF THE INDEX FINGERS

Congenital onychodysplasia of the index fingers (COIF), also known as Iso and Kikuchi syndrome, was first described in 1969.[45,46] Original cases were congenital, limited mainly to the index fingers, and characterized by anonychia, micronychia, and/or polyonychia (Fig. 27-5). They were nonfamilial and nonhereditary and without underlying bone or joint abnormalities. Since that time, clinical criteria have been changed or expanded to encompass a number of additional observations.[47]

Although the index fingers are most commonly affected, onychodystrophy has been reported on other fingers and toes.[48,49] Malalignment, "rolled micronychia," hemionychogryphosis, onychoheterotopia, and polyonychia with syndactyly have also been detailed. Unlike nail-patella syndrome, abnormalities in the nail unit are more prominent on the radial aspects of the digits. A Y-shaped bifurcation of the distal phalanx on lateral radiograph views is frequent and is characteristic of the condition.[50] Familial cases have also been documented.[51]

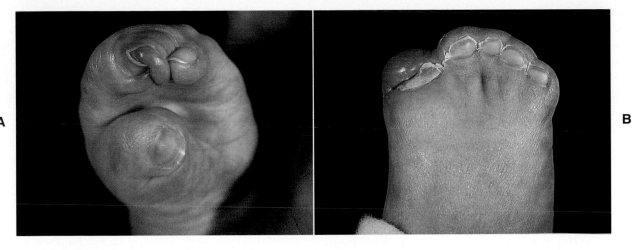

FIG. 27-6
A, Fused second to fourth digits of the hand of a patient with Apert syndrome had a single circumferential nail. **B,** Synonychia and syndactyly of the toes in a patient with Apert syndrome.

The pathogenesis of congenital onychodysplasia is poorly understood. An abnormal vascular supply, anomalies from an abnormal grip, external deformation from pressure against the cranium, teratogen exposure, and genetic influences have been implicated by a number of authors.[52] It is quite possible that the clinical findings may be explained by any of these theories if the inciting event occurs at a specific time during the embryologic development of the nail unit.

ONYCHOATROPHY

Onychoatrophy refers to a progressive reduction in size and thickness of the nail unit. The term is usually used to describe acquired dissolution of ungual structures and should not be used synonymously with micronychia, although some authors do so. Inflammatory disorders, which are observed in older children and adults and rarely documented in newborns, such as Stevens-Johnson syndrome or graft-vs-host disease, may result in onychoatrophy. Infants with congenital disorders that have a progressive phenotype, such as acrogeria or dyskeratosis congenita, can have onychoatrophy as well. Digital artery occlusion from emboli may result in phalangeal necrosis and destruction of nail structures. Other postnatal vascular insults such as extensive aplasia cutis congenita or disseminated intravascular coagulation from homozygous protein C deficiency could potentially have similar effects.

ECTOPIC NAILS

Onychoheterotopia, or ectopic nails, occurs when ungual tissue develops on areas other than the dorsal aspect of the distal phalanx.[53] Cases that have been reported tend to involve the palmar surface of the fifth fingers.[54-57] They have been both sporadic and reported in siblings, suggesting possible autosomal recessive inheritance. Other abnormalities of the hand may also be present, including underlying osseous malformations. A circumferential nail of the fifth finger has been documented in association with a deletion in the long arm of chromosome 6.[58] This tubular defect may occur on other digits as well.[59] The presence of a circumferential nail is frequently observed at the tip of the fused digits of the hand in acrocephalosyndactyly or Apert syndrome (OMIM 101200).[60] Synonychia and fusion of all of the toes are also observed in this sporadic condition, which is caused by mutations in the gene encoding fibroblast growth factor receptor-2 (FGFR-2) found on the chromosomal locus 10q26[61] (Fig. 27-6).

HYPERTROPHY OF THE NAIL

Large nails with anatomically normal nail units may be observed in newborns with macrodactyly. Conditions that display macronychia include epidermal nevus syndrome, Proteus syndrome, Maffucci syndrome, Klippel-Trenaunay-Weber syndrome, and gigantism. Patients with the ectrodactyly-ectodermal dysplasia–cleft lip/palate (EEC) syndrome also may have a large nail on the fused digits. Several terms are used to describe different types of enlarged nails. *Onychauxis* refers to nails that exhibit thick nail plates and retain a normal overall size and shape. *Onychogryphosis* is present when the nail plate thickens and develops an inferior overcurvature. If nail growth is uneven, the plate deviates obliquely and takes on the appearance of a ram's horn. The nail plates are usually discolored and display oyster-like striations across the surface. Although onychogryphosis is usually observed on toenails in the elderly or on digits that have been permanently injured, hereditary autosomal dominant and congenital forms involving both the fingernails and toenails have been reported.[62,63] Hemi-onycho-gryphosis has been seen in cases of congenital malalignment of the great toe nails and COIF. *Pachyonychia* refers to thickening and superior deviation of the nail plate from accumulation of subungual hyperkeratosis. This may be observed in older patients with psoriasis or onychomycosis, but the term is classically used to describe the inherited condition, pachyonychia congenita.

PACHYONYCHIA CONGENITA

Pachyonychia congenita is characterized by hard, thick nails that angle upward at their distal free edge because of massive accumulation of keratin in the ventral nail plate. The lateral borders curve under and give the plates a pincer appearance (Fig. 27-7). Unlike onychogrypho-

sis, the nails of pachyonychia congenita have a smooth surface. Although pachyonychia congenita syndrome is transmitted as an autosomal dominant trait with a high degree of penetrance, full expressivity may not become evident until later childhood or adulthood. Infants with pachyonychia congenita initially display a yellowish brown discoloration of their nails. Thickening from subungual hyperkeratosis occurs gradually over months to years.

It is now accepted that patients with pachyonychia congenita can be classified into one of two syndromes[64] that have one of several genetic defects in hard keratin.[65] Mutations in keratin 16 (located on chromosome 17) or in keratin 6A (located on chromosome 12) have been found in type I, the Jadassohn-Lewandowski variant. As newborns, these patients may have foamy white mucosal plaques of oral leukokeratosis (Fig. 27-8). During childhood debilitating palmoplantar keratoderma, hyperhidrosis, and secondary bullae develop. Clusters of rough, dry, spiny papules become evident over the body, particularly on the elbows and knees, similar to psoriasis. Later, there may be eruption of epidermoid cysts. Type II patients with the Jackson-Lawler form of the disease have abnormalities in the keratin 17 gene (found on chromosome 17) or keratin 6B (found on chromosome 12).[66,67] Natal teeth with minimal oral leukokeratosis, cylindromas, steatocystomas, and milder keratoderma are present in these cases.

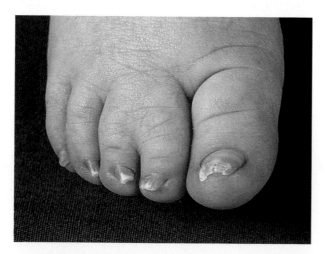

FIG. 27-7
Pachyonychia congenita. Pincer appearance of nails.

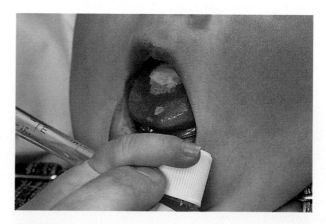

FIG. 27-8
Pachyonychia congenita. White oral mucosal leukokeratotic plaques.

INGROWN TOENAILS

There are three types of ingrown toenails in neonates. Congenital malalignment of the great toe nails presents with a trapezoid-shaped nail plate that deviates laterally with respect to the longitudinal axis of the distal phalanx[68] (Fig. 27-9). Cases may be unilateral, bilateral, sporadic, or inherited as an autosomal dominant trait.[69] Recurrent damage to the nail matrix occurs when the child is old enough to crawl and walk. This damage is manifested by multiple transverse ridges, discoloration caused by infection and hemorrhage, paronychia, onycholysis, and nail loss.[70] Mild degrees of malalignment may improve over time.[71] However, when marked deviation of the nail plate results in the distal free edge embedding into the soft tissues of the hyponychium, surgical rotation of the misdirected matrix may be necessary to prevent chronic long-term disability.[72]

Congenital hypertrophy of the lateral nail folds of the hallux may present at birth or in the first month of life as red, firm, enlarged masses of tissue that may cover significant amounts of the nail plate.[73] If the induration persists, it may become painful or infected when the infant begins to crawl or walk. The condition usually remits spontaneously. A 2-week trial of a potent topical steroid solution (e.g., fluocinonide twice daily) would not be unreasonable if surgical reduction of the excess tissue is contemplated.

Embedding of the distal free margin of the nail plate into the soft tissue of the hyponychium is not uncommon. A prominent ridge of tissue may form a wall that results in embedding or superior deflection of the nail plate. Most neonates outgrow these findings by 6 months of age.[74] Some authors believe that factors such as sleeping prone, especially when the child begins to kick actively, and tight-fitting sleepers may predispose the older infant to paronychia.[75]

PARONYCHIA AND INFECTIOUS NAIL DYSTROPHY

Infections of the nail unit in neonates are extremely important to identify and treat promptly because of the possibility of irreversible damage to the nail matrix. Acute paronychia presents with red, swollen, tender nail folds. Purulent material accumulates in the periungual groove and can extend under the nail plate. Chronic paronychia manifests with painless swelling of the nail fold, loss of the cuticle, and development of granulation tissue. Organisms responsible for paronychia include *Candida* spp.,[76] *Staphylococcus, Streptococcus, Veillonella* (in neonates),[77] anaerobes, saprophytes, and herpes simplex. Paronychia is most common on the fingers as a result of developmentally appropriate sucking or mouthing of the digits. Systemic diseases associated with paronychia include mucocutaneous candidiasis, DiGeorge syndrome, acrodermatitis enteropathica, Langerhans' cell histiocytosis,[78] and HIV infections.[79] Once diagnostic tests have been completed (e.g., cultures, Gram stain, potassium hydroxide preparation, and Tzanck preparation), treatment can be started. Burow's solution soaks aid in gentle debridement of infected tissues. In mild cases, twice daily use of topical solutions such as clindamycin or clotrimazole is indicated. Several days of concomitant applications of a topical steroid solution may reduce any pain and swelling. In more severe cases, purulent material may have to be surgically drained and granulation tissue may need to be cauterized.

Onychomycosis is extremely rare in neonates. Congenital candidiasis localized to the nails has been reported once[80] (Fig. 27-10). Presumed candidal onychomycosis without paronychia developed in a 2-week-old, and *Trichophyton rubrum* was isolated from the nails of a 4-month-old who may have acquired the organism as a neonate.[81,82]

ONYCHOLYSIS

Separation of the nail plate from the nail bed is known as onycholysis. This usually occurs at the distal free edge of the nail plate but may be observed laterally as well. The

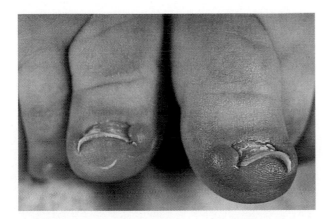

FIG. 27-9
Ingrown nails characterized by erythema and swelling of the medial nail folds in a case of congenital malalignment of the great toe nails.

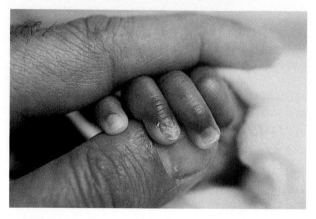

FIG. 27-10
Onychomycosis due to congenital candidiasis is characterized by punctate leukonychia, pits, brittleness, and chipping of the surface of the nail plate. (Courtesy Dr. Lloyd Krammer, INOVA Fairfax Hospital for Children.)

BOX 27-2

Causes of Onycholysis

Systemic
Thyroid disease
Iron deficiency
Erythropoietic
   protoporphyria

**Congenital/
Hereditary**
Partial hereditary
   onycholysis
Ectodermal dysplasias
Periodic shedding
   of the nails
Leprechaunism

Primary Skin Diseases
Epidermolysis bullosa
Psoriasis

Medications*
Indomethacin
Retinoids
Antibiotics
Chemotherapy

Local Causes
Thermal injury
   (pulse oximeters)
Trauma

Infections
Candida

Modified from Baran R, Dawber RPR. Diseases of the nails and their management, 2nd edition. Oxford: Blackwell Scientific Publications, 1994: p 59.
*Directly or in combination with ultraviolet light (photoonycholysis).

---

separation creates a narrow space that can fill with keratin, exogenous debris, or fluids such as water or saliva. The air pocket of the cleft gives an onycholytic nail a grayish white color. Onycholysis is a physical sign for which there are numerous causes (Box 27-2).

CHROMONYCHIA

Nail dyschromia may be due to discoloration of the nail plate or nail bed[83] (Table 27-2). The causes of nail discoloration may be exogenous, secondary to local infectious agents, systemic drugs or diseases, primary skin diseases, or ungual neoplasms (Fig. 27-11). The shape of the discolored area depends upon how and where in the nail unit the pigment is deposited, and the duration of the pigment deposition.

Leukonychia (white nails) is the most common type of nail dyschromia.[84] It should not be confused with onycholysis. Total or subtotal leukonychia may be inherited as an autosomal dominant trait.[85] Partial leukonychia on the distal portion of the nail apparatus may be a sign of congenital candidiasis limited to the nail plates.[86] Transversely striated leukonychia in a longitudinal band may be observed after a febrile illness similar to Beau's lines. Multiple striations are associated with successive events that affect the matrix, including administration of chemotherapeutic agents,[87] the classic Mees' lines of heavy metal intoxication, or Muehrcke's paired lines of hypoalbuminemia. Muehrcke's lines have also been described in the presence of zinc deficiency. Partial leukonychia in which the proximal portion of the nail is white has several eponyms. They include Lindsay's half-and-half nails of uremia and Terry's nails secondary to cirrhosis or congestive heart failure. Leukonychia may also be a sign of malnutrition or iron deficiency anemia. Punctate leukonychia is manifested by small, irregular white spots. It is usually caused by repeated minor trauma to the nail matrix.

Single longitudinal pigmented bands of the nail in children are due to melanocytic nevi located in the nail matrix (Fig. 27-12). Multiple longitudinal pigmented bands are common in dark-skinned persons but are unusual in children. Multiple brown bands may be observed in fetal hydantoin syndrome, Addison and Cushing disease, Peutz-Jegher syndrome, HIV, and after exposure to maternal chlorpromazine ingestion or other maternally ingested drugs.[88] A study of longitudinal pigmented bands in 100 individuals found that 22 persons had nail matrix nevi.[89] Twelve patients had lesions present at birth, and most were located on the fingernails. The bands were different shades, from light tan to black, and their width varied from 2 mm to the breadth of the entire nail plate.

TABLE 27-2

Chromonychia (Nails With Abnormal Color)

Condition	Color	Other features
Hematomas	Purple	Observed on fingers, similar to sucking blisters (Fig. 27-9)
Endocarditis	Purple	Splinter shaped
Phototoxicity	Purple	Drugs, porphyrias
Hyperbilirubinemia	Yellow-brown	Scleral icterus
Yellow nail syndrome	Yellow	Lymphedema, respiratory disease, nephrotic syndrome[71]
Pernicious anemia	Blue-gray	Macrocytosis
Onychomycosis	Gray-green	*Aspergillus, Pseudomonas*
Candidiasis	White	
PCB exposure	Brown-gray	
Addison's/Cushing's disease	Brown	

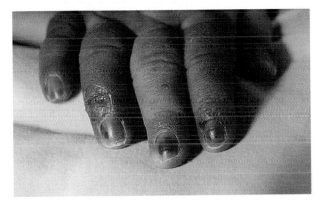

FIG. 27-11
A dusky violaceous hue of the nail beds resulting from ecchymoses and an eroded blister caused by vigorous intrauterine sucking.

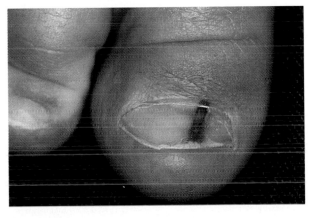

FIG. 27-12
A longitudinal pigmented band of the nail plate develops from a nevoculluar nevus in the nail matrix.

Periungual pigmentation (Hutchinson's sign) was present in many of these benign lesions. In a series of eight cases of longitudinal melanonychia in children, four were present at birth.[90] No cases of melanoma were documented in either series. There have even been isolated reports of spontaneous regression of ungual nevi.[91] Only two well-documented cases of melanoma of the nail unit in young children have been reported.[92,93] Most cases of suspected ungual melanomas are probably benign Spitz nevi. Their pathology should be interpreted with caution, even by dermatopathologists. Most experts in nail diseases do not recommend biopsy of longitudinal pigmented bands unless a previously stable lesion undergoes progressive, rapid change. Biopsy specimens should be obtained from children who are predisposed to develop malignancies (e.g., xeroderma pigmentosum or dysplastic nevus syndrome). Improperly performed biopsies can lead to permanent nail dystrophy.

REFERENCES

1. Baran R, Dawber RPR: Diseases of the nails and their management, Oxford: Blackwell Scientific Publications, 1994.

2. Silverman R: Nail and appendageal abnormalities. In Schachner LA, Hansen RC, eds. Pediatric dermatology, 2nd edition. London: Churchill Livingstone, 1995: pp 617-618.

3. Turano AF: Transverse nail ridging in early infancy. Pediatrics 1968;41:996-997.

4. Wolf D, Wolf R, Goldberg MD: Beau's lines, a case report. Cutis 1982;29:191-194.

5. Yinnon AM, Matalon M: Koilonychia of the toenails in children. Int J Dermatol 1988;27:685-687.

6. Hogan GR, Jones B: The relationship of koilonychia and iron deficiency in infants. J Pediatr 1970;77:1054-1057.

7. Crosby DL, Petersen MJ: Familial koilonychia. Cutis 1989; 44:209-210.

8. Bumpers RD, Bishop ME: Familial koilonychia: a current case. Arch Dermatol 1980;116:845-846.

9. Chapman RS: Overcurvature of the nails: an inherited disorder. Br J Dermatol 1973;89:211-213.

10. Egawa T: Congenital claw-like fingers and toes. Plast Reconstr Surg 1977;59:569-574.

11. Takeshi M, Tadao K, Ogawa Y, et al: Claw nail deformity of the toe accompanied with cleft hand. J Plast Reconstr Surg 1998;101:427-430.

12. Johnson CF: Broad thumbs and broad great toes with facial abnormalities and mental retardation. Pediatrics 1966;68:942.

13. Baran R, Dawber RPR: Diseases of the nails and their management, 2nd edition. Oxford: Blackwell Scientific Publications, 1994: pp 324-327.

14. Silverman RA: Nail and appendageal disorders. In Schachner LA, Hansen RC, eds. Pediatric dermatology, 2nd edition. London: Churchill Livingstone, 1995: p 629.

15. Katz BZ: Finger clubbing as sign of HIV infection in children [letter]. Lancet 1997;349:575.

16. Hopsu-Havu VK, Jansen CT: Anonychia congenita. Arch Dermatol 1973;107:752-753.

17. Teebi AS, Kaurah P: Total anonychia congenita and microcephaly with normal intelligence: a new autosomal-recessive syndrome? Am J Med Genet 1996;66:257-260.

18. Nevin NC, Thomas PS, Eady DJ, et al: Anonychia and absence/hypoplasia of distal phalanges (Cook's syndrome): report of a second family. J Med Genet 1995;32:638-641.

19. Rahbari H, Heath L, Chapel TA: Anonychia with ectrodactyly. Arch Dermatol 1975;111:1482-1483.

20. Verbov, J: Anonychia with bizarre flexural pigmentation—an autosomal dominant dermatosis. Br J Dermatol 1975;92:469-474.

21. Strandskov HH: Inheritance of absence of thumb nails. J Hered 1939;30:53-54.

22. Robinson GC, Miller JR, Bensimon JR: Familial ectodermal dysplasia with sensorineural deafness and other anomalies. Pediatrics 1962;30:797-802.

23. Lin, HJ, Kakkis ED, Eteson, DJ, et al: DOOR syndrome (deafness, onycho-osteodystrophy, and mental retardation): a new patient and delineation of neurologic variability among recessive cases. Am J Med Genet 1993;47:534-539.

24. Qazi QH, Heckman LS, Markouizos D, et al: The Coffin-Siris syndrome. J Med Genet 1990;27:333-336.

25. Bruckner-Tuderman L, Schnyder UW, Baran R: Nail changes in epidermolysis bullosa: clinical and pathogenic considerations. Br J Dermatol 1995;132:339-344.

26. Crain LS, Fitzmaurice NE, Mondry C: Nail dysplasia and fetal alcohol syndrome. Am J Dis Child 1983;137:1069.

27. D'Souza SW, Robertson IG, Donnai D: Fetal phenytoin exposure, hypoplastic nails, and jitteriness. Arch Dis Child 1990;65:320.

28. Hsu MM, Mak CP, Hus CC: Follow-up of skin manifestations in Yu-Cheng children. Br J Dermatol 1995;132:427-432.

29. Thakker JC, Kothari SS, Deshmu KL, et al: Hypoplasia of nails and phalanges: a teratogenic manifestation of phenobarbitone. Indian Pediatr 1991;28:73.

30. Jåger-Roman E, Deichl A, Jakob S, et al: Fetal growth, major malformations, and minor anomalies in infants born to women receiving valproic acid. J Pediatr 1986;108:997.

31. Duester GA: Hypothetical mechanism for fetal alcohol syndrome involving ethanol inhibition of retinoic acid synthesis at the alcohol dehydrogenase step. Alcohol Clin Exp Res 1991;15:568-572.

32. Fex G, Larsson K, Andersson A, et al: Low serum concentration of all-trans and 13-cis retinoic acids in patients treated with phenytoin, carbamazepine, and valproate: possible relation to teratogenicity. Arch Toxicol 1995;69:572-574.

33. Lucas GL, Opitz JM: The nail-patella syndrome: clinical and genetic aspects of 5 kindreds with 38 affected family members. J Pediatr 1966;68:273-288.

34. Simila S, Vesa L, Wasz-Hockert O: Hereditary onycho-osteodysplasia (the nail-patella syndrome) with nephrosis-like renal disease in a newborn boy. Pediatrics 1970;46:61-65.

35. Daniel CR III, Osment LS, Noojin RO: Triangular lunulae: a clue to nail-patella syndrome. Arch Dermatol 1980;116:448-449.

36. Carbonara P, Kane AC, Alpert M: Hereditary osteo-onychodysplasia (HOOD). Am J Med Sci 1964;248:139-151.

37. Browning MC, Weidner N, Lorentz WB Jr: Renal histopathology of the nail-patella syndrome in a two-year-old boy. Clin Nephrol 1988;29:210-213.

38. Looij BJ Jr, Te Slaa RL, Hogewind BL, et al: Genetic counselling in hereditary osteo-onychodysplasia (HOOD, nail-patella syndrome) with nephropathy. J Med Genet 1988;25:682-686.

39. Drut RM, Chandra S, Latorraca R, et al: Nail-patella syndrome in a spontaneously aborted 18-week fetus: ultrastructural and immunofluorescent study of the kidneys. Am J Med Genet 1992;43:693-696.

40. Lichter PR, Richards JE, Downs CA, et al: Cosegregation of open-angle glaucoma and the nail-patella syndrome. Am J Ophthalmol 1997;124:506-515.

41. Gilula LA, Kantor OS: Familial colon carcinoma in nail-patella syndrome. Am J Roentgenol 1975;123:783-790.

42. Burkhart CG, Bhumbra R, Iannone AM: Nail-patella syndrome: a distinctive clinical and electron microscopic presentation. J Am Acad Dermatol 1980;3:251-256.

43. Greenspan DC, Byers MG, Eddy RL, et al: Human collagen gene COL5A1 maps to the q34.2 q34.3 region of chromosome 9, near the locus for nail-patella syndrome. Genomics 1992;12:836-837.

44. Dreyer SD, Zhou G, Baldini A, et al: Mutations in LMX1B cause abnormal skeletal patterning and renal dysplasia in nail patella syndrome. Nat Genet 1998;19:47-50.

45. Iso R: Congenital nail defects of the index finger and reconstructive surgery. Orthop Surg (Tokyo) 1969;20:1383-1384.

46. Baran R, Stroud JD: Congenital onychodysplasia of the index fingers. Iso and Kikuchi syndrome. Arch Dermatol 1984;120:243-244.

47. Prais D, Horev G, Merlob P: Prevalence and new phenotypic and radiologic findings in congenital onychodysplasia of the index finger. Pediatr Dermatol 1999;16:201-204.

48. Youn SH, Kwon OS, Park KC, et al: Congenital onychodysplasia of the index fingers—Iso-Kikuchi syndrome. A case involving the second toenail. Clin Exp Dermatol 1996;21:457-458.

49. Kikuchi I: Congenital onychodysplasia of the index fingers: a case involving the thumbnails. Semin Dermatol 1991;10:7-11.

50. Miura T, Nakamura R: Congenital onychodysplasia of the index fingers. J Hand Surg 1990;15A:793-797.

51. Millman AJ, Strier RP: Congenital onychodysplasia of the index fingers. Report of a family. J Am Acad Dermatol 1982;7:57-65.

52. Kikuchi I: Congenital onychodysplasia of the index fingers: a case involving the thumbnails. Semin Dermatol 1991;10:7-11.

53. Muraoka M, Yoshioka N, Hyodo T: A case of double fingernail and ectopic fingernail. Ann Plast Surg 1996;36:201-205.

54. Miura T: Two families with congenital nail anomalies: nail formation in ectopic areas. J Hand Surg 1978;61:348-351.

55. Katayama I, Maeda M, Nishioka K: Congenital ectopic nail of the fifth finger. Br J Dermatol 1984;111:231-233.

56. Aoki K, Hataba Y: A case of congenital onychoheterotopia on both fifth fingers. Clin Exp Dermatol 1991;16:285-286.

57. Tomita K, Inoue K, Ichikawa H, et al: Congenital ectopic nails. Plast Reconstr Surg 1997;100:1497-1499.

58. Kalisman M, Kleinert HE: A circumferential fingernail—fingernail on the palmar aspect of the finger. J Hand Surg 1983;8:58-60.

59. Alves GF, Poon E, John J, et al: Circumferential fingernail. Br J Dermatol 1999;140:960-962.

60. Cohen MM Jr, Kreiborg S: Hands and feet in the Apert syndrome. Am J Med Genet 1995;57:82-96.

61. Wilkie AO, Slaney SF, Oldridge M, et al: Apert syndrome results from localized mutations of FGFR2 and is allelic with Crouzon syndrome. Nat Genet 1995;9:165-172.

62. Schmidt H: Total onychogryphosis traced during six generations. Proc Fenno Scand Assoc Dermatol 1965;36-37.

63. Lubach D: Erbliche onychogryphosis. Hautarzt 1982;33:331.

64. Gorlin RJ, Pindborg JJ, Cohen MM Jr: Syndromes of the head and neck, 2nd edition. New York: McGraw-Hill, 1976: pp 600-603.

65. McLean WHI, Rugg EL, Lunny DP, et al: Keratin 16 and keratin 17 mutations cause pachyonychia congenita. Nat Genet 1995;9:273-278.

66. Smith FJ, Corden LD, Rugg EL, et al: Missense mutations in keratin 17 cause either pachyonychia congenita type 2 or a phenotype resembling steatocystoma multiplex. J Invest Dermatol 1997;108:220-223.

67. Smith FJ, Jonkman MF, van Goor H, et al: A mutation in human keratin K6b produces a phenocopy of the K17 disorder pachyonychia congenita type 2. Hum Molec Genet 1998;7:1143-1148.

68. Baran R, Bureau H: Congenital malalignment of the big toenail as a cause of ingrowing toenail in infancy: pathology and treatment (a study of thirty cases). Clin Exp Dermatol 1983;8:619-623.

69. Harper KJ, Beer WE: Congenital malalignment of the great toe-nails—an inherited condition. Clin Exp Dermatol 1986;11:514-516.

70. Cohen JL, Scher RK, Pappert AS: Congenital malalignment of the great toenails. Pediatr Dermatol 1991;8:40-42.

71. Dawson TAJ: Great toe-nail dystrophy. Br J Dermatol 1989;20:139.

72. Baran R: Significance and management of congenital malalignment of the big toenail. Cutis 1996;58:181-184.

73. Hammerton MD, Shrank AB: Congenital hypertrophy of the lateral nailfolds of the hallux. Pediatr Dermatol 1988;5:243-245.

74. Honig PJ, Spitzer A, Bernstein R, Leyden JJ: Congenital ingrown toenails. Clin Pediatr 1982;21:424-426.

75. Bailie FB, Evans DM: Ingrowing toenails in infancy. Br Med J 1978;2:737-738.

76. Raval DS, Barton LL, Hansen RC, et al: Congenital cutaneous candidiasis: case report and review. Pediatr Dermatol 1995;12:355-358.

77. Sinniah D, Sandiford BR, Dugdale AE: Subungual infection in the newborn: an institutional outbreak of unknown etiology, possibly due to Veillonella. Clin Pediatr 1972;11:690-692.

78. De Berker D, Lever LR, Windebank K: Nail features in Langerhans cell histiocytosis. Br J Dermatol. 1994;1304:523-527.

79. Russo F, Collantes C, Guerrero J: Severe paronychia due to zidovudine-induced neutropenia in a neonate. J Am Acad Dermatol 1999;40:322-324.

80. Arbegast KD, Lamberty LF, Koh JK, et al: Congenital candidiasis limited to the nail plates. Pediatr Dermatol 1990;7:310-312.

81. Kurgansky D, Sweren R: Onychomycosis in a 10-week-old infant. Arch Dermatol 1990;126:1371.

82. Jewell FW: Trichophyton rubrum onychomycosis in a 4-month-old infant. Cutis 1970;6:1121-1122.

83. Paradisio M, Van Asperen P: Yellow nail syndrome in infancy. J Paediatr Child Health 1997;33:454-457.

84. Zaun H: Leukonychias. Semin Dermatol 1991;10:17-20.

85. Kates SL, Harris GD, Nagle DJ: Leuconychia totalis. J Hand Surg 1986;11:465-466.

86. Arbegast KD, Lamberty LF, Koh JK, et al: congenital candidiasis limited to the nail plates. Pediatr Dermatol 1990;7:310-312.

87. Shelly WB, Humphrey GB: Transverse leukonychia (Mees' lines) due to daunorubicin chemotherapy. Pediatr Dermatol 1997;14:144-145.

88. Silverman RA: Nail and appendageal abnormalities. In Schachner LA, Hansen RD, eds: Pediatric dermatology, 2nd edition. New York: Churchill Livingston, 1994: pp 635-636.

89. Tosti A, Baran R, Piraccini BM, et al: Nail matrix nevi: A clinical and histopathologic study of twenty-two patients. J Am Acad Dermatol 1996;34:765-71.

90. Léauté-Labreze C, Bioulac-Sage P, Taïeb A: Longitudinal melanonychia in children: a study of eight cases. Arch Dermatol 1996;132:167-169.

91. Tosti A, Baran R, Morelli R, et al: Progressive fading of a longitudinal melanonychia due to a nail matrix melanocytic nevus in a child. Arch Dermatol 1994;130:1076-1077.

92. Lyall D: Malignant melanoma in infancy. JAMA 1967;202:93.

93. Kiryu H: Malignant melanoma in situ arising in the nail unit of a child. J Dermatol 1998;25:41-44.

Index

A

Aagenaes syndrome, 334-335
Abscess
  in AIDS, 213
  breast, 182-183
  described, 38*t*, 181-182, 182*f*
  scalp, 104, 183
Absorption, percutaneous
  of hazardous compounds, 52*t*
  hazards of, 63*t*
  of neonatal skin, 62-63
  of xenobiotics, 51-53
Acanthosis, in atopic dermatitis, 260
Acanthosis nigricans, 431, 460
Acatalasemia, 480-481
Acetylcholinesterase, in EB diagnosis, 165
N-acetyl-glucosamine-1-phosphotransferase defect, 446
Achromobacter, 193
Acidemia, methylmalonic (MMA), 171, 266
Acinetobacter, 193
Acne
  diagnosis of, 145*t*
  infantile, 94*f*, 94-95
  neonatal, 94, 94*f*, 95, 154, 154*f*
Acquired immunodeficiency disease syndrome (AIDS)
  cancer as presenting sign for, 213
  chemoprophylaxis for, 214
  cutaneous findings in, 212
  infectious disorders associated with, 212-213
  inflammatory disease with, 213-214
Acrochordons, 125, 125*f*
Acrocyanosis, 98-99, 99*f*
Acrodermatitis enteropathica (AE), 150*t*, 171, 253-254, 267
Acropustulosis of infancy, 38*t*
  diagnosis of, 146*t*
  lesions of, 155*f*, 155-156
  vs. transient neonatal pustular melanosis (TNPM), 93
Acute hemorrhagic edema (AHE)
  clinical findings in, 308
  management of, 309
  pathogenesis of, 308
Acute intermittent porphyria (AIP), 310*t*
Acyclovir
  for HSV, 206
  for varicella, 208
Adams-Oliver syndrome, 126*t*, 330*t*, 331, 335
Addison disease, 382
Adhesions, labial, 482-483
Adhesives
  hydrophilic gel-based, 62
  injuries associated with, 113, 113*f*
  minimizing contact with, 166-167
  wounds from, 54
Adnexal polyp, 130, 139*f*
A&D ointment, 65*t*
Adolescence, hormonal changes of, 11
Adrenocortical unresponsiveness syndrome, 382
AEC (ankyloblepharon-ectodermal dysplasia-cleft palate) syndrome, 468*f*, 468-469, 492-493
Aeromonas spp., 193
Aerosol tents, to limit TEWL, 69
Albinism. *See also* Hypopigmentation disorders
  in Chediak-Higashi syndrome, 356*f*, 356-357
  clinical characteristics of, 354*t*
  Cross-McKusick-Breen syndrome, 356
  diagnosis of, 356
  in fetal skin development, 6
  Hermansky-Pudlak syndrome, 356
  hypopigmentation in, 98

Albinism—cont'd
  incidence of, 353, 355
  oculocutaneous, 353
Albright hereditary osteodystrophy (AHO)
  clinical findings in, 407, 407*f*
  osteoma cutis associated with, 405, 406
Alcaligenes faecalis, 193
Alcohol
  as fetal teratogen, 507*t*
  as topical antiseptic, 68
Alezzandrini syndrome, 365
Allergies, and atopic dermatitis, 244
Aloe vera protective ointment, 65*t*
Alopecia
  in acrodermatitis enteropathica (AE), 171
  areata, 495
  "black dot tinea," 230
  clinical findings in, 409*f*, 409-410
  diffuse, 491-494, 492*t*
  in focal dermal hypoplasia (FDH), 465
  halo scalp ring, 106, 106*f*
  in ichthyosis disorders, 280, 286
  in incontinentia pigmenti, 462
  from ischemia, 106, 106*f*
  with lamellar ichthyosis, 493, 493*f*
  localized, 494*b*, 494-495
  neonatal occipital, 494, 494*f*
  and nevus sebaceus, 409, 409*f*
  triangular, 494
  in Turner syndrome, 461
Alpha-fetoprotein, in EB diagnosis, 165
α-6/β-4 integrin, 22
Alveolar cysts, 88-89
Ambras syndrome, 496
Amebiasis, characteristics of, 234*t*
Aminoglycoside, for ecthyma gangrenosum, 194
Ammonium lactate, cautious use of, 67*t*
Amniocentesis, 84
  for harlequin ichthyosis, 276
  scars from, 103, 104*f*
Amnion rupture malformation sequence, 131, 131*f*
Amniotic bands, micronychia with, 507*t*
Amphotericin B
  for *Candida* infections, 226
  for fungal infections, 229, 230
Anagen
  in fetal development, 10
  loose anagen syndrome, 77
Anatomy, of skin, 19*f*
Androgens, neonatal, 94-95
Anemia, parvovirus in, 215
Anesthesia
  EMLA, 73, 80*t*, 80-81, 81*f*
  lidocaine toxicity, 81, 81*t*
Anetoderma, of prematurity, 105, 113
Angelman syndrome, 356
"Angel's kiss," 100, 324
Angioedema, 300
Angiofibromas
  in tuberous sclerosis, 455, 456, 456*f*
Angiogenesis
  defined, 341
  in fetal skin development, 8
Angioma, sudoriparous, 348
Angiomyolipomas, with tuberous sclerosis, 455
Annular configuration, 43*t*
Annular erythemas
  centrifugum, 294, 295*t*, 296
  diagnosis of, 296

Annular erythemas—cont'd
  familial, 296
  of infancy, 294, 295*t*, 296
  persistent forms, 295*t*
  transient forms, 295*t*
Annulus migrans, 479
Anonychia, of nails, 506*f*, 506-507, 507*f*
Ant bites, 235*t*
Antibacterial scrubs, 247
Antibiotics
  in atopic dermatitis, 247
  for coagulase negative staphylococci (CONS), 191
  diaper rash due to, 252
  for gram-negative infections, 193
  for nonnecrotizing subcutaneous infections, 184, 185
  for problematic hemangiomas, 344
  for *S. aureus* infections, 184
  for tuberculosis, 192
Antibiotic therapy
  for group A β-hemolytic streptococcal infections, 188-189
  for necrotizing subcutaneous infections, 186, 188
  for purpura fulminans, 195
Antifungal agents, for *Candida* diaper dermatitis, 253
Antihistamines, for pruritus, 233
Antimicrobial qualities, of newborn skin, 21
Antimicrobial washes, 67
Antisepsis, for newborns, 67-68
Apert's syndrome, 34
Aplasia cutis, 5
  bullous, 127, 127*f*
  chromosomal defects reported with, 126*t*
  congenita (ACC), 39*t*, 40*t*, 172. *See also* congenital localized absence of skin
  described, 125-126
  diagnosis of, 129, 150*t*
  etiology of, 128
  in focal dermal hypoplasia, 465
  linear facial defects of, 127, 127*f*
  in lumbosacral region, 125
  malformations associated with, 126*t*
  membranous, 127, 127*f*
  proposed etiology for, 126*t*
  scalp defect of, 128, 128*f*
  truncal, 128, 128*f*
Aplastic nevus, 495
Apligraft, for EB, 166
Apocrine glands
  fetal development of, 11-12
  in newborn skin, 24
Appendages, development of fetal, 10
Aquaphor
  composition of, 65*t*, 67
  for red scaly baby, 271
  to reduce infection, 54
  and TEWL, 51
Arachnodactyly, Beals contractural, 459
Arachnoid cyst, 340
Arciform configuration, 44*t*
Arteriovenous malformations (AVMs), 329*f*, 329-330
Arthritis
  juvenile, 303
  in Kawasaki disease, 307
Arthropathy, in NOMID, 302
Artificial skin substitutes, for EB, 166
Ascites, parvovirus in, 215
Aspergillosis
  primary cutaneous, 228-229, 229*f*
  systemic, 229

Aspergillus infection
  clinical presentation of, 142
  diagnosis of, 144*t*, 147*t*
Ataxia-telangiectasia (AT) syndrome, 326, 370
Atopic dermatitis (AD), 40*t*, 42*t*
  allergen avoidance in, 247
  classic infantile, 260
  cutaneous findings in, 241-244, 242*f*, 243*f*
  diagnosis of, 243, 244-245
  environmental control for, 245
  etiology of, 244
  evaluation of, 272*t*
  extracutaneous findings in, 244
  in HIV-infected patients, 213
  incidence of, 241
  inflammation of, 260
  management of, 272*t*
  new therapies for, 247
  prognosis for, 245
  pruritus in, 246
  treatment of, 245
  xerosis in, 246
Atrichia
  congenital, 493
  with papular lesions, 492
Atrophoderma, follicular, 493
Atrophy, described, 40*t*
Avermectin, in scabies, 233

B

Baby Magic Baby Lotion, 65*t*
Bacteremia
  in coagulase negative staphylococci (CONS), 190
  ecthyma gangrenosum with, 194
Bacterial cultures, 73, 74-75
Bacterial skin infections
  ecthyma gangrenosum, 193-194, 194*f*
  gram-negative, 192-198
  gram-positive, 179-190
  Haemophilus influenzae, 140
  initiation of, 179
  Listeria monocytogenes, 140, 191, 193
  Mycobacterium tuberculosis, 192
  Neisseria meningitidis, 194-196
  Pseudomonas, 140
  staphylococcal, 180-188
  staphylococcal scalded skin syndrome, 137-138
  Staphylococcus aureus pyoderma, 157
  streptococcal, 138, 140, 188-191
"Ball-and-socket deformity," in ichthyosis disorders, 283
Balmex diaper rash ointment, 65*t*
Bamboo hairs, 283
Bannayan-Riley-Ruvalcaba (BRR) syndrome, 330*t*, 335, 385, 466
Bannayan-Zonana syndrome, 335
Barber-Say syndrome, 498
Barrier failure, 57
Barrier functions, of skin, 46
Bart's syndrome, 160
Basal cell nevus syndrome, 370
Basement membrane, in DEJ, 8
Basic fibroblast growth factor (bFGF), 341
Bathing
  in atopic dermatitis, 246
  of newborns, 63-64
Bazex-Dupre-Christol syndrome, 493
Bazex syndrome, 489
Beare-Stevenson syndrome, 462
Bean syndrome, 330*t*, 334
Beau's lines, 505*f*, 505-506
Becker nevus syndrome, 415
Beckwith-Wiedemann syndrome, 330*t*, 335*f*, 480
Bedbug bites, 235*t*
Bee bites, 235*t*
Beetle bites, 236*t*
Behçet's disease, 483
  diagnosis of, 146*t*, 158
Benign cephalic histiocytosis, 404
Benign neonatal hemangiomatosis, 339
Benzethonium chloride, 67*t*
Benzoyl peroxide, topical, 95
Beta-hemolytic streptococci (GBS), 140, 189-190
BIDS, 489
Bilirubin, phototherapy for unconjugated, 109
Biooclusive dressings, for problematic hemangiomas, 344

Biopsy, skin, 73, 78
  in bullous pemphigoid, 169
  for cystic medial necrosis (CMN), 389
  for deep fungus, 74
  for dermatitis, 261
  for dermatosis, 170
  for diffuse mastocytosis, 262
  of encephalocraniocutaneous lipomatosis (ECL), 427
  in erythropoietic protoporphyria (EPP), 311
  fetal, 12, 84
  in GVHD, 270
  in ichthyosis disorders, 281, 282, 283, 285, 287
  in incontinentia pigmenti, 378
  for infectious panniculitis, 425
  in LEOPARD syndrome, 383
  in maternal bullous disease, 168
  for nevus of Ota, 374
  in protein C and S deficiency, 316
  for psoriasis, 262
  punch biopsy for, 78, 78*b*
  for red scaly baby, 271
  specialized tests, 79
  in SSSS, 138
  in transient porphyrinemia, 110
  in universal melanosis, 381-382
  for urticaria, 302
Biotin deficiency, 254-255
Birthmarks, vascular
  classification of, 324
  diagnosis of, 150*t*
Bite reactions, 237-238*t*
Bites
  arthropod, 236*t*-237*t*, 236-238
  described, 238
Black fly bites, 235*t*
Blanching, phenylephrine-induced, 48*f*
Blaschko lines, 7, 157
  in CHILD syndrome, 285
  in hyperpigmentation, 376*b*
  in ichthyosis disorders, 281, 282
  in incontinentia pigmenti, 462, 462*f*
  in mosaic conditions, 358
  nevus depigmentosus, 361-362
Blepharitis, seborrheic, 485
Blistering diseases and disorders, 9-10
  bullous dermatosis, 169
  evaluating, 82
  of premature infant skin, 56
Blisters
  diagnosis of, 148*t*
  in diffuse cutaneous mastocytosis, 443*f*
  in epidermolysis bullosa, 158, 158*t*, 160, 160*f*
  in mastocytosis, 167*f*, 262
  of maternal bullous disease, 168*f*, 168-169
  sucking, 148*t*, 95, 95*f*
  with TEN, 169
  transillumination, 113, 114*f*
Blood gas monitoring
  complications of, 112-113, 113*f*, 114*f*
  fetal scalp puncture for, 104
Bloom syndrome, 370, 467
Blueberry muffin baby, 312, 313*f*, 314, 440
Blue nevus, congenital, 375*f*, 375-376
Blue rubber bleb nevus syndrome, 330*t*, 334
Bockenheimer syndrome, 327, 327*f*
Body heat, escape of, 55
Bohn's nodules, 88-89, 473, 474*f*, 474*t*
Bone abnormalities. *See also* Skeletal abnormalities
  in CHILD syndrome, 285
  in desmoid fibromatosis, 399, 399*f*
  in Proteus syndrome, 466
Bone marrow transplantation (BMT)
  for Chediak-Higashi syndrome, 357
  for Griscelli syndrome, 358
Bonnet-Dechaume-Blanc syndrome, 334
Boric acid poisoning, 262
Bowel atresia, aplasia cutis associated with, 128
Brachmann-de Lange syndrome, 487
Brain tissue, heterotopic, 121, 499, 499*f*, 500*f*
Branchial cysts, 119, 119*f*
Brancial clefts
  characteristics of, 119-120
  "hemangiomatous," 335
Breast abscess
  diagnosis of, 182
  management of, 182-183
Brégeat syndrome, 334
Bronchogenic cysts, 120

Bronze baby syndrome, 110, 110*f*
Brown fat, in neonate, 23
Bruton's hypogammaglobulinemia, 271
"Bubble wrap," to limit TEWL, 69
Buffy coat smear microscopy, for *Candida* infection, 226
Bullae
  chronic bullae, disease of childhood, 169
  conditions presenting with, 138*b*
  of congenital syphilis, 196
  described, 148*t*
  diagnosis of, 147*t*
  diagnosis of bullous disease, 148*t*
  ichthyosis, 171
  impetigo, 138*b*
  in diffuse cutaneous mastocytosis, 443
  of incontinentia pigmenti, 157, 157*f*
  of staphylococcal pustulosis, 180, 180*f*
  in STSS, 189
  pemphigoid, 149*t*, 169
Bullous pemphigoid (BP) antigens, 22
Buphthalmos, 484
Burns
  chemical, 107-108, 108*f*
  due to phototherapy UVA, 109
  scald, 155
  thermal, 114*f*
Buschke-Ollendorff syndrome, 416
Butterfly-shaped mark, 324-325
Buttock, perinatal gangrene of, 108-109, 173

C

Cadherin adhesion molecules, 3
Café au lait macules, 370, 371*t*, 372*f*, 373*f*
  in neurofibromatosis, 451, 452*f*, 453
  in Proteus syndrome, 466
  in Turner syndrome, 461
Calcification, iatrogenic, 406
Calcifying disorders, 404
  dystrophic calcification, 405
  idiopathic, 405-406
  metastatic calcification, 405
Calcinosis
  metastatic, 405
  tumoral, 406
Calcinosis cutis, 110-111, 404
  from calcium salts, 111, 111*f*
  with subcutaneous fat necrosis, 111
Calciphylaxis, 405
Calluses, sucking, 40*t*, 95, 478, 479*f*
Calvarial defects, 120
Cancer. *See also* Melanoma; Neoplastic disorders
  AIDS associated with, 213
  PCR for detection of, 83
  Peutz-Jeghers syndrome associated with, 384
  testicular, 279
  xeroderma pigmentosum associated with, 380-381
Candida infection, 223
  clinical presentation of, 223
  diagnosis of, 226
  diaper rash resulting from, 252*f*
  evaluation of, 272*t*
  management of, 272*t*
  of nail, 226
  treatment of, 226-227
Candidiasis
  AIDS associated with, 212
  congenital, 141, 224, 224*f*
  diagnosis of, 144*t*
  epidemiology of, 223
  erythroderma in, 262-263
  in KID syndrome, 285
  invasive fungal dermatitis (IFD), 225
  oral (thrush), 225, 225*f*
  postnatally acquired, 141-142
  with psoriasiform Id, 250
  systemic, 224-225, 225*f*
  vs. transient neonatal pustular melanosis (TNPM), 93
Capillary blood cell velocity (CBV), 26
Capillary ectasias, 100
Capillary malformations
  butterfly-shaped mark, 324-325
  port wine stains, 325*f*, 325-326
  salmon patch, 324, 325*f*
  telangiectasia, 326
Caput succedaneum, artificial, 107
Carbohydrate-deficient glycoprotein syndrome, 432
Carbon baby, 381

Carcinoma, nevus sebaceus associated with, 410. *See also* Cancer
Cardiac conditions
  Kawasaki disease associated with, 307
  LEOPARD syndrome associated with, 382
Carney syndrome, 371*t*, 375, 383, 384
Catagen, in fetal development, 11
Cataracts, in ichthyosis disorders, 286. *See also* Ocular problems
Caterpillar bites, 235*t*
Catheterization, of umbilical arteries, 108, 108*f*
Cellulitis, 42*t*, 182*f*
  in AIDS, 213
  clinical findings in, 184-185
  diagnosis of, 185
  erysipelas, 188
  management of, 185
Centipede bites, 235*t*
Central nervous system (CNS)
  malformations, 340
  toxicity, 52
Cephalhematoma, 106, 107, 107*f*
Cephaloceles, 121
Ceramides, in epidermal barrier, 20-21
Ceruloplasmin therapy, 365
Cervical tabs, 118-119, 119*f*
Cesarean section
  and HPV, 218
  scalpel lacerations from, 107
Chagas disease, 234*t*
Chanarin-Dorfman syndrome, 265, 277*t*, 280, 282
Chediak-Higashi syndrome (CHS), 356*f*, 356-357
  hair examination in, 78*t*
  hypopigmentation in, 98
Cheilitis, AIDS associated with, 212
Chemotherapy
  for fibrosarcoma, 439
  for Langerhans' cell histiocytosis, 438
Chickenpox. *See* Varicella
CHILD (congenital hemidysplasia with ichthyosiform nevus and limb defects) syndrome, 277*t*, 285*f*, 285-286, 411, 412
Chimerism, human, 376
CHIME syndrome, 277*t*, 287-288
Chlorhexidine gluconate, for skin antisepsis, 68
Cholesterol
  in epidermal barrier, 20-21
  in ichthyosis disorders, 279
Cholestyramine in Aquaphor, 65*t*
Chondrodysplasia punctata, 265, 265*f*
Chondroectodermal dysplasia, 478*t*
Chorionic villus sampling (CVS), 84, 103-104
Christ-Siemens-Touraine syndrome, 469, 469*f*
Chromonychia, 512-513, 513*f*, 513*t*
Chromosomal abnormalities. *See also* Genetics; Mutations
  chromosome 16-18 defect, 126*t*
  hypomelanosis of Ito with, 359
  micronychia in, 507*t*
Circumcision, meatal ulceration following, 114
Clawlike nails, 506
Cleft palate
  in ankyloblepharon, ectodermal defects and cleft lip (AEC) syndrome, 468
  in ectrodactyly-ectodermal dysplasia-clefting (EEC) syndrome, 469
Clefts
  branchial, 119-120, 335
  midline cervical, 120
  supraumbilical, 120
Clostridium perfringens, 193
Clouston syndrome, 469
Clubbing, of nails, 506
Coagulase-negative staphylococci (CONS), 190-191
Coal tar, cautious use of, 67*t*
"Coast of Maine" appearance, 372, 373
Cobalamin deficiency, 267
"Cobblestone" appearance, 416
Cobb syndrome, 330*t*, 334
Cockayne syndrome, 380
Coffin-Siris syndrome, 487, 497, 507, 507*t*
Cold temperature
  exposure to, 98-99, 99*f*
  panniculitis from, 423
  resistance to, 423
Collagenomas, in tuberous sclerosis, 455, 456*f*

Collagens, 22
  dermal, 22
  in newborn DEJ, 22
Collodion baby, 276, 278-277*t*, 278-279, 279*f*, 280, 493, 493*f*
Colobomata, 483-484
Colony-stimulating factors (CSFs), 28
Color changes
  pigmentary abnormalities, 96*f*, 96-98, 97*b*, 97*f*-100*f*
  from vascular abnormalities, 98-100, 99*f*, 100*f*
Comedonicus nevus, 412-414, 413*f*
Complement deficiency, 196
Computed tomography (CT)
  in cellulitis, 185
  for dermoid cysts, 123
  in neuroblastoma, 440
Condyloma acuminata, in HPV infection, 217
Condyloma lata, *vs.* syphilis diagnosis, 218
Congenital adrenal hyperplasia (CAH), 98
Congenital blue nevi, 375*f*, 375-376
Congenital eccrine angiomatous hamartoma, 348
Congenital erythropoietic porphyria (CEP), 309, 310*t*, 311
Congenital generalized lipodystrophy (CGL), 431-432
Congenital ichthyosiform erythroderma (CIE), 263, 264*f*
Congenital localized absence of skin (CLAS), 160, 161*f*
Congenital melanocytic nevi (CMN), 386-391, 495
Congenital milia syndrome, 151*t*
Congenital nonbullous ichthyosiform erythroderma (CIE), 277*t*, 280
Congenital onychodysplasia of index fingers (COIF), 508*f*, 508-509
Congenital varicella syndrome, 206
Congestive heart failure. *See also* Cardiac conditions
  hemangiomas associated with, 343
  in I-cell disease, 447
Connective tissue nevus, 416*f*, 416-417
Conradi-Hünermann syndrome, 265, 265*f*, 277*t*, 286, 286*f*
Contact dermatitis
  allergic, 67
  cutaneous findings in, 253
  management of, 253
  pathogenesis of, 253
Copper histidine therapy, 365
Copper-transporting P-type ATP-ase, 488
Coproporphyria, 312
Cord care regimens, 67
Corneal lesions, in ichthyosis disorders, 289. *See also* Ocular problems
Cornelia de Lange syndrome, 45, 487, 497, 497*f*
Corneocytes, 20-21
Cornification, disorders of. *See* Ichthyosis
Coronary artery aneurysms, Kawasaki disease associated with, 307. *See also* Cardiac conditions
Corticosteroids
  for atopic dermatitis, 246, 260
  for problematic hemangiomas, 344-345, 345*f*
  for pruritus, 233
  for psoriasis, 250, 262
  for pyoderma gangrenosum, 170
  scabies associated with, 232
  side effects of, 345
Corymbiform configuration, 44*t*
Costello syndrome, 458, 460, 487
Covermark, 359
Cowden syndrome, 466
Cowlick, 487
Cradle cap, 242*f*, 248
Crandall syndrome, 489, 489*f*
Cranial dysraphism
  cephaloceles, 121
  dermoid cyst and sinus, 122*f*, 122-123
  nasal gliomas, 122, 122*f*
Critic-Aid, composition of, 65*t*
Cronkhite-Canada syndrome, 385
Cross-McKusick-Breen syndrome, 356
Crusts
  described, 38
  eczematous dermatitis with, 253*f*
  in Sweet syndrome, 305*f*
Curth-Macklin disorder, 277*t*, 281
Cutis laxa, 457*f*, 457-458
Cutis marmorata, 44*t*, 98-99, 99*f*
Cutis marmorata telangiectatica congenita (CMTC), 44, 172, 330-331, 331*f*

Cutis verticis gyrata, 460, 461-462
Cystic fibrosis (CF)
  erythematous lesions in, 267, 267*f*
  zinc abnormalities in, 255
Cystic hygroma, 328, 328*f*. *See also* Lymphangiomas
Cysts
  arachnoid, 340
  branchial, 119, 119*f*
  bronchogenic cysts, 120
  dermoid, 36, 122*f*, 122-123
  epidermal inclusion, 89
  eruption, 474*t*, 475, 475*f*
  foreskin, 89
  median raphe, 89, 120, 120*f*
  mucous retention, 473
  of omphalomesenteric duct, 130-131
  palatal, 88-89
  preauricular, 117-118, 118*f*
  renal, 455
  thyroglossal duct, 482
  urachal, 130, 130*f*
  urethral retention, 483
Cytokines
  in atopic dermatitis, 244
  in neonates, 28
Cytomegalovirus (CMV) infection, 141
  clinical findings of, 211
  dermal erythropoiesis with, 314
  diagnosis of, 203*t*, 211
  therapy for, 211

D

Dandy-Walker malformation, 340
Darier's sign, 82-83, 167, 262, 442*f*, 443
Darkfield examination, for treponemal antigen, 141
De Barsy syndrome, 460
Deerfly bites, 236*t*
Dellman syndrome, 427
Demarcation lines, pigmentary, 385-386
Demodicidosis, 233, 234*t*
Dennie-Morgan fold, 243
Depigmentation. *See* Albinism; Hypopigmentary disorders
Depigmentosus, 361
Dermablend, 359
Dermabrasion, for epidermal nevus, 412
Dermal-epidermal junction (DEJ)
  in fetal development, 8-9
  in newborn skin, 21-22
Dermal hypoplasia, focal facial, 127, 127*f*
Dermal immune system (DIS), 27
Dermal melanosis (Mongolian spots), 96, 96*f*. *See also* Mongolian spots
Dermal microvascular unit (DMU), 27
Dermal ridge patterns, absent, 173
Dermatitis. *See also* Atopic dermatitis; Contact dermatitis; Irritant diaper dermatitis; Seborrheic dermatitis
  "ammoniacal," 63
  Candida diaper, 225*f*, 225-226
  described, 241
  distribution of, 260-261
  nickel, 253
Dermatofibrosarcoma protuberans (DFSP), 239-440, 439*f*, 440*f*
Dermatoglyphics, absence of, 470
Dermatomal configuration, 43*t*
Dermatophyte test medium (DTM), 74
Dermatophytosis
  diagnosis of, 231
  tinea capitis, 230, 230*f*
  tinea corporis, 230
  tinea faciei, 230
  Trichophyton spp., 230
Dermatosis
  chronic, 149*t*
  congenital erosive and vesicular, 170
  diagnosis of, 149*t*
Dermis
  anatomy of, 19*f*
  in fetal skin development, 6-8
  in newborn skin, 22
  specialized components of, 7-8
Dermographism, familial, 302
Dermoid cysts, 36, 122*f*, 122-123
Dermopathy, restrictive, 7, 150*t*, 171-172, 289*f*, 289-290

Desitin diaper rash ointment, 65t
Desmoid fibromatoses, 396t, 398-399, 399f
Desquamation
    neonatal, 99f, 101
    of SSSS, 187f
Developmental abnormalities, 123-125, 124f, 125f
    accessory tragi, 118, 118f
    adnexal polyp, 130, 139f
    amnion rupture malformation sequence, 131, 131f
    aplasia cutis, 125-129, 127f, 128f
    branchial cysts, 119, 119f
    bronchogenic cysts, 120
    cervical tabs, 118-119, 119f
    cranial dysraphism, 121
    cutaneous dimples, 129-130
    median raphe cysts, 120, 120f
    midline cervical clefts, 120
    neural tube dysraphism, 120
    preauricular pits and sinuses, 117-118, 118f
    supernumerary digits, 119, 119f
    supernumerary mammary tissue, 117, 118f
    supraumbilical cleft, 120
    of umbilicus, 130f, 130-131, 131f
Diabetes, gestational, 33
Diagnostic procedures. See also specific disorders
    bacterial cultures, 73, 74-75
    Darier's sign, 82-83
    darkfield examination, 83, 83b
    direct fluorescent antibody (DFA), 75-76
    EMLA in, 80t, 80-81, 81f
    fluorescence in situ hybridization, 73, 84
    for herpesvirus infection, 73, 75-76
    immunofluorescence, 73, 79-80
    microscopic hair exam, 77-78
    Nikolsky sign, 82, 262
    polymerase chain reaction, 73, 76, 83-84, 235
    postoperative wound care, 73, 81-82
    potassium hydroxide examination, 73-74, 74b, 74f
    prenatal, 84-85
    for scabies, 73, 77b, 77f
    skin biopsy, 73, 78b, 78-79
    Tzanck preparation, 73, 74, 75, 75b, 76t
    viral culture, 73, 76
    Wood's light exam, 83
Diaper care products, 64, 65t-66t, 66-67, 250
Diaper dermatitis
    Candida, 252
    cutaneous findings in, 251, 251f, 252f
    incidence of, 250-251
    irritant (IDD), 251, 251f
    management of, 252
    pathogenesis of, 251-252
    in premature infant, 54
Diaper erosions, 154
Diapering, in neonatal nursery, 64
Diarrhea, in AE, 171
Diazoxide, hypertrichosis induced by, 498
Dietary measures, for lipodystrophy, 432
Diffuse cutaneous mastocytosis, 443f, 443-444
DiGeorge syndrome, 271
Digital fibromatoses, infantile, 396t, 400, 400f
Digits, supernumerary, 119, 119f
Dilantin, effect on nails of, 12
Dimples, cutaneous
    etiology of, 130
    genetic disorders associated with, 129b
    location of, 129
    lumbosacral, 125, 125f
Direct fluorescent antibody (DFA) test
    for herpesvirus infection, 73, 75-76
    for treponemal antigen, 141
Disseminated intravascular coagulation (DIC)
    bullae due to, 173
    purpura fulminans in, 315
DNA, detection of foreign, 83
Dr. Danis buttocks cream, 65t
Dohi, reticulate acropigmentation of, 385
DOOR (deafness, onycho-osteodystrophy, retardation)
    syndrome, 506
Dowling-Meara EB, 160, 160f, 161, 163, 164
Down syndrome, 33, 34
    leukemoid reaction in, 157
    milia-like lesions associated with, 405
Drug eruptions, cutaneous, 299f, 299-300
Dyprotex, 65t
Dyschromatosis symmetrica hereditaria, 385
Dyschromatosis universalis hereditaria, 385

Dyskeratosis congenita
    micronychia in, 507t
Dysraphism
    cranial, 120-123, 121f, 122
    neural tube, 120-123, 121f, 122
    spinal, 123-125, 124f, 125f
Dystrophic Epidermolysis Bullosa Research Association
    (DebRA), 167

E

Ear
    calcified nodule of, 405, 405f
    preauricular pits and sinuses, 117-118, 118f
Ecchymoses, perinatal, 105
Eccrine duct, obstructions of, 89
Eccrine glands
    fetal development of, 11
    in newborn, 25
    in premature infant skin, 55
Echovirus 19 infection, 141
Ecthyma gangrenosum, 193-194, 194f
Ectodermal dysplasias, 172-173, 290, 468-470, 507t
    hidrotic ectodermal, 492
    hypohidrotic ectodermal, 492
    X-linked hypohidrotic ectodermal, 265-266, 266f
Ectoparasitic infestations, 231-233. See also Parasitic
    infestations
Ectropion, in ichthyosis disorders, 280
Eczematous disorders
    biotin deficiency with, 254
    contact dermatitis, 253
    described, 241
    diaper dermatitis, 250-253
    hand and foot, 40t
    in Hartnup disease, 255
    hyper-IgE syndrome, 256
    Job syndrome, 256
    nummular, 43t
    in Omenn syndrome, 255
    phenylketonuria associated with, 255
    psoriasis, 249-250
    seborrheic dermatitis, 247-249
    Wiscott-Aldrich syndrome, 255f, 255-256
    zinc deficiency, 253
EDA gene, 12
Edema
    acute hemorrhage, 308f, 308-309
    parvovirus associated with, 215
    in Turner's syndrome, 460
EEC (ectrodactyly-ectodermal dysplasia-clefting) syn-
    drome, 469
Effusions, parvovirus in, 215
Ehlers-Danlos syndrome (EDS), 458-459, 459f
Elase ointment, 65t
Elastic stockings, 333-334
Elastin (ELN) gene, 458
Electron microscopic (EM) studies, 73, 79
    in EB, 164
    of embryonic dermal development, 7
    in epidermolytic hyperkeratosis, 281
    in Farber disease, 467
    in hair shaft abnormalities, 490, 490f, 491
    of hypopigmented macules, 363
    in lipoblastoma, 429-430
Elejalde syndrome, 358
Ellis-van Creveld syndrome, 478t
Embryology
    cutaneous, 18
    of dermis, 7
    of epidermis, 3-4
Embryopathy, varicella, 206
EMLA (eutectic mixture of local anesthetics), 80-81
    for drug eruptions, 299
    petechial eruption with, 81f
    safe use of, 80t
Emollients, 57
    for AEC syndrome, 468-469
    for atopic dermatitis, 260
    in ichthyosis, 276
    for psoriasis, 262
    for red scaly baby, 271
    to reduce infection, 54
    use of, 64-67, 65t-66t

Encephaloceles, 121f, 495
    vs. deep hemangiomas, 342
    evaluation of, 121
    with hypertrichosis, 499
Encephalocraniocutaneous lipomatosis (ECL),
    427-428
Endovascular embolization, for AVMs, 330
Enteroviral infections, 141
    clinical findings in, 216f, 216-217
    diagnosis of, 203t, 217
    vs. HSV diagnosis, 205-206
    treatment for, 217
Enzyme-linked immunosorbent assay (ELISA)
    in NLE, 298
    for toxoplasmosis, 235
    for varicella, 208
Eosinophilia, peripheral, of erythema toxicum, 91
Eosinophilic gastroenteritis, 271
Eosinophilic pustular folliculitis, 146t, 156, 156f
Epidermal necrosis, 149t
"Epidermal nevus syndrome," 411
Epidermis
    anatomy of, 19f
    basal cell layer, 20
    components of, 2-3
    embryonic development of, 3-4
    fetal development of, 4-5, 18-19
    in newborn skin, 21
    specialized cells within, 5-6
Epidermolysis bullosa (EB), 148t, 19, 39t
    anonychia with, 507
    classification system for, 164
    cutaneous findings in, 158, 158f, 160, 160f
    described, 158
    diagnosis of, 79, 148t, 165
    dystrophic, 162-163
    etiology of, 163-164
    extracutaneous findings in, 160-161, 162, 166
    junctional, 160, 162
    Kindler syndrome, 163
    Koebner, 161, 163
    laboratory evaluation of, 164-165
    management of, 165-167, 166t
    milia associated with, 88
    neonatal complications of, 165, 166t
    pathogenesis of, 163-164
    prenatal diagnosis of, 164-165
    recessive dystrophic, 160
    simplex, 161f, 161-162
    subtypes for, 159t
    superficialis, 163
    Weber-Cockayne, 161, 163
Epidermolysis bullosa acquisita (EBA) antigen, in new-
    born DEJ, 22
Epidermolysis bullosa simplex, with mottled pigmenta-
    tion (EBS-MP), 162
Epidermolytic hyperkeratosis, 277t, 280 281, 281f, 282
Epilepsy, in tuberous sclerosis, 454
Epiluminescent microscopy (ELM), 77
Epstein pearls, 88, 89t, 474t, 474-475, 475f
Epulis, congenital, 473
Erosions, 95
    in AEC, 468f
    conditions presenting with, 139b
    described, 39t
    diagnosis of, 147t, 151t
    diaper, 154
    of HSV, 204-205, 205f
    iatrogenic causes of, 155
    of linear porokeratosis, 172
    in maternal bullous disease, 168, 168f
    in NLE, 169
    overlying giant nevi, 172
    of SSSS, 137-138, 187f
    with TEN, 169
Eruption cysts, 474t, 475, 475f
Eruptions
    of congenital syphilis, 196
    drug-related, 299
    phototherapy-induced, 109-110, 110f
    purpuric phototherapy-induced, 316
Erysipelas, 188
Erythema
    annular, 294, 295t, 296, 296t
    of SSSS, 137
    from umbilical artery catheterization, 108, 108f

Erythema multiforme (EM)
  clinical findings in, 303f, 303-304
  diagnosis of, 304
  etiology of, 304
  laboratory evaluation of, 304
  management of, 304
Erythema toxicum neonatorum, 38t, 91, 93, 152
Erythroderma. See also Inflammatory diseases
  bullous congenital ichthyosiform, 277t, 280-281, 281f
  congenital ichthyosiform, 263, 264f, 277t, 280
  described, 260
  differential diagnosis for, 261b
  of GVHD, 269f, 269-270, 270f
  ichthyosiform, 278
  scaling, 276
Erythrokeratoderma progressive symmetrica, 287
Erythrokeratoderma variabilis, 286-287, 287f
Erythromycin, for infantile acne, 95
Erythropoiesis, dermal, 312, 313f, 314
Erythropoietic porphyria, congenital, 309, 310t, 311
Erythropoietic protoporphyria, 310t, 311f, 311-312
Escherichia coli, 193
Essential fatty acid (EFA) deficiency, 268
Estimated gestational age (EGA), 1
Eucerin cream, 65t, 66
Eumelanin, 20
Evaporimeter, 50
Extracorporeal membrane oxygenation (ECMO) therapy, complications of, 106, 106f
Extramedullary hematopoiesis (EMH), 212. See also Erythropoiesis, dermal

F

Failure to thrive
  in ichthyosis disorders, 283
  in Leiner's phenotype, 268-269
  in Riley-Day syndrome, 457
Familial cold urticaria, 301
Familial hemophagocytic lymphohistiocytosis (FHL), 438
Familial peeling skin syndrome, 282
Familial progressive hyperpigmentation, 381
Fanconi syndrome, 487
Farber disease, 433, 445-446, 467
Fasciitis, necrotizing, 185-186
Fat, subcutaneous, 420. See also Subcutaneous fat disorders
Feet. See also Soles
  congenital nodules of, 428-429, 429f
  multiple anomalies of, 131, 131f
  in Turner syndrome, 461f
Fetal alcohol syndrome, 33, 498
Fetal hydantoin syndrome, 487
Fetal varicella syndrome, 141, 206f, 206-209, 207f
Fetoscopy, 84
Fetus papyraceus, aplasia cutis with, 128, 128f
Fibrolipomas, polypoid, 426
Fibromas
  vs. NLCS, 426
  periungual, 456
  warty, 431
Fibromatoses
  adult-type, 401f, 401-402
  classification of, 395, 395b, 396t
  colli, 396t, 399-400
  desmoid-type, 396t, 398-399, 399f
  gingival, 396t, 401
  hamartoma of infancy, 396t, 400-401
  infantile digital, 396t, 400, 400f
  infantile myofibromatosis, 395, 396t, 397f, 397-398, 398f
  juvenile, 396t
  juvenile hyaline, 444-445
  of skin and soft tissues, 395b
Fibronectin, 23
Fibrosarcoma, congenital/infantile, 438, 439f
Fibrosis, focal dermal cicatricial, 113
Filaggrin, 20
Fingertips, blisters of, 173
Fissure, described, 40t
Fistulae, of lower lip, 478-479
5-fluorocytosine (5-Fc), 227
Flea-bite dermatitis, 91
Flea bites, 235t, 236f

Fluconazole
  for Candida infections, 226, 227
  for candidal infection, 227
Fluid intake, in ichthyosis disorders, 276, 278
Fluorescence in situ hybridization (FISH), 84
Fluorescent antibody-to-membrane antigen assays (FAMA), for varicella, 208
Fly bites, 236t
Focal dermal hypoplasia, 40t, 151t, 172
Follicularis, ichthyosis, 493
Folliculitis, 181-183
  in AIDS, 213
  eosinophilic pustular, 156, 156f
  management of, 181
  pathogenesis of, 181
Food, and atopic dermatitis, 244
Forceps injury
  fat necrosis of temple secondary to, 421f, 421
  marks from, 105, 106f
Fordyce condition, 24
Fordyce spots, 479, 479f
Foreskin cysts, 89
4p(-) syndrome, aplasia cutis associated with, 127t
Freckling, in neurofibromatosis, 452f, 453
Free fatty acids, in epidermal barrier, 20-21
Fresh frozen plasma, for purpura fulminans, 316
Fungal culture
  media for, 74
  samples, 74
Fungal infections
  aspergillosis, 142, 228-229, 229f
  candidiasis, 141-142, 223-225
  dermatophytosis, 230f, 230-231, 231f
  diagnosis of, 73
  Malassezia, 54, 227, 227f, 228
  mucormycosis, 229f, 229-320
  onychomycosis, 231
  phycomycosis, 229f, 229-230
  trichosporosis, 142, 228
  zygomycosis, 142, 229
Fungemia, Malassezia, 228
Funisitis, 184

G

Gait, in CHIME syndrome, 287
Gallstones, protoporphyrin-rich, 311
Gangrene
  of buttock, 108-109, 151t
  diagnosis of, 151t
  perinatal, 108, 108f, 173
Gardnerella vaginalis, 193
Gastroenteritis, eosinophilic, 271
Gastrulation, 3
Gaucher's disease, 277t, 288, 370
Generalized atrophic benign epidermolysis bullosa (GABEB), 162, 163
GeneTest, 13
Gene therapy
  for EB, 167
  in X-linked recessive ichthyosis, 279-280
Genetic counseling, 12
Genetic disorders. See also Mutations; specific disorders
  cutaneous dimples associated with, 129b
  prenatal diagnosis of, 73
Genetics
  of albinism, 353, 354t, 355-356
  of atopic dermatitis, 244
  for Bannayan-Riley-Ruvalcaba syndrome, 385
  of Bloom syndrome, 467
  of CEP, 309
  for chondrodysplasia punctata, 286
  of cutis laxa, 457-458
  for EEC, 470
  of epidermolytic hyperkeratosis, 281
  of erythrokeratoderma variabilis, 287
  for Griscelli syndrome, 358
  of hypopigmentation disorders, 360, 365
  of incontinentia pigmenti, 378, 463
  for KID syndrome, 284
  of lamellar ichthyosis, 280
  of mastocytosis, 444
  of McCune-Albright syndrome, 373
  of nail-patella syndrome, 508
  for neonatal purpura fulminans, 315
  of Netherton syndrome, 283

Genetics—cont'd
  neuroblastoma, 440
  for neurofibromatosis, 372, 453
  of psoriasis, 250
  of Riley-Day syndrome, 457
  of Sjögren-Larsson syndrome, 282
  of subcutaneous fat disorders, 427, 428, 431, 432
  of TTD, 284
  of tuberous sclerosis, 457
Genital mucous membrane disorders
  labial adhesions, 482-483
  perianal pyramidal protrusion, 483, 483f
  pyoderma gangrenosum, 483
  urethral retention cyst, 483
Genitourinary malformations, in EEC, 469-470
Gentian violet, 67
Geographic tongue, 479
Gigantism, 509
Glaucoma
  congenital, 484, 484f
  infantile, 484
  signs of, 484
Glioma, nasal, 122, 122f, 342
"Glistening dots," 282
Glomangiomas, 348
Glomangiomatosis, familial, 348
Glomus tumors, 348
Glucocorticoid treated mothers, preterm infants of, 47
Glycerin, cautious use of, 67t
Glycosaminoglycans (GAGs), 23
Goldenhar syndrome, 118, 427
Goltz syndrome, 7, 40, 151, 172-173, 426, 427
  focal dermal hypoplasia of, 456f, 464-465
Gorham syndrome, 334
Gorlin syndrome, 12
Graft-versus-host disease (GVHD)
  clinical manifestations of, 269f, 269-270, 270f
  onychoatrophy associated with, 509
Granular cell tumor, 474, 474t
Granules
  in Chediak-Higashi syndrome, 357
  Fordyce, 479, 479f
Granuloma
  injection site, 424
  pyogenic, 348
  umbilical, 131, 131f
Griscelli syndrome
  clinical findings in, 357-358
  hair examination in, 78t
Group A streptococcal (GAS) infections, 138, 140, 189
  diagnosis of, 144t
  impetigo, 188-189
  necrotizing fasciitis, 188-189
  toxic shock syndrome, 189
Group B streptococcal (GBS) infections
  clinical findings in, 189-190
  diagnosis of, 144t, 147t
  management of, 190
  pathogenesis of, 190
Grouped configuration, 44t
Growth factors (GFs), 28
Gunther disease, 173
Guttate (teardrop) lesions, 250
Gyrate configuration, 44t

H

Haemophilus influenzae infection, 140, 144t
Hair, 10
  in AEC syndrome, 468
  bamboo, 283
  disorders of hairline, 487
  hair shaft abnormalities, 487-491
  heterochromia of scalp hair, 487
  in CHIME syndrome, 287
  examination of, 35
  microscopic examination of, 77
  in newborn evaluation, 45
  scalp hair whorls, 487
  scrotal, 500
  in TTD, 284
  uncombable, 490
Hair collar sign, 121, 127f

Hair follicles
  embryonic development of, 4f
  fetal development of, 10-11
  in newborn skin, 23-24, 24f
Hairline, displacement of, 487
Hair shaft, composition of, 10
Hair shaft abnormalities
  hypotrichosis with, 491
  monilethrix, 487-488, 488f
  pili annulati, 491
  pili torti, 488f, 488-489, 489f
  trichorrhexis invaginata, 491, 491f
  trichorrhexis nodosa, 489, 489f
  trichothiodystrophy, 489f, 489-490, 490f
  uncombable hair, 490
  woolly hair, 490
Hair whorls, of scalp, 487
Hairy patch, 123-124, 124f
Hallermann Streiff syndrome, 478t, 495
Hallopeau-Siemens EB, 162
Halo nevus, 364
Halo scalp ring, 106, 106f
Hamartomas, 125
  congenital nevi as, 388
  congenital smooth muscle, 414f, 414-415, 499
  connective tissue nevus, 416f, 416-417
  described, 408
  of eccrine ducts, 414
  epidermal nevus, 410-412
  fibrous, 396t, 400-401
  Michelin tire baby, 415
  nevus comedonicus, 412-414, 413f
  nevus lipomatosus, 416, 416f
  nevus sebaceus, 409f, 409-410
  in Proteus syndrome, 466
Hands. See Palms
Happy Hiney, 66t
Harderoporphyria, 312
Harlequin ichthyosis, 276, 277t, 278, 278f
Hartnup disease, 255
Hashimoto-Pritzker disease, 437
Hay Wells syndrome, 468f, 468-469, 492-493
Hazardous compounds, percutaneous absorption of, 52, 63, 63t
Head cover, to limit TEWL, 69
Hearing deficits, screening for, 117
Heart block, NLE associated with, 297, 298. See also Cardiac conditions
"Heat rash," 90
Heel pricks
  calcified nodules from, 111-112, 112f
  complications of, 105, 105f
Hemangioendothelioma, spindle cell (SCHE), 348
Hemangiomas, 37t, 39t
  clinical course for, 342-344, 343f
  common, 338-339, 339f
  congenital, 336, 338, 338f
  CVS associated with, 104
  diagnosis of, 341-342
  differentiated from vascular malformations, 337t
  facial, 340f, 340-341
  of head and neck, 343
  management of, 344-346
  multiple neonatal, 339-340, 340f
  of oral mucosa, 474, 475, 475f
  pathogenesis of, 341
  precursors for, 336, 336f, 338f
  of premature infant skin, 56-57
  with spinal dysraphism, 124f, 124-125
  strawberry, 338, 339f
  structural malformations associated with, 340f, 340-341, 341f
  ulcerations associated with, 39t, 172
  visceral, 338f, 339
Hemangiomatosis, visceral, 343
Hemangiopericytoma, infantile, 348
Hemidesmosomes, in newborn DEJ, 22f
Hemionychogryphosis, 510
Hemiplegia, in incontinentia pigmenti, 462
Hennekam syndrome, 334
Henoch-Schönlein purpura, 309
Hepatoerythropoietic porphyria (HEP), 312
Hepatomegaly, in NLE, 297
Hereditary diseases and disorders
  Beare-Stevenson syndrome, 462
  Costello syndrome, 460
  cutis verticis gyrata, 461-462

Hereditary diseases and disorders—cont'd
  cutix laxa, 457f, 457-458
  de Barsy syndrome, 460
  ectodermal dysplasia syndromes, 468-470
  Ehlers-Danlos syndromes, 458
  ichthyosis, 263-266
  Marfan syndrome, 459-460
  mosaic disorders, 462-467
  neurocutaneous syndromes, 451-455
  Noonan syndrome, 461
  photosensitivity disorders, 467-468
  Turner syndrome, 460-461, 461f
Hereditary osteoonchodysplasia (HOOD), 508
Herlitz (gravis) EB, 162, 163
Hermansky-Pudlak syndrome (HPS)
Herpes gestationis, 168
Herpes simplex virus (HSV) infection, 37t, 39t, 142-143
  diagnosis of, 144t-145t, 147t, 202, 203t, 205
  epidemiology of, 200
  erythema with, 263
  evaluation of, 272t
  intrapartum inoculation of, 104
  intrauterine, 202, 204
  management of, 202, 202t
  neonatal (perinatal), 204
  prognosis for, 202, 204, 205
Herpes zoster, diagnosis of, 145t. See also Chickenpox
Herpetiform configuration, 44t
Heteroplasia, progressive osseous, 407, 407f, 408
Hibiclens, 68
Hidrotic ectodermal dysplasia, 469
Hip joints, tumoral calcinosis of, 406
Histiocytoses
  benign cephalic, 404
  congenital "self-healing," 146t, 156
  Langerhans' cell, 436-438, 437f, 438f
  non-Langerhans' cell, 402-404, 403f, 404f
Hives. See Urticaria
Hornet bites, 235t
Horsefly bites, 236t
Human immunodeficiency virus (HIV) infection
  diagnosis of, 203t
  perinatal transmission of, 213
  TB associated with, 192
Human papilloma virus (HPV) infection
  clinical findings in, 217, 217f, 218f
  diagnosis of, 218-219
  pathogenesis of, 217-218
  treatment for, 219
Hunter syndrome, 370
Hurler syndrome, 447
Hutchinson's sign, 513
Hyaluronic acid, 23
Hydantoins, micronychia with, 507t
Hydrocephalus
  NCM associated with, 389
  transillumination devices for detection of, 113
Hydrops, secondary to parvovirus, 215
Hydroxyzine hydrochloride, cutaneous reactions associated with, 300
Hyperbilirubinemia
  history in, 34
  phototherapy for, 55, 57
Hyperimmunoglobulin E syndrome
  clinical findings in, 157
  diagnosis of, 146t
Hyperinsulinemia, 498
Hyperkeratosis (scaling)
  epidermolytic, 171, 277t, 280-281, 281f
  impaired barrier function associated with, 56
Hypermelanosis
  epidermal, 371t, 376-377, 377f
  linear and whorled nevoid, 371t, 376f, 376-377, 377f, 464
Hypernatremia, risk for, 56
Hyperpigmentation
  of atopic dermatitis, 242-243, 243f
  epidermal, 96, 97b, 97f, 98, 98f
  evaluation of, 41t
  in incontinentia pigmenti, 464f
Hyperpigmentation disorders
  blue-gray, 371t, 373, 376
  chimerism, 376
  cutaneous mastocytosis, 381
  demarcation lines, 385-386
  dyschromatosis, 385
  hypermelanosis, 371t, 376f377f, 376-377

Hyperpigmentation disorders—cont'd
  incontinentia pigmenti, 371t, 376, 377-378
  lentigines, 382-385
  localized flat lesions, 370-376
  melanocytic nevi, 386-391
  metabolic causes of, 382
  mosaic conditions, 371f, 376, 376f
  Naegeli-Franceschetti-Jadassohn syndrome, 379
  neurocutaneous melanosis, 389-390
  phakomatosis pigmentokeratotica, 379
  phakomatosis pigmentovascularis, 371t, 378-379, 379f
  poikiloderma, 382
  postinflammatory, 381
  striped hyperpigmentation of torso, 379f, 379-380
  tan-brown lesions, 370-373, 371t, 372f, 373f
  universal melanosis, 381
  xeroderma pigmentosum, 380-381
Hypersensitivity syndrome reaction, 300
Hypertrichosis, 121, 121f, 123-124, 124f
  in Ambras syndrome, 496
  anterior cervical, 500
  in Barber-Say syndrome, 498
  in Coffin-Siris syndrome, 497
  in Cornelia de Lange syndrome, 497, 497f
  with cranial meningoceles, 499
  diffuse, 495f, 495-498
  drug induced neonatal, 498
  encephalocele with, 499, 499f
  and facial anomalies, 497
  familial cervical, 499
  with gingival fibromatosis, 496
  hamartoma with overlying, 414f
  hemihypertrophy with, 500
  lanuginosa, 45, 496, 496f
  localized congenital, 498b, 498-500
  nevoid, 500
  with osteochondrodysplasia, 497
  prepubertal, 496
  primary, 495
  in Rubenstein Taybi syndrome, 498
  in Seip-Berardinelli syndrome, 498
  with spinal fusion abnormalities, 499
  X-linked dominant, 496
Hypertriglyceridemia, in lipodystrophy, 431
Hypohidrotic ectodermal dysplasia, 457, 469, 469f
Hypoimmunoglobuulin-E syndrome, 256, 256f
Hypomelanosis of Ito
  clinical findings in, 358-360, 359f, 360f
  detection of, 83
Hypopigmentation, 98
  of atopic dermatitis, 242, 243f
  evaluation of, 41t
  in incontinentia pigmenti, 464f
  postinflammatory, 364, 364f
  segmental, 360f
Hypopigmentation disorders
  Alezzandrini syndrome, 365
  congenital giant halo nevi, 364
  generalized depigmentation, 353-356
  generalized pigment dilution, 356
  Menkes kinky hair syndrome, 364-365
  mosaic conditions, 358-360, 359f, 360f
  nevus anemicus, 363f, 363-364
  nevus depigmentosus, 361-362
  piebaldism, 360f, 360-361
  tuberous sclerosis complex, 362-363
  Waardenburg syndrome, 361
  Ziprkowski Margolis syndrome, 365
Hypoplasia
  focal dermal, 456f, 464-465
  of nails, 506
Hypothalamic hamartoblastoma, 478t
Hypothermia
  in newborn, 27
  preventing, 35
Hypothyroxinemia, in premature infants, 67-68
Hypotrichosis
  diffuse, 45
  with ectodermal dysplasias, 492-493
  with hair shaft abnormalities, 491
  with ichthyoses, 493, 493f
  with immunodeficiency syndromes, 493-494
  isolated congenital, 491
  Marie Unna, 492
  and milia, 492
  with premature aging syndromes, 493

I

Iatrogenic injuries
  from blood gas monitoring, 112-113, 113f, 114f
  calcinosis cutis, 110-111, 111f
  diagnosis of, 148t
  heel prick nodules, 111-112, 112f
  meatal ulceration, 114
IBIDS syndrome, 277t, 283-284, 489
I-cell disease, 446-447
Ichthyoses
  bullous, 171, 263
  chondrodysplasia punctata, 265, 265f
  erythrodermas with, 263, 264f, 265
  evaluation of, 273t
  follicularis, 277f, 287
  harlequin, 5, 276, 277t, 278, 278f
  hypotrichosis with, 493, 493f
  hystrix, 277t, 281
  impaired barrier function associated with, 56
  lamellar, 263, 277t, 280, 280f, 493, 493f
  management of, 273t
  Sjögren-Larsson syndrome, 265
  vulgaris, 279
  X-linked, 5, 279f, 279-280
Ichthyosis disorders
  CHILD syndrome, 277t, 285f, 285-286
  CHIME syndrome, 277t, 287-288
  colloidion baby, 278-277t, 278-279, 279f
  Conradi-Hünerman syndrome, 277t, 286, 286f
  ectodermal dysplasias, 290
  erythrokeratoderma progressive symmetrica, 287
  erythrokeratoderma variabilis, 286-287, 287f
  familial peeling skin syndrome, 282
  Gaucher's disease, 277t, 288
  KID syndrome, 277t, 284f, 284-285
  ichthyosis follicularis (IFAP) syndrome, 277f287
  linearis circumflexa, 283
  Netherton's syndrome, 277t, 282-283, 283t
  Neu-Laxova syndrome, 290
  neutral lipid storage disease, 277t, 282
  Olmsted syndrome, 289
  palmoplantar keratodermas, 288f, 288-289
  restrictive dermopathy, 289f, 289-290
  Sjögren-Larsson syndrome, 282
  trichothiodystrophy, 277t, 283-284
  tyrosinemia II, 289
Ilex paste, 66t
Immunodeficiency
  of Bloom syndrome, 467
  of Griscelli syndrome, 357
  oral and genital ulcerations with, 481, 482f
Immunodeficiency syndromes. *See also* Acquired
    immunodeficiency disease syndrome
  Bruton hypogammaglobulinemia, 271
  DiGeorge syndrome, 271
  eosinophilic gastroenteritis, 271
Immunofluorescence studies
  in annular erythema, 294
  in EB, 164
  immunohistochemistry, 80
  in maternal bullous disease, 168
  technique for, 79b
  types of, 73, 79-80
  for varicella, 208
Immunologic diseases
  graft-*versus*-host disease, 269f, 269-270, 270f
  Leiner phenotype, 268f, 268-269
  Omenn syndrome, 269, 269f
Immunosorbent agglutination assay (ISAGA), for
    toxoplasmosis, 235
Immunosurveillance, cutaneous, 27
Immunotherapies, for purpura fulminans,
    195-196
Impetigo, 148t
  in AIDS, 213
  cutaneous findings in, 180f, 180-181
  diagnosis of, 180-181
  extracutaneous findings in, 180
  management of, 181
  pathogenesis of, 180
  S. pyogenes, 188
Incontinentia pigmenti, 42t, 371t, 376, 377-378,
    462-464, 463f, 464f
  clinical features of, 156-157, 157f
  diagnosis of, 146t
  vs. HSV diagnosis, 206

Infectious diseases. *See also* Bacterial infections; Fungal
    infections; Viral infections
  atopic dermatitis associated with, 246-247
  candidiasis, 262-263
  congenital syphilis, 196, 263
  cutaneous barrier to, 54
  diagnosis of, 147t
  herpes simplex, 263
  staphylococcal scalded skin syndrome, 262
Infestations
  demodicidosis, 233
  myiasis, 233
  scabies, 152, 231
Inflammatory diseases, 292-323
  atopic dermatitis, 246, 260
  boric acid poisoning, 262
  diffuse mastocytosis, 262
  evaluation of, 272t
  management of, 272t
  neonatal onset multisystem inflammatory disease
    (NOMID), 302f, 302-303
  psoriasis, 261-262
  seborrheic dermatitis, 260-261, 261f
Inflammatory linear verrucous epidermal nevus
    (ILVEN), 410, 412f
Influenza, *vs.* HSV diagnosis, 206
Injuries
  alopecia from ischemia, 106, 106f
  burns, 107-108, 108f
  caput succedaneum, 105-106
  cephalhematoma, 107, 107f
  effects of vacuum extraction, 107
  halo scalp ring, 106, 106f
  iatrogenic, 112-113, 114, 148t
  lacerations, 107
  perinatal soft tissue injury, 105, 106f
  puncture wounds, 103-105
Insect bites, 236t-237t
Insensible water loss (IWL), 69. *See also* Transepidermal
    water loss
Interferon treatment of hemangiomas (IFNs), 28, 346
Interleukins (ILs), 28
Internet, databases on, 84-85
Intracranial hemorrhage, in premature infant, 53
Intraspinal lipomas, 425-426, 426f
Intrauterine epidermal necrosis, 170
Intravenous immune globulin (IVIG), in Kawasaki dis-
    ease, 308
Intraventricular hemorrhage (IVH), in premature in-
    fant, 53
Invasive fungal dermatitis (IFD), 225
Iodine, exposure to, 67
Iris configuration, 44t
Isoniazid, 192
Ito, hypomelanosis of, 83, 358-360, 359f, 360f
Itraconazole, for *Candida* infections, 226
Ivermectin, in scabies, 233

J

Jackson-Lawler syndrome, 478t
Jadassohn-Lewandowsky syndrome, 478t
Jaffe-Campanacci syndrome, 370, 373
Jaundice, physiologic, 98, 98f
Jentigo pattern, 383
Job syndrome, 256. *See also* Hyperimmunoglobulin E
    syndrome
Johanson-Blizzard syndrome, 126t
Joint flexion contractures, of JHF, 445
Joint swelling, of Farber disease, 445
Junctional EB (JEB), 160
Juvenile arthritis, 303
Juvenile hyaline fibromatosis (JHF), 444-445
Juvenile xanthogranuloma, 402-404, 403f, 404f

K

Kala azar, 234t
"Kangaroo mother care," 56
Kaposiform hemangioendothelioma, 344, 347
Kaposi sarcoma, 213
Kasabach-Merritt syndrome, 343, 344, 346, 347f,
    347-348
Kawasaki disease
  clinical findings in, 306f, 306-307
  diagnostic criteria of, 307b

Kawasaki disease—cont'd
  incidence of, 306
  management of, 308
  pathogenesis of, 307
Keloid formation, in Turner syndrome, 461
Keratinization, 5
Keratinocytes, 1, 18
  of epidermis, 3
  in ichthyosis disorders, 281
  in stratum granulosum, 20
  in stratum spinosum, 20
Keratins, function of, 19
Keratodermas
  described, 40t
  palmoplantar, 288f, 288-289
Keratosis-ichthyosis-deafness (KID) syndrome, 265,
    277t, 284f, 284-285, 493
Kerion formation, tinea capitis associated with, 230
KID syndrome, 265, 277t, 284f, 284-285, 493
Killer cell function, in Chediak-Higashi syndrome, 357
Kindler syndrome, 163
Kissing bug bites, 235t
Klebsiella pneumoniae, 193
Kleinfelter syndrome, 286
Klippel-Trénaunay syndrome, 8, 327, 330t, 333f, 333-
    334, 466, 509
Koebner EB, 161, 163
Koebner phenomenon, 249
Koilonychia, 506
Kyphoscoliosis, familial cervical hypertrichosis with,
    499

L

Labia, adhesions of, 482-483
Lacerations, scalpel, 107. *See also* Injuries
Lacrimal sac, mucocele of, 485
LAMB syndrome, 383, 384
Lamellar bodies, 20
Lamellar ichthyosis (LI), 277t, 280, 280f, 493, 493f
Langerhans' cell histiocytosis (LCH), 248-249, 436-
    438, 437f, 438f
  diagnosis of, 79
  "self-healing" variant of, 438f
Langerhans' cells, 20
  of epidermis, 3
  fetal development of, 6
  in neonates, 27-28
Lanugo hairs, 18
Laryngeal involvement
  in EB, 161
  in HPV, 217
Laser treatment
  for AVMs, 330
  bare fiber Nd:YAG, 346
  for congenital nevi, 387
  for epidermal nevus, 412
  for phakomatosis pigmentovascularis, 378
Latex agglutination (LA) test, for varicella, 208
"Leather-grain" appearance, 416
Leiner's disease, 249, 268
  phenotype, 268f, 268-269
  evaluation of, 273t
  management of, 273t
Leishmaniasis, 235-236
  characteristics of, 234t
  cutaneous, 235
  treatment for, 235-235
  visceral, 235-236
Lentigines neonatorum. *See* Transient neonatal pustu-
    lar melanosis
Lentiginosis
  centrofacial, 371t, 384
  mosaicism, 371t, 384
  segmental, 371t, 384
LEOPARD syndrome, 371t, 382-383
Leprechaunism, 430f, 431-431, 497-498
Leptomeningeal melanocytosis, malignant melanoma
    arising from, 441
Leptomeningeal melanosis (LMM), 387
Lesions. *See also specific lesions*
  blueberry muffin, 312, 313f, 314, 314b
  borders of, 42t
  of candidiasis, 141-142
  classification of, 35
  color of, 41t

Lesions—cont'd
  configuration of, 42t
  of congenital histiocytosis, 156
  diagnosis using, 371t
  fungal, 141-142
  in *H. influenzae* infection, 140
  herpetic, 142-143
  of HPV, 217, 217f, 218f
  of incontinentia pigmenti, 156-157, 157f
  of neonatal purpura fulminans, 315, 315f
  primary, 35t-38t
  secondary, 38t-41t
  in tuberous sclerosis, 455, 456f
Lesions, benign transient, 145t
  acne, 94f, 94-95
  color changes involved in, 96-100
  diagnosis of, 148t
  diaper erosions, 154
  erythema toxicum neonatorum, 152
  iatrogenic causes of, 155
  incidence of, 89t
  miliaria, 153-154
  neonatal acne, 154, 154f
  neonatal pustular melanosis, 152-153, 153f
  neonatal pustulosis, 153
  papules, 88-91
  pustules, 91-94
  sucking blisters, 95, 95f, 154
  umbilical granuloma, 95f, 95-96
Leukemia, congenital, 436, 437f
Leukemoid reaction, Down syndrome associated with, 157
Lice, bites of, 236t
Lichenification
  in atopic dermatitis, 243f
  described, 40t
Lidocaine toxicity, 81, 81t
Lighting, limiting nursery, 55
Linear configuration, 42t
Linear IgA disease, 169
Linear porokeratosis, 172
Lip. *See also* Oral mucous membrane disorders
  fistulae of, 478-479
  sebaceous hyperplasia of, 479, 479f
Lipids
  as barrier to infection, 54
  in epidermal barrier, 20-21
  and permeability barrier function, 51
Lipid storage disease, 280. *See also* Subcutaneous fat disorders
Lipoblastoma, 429f, 429-430
Lipoblastomatosis, 429f, 429-430
Lipodystrophies
  carbohydrate-deficient glycoprotein syndrome, 432
  congenital generalized, 431-432, 498
  leprechaunism, 430f, 431-431
Lipogranulomatosis, 433, 445-446, 467
Lipoid proteinosis, in Costello syndrome, 460
Lipoma, 37t
  associated with spinal dysraphism, 124
  clinical findings with, 425-426, 426t
Lipomatosis
  congenital diffuse, 428, 428f
  encephalocraniocutaneous, 427-428
Lipomatosus, nevus, 415-416, 416f
Listeria infection
  clinical findings in, 140
  diagnosis of, 144t
Listeria monocytogenes, 191, 193
Liver disease, in NLE, 297
LMX1B genes, 10, 12
Lobster claw deformity, in EEC, 469
Loose anagen syndrome, 77
Lubricating agents, for EB, 166. *See also* Emollients
Lumbosacral lipomas, 425-426, 426f
Lupus erythematosus, neonatal (NLE), 33, 43t, 44t
  clinical findings in, 296-297, 297f, 298f
  diagnosis of, 298
  management of, 298-299
  pathogenesis of, 297-298
Lymphadenopathy, with scalp abscess, 183
Lymphangiomas, 374t, 476, 776f
  circumscriptum, 328
Lymphatic malformations (LMs), 374t, 476, 776f
  clinical findings in, 328f, 328-329
  treatment of, 329

Lymphedema
  hereditary cholestasis with, 334-335
  in Turner syndrome, 460
Lymphohistiocytosis, familial hemophagocytic, 438
Lysosomal storage disorders, 447-448

M

Macrocephaly
  in Bannayan-Riley-Ruvalcaba syndrome, 385
  neurocutaneous melanosis (NCM) associated with, 389
Macroglossia, 480, 480f
  causes of, 480b
  defined, 479
Macrosomia, in Bannayan-Riley-Ruvalcaba syndrome, 385
Macular pigmentation, 480, 481f
Macules
  ash leaf, 35t
  café au lait, 370, 371t, 372f, 373f
  of congenital syphilis, 196
  described, 35t
  in erythema toxicum neonatorum, 152
  hyperpigmented penile, 385
  hypopigmented, 362, 362f, 363, 363f
  lingual melanotic, 480
  in transient neonatal pustular melanosis (TNPM), 152, 152f
Maffucci syndrome, 334, 466, 509
Magnetic resonance imaging (MRI)
  for dermoid cysts, 123
  with gadolinium enhancement, 332, 332f
  for NCM, 389
  of pseudotail, 125
  for venous malformations, 476
Malassezia infection
  diagnosis and treatment of, 228
  neonatal cephalic pustulosis, 227-228
  in premature infant skin, 54
  sepsis, 228
  skin colonization with, 227
  tinea versicolor, 227, 227f
Mal de Meleda, 289
Malformations, in Proteus syndrome, 466. *See also* Vascular malformations; Venous malformations
Mammary glands, 10
Mammary tissue, supernumerary, 117, 118f
Maple syrup urine disease (MSUD), 267
"Marble-cake" pattern, of incontinentia pigmenti, 157
Marfan syndrome, 459-460
Marie Unna hypotrichosis, 490, 492
Marinesco-Sjögren syndrome, 489
Mastocytomas, 36, 167, 167f
  clinical presentation of, 442, 442f
  solitary, 444
Mastocytosis, 167, 168f, 442-444
  cutaneous, 381
  diagnosis of, 148t
  diffuse, 262
  diffuse cutaneous, 443f, 443-444
  evaluation of, 272t
  histamine-releasing triggers to avoid in, 444b
  management of, 272t
  urticaria pigmentosa, 442, 443f
Maternal bullous disease, blistering caused by, 168f, 168-169
Maternal history
  in HSV, 142
  key points of, 139b
  NLE in, 297, 298
Maternal infection
  HIV, 213-214
  with HPV, 218
  with HSV, 290-292
  varicella, 207-208
Maternal melanoma, 441
McCune-Albright syndrome, 370, 372-373, 373f, 454
Mechanobullous diseases, of premature infant skin, 56
Meckel diverticulum, 96
Meconium
  prepartum passage of, 100
  staining, 98, 99f
Median raphe cysts, 89, 120, 120f
Meibomian glands, 24

Melanin
  fetal development of, 6
  protective role of, 20
Melanin abnormalities. *See also* Hyperpigmentation disorders; Hypopigmentation disorders
  epidermal hyperpigmentation, 96, 97b, 97f, 98, 98f
  Mongolian spots, 96, 96f, 97b
Melanocytes, 1, 6
  during embryogenesis, 20
  of epidermis, 3
Melanocytosis, dermal, 371t, 373, 376
  blue-gray color associated with, 374f
  etiology of, 373
Melanocytosis, leptomeningeal, 441
Melanoma
  "benign juvenile," 390-391
  congenital malignant, 390, 441f, 441-442
  from LCMN, 388, 389
  in NCM, 289
  prepubertal, 386
  and UVA, 55
Melanosis
  leptomeningeal, 387
  neonatal pustular, 145t
  neurocutaneous (NCM), 387, 389-390
  universal acquired, 381
Melanosomes, 20
Meningoceles, 107, 120-121, 121f, 342
  cranial, 495
  hypertrichosis with, 499
Meningococcemia, purpura fulminans with, 195
Menkes kinky hair syndrome, 364-365, 488, 488f
  examination in, 78t
  hypopigmentation in, 98
  pili torti in, 488f
Menstrual age, 1
Mental retardation
  in Costello syndrome, 460
  hypocalcemia related to, 408
  in incontinentia pigmenti, 462
  PKU associated with, 357
Merkel cells, fetal development of, 6
Metabolic diseases
  cystic fibrosis, 267, 267f
  essential fatty acid deficiency, 268
  maple syrup urine disease, 267
  methylmalonic acidemia, 266
Methylmalonic acidemia, 171
  diagnosis of, 150t
  erythroderma in, 266
Michelin tire baby, 415, 427, 428. *See also* Lipomatosis
Micronychia, 507, 507t
MIDAS (microphthalmia, dermal aplasia, and sclerocornea), 466f, 466-467
Midge bites, 235t
Milia, 36t
  characteristics of, 88, 89f
  congenital, 173
  diagnosis of, 88
  hypotrichosis and, 492
Miliaria
  crystallina, 145t, 89, 153
  defined, 89
  diagnosis of, 145t, 154
  profunda, 90
  pustulosa, 90
  rubra, 90, 90f, 153, 153f
  vs. TNPM, 93
Millipede bites, 235t
Minoxidil, maternal, 498
Mite bites, 235t
"Mitten" deformities, 162
MLS (microphthalmia and linear skin defects), 466, 466f
Moisturizing agents, for atopic dermatitis, 246. *See also* Emollients
Moll glands, 24
Molluscum contagiosum
  cutaneous findings in, 219
  diagnosis of, 219
  lesions of, 218-219
  pathogenesis of, 219
  treatment of, 219-220
Molluscum dermatitis, 219
Mongolian spots, 36t, 96, 96f, 371t, 373-374, 374f
Monilethrix, 487-488, 488f

Monitoring, blood gas
  complications of, 112-113, 113*f*, 114*f*
  fetal scalp puncture for, 104
Montgomery tubercles, 24
Morphogenesis, epidermal, 4*f*
Morphology
  diagnosis using, 371*t*
  zosteriform, 416
Mosaic disorders, 371*f*, 376, 376*f*
  focal dermal hypoplasia of Goltz, 456*f*, 464-465
  hypomelanosis of Ito, 358-360, 359*f*, 360*f*
  incontinentia pigmenti, 462-464, 463*f*, 464*f*
  MIDAS, 466*f*, 466-467
  mosaicism, 5, 462
  Proteus syndrome, 465-466, 466*f*
Mosaicism
  defined, 462
  somatic, 5
Mosquito bites, 236*t*
Moth bites, 235*t*
Mouse hairless genes, 10
Moynahan syndrome, 371*t*, 382-383
Mucocele, of lacrimal sac, 485
Mucolipidosis, 446-447, 448
Mucopolysaccharidoses, 45
  classification of, 448*t*
  clinical findings in, 447
  diagnosis of, 447-448
Mucormycosis, 142, 229
Mucous membrane disorders. *See* Genital mucous
    membrane; Ocular mucous membrane; Oral mu-
    cous membrane
Mucous membranes, examination of, 35
Mutational DNA analysis, in EB, 164
Mutations. *See also* Genetics
Mycobacterium tuberculosis, 192
Myiasis, 233, 234*t*
Myocarditis, parvovirus associated with, 215. *See also*
    Cardiac conditions
Myofibromatosis, infantile, 348, 395, 396*t*
  clinical findings in, 397*f*, 397-398, 398*f*
  treatment of, 398

N

Naegeli-Franceschetti-Jadassohn syndrome, 379
Nail dystrophy
  in AEC syndrome, 468
  in ichthyosis disorders, 289
  in incontinentia pigmenti, 462
Nail growth, pathologic factors affecting, 504*b*
Nail-patella syndrome, 12, 45, 507*t*, 508
Nails, 10
  alterations in shape of, 506
  alterations in size of, 506-507
  Beau lines, 505*f*, 505-506
  Candida infection of, 226, 511, 512*f*
  dyschromia of, 512-513, 513*f*, 513*t*
  ectopic, 509, 509*f*
  examination of, 35
  function of, 504
  hypertrophy of, 509-510
  ingrown toenails, 511, 511*f*
  micronychia, 507, 507*t*
  in newborn evaluation, 45
  onychomadesis, 506
  pachyonychia congenita of, 510, 510*f*
  psoriasis in, 249
Nail unit
  composition of, 504, 505*f*
  infections of, 511
  in newborn, 24, 25*f*
  onychoatrophy of, 509
NAME syndrome, 383, 384
Nasal carriage, as reservoir for skin infections, 180
Nasolacrimal duct, obstruction of, 484
National Center for Biotechnical Information (NCBI), 85
National Epidermolysis Bullosa Registry (NEBR), 167
Necrolysis, toxic epidermal. *See* Toxic epidermal
    necrolysis
Necrosis, intrauterine epidermal, 170
Necrotizing enterocolitis (NEC), in premature infant, 53
Necrotizing fasciitis
  defined, 185
  diagnosis of, 185-186
  S. pyogenes, 188-189

Needle marks, 104-105
Neisseria meningitidis, 194-196
Neonatal lupus erythematosus (NLE), 169, 296-299,
    297*f*, 298*f*
Neonatal noma, 149*t*, 171, 481
Neonatal onset multisystemic inflammatory disease
    (NOMID), 301
Neonatal skin
  characteristics of, 62
  injury to, 62
  percutaneous absorption of, 21, 62-63
Neoplastic disorders
  congenital melanoma, 441*f*, 441-442
  congenital teratoma, 442
  dermatofibrosarcoma protuberans, 239-440, 439*f*,
    440*f*
  familial hemophagocytic lymphohistiocytosis (FHL),
    438
  Farber disease, 445-446
  fibrosarcoma, 438, 439*f*
  juvenile hyaline fibromatosis, 444-445
  Langerhans' cell histiocytosis, 436-438, 437*f*, 438*f*
  leukemia, 436, 437*f*
  mastocytosis, 442-444
  melanocytic, 391
  neuroblastoma, 440*f*, 440-441
  rhabdomyosarcoma, 441, 441*f*
Nerve growth factor receptor (NGFR), 10
Nerves, in newborn skin, 25-26
Netherton syndrome, 263, 264*f*, 265, 276, 277*t*, 282-
    283, 283*t*
  compared with atopic dermatitis, 245
  diagnosis of, 77, 78*t*
  hair shaft abnormality of, 491
Neu-Laxova syndrome, 290
Neural crest cells, in fetal skin development, 5
Neural tumors, 402, 402*f*
Neurolemmomatosis, 402
Neuroblastoma, 36, 440*f*, 440-441
Neurocutaneous melanosis (NCM), 387, 389-390
Neurofibromas, 402, 402*f*
  of oral mucosa, 474*t*, 476
  pacinian, 402
  peripheral, 452*f*, 453
  plexiform, 499
Neurofibromatosis, 1, 370-372, 371*t*
  café au lait spots in, 452*f*
  consensus criteria for, 451, 452*b*
  diagnosis of, 453-454
  ocular disorders associated with, 484
  and rhabdomyosarcoma, 441
Neurotoxicity, of antimicrobial cleansing agents, 64
Neutral lipid storage disease, 277*t*, 282
Nevus
  achromicus, 362*f*
  anemicus, 363*f*, 363-364
  aplastic, 495
  basal cell carcinoma, 12
  Becker, 415
  of CHILD syndrome, 285-286
  clinical findings in epidermal, 410-411, 411*f*, 412*f*
  comedonicus, 412-414, 413*f*
  congenital intermediate, 371*t*, 386*f*, 386-387
  congenital large, 387*f*, 387-389, 388*f*
  congenital melanocytic, 495, 498, 498*f*
  congenital small, 371*t*, 386*f*, 386-387
  connective tissue, 416*f*, 416-417
  depigmentosus, 36*t*, 361-362
  faun tail, 124
  "flammeus," 325
  fuscoceruleus
    acromiodeltoideus, 375
    ophthalmomaxillaris, 371*t*, 374*f*, 374-375
  halo, 364
  large melanocytic (LCMN), 387*f*, 387-389, 388*f*
  linear epidermal, 42*t*
  melanocytic, 441
  in nail matrix, 512, 513*f*
  nevus lipomatosus cutaneous superficialis (NLCS),
    426-427
  of Ota, 371*t*, 374*f*, 374-375
  pathogenesis of epidermal, 411-412
  sebaceous, 36*t*, 409*f*, 409-410, 495
  simplex, 36*t*, 100
  spilus, 371*t*, 390, 390*f*
  Spitz, 513
  treatment of epidermal, 412

Nevus—cont'd
  in Turner syndrome, 461
  white sponge, 474*t*, 477
  woolly hair, 490
Nickel dermatitis, 253
Nikolsky sign, 82, 262
Nipple, accessory, 117, 118*f*
Nodules
  Bohn nodules, 473, 474*f*, 474*t*
  calcified ear, 405, 405*f*
  congenital pedal, 428-429, 429*f*
  described, 36*t*
  in Farber disease, 467
  in infantile myofibromatosis, 397, 397*f*
  in Langerhans' cell histiocytosis, 436
  mastocytomas, 167, 168*f*
  of panniculitis, 423
  of scabies, 232, 232*f*
  of subcutaneous fat necrosis (SCFN), 420
  in Sweet syndrome, 305
Noma neonatorum, 149*t*, 171, 481
Noonan syndrome, 461, 507*t*
"Norwegian scabies," 213, 232
Nova syndrome, 336
Nummular configuration, 43*t*
Nutrition
  in EB, 165-166
  in lipodystrophy, 165-166
Nutritional deficiencies, compared with atopic dermati-
    tis, 245
Nystatin 66,*t*226

O

Oatmeal baths, for seborrheic dermatitis, 249
Ocular mucous membrane disorders
  Behçet's disease, 483
  colobomata, 483-484
  glaucoma, 484, 484*f*
  mucocele of lacrimal sac, 485
  nasolacrimal duct obstruction, 484
  seborrheic blepharitis, 485
Ocular problems
  in CEP, 309
  in epidermolysis bullosa, 162, 163
  in focal dermal hypoplasia, 465
  in KID syndrome, 285
  woolly hair associated with, 490
Oculoauriculovertebral syndrome, 118
Oculocerebrocutaneous syndrome, 126*t*, 427
Oculocutaneous albinism (OCA), 353-356, 355*f*
Ogna variant, of EB, 161-162
Olmsted syndrome, 289
Omenn syndrome, 255, 269, 269*f*
Omphalitis, 184
Omphalomesenteric duct, anomalies of, 130-131, 131*f*
Onychauxis, 510
Onychoatrophy, 509
Onychodysplasia
  clinical manifestations of, 507*t*
  of index fingers, 508*f*, 508-509
Onychodystrophy, *Candida*, 224
Onychogryphosis, 510
Onychoheterotopia, 509, 509*f*
Onycholysis, 511-512, 512*b*
Onychomadesis, 506
Onychomycosis, 231, 511, 512*f*
Opitz syndrome, 126*t*
Opportunistic infections
  in HIV-infected children, 213
  in premature infant skin, 54
Oral-facial-digital (OFD) syndrome, 88, 481, 481*f*, 490
Oral mucous membrane disorders
  acatalasemia, 480-481
  annulus migrans, 479
  benign papular lesions, 474*t*
  Bohn nodules, 473, 474*f*, 474*t*
  congenital epulis, 473
  congenital ranula, 473, 474*t*
  ectopic thyroid tissue, 481-482
  Epstein pearls, 474*t*, 474-475, 475*f*
  eruption cysts, 474*t*, 475*f*
  fistulae of lower lip, 478-479
  granular cell tumor, 474, 474*t*
  hemangiomas, 474, 475, 475*f*
  with immunodeficiency, 481, 482*f*
  lingual melanotic macule, 480

Oral mucous membrane disorders—cont'd
  lymphangiomas, 374t, 476, 776f
  macroglossia, 479-480, 480f
  macular pigmentation, 480, 481f
  natal teeth, 477-478, 478t
  neurofibromas, 474t, 476
  oral-facial-digital syndrome, 481, 481f, 490
  sebaceous hyperplasia of lip, 479, 479f
  sucking calluses, 478, 479f
  venous malformations, 474t476-477
  white sponge nevus, 474t, 477
Organogenesis, in fetal skin development, 1
Osler-Weber-Rendu syndrome, 8
Osteoma
  congenital plate-like cutaneous, 408
  cutis, 406
Osteopoikilosis, 416
Ota, nevus of, 371t, 374f, 374-375

P

Pachyonychia congenita, 478t, 510, 510f
Pads, sucking, 95
Palatal cysts, 88-89
Pallister-Hall syndrome, 478t
Palmoplantar keratodermas, 288f, 288-289
Palms
  hairy cutaneous malformations of, 500
  keratodermas of, 288, 288f
Panniculitis
  cold, 423f, 423-424
  due to mechanical trauma, 424
  with E. coli sepsis, 425f
  infectious, 424-425, 425f
  injection-site granuloma, 424
  post-steroid, 424
Papillomas, in FDH, 465
Papules. See also Cysts, Hamartomas
  of Candida diaper dermatitis, 252
  congenital, 89
  of congenital syphilis, 196
  described, 36t
  in erythema toxicum, 152, 635
  HPV, 217, 218f, 287f
  milia, 88, 89f
  of miliaria, 89-90, 90f
  oral mucosal cysts, 88-89
  of PCA, 229
  of scabies, 232, 232f
  sebaceous hyperplasia, 90, 91f
Parasitic infections
  characteristics of, 234t
  leishmaniasis, 235-236
  toxoplasmosis, 233, 234t, 235
Parkes Weber syndrome (PaWS), 330t, 333
Paronychia, 511
  acute, 183f, 183-184
  Candida, 224, 226, 226f
Parvovirus infections, 203
  cutaneous findings in, 214
  diagnosis of, 215
  etiology of, 214-215
  treatment for, 215-216
Patches
  of atopic dermatitis, 242f
  described, 36t
  Shagreen, 362, 416, 455, 456f
Patent ductus arteriosus (PDA). See also Cardiac
      conditions
  and natal teeth, 478t
  in premature infant, 53
"Peau d'orange" appearance, 416
Pemphigus foliaceus, 168
Pemphigus vulgaris, 168
Penicillin, for ecthyma gangrenosum, 194
Pentachlorophenol, as laundry product, 64
Pentavalent antimonials, 236
Peptides, as barrier to infection, 54
Perianal pyramidal protrusion, 483, 483f
Periderm cells
  in developing skin, 18
  of embryonic epidermis, 3
Periorificial areas, in Olmsted syndrome, 289
Permeability barrier
  development of competent, 47
  epidermal, 20-21
  fluid and electrolyte imbalance in immature, 49-51
  regulatory signals for formation of, 49t

Permethrin, for scabies, 233
Petechiae
  of congenital syphilis, 196
  in Langerhans' cell histiocytosis, 436
  perinatal, 105
Petrolatum. See also Emollients
  for red scaly baby, 271
  and TEWL, 51, 69
Petroleum, white, as skin barrier, 64
Peutz-Jeghers syndrome, 384, 384f
PHACE syndrome, 340
Phakomatosis pigmentokeratotica, 379
Phakomatosis pigmentovascularis, 371t, 378-379,
    379f
  classification of, 378t
  diagnosis of, 378
Phenol, as laundry product, 64
Phenylketonuria (PKU), 98, 255, 357
Phenytoin, in treatment of RDEB, 167
Pheomelanins, 20
Philtrum, long, 497
Photophobia, congenital, 493
Photoprotection, in albinism, 356
Phototherapy
  bronze baby syndrome from, 110, 110f
  complications of, 109-110, 110f
  and fluid requirements, 49
  for hyperbilirubinemia, 55, 57
  purpuric eruption induced by, 316
  and TEWL, 62
Phototoxicity, 55
  clinical manifestations of, 311
  drug-induced, 109, 316
Phycomycosis, 229f, 229-230
PIBIDS syndrome, 277t, 283-284
Piebaldism, 6, 360f, 360-361
Pigmentary abnormalities. See also Hyperpigmentation
      disorders; Hypopigmentation disorders
  localized, spotty, 383-385, 384f
  meconium staining, 98, 99f
  melanin abnormalities, 96f-98f, 96-98, 97b
  physiologic jaundice, 98, 99f
Pigmentation, macular, 480, 481f
Pili annulati, 491
Pili torti, 488f, 488-489, 489, 489f
Pincer appearance, of nails, 506, 510, 510f
Pityriasis Alba, 364
Placode, of pregerm-stage follicle, 10
Plaques
  of atopic dermatitis, 242f
  of congenital syphilis, 196
  described, 36t
  due to panniculitis, 423
  of subcutaneous fat necrosis (SCFN), 420
  in Sweet syndrome, 305
Plastic wraps, to limit TEWL, 69
Plexiform neurofibroma, 499
Pneumocystis carinii pneumonia, in HIV-infected chil-
    dren, 213
Poikiloderma
  described, 382
  in Rothmund-Thomson syndrome, 467
Poisoning, boric acid, 262
Pollitt syndrome, 489
Polychlorinated biphenyls, micronychia with, 507t
Polycyclic configuration, 44t
Polydactyly, rudimentary, 119, 119f
Polymerase chain reaction (PCR), 73, 83-84
  for toxoplasmosis, 235
  in viral infection diagnosis, 76
Polyostotic fibrous dysplasia, 372, 373
Polyps
  adnexal, 130, 139f
  umbilical, 131, 131f
Polythelia, 117
Porokeratosis, linear
  clinical manifestations of, 172
  diagnosis of, 151t
Porphyrias, 173
  acute intermittent, 310t
  ALA dehydratase, 310t
  characteristics of, 309
  classification of, 310t
  congenital erythropoietic, 309, 310t, 311
  cutanea tarda (PCT), 310t
  diagnosis of, 151t
  erythropoietic protoporphyria, 310t, 311f, 311-312
  hepatoerythropoietic, 312

Porphyrias—cont'd
  homozygous variegate, 312
  variegate, 312
Porphyrinemias, 173
  phototherapy and, 109-110, 110f
  transient, 312
Port-wine stains (PWS)
  vs. capillary ectasias, 100
  characteristics of, 325f, 325-326
  management of, 326
Positron electron tomography (PET), in Sturge-Weber
      syndrome, 332
Postmature infant, desquamation in, 99f, 101
Postoperative wound care, 78, 81-82
Potassium hydroxide preparation, 73-74, 74b, 74f
Povidone-iodine, 67
Prader-Willi syndrome, 356
Preauricular pits and sinuses, 117-118, 118f
Preimplantation genetic diagnosis (PGD), 84
Premature infants
  consequences of skin immaturity for, 46
  hemangiomas in, 34
  major complications of, 53
  skin care recommended for, 70b
Premature infant skin
  affect of light on, 54-55
  anetoderma of, 105, 105f
  care of, 57
  characteristics of, 18, 46
  diseases of, 56-57
  hemangiomas of, 56
  increased permeability of, 52-53
  and infection, 54
  mechanical injury to, 53-54
  neurocutaneous development in, 56
  permeability of, 21
  scarring of, 56
  and thermal homeostasis, 55-56
Prenatal diagnosis
  of epidermolytic hyperkeratosis, 281
  of Griscelli syndrome, 358
  of Sjögren-Larsson syndrome, 282
Preterm infants. See also Premature infants
  cutaneous water losses in, 50
  permeability barrier in, 46-47, 48f
  phenylephrine-induced blanching in, 48f
  topical medications for, 53
Prickly heat, 90, 153-154
Primary cutaneous aspergillosis (PCA), 228-229, 229f
Profilaggrin, 20
Proflavine hemisulfate, 67
Progressive osseous heteroplasia (POH), 407f, 408
Properdin deficiency, 196
Proprionobacteria, in premature infant skin, 54
Propylene glycol, cautious use of, 67t
Proshield, 66t
Protein C concentrate, 316
Protein C deficiency, 315-316
Protein S concentrate, 316
Protein S deficiency, 195, 315-316
Protcoglycans (PGs), 23
Proteus syndrome, 330t, 335f, 378, 385, 412, 427, 465-
    466, 466f, 509
Prothrombin complex concentrate, 316
Pruritus. See also Urticaria
  of atopic dermatitis, 241, 246, 260
  in diffuse cutaneous mastocytosis, 443, 444
  of scabies, 231
  in seborrheic dermatitis, 248
Pseudoanuria, 64
Pseudoarthrosis, congenital, 453
Pseudoclefts, of lip, 335
Pseudo-Darier's sign, 82-83, 499
Pseudohypoparathyroidism (PHP), 407, 408
Pseudomonas aeruginosa, 193, 481
Pseudomonas infection, 140
  diagnosis of, 144t, 147t
  ecthyma gangrenosum, 193-194, 194f
Pseudomonas mirabilis, 193
Pseudopseudohypoparathyroidism (PPHP), 407
Pseudotail, 125
Psoriasis
  characteristics of, 261-262
  compared with atopic dermatitis, 245
  compared with SD, 248, 249f
  cutaneous findings in, 249f, 249-250
  diagnosis of, 146t, 250
  evaluation of, 272t

Psoriasis—cont'd
  generalized, 262
  in HIV-infected patients, 213
  incidence of, 249
  management of, 250, 272t
  pathogenesis of, 250
  pustular, 157-158
Pulse oximetry, complications of, 112
Punch biopsy, 78, 79. See also Biopsy
    for EB
  technique for, 78b
Puncture wounds
  amniocentesis scars, 103, 104f
  anetoderma, 105, 105f
  chorionic villus sampling (CVS), 103-104
  for fetal blood sampling, 104
  from fetal monitoring, 104
  needle marks, 104-105
Purpura
  Henoch-Schönlein, 309
  in newborn, 312, 313b
Purpura fulminans (PF), 315f, 315-316
  clinical findings in, 194-195, 195f
  diagnosis of, 151t, 195
  management of, 195-196
  neonatal, 173
Purpuric phototherapy-induced eruption, 316
Pustules
  acropustulosis of infancy, 155
  conditions presenting, 137b
  of congenital candidiasis, 263
  congenital leukemoid reaction, 157
  described, 38t
  of eosinophilic pustular folliculitis, 156, 156f
  of erythema toxicum neonatorum, 91, 92f, 152
  of PCA, 229
  scabies, 232, 232f
  staphylococcal, 262
  in Sweet syndrome, 304
  in TNPM, 152, 152f
  transient neonatal pustular melanosis, 91-94, 93f
Pustulosis, neonatal cephalic, 154, 154f, 227-228
Pyloric atresia, EB with (PA-JEB), 162, 163
Pyoderma gangrenosum (PG), 483
  clinical findings in, 170, 171f
  diagnosis of, 149t
Pyodermas, 38t
Pyogenic granuloma, 348
Pyrazinamide, 192

R

"Raccoon facies," 63
Radiologic examination
  for aplasia cutis, 129
  in Farber disease, 446
  in NOMID, 303
  of pseudotail, 125
Ranula, congenital, 473, 474t
Rapp-Hodgkin syndrome, 490, 492-493
Reaction patterns, in newborns, 45
Recessive dystrophic EB (RDEB), 160, 162
Red scaly baby, evaluation of, 271, 271b. See also Ery-
    throdermas
Renal disease
  nodular calcification associated with, 405
  nail-patella syndrome in, 508
Rendu-Osler-Weber disease, 8, 326
Respiratory tract infection, in I-cell disease, 447
Restrictive dermopathy, 7, 150t, 171-172, 289, 289f,
    290
Reticulate configuration, 44t
Retiform configuration, 44t
Retinoids, for harlequin ichthyosis, 276
Retinopathy, pigmentary, 497
Rhabdomyomas, cardiac, 455
Rhabdomyosarcomas, 441, 441f
Rh incompatibility, dermal erythropoiesis in, 314f
Richner-Hanhart syndrome, 289
Rifampin, 192
Riley-Day syndrome, 457
Riley-Smith syndrome, 335
Rothmund-Thomson syndrome, 467
Rubella
  dermal erythropoiesis in, 314
  diagnosis of, 203t
  congenital, 211-212

Rubenstein Taybi syndrome, 498
Rubor, from excessive hemoglobin, 100
Ruvalcaba-Myhre-Smith syndrome, 335

S

Sabinas brittle hair syndrome, 489
Sabin-Feldman dye test, 235
Sack-Barabas type, of EDS, 459f, 4458-459
Sacral medial telangiectatic vascular nevi, 325
Salmon patch, 89t, 100f, 324, 325f
Sand flea bites, 235t
Sand fly bites, 235t
Sarcoptes scabiei mite, 232, 232f
Scabies, 152, 231-233, 232f
  vs. acropustulosis of infancy, 155
  in AIDS, 213
  characteristics of, 234t
  compared with atopic dermatitis, 245
  diagnosis of, 145t, 232
  neonatal, 232
  pathognomonic sign of, 232
  treatment for, 233
Scabies preparation, 77, 77f
Scald burns, 155
Scaling, 10
  described, 39t
  in X-linked hypohidrotic ectodermal dysplasia, 290
Scalp
  abscess of, 183
  ACC of, 172
  NLE lesions of, 297
  swelling of, 105-106
Scalp hair
  heterochromia of, 487
  parietal whorls, 487
Scars
  amniocentesis, 103, 104f
  described, 41t
  in focal dermal hypoplasia, 465
  intrauterine, 40t
  of prematurity, 56
  in Turner syndrome, 461
Schimmelpenning syndrome, 427
Schwannomas, 402
SCID, 270f
Sclerema
  clinical findings in, 422
  distinguished from subcutaneous fat necrosis
    (SCFN), 422
  pathogenesis of, 422
  treatment of, 422
Scleroderma, distinguished from subcutaneous fat
    necrosis (SCFN), 420, 421
Sclerotherapy, for lymphatic malformations, 329
Scoliosis, in Marfan syndrome, 459
Scorpion bites, 235t
Scrotum
  calcification of, 405
  hair on neonatal, 500
Sebaceous glands
  fetal development of, 10-11
  hypertrophy of, 90, 91f
  maturation of, 11
  in newborn skin, 24
Sebaceous hyperplasia
  clinical presentation of, 90, 91f
  of lip, 479, 479f
Sebaceous nevus, 36t, 409-410, 410f, 495
Seborrheic dermatitis (SD)
  in children with AIDS, 213
  compared with atopic dermatitis, 245
  cutaneous findings in, 247, 247f, 248f
  diagnosis of, 248-249
  evaluation of, 272t
  inflammation of, 260-261, 261f
  management of, 249, 272t
  pathogenesis of, 247-248
Seip-Berardinelli syndrome, 431-432, 498
Seizures
  in CHIME syndrome, 287
  in incontinentia pigmenti, 462
  in tuberous sclerosis, 454
Selenium deficiency, 161
Sepsis, risk factors for, 34
Serpiginous configuration, 44t
Serratia marcescens, 193

Serum-sickness-like reaction, 300
Servelle-Martorell syndrome, 330t, 333-334
Sexually transmitted diseases, HPV as, 218. See also
    Syphilis
Shagreen patches, in tuberous sclerosis, 362, 416, 455,
    456f
Short stature
  in focal dermal hypoplasia, 465
  in Rothmund-Thomson syndrome, 467
  in Turner syndrome, 461
Shoulders, tumoral calcinosis of, 406
SIBIDS syndrome, 277t, 283-284
Silver-Russell syndrome, 370, 373
Silver sulfadiazine (Silvadene), 82
Single photo emission tomography (SPECT), in Sturge-
    Weber syndrome, 332
Sinuses
  branchial, 119-120
  bronchogenic, 120
  cranial dermal, 122
  preauricular, 118f
Sjögren-Larsson syndrome, 265, 282
Skeletal abnormalities
  in CHILD syndrome, 285
  in focal dermal hypoplasia, 465
  nail-patella syndrome with, 508
Skin-associated lymphoid tissues (SALT), 27
Skin care
  antisepsis, 67-68
  bathing, 63-64
  control of transcutaneous water loss, 68-69, 70/ib/I
  diapering, 64
  emollients, 64-67, 65t-66t
  of premature newborn, 70b
Skin immune system (SIS), 27
Skin stripping, by removal of adhesive-backed prod-
    ucts, 62
Sleeping sickness, 234t
Smooth muscle hamartoma, 414f, 414-415
Sodium hypochlorite, as laundry product, 64
Soles
  hairy cutaneous malformations of, 500
  keratodermas of, 288, 288f
Spangled appearance, of uncombable hair, 490
Speckled lentiginous nevus, 371t, 390, 390f
Spider bites, 235t
Spinal dysraphism, 123
  acrochordon, 125, 125f
  cutaneous lesions associated with, 123b
  dimples with, 125, 125f
  hemangiomas associated with, 124f, 124-126, 341,
    341f
  hypertrichosis, 123-124, 124f
  lipomas, 124
  pseudotails, 125, 125f
Spindle and epithelioid nevus, 390-391
Spindle cell hemangioendothelioma (SCHE), 348
Spitz nevus, 390-391
Spongiosis, in atopic dermatitis, 260
Staphylococcal infections
  abscesses, 181-184
  in atopic dermatitis, 246-247
  bacterial folliculitis, 181-183
  cellulitis, 184-185
  coagulase-negative, 190-191
  funisitis, 184
  impetigo, 93, 180-181
  necrotizing fasciitis, 185-186
  omphalitis, 184
  in premature infant skin, 54
  paronychia, 183f, 183-184
  pyoderma, 137, 144t
  toxin-mediated diseases, 186-188, 187f
Staphylococcal scalded skin syndrome (SSSS),
    137-138
  clinical findings in, 186, 187f
  diagnosis of, 147t, 186, 187f, 188
  erythroderma in, 262
  evaluation of, 272t
  management of, 188, 272t
Sterile transient neonatal pustulosis, 153
Stevens-Johnson syndrome, 509
Stings
  arthropod, 236t-237t, 236-238
  vs. bites, 238
"Stork bites," 100, 324
Stratum basale, 19f, 18, 19-20, 20f

Stratum corneum, 19f, 18, 19, 20
  as barrier to infection, 54
  of fetus, 46
  immaturity of, 5
  integrity of, 63
  in newborn skin, 21, 62
Stratum granulosum, 19f, 18, 19, 20
Stratum lucidum, 19f, 18, 19, 20
Stratum spinosum, 19f, 18, 19, 20
Strawberry hemangioma, 338, 339f
Streptococcal infections, 138, 140
  diagnosis of, 144t
  group A β-hemolytic, 188-189
  group B (GBS), 189-190
Streptococcal toxic shock syndrome (STSS)
  diagnoses of, 189
  management of, 189
  pathogenesis of, 189
Sturge-Weber Foundation, 333b
Sturge-Weber syndrome (SWS), 8, 324, 325f, 331-333, 340
  ocular disorders associated with, 484
  vascular anomalies in, 330t
Subcutaneous fat
  anatomy of, 19f
  function of, 420
  necrosis, 45
  in newborn skin, 23
Subcutaneous fat disorders
  de Barsy syndrome, 460
  Farber disease, 433
  lipodystrophies, 430-433
  necrosis, 420-422
  panniculitis, 423-425
  sclerema neonatorum, 422
  tumors, 425-430
Subcutaneous fat necrosis of the newborn (SCFN)
  clinical findings in, 420, 421f
  diagnosis of, 421-422
  pathogenesis of, 420-421
  treatment of, 422
Subcutis, in fetal skin development, 6-8
Substance abuse, cutaneous findings of, 33
Sucking
  calluses, 478, 479f
  pads, 95
  in utero, 95
Sulfones, for pyoderma gangrenosum, 170
Sunlight exposure, and EPP, 311-312
Super Dooper Diaper Doo, 66t
Surfactant replacement therapy, 57
Surfactants, in bathing products, 64
Surgical intervention
  for AEC syndrome, 468
  for cutaneous zygomycosis, 230
  for cutis laxa, 458
  for hemangiomas, 346
Sweat ducts, obstruction of, 89-90, 90f
Sweat glands, fetal development of, 10, 11
Sweating, neonatal, 25
Sweating abnormalities, 457
Sweet syndrome
  clinical findings in, 304-306, 305f
  diagnosis of, 306
  laboratory evaluation of, 305
  management of, 306
  pathogenesis of, 305
Syphilis, congenital (CS)
  clinical findings in, 196f, 196-197
  condyloma lata in differential diagnosis of, 218
  diagnosis of, 147t, 197
  erythema with, 263, 264f
  evaluation of, 273t
  lesions associated with, 43t, 140-141
  management of, 198, 273t

T

Tabby genes, 10, 469
Tail, persistent vestigial, 125
Tardive congenital nevi, 388
Targetoid configuration, 44t
Tar shampoo, for seborrheic dermatitis, 249
Tay syndrome, 265, 277t, 283-284, 489
Teeth, examination of, 35

Teeth, natal, 477-478, 478t
  etiology for, 477
  in restrictive dermopathy, 289-290
  syndromes associated with, 478t
Telangiectasia, 326
Telogen, in fetal development, 11
Temperature, and erythroderma, 260. See also Cold temperature
Teratoma
  congenital, 442
  in differential diagnosis, 342
Thermoregulation
  in neonates, 26-27
  of newborn skin, 21
  in premature infant skin, 55-56
Thrombocytopenia, transient, 421, 421f
Thrombocytopenic consumptive coagulopathy, 343-344
Thromboses, in umbilical artery catheterization, 108
Thrush, oral, 225, 225f
Thyroglossal duct cysts, 482
Thyroid tissue, ectopic, 481-482
Tick bites, 235t
Tiger-tail pattern in trichothiodystrophy, 284
Tinea capitis, 230, 230f, 231
Tinea corporis, 43t, 230, 231
Tinea diaper dermatitis, 230-231, 231f
Tinea faciei, 230, 231
Tinea unguium, 231
Tinea versicolor (pityriasis versicolor), 227, 227f
Toenails, ingrown, 511, 511f
Tongue
  benign papular lesions of, 474t
  geographic, 479
  macroglossia, 479-480, 480f
Topical medication
  for newborn, 21
  systemic absorption of, 56
  and TEWL, 51
TORCH syndromes, 33, 484
Toxic epidermal necrolysis (TEN), 169
  compared with SSSS, 262
  diagnosis of, 149t
Toxic shock syndrome, 179. See also Streptococcal toxic shock syndrome
Toxoplasmosis
  characteristics of, 234t
  congenital, 233, 235
  diagnosis of, 235
  etiology of, 233
  treatment for, 235
Tragi, accessory, 118, 118f
Transcutaneous oxygen monitoring, complications of, 112-113, 114f
Transdermal drug delivery, 53
Transepidermal water loss (TEWL)
  causes of, 50
  control of, 68
  effects of radiant heating on, 49, 50f
  measurement of, 50
  in preterm infant, 21, 47
  prevention of excessive, 20
  strategies to reduce, 50-51
Transient dermolytic disease of the newborn (TBND), 163
Transient neonatal pustular melanosis (TNPM), 38t, 91, 152-153, 153f
  clinical features of, 92f, 93f, 93-94
  diagnosis of, 92-93
Transillumination blisters, 113, 114f
Transmission EM (TEM), 79
Transplant studies, hair follicle development in, 10
Trauma. See also Injuries
  alopecia related to, 494b, 494-495
  diagnosis of perinatal, 148t
  to preterm infants' skin, 47f
Treponema pallidum, 83, 196-198
Tretinoin, for infantile acne, 95
Trichophyton spp., 230
Trichorrhexis invaginata
  in ichthyosis disorders, 283
  in Netherton syndrome, 491, 491f
Trichorrhexis nodosa, 489, 489f
Trichosporosis
  clinical features of, 228
  diagnosis of, 147t

Trichothiodystrophy (TTD), 265, 277t, 283-284, 380
  clinical features of, 489f, 489-490, 490f
  hair examination in, 78t
Triclosan, cautious use of, 67t
Trigeminal nerve, branches of, 332f
Trimethroprim/sulfamethoxazole, cutaneous reactions associated with, 300
Triple dye, 67
Trisomies
  aplasia cutis associated with, 126t
  aplasia cutis in, 126, 127f
  micronychia in, 507t
Tryosinemia II, 289
Trypanosomiasis, 234t
Tuberculosis, congenital (CT), 192
Tuberous sclerosis
  ash leaf spots of, 456
  clinical findings in, 454-455
  criteria for, 362b, 454, 454b, 455b
  hypopigmented macules in, 363f
Tufted angioma (TA), 346, 347f
Tumor necrosis factors (TNFs), 28
Tumors. See also Vascular tumors, Hamartomas
  congenital pedal nodules, 428
  described, 37t
  in desmoid fibromatosis, 399, 399f
  epulis, congenital, 473
  fat, 425-430
  glomus, 348
  granular cell, 474, 474t
  lipoblastoma, 429f, 429-430
  lipoma, 425-426, 426f
  lipomatosis, 427-428
  neural, 402, 402f
  nevus lipomatosus cutaneous superficialis, 426-427
Turner syndrome, 370
  clinical features of, 460-461, 461f
  micronychia in, 507t
Twin spot phenomenon, 378
Twin transfusion, 100
Tyndall effect, 373-374
Tyrosinase, 353, 354t
Tyson's glands, 24
Tzanck preparation, 73, 75
  findings on, 76f
  multinucleated giant cell on, 76f
  technique for, 75b

U

Ulcerations, 139b
  within CMTC, 330
  of congenital syphilis, 196
  crusted, 106, 106f
  described, 39t
  diagnosis of, 147t
  hemangioma associated with, 172
  iatrogenic causes of, 155
  liponecrosis leading to, 424
  meatal, 114
  of noma neonatorum, 171
  overlying giant nevi, 172
  of pyoderma gangrenosum, 170, 171f
  of vascular malformation, 172
Ultrasonography
  and amniocentesis, 103
  of pseudotail, 125
Ultraviolet (UV) light
  burns caused by, 62, 109
  newborns exposed to, 21
  and premature infant skin, 54
  xeroderma pigmentosum and, 380
Umbilical anomalies
  granuloma, 131, 131f
  of omphalomesenteric duct, 130-131, 131f
  of urachus, 130, 130f
Umbilical artery catheterization, 108, 108f
Umbilical cord, funisitis of, 184
Umbilical granulomas, 95f, 95-96
Urachal cyst, 130, 130f
Urine output, diapering and, 64
Urticaria (hives), 37t, 44t
  clinical findings in, 300, 300f, 301f
  diagnosis of, 301
  etiology of, 301
  familial physical, 301-302

Urticaria (hives)—cont'd
  giant, 300
  management of, 301
Urticaria pigmentosa, 381, 442, 443f

V

Valacyclovir, 210
Vancomycin, cutaneous reactions associated with, 299
Van der Woude syndrome, 479
Varicella (chickenpox) infection, 141, 206
  congenital, 206f, 206-209, 207f
  diagnosis of, 145t, 147t
  vs. HSV diagnosis, 206
  infantile herpes zoster, 210
  neonatal, 209f, 209-210
  prenatal diagnosis of, 208
  prophylaxis for, 210-211
  treatment for, 208
Varicella zoster immunoglobulin (VZIG), 208, 210
Varicella zoster virus (VZV)
  DFA for, 75-76
  diagnosis of, 203t
Vascular endothelial growth factor (VEGF), 341
Vascular malformations, 172
  arteriovenous, 329f, 329-330
  capillary, 324-326, 325f
  hemangiomas differentiated from, 337t
  lymphatic, 328f, 328-329
  syndromes associated with, 330t, 330-336
  venous, 326f, 326-328, 327f
Vascular networks, in newborn skin, 25-26, 26f
Vascular tumors
  congenital eccrine angiomatous hamartoma, 348
  glomus, 348
  hemangiomas of infancy, 336-346, 337t
  infantile hemangiopericytoma, 348
  kaposiform hemangioendothelioma, 347
  in Kasabach-Merritt syndrome, 347f, 347-348
  pyogenic granuloma, 348
  spindle cell hemangioendothelioma, 348
  tufted angioma, 346, 347f
Vasculogenesis, 8, 341
Vaseline, 66t. See also Petrolatum
Vasomotor instability, cutaneous, 98-99, 99f
Vasomotor tone, in neonates, 26
Vasospasm, in umbilical artery catheterization, 108
Venous malformations (VMs), 474t476-477
  clinical findings in, 326f, 326-327, 327f
  diagnosis of, 327
  treatment for, 327-328

Vernix caseosa, 18, 100, 100f
Verrucae, 36t, 44t
Very low birth weight (VLBW) infants, 223
Vesicles
  in diffuse cutaneous mastocytosis, 443
  of HSV, 204, 204f
  of hyperimmunoglobulin E syndrome, 157
  of incontinentia pigmenti, 157, 157f
  in newborn, 45
  of scabies, 232, 232f
  of staphylococcal pustulosis, 180, 180f
  in STSS, 189
Vesiculopustular diseases, differential diagnosis of, 144t-146t
Vesiculopustules
  acropustulosis of infancy, 155
  in Langerhans' cell histiocytosis, 436
Viral culture, 73, 76
Viral infections
  AIDS, 212-214
  culture of, 73, 76
  cutaneous manifestations of, 200
  cytomegalovirus, 141, 211
  enteroviruses, 141, 216-217
  herpes simplex, 142-143, 200
  human papilloma virus, 217-219
  human parvovirus B19, 214-216
  molluscum contagiosum, 219-220
  rubella, 211-212
  Tzanck smear for, 73, 75, 75b, 76f, 76t
  varicella, 141, 206-211
Vitiligo, in Turner syndrome, 461
Vohwinkel syndrome, 288-289
Vorner palmoplantar keratoderma, 288

W

Waardenburg syndrome, 360
  in fetal skin development, 6
  types of, 361b
Warfarin, micronychia with, 507t
Warts. See also Human papilloma virus
  anogenital, 218, 218f, 483
Wasp bites, 235t
Watson syndrome, 370
Weber-Cockayne EB, 161
Weidemann-Rautenstrauch syndrome, 478t
Wells syndrome, 185
Wheals
  in erythema toxicum neonatorum, 152
White sponge nevus, 474t, 477

Winer, nodular calcification of, 405, 405f
Wiskott-Aldrich syndrome, 255f, 255-256
Wood's light examination, 83
  in CEP, 309
  to detect freckling, 453
  of hypopigmentation, 364
Woolly hair, 490
Wound care, 73, 81-82, 165
Wrinkling, in Turner syndrome, 461
Wyburn-Mason syndrome, 330t, 334

X

Xanthogranulomas, juvenile, 36t
  clinical findings in, 402-404, 403f, 404f
  ocular disorders associated with, 484
Xenobiotics, percutaneous absorption of, 46, 51-53
Xeroderma pigmentosum, 380-381
Xerosis (dry skin)
  of atopic dermatitis, 244, 246
  in seborrheic dermatitis, 248
X-linked dominant conditions, 34
  alopecia associated with, 495
  chondrodysplasia punctata, 277t, 286, 286f
  hypohidrotic ectodermal dysplasia, 265-266, 266f
  recessive ichthyosis (RXLI), 279f, 279-280
X-p22 microdeletion syndrome, 126t

Y

Yeast infections. See also Candidiasis
Yeast opsonization defect, 268
Yellow mutant albinism, 353
Yellow nail syndrome, 513t

Z

Zinc deficiency
  AE associated with, 171
  clinical findings in, 254, 254f
  etiology of, 253-254
  management of, 254
Zinc oxide ointment, 66t
Ziprkowski-Margolis syndrome, 365
Zosteriform configuration, 43t
Zosteriform lentiginous nevus, 383
Zygomycosis, 229-230
  diagnosis of, 147t
  neonatal, 229-230
  treatment for, 230